ESTIMATED MINIMUM SODIUM, CHLORIDE, AND POTASSIUM REQUIREMENTS FOR HEALTHY PERSONS

Age	Weight (kg)	Sodium (mg)*†	Chloride (mg)*†	Potassium (mg)‡
MONTHS				
0-5	4.5	120	180	500
6-11	8.9	200	300	700
YEARS				
1	11	225	350	1000
2-5	16	300	500	1400
6-9	25	400	600	1600
10-18	50	500	750	2000
>18§	70	500	750	2000

*No allowance has been included for large, prolonged losses from the skin through sweat.
†There is no evidence that higher intakes confer any additional health benefit.
‡Desirable intakes of potassium may considerably exceed these values (~13,500 mg for adults).
§No allowance has been included for growth. Values given for people under 18 years of age assume a growth rate corresponding to the 50th percentile reported by the National Center for Health Statistics and averaged for males and females.

ESTIMATED SAFE AND ADEQUATE DAILY DIETARY INTAKES (ESADDI) OF SELECTED VITAMINS AND MINERALS*

Category	Age (years)	VITAMINS		TRACE ELEMENTS†				
		Biotin (µg)	Pantothenic acid (mg)	Copper (mg)	Manganese (mg)	Fluoride (mg)	Chromium (µg)	Molybdenum (µg)
Infants	0- 0.5	10	2	0.4-0.6	0.3-0.6	0.1-0.5	10-40	15-30
	0.5-1	15	3	0.6-0.7	0.6-1	0.2-1	20-60	20-40
Children and adolescents	1-3	20	3	0.7-1	1-1.5	0.5-1.5	20-80	25-50
	4-6	25	3-4	1-1.5	1.5-2	1-2.5	30-120	30-75
	7-10	30	4-5	1-2	2-3	1.5-2.5	50-200	50-150
	11+	30-100	4-7	1.5-2.5	2-5	1.5-2.5	50-200	75-250
Adults		30-100	4-7	1.5-3	2-5	1.5-4	50-200	75-250

*Because there is less information on which to base recommendations for allowances of minerals, these figures are not given in the main table of RDAs and are provided here in the form of ranges of recommended intakes.
†Since toxic levels for many trace elements may be reached with only several times usual intakes, the upper levels for the trace elements given in this table should not be habitually exceeded.

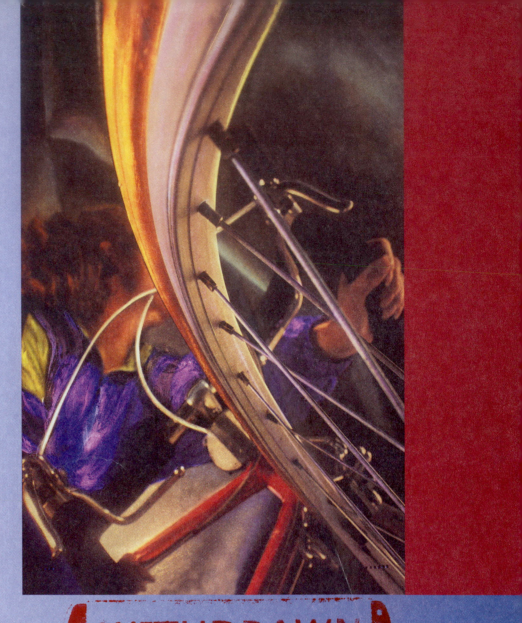

Exercise Physiology

EXERCISE, PERFORMANCE, AND CLINICAL APPLICATIONS

Exercise Physiology

EXERCISE, PERFORMANCE, AND CLINICAL APPLICATIONS

ROBERT A. ROBERGS, Ph.D.

Center for Exercise and Applied Human Physiology
The University of New Mexico
Albuquerque, New Mexico

SCOTT O. ROBERTS, Ph.D.

Department of Health, Physical Education, and Recreation
Texas Tech University
Lubbock, Texas

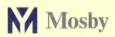 Mosby

St. Louis   Baltimore   Boston
Carlsbad   Chicago   Naples   New York   Philadelphia   Portland
London   Madrid   Mexico City   Singapore   Sydney   Tokyo   Toronto   Wiesbaden

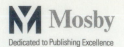

Mosby
Dedicated to Publishing Excellence

A Times Mirror
Company

Vice President and Publisher: James M. Smith
Senior Acquisitions Editor: Vicki Malinee
Senior Development Editor: Michelle Turenne
Project Manager: Patricia Tannian
Production Editor: Melissa Mraz
Book Design Manager: Gail Morey Hudson
Manufacturing Supervisor: Karen Lewis
Internal and Cover Design: William Seabright and Associates
Cover Art: Peter J. Coe

Credits for all materials used by permission appear after the Index.

Printed in the United States of America
Composition and Color Separation by Accu-Color Inc./Beaumont
Printing/binding by Von Hoffmann Press, Inc.

Mosby–Year Book, Inc.
11830 Westline Industrial Drive
St. Louis, Missouri 63146

Library of Congress Cataloging in Publication Data

Robergs, Robert A.
    Exercise physiology: exercise, performance, and clinical
applications / Robert A. Robergs, Scott O. Roberts.
        p.   cm.
    Includes bibliographical references and index.
    ISBN 0-8151-7241-9
    1. Exercise—Physiological aspects.   I. Roberts, Scott O.
II. Title.
QP301.R545   1996
612'.044—dc20   96-17003
                                            CIP

96 97 98 99 00 / 9 8 7 6 5 4 3 2

Preface

*I*n undertaking the preparation and development of *Exercise Physiology: Exercise, Performance, and Clinical Applications,* we wanted to provide some background on why we decided to take on the challenge of writing a textbook of this magnitude.

Why write another exercise physiology text?

As recent graduates of both the pure and applied fields of exercise science, our experiences showed us the ever increasing need for presenting more advanced content within exercise physiology. Our experiences as academic professionals reinforced this need: instructing advanced undergraduate and graduate students requires the careful integration of information from both textbooks and recent research to present a timely and logical progression of both knowledge and data.

Before taking their first exercise physiology class, most universities require students to complete classes in kinesiology, introductory anatomy and physiology, and in some cases, introductory courses in chemistry, physics, and biochemistry. Given this preparation, why is it that the typical exercise physiology text presents fundamental anatomy and physiology sections? Many times the level of content in these chapters is lower than that of the introductory anatomy and physiology texts that the students use in their prerequisite classes. This indicated to us that we either had to increase the academic level of writing and content in this text or devote space used in relating simple physiology to more topical content in exercise physiology. As you will see, we chose to do both.

Who is this text written for?

We wanted to write a textbook for the advanced undergraduate and graduate courses offered in exercise physiology. Many universities offer two or more classes in exercise physiology, with senior level classes also addressing the needs of Masters Degree students. Our goal was to write a textbook that serves the advanced undergraduate, but with enough detail, currentness, and focus to also serve the more advanced needs of graduate students.

Unlike exercise physiology students of the 1970s and 1980s who usually went into teaching physical education, today's students are pursuing careers in corporate and public health centers, personal training, and rehabilitation programs within hospitals. Clinical programs such as physical therapy, occupational therapy, and dietetics are also becoming increasingly interested in exercise science. In the near future exercise physiology may also become a part of the medical curriculum. In fact, the Exercise Science Program and related university fitness testing programs at the University of New Mexico offer rotations in the supervision of clinical exercise testing for medical students and interns. Exercise physiology is no longer a discipline that is structured solely within physical education. The optimal text needs to address the content required by the physical education student, while stimulating the increasing population of students outside of physical education who require exercise physiology training and education.

What is the academic level of this text?

Based on our own personal experiences as researchers and educators in exercise physiology, our intent has been to write a text that is succinct in its coverage of the major topics and issues, but *does not minimize exercise physiology as an advanced topic of study*. This point is especially important to us in light of the misconceptions about just exactly what the study of exercise physiology truly entails.

In the traditional exercise physiology course, there is usually little or no time for in-depth coverage of physiology, biochemistry, and applied topics. Nor is there room to write on all these topics in one text. However, our textbook restructures the usual exercise physiology content by presenting more advanced descriptions of important topics, rather than concentrating on topics that have developed into separate sciences (such as body composition, exercise prescription, and sports physiology). Instead, we focus on pertinent and current topics not usually included in exercise physiology texts, such as central versus peripheral determinants of VO$_2$max, fatigue, and applications of magnetic resonance to exercise physiology.

The format and structure of many of the existing exercise physiology texts show strong connections with sport, athletic performance, and the discipline of physical education, whereas other texts are known for their more advanced presentation of material. Our intent is to create a text that provides a new approach to the knowledge base in exercise physiology, while addressing developments that will assist in carrying the field into the 21st century.

What makes this text unique?

In improving on the structure and organization of material, it is important that the content be as current as possible, while simultaneously addressing the increasingly diverse needs of the exercise physiology student. In *Exercise Physiology,* we address *how the body adapts to exercise during acute and chronic timeframes* as the fundamental knowledge base of exercise physiology.

In the past, texts have divided content based on systems physiology and have presented specific examples of how exercise affects physiology. For example, a text may present pure physiology, applied physiology, other physiologic systems, and the physiologic changes based on training. However, the student may still be struggling to simply understand the basic concepts. Acute and chronic adaptations to exercise may be dispersed throughout the text, further leaving their importance underemphasized and vague. Consequently, confusion and frustration can be the result.

Rather, adaptation of exercise during acute and chronic timeframes provides a knowledge base that is a logical extension of pure physiology, as well as a logical format in which to present research findings. Similarly, applications of exercise physiology to exercise testing and clinical populations are also addressed since these represent areas for growth, as well as the future directions, for the field of exercise physiology.

How does our text meet the future needs of exercise physiology and the future needs of student populations?

We have developed a text that provides the instructor with structured coverage of the content in exercise physiology but with a uniqueness that we hope you will find appealing. The success of our text will depend on how accurate we are in foreseeing the future of our discipline, and how our perceptions mirror those of instructors of exercise physiology. It is our hope that this text will raise not only the academic standards of exercise physiology, but also the standards by which our discipline is viewed within the clinical and scientific communities. The presentation of more advanced knowledge, the focus on acute and chronic adaptations to exercise, and the descriptions and examples of the applied and clinical importance of exercise will educate the student at a level required in a discipline that is exploding in growth from both research and the awareness by the medical community that exercise is a viable and successful prescription.

Organization

You will find that this text is written in six parts:

Part 1—Fundamentals presents a brief history of the development of exercise physiology as a separate scientific discipline, and provides the necessary content of cellular metabolism, muscle contraction, and neuromuscular function for enhanced understanding of acute and chronic adaptations to exercise.

Part 2—Systemic Responses to Exercise presents the contents of systems physiology and how each system acutely and chronically adapts to exercise.

Part 3—Aids to Exercise Performance presents material on topics that are known to either improve or impair exercise performance.

Part 4—Measurements of Physiologic Composition and Capacities explains how researchers measure such things as endurance and intense exercise capacities, lung function, and body composition.

Part 5—Special Topics Within Exercise Physiology describes the latest research findings for applied topics of particularly high interest in exercise physiology and biochemistry such as exercise and: fatigue, aging, gender, children, and environmental concerns.

Part 6—Exercise and Health presents information that explains the importance of exercise to optimal health and well-being, as well as detailing the use of exercise as a diagnostic and rehabilitative tool for many clinical populations.

Unique Features

This textbook presents material in a unique format and also includes material on topics not typically presented in an exercise physiology text. These unique features include:

- More detail on bioenergetics and thermodynamics in Chapter 2, with examples that pertain to exercise physiology rather than physics.

- Chapter 3 is solely devoted to explaining enzyme function and nomenclature.

- Detailed coverage of metabolism. Coverage has been separated into two chapters: catabolism and anabolism (Chapters 4 and 5). The specific regulation of catabolism and anabolism in skeletal muscle, the liver, and adipose tissue is emphasized while exercising and recovering from exercise.

- Calorimetry and ergometry are presented in Chapter 6 with more complete coverage of the limitations and applications of the procedures. A description of the historical development of the science of calorimetry is also provided.

- Muscle contraction is presented separately in Chapter 7 and covers the three muscle types: skeletal, cardiac, and smooth muscles. Also, comparative physiology of contraction in the three different types of muscle is presented, and detailed information on the molecular biology of contractile proteins in skeletal muscle is also included.

- Neuromuscular physiology is presented in Chapters 8 and 9. Chapter 8 is solely concerned with the importance of neuromuscular physiology and movement, and the differences between motor units in human skeletal muscle. Chapter 9 discusses how neuromuscular function changes during exercise and in response to exercise training.

- Chapter 10 presents research findings about how the body adapts to different types of exercise, with an emphasis on muscle metabolism.

- Cardiovascular and pulmonary physiology, Chapters 11 and 12, are structured around acute (immediate responses) and chronic adaptations (training responses) to exercise.

- Rather than following the more traditional gland-by-gland approach, the neuroendocrine regulation of physiology is presented in Chapter 13 and is organized by important body functions during exercise such as energy metabolism, substrate selection, cardiorespiratory function, fluid balance, and blood pressure.

- Chapter 14 presents coverage of skeletal function and adaptation, and provides an emphasis on prevention.

- Immune adaptations and the impact of exercise on immune function are covered in Chapter 15.

- Procedures used to measure exercise performance and functional capacities are included in Part 4, Measurements of Physiologic Composition and Capacities, and evaluate how and why some individuals perform better than others.

- Carbohydrate nutrition before, during, and after exercise, and to enhance exercise endurance, is detailed in Chapter 17.

- Chapter 22 examines fatigue and attempts to explain the causes of the multiple types of fatigue, such as fatigue that follows long-duration exercise versus fatigue that results from intense, short-duration exercise.

- Gender differences both during and in response to exercise are examined in Chapter 23.

- Separate chapters are also devoted to the emerging fields of exercise and aging (Chapter 24) and pediatric exercise physiology (Chapter 25).

- Exercise at different altitudes, exercise in hot and in humid environments, exercise in air pollution, and unique coverage of exercise during exposure to altered gravitational forces are given detailed coverage (Chapter 26).

- Clinical Applications of content are integrated in selected chapters to provide greater relevance to a diverse audience.

- An attractive full-color design is used throughout the text and illustration program to enhance the teaching-learning process.

Pedagogic Features

Numerous pedagogic tools are included in every chapter to enhance the learning process. These include chapter objectives, key terms, definition boxes (with pronunciation guides when appropriate), Focus Boxes of supplemental content related to the text, Clinical Application boxes in selected chapters, bulleted chapter summaries, review questions, application questions, thorough references, and recommended readings.

Additionally, a comprehensive appendix of useful conversion charts, normal values for blood and muscle compounds, equations of indirect calorimetry, and Recommended Nutrient Intake (RNI) is provided. A comprehensive glossary concludes the text.

Finally, Recommended Dietary Allowances (RDA) and helpful reference and conversion materials are located inside the front and back covers of the text for convenience of use.

The Ancillary

The ViewStudy Image Disc for Exercise Physiology. This unique, new CD-ROM software includes photographs and illustrations with accompanying captions from *Exercise Physiology.* Cross-referenced by topic, concept, and figure number, the figures and captions can be printed at full size for use as transparency acetates. The images can also be imported into common word processing programs. The innovative slide show feature allows selected images to be arranged for presentation on computer screens, video projectors, overhead projection panels, or transparency acetates. This software can be used on Macintosh and Windows platforms and is free to qualified adopters of the textbook.

Acknowledgments

We would like to acknowledge and thank our reviewers whose comments, suggestions, support, and enthusiasm were valuable to us in improving the manuscript.

James L. Webb
California Polytechnic State University
San Luis Obispo

Robert Gotshall
Colorado State University

Douglas S. King
Iowa State University

Jeffrey A. Potteiger
University of Kansas

Stanley P. Brown
University of Mississippi

Ethel M. Frese
Saint Louis University

Serge P. von Duvillard
William Paterson College

William S. Barnes
Texas A&M University

Julie Felix
Virginia Tech State University

William Thorland
Washington State University

Dan Fitzsimons
University of Wisconsin at Madison

Carol D. Rodgers
University of Toronto

The following individuals have inspired us personally, academically, and professionally, and we wish to express our gratitude to them.

from Robert Robergs

Alan Morton, Ph.D., at the University of Western Australia reassured me of my competencies, recognized and addressed my weaknesses, and supported my initial efforts in preparing to become a research scientist and academic professional.

Paul Ribisl, Ph.D., at Wake Forest University provided me with the opportunity to prove myself in the American academic market.

David Costill, Ph.D., at Ball State University opened the doors to a future as a research professor in the American university system, and represents to me what an exercise physiologist should be: a person competent in many areas of human physiology, proven by research, publications, and public speaking; and who is simply a "bonza bloke."

William Fink at Ball State University is the assistant laboratory director and biochemical "wizard" who supports David Costill. Bill taught me about life, friendship, and how to prioritize a passion for golf during busy academic, research, and administration schedules.

Clyde Williams, Ph.D., at Loughborough University, England, represents the model of a university professor and scientist that I strive to become.

Unending thanks are directed to my family in Australia, who supported my departure for the United States in 1985, and have remained fully supportive ever since. Thank you, **Mum, Dad,** and **Helen.** I want to make you proud.

Finally, I need to express love and thanks to **Sharon** and **Bryce.** I have shared my life with both of you during the writing of this text and part of this achievement is because of your love and support.

from Scott Roberts

Bill Colvin, Ed.D., at California State University at Chico taught me how to be a dedicated teacher and the importance of always putting your students first.

Tom Fahey, Ed.D., at California State University at Chico inspired me to become a writer, and also taught me the importance of balancing work and play.

William Bynum, Ph.D., at California State University at Sacramento encouraged me to pursue a career as a researcher and college professor.

Irv Faria, Ph.D., at California State University at Sacramento taught me how to conduct research.

My early clinical experiences were greatly influenced by **Bob Holly, Ph.D.,** and the terrific staff at the University of California at Davis, as well as all of the individuals involved in the American College of Sports Medicine Exercise Test Technologists Workshops at UC: Davis.

I would also like to acknowledge those from whom I have learned through their writing, research, and presentations, including **Jack Wilmore, Michael Pollock, William Haskell, Oded Bar-Or,** the late **Ed Fox,** and **David Costill** to name just a few.

I would also like to offer my warmest and most sincere thanks to my mentor, colleague, and friend **Robert Robergs.** I am greatly appreciative of everything you have done for me and the opportunities you have given me.

Lastly, heartfelt love and appreciation to my wife **Julia** and our children **Andrew, Daniel,** and **Michael** for their unending love and support during graduate school and throughout the writing of this book.

ROBERT A. ROBERGS
SCOTT O. ROBERTS

Contents

Contents

Focus Boxes

To provide students with greater depth of coverage of important topics, *Focus Boxes* are included in the text to present additional content that supplements the main narrative. The Focus Boxes can be found on the following pages:

Clinical Applications

With the diversity of student populations enrolled in exercise physiology courses, the Clinical Applications boxes present additional depth of coverage about various research topics and findings that are applicable to situations related to the field of medicine. Clinical Applications are located on the following pages:

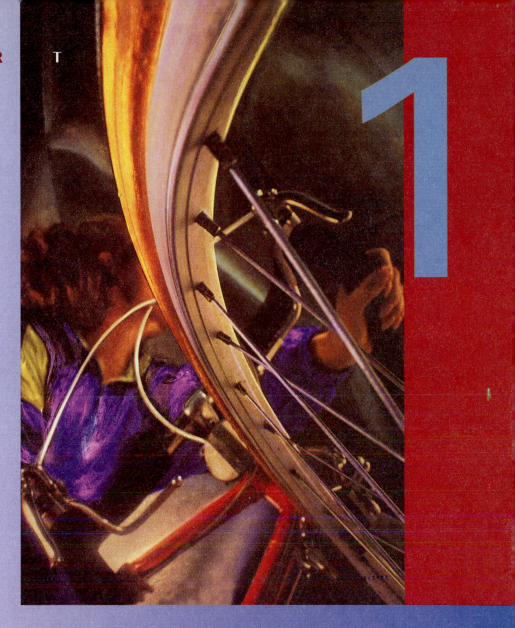

Fundamentals

Exercise Physiology: Past, Present, and Future

After studying this chapter you should be able to:

■ Describe the research that established the field of exercise physiology.

■ Describe how the field of exercise physiology has developed during the twentieth century.

■ Explain the more important scientific achievements that have developed the discipline of exercise physiology.

■ Identify scientists who have contributed to the academic and research base of exercise physiology.

■ Identify the current and future directions of exercise physiology, and the implications these directions may have for the academic content and practice in clinical, pure, and applied sciences.

■ Demonstrate your knowledge of an academic library and know which research journals to inspect for research or review articles about exercise physiology.

exercise physiology

clinical exercise physiology

pure research

applied research

The science of exercise physiology has a long history, which in more recent times was academically founded in the discipline of physical education. As a class in physical education, exercise physiology was primarily applied to further understanding of participation in sports and athletics. Today, exercise physiology is a discipline that has expanded beyond the boundaries of traditional physical education. The widely accepted medical recognition of exercise's role in preventive, rehabilitative, and diagnostic applications has further developed the field, has altered the application of this knowledge, and, some may argue, has redefined the science of exercise physiology. Despite these changes the student must remember the physical education heritage of exercise physiology, since this is the base from which this science began. Furthermore, the fundamental objective of physical education, to increase the health and quality of life by participation in exercise throughout the lifespan, is even more applicable in today's society. Whether exercise physiology remains within the field of physical education is a contentious issue between the traditional and "new breed" exercise physiologists. However, this issue is not the focus of this chapter. The purpose of this chapter is to introduce the science of exercise physiology as a complex and advanced field of inquiry. Important clinical, sport, athletic, environmental, and academic issues are identified, and documentation of major research findings during the twentieth century is presented. The identification of these broad research inquiries reveals how this discipline has developed, enables projections to the future research and application of knowledge within the discipline, and in concert with the content of this textbook, fosters the development of the science of exercise physiology into the twenty-first century.

What is Exercise Physiology?

Exercise physiology is a discipline that has traditionally focused on the study of how exercise alters the structure and function of the human body. Such a broad definition is problematic, since academic and research inquiry of exercise and the structure and function of the human body can be done at the level of the total body, body systems, organs, tissues, cells, and subcellular molecules. Thus exercise physiology requires understanding of anatomy, physiologic systems, cellular biology, chemistry and biochemistry, and molecular biology. Discussion of the increasingly demanding knowledge base of exercise physiology occurs later in this chapter.

Development of Exercise Physiology

Many students are told to focus on recent research, with the intent that this will enable students to remain abreast of new research findings and current topics of interest. These justifications are true, but students who ignore the wealth of research published since the early 1890s, much of which is high in qual-

---

exercise physiology

study of how exercise alters the structure and function of the human body

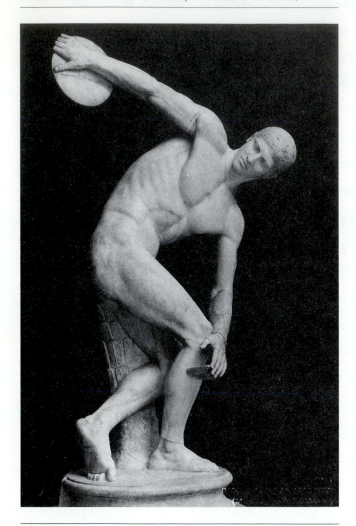

FIGURE 1.1

A Roman discus thrower. (Courtesy The Bettman Archive.)

ity (see Chapter 6), are unable to critically evaluate recent research for how it adds a unique contribution to the field. A student who wants to pursue a career as an exercise physiologist should try to devote library time solely to perusing topics of interest in the older published literature. Students will be amazed at what was accomplished and what was known so long ago.

The use of exercise as a condition from which to investigate bodily function can be dated back to the first Olympics, when the athletic feats that could be performed by the body were observed, and specific training programs were devised to foster improvements in either muscle hypertrophy and strength or endurance (Figure 1.1). The story of Pheidippides, a trained Greek runner who ran 150 miles from Athens to Sparta and a few days later ran the 22 miles from Marathon to Athens (the origin of the marathon race),[5] is a classic example of the presence of "exercise" in life hundreds of years ago. The argument can also be made that in many aboriginal cultures the benefits of exercise were apparent for

success in hunting, during war, and in longevity and that these benefits date back thousands of years. The belief that regular exercise may contribute to health and improve physical performance is not a state of mind confined to the twentieth century!

Organized research to specifically learn more about how the body functions during exercise has a history in chemistry and nutrition.[20] During the 1800s Antoine-Laurent Lavoisier and Pierre-Simon Laplace proposed that metabolism and life itself were dependent on an essential component in the air that they termed "oxygene."[5,17] Although this theory was in opposition to the general belief that blood was the most important life-giving substance, it was not until the early 1900s, when exercise was used by chemists to study the macronutrients used during exercise, that the role of oxygen was proven.[20] At the same time the ability of the body to combust foodstuffs during exercise was researched, and allowed calculations of efficiency, the energy expended during exercise, and the principles of using energy expenditure as a measure of exercise intensity.[20]

During the early decades of the twentieth century, additional research unrelated to exercise was being completed that was to influence subsequent research involving exercise. Many of these achievements were accomplished by Europeans. For example, August Krogh of Denmark researched the circulation of blood through capillaries and designed several pieces of laboratory equipment, including a carbon dioxide analyzer and a precision weight scale. Krogh's achievements were recognized by Denmark with the establishment of the August Krogh Institute, which remains a productive research institute today.[2] The German scientists Rubner and Voit pioneered the development of direct and indirect calorimetry and applied these technologies to human metabolism.[20] C.G. Douglas and John S. Haldane studied the role of oxygen and metabolic acidosis on the control of ventilation. The gas collection bags used by these researchers are named Douglas bags after Douglas (Figure 1.2), and the effect of oxygen on carbon dioxide transport in the blood and the control of ventilation is termed the Haldane effect because of his work in this area (see Chapter 6 and Appendix B).

Christian Bohr of Denmark studied the influence of oxygen availability on the oxygen–hemoglobin dissociation curve as early as 1904, and the alteration of this sigmoidal relationship and the conditions that foster the alteration is termed the Bohr effect.[5] Another great scientific achievement resulted from the work of Otto Frank of Germany and Henry Starling of Britain. These scientists experimented on animal hearts and determined that increasing the flow of blood through the chambers of the heart increased the ability of the heart to eject blood. This relationship has been termed the Frank-Starling law (see Chapter 11).

A surprisingly large volume of research was also being conducted using exercise during the first three decades of the twentieth century. Archibald V. Hill of Great Britain studied oxygen consumption during exercise and from these studies

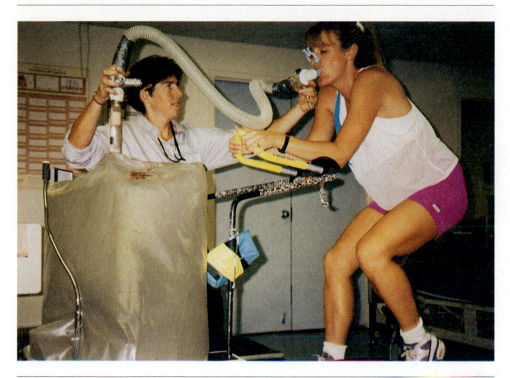

Students using Douglas bags to collect expired air for later analysis of carbon dioxide and oxygen content and expired volume, which are required variables in the calculations of indirect calorimetry.

introduced the term "maximal oxygen consumption" as a measure of the maximal cardiorespiratory capacity of the body and an indicator of the potential for endurance exercise. Subsequent research documented the importance and meaning of this measure.[13,21,26] Rubner and Voit extended the theoretical findings of Lavoisier with human research of indirect calorimetry in differing nutritional, environmental, and exercise conditions.[20] Furthermore, it was in the late 1920s that Hill and Otto Meyerhof published extensive findings of carbohydrate catabolism and the production of lactic acid in skeletal muscle.[20] These findings led to introduction of the terms *oxygen deficit* and *oxygen debt,* which were utilized to explain the metabolic energy from anaerobic sources used at the start of exercise, and the subsequent metabolism required to replenish these energy stores during the recovery, respectively. The work of Hill, Krogh, and Meyerhof was rewarded by the scientific community, since each man received a separate Nobel Prize for his contribution to the understanding of muscle metabolism. As discussed in Chapter 10, more recent research has shown that the oxygen debt term and assumptions are no longer valid.

In the United States an organized effort at investigating the effects of exercise on the human body began after the formation of the Harvard Fatigue Laboratory by L.J. Henderson in 1927. David Bruce Dill was the research director of the lab and remained in this position until the laboratory closed in 1947. Research from the Harvard Fatigue Laboratory was initially conducted to increase knowledge of how different employment conditions affected the body. This initial purpose complemented the area of environmental physiology, which was the specialty of Bruce Dill. Subsequent research from the lab was focused on human physiology at altitude and in dry and moist heat. Additional research interests included metabolism during exercise, the effects of aging on metabolism at rest and during exercise, blood gas transport and acid-base balance, and nutrition.[4,6,13]

The impact of the Harvard Fatigue Laboratory to the development of exercise physiology was probably more important for the subsequent contributions of the scientists who either visited the lab or were trained within the lab for a career in research of human physiology. August Krogh, E. Asmussen, P.F. Scholander, and R. Margaria all visited the lab and conducted research. Similarly, the American products of the lab extended the focus of research of exercise physiology into other universities and set the stage for the spread of the interest and the ability to conduct quality research in exercise-related topics within the fields of physiology and biochemistry. The development of the field of exercise physiology throughout the world is indicated in Table 1.1, which lists examples of major research interests for given dates.

The research of exercise physiology has undergone several transitions, which we have identified as "the beginnings,"

TABLE 1.1

Development of research and interest areas involving exercise

HISTORICAL CATEGORY	IMPORTANT RESEARCH TOPICS	DATES
BEGINNINGS		**?-1960**
Nutrient needs that accompany exercise		
Body's cardiorespiratory responses to exercise		
Potential causes of muscle fatigue during exercise		
Body's responses to exercise in hot and cold environments		
Regulation of chemical reactions in skeletal muscle and liver		
ERA OF SPORTS AND ATHLETICS		**1960-1980**
Influence of diet and exercise on muscle carbohydrate stores		
Muscle metabolic demands of different exercise intensities		
Motor unit and muscle fiber type determinants of exercise performance		
Muscle and cardiorespiratory predictors of strength and endurance		
Effects of training on cardiovascular and muscle function		
Effects of training on exercise performance		
Effects of exercise performed in different environments		
ERA OF MEDICAL AWAKENING		**1970-PRESENT**
Effects of exercise training on health and quality of life		
Effects of exercise training on cholesterol		
Effects of exercise training on heart function in diseased populations		
Effects of exercise training on disease prevention and rehabilitation		
Role of exercise in health promotion		
PRESENT STATUS OF EXERCISE RESEARCH AND KNOWLEDGE		**1990-PRESENT**
Role of exercise in supporting body functions in microgravity		
Exercise as an independent risk factor for heart disease		
Benefit of exercise for special populations: disabled, elderly, children, pregnant women, etc.		
Molecular adaptations of skeletal muscle to exercise		
Regulation of blood flow through skeletal muscle during exercise		

"the era of sports and athletics," and "the era of medical awakening." It is difficult to detect a true beginning to either of these transitions, and the dates should be viewed as approximate. Research into nutrition and muscle metabolism were good examples of topics that progressed from resting conditions, to the condition that provides the greatest challenge to homeostasis in each example: exercise. This early research soon provided adequate knowledge from which scientists could begin to ask and answer applied questions that concerned exercise. For example, studying the acute responses of body systems to exercise stresses stimulated the need to know why these responses occurred, if they differed among individuals, and what factors altered these responses. The individuals most interested in this information at this time period were athletes and their coaches. Not surprisingly, research interest using exercise was primarily focused on these needs. This development lead to the "era of sports and athletics."

During the 1960s and 1970s, research findings indicating the potential for exercise to aid not only the athlete, but also the average citizen, were presented. Athletes were healthier than the average citizen, had fewer signs of degenerative diseases, and arguably had a higher quality of life. Indirect research evidence linked these differences to the adaptations of the body to continued exercise stress. Nevertheless, medical and public sentiment was skeptical, since those who exercised regularly in Western societies during these dates were generally regarded as eccentric or antisocial. Despite the research indicating the benefits of exercise, the medical community was still skeptical about the roles of exercise in preventive and rehabilitative medicine. However, the voices of George Sheehan and Kenneth Cooper, physicians hooked on exercise, were about to awaken the medical community.

A significant development that catalyzed the medical recognition of exercise's importance was the growing voice of the members of the American College of Sports Medicine, founded in 1954. In conjunction with the known deteriorating fitness of the children of most Western societies, with those of the United States being a notable example, and the increasing incidence of mortality from coronary artery disease, the role of exercise in health maintenance and disease prevention was given increased attention.[17] Exercise was shown to lower serum cholesterol concentrations, and the known reductions in body fat and total body weight that accompany regular exercise with a healthy diet were also shown to decrease the risk for diabetes, hypertension, and musculoskeletal deterioration. The rest of the story is presented in several chapters of this book. However, it is clear that exercise in today's society is more than recreation. Comments of two knowledgeable scientists come to mind. The first is from Covert Bailey, who has claimed that if exercise could be packaged into a pill, it would be the most prescribed medication in all of history. The second comment is from Åstrand's textbook,[1] which identified the irony of the medical recommendation of requiring a physical examination before commencing an exercise training program. Åstrand stated that this reasoning is backward, for if a medical examination is required, it should be for all those individuals who refuse to regularly partake in physical activity! Åstrand's commentary, made before 1970, may make him a prophet because it may not be long before insurance companies make deductions for those individuals who give proof of regular physical activity.

Scandinavian Influence

A brief history of exercise physiology would be incomplete without recognition of the many Scandinavian scientists who have contributed to the development of the field. The Harvard Fatigue Laboratory hosted several Scandinavian researchers. During the 1930s, three notable Norwegians conducted research at Harvard: Erik Hohwu-Christensen, Erling Asmussen, and Marius Nielsen.[2] After his return to Stockholm, Hohwu-Christensen was mentor to Per-Olaf Åstrand. Åstrand developed into a prolific researcher during the 1950s and 1960s and was the primary author of one of the most influential textbooks detailing the body's responses to exercise and helping to establish exercise physiology as a valid topic of scientific inquiry.[1] Since the 1960s, prominent physiologists have emerged from Scandinavia. Bengt Saltin (Table 1.2) has researched muscle metabolism, training adaptations to exercise, and more recently the change in blood flow to skeletal muscle during exercise.[3,7] Lars Hermansen researched muscle training adaptations to exercise, and Eric Hultman and Kent Sahlin have been widely published in the area of muscle biochemistry and metabolic acidosis. Women have also been prominent in exercise research in Scandinavia. Nina Vollestad has completed important studies of muscle glycogen use dur-

ing exercise, Karen Piehl has studied the replenishment of muscle glycogen after exercise, and Brigetta Essen has completed numerous studies of muscle metabolic adaptations to training. The contributions of these and other Scandinavian researchers to exercise physiology can be appreciated by perusing through the many supplement issues of *Acta Physiologica Scandinavica*.

Recent Status of Exercise Physiology

Today exercise is used as a therapy during rehabilitation from injury and illness and as a preventive strategy to combat atherosclerotic cardiovascular disease. Table 1.3 lists the various disciplines that have used exercise as a condition from which to further evaluate physiologic or cellular function. The medical interest in exercise physiology is developing into a separate field, **clinical exercise physiology,** and textbooks are being written to satisfy this need.

The recent history of exercise physiology is best categorized into the divisions of pure research and applied research. Brooks[3] has succinctly defined these two divisions of exercise-related research:

Pure research uses exercise to further understand physiology

Applied research uses physiology to further understand exercise

Pure Research

The field of exercise physiology has expanded considerably because of the unique role of exercise in presenting challenges to bodily function, and the opportunities these challenges provide to learn more about how the body functions and is regulated. Focus Box 1.1 lists examples of questions that pure exercise-related research has attempted to answer. Of course, this list presents a sampling of literally thousands of selected questions that have been addressed.

The role of pure research in the development of a discipline cannot be overemphasized. During the 1960s, research on muscle glycogen biochemistry was pivotal in providing the knowledge necessary to allow applied questions to be asked concerning carbohydrate nutrition, muscle glycogen,

clinical exercise physiology
study of exercise use in the treatment or rehabilitation of clinical disorders

pure research
uses exercise to further understand physiology

applied research
uses physiology to further understand exercise

TABLE 1.2

Prominent researchers in exercise-related topics since the 1970s

NAME	RESEARCH INTERESTS	RESEARCH AFFILIATION
Ken Baldwin	Muscle molecular biology	University of California–Irvine (U.S.A.)
George Brooks	Lactate metabolism; muscle biochemistry	University of California–Berkeley (U.S.A.)
David Costill	Fluid balance, carbohydrate metabolism, muscle histology	Ball State University (U.S.A.)
Eddie Coyle	Carbohydrate metabolism	University of Texas–Austin (U.S.A.)
Jerry Dempsey	Pulmonary function	University of Wisconsin (U.S.A.)
Barbara Drinkwater	Bone metabolism	Pacific Medical Center–Seattle (U.S.A.)
Carl Gisolfi	Intestinal absorption of water and carbohydrate	Iowa State University (U.S.A.)
Phil Gollnick	Muscle biochemistry	Deceased
Bill Haskell	Health, cholesterol	Stanford University (U.S.A.)
John Holloszy	Muscle biochemistry, diabetes	Washington University, St. Louis (U.S.A.)
Jere Mitchell	Cardiovascular function	Harry S. Moss Heart Center (U.S.A.)
Timothy Noakes	Exercise performance, fluid balance	University of Capetown (S. Africa)
Ralph Paffenberger	Health, epidemiology	Stanford University (U.S.A.)
Larry Rowell	Cardiovascular function	University of Washington–Seattle (U.S.A.)
Kent Sahlin	Muscle biochemistry	Karolinska Institute (Sweden)
Bengt Saltin	Training adaptations; peripheral blood flow	Karolinska Institute (Sweden)
John Sutton	Muscle biochemistry; high altitude	University of Sydney (Australia)
Charles Tipton	Exercise performance	University of Arizona (U.S.A.)
Peter Wagner	Respiration	University of California–San Diego (U.S.A.)
Brian Whipp	Control of ventilation	St. George's Hospital Medical School (Britain)
Clyde Williams	Muscle biochemistry	Loughborough University (Britain)

and exercise performance. Similarly, the pure research of Frank and Starling on myocardial ventricular filling and ejection has been the basis for the development of pharmacologic agents to treat heart failure, hypertension, atherosclerotic heart disease and to emphasize the importance of venous return in the function of the heart and central circulation during exercise. In more recent years, the molecular research on genetic regulation has been applied to exercise to identify the molecular events in the regulation of protein synthesis after exercise, in the regulation of membrane receptor movement to and from the sarcolemma of muscle in response to exercise and specific hormones, and in the effects of exercise

on the immune system. History has shown that the answers obtained from pure research are used to frame questions of an applied nature and that they therefore fuel applied research.

Applied Research

Despite the overwhelming medical interest in exercise physiology, applied research remains an important, if not the primary, component of the discipline.[6] The quest for fostering optimal athletic performance remains the driving force for this research. However, today the focus of the research is not just for elite athletes, but also for the increasing popula-

TABLE 1.3

Academic disciplines that have used exercise to further evaluate human function or used exercise as a clinical diagnostic tool

DISCIPLINE/TOPIC	EXAMPLE APPLICATIONS
Anatomy/body composition	Role of exercise in changing lean and fat body mass
Biochemistry	Metabolic responses to muscle contraction and training
Biology	Alterations to the morphology of muscle after training
Biomechanics	Kinetics and kinematics of movement
Cardiology	Diagnostic, rehabilitative, and preventive uses
Endocrinology	Diabetes research
Immunology	Immune responses; treatment of individuals with AIDS
Nephrology	Reversal of cardiovascular risk factors; possibility of improved renal function?
Neurology	Effects of exercise on nerve function
Nutrition	Macronutrient and micronutrient needs during exercise
Occupational therapy	Injury rehabilitation/prevention
Orthopedics	Effects of exercise on bone remodeling
Physical therapy	Injury rehabilitation/prevention
Psychiatry	Stress reduction
Pulmonology	Respiratory muscle training

FOCUS BOX 1.1

Examples of specific exercise-related pure research questions since 1950

What regulates cardiac, vascular, and respiratory function during exercise?

What regulates microvascular blood flow?

How does exercise influence the regulation of blood glucose?

What are the contributions of the macronutrients (carbohydrate, fat, protein) to muscle energy production during exercise of different intensities and during recovery?

What are the main sources of the endogenous macronutrients used during exercise?

Why does carbohydrate ingestion during exercise delay fatigue?

What are the biochemical exchanges that occur between skeletal muscle and the liver during exercise, and why?

How do lactate and free protons leave skeletal muscle during exercise?

What are the roles of cAMP in the muscle fibers' intracellular responses to contraction?

What are the molecular determinants of muscle injury and the repair process?

Are the oxygen consumption responses of working muscle and the total body similar during exercise?

What are the causes of arterial hypoxemia during intense exercise in well-trained athletes?

What factors regulate the emptying of the stomach and uptake of water and nutrients by the small intestine?

FOCUS BOX 1.2

Examples of specific exercise-related applied research questions since 1950

Does exercise training alter the proportion of muscle fiber types?

What are the best physiologic predictors of strength, endurance, and sprint exercise performance?

What combination of nutrition and exercise best increases muscle glycogen stores?

What cardiovascular and neuromuscular adaptations occur during endurance training?

Which of the central or peripheral adaptations are most important in increasing $\dot{V}O_2$max after training?

What factors contribute to the increase in lactate production during exercise?

What factors contribute to the increase in blood lactate during exercise?

What is the role of exercise in the process of acclimation to a hot environment?

What is the best way to become heat acclimated?

Does training at altitude improve sea level or altitude exercise performance?

How much endurance exercise is needed to induce significant adaptations?

How much and what type of exercise best prevents the development of atherosclerotic cardiovascular disease?

Can ingesting carbohydrates during exercise spare muscle glycogen and improve exercise performance?

What types of exercise best retain bone mineral in the elderly and amenorrheic female?

What beverages best hydrate the body during or following exercise?

What are the causes of gender differences in acute and chronic responses to exercise?

What beverages best provide carbohydrates to the body during exercise?

---

tion of individuals who are now participating in regular physical activity. Increased involvement in exercise by the young, elderly, and female populations has presented additional research questions specific to the needs of these individuals.

Applied research has also developed because of the increased medical recognition of the benefits of physical activity. What types of exercise are best for which populations? Is exercise prescription for fitness different for different populations? Do the different populations respond differently to exercise when in different environments? These and other questions are all relevant and have been or still need to be answered. (see Focus Box 1.2)

Academic Development of Exercise Physiology

An interesting means to evaluate how the importance of exercise physiology has developed over the latter part of the twentieth century is to compare the academic programs that have incorporated the science of exercise physiology. Such a comparison is provided in Figure 1.3. During the 1970s, exercise physiology was one of many core courses in physical educa-

tion. At the time the main employment options for graduates in physical education were teaching, coaching, corporate fitness, community recreation programs, and fitness clubs. Today the academic structure comprising exercise physiology courses is totally different. Students from diverse backgrounds and equally diverse intended careers are taking classes in exercise physiology. Ironically, despite the recognized importance of exercise in the medical community, most medical programs throughout the United States do not require completion of a course in exercise physiology, although it probably will not be long before this changes (see Table 1.3).

New Frontiers of Exercise-Related Research

In the last 50 years, tremendous achievements have been possible in both pure and applied research as a result of the application of new or improved research techniques or the application of techniques to new conditions. The percutaneous needle biopsy technique to sample human skeletal muscle before, during, and after exercise is an example of a revolutionary advancement that has influenced both exercise physiology and muscle biochemistry

FIGURE 1.3

A comparison of the academic function of exercise physiology between the 1970s and the 1990s. During the 1970s, exercise physiology was a course required for students of physical education. During the 1990s, exercise physiology is a required or recommended course for students from diverse educational backgrounds and for diverse vocational fields.

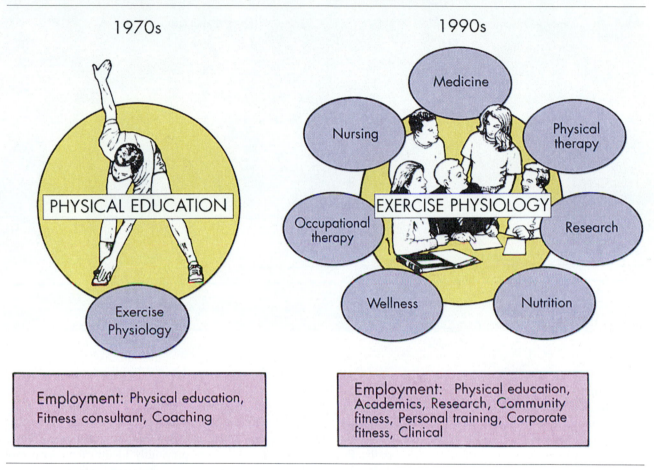

research[3,7] (see Chapters 8 and 9). In recent years similar advances have been made because of new equipment, technologies, and research techniques. The use of stable isotopes to study cellular metabolism in humans during rest, exercise, and postexercise conditions has contributed to the further understanding of substrates used during exercise. Similarly, noninvasive techniques such as magnetic resonance (MR) imaging and MR spectroscopy are providing insight into the function and adaptability of skeletal muscle metabolism to different exercise intensities[10] (see Chapter 10).

The future of research in exercise physiology is more and more dependent on the use of sophisticated equipment and academic and research skills that span applied approaches, as well as the pure fields of molecular biology, biochemistry, neurophysiology, cardiology, pulmonary physiology, and endocrinology. The enormous amount of exercise-related research published in journals (Focus Box 1.3) makes acquiring a broad knowledge base a more difficult task and the future of the field more challenging and more rewarding.

What is exercise physiology today?
How will exercise physiology develop in the future?
What are the future directions in which exercise related research are focused?

These all are important questions. In the introductory remarks of this chapter, concern was expressed about the ever expanding academic information contained within the general definition of the discipline. As with other disciplines, the splitting of the field into separate but related areas of interest is inevitable. For example, chemistry has developed into biochemistry, inorganic chemistry, and organic chemistry. In fact, evidence of the separation of traditional exercise physiology topics is already present. The field of body composition has grown and become a separate area of inquiry, as have exercise prescription, clinical exercise physiology, exercise nutrition, exercise biochemistry, and training for sports and athletic performance. Today separate textbooks are written for the specific courses that have been developed for these topics. How

FOCUS BOX 1.3

Journals that publish exercise-related research and reviews

Acta Physiologica Scandinavica

American Journal of Clinical Nutrition

American Journal of Physiology

American Journal of Sports Medicine

Biochemistry

Canadian Journal of Applied Sports Sciences

Circulation

European Journal of Applied Physiology

International Journal of Sports Medicine

International Journal of Sports Nutrition

Journal of Applied Physiology

Journal of Biochemical Research

Journal of Biochemistry

Journal of Clinical Investigation

Journal of Physiology

Journal of Sports Medicine and Physical Fitness

Journal of Sports Sciences Research

Medicine and Science in Sports and Exercise

Metabolism

Pediatric Exercise Science

Pflugers Archives

Physiological Reviews

Research Quarterly For Exercise and Sport

Sports Medicine

The Physician and Sports Medicine

this development has influenced exercise physiology is unclear, because textbooks developed for the field have changed minimally in structure, content, and presentation over the last 20 years.

These facts are some of the fundamental reasons that this text differs from those already used in exercise physiology. We have not only written the book based on a more advanced coverage of information, but altered the structure and presentation of the material to reflect recent and hopefully future trends in exercise-related research. Topics of exercise and its relationship to aging, fatigue, gender differences, children, skeletal function, immune function, as well as the subjects of exercise nutrition, and exercise in extreme environments, have been given increased attention, although topics that have emerged as separate disciplines have received less attention (e.g., body composition, exercise prescription, training strategies).

The future of exercise physiology seems destined to be one of continued increased interest and diversity. The new disciplines that were previously identified to have evolved from traditional exercise physiology will probably firmly establish themselves as separate courses in graduate programs catering to exercise-related topics throughout the world. How all these changes will affect the academic material presented in exercise physiology is unclear. However, what is clear is that current courses in exercise physiology need to change to meet the needs of the students who must be trained for the present and the future. We feel that the new approach adopted in this text is congruent with the future development of the discipline.

SUMMARY

■ **Exercise physiology** can be defined as the study of how exercise alters the structure and function of the human body. In the early twentieth century, exercise was used by chemists to study the macronutrients used during exercise. At the same time, the ability of the body to combust foodstuffs during exercise was researched, and allowed calculations of efficiency, the energy expended during exercise, and the principles of using energy expenditure as a measure of exercise intensity.

■ A surprisingly large volume of research was also being conducted using exercise during the first three decades of the twentieth century. Hill of Great Britain studied oxygen consumption during exercise, Rubner and Voit extended the theoretic findings of Lavoisier with human research of indirect calorimetry in differing nutritional, environmental, and exercise conditions, and Hill and Meyerhoff published extensive findings of carbohydrate catabolism and the production of lactic acid in skeletal muscle.

■ In the United States an organized effort investigating the effects of exercise on the human body began after the formation of the Harvard Fatigue Laboratory in 1927. David Bruce Dill was the research director of the lab; he remained in this position until the laboratory closed in 1947. Research from the Harvard Fatigue Laboratory was conducted in the areas of environmental physiology (altitude, dry, and moist heat), skeletal muscle metabolism during exercise, the effects of aging on metabolism at rest and during exercise, blood gas transport and acid-base balance, and nutrition.

■ Research in exercise physiology has undergone several transitions, identified as "the beginning," "the era of sports and athletics," and "the era of medical awakening." Nutrition and muscle metabolism are good examples of topics in which research progressed from resting conditions to the condition that provides the greatest challenge to homeostasis in each example: exercise. This early research soon provided adequate knowledge from which scientists could begin to ask and answer applied questions that concerned exercise.

■ During the 1960s and 1970s, research findings were presented that indicated the potential for exercise to aid not only the athlete, but also the average citizen. Athletes were healthier than the average citizen, had fewer signs of degenerative diseases, and arguably had a higher quality of life. Indirect research evidence linked these differences to the adaptations of the body to continued exercise stress. The vocalization of the medical doctors who were hooked on exercise, such as George Sheehan and Kenneth Cooper, assisted the recognition of the important health benefits of exercise by the medical community.

■ In conjunction with the known deteriorating fitness of Western societies' children, with those of the United States being a notable example, and the increasing incidence of and mortality from coronary artery disease, the role of exercise in health maintenance and disease prevention was given increased attention.

■ Today, exercise is used as a therapy during rehabilitation from injury and illness and as a preventive strategy to combat atherosclerotic cardiovascular disease. The medical interest in exercise physiology is developing a separate discipline, **clinical exercise physiology,** and textbooks are being written to satisfy this need.

■ The recent history of exercise physiology is best categorized into the divisions of pure research and applied research. **Pure research** uses exercise to further understand physiology, whereas **applied research** uses physiology to further understand exercise.

■ Despite the overwhelming medical interest in exercise physiology, applied research remains an important, if not the primary, component of the discipline. The quest for fostering optimal athletic performance remains the driving force for this research. However, today the focus of the research is not just on elite athletes, but also the increasing population of individuals now participating in regular physical activity.

■ In the last 50 years, tremendous achievements have been possible in both pure and applied research because of the application of new or improved research techniques or the application of techniques to new conditions. During the 1960s the application of the needle biopsy of percutaneous muscle to research of muscle biochemistry stimulated a wealth of research. Today, the use of stable isotopes to study cellular metabolism in humans during rest, exercise, and postexercise conditions has contributed to the further understanding of substrates used during exercise. Similarly, noninvasive techniques such as magnetic resonance (MR) imaging and MR spectroscopy are providing insight into the function and adaptability of skeletal muscle metabolism to different exercise intensities.

REVIEW QUESTIONS

1. What is the history of the science of exercise physiology?

2. What are the names of several scientists who were influential in providing research findings that are important in the development of knowledge in exercise physiology? What were the topics researched?

3. Why was the Harvard Fatigue Laboratory important for the development of exercise physiology in the United States and Scandinavia?

4. Why has there been increased clinical recognition of exercise?

5. Explain the difference between pure and applied research.

6. Be able to give the names of important pure and applied researchers in exercise physiology and explain their research.

REFERENCES

1. Åstrand PO: *Textbook of work physiology: physiological bases of exercise,* New York, 1986, McGraw-Hill.

2. Åstrand PO: Influence of Scandinavian scientists in exercise physiology, *Scand J Med Sci Sports* 1:3-9, 1991.

3. Brooks GA: Basic exercise physiology. *American College of Sports Medicine-40th anniversary lectures,* Indianapolis, 1994, American College of Sports Medicine.

4. Buskirk ER: From Harvard to Minnesota: keys to our history, *Exerc Sports Sci Rev* 20:1-26, 1992.

5. Chapman CB, Mitchel JH: The physiology of exercise, *Sci Am* 212:88-96, 1965.

6. Chapman CB: The long reach of Harvard's Fatigue Laboratory: 1926-1947, *Perspect Biol Med* 34:17-33, 1990.

7. Costill DL: Applied exercise physiology. *American College of Sports Medicine-40th anniversary lectures,* Indianapolis, 1994, American College of Sports Medicine.

8. DeJours P: Control of respiration in muscular exercise. In Fenn WO, Rahn H, editors: *Respiration,* vol 1, section 3, Washington D.C., 1964, American Physiological Society.

9. Dill DB: *Heat, life and altitude,* Cambridge, 1938, Harvard University Press.

10. Fleckenstein JL, Watamull D, McIntire DD et al: Muscle prton T2 relaxation tims during work and during repetitive voluntary exercise, *J Appl Physiol* 74(60): 2855-2859, 1993.

11. Gollnick PD, Armstrong RB, Saubert CW et al: Enzyme activity and fiber composition in skeletal muscle of untrained and trained men, *J Appl Physiol* 33:312-319, 1972.

12. Gollnick PD: Metabolism of substrates: energy substrate metabolism during exercise and as modified by physical training, *Fed Proc* 44:353-357, 1985.

13. Hill AV: Muscular exercise, lactic acid, and the supply and utilization of oxygen, *Q J Med* 16:135-171, 1923.

14. Horvath SM, Horvath EC: *The Harvard Fatigue Laboratory: its history and contributions,* Englewood Cliffs, NJ, 1973, Prentice Hall.

15. Jackson MA: Bruno Balke welcomes and creates avalanches, *Phys Sports Med* 7:93-98, 1977.

16. Karpovich PV: *Physiology of muscular activity,* Philadelphia, 1965, WB Saunders.

17. Kennedy JF: The soft American, *Sports Illustrated* 13:14-17, 1960.

18. Keys A: From Naples to seven countries: a sentimental journey, *Prog Biochem Pharmacol* 19:1-30, 1983.

19. Keys A: Physical performance in relation to diet, *Fed Proc* 2:164-187, 1943.

20. Lusk G: *The elements of the science of nutrition,* Philadelphia, 1928, WB Saunders.

21. Mitchell JH, Sproule WC, Chapman CB: The physiological meaning of the maximal oxygen uptake test, *J Clin Invest* 37:538-547, 1958.

22. Morehouse LE, Miller AT: *Physiology of exercise,* St. Louis, 1971, Mosby.

23. Pipe AL: Sport, science, and society: ethics in sports medicine, *Med Sci Sports Exerc* 25(8):888-900, 1993.

24. Raven PB, Squires WG: What is science? *Med Sci Sports Exerc* 21(4):351-352, 1989.

25. Sahlin K, Katz A, Broberg S: Tricarboxylic acid cycle intermediates in human muscle during prolonged exercise, *Am J Physiol* 259(28):C834-C841, 1990.

26. Taylor HL, Buskirk ER, Henschel A: Maximal oxygen intake as an objective measure of cardiorespiratory performance, *J Appl Physiol* 8:73-80, 1955.

RECOMMENDED READINGS

■ Åstrand PO: *Textbook of work physiology: physiological bases of exercise,* New York, 1986, McGraw-Hill.

■ Åstrand PO: Influence of Scandinavian scientists in exercise physiology, *Scand J Med Sci Sports* 1:3-9, 1991.

■ Chapman CB, Mitchell JH: The physiology of exercise, *Sci Am* 212:88-96, 1965.

■ Chapman CB: The long reach of Harvard's Fatigue Laboratory: 1926-1947, *Perspect Biol Med* 34:17-33, 1990.

■ Costill DL: Applied exercise physiology. *American College of Sports Medicine-40th anniversary lectures,* Indianapolis, 1994, American College of Sports Medicine.

■ Dill DB: *Heat, life and altitude,* Cambridge, 1938, Harvard University Press.

■ Horvath SM, Horvath EC: *The Harvard Fatigue Laboratory: its history and contributions,* Englewood Cliffs, NJ, 1973, Prentice Hall.

■ Kennedy JF: The soft American, *Sports Illustrated* 13:14-17, 1960.

■ Lusk G: *The elements of the science of nutrition,* Philadelphia, 1928, WB Saunders.

CHAPTER 2

Bioenergetics and the Design of Cellular Metabolism

OBJECTIVES

After studying this chapter you should be able to:

- Identify the different forms of energy in biologic systems.

- Define the terms thermodynamics, energetics, and bioenergetics.

- Describe the laws of thermodynamics.

- Explain reactions in terms of changes in enthalpy and entropy.

- Explain the differences between the standard and absolute ΔG for a given reaction.

- Describe why adenosine triphosphate (ATP) is an important molecule in energy transfer reactions.

- Explain why substrate and product concentrations can influence the free energy release during chemical reactions.

- Identify the importance of "activated" molecules in metabolism.

- Describe the involvement of electrons in catabolism and anabolism.

- Identify the molecules that are involved in the exchange of electrons and protons during chemical reactions.

- Describe the interrelationships between the catabolic pathways and between catabolism and anabolism during metabolism.

KEY TERMS

thermodynamics	equilibrium
energetics	endergonic
bioenergetics	equilibrium constant (K'eq)
enthalpy	mass action ratio (L)
exothermic	metabolism
endothermic	catabolism
entropy	anabolism
free energy	oxidation
exergonic	reduction

The controlled conversion of energy from one form to another characterizes the function of the body at the cellular level. The expenditure of energy during muscle contraction exemplifies the conversion of chemical energy released in the breakdown of adenosine triphosphate (ATP) to the production of mechanical energy. Other forms of energy transfer exist in the body. Solar radiation is converted to chemical energy in the retina of the eye, and this energy is then converted to electrical energy in the form of a nerve action potential as information is directed to the brain to provide the cognitive sensation of sight. The ability for energy to be transferred from one form to another and the direction in which this exchange occurs can be explained and predicted by application of the laws of thermodynamics. Furthermore, the application of these laws to cellular metabolism can explain why a certain reaction proceeds in one direction, yet under different cellular conditions may proceed in the reverse direction. This is not a minor point, because the ability for cells to control reaction rates and directions is a fundamental concept that must be understood before the process of the breakdown of molecules (catabolism) or their synthesis (anabolism) can truly be appreciated and understood. The purpose of this chapter is to introduce the laws governing the completion and direction of chemical reactions in the body, to explain the directionality of specific chemical reactions, and to provide an overview of the design of cellular metabolism.

Energy Transfer

The processes of life, electronics, and mechanization exist because of the organized and controlled transfer of energy from one form to another. We exploit the controlled transfer of energy in everyday life by using electricity and gas to run our household appliances, petroleum products to fuel our combustion engines, and solar energy, in combination with water and fertile soil, to grow plants. Many other examples of energy transfer are shown in Figure 2.1, and the form of energy in these transfers can be thermal, chemical, mechanical, electrical, radiant, or a combination of several forms. The science that explains and quantifies energy transfer has historically been called **thermodynamics**, however, because not all energy transfer is thermal, another accepted name is **energetics**.[9]

Not all principles in energetics are explained in detail in this text. These principles are based on mathematic derivations more suited to the advanced study of physical chemistry.[1] Nevertheless, some underlying concepts should be identified to appreciate how the principles of energetics can be applied to living biologic systems, such as the human body. The science that applies the principles of energetics to living systems is called **bioenergetics**.[1,8]

thermodynamics (ther'mo-di-nam'iks)
the branch of physicochemical science concerned with energy transfer between heat and mechanical work

energetics (en-er-jet'iks)
the study of energy transfer in physical and chemical changes

bioenergetics (bi'o-en-er-jet'iks)
the study of energy transfer in chemical reactions within living tissue

FIGURE 2.1

Interconversion among the differing forms of energy.

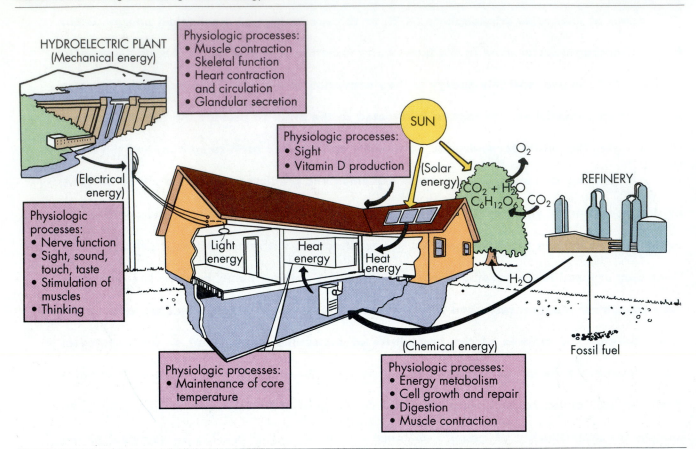

HYDROELECTRIC PLANT
(Mechanical energy)

Physiologic processes:
• Muscle contraction
• Skeletal function
• Heart contraction
  and circulation
• Glandular secretion

Physiologic processes:
• Sight
• Vitamin D production

SUN

(Solar energy)

O_2

$CO_2 + H_2O$
$C_6H_{12}O_6$ CO_2

REFINERY

(Electrical energy)

Physiologic processes:
• Nerve function
• Sight, sound, touch, taste
• Stimulation of muscles
• Thinking

Light energy

Heat energy

Heat energy

H_2O

Physiologic processes:
• Maintenance of core temperature

(Chemical energy)

Fossil fuel

Physiologic processes:
• Energy metabolism
• Cell growth and repair
• Digestion
• Muscle contraction

The human body is an excellent example of the importance of bioenergetics. Table 2.1 lists the many forms of energy and provides examples of physiologic processes within the human body that use them. Of the processes listed, two appear in multiple energy forms—sight and muscle contraction. Sight occurs from the transfer of energy from a radiant to an electrical form. Similarly, the mechanical consequences of muscle contraction stem from the transfer of electrical energy to chemical energy and chemical energy to mechanical energy. The exchange of energy between forms is the foundation on which the specialized and complex functions of biologic life exist.

First Law of Thermodynamics: Conservation of Energy

An understanding of the first law of thermodynamics is crucial to the understanding of bioenergetics. *Energy cannot be created or destroyed, but it can be changed from one form to another.*

The human body is an example of a system that can have energy transfer between it and the surrounding environment and also in systems within itself. The words energy, work, system, surroundings, and universe have their own meanings in bioenergetics, as indicated in Figure 2.2. These terms are

TABLE 2.1

Energy forms within the human body and examples of physiologic processes that use them

ENERGY FORM	PHYSIOLOGIC PROCESSES
Solar (radiant)	Sight
	Vitamin D production
Electrical	Nerve function
	Sight, sound, touch, taste
	Stimulation of muscle
	Thinking
Chemical	Energy metabolism
	Cell growth and repair
	Digestion
	Muscle contraction
Thermal (heat)	Maintenance of core temperature
Mechanical	Muscle contraction
	Skeletal function and movement
	Heart contraction and circulation
	Glandular secretion

FIGURE 2.2

The association among the system, surroundings, and universe during exergonic reactions when there is an increase in entropy.

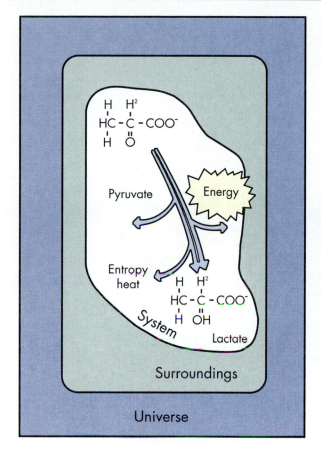

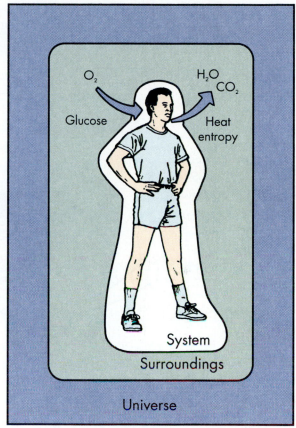

important to define when accounting for energy transfer.[8] Figure 2.3 illustrates common examples of energy transfer in the body that should be recognized. Based on the first law of thermodynamics, no energy is lost in any of these transfers. Evaporation of water from the skin to a vapor releases energy equivalent to that stored in the hydrogen bonds that made it a liquid. Similarly, the chemical energy in the fuel used by muscle to eventually cause contraction can be accounted for by the major by-products of contraction, which are mainly mechanical work (contraction) and heat.

A reaction can be viewed as energy transfer. If no work is done in a reaction (e.g., if it occurred in a test tube), all of the enthalpy change is heat. Conversely, if the same reaction(s) occurred in the body, part of the change in energy can be harnessed to accomplish mechanical or chemical work (e.g., muscle contraction), with less heat absorbed or released.[9] The relationships between a change in total heat or energy content (ΔH), work done by a reaction (w), and heat absorbed (+q) and released (-q) in a reaction are expressed in the following equation:

$$2\text{-}1 \qquad \Delta H = q - w$$

ΔH is termed the change in **enthalpy**.[1,5] The component of energy that can be used to perform work is called *free energy,* and is discussed later. Reactions that produce heat result in a negative ΔH and are termed **exothermic.** Reactions that absorb heat result in a positive ΔH and are termed **endothermic** (Figure 2.5).

Weight gain or loss is based on the first law of thermodynamics. Assuming that body mass represents a total store of

---

enthalpy (en'thal'py)
a thermodynamic function concerning heat content

exothermic (eks-o-ther'mik)
denotes a chemical reaction that releases heat

endothermic (end-o-ther'mik)
denotes a chemical reaction that absorbs heat

FIGURE 2.3

Two examples of enthalpy changes during exercise. In muscle, adenosine triphosphate (ATP) is hydrolyzed to provide the free energy for contraction, releasing heat and increasing entropy. During exercise, most of this heat is transferred from the contracting muscles to the skin via blood flow. The heat of the body can then be absorbed in the transformation of liquid water to a vapor, and increasing entropy. In each example, there is a system involved in the energy transfer, and a surroundings that is affected by the energy transfer. The system and surroundings combine to equal the universe.

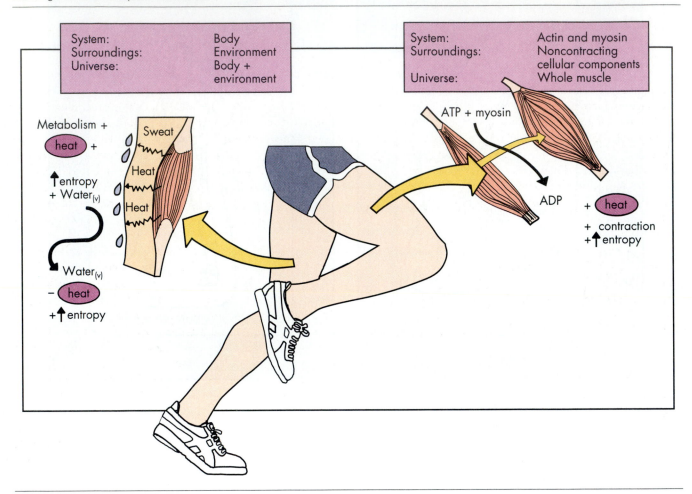

potential chemical energy (enthalpy), energy balance exists when energy expenditure (w) equals energy intake (+q) (i.e., the caloric balance equation). Consequently, weight loss can occur only if w exceeds q. Therefore stored energy reserves must be used to replace a deficit in caloric intake. The difficulties with weight loss and the roles of exercise and diet in weight loss are explained in Chapter 28.

Another important lesson depicted in Figure 2.3 is that both evaporation and muscle contraction occur in biologic life, yet the processes have differing ΔH characteristics. Evaporation of water absorbs heat, and since no work is performed, ΔH is positive. Conversely, not only is heat released during muscle contraction, but also work is performed and ΔH is negative. Consequently, quantifying the change in enthalpy does not provide sufficient information to state whether a reaction will proceed in one direction or another. If all reactions were

to proceed with heat release, evaporation would not occur. Of course, this situation would be disastrous for body heat regulation during exercise (see Chapters 13 and 26).

If we apply common sense to the issue of energy transfer, we realize that reactions always seem to proceed in the direction that results in less *usable energy*. The generation of electricity, whether by coal combustion, solar energy, or nuclear fission, never produces energy equal to the energy provided in the original sources. In many machines less than 25% of the input energy is released in the form of useful work. The ratio of energy input to output for a given amount of work is termed *efficiency*. As explained in Chapter 4, the efficiency of the body's metabolic pathways can vary between 25% and 40%. Chapter 7 reveals that the body is approximately 30% efficient in converting chemical energy into mechanical energy during exercise.

Second Law of Thermodynamics: Directionality

To determine why, or in which direction, a reaction is to proceed, we need to understand the second law of thermodynamics. *Energy transfer always proceeds in the direction of increased entropy.*

If we turn again to Figure 2.3, an additional by-product (other than work and heat) in energy transfer reactions in biologic systems is **entropy**. Entropy is a term for increased randomness or disorder.[5,8,9] The need to define the system and surroundings is crucial to identifying entropy changes during a reaction. Entropy can be visualized in many different ways in biologic systems. Gases generally have more entropy than liquids, and liquids have more entropy than solids. Similarly, certain molecules have a higher degree of order (less entropy) than others. Protein molecules, with very specific three-dimensional structures, denature to a more random structure, thus increasing entropy. Students should not immediately associate increased entropy with simply an increase in the number of molecules formed during reactions.

Water evaporation and muscle contraction are two examples in which the ΔH values are in opposition, yet the increase in entropy is a consistent feature of the energy transfer. For changes in enthalpy, temperature (T), and entropy (ΔS for the universe [system + surroundings]) at constant temperature and pressure, the following relationship exists:

$$2\text{-}2 \qquad \Delta H - T\Delta S < 0$$

For a reaction to proceed, the change in the product of T and ΔS must exceed ΔH. In the previous example of evaporation, the increase in entropy must have been greater than the positive change in enthalpy. In biologic systems, the ability to utilize the energy released in reactions is the basis for metabolism. The difference between enthalpy and entropy for a given reaction must therefore represent an energy source (**free energy**) that is available for an additional source of work. In humans, this work is most often chemical or mechanical, but in other biologic systems this energy can also be used in other ways (for example, the light in the tail of the firefly). The difference between enthalpy and entropy for a reaction is called a change in free energy and is denoted *Gibbs' free energy* (ΔG).[1,5,8,9] Equation 2-2 can then be written as:

$$2\text{-}3 \qquad \Delta G = \Delta H - T\Delta S$$

All biologic reactions proceed in the direction that results in a negative ΔG, and are termed **exergonic** reactions. If ΔG is zero, the reaction is at **equilibrium** and no net change in energy transfer occurs. If ΔG is positive, by convention the reaction is termed **endergonic** (Figure 2.4).

At this time it is important to realize the characteristics of the entropy change during exergonic reactions. The increase in entropy does not have to be of the system but can be within the surroundings. For example, energy metabolism during growth and development results in an increased organization of the human body (decreased entropy), yet as we previously explained, each of these reactions must have been exergonic, releasing free energy and increasing the entropy of the surroundings. Consequently, to uphold the second law of thermodynamics in bioenergetics, entropy increases in the surroundings must exceed the decreased entropy of the biologic system. Living organisms order (decrease entropy) their internal milieu by releasing heat and entropy to their surroundings, thereby increasing the net entropy of the universe.

How do reactions exist that decrease randomness of the system, yet increase the entropy of the surroundings? Similarly, how can molecules be synthesized if there is no such thing as an endergonic reaction in biologic systems? The answer to these questions is relatively simple. Reactions that would be endergonic occur by their coupling to exergonic reactions. Thus the formation of ATP (Figure 2.5), which requires energy input, is coupled to a reaction that releases more free energy than is required for ATP synthesis.

Table 2.2 lists the change in enthalpy and free energy for glucose and palmitic acid (the main free fatty acid metabolized in skeletal muscle) under standard conditions (298° K, 760 mm Hg, pH = 7 (°K = 273 + °C). Compared with glucose, palmitic acid has a larger store of chemical energy that can be released as heat (-ΔH) and a larger amount of free energy (ΔG) that is harnessed during energy metabolism. Despite the differences in enthalpy and free energy between glucose and palmitic acid, glucose is the preferred fuel during moderate to intense exercise intensities. The biochemical reasons for this discrepancy are explained in Chapter 4.

It is important to understand the conditions at which the change in ΔG is determined. Under standard conditions (pH=7.0, T=25°C [298 °K]), initial product and substrate concentrations each equaling 1 mol/L, the standard Gibbs'

entropy (en′tro-pi)
the fraction of energy from a reaction that is unable to be used to perform work because of its use in increasing randomness or disorder

free energy
the energy from a reaction that can be used to perform work

exergonic (eks-er-gon′ik)
referring to a reaction that takes place with a release of free energy to its surroundings

equilibrium (e′kwi-lib′ri-um)
a state of dynamic balance in one or more reactions that proceed in opposing directions

endergonic (en-der-′gon-ik)
referring to a reaction that takes place with absorption of free energy from its surroundings

FIGURE 2.4

The change in free energy during exergonic and endergonic reactions. As explained in the text, endergonic reactions are converted to exergonic reactions in biologic systems by coupling to the hydrolysis of a high energy phosphate compound (e.g., ATP). Also, by convention, an endergonic reaction in vivo proceeds in the reverse direction, and therefore is then exergonic.

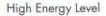
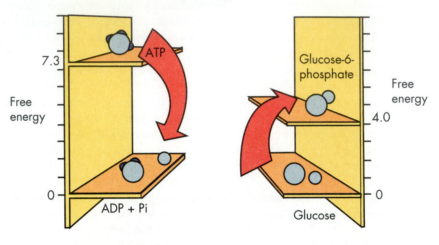
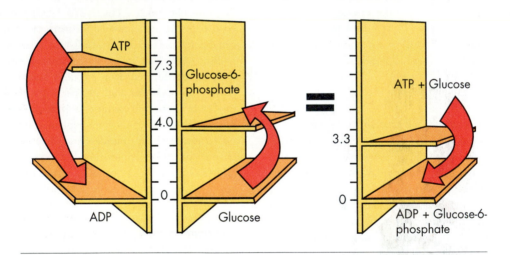

FIGURE 2.5

The structure of ATP and its metabolite products ADP and AMP. At pH = 7.0, the phosphate groups are completely ionized. (Courtesy Olmstead J, and Williams GM: *Chemistry: the molecular science*, St. Louis, 1994, Mosby.)

TABLE 2.2

The change in enthalpy and free energy from the complete catabolism of glucose and palmitic acid

	ΔH		ΔG°'	
CHEMICAL FORMULA	**Kcal/mol**	**Kj/mol**	**Kcal/mol**	**Kj/mol**
$C_6H_{12}O_6 \leftrightarrow$ CH3-CHOH-COOH*	-47	-196	-14.6[†]	-61
$C_6H_{12}O_6 + 6O_2 \leftrightarrow 6H_2O + 6CO_2$	-686	-2860	-277	-1157
$CH_3(CH_2)_{14}COOH$[‡]	-2340	-9753	-942	-3994

From Lehninger AL: *Principles of biochemistry,* New York, 1993, Worth; and Newsholme EA, Leech ER: *Biochemistry for the medical sciences,* Chichester, Eng, 1983, John Wiley & Sons.
* Lactic acid.
[†] Assumes 2 net ATP from glucose flux through glycolysis.
[‡] Palmitic acid.

free energy change (ΔG°') can be calculated from the measurement of the ratio of products and substrates after reaching equilibrium.

$$2\text{-}4 \qquad \Delta G°' = -R\,T\,\ln\frac{[products]}{[substrates]} \text{ (Kcal/mol)}$$

$$2\text{-}5 \qquad \Delta G°' = -R\,T\,\ln K'eq$$

NOTE: ln = 2.303 log
R = 0.001987 Kcal/mol/°K
T = 298 °K
$$K'eq = \frac{[products]}{[substrates]}$$

For reactions having multiple substrates (A + B) and products (C + D), their concentrations are used to calculate K'eq as follows:

$$A + B \leftrightarrow C + D$$

$$2\text{-}6 \qquad K'eq = \frac{[C]\,[D]}{[A]\,[B]}$$

The ratio of [products]/[substrates] is also termed the **equilibrium constant (K'eq),** because this value represents the resulting concentrations after the reaction reaches equilibrium (i.e., rates of forward and reverse reactions are equal). It is important to note that all biologic reactions are potentially reversible. The factors that determine whether a reaction proceeds in the reverse direction are discussed in the sections to follow. If the reaction has an inherent favoring of product formation, given equal substrate and product to begin with, the reaction spontaneously proceeds in the direction written. This result produces a K'eq greater than one, a positive logarithm, and therefore a negative ΔG°' (equation 2-4). Consequently, a K'eq less than one and a positive ΔG°' occur when the reaction favors substrate formation under standard conditions. Remember that the Keq is strictly a the-

oretic constant obtained under standard conditions, and is important for providing a standard reference condition from which different reactions can be compared.

Energy Transfer Within Cells

Table 2.3 lists the concentrations of many of the important molecules of energy metabolism within skeletal muscle at rest and after short-duration intense exercise to fatigue. It is clear that concentrations are well below 1 M, even if expressed relative to intracellular water, and also that substrate and product concentrations are not equal. Furthermore, depending on the exercise, rest, and environmental conditions, muscle temperatures can vary between 35° and over 40° C and muscle pH could vary between 7.0 and 6.0.[2] It is apparent that the ΔG°' must be altered to represent in vivo conditions.

The reaction of ATP hydrolysis is used as an example to identify the change in free energy release between standard (ΔG°') and absolute (ΔG) conditions (Figure 2.5).

$$ATP \leftrightarrow ADP + Pi$$

The ΔG°' for ATP hydrolysis is –7.3 Kcal/mol. Table 2.5 indicates that the known concentrations of the products and substrates of this reaction are very different from each other and much lower than 1 M, so that within the cell the expression of products/substrates is less than 1.

$$2\text{-}7 \qquad \text{mass action ratio (L)} = \frac{[products]}{[substrates]}$$

equilibrium constant (K'eq)

the product of product concentrations divided by the product of substrate concentrations for a reaction when at equilibrium

TABLE 2.3

The concentrations of molecules that are important in energy metabolism within skeletal muscle at rest and after intense exercise to fatigue

MOLECULE	REST	FATIGUE
	(mmol/kg wet wt)*	
CrP	24.0	3.0
ATP	5.0	4.5
ADP	0.05	0.5
Cr	4.0	25.0
Pi	3.0	24.0
H$^+$	1.0×10^{-4}	4×10^{-3}
Lactate	1.0	25.0
Glycogen	200.0	75.0

Data are from references 3,4,6,7, and 11.
* These concentrations apply to molecules in solution in the cytoplasm of the cell. For a concentration unit applicable for precise bioenergetic calculations, the metabolites would be expressed relative to muscle water, which is estimated at approximately 78% of wet weight muscle, hence increasing the concentration shown by a factor of 1.3.

The expression of in vivo products divided by substrates is termed the **mass action ratio**.[9] The mass action ratio is almost always very different from the K'eq for a given reaction, which indicates the very different bioenergetic cellular conditions compared with standard. Under physiologic conditions the differences in substrate and product concentrations from standard conditions result in either a greater or lesser release of free energy during chemical reactions. The mass action ratio is then used in a modified version of equation 2-4 to calculate the ΔG.

2-8
$$\Delta G = \Delta G^{\circ\prime} + RT \ln L$$

For ATP,
$$\Delta G = -7.3 + [0.001987 \times 311 \times (\ln 0.00003)]$$
$$\text{where, } R = 0.001987$$
$$T = 311^\circ K$$
$$0.00003 = L = [ADP] / [ATP]$$
$$\ln = 2.303 \log$$
$$= -7.3 + (0.001987 \times 311 \times -10.4143)$$
$$= -7.3 + -6.43$$
$$= -13.7 \text{ Kcal/mol}$$

The ΔG for ATP hydrolysis calculates to be more negative than the ΔG°′, indicating that there is more free energy released during this reaction in vivo than under standard conditions. Furthermore, the ΔG of -13.7 Kcal/mol for ATP hydrolysis calculates very close to the experimentally deter-

mined value of -14.2 Kcal/mol reported by Veech et al.[11] for rat muscle. It should be understood that the calculation of ΔG for a given reaction is different in differing tissues because of dissimilar concentrations of substrates and products and that dissimilar proportions of the metabolites can be bound to proteins or "free" in solution in the cytosol.[8] Furthermore, the ΔG of a given reaction changes under metabolic conditions that influence the substrate or product concentrations of the reaction.

Values for each of ΔG°′ and ΔG for several important phosphate molecules and reactions involved in energy metabolism in skeletal muscle are listed in Table 2.4. For many of these molecules and reactions there is a large difference between ΔG°′ and ΔG, which in many circumstances does not favor an increased release of free energy. The release of large amounts of free energy from the splitting of terminal phosphate bonds has led to the terminology of a "high-energy phosphate" bond. There is controversy concerning the chemical correctness of a high-energy bond, since the free energy of hydrolysis of the high-energy phosphate molecules does not come only from the bond.[9] Consequently, it is more correct to use the term *high-energy phosphate* than high-energy bond.

Not all reactions in cells have a large negative ΔG. Reactions that have a ΔG close to zero are termed *near equilibrium reactions,* are potentially reversible under in vivo conditions, and are important in energy metabolism because of their regulation by substrate and product concentrations. As explained in Chapter 6, the reversibility of the creatine phosphate (CrP) reaction, catalyzed by the enzyme creatine kinase, is crucial to the roles of CrP in energy metabolism during skeletal muscle contraction.

Design of Cellular Metabolism

Developing an understanding of energy metabolism is like trying to complete a jigsaw puzzle for which you do not know the intended outcome. If you start with the pieces of a puzzle already dismantled and therefore have no knowledge of how the puzzle looks when complete, it will be nearly impossible to put the puzzle together. If you study energy metabolism one pathway at a time, it is difficult to comprehend the overall purpose of metabolism and the diverse regulation that exists between pathways and between different tissues. The complete picture of energy metabolism encompasses how multiple pathways influence one another within a given cell and how similar pathways of cells in different tissues function differently to result in a well-organized whole body response to varied metabolic conditions.

Metabolism can be defined as the sum of all chemical reactions in the body. The complete picture of metabolism in the typical eukaryotic cell is a tremendous example of energy transfer and the role of several important molecules that serve

TABLE 2.4

The standard Gibbs' free energy change ($\Delta G^{\circ\prime}$) for the hydrolysis of several high-energy phosphate molecules, and the $\Delta G^{\circ\prime}$ and absolute Gibbs' free energy change (ΔG) for several coupled reactions in energy metabolism within skeletal muscle during resting conditions

MOLECULE/REACTION	$\Delta G^{\circ\prime}$		ΔG^{*}	
	Kcal/mol[†]	Kj/mol	Kcal/mol[†]	Kj/mol
Phosphoenolpyruvate (PEP)	-14.8	-61.9	—	—
3-Phosphoglyceroyl phosphate (PG3P)	-11.8	-49.3	—	—
Creatine phosphate (CrP)	-10.3	-43.1	0	0
Adenosine triphosphate (ATP)	-7.3	-30.5	-14.2	-59.4
Glucose 1-phosphate (G1P)	-4.9	-20.9	—	—
Glucose 6-phosphate (G6P)	-3.3	-13.8	—	—
Fructose 6-phosphate (F6P)	-3.8	-15.9	—	—
CrP + ADP + H$^+$ ↔ Cr + ATP + H$_2$0	-3.0	-12.5	0	0
G1,3P + ADP ↔ G3P + ATP	-4.5	-18.8	0.3	1.2
Glucose + ATP ↔ G6P + ADP	-4.0	-16.7	-8.0	-33.5
F6P + ATP ↔ F1,6P + ADP + H$^+$	-3.4	14.2	-5.3	22.2

Data are from references 8, 9, 10, and 11.

* ΔG values are not provided for reactions where in vivo substrate and product concentrations are uncertain.

† 1 Kcal = 4.1855 Kj.

as coupling agents in the transfer of free energy within and between metabolic pathways. A metabolic pathway consists of a series of individual reactions that result in the formation of an end product. Figure 2.6 illustrates the relationships between the two main functions of metabolism—**catabolism** and **anabolism**. Catabolism involves the breakdown of energy-yielding nutrients, the release of free energy and electrons and their coupled transfer to intermediary molecules (ATP, NADH, FADH, acetyl-CoA, and NADPH), and the formation of low–energy end products. The intermediary molecules can be used in a controlled and regulated manner to provide free energy to make the reactions of anabolism exergonic. Anabolism involves the covalent bonding of electrons, protons, and small molecules to produce larger molecules. Thus the free energy cost of building new and larger molecules occurs at the expense of the increased heat and entropy released from catabolism, as explained previously by the laws of thermodynamics.

Catabolic Reactions and Adenosine Triphosphate Regeneration

The formation of ATP during catabolism does not always involve the complete synthesis of new ATP molecules. During intense exercise, some ATP molecules are broken down to form molecules that do not have an adenine base

(e.g., IMP; see Chapter 5), and therefore new ATP must be synthesized to restore the normal cellular concentration. However, most ATP is reformed in cells, especially skeletal muscle fibers, by adding Pi to ADP. Thus use of the phrase *ATP regeneration* is more appropriate.

The substrates used by cells in catabolism for the formation of ATP are carbohydrates, free fatty acids, and amino acids (Figure 2.7). These molecules are catabolized during specific chemical pathways that release free energy stored as either ATP or NADPH and electrons and protons that become attached to certain molecules (NAD$^+$↔NADH,

mass action ratio
the product of product concentrations divided by the product of substrate concentrations for a reaction under physiologic conditions

metabolism (me-**tab'o**-lizm)
the sum of all reactions of the body

catabolism (ca-**tab'o**-lizm)
the reactions of the body that decrease the size of molecules

anabolism (a-**nab'o**-lizm)
the reactions of the body that increase the size of molecules

F I G U R E   2 . 6

The association between the reactions of catabolism and anabolism. (Modified from Atkinson DE: *Cellular energy metabolism and its regulation*, NY, 1977, Academic Press.)

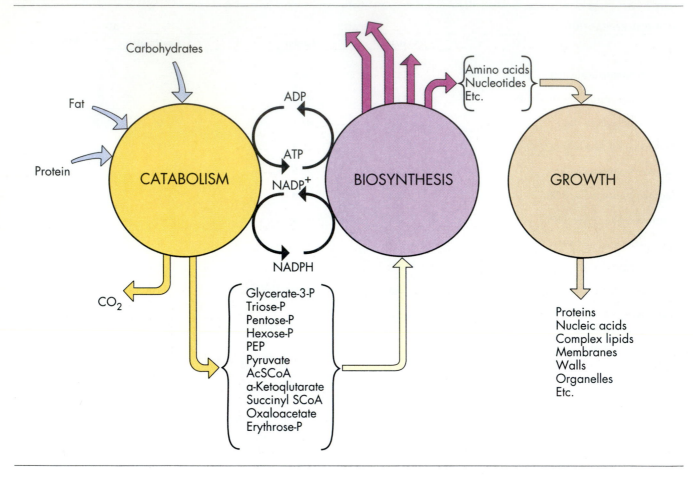

FAD$^+$↔FADH, NADP$^+$↔NADPH). The metabolic pathways specific for each of carbohydrate, free fatty acids, and amino acids are glycolysis, ß-oxidation, and transamination, respectively. Carbon backbones from each substrate eventually enter into the tricarboxylic acid cycle (TCA cycle) of the mitochondria, where additional electrons and protons are removed and the majority of carbon dioxide is produced.

Glycolysis therefore provides acetyl-CoA, which can enter into the TCA cycle; ß-oxidation provides acetyl-CoA, which also enters into the TCA cycle; and depending on the carbon numbers of the amino acid side chains, amino acid transamination can provide carbon molecules that can enter into glycolysis, form acetyl-CoA, or form molecules of the TCA cycle. The amine (NH$_2$) groups removed from amino acids are added to other carbon molecules (mainly pyruvate in skeletal muscle), removed from the cell and circulated to the liver, and processed to form urea, which is filtered from the blood by the kidney and removed from the body in urine (see Chapter 4).

Importance of Adenosine Triphosphate

The molecule ATP is illustrated in Figure 2.5. ATP consists of a backbone structure containing a modified nucleotide and a ribose sugar, from which a linear chain of three phosphate groups is attached.[8] Each of the three phosphate groups provides a $\Delta G°' = 7.3$ Kcal/mol. Consequently, conversion of ADP to AMP has a $\Delta G°' = -7.3$ Kcal/mol, and removal of two of the phosphates (for example, ATP↔AMP + 2Pi) has a $\Delta G°' = -14.6$ Kcal/mol.

The hydrolysis of ATP provides free energy for such biologic processes as molecular transport across cell membranes, the generation of concentration gradients, growth and development, the genetic regulation of cell function, and muscle contraction. Consequently, ATP is a molecule that transfers free energy between the reactions breaking down molecules (catabolism) and those that utilize free energy. Given the role of ATP in transferring free energy, it is understandable that the $\Delta G°'$ of ATP is intermediary to the other phosphate molecules involved in energy metabolism (Table 2.5). ATP can

FIGURE 2.7

The substrates used in catabolism. During the catabolic reactions, molecules are produced, free energy is stored, electrons and protons are stored, and heat is released. (Modified from Lehninger AL, et al: *Principles of biochemistry*, NY, 1993, Worth.)

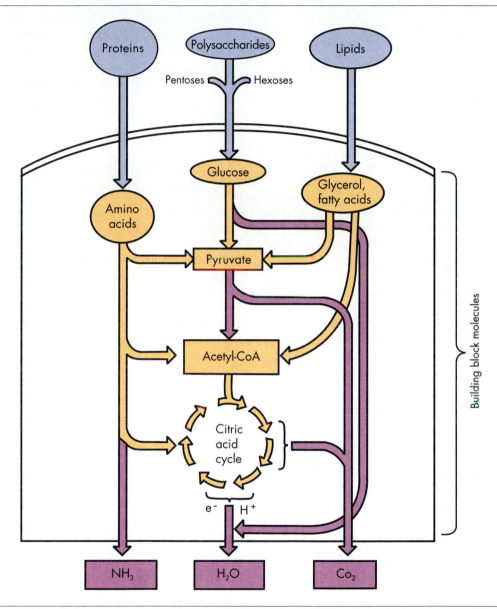

therefore be formed if the reaction ADP + Pi↔ATP is *coupled* to reactions releasing free energy in amounts greater than that required to add the phosphate group to ADP (that is, ΔG = –14.2 Kcal/mol). Similarly, the coupling of ATP hydrolysis to endergonic reactions provides free energy to drive the reaction to completion. The concept of free energy coupling is important for a complete understanding of energy metabolism. In coupling, free energy is transferred from one reaction to another, as indicated in the example of creatine phosphate and ATP under standard conditions.

Equation

$$CrP + H_2O \leftrightarrow Cr + Pi$$
$$\Delta G^{\circ\prime} = -10.3 \text{ Kcal/mol}$$
$$ATP + H_2O \leftrightarrow ADP + Pi + H^+$$
$$\Delta G^{\circ\prime} = -7.3 \text{ Kcal/mol}$$

Coupling

$$CrP + ADP + H^+ \leftrightarrow Cr + ATP + H_2O$$
$$\Delta G^{\circ\prime} = -3.0 \text{ Kcal/mol}$$
$$(-10.3 + 7.3 = -3.0)$$

TABLE 2.5

The free energy release from the dephosphorylation of certain phosphorylated compounds in skeletal muscle

COMPOUND	$\Delta G^{\circ\prime}$ (Kcal/mol)
Phosphoenolpyruvate	-14.8
Creatine phosphate	-10.3
ATP $\leftrightarrow$ ADP	-7.3
Glucose-1-phosphate	-5.0
Glucose-6-phosphate	-3.3

Adapted from Lehninger AL: *Principles of biochemistry*, New York, 1993, Worth.

The coupling of free energy is not confined to single reactions. When reactions exist that sequentially provide products that are substrates for other reactions, such as in a pathway, the free energy exchange of each reaction in a pathway can be summed to provide an overall $\Delta G^{\circ\prime}$ and ΔG.

The utility of ATP in energy transfer is the reason for it to be termed the *energy currency of the cell*. However, unlike real money, ATP cannot be stored. As discussed in Chapter 5, the design of energy metabolism is not to increase the concentration of ATP in cells, but to respond to its use by increasing the rate at which ATP is formed.

Other Molecules That Transfer Free Energy and Chemical Groups

ATP has been presented as a molecule that transfers a phosphate group to other molecules and in the process provides the free energy needed to make this transfer exergonic. Other molecules also exist that enable the transfer of chemical groups to other molecules—an exergonic process. These molecules are collectively termed high-energy or "activated" intermediates.

Table 2.6 lists examples of several activated intermediates in metabolism. Coenzyme A (CoA) is a common activated carrier. It is involved in the entry of two carbon groups from glycolysis into the TCA cycle in the form of acetyl-CoA. Similarly, acetyl–CoA can be reverted to the synthesis of free fatty acids or cholesterol. Biotin is a carrier that facilitates the fixation of carbon dioxide during certain chemical reactions. The best example is in the formation of oxaloacetate from pyruvate in the liver. This is an exergonic reaction that does not require the dephosphorylation of ATP. However, ATP dephosphorylation is required to add the carbon dioxide to the biotin carrier.

Molecules That Harness Electrons and Protons

An important characteristic of catabolism is the harnessing not only of free energy in the regeneration of ATP, but also the harnessing of electrons and protons that are removed from molecules during **oxidation** reactions. Oxidation refers to the removal of electrons during a chemical reaction. When a molecule becomes oxidized, it usually releases electrons that are added to another molecule. The molecule that gains electrons is said to be reduced and is able to then bind other atoms. Oxidation reactions occur in concert with **reduction** reactions, hence the term *oxidation-reduction* reactions (see Focus Box 2.1).

The molecules that receive electrons, and therefore become reduced, are important for the ability to generate large amounts of ATP from catabolism, and also for the electrons (reducing power) that are needed in the synthesis of molecules in anabolism. Figure 2.8 illustrates the molecules formed in the harnessing of electrons from catabolism. The molecules NADH and FADH are predominantly used in the regeneration of ATP in mitochondrial respiration. NADPH is an important molecule that provides the reducing power needed during anabolism.

TABLE 2.6

Molecules that transfer chemical groups and influence the free energy change of chemical reactions

MOLECULE	GROUP TRANSFERRED	CHEMICAL FORMULA
ATP	Phosphate	$-PO_3^-$
NADH, NADPH	Electron and proton	e^-, H^+
FADH	Electron and proton	e^-, H^+
Coenzyme A	Acetyl	$-CH_2CH_3$
Biotin	Carboxyl	$-COO^-$
S-Adenosylmethionine	Methyl	$-CH_3$
UDP-glucose	Glucose	$-C_6H_{12}O_6$

Electrons, protons, and oxidation-reduction reactions

Electrons are negatively charged subatomic particles that circulate around the atom nucleus. Electrons are essential for atoms to form covalent (electron-sharing) bonds. During many chemical reactions, electrons are either removed or added to molecules. Molecules that lose one or more electrons are said to be *oxidized*, whereas molecules that gain electrons are said to be *reduced*. Consequently, oxidation involves the loss of electrons, and reduction involves the gaining of electrons. Because oxidation and reduction reactions occur together, they are often termed *oxidation-reduction* or *redox* reactions.

$$A{:}e + B \leftrightarrow A + B{:}e$$

There are many examples of oxidation-reduction reactions in metabolism (Figure 2.9). The enzymes that catalyze these reactions are termed dehydrogenases. There are important examples of oxidation-reduction reactions in glycolysis, in which NAD^+ and NADH either receive or donate electrons, respectively (see Chapter 3). The same is true for the electron carrier oxidation-reduction pair FAD^+ and FADH, which is used in mitochondrial respiration.

A proton is a hydrogen atom that has lost its electron. Protons are symbolized H^+ and, like electrons, are integral to the design of energy metabolism. The concentration of protons ($[H+]$) in solution determines the acidity of the solution and is represented numerically by the negative log of the $[H^+]$ (pH). The movement of protons across the inner mitochondrial membrane during the electron transport chain is the driving force that eventually provides the free energy to phosphorylate ATP in the process of oxidative phosphorylation.

Anabolic Reactions and Reducing Power

Many of the reactions of the body that are involved in the synthesis of larger molecules require the input of electrons, protons, and free energy. To provide these additions, a specialized pathway of catabolism exists. This pathway is called the *pentose phosphate pathway* and involves the catabolism of glucose to a phosphorylated ribose sugar (see Figure 2.7). The ribose sugar is then used as a subunit in the synthesis of nucleotides (bases in the structure of DNA and RNA).

Electrons and protons are added to $NADP^+$ during the pentose phosphate pathway, resulting in two NADPH molecules for each conversion of glucose-6-phosphate to ribose-5-phosphate (see Chapter 5).

NADPH is essential for the synthesis of many molecules, including free fatty acids. Because skeletal muscle has only minimal activity of this pentose phosphate pathway, the majority of free fatty acids are synthesized in adipose tissue and the liver, which both have high activity (possess higher concentrations of the enzymes) of this pathway.

Interrelationships Between Catabolism and Anabolism

Catabolism can now be viewed as a series of reactions that breaks down molecules. During catabolism, other molecules are produced that can be used as components to synthesize larger molecules; free energy is released and harnessed in the form of ATP; electrons and protons are released and harnessed in the form of NADH, FADH, and NADPH; and heat is produced.

Some of the main molecules produced from catabolism that are incorporated into anabolic reactions are illustrated in Figure 2.10. As previously mentioned, glucose-6-phosphate can be converted to ribose-5-phosphate, which is then used as a component of nucleotide synthesis. Several of the glycolytic and TCA cycle intermediates can be used to form amino acids, which are then available for protein synthesis. In cells of the liver, acetyl-CoA can be incorporated into free fatty acid or cholesterol synthesis.

Many of the catabolic and anabolic reactions of metabolism occur together. Greater stimulation for catabolism increases catabolism and reduces anabolism, and vice versa. Catabolism and anabolism therefore function in a *dynamic balance,* and the diversity of cell function is dependent on the molecular balance and interactions between catabolism and anabolism.

oxidation (ok-si-da'shun)
the process of removing electrons from a molecule during a chemical reaction

reduction (re-duk'shun)
the process of adding electrons to a molecule during a chemical reaction

FIGURE 2.8

The molecules that are used to harness electrons and protons during catabolism.

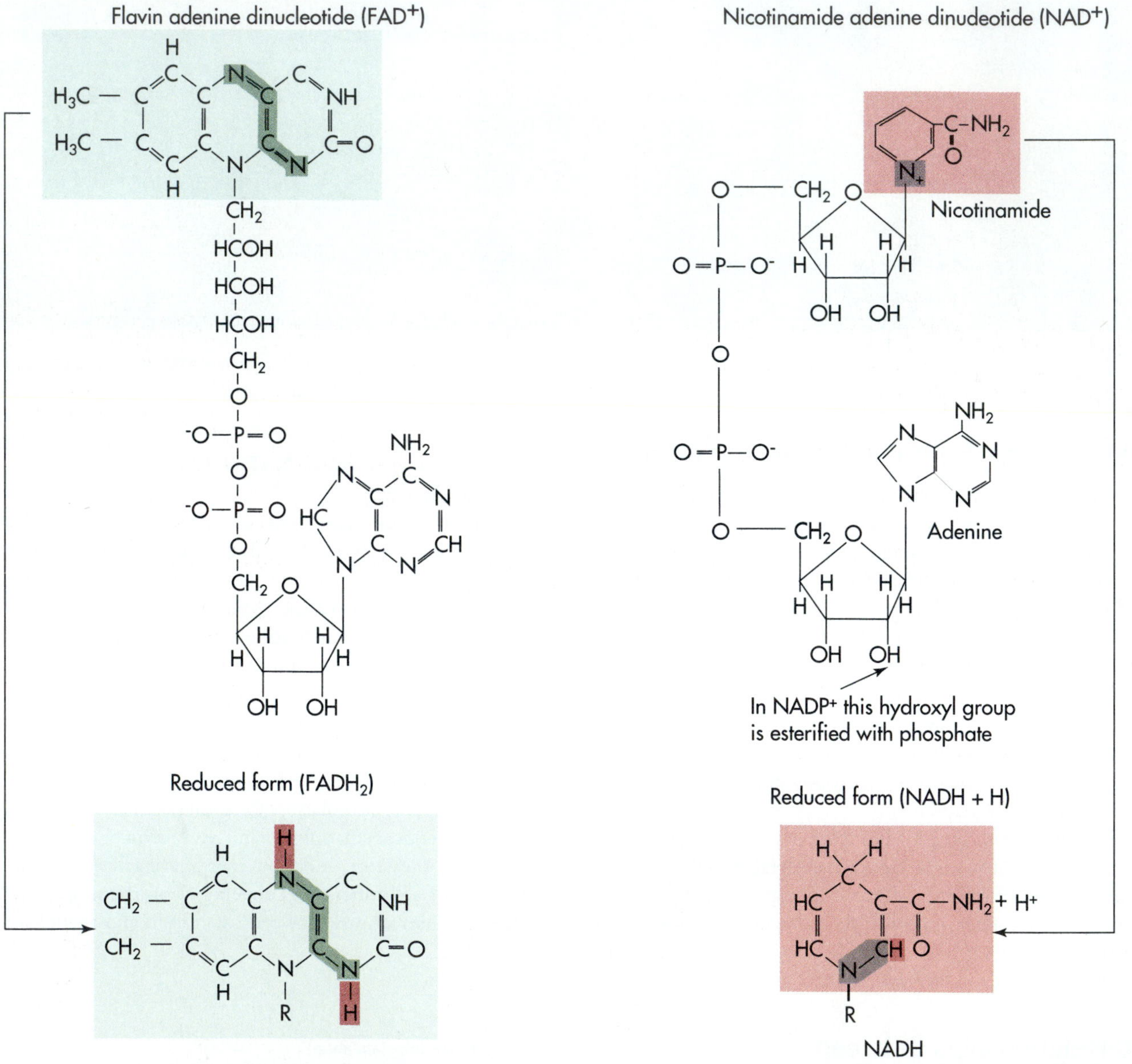

Flavin adenine dinucleotide (FAD⁺)

Nicotinamide adenine dinudeotide (NAD⁺)

Nicotinamide

Adenine

In NADP⁺ this hydroxyl group
is esterified with phosphate

Reduced form (FADH₂)

Reduced form (NADH + H)

NADH

FIGURE 2.9

The reaction catalyzed by lactate dehydrogenase. Conversion of pyruvate to lactate involves the reduction of pyruvate and oxidation of NADH. Conversion of lactate to pyruvate requires the oxidation of lactate and the reduction of NAD+ to NADH.

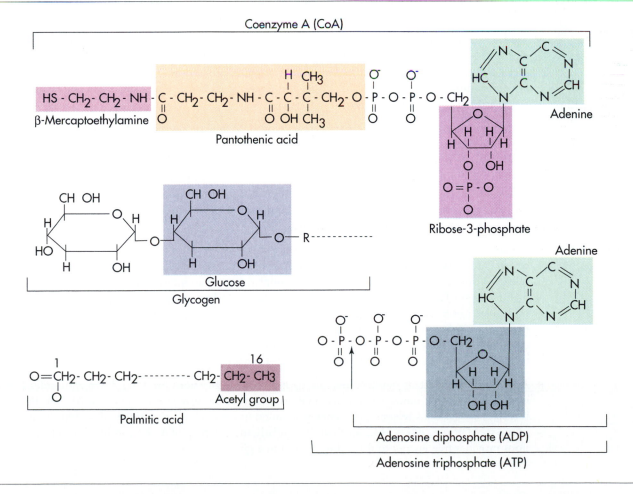

FIGURE 2.10

Many of the molecules produced catabolism are used as chemical components that are added to other molecules in anabolism, resulting in larger, more complex molecules. (From Lehninger AL et al: *Principles of biochemistry*, NY, 1993, Worth.)

SUMMARY

- The science that explains and quantifies energy transfer has historically been called **thermodynamics,** or **energetics.** The science that applies the principles of energetics to living systems is called **bioenergetics.** The ability for energy to be transferred from one form to another and the direction in which this exchange occurs can be explained and predicted by application of the two laws of thermodynamics.

- Based on the first law of thermodynamics, no energy is lost in any energy transfer. The change in total heat or energy content (ΔH) is termed the change in **enthalpy.** The component of energy that can be used to perform work is called "free energy." Reactions that produce heat result in a negative ΔH and are termed **exothermic.** Reactions that absorb heat result in a positive ΔH and are termed **endothermic.**

- A reaction proceeds in the direction of increased **entropy.** Entropy is a term for increased randomness or disorder. The difference between enthalpy and entropy for a given reaction represents an energy source (termed **free energy**) that is available for an additional source of work, and is denoted *Gibb's free energy* (ΔG). In humans this work is most often chemical, electrical, or mechanical.

- All biologic reactions proceed in the direction that results in a negative ΔG and are termed **exergonic** reactions. If ΔG is zero, the reaction is at **equilibrium** and no net change in energy transfer occurs. If ΔG is positive, by convention the reaction is termed **endergonic.** However, the student must realize that in biologic systems there are no endergonic reactions.

- To uphold the second law of thermodynamics in bioenergetics, entropy increases in the surroundings must exceed the decreased entropy of the biologic system. Living organisms order (decrease entropy) their internal milieu by releasing heat and entropy to their surroundings, thereby increasing the net entropy of the universe.

- Under standard conditions (pH=7.0, T=25°C [298 °K]), initial product and substrate concentrations each equaling 1 mol/L), the standard Gibbs' free energy change ($\Delta G°'$) can be calculated from the measurement of the ratio of products and substrates after reaching equilibrium. The ratio of [products]/[substrates] at equilibrium (i.e., rates of forward and reverse reactions are equal) under standard conditions is termed the **equilibrium constant (K'eq).**

- Substrate concentrations inside cells are well below 1 M and are not equal. Furthermore, depending on the exercise, rest, and environmental conditions, muscle temperatures can vary between 35° and over 40° C and muscle pH can vary between 7.0 and 6.0. It is apparent that the $\Delta G°'$ must be altered to represent in vivo conditions. The expression of in vivo products divided by substrates is termed the **mass action ratio.** The mass action ratio is almost always different from the K'eq for a given reaction, which indicates the different bioenergetic cellular conditions compared with standard. The mass action ratio is used in a modification of the $\Delta G°'$ equation to calculate ΔG.

- **Metabolism** can be defined as the sum of all chemical reactions in the body, which can be grouped as either **catabolism** or **anabolism.** Catabolism involves the breakdown of energy-yielding nutrients, the release of free energy and electrons and their coupled transfer to intermediary molecules (ATP, NADH, FADH, acetyl-CoA, and NADPH), and the formation of low-energy end products. The intermediary molecules can be used in a controlled and regulated manner to provide free energy to make the reactions of anabolism exergonic. Anabolism involves the covalent bonding of electrons, protons, and small molecules to produce larger molecules. Thus the free energy cost of building new and larger molecules occurs at the expense of the increased heat and entropy released from catabolism.

- ATP is a molecule that transfers free energy between the reactions breaking down molecules (catabolism) and those that utilize free energy. ATP can therefore be formed if the reaction ADP + Pi $\leftrightarrow$ ATP is *coupled* to reactions releasing free energy in amounts greater than that required to add the phosphate group to ADP (i.e., ΔG = -14.2 Kcal/mol). Similarly, the coupling of ATP hydrolysis to endergonic reactions provides free energy to drive the reaction in a given direction.

SUMMARY—Cont'd

■ Other molecules also exist that enable the transfer of chemical groups to other molecules, an exergonic process. These molecules are collectively termed high-energy or "activated" intermediates. The molecules that receive electrons, and therefore become reduced in what are called **oxidation** and **reduction** reactions, are important for the ability to generate large amounts of ATP from catabolism and also for the electrons (reducing power) that are needed in the synthesis of molecules in anabolism.

REVIEW QUESTIONS

1. Define the terms thermodynamics, energetics, and bioenergetics.

2. What are three examples of biologic processes that involve the transfer of energy from one form to another?

3. What are the differences between enthalpy, entropy, and free energy?

4. How are endergonic reactions different from exergonic reactions?

5. When concerned with chemical reactions, what is "coupling," and how does this phenomenon explain why all the chemical reactions in the body are exergonic?

6. Why is the free energy change of a chemical reaction in the body almost always different from the free energy change of the same reaction under standard conditions?

7. How are the reactions of catabolism to anabolism connected?

8. What is "reducing power," and how is it obtained and used in metabolism?

APPLICATIONS

1. What would be the implications to the design of metabolism if our cells could break down large molecules to end products such as carbon dioxide, water, and energy in just one or two reactions?

2. Be creative and try to design another metabolic design that enables the controlled collection of free energy release for later use in cell function.

3. The second law of thermodynamics explains why concentrations of substrates and products can alter the directionality of chemical reactions. What problems would exist for cells if they solely relied on substrate and product concentrations for the regulation of the rate and directionality of chemical reactions?

REFERENCES

1. Atkinson DE: *Cellular energy metabolism and its regulation,* New York, 1977, Academic Press.

2. Bangsbo J, Johansen L, Quistorff B, Saltin B: NMR and analytical biochemical evaluation of CrP and nucleotides in the human calf during muscle contraction, *J Appl Physiol* 74(4):2034-2039, 1993.

3. Chasiotis D: Role of cyclic AMP and inorganic phosphate in the regulation of muscle glycogenolysis during exercise, *Med Sci Sports Exerc* 20(6):545-550, 1988.

4. Cheetham ME, Boobis LH, Brooks S, Williams C: Human muscle metabolism during sprint running, *J Appl Physiol* 61(1):54-60, 1986.

5. Harold F: *The vital force: a study of bioenergetics,* New York, 1986, WH Freeman.

6. Harris RC, Hultman E, Sahlin K: Glycolytic intermediates in human muscle after isometric contraction, *Pflugers Arch* 389:277-282, 1981.

7. Jones NL, McCartney N, Graham T et al: Muscle performance and metabolism in maximal isokinetic cycling at slow and fast speeds, *J Appl Physiol* 59(1):132-136, 1985.

8. Lehninger AL: *Principles of biochemistry,* New York, 1993, Worth.

9. Newsholme EA, Leech ER: *Biochemistry for the medical sciences,* Chichester, England, 1983, John Wiley & Sons.

10. Stryer L: *Biochemistry,* New York, 1981, WH Freeman.

11. Veech RL, Randolph Lawson JW, Cornell NW, Krebs HA: Cytosolic phosphorylation potential, *J Biol Chem* 254(14):6538-6547, 1979.

12. Young DS: Implementation of SI units for clinical laboratory data: style specifications and conversion tables, *Ann Intern Med* 106:114-120, 1987.

RECOMMENDED READINGS

■ Atkinson DE: *Cellular energy metabolism and its regulation,* New York, 1977, Academic Press.

■ Bangsbo J, Johansen L, Quistorff B, Saltin B: NMR and analytical biochemical evaluation of CrP and nucleotides in the human calf during muscle contraction, *J Appl Physiol* 74(4):2034-2039, 1993.

■ Cheetham ME, Boobis LH, Brooks S, Williams C: Human muscle metabolism during sprint running, *J Appl Physiol* 61(1):54-60, 1986.

■ Jones NL, McCartney N, Graham T et al: Muscle performance and metabolism in maximal isokinetic cycling at slow and fast speeds, *J Appl Physiol* 59(1):132-136, 1985.

■ Veech RL, Randolph Lawson JW, Cornell NW, Krebs HA: Cytosolic phosphorylation potential, *J Biol Chem* 254(14):6538-6547, 1979.

CHAPTER 3

Enzyme Function and Regulation

OBJECTIVES

After reading this chapter you should be able to:

- Explain why enzymes regulate energy metabolism.

- Describe the complex structure of enzymes.

- Explain the roles of the binding and active sites.

- Explain how enzymes increase the rate of reactions.

- List and explain the factors that influence enzyme activity.

- Describe how two important enzymes of metabolism are regulated.

- Identify the nomenclature of enzymes.

KEY TERMS

biologic catalysts	coenzymes
primary structure	Q_{10} value
isozymes	International Unit
transition state	specific activity
activation energy	V_{max}
binding site	allosteric enzymes
active site	$S_{0.5}$
cofactors	

From previous study of physiology and chemistry, you should know that enzymes are *biologic catalysts* that increase the rates of reactions without participating in the transfer of energy. From your knowledge of bioenergetics you should also be aware that all reactions are potentially reversible and that the factors controlling the directionality of reactions are the substrate and product concentrations of the reaction. Enzymes do not alter the energetics, and therefore the directionality, of biologic reactions. Nevertheless, the regulated function of enzymes is crucial to the control of metabolism and to the body's ability to respond quickly to conditions that perturb its internal milieu. The purpose of this chapter is to explain how enzymes increase rates of reactions, to identify factors that can influence enzyme activity, and to explain why the regulation of enzyme activity can regulate the chemical reactions of metabolism.

Why Enzymes Regulate Metabolism

Chapter 2 discussed substrate and product concentrations in the body tissues that are considerably smaller than 1 mol/L and in fact are measured in a µmol to mmol/kg wet wt range. If we assume that a muscle fiber weighs approximately 100 µg, there would be 10 million fibers/kg of muscle in which the approximately 1 mmol (6.03×10^{20} molecules) of substrate and product is distributed. Thus for just one of the hundreds of enzyme-catalyzed reactions in a cell, there would be 6.03×10^{13} substrate molecules distributed throughout the fiber, which is minor considering the atomic size of the molecules compared with the visual dimensions and volume of a muscle fiber.

The purpose of the previous calculations was to show that the concentrations and the numbers of molecules are very low within cells. Consequently, if reactions were only to proceed from random association of substrates allowing product formation, the rate of chemical reactions would be extremely low. It would be hard to imagine living when able to move only at speeds similar to the sloth or to function without the internal ability to respond quickly to stimuli.

As a result of the low substrate concentrations of biologic reactions, an exergonic reaction ($-\Delta G$) that is not catalyzed by an enzyme does not produce product at a physiologically measurable rate.[2,16] Therefore the control of enzyme function is a means to regulate the rate of exergonic chemical reactions and therefore regulate cellular and bodily function. Given this, it is obviously important to understand how enzymes work and how they are regulated.

---

biologic catalyst
molecules that enhance the rate of chemical reactions

Enzyme Structure

Enzymes are protein molecules and like other proteins have large molecular weights that can range from 12,000 to greater than 1 million.[13] The size of enzymes is therefore very large compared with substrates, products, and regulating molecules. As with all proteins, enzymes are composed of amino acid molecules linked together by *peptide bonds,* a special type of covalent bond. The amino acid composition and structural order of a protein are termed the **primary structure**. The *polypeptide* chains of an enzyme form a backbone from which the diverse side chains of the 20 amino acids commonly found in proteins extend. Because the amino acid side chains can be positively charged, negatively charged, or neutral, interactions and repulsion between these groups cause the enzyme structure to become nonlinear and to fold into a three-dimensional structure (Figure 3.1). The interactions between side chains can cause very weak bonds to occur, such as *hydrogen* or *ionic bonds*. Despite these bonds having less than one tenth the energy of a covalent bond, the large number of these bonds combine to give structural stability and a specific three-dimensional shape to the enzyme. Shape and structural stability are also aided by covalent bonds that can form between the sulfur atoms *(disulfide bonds)* of certain amino acid side chains.

On the surface of an enzyme are specific binding sites for substrates and, depending on the enzyme, other binding sites for molecules that either decrease or increase enzyme activity. As discussed in subsequent sections, the location and function of these binding sites are important for understanding the function and regulation of specific enzymes.

For many, but not all, enzymes there are several different primary structures termed **isozymes** (or isoenzymes). The isozymes of a given enzyme exhibit a high degree of amino acid sequence homology and may differ by only a few amino acid residues. Nevertheless, because of the important

---

FIGURE 3.1

The three dimensional structure of phosphorylase-a (EC: 2.4.1.1). The active site, phosphorylation site, and binding sites for inorganic phosphate and glycogen are shown. (Adapted from Stryer L: *Biochemistry,* NY, 1981, WH Freeman.)

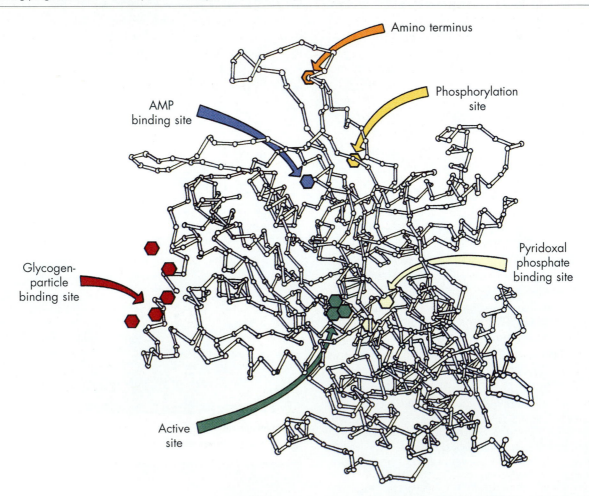

charge characteristics of the amino acid side chains, such small differences can have a profound influence on enzyme function if their location alters the charge characteristics of binding sites.

Enzyme Function

In a chemical reaction the substrates must pass through several unstable structures (the least stable being termed the **transition state**) before product formation. The change of substrates to the transition state requires an input of free energy, termed the **activation energy** $(\Delta A^+)^*$ of a reaction (Figure 3.2). Enzymes increase the rate of a chemical reaction by providing an alternate reaction mechanism in the formation of the transition state. The enzyme-catalyzed mechanism has a lower ΔA^+ than the non-catalyzed reaction.

Several mechanisms have been proposed to account for how enzymes can lower the ΔA^+. The most simple is termed the *"lock and key"* mechanism (Figure 3.3), which implies that a specific **binding site** (lock) exists on the enzyme for the substrate (key) and that when the substrate binds, the reaction is facilitated. In this example the binding site and the **active site** are synonymous. The active site is the region on an enzyme that provides the alternate reaction mechanism that decreases ΔA^+.

Organic and physical chemistry research performed as early as the 1950s[3,7,14,19,21] has shown that the mechanisms of enzyme catalysis must be more complex than illustrated by the lock and key example. The lock and key model indicates that the *enzyme-substrate complex* is a fixed structure, with a well-defined active site that is synonymous with a binding site. This is not always true because after the substrate binds to the enzyme, the enzyme can undergo a conformational change that develops the active site. The enzyme-substrate complex can be a very dynamic structure, and the binding site can be distinct from the active site. The chemical interaction between the substrate and active site are not covalent bonds but are generally weak ionic interactions or hydrogen bonds. The ionic and hydrogen bonds enable the enzyme and substrate to bind easily and allow the enzyme and product to release easily. The same principles are true for multiple-substrate enzyme-catalyzed reactions. However, depending on the enzyme, substrates bind either in sequence or together.

The additional mechanisms that explain the lower ΔA^+ in enzyme-catalyzed reactions are based on how the active site can facilitate the formation of the transition state and product and are explained in detail by Fersht.[7] Essentially, the binding of the substrates on the enzyme greatly increases the probability of interaction and effectively increases the concentration of substrates at the active site by a factor between 100 and 10,000.[19] The term used to describe this mechanism is *proximity*.

Enzymes not only increase the proximity of substrates at the active site, but also enable the substrates to bind in a specific *orientation* that facilitates the chemical reaction. Another term used to describe this mechanism is *orbital steering*, since the orientation causes overlap of the orbitals of specific atoms within the substrates and active sites that are involved in the chemical reaction.[21]

A final proposed mechanism of enzyme function is based on the development of *strain* in the substrates. After the substrates bind to the enzyme, minor conformational changes may occur in the substrates, causing them to adopt a structure facilitating the formation of the transition state. This mechanism has also been termed *induced fit*.[16]

From the proposed mechanisms of enzyme function, it is clear that the decrease in ΔA^+ during enzyme-catalyzed reactions can be explained by chemical theories. These mechanisms identify the dynamic nature and the three-dimensional structure of the enzyme-substrate complex, making it easier for the student to appreciate the *specificity* that exists between enzyme and substrates. Understanding the mechanisms of enzyme function also enables the student to increase his or her appreciation for the metabolic conditions that can either inhibit or activate the mechanisms that decrease ΔA^+. For any given concentration of substrate and product, a change that makes ΔA^+ less positive increases the rate of enzyme catalysis and vice versa.

---

primary structure

the sequence of amino acids that forms the covalent backbone structure of proteins

isozymes (i'so-zyms)

different structures of a specific enzyme that often have different kinetic characteristics

transition state

the temporary activated structure of a substrate that exists before product formation

activation energy

the amount of energy required to convert 1 mole of substrate to the transition state

binding site

the location on or within an enzyme responsible for the noncovalent binding of substrates

active site

the location on or within an enzyme responsible for the reaction mechanism

---

* The conventional symbol for activation energy is ΔG^+, however, because this may cause confusion with the application of Gibbs' free energy to energetics, the symbol ΔA^+ is used.

FIGURE 3.2

An illustration of the difference in ΔA^+ between uncatalyzed and enzyme-catalyzed reactions.

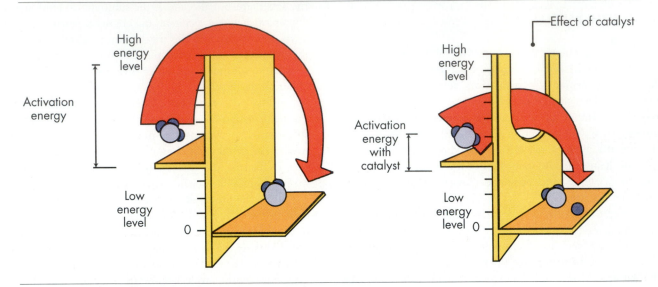

FIGURE 3.3

The early model of enzyme-substrate complexes was synonomous with a lock and key mechanism; however, many enzymes undergo an altered structure after binding to the substrate(s) that is important for developing the ability for the reaction mechanism to operate. In the same manner, inhibitor and/or activator molecules can alter the reaction mechanism, thus influencing the catalytic effectiveness of the enzyme. Not all enzymes are influenced by inhibitors, activators, or cofactors.

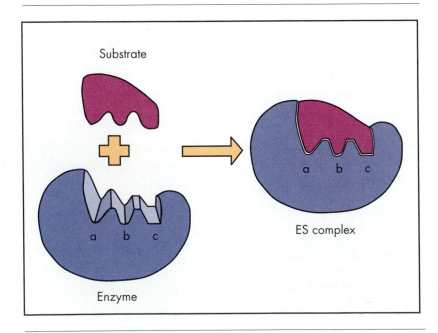

TABLE 3.1

The important cofactors and coenzymes of energy metabolism

	FUNCTION	ENZYME/METABOLIC EXAMPLE
COFACTORS		
Fe^{++}	Enzyme activity	Cytochrome-*c* oxidase
Mg^{++}	Enzyme activity	Myosin ATPase
Zn^{++}	Enzyme activity	Carbonic anhydrase
Mn^{++}	Enzyme activity	Arginase
Cu^{++}	Enzyme activity	Cytochrome-*c* oxidase
COENZYMES		
Biocytin	Transfer of CO_2	Pyruvate carboxylase
Coenzyme A (CoA)	Enzyme activity	Pyruvate carboxylase
NAD/NADH	Transfer H^+ and e^-	Lactate dehydrogenase
FAD/FADH	Transfer H^+ and e^-	Acyl-CoA dehydrogenase
NADP dehydrogenase	Transfer H^+ and e^-	Glucose-6-phosphatase
Ubiquinone	Transfer H^+ and e^-	Electron transport chain

Factors That Change Enzyme Function

Cofactors and Coenzymes

Cofactors are molecules or compounds that are necessary for the reaction mechanism between an enzyme and a substrate to proceed.[5] Cofactors can be inorganic, such as Fe^{++} or Mg^{++}, or an organic molecule. Organic cofactors are termed **coenzymes** and usually transfer specific atoms or functional groups during enzyme-catalyzed reactions. In some enzymes the cofactor is tightly bound to the enzyme and is termed a *prosthetic group*. A complete and active enzyme with its cofactors is a *holoenzyme,* whereas the protein component of the holoenzyme (the true enzyme) is an *apoenzyme.*[13]

Table 3.1 lists the important cofactors and coenzymes, with examples of an enzyme and its role in metabolism. Focus Box 3.1 lists the various types of cofactor functions and, where pertinent, provides examples within energy metabolism.

Temperature

An increase in temperature increases the rate of both enzyme catalyzed and noncatalyzed chemical reactions. Increased temperatures do not make ΔA^+ less positive but increase the number of molecules having sufficient kinetic energy to overcome the ΔA^+ and proceed to the transition state. However, for most enzymes, temperature increases above 60° C can disturb the ionic and hydrogen bonds that maintain the structure and function of an enzyme, thereby causing the enzyme to *denature.* The duration at which the enzyme is exposed to the temperature is also important, because *thermal denaturation* is both a temperature- and a time-dependent process. The relationship between increasing temperatures and enzyme activity is presented in Figure 3.4.

An expression used for the relationship between the rate of a reaction and the temperature is the Q_{10} **value**. The Q_{10} value is the ratio of a reaction rate at ([T° C + 10° C]/T° C). The Q_{10} value for most enzyme-catalyzed reactions is within the range of 1.5 to 2.5,[16] indicating that an increase in temperature of 10° C approximately doubles the rate of an enzyme-catalyzed reaction.

pH

The side chains of the amino acids of an enzyme can be charged or uncharged. The pH ($-\log[H^+]$) of a solution can alter the charge characteristics of amino acid side chains and

---

cofactors (co-fak-tors)
additional chemical compounds that are required to bind to enzymes to give catalytic activity

coenzymes (co-en'zyms)
cofactors that are organic molecules

Q_{10} value
the relative increase in enzyme activity with a 10-degree increase in temperature

FOCUS BOX 3.1

The various functions of enzyme cofactors/coenzymes

Where pertinent, examples are provided from energy metabolism.

Interenzyme carriers

Involves the transfer of a substrate between two enzymes and is the most usual type of cofactor.

NAD^+ coenzyme carries electrons (e^-) and protons (H^+)
Glyceraldehyde-3-phosphate dehydrogenase

Glyceraldehyde-3-phosphate $\leftrightarrow$ 3-Phosphoglycerolyl phosphate
$NAD^+ \leftrightarrow NADH + H^+$

$NAD^+ \leftrightarrow NADH + H^+$
Lactate $\leftrightarrow$ Pyruvate
Lactate   dehydrogenase

A prosthetic group

A special chemical compound bound to the enzyme that is essential for enzyme function. Usually the prosthetic group is part of the active site.

Mg^{++} − Hexokinase

Alters the shape of the enzyme molecule

The cofactor is necessary for causing a structural modification to the enzyme that is important for enzyme activity.

Subunit aggregation

Enzyme subunits can rely on a cofactor for proper alignment and association with each other, resulting in optimal activity.

Stabilizers

Some enzymes rely on cofactors for structural stability and activity.

Templates

Some enzymes require a sequence of molecules from which a new series of units within a molecule are synthesized.

DNA
RNA polymerase

Primers

Some enzymes require a short length of a molecular chain to perform their catalytic or synthesizing function.

$Glycogen_{n>4} \leftrightarrow Glycogen_{n-1}$ + Glucose-1-phosphate
phosphorylase

Intermediates

Enzymes may use a cofactor in the reaction and in the process produce another cofactor molecule.

---

therefore potentially alter the three-dimensional structure of the active site, the entire enzyme, or the charge distribution of the substrates. Either condition could decrease enzyme activity.

For most enzymes the plot of pH and enzyme activity (Figure 3.5) gives a bell-shaped curve; however, the pH range of this curve and the pH corresponding to optimal enzyme activity are specific to the enzyme. For example, the gastric enzymes of digestion must remain functional at pH values approximating 2.0, whereas intracellular enzymes must operate at a pH close to 7.0.

Enzyme Concentration

In the human body, and all biologic systems, the concentration of enzymes in cells can change in response to both acute and chronic stimuli. Of particular interest to exercise physiologists is the increase in specific enzyme concentrations after exercise training. An increase in enzyme concentration increases the rate of a chemical reaction for a given reaction condition. The activity of an enzyme is measured under optimal conditions (optimal pH, T = 298° or 310° K, near saturating substrate concentrations, with necessary cofactors.

Under ideal conditions the reaction rate is proportional to enzyme concentration. The unit of measurement for enzyme activity is called the **International Unit (IU).** One IU of enzyme activity is equal to the amount of enzyme causing transformation of one micromole (μmol) of substrate to product per minute (1 μmol/min). Another commonly used unit of enzyme activity is **specific activity.** The specific activity is the number of enzyme units/mg of protein.

Endurance training is known to cause large increases in the activity of key mitochondrial enzymes, such as citrate synthase of the TCA cycle, and ß-hydroxyacyl-CoA dehydrogenase of the ß-oxidation pathway (Figure 3.6). Results such as these are interpreted to indicate an increased mitochondrial mass after endurance training, along with greater concentrations of mitochondrial enzymes. The metabolic adaptations to exercise are described in Chapter 10.

Substrate Concentration

When the enzyme concentration is constant, the rate of an enzyme-catalyzed reaction increases with an increase in substrate. The relationships between the substrate concentra-

FIGURE 3.4

The effect of increased temperature on enzyme activity. Over a specific range of temperatures, enzyme activity increases with an increase in temperature. If the temperature is too high, denaturation occurs and enzyme activity decreases. (Adapted from Newsholme EA, Leech ER: *Biochemistry for the Medical Sciences,* Chichester, England, 1983, John Wiley & Sons.)

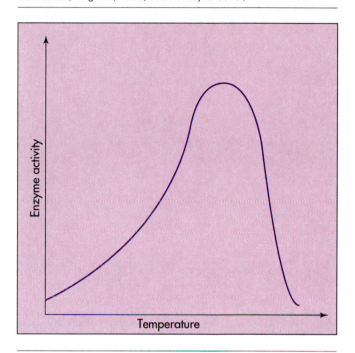

FIGURE 3.5

The effect of changing pH on enzyme activity. Specific enzymes have a specific pH range in which they have optimal activity (Adapted from Newsholme EA, Leech ER: *Biochemistry for the Medical Sciences,* Chichester, England, 1983, John Wiley & Sons.)

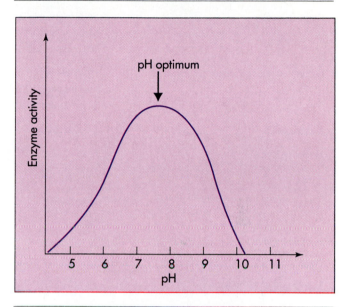

FIGURE 3.6

The increased activity (concentrations) of specific mitochondrial enzymes after an intensive endurance training program. (Adapted from Hurley BF, et al: *J Appl Physiol* 60 (2):562-567, 1982.)

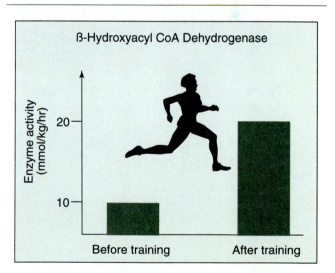

tions and the initial rate of a reaction are depicted for two differing hypothetical enzymes in Figure 3.9 (see Focus Box 3.2). The *maximal rate of catalysis* for each enzyme **(V$_{max}$)** is similar; however, the two enzymes differ in activity for substrate concentrations far less than at V$_{max}$. For example, compared with enzyme A, enzyme B requires twice the substrate concentration to provide half maximal activity (see Focus Box 3.2). Consequently, enzyme A would require a lesser increase in substrate concentration for increased activity. Enzyme activity at low substrate concentrations is important for biologic function because of the low substrate concentrations in cells. The difference between the substrate concentration at half maximal activity for hexokinase (skeletal muscle) and glucokinase (liver), is important for explaining the differing functions of glucose metabolism in the two different tissues (see Chapters 4 and 5). An explanation of enzyme terminology is provided in Focus Box 3.3.

Students should remember that energetics and the magnitude of –ΔG have no direct influence on reaction rates in biologic systems. The rate of reactions is determined by enzyme function, and it is both coincidental and beneficial to metabolism that enzymes have increased activity as substrate concentrations increase and that reactions become more exergonic.

International Unit
the recognized unit of enzyme activity

specific activity
enzyme activity expressed relative to total protein

V$_{max}$
the maximal rate of catalysis of an enzyme

TABLE 3.2

Examples of enzymes that have multiple isozymes

ENZYME	ISOZYMES	DIFFERENCES
Creatine kinase	Skeletal muscle (MM or CK-3)	No kinetic differences
	Myocardium (MB or CK-2)	
	Brain (BB or CK-1)	
Lactate dehydrogenase	Heart (HHHH)	Lower $S_{0.5}$* for pyruvate
	Intermediate (HHMM and other variations)	
	Muscle (MMMM)	Higher $S_{0.5}$ for pyruvate
Hexokinase	Four isozymes	
Myosin ATPase	Fast	Stable high pH (10)
		Unstable low pH (4.3)
		High V_{max}
	Intermediate	Unstable low pH (4.6)
	Slow	Unstable high pH (10)
		Stable low pH (4.3)
		Low V_{max}

*See Focus Box 3.2 for a definition.

CLINICAL APPLICATION

Alterations in Serum Creatine Kinase: Myocardial Infarction or Exercise-Induced Skeletal Muscle Damage

An increase in serum creatine kinase (CK) is used clinically as a biochemical marker of myocardial injury, like that of ischemia causing myocardial damage during a myocardial infarction (MI). An increase in serum CK also results from damage to skeletal muscle. Skeletal muscle damage can result from muscle injury (e.g., a tear) or the more common microscopic damage resulting from exercise, especially when the exercise involves eccentric contractions or the individual is unaccustomed to the exercise intensity or duration.

Figure 3.7 presents changes in known isozymes of CK (see Table 3.3) in serum from humans for different conditions. Severe eccentric exercise can cause extremely high serum CK levels, which typically peak between 24 and 48 hours after exercise. Although an increase in total serum CK following exercise has been interpreted as a sign of muscle damage, the fact that even short-duration intense exercise in well-trained individuals also raises CK indicates that even undamaged or minimally damaged muscle fibers release CK.[10]

After myocardial injury, total CK activity in the serum increases. When this activity is differentiated into CK isozymes, an increase in the MB (CK-2) isozyme of the heart is evident. Typically, an increase in the CK-2 isozyme causing greater than 3% to 5% of total activity is used to indicate a myocardial infarct.[10] Episodes of brain ischemia, like that during stroke, cause increases in the brain isozyme of CK (CK-1).

Myocardial infarction and stroke are not the only clinical conditions in which CK increases. Muscular dystrophies and myopathies are also characterized by elevated serum CK values at rest.[10] Alcoholic intoxication, hypothyroidism, and hyperthermia increase the CK-2 isozyme. Ironically, exercise also increases the CK-2 isozyme activity in serum, and Apple et al.[1] have noted the similarity in serum CK profiles between marathon runners and individuals recovering from MI. It is accepted that the exercise-induced release of CK-2 in healthy individuals is not from the heart but from skeletal muscle, thereby indicating that CK-2 exists in skeletal muscle.[10]

FIGURE 3.7

The multiple factors involved in increasing the rate of the phosphorylase-catalyzed reaction.

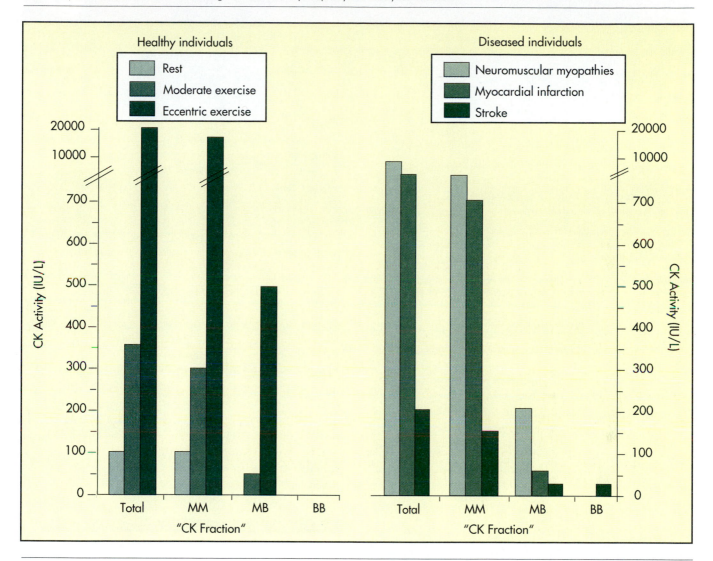

Isozymes

A given enzyme may have several different primary structures, termed *isozymes*. Not all enzymes have isozymes; however, the presence of different isozymes of a given enzyme is usually accompanied by slight differences in the kinetics of catalysis.

Table 3.2 lists examples of enzymes known to have different isozymes that are important to energy metabolism or muscle contraction. For creatine kinase, the different isozymes are tissue specific and do not seem to have markedly different enzyme kinetics (see Clinical Application 3.1). Heart-type lactate dehydrogenase (LDH) has a lower pyruvate concentration required for half maximal activity than does the muscle type. Heart-type LDH is also present in kidney and liver tissue, and this explains why these tissues can readily take up lactate for subsequent conversion to pyruvate, which can be further catabolized or incorporated into glyconeogenesis (see Chapter 5).

Inhibition and Activation

The regulation of enzyme activity by substrate and product concentrations applies mainly to enzymes that are not inhibited or activated when other molecules bind to the enzyme. Molecules other than substrates that bind to enzymes and affect their activity are called *allosteric regulators,*

FOCUS BOX 3.2

Enzyme kinetics

In 1913 Leonor Michaelis and Maude Menten postulated that the rate-limiting step in enzyme catalysis is the conversion of a bound substrate and enzyme (ES) to product (P).

$$E + S \leftrightarrow ES \leftrightarrow E + P$$

Thus if there is an increase in the substrate concentration, there is an increase in the number of enzyme molecules bound to substrate (ES), as well as an overall increase in product formation. If the substrate concentration increased to levels that immediately reform enzyme-substrate complexes after product release, thus saturating the enzyme, the enzyme would function at its maximal catalytic rate in converting substrates to products. The maximal rate of an enzyme-catalyzed reaction is termed V_{max} (Figure 3.8). For enzymes that do not exhibit cooperativity and are not regulated by activators (not allosteric enzymes), the relationship between the substrate concentration and enzyme activity is a rectangular hyperbola.

The V_{max} value of enzymes is not very meaningful, for as previously explained, substrate concentrations within cells are very small. Consequently, in vivo enzymes operate far below their V_{max} capabilities. A more physiologically meaningful indication of enzyme function would be one that exists at smaller substrate concentrations. Michaelis and Menten defined such a value and termed it the *Michaelis-Menten constant* (K_M), which equals the substrate concentration for an enzyme at one half V_{max} activity.

From the kinetic relationships between enzyme activity and substrate concentrations, Michaelis and Menten developed an equation, termed the *Michaelis-Menten equation.*

3-1A
$$V_O = \frac{V_{max}\,[S]}{[S] + K_M}$$

Where V_O = the initial rate of catalysis.

When both sides of the equation are reciprocated, the equation can be transformed to one that fits a straight line of the form $y = bx + c$; where y equals a y-axis value, b equals the slope, x equals an x-axis value, and c equals the y-intercept.

3-1B
$$\frac{1}{V_O} = \frac{K_M + [S]}{V_{max}\,[S]}$$

which simplifies to

3-1C
$$\frac{1}{V_O} = \frac{K_M}{V_{max}}\frac{1}{[S]} + \frac{1}{V_{max}}$$

Where $1/V_O$ equals the y-axis, K_M/V_{max} equals the slope, $1/[S]$ equals the x-axis, and $1/V_{max}$ equals the y-intercept. From a graph of this plot for several values of V_O, the exact values for each of V_{max} and K_M for the enzyme of concern (Figure 3.9) can be calculated. Table 3.3 lists the K_M and V_{max} values for several enzymes of the body. All of the listed enzymes of Table 3.3 have a relatively low K_M for their main substrate. Enzymes that have a low K_M for a substrate have a high affinity for the substrates, have increased catalysis for small changes in substrate, and are therefore more sensitive to changing conditions.

Since enzymes upholding Michaelis-Menten kinetics can be inhibited by certain molecules, with the K_M increased if the inhibitor molecule binds to the enzyme at a location other than the substrate binding site (termed a noncompetitive inhibitor), the K_M is not really a true constant (Figure 3.10). Consequently, Atkinson[2] has proposed that the term $\mathbf{S_{0.5}}$ be used rather than K_M. Furthermore, the term $S_{0.5}$ is also suited to allosteric enzymes, where enzyme activity can be influenced not only by substrate and inhibitor concentrations, but also by concentrations of activators. The shape of the substrate concentration enzyme activity curves for allosteric enzymes is sigmoidal and is represented by a family of curves depending on substrate, inhibitor, and activator concentrations (Figure 3.10).

TABLE 3.3

Substrate concentration at half V_{max} (K_M) for several enzymes of metabolism

ENZYME	SUBSTRATE	K_M*
Hexokinase	ATP	0.4
Carbonic anhydrase	HCO_3.	9.0
Pyruvate carboxylase	Pyruvate	400

*K_M units are mmol/L.

and these enzymes are termed **allosteric enzymes.** Enzymes that are not activated by allosteric regulators uphold the assumptions of *Michaelis-Menten kinetics* and are termed *Michaelis-Menten enzymes.* A description of the study of the rates of enzyme–catalyzed reactions, Enzymes Kinetics, is provided in Focus Box 3.2.

The existence of enzymes that are inhibited or activated is important for the regulation of metabolism. Inhibition of an enzyme would prevent increases in substrate from increasing enzyme activity, thus allowing the substrate to be directed through another metabolic pathway (Figure 3.11). Conversely, the activation of an enzyme would favor a reaction

The effects of an increase in substrate concentration on the activity of two differing enzymes. Both enzymes have a similar V_{max}, yet very different $S_{0.5}$ values.

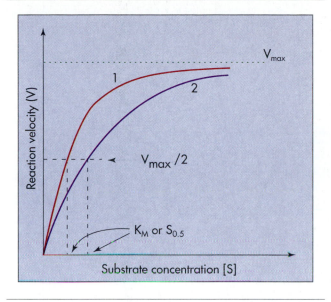

Sigmoidal curves of the allosteric enzyme glycogen synthase when exposed to different concentrations of the activator glucose-6-phosphate.

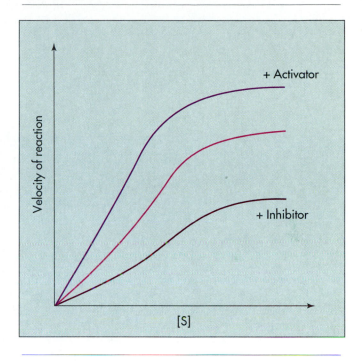

A recipricol plot of enzyme activity without inhibition, with competitive inhibition, and with noncompetitive inhibition. Competitive inhibition decreases V_{max}, but K_M remains unchanged. Conversely, noncompetitive inhibition does not affect V_{max}, but increases K_M.

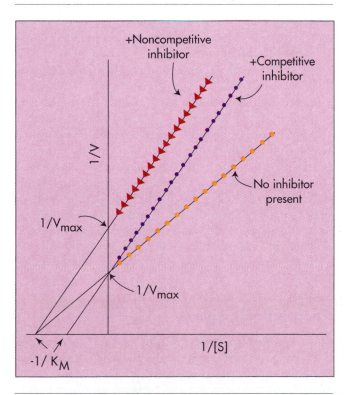

and potentially the operation of an entire metabolic pathway.[17] The formation of inhibitors and activators is specific to metabolic conditions; and in many instances a molecule is an activator of one enzyme and an inhibitor of another. Two examples of allosteric enzymes important for energy metabolism are provided later in the next section.

Examples of Enzyme Regulation

Phosphorylase

Phosphorylase (EC: 2.4.1.1) is the main enzyme of the three involved in the catabolism of glycogen *(glycogenolysis)*, the glucose storage molecule within many different metabolically active tissues of the body. The two tissues of primary interest to glycogenolysis during and after exercise are skeletal muscle and the liver.

allosteric enzymes

enzymes that have increased activity at a given substrate concentration when bound to specific molecules

$S_{0.5}$

the substrate concentration at half V_{max} for a given reaction condition

FIGURE 3.11

The regulation of enzymes that catalyze reactions early in pathways can redirect substrate to other connecting pathways. In this example, depending on which enzymes are inhibited or activated, glucose entering a muscle cell can be directed to either glycogen synthesis, pentose phosphate formation, or catabolism in glycolysis.

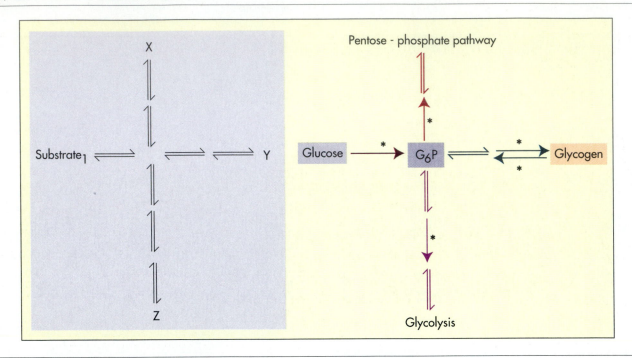

Glycogen$_n$ + Pi ↔ Glycogen$_{n-1}$ + Glucose-1-phosphate

Skeletal muscle phosphorylase has a molecular weight of 190,000 g/m and consists of two identical subunits, each of which can bind a phosphate group.[13] When the two subunits are phosphorylated, the enzyme is most active and is termed phosphorylase-a. The unphosphorylated enzyme is termed phosphorylase-b. However, phosphorylase-b can have increased activity when bound to specific allosteric activators, of which AMP is the main activator (Figure 3.1). A series of enzymes exist that regulate the addition of the phosphate to phosphorylase, and evidence exists to indicate that all of the enzymes of muscle glycogen metabolism exist bound to the glycogen molecule as a large enzyme complex.[16] Consequently, when muscle glycogen concentrations are large, the proximity of the enzymes increases the sensitivity of phosphorylase-a formation and the potential for rapid glycogenolysis. Interestingly, maximal rates of glycogenolysis during exercise have been reported between 0.4 and 0.65 mmol/kg wet wt.[20]

In resting muscle almost 99% of phosphorylase is in the inactive structure.[16,18] During muscle contraction the increase in cytosolic Ca^{++} activates an enzyme (phosphorylase kinase) that catalyzes the addition of the phosphates to phosphorylase. Increased circulating concentrations of the hormone epinephrine also increase the potential activity of phosphorylase by activating phosphorylase kinase by a cAMP mechanism[15] (Figure 3.12). Regardless of the potential activ-

ity of phosphorylase, little in vivo activity results until the cellular concentration of inorganic phosphate increases.[4] As previously indicated, inorganic phosphate is a substrate for the phosphorylase reaction, and until its concentration approaches the $S_{0.5}$ for phosphorylase (26.2 mmol/L), minimal activity results from the conversion of phosphorylase-b to the phosphorylase-a structure.[4,18]

During intense muscle contraction the inorganic phosphate concentration increases and metabolic activators are produced (present) that increase the conversion of phosphorylase-b to phosphorylase-a (Ca^{++}, cAMP) or provide additional allosteric activation of both phosphorylase-a and phosphorylase-b (AMP) (Figure 3.13, Table 3.4). This activation lowers the $S_{0.5}$ for Pi, and the catabolism of glycogen can then occur at a rapid rate to eventually provide substrate for the central pathways of energy metabolism. Obviously, the presence of glycogen and its regulated catabolism during exercise is important for prolonged and intense muscle contractions and optimal exercise performance. A list of molecules that influence phosphorylase activity is presented in Table 3.4.

Phosphofructokinase

Phosphofructokinase (PFK) (EC: 2.7.1.11) is recognized as the main allosteric enzyme regulating the first central pathway of energy metabolism, *glycolysis*. PFK catalyzes the addition of a phosphate to fructose 1-phosphate, which requires

FIGURE 3.12

The sequence of biochemical events that occurs during the increase in cAMP within a cell, and the resultant activation and inhibition of specific enzymes involved in glycogen metabolism. (Modified from Stryer L: *Biochemistry*, NY, 1981, WH Freeman.)

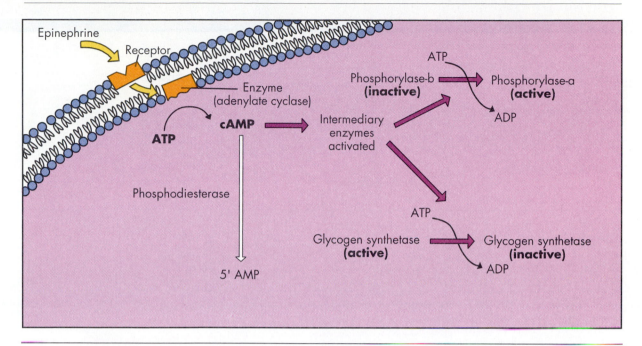

FIGURE 3.13

The multiple factors involved in increasing the rate of the phosphorylase-catalyzed reaction.

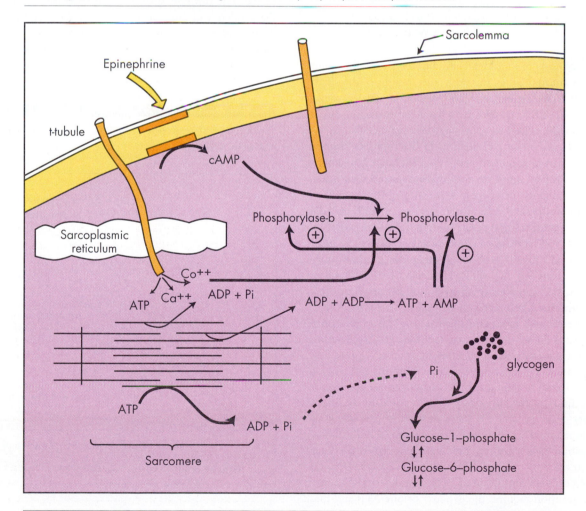

TABLE 3.4

Allosteric regulators of phosphorylase and phosphofructokinase

ENZYME	INHIBITORS	ACTIVATORS
Phosphorylase-b (unphosphorylated)	ATP	Pi (substrate)
	Glucose-6-phosphate	AMP
		IMP
Phosphorylase-a (phosphorylated)	ATP	Pi (substrate)
	Glucose-6-phosphate	AMP
	Ca++	IMP
Phosphofructokinase	ATP*	AMP
	citrate	ADP*
	H+	

*Atkinson[1] proposes that it is not ATP, ADP, or Pi that independently effects enzyme function, but that their mass action ratio ([ADP] [Pi]/[ATP], often termed phosphorylation potential) is more important.

the coupled free energy and phosphate of ATP dephosphorylation to ADP.

$$\text{Fructose-1-phosphate} + \text{ATP} \leftrightarrow \text{Fructose-1,6-bisphosphate} + \text{ADP}$$

PFK consists of four identical subunits. Although subunit size differs among tissues, the molecular weight of the smallest subunit is approximately 50,000 g/M.[2,7,22] Two isozymes of PFK exist, PFK1 and PFK2. PFK1 is the main isozyme in skeletal muscle, whereas both isozymes are present in the liver. PFK2 catalyzes the formation of fructose 2,6–bisphosphate, which is a potent activator of PFK1.[22] Each subunit can bind substrate, activator, and inhibitor molecules, resulting in a complex tissue-specific regulation of PFK.

The activator and inhibitor molecules of PFK and the metabolic conditions that result in their formation are listed in Table 3.4. PFK activity can be reduced during severe intracellular acidosis (pH < 6.6) as a result of an increase in the inhibition provided by ATP. However, the increase in allosteric activator molecules during muscle contraction offsets this inhibition and retains high catalytic activity.[6] As previously mentioned, production of fructose 2,6-bisphosphate also increases PFK1 activity, and fructose 2,6-bisphosphate production is stimulated by increases in fructose 6–phosphate. Interestingly, ATP, a substrate is also an inhibitor and fructose 1,6–bisphosphate, a product, is also an activator. These conditions are unusual for enzymes and are caused by additional regulatory binding sites for these molecules that affect the structural relationships between the subunits of PFK. As with most multiple-unit enzymes, PFK displays cooperatively and is characterized by a sigmoidal activity curve (Figure 3.14).

The complex regulation of PFK is understandable, since the PFK reaction requires the expense of one ATP and must be activated in concert with phosphorylase to allow the glucose 6-phosphate produced from glycogenolysis to be catabolized through glycolysis. As discussed in Chapter 4, the sudden and large increase in muscle glycolytic activity during intense exercise is necessary to support continued contraction when creatine phosphate stores decline to low levels.

FIGURE 3.14

The sigmoidal activity curve of PFK, and the affect of increased AMP on this curve.

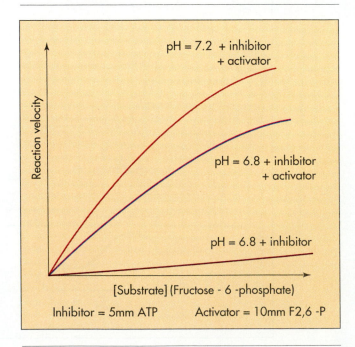

pH = 7.2 + inhibitor + activator

pH = 6.8 + inhibitor + activator

pH = 6.8 + inhibitor

Reaction velocity

[Substrate] (Fructose - 6 -phosphate)

Inhibitor = 5mm ATP   Activator = 10mm F2,6 -P

FOCUS BOX 3.3

Enzyme nomenclature

In 1961 the International Union of Biochemistry adopted a system of nomenclature for enzymes prepared by the Enzyme Commission (EC).[12] The EC proposed a systematic name and a corresponding numeric code for each enzyme. Since these names are often complex and the numeric code is difficult to remember, specific generic names were also proposed for enzymes. For example, the enzyme acyl-CoA:malonyl-CoA C-acyltransferase (EC: 2.3.1.85) has the generic name of fatty acid synthase and the enzyme ATP pyrophosphate-lyase (cycling) (EC: 4.6.1.1) has the generic name of adenylate cyclase. The four numbers of each enzyme code denote the main enzyme division, subclass, sub-subclass, and serial number, respectively.

Table 3.5 lists the six major divisions of enzymes classified by the EC system, as well as the terminology and meanings of many names and syllables used in generic nomenclature. With the generic names, the suffix -ase is used to designate that the molecule is an enzyme. However, there are examples of enzyme trivial names that do not end in -ase (e.g., pepsin, lysozyme). The syllables and words of the name (e.g., *kin*ase, *dehydrogen*ase, *lip*ase) identify the enzyme's catalytic role in the reaction, although many generic names also state the substrate of the reaction (e.g., glucose 6-phosphate dehydrogenase, pyruvate kinase).

The EC system is not perfect. Although enzymes can have the same function, and therefore the same systemic and trivial name, their kinetic properties and molecular structures may differ depending on which organism and tissue they are from. Horse liver alcohol dehydrogenase has half the molecular weight of yeast alcohol dehydrogenase. Another difficulty is that even within the same organism and tissue, one reaction can be catalyzed by differing isozymes of the same enzyme. The EC recommends that isozymes be designated by Arabic numerals. The ability of exercise training to alter the isozyme distribution of specific enzymes in specific types of muscle, and how these changes can alter energy metabolism, are major research interests in exercise physiology.

TABLE 3.5

Scheme of classification and numbering of enzymes, as recommended by the Nomenclature Committee of the International Union of Biochemistry and Molecular Biology, 1992. Examples are provided within each division. Explanations of the terminology used in "trivial" names are listed.

SYSTEMATIC NAME EXAMPLE	TYPES OF ENZYMES	TRIVIAL NAME
1. OXIDOREDUCTASES EC:1.1.1.27	Enzymes catalyzing oxido-reduction reactions $Pyruvate + NADH + H^+ \leftrightarrow Lactate + NAD^+$	Lactic acid dehydrogenase Lactate dehydrogenase
2. TRANSFERASES EC:2.4.1.1	Enzymes catalyzing the transferring of a chemical group from one compound to another $Glycogen_n + Pi \leftrightarrow Glycogen_{n-1} + Glucose\text{-}1\text{-}phosphate$	Glycogen phosphorylase
3. HYDROLASES EC:3.1.1.7	Enzymes that catalyze the cleavage of certain bonds producing water as a byproduct $Acetycholine + H_2O \leftrightarrow Choline + Acetate$	Acetylcholine acetylhydrolase Acetylcholinesterase

Continued.

FOCUS BOX 3.3—Cont'd

Enzyme nomenclature

TABLE 3.5—Cont'd

SYSTEMATIC NAME EXAMPLE	TYPES OF ENZYMES	TRIVIAL NAME
4. LYASES EC:4.1.3.7	Enzymes that catalyze the cleavage of certain bonds leaving double bonds or rings, or catalyze the addition of groups to double bonds	Citrate oxaloacetate-lyase Citrate synthase
	Citrate + CoA $\leftrightarrow$ Acetyl-CoA + H_2O + Oxaloacetate	
5. ISOMERASES EC:5.3.1.9	Enzymes that catalyze geometric or structural changes within one molecule	Glucose-6-phosphate isomerase
	Glucose-6-phosphate $\leftrightarrow$ Fructose-6-phosphate	
6. LIGASES EC:6.4.1.1	Enzymes catalyzing the joining of two molecules coupled with the hydrolysis of a pyrophosphate bond of a triphosphate	Pyruvate carboxylase
	ATP + Pyruvate + HCO_3 $\leftrightarrow$ ADP + Pi + Oxaloacetate	

TRIVIAL NAME TERMINOLOGY

Kinase	Transfer of a phosphate
Phosphatase	Removal of a phosphate
Dehydrogenase	Removal of electrons and protons
Mutase	Altered position of a side group within the same molecule
Isomerase	Altered geometric structure of the same molecule
Transferase	Transferring of a side group from one molecule to another
Synthase	Joining together of two molecules
Lipase	Cleavage of acyl groups from fatty acid chains

SUMMARY

■ Enzymes are **biologic catalysts** because they increase the rates of chemical reactions without participating in the transfer of energy or affecting the directionality of the reaction. However, since concentrations of substrates and products within cells are extremely small, the regulation of enzyme activity essentially regulates the rates of chemical reactions and the function of metabolic pathways within biologic systems.

■ Enzymes are protein molecules, consisting of a **primary structure** of amino acids that have a three-dimensional structure within which exist **binding sites** for substrates and cofactors, an **active site** for facilitating the reaction, and possible additional binding sites for activator and inhibitor molecules. Enzymes that bind and are influenced by activator molecules are termed **allosteric enzymes**.

SUMMARY—Cont'd

- Enzymes increase the rates of chemical reactions by providing an alternate reaction mechanism that facilitates the conversion of substrate to product. This alternate mechanism provides sufficient free energy to overcome the **activation energy** needed to convert a substrate to a **transition state** that favors product formation.

- Enzyme activity is influenced by the need for **cofactors** and **coenzymes,** substrate concentrations, enzyme concentrations, temperature, pH, inhibitor concentrations, the type of **isozyme,** and if allosteric, activator concentrations. An increase in temperature is a powerful means to increase enzyme activity, as indicated for many enzymes by the doubling of the rate of catalysis with a 10-degree increase in temperature **(Q_{10} value).**

- Important measures of enzyme function are the maximal rate of catalysis **(V_{max})** and the substrate concentration at one half V_{max} (K_M or $S_{0.5}$). Enzyme activity is usually expressed as the rate of formation of product expressed per minute **(International Unit).** Another expression of enzyme activity is the rate of product formation relative to the protein concentration of the enzyme, called **specific activity.** The study of enzymes is called enzymology, and the specific study of enzyme catalysis is called enzyme kinetics.

- Two important allosteric enzymes of energy metabolism in skeletal muscle are phosphorylase and phosphofructokinase. Each enzyme has specific activator and inhibitor molecules that influence the rate of enzyme catalysis. In turn the increased product formed influences the thermodynamics of the reactions that follow in their respective pathway.

- Multiple names exist for almost all enzymes. The Enzyme Commission (EC) has categorized all enzymes and provided each with a specific four-number code, a systematic name, and a trivial name. The trivial name is used most and usually denotes the substrate and the type of reaction involved.

REVIEW QUESTIONS

1. Why do enzymes essentially regulate chemical reactions if they do not alter the thermodynamics of reactions?

2. Explain the general structure and function of an enzyme.

3. What are the proposed processes for how enzymes increase the rate of catalysis?

4. What is the activation energy of a reaction?

5. What are cofactors and coenzymes?

6. How do changes in temperature and pH affect enzyme activity?

7. Why are allosteric enzymes important in the control of energy metabolism?

8. How do the activity curves of Michaelis–Menten and allosteric enzymes differ? Draw these curves to show how enzyme activity changes with an increase in substrate concentration.

9. Understand the meaning of the main trivial name terminology for enzyme catalysis.

APPLICATIONS

1. During metabolism, some enzymes must be inhibited, whereas other enzymes must be activated. Propose explanations for how this contradictory scenario may be regulated to allow for optimal cell function.

2. Many individuals with abnormally high serum cholesterol have this condition because of the inability to inhibit the enzyme that synthesizes cholesterol (HMG CoA reductase). Propose a strategy that could be used by medical researchers and doctors to help treat this deadly disorder.

3. If allosteric enzymes are potentially more beneficial because of improved regulation, why are not all enzymes of the body allosteric enzymes?

4. List the known causes for the release of creatine kinase from skeletal muscle. Why might there be clinical concern over the similar release of CK-2 from skeletal muscle after exercise and cardiac muscle after an MI?

REFERENCES

1. Apple FS, Sherman WM, Ivy JL: Comparison of serum creatine kinase and creatine kinase MB activities post marathon race versus post myocardial infarction, *Clin Chim Acta* 138:111-118, 1984.

2. Atkinson DE: *Cellular energy metabolism and its regulation,* New York, 1977, Academic Press.

3. Bruice TC, Brown A, Harris DO: On the concept of orbital steering in catalytic reactions, *Proc Nat Acad Sci USA* 68(3):658-661, 1971.

4. Chasiotis D: Role of cyclic AMP and inorganic phosphate in the regulation of muscle glycogenolysis during exercise, *Med Sci Sports Exerc* 20(6):545-550, 1988.

5. Dixon M, Webb EC, Thorne CJR, Tipton KF: *Enzymes,* New York, 1979, Academic Press.

6. Dobson GP, Yamamoto E, Hochachka PW: Phosphofructokinase control in muscle: nature and reversal of pH-dependent ATP inhibition, *Am J Physiol* 259(19):R71-R76, 1986.

7. Ferscht A: *Enzyme structure and mechanism,* San Francisco, 1977, WH Freeman.

8. Hammes GG, Wu CW: Regulation of enzyme activity, *Science* 172:1205-1211, 1971.

9. Harold F: *The vital force: a study of bioenergetics,* New York, 1986, WH Freeman.

10. Hortobagyi T, Denahan T: Variability in creatine-kinase: methodological, exercise, and clinically related factors, *Int J Sport Med* 10:69-80, 1989.

11. Hurley BF, Nemeth PM, Martin III WH et al: Muscle triglyceride utilization during exercise: effect of training, *J Appl Physiol* 60(2):562-567, 1982.

12. International Union of Biochemistry and Molecular Biology Nomenclature Committee: *Enzyme nomenclature 1992: recommendations of the nomenclature committee of the International Union of Biochemistry and Molecular Biology on the nomenclature and classification of enzymes,* San Diego, 1992, Academic Press.

13. Lehinger AL: *Principles of biochemistry,* New York, 1993, Worth.

14. Lienhard GE: Enzymatic catalysis and transition-state theory, *Science* 180:149-154, 1973.

15. Meinke MK, Edstorm RD: Muscle glycogenolysis: regulation of the cyclic interconversion of phosphorylase-a and phosphorylase-b, *J Biol Chem* 266(4):2259-2266, 1991.

16. Newsholme EA, Leech ER: *Biochemistry for the medical sciences,* Chichester, England, 1983, John Wiley & Sons.

17. Newsholme EA, Crabtree B, Parry-Billings M: The energetic cost of regulation: an analysis based on the principles of metabolic-control-logic. In Kinney JM, Tucker HN, editors: *Energy metabolism: tissue determinants and cellular corollaries,* New York, 1991, Raven Press.

18. Ren JM, Hultman E: Regulation of phosphorylase: an activity in human skeletal muscle, *J Appl Physiol* 69(3):919-923, 1990.

19. Reuben J: Substrate anchoring and the catalytic power of enzymes, *Proc Nat Acad Sci* 68(3):563-565, 1971.

20. Robergs RA, Pascoe DD, Costill DL et al: Effects of warm up on muscle glycogenolysis during intense exercise, *Med Sci Sports Exerc* 23(1):37-43,1991.

21. Storm DR, Koshland DE: A source for the special catalytic power of enzymes: orbital steering, *Proc Nat Acad Sci USA* 66(2):445-452, 1970.

22. Stryler L: *Biochemistry,* New York, 1981, WH Freeman.

23. Watson JD, Hopkins NH, Roberts JW et al: *Molecular biology of the gene,* ed 4, Menlo Park, California, 1987, Benjamin Cummings.

RECOMMENDED READINGS

▪ Bruice TC, Brown A, Harris DO: On the concept of orbital steering in catalytic reactions, *Proc Natl Acad Sci USA* 68(3):658-661, 1971.

▪ Chasiotis D: Role of cyclic AMP and inorganic phosphate in the regulation of muscle glycogenolysis during exercise, *Med Sci Sports Exerc* 20(6):545-550, 1988.

▪ Dobson GP, Yamamoto E, Hochachka PW: Phosphofructokinase control in muscle: nature and reversal of pH-dependent ATP inhibition, *Am J Physiol* 259(19):R71-R76, 1986.

▪ Hammes GG, Wu CW: Regulation of enzyme activity, *Science* 172:1205-1211, 1971.

▪ Hortobagyi T, Denahan T: Variability in creatine-kinase: methodological, exercise, and clinically related factors, *Int J Sports Med* 10:69-80, 1989.

▪ International Union of Biochemistry and Molecular Biology Nomenclature Committee: *Enzyme Nomenclature 1992: recommendations of the nomenclature committee of the International Union of Biochemistry and Molecular Biology on the nomenclature and classification of enzymes,* San Diego, 1992, Academic Press.

▪ Meinke MH, Edstrom RD: Muscle glycogenolysis: regulation of the cyclic interconversion of phosphorylase-a and phosphorylase-b, *J Biol Chem* 266(4):2259-2266, 1991.

▪ Ren JM, Hultman E: Regulation of phosphorylase-a activity in human skeletal muscle, *J Appl Physiol* 69(3):919-923, 1990.

▪ Reuben J: Substrate anchoring and the catalytic power of enzymes, *Proc Natl Acad Sci USA* 68(3):563-565, 1971.

▪ Storm DR, Koshland DE: A source for the special catalytic power of enzymes: orbital steering, *Proc Natl Acad Sci USA* 66(2):445-452, 1970.

CHAPTER 4

Catabolism: Skeletal Muscle, the Liver, and Adipose Tissue

OBJECTIVES

After studying this chapter you should be able to:

- Explain the metabolic roles of the creatine kinase and adenylate kinase reactions in skeletal muscle.

- Tabulate the ATP production that occurs from the catabolic pathways of carbohydrate and lipid metabolism.

- Describe the regulation of the key enzymes of glycolysis and the TCA cycle.

- Explain how the function and regulation of the catabolic pathways differ in skeletal muscle, the liver, and adipose tissue.

- Detail how amino acid catabolism can be beneficial for the catabolism of carbohydrate in skeletal muscle.

- Detail how carbohydrate catabolism can be beneficial for the catabolism of FFA in the liver.

- Explain how skeletal muscle, the liver, and adipose tissue interact during prolonged exercise.

KEY TERMS

- catabolism
- anaerobic metabolism
- aerobic metabolism
- phosphagen system
- glycolytic metabolism
- mitochondrial respiration
- glucose
- fructose
- glycogen
- triacylglycerols
- fatty acids
- glycerol
- amino acids
- purine nucleotide cycle
- creatine phosphate shuttle
- glycogenolysis

- glycolysis
- GLUT proteins
- redox potential
- lactate
- mass action effect
- acetyl-CoA

- tricarboxylic acid cycle
- electron transport chain
- oxidative phosphorylation
- reduction potential
- lipolysis
- ß-oxidation
- carnitine shuttle
- ketone bodies
- Cori cycle

- Alanine cycle

The main tissues that influence energy metabolism during exercise are the contracting skeletal muscle, the liver, and the adipocytes. During exercise molecules need to be made more available to fuel the metabolic pathways in contracting muscle. To accomplish this, some pathways of metabolism need to have decreased activity, while others need increased activity. The extent to which certain pathways are activated or hindered depends on the tissue and the duration and intensity of the exercise. Furthermore, the functions of the contracting skeletal muscle, the liver, and the adipocytes often support the metabolic functions of one another, to ensure an adequate availability of energy substrate. The function of the three tissues, and their interactions in metabolism during and even after exercise, necessitates that they be studied not only separately, but also as a collective whole, so that their combined implications to energy metabolism during exercise can be appreciated. The purpose of this chapter is to apply concepts of bioenergetics and enzyme function to explain the function and regulation of metabolic pathways during and following exercise. By learning the metabolic roles in multiple tissues, the student will develop a more thorough understanding of the body's metabolic response to exercise.

Metabolism: Catabolism and Anabolism

Metabolism can be defined as the sum of all chemical reactions in the body (see Chapter 2). The complete picture of metabolism in the typical cell from multicellular organisms is a tremendous example of energy transfer and of the role of several important molecules that transfer free energy, electrons, and protons within and between metabolic pathways. Remember that *a metabolic pathway consists of a series of individual reactions that result in the formation of an end product.* These reactions can be divided into **catabolism** and *anabolism*. Catabolism consists of the reactions that break down molecules and release free energy, electrons, and protons. Anabolism consists of reactions that combine smaller molecules into larger molecules by the use of free energy and the electrons and protons released during catabolism. As explained in Chapter 2, the free energy cost of building new and larger molecules occurs at the expense of the increased heat and entropy released from catabolism.

Although the presentation of catabolism and anabolism is separated in this text, these processes are not always occurring separately. Most of metabolism occurs with catabolic and anabolic reactions occurring simultaneously, forming a dynamic balance between degradation and synthesis. As discussed, simultaneous catabolism and anabolism can occur in the same tissue (e.g., skeletal muscle glycogen degradation and synthesis in different muscle fiber types), as well as in different tissues during the same rest or exercise conditions (e.g., skeletal muscle versus the liver). These facts should be kept in mind when studying energy metabolism.

catabolism (ca-**tab**'o-lizm)
a part of metabolism that involves the breakdown of relatively complex molecules with the release of energy

TABLE 4.1

Metabolic and structural differences between skeletal muscle, the liver, and adipose tissue

SKELETAL MUSCLE FIBER	HEPATOCYTE	ADIPOCYTE
CELLULAR APPEARANCE		
Long, cylindric, and multinucleated cells; obvious striations	Small, loosely packed parenchymal cells	Nucleus pushed to the side of a large lipid vacuole; transparent
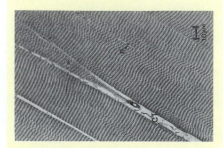	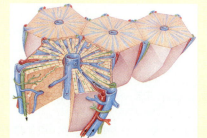	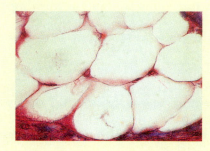
SUBCELLULAR APPEARANCE		
Striated appearance; structurally organized proteins	Random and numerous circular structures (see above)	Opaque, except for nucleus (see above)
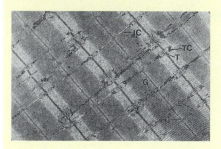		
MAIN FUNCTIONS		
Contractions/movement; glucose uptake; heat production; glycogen storage	Blood lipid metabolism; glycogen stores; blood glucose regulation; iron metabolism; catabolizes wastes, alcohol, hormones, and certain drugs	Stores lipid; glucose uptake; thermal and mechanical insulation
METABOLIC FUNCTIONS DURING EXERCISE		
Carbohydrate and lipid catabolism; glucose uptake; lactate and alanine release	Glycogenolysis and gluconeogenesis; glucose release into circulation	Lipolysis causing release of FFA and glycerol into circulation
METABOLIC FUNCTIONS AFTER EXERCISE		
Glucose uptake; glycogen synthesis; triglyceride synthesis	Glucose uptake, lipid and glycogen synthesis; lipoprotein metabolism	Triglyceride synthesis

(*Top left,* From Eisenburg BR: Quantitative structure of mammalian skeletal muscle. In *Handbook of physiology,* 1983, American Physiological Society. *Top middle,* From Seeley RR, Stephans TD, Tate P: *Anatomy & physiology,* St Louis, 1995, Mosby. Art by Barbara Cousins. *Bottom left,* From Thibodeau GA, Patton KT: *Anatomy & physiology,* St Louis, 1996, Mosby. Art by Ed Reschke.)

Catabolism During Exercise

*T*he main tissues of the body that are involved in catabolism during and following exercise are skeletal muscle, the liver, and adipose tissue. The electron micrographs of the cellular and subcellular organization of skeletal muscle, the liver, and adipose tissue are presented in Table 4.1. It is obvious that the cells of skeletal muscle, the liver, and adipose tissue are very different in *subcellular organization, organelle content, appearance,* and *function.*

Skeletal Muscle

Details of the structure and function of skeletal muscle are presented in Chapter 7. Essentially, the structure and function of skeletal muscle are to support contraction. Muscle contraction can cause more than a 100-fold increase in the cellular demand for ATP within skeletal muscle. Consequently, the design and function of metabolism in skeletal muscle are to produce ATP in rates that meet the ATP demand as well as possible. Skeletal muscle therefore must have sensitive biochemical control of metabolic pathways involving the sudden activation and inhibition of specific enzymes and must be primarily suited to catabolism. The main catabolic pathways of skeletal muscle (Figure 4.1) are *glycogenolysis,* the breakdown of glycogen to glucose-1-phosphate; *glycolysis,* the breakdown of glucose to either pyruvate or lactate; *lipolysis,* the breakdown of triacylglycerol molecules to free fatty acids (FFAs) and glycerol; *β-oxidation,* the breakdown of activated free fatty acid molecules to acetyl-CoA units within the mitochondria; and *cellular respiration,* interactions between pathways within the mitochondria that end in the use of oxygen and the production of large amounts of ATP. (See Focus Box 4.1.)

Liver

The liver is the body's largest gland, but its functions are not confined to glandular activity. The cells of the liver are called *hepatocytes,* are very small compared with a skeletal muscle fiber, and radiate outward from a central vein to form hexagonal structures called lobules. The liver lobule would be anatomically synonymous with the skeletal muscle fascicle. The important functions of the liver during exercise are its capacity to take up nutrients from the blood and to respond to the hormonal regulation of blood glucose by releasing glucose when blood glucose levels decrease below normal (~3 to 4 mmol/L). For example, the liver removes large amounts of *lactate* and *alanine* from the blood during exercise (by-products of glycolysis and amino acid catabolism in skeletal muscle) and these molecules are taken up by the liver and reconverted to glucose via the pathway of *gluconeogenesis.* Glucose is then either released into the blood or used to synthesize glycogen or lipid. Thus the liver can release glucose into the blood from stored glycogen or from the pathway of gluconeogenesis.

Adipose Tissue

Adipose tissue is composed of cells called *adipocytes,* which contain a lipid droplet surrounded by a thin layer of cytoplasm, a compressed nucleus, and cell membranes. Adipocytes can take up glucose from the blood during times of high blood glucose concentrations and increased insulin and convert glucose to glycerol. Adipocytes can also take up FFA from circulating *lipoprotein* molecules in the blood and with glycerol can form triacylglycerols for storage. Furthermore, adipocyte metabolism responds to exercise by catabolizing triglycerides and releasing free fatty acid molecules into the blood for use by the contracting muscle. Despite the simplistic appearance of the adipocyte, these metabolic processes indicate that adipocytes contain the enzymes necessary for glycolysis, triacylglycerol synthesis and catabolism and the biochemical molecules involved in the regulation of these pathways during different metabolic conditions.

Catabolism in Skeletal Muscle

*S*keletal muscle can produce the ATP required to support muscle contraction from one or a combination of three metabolic reactions or pathways: the transfer of the phosphate from creatine phosphate (CrP) to ADP to form ATP, glycolysis, and the use of oxygen in the mitochondria. The production of ATP from CrP and glycolysis does not require the presence of oxygen and has been referred to as **anaerobic metabolism**. Conversely, the ATP production from cellular respiration in mitochondria, which uses oxygen, has been termed **aerobic metabolism**. These terms are not entirely accurate for describing energy metabolism. Aerobic metabolism is not 100% aerobic because ATP from glycolysis is still produced. It is inappropriate to differentiate two extremes of energy metabolism when they can share a common central pathway (e.g., glycolysis in carbohydrate catabolism). Terms that are gaining increased acceptance for qualifying the source of ATP production are

anaerobic metabolism
reactions of metabolism that do not require the presence of oxygen. However, this term is also used loosely to refer to the reactions of creatine kinase, adenylate kinase, and glycolysis

aerobic metabolism
reactions that are involved in the use of oxygen. However, this term loosely refers to mitochondrial respiration, and in particular, to the combined reactions of pyruvate oxidation, the TCA cycle, and the electron transport chain

F I G U R E   4 . 1

The metabolic relationships between the main nutrients and the pathways of catabolism. The amino acid, carbohydrate, and fat metabolism share common intermediates and pathways. However, as can be seen, the intracellular locations of these pathways differ.

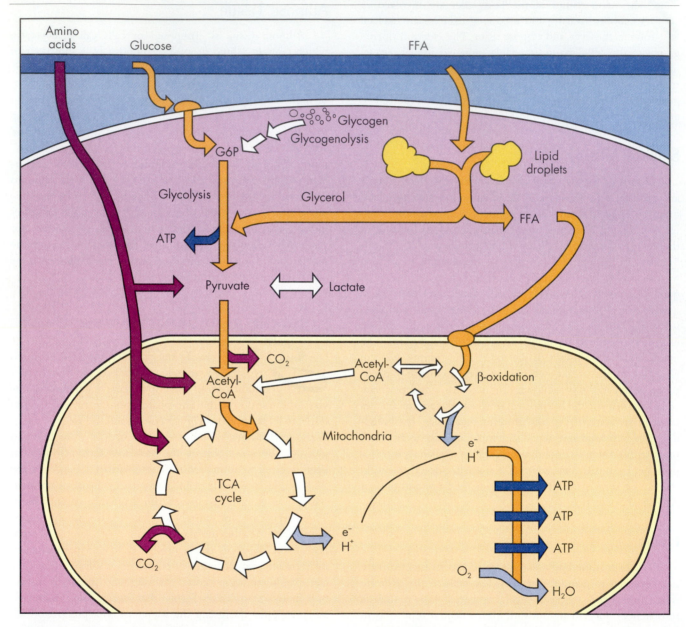

the **phosphagen system, glycolytic metabolism,** and **mitochondrial respiration,** respectively.

Phosphagen System

The CrP reaction is the most rapid means to regenerate ATP and is catalyzed by creatine kinase (EC: 2.7.3.2). Approximately 4% of skeletal muscle creatine kinase is located on the outer mitochondrial membrane, with 3% being bound to the myofibrillar proteins of the sarcomere and the remainder remaining free in cytosolic solution.[13] The

phosphagen system
the regeneration of ATP via creatine phosphate hydrolysis and ADP

glycolytic metabolism
reactions of the glycolytic pathway

mitochondrial respiration
reactions of the mitochondria, which ultimately lead to the consumption of oxygen

FOCUS BOX 4.1

Main nutrients involved in energy metabolism

The main nutrients of the body used in energy metabolism are *carbohydrates, lipids,* and *amino acids* (Figure 4.2). The nutrient most important to energy metabolism during moderate to intense exercise is carbohydrate. There are many different types of carbohydrate molecules; however, **glucose** is the favored carbohydrate for metabolism in skeletal muscle, the liver, and adipose tissue. **Fructose** can also be incorporated into the glycolytic pathway; however, the liver is the major tissue involved in fructose metabolism. **Glycogen** consists of a protein core (glycogenin) to which chains of glucose molecules are attached.[11,23,34] The glucose chains (alpha 1-4 bonds) branch from themselves (alpha 1-6 bonds), resulting in a large structure with the ends of many glucose polymer chains exposed to the surrounding cellular medium. Glycogen molecules in skeletal muscle are visualized in electron microscopy as darkly stained circular structures dispersed throughout the cytosol, hence the term "glycogen granule"[11] (see Glycogenolysis).

Many types of lipid molecules exist within cells. The main lipids of interest to energy metabolism are those that comprise **triacylglycerols**. A triacylglycerol consists of three **fatty acid** (FA) molecules attached to a carbohydrate backbone called **glycerol.** Fatty acid molecules vary in the number of carbon atoms they contain, in the presence and location of double bonds between carbons, and in whether they are bound to a glycerol backbone. FA molecules that are bound to glycerol are termed *esterified* fatty acids, whereas FAs free from glycerol are termed *nonesterified* fatty acids, or *free fatty acids* (FFAs). The FFA molecule is catabolized in muscle during muscle contraction.

Fatty acid molecules that contain no double bonds are termed *saturated,* whereas FA molecules with double bonds are termed *unsaturated.* The main FAs used in energy metabolism are palmitic acid *(palmitate),* stearic acid *(stearate,* 18 C, saturated), and oleic acid *(oleate,* 18 C, monounsaturated). Palmitate is a saturated FA consisting of 16 carbon atoms attached end to end to form a backbone to which hydrogen and oxygen molecules are also attached. Palmitate is the predominant FA in the body and is therefore used to represent the reactions and energy liberated from FFA catabolism.

Amino acid molecules differ from carbohydrate and lipid molecules in that they contain nitrogen atoms. There are 20 amino acids within the body,[45] and all have a structure comprising an acid (COOH), amine (NH_2), CH, and R group (side chain) attached to a central carbon atom. Amino acids differ by the structure of the R group and can be classified by the characteristics of the R group or by the charge of the R group. Amino acids can be incorporated into catabolism by removing the amine group *(deamination)* and converting the remaining structure into a molecule of either the glycolytic or citric acid cycle pathways. Similarly, pyruvate produced from glycolysis can have an amine group added *(transamination)* from the deamination of another amino acid, producing alanine. Alanine then leaves the muscle and circulates to other tissues such as the liver (see Chapter 5).

During times of low carbohydrate nutrition, when FFA catabolism is the predominant substrate, the liver can produce *ketone bodies* from acetyl-CoA molecules. Ketone bodies comprise three different molecules: acetoacetate, ß-hydroxybutarate, and acetone, with the main ketone body being acetoacetate. Once in the circulation, acetoacetate and ß-hydroxybutarate can be used by contracting muscle, the heart, and the kidney for substrate in catabolism.

Glucose (glu-kos)
the form of sugar by which carbohydrate is metabolized in animals

fructose (fruc-tos)
the form of sugar predominantly found in fruit and honey

glycogen (gli'ko-jen)
a sugar polysaccharide that is the form of carbohydrate storage in animal tissues

triacylglycerol (tri-as'il-glis'er-ol)
a lipid consisting of a glycerol backbone and three free fatty acid molecules; the principal form of fat storage in the body

fatty acids
the lipid components of triacylglycerols, which are catabolized in tissues

glycerol (gli-ser-ol)
an alchohol, which is the structural backbone of triacylglycerols

amino acids
amine (NH_2) containing molecules that are the primary components of proteins

FIGURE 4.2

The structures of key substrates involved in the pathways of metabolism. Glycogen consists of glucose molecules connected together and is a highly branched and structurally organized molecule. Fructose, like glucose, is another monosaccharide. Triacylglycerols comprise fatty acids and a glycerol molecule. Fatty acids can differ in carbon numbers and the degree of saturation. Palmatite is the main free fatty acid used in lipid catabolism. Amino acids (e.g., alanine) are named for their amine group located on a central carbon atom and differ in their side chain length, structure, and charge.

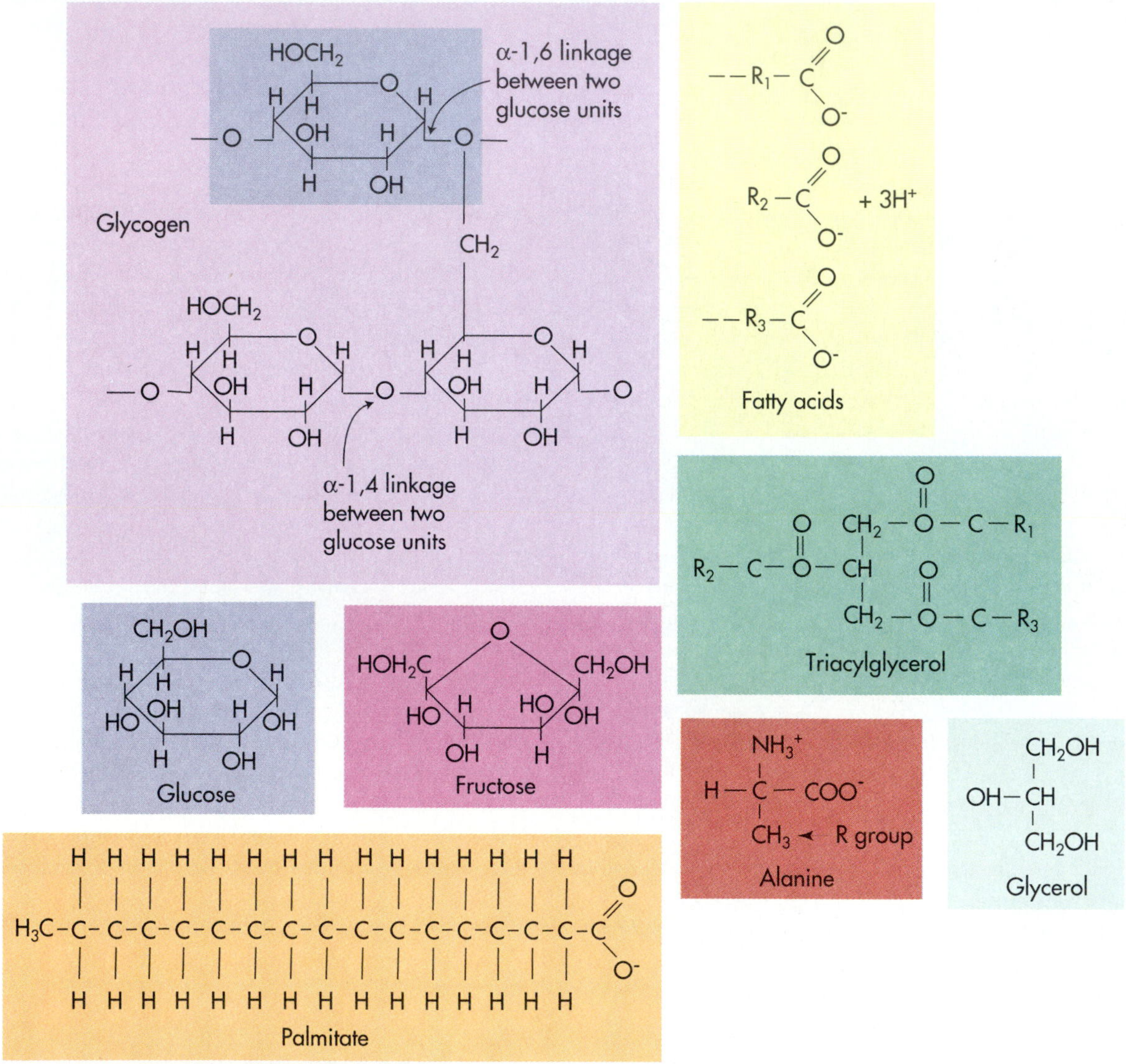

distribution of creatine kinase enables the rapid synthesis of ATP in the regions where it is needed. Furthermore, as explained later in this section, the mitochondrial bound enzyme is essential for the operation of the *creatine phosphate shuttle*.

$$CrP + ADP + H^+ \leftrightarrow ATP + Cr$$

During muscle contraction when there are transient increases in ADP in the locations of the contractile filaments,

the direction of the creatine kinase reaction favors ATP production (Figure 4.3). However, the ATP production capacity of the creatine kinase reaction relies on a store of CrP, which approximates 24 mmol/kg wet wt (see Table 2.3). Another name for this system is the ATP-PC system. However, this name is inappropriate, since energy metabolism in skeletal muscle is designed to maintain a constant intracellular ATP concentration. The convention to regard ATP as a store of potential free energy available for energy metabolism should be avoided. Data presented in Chapter 10 show that only

FIGURE 4.3

The creatine kinase and adenylate kinase reactions that cause rapid (ATP) regeneration in the vicinity of the contractile proteins.

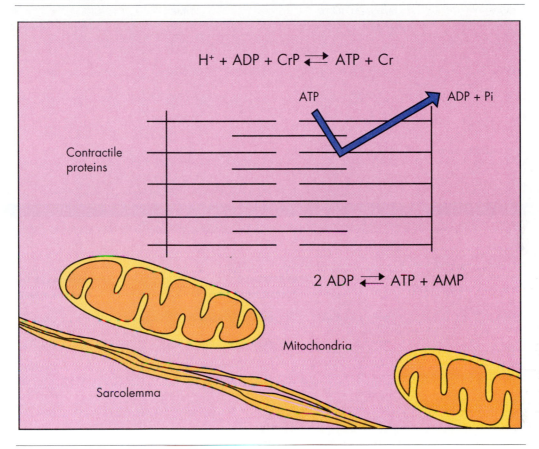

extreme exercise can cause minor decreases in the ATP concentration within skeletal muscle.

An additional one-enzyme-catalyzed reaction exists to regenerate ATP, and the enzyme involved is *adenylate kinase* (EC: 2.7.4.3) (Figure 4.3). The adenylate kinase reaction is similar to the creatine kinase reaction in that it is near equilibrium. This reaction also serves to produce the allosteric activator (AMP) of phosphorylase and phosphofructokinase (see Chapter 3), thus stimulating increased glycogenolysis and glycolysis.

$$ADP + ADP \leftrightarrow ATP + AMP$$

Continued increases in AMP would decrease the phosphorylation potential of the cell. This is partially prevented by the conversion of AMP to inosine monophosphate (IMP) by the *AMP deaminase*–catalyzed reaction of the **purine nucleotide cycle**. This reaction is stimulated during acidic conditions, with an ammonium ion (NH_4^+) produced as a by-product.[47] The ammonium ion is very toxic to the cell and is removed into circulation for metabolism by the liver, excretion by the kidney, or loss through sweat.

The importance of the phosphagen system is that it can regenerate ATP at a high rate (Table 4.2). During exercise that demands ATP production in excess of ATP supply from mitochondrial respiration or glycolysis, the creatine kinase reaction enables ATP to be produced to meet the ATP demand of muscle contraction. However, the finite intramuscular store of CrP can be depleted during intense exercise in as little as 10 seconds, which would provide ATP at approximately 2.4 mmol/kg wet wt/s of muscles, or $1.44 + 10^{21}$ molecules of ATP each second. Table 4.3 lists activities that would rely heavily on ATP regeneration from CrP hydrolysis, glycolysis, and oxidative phosphorylation.

purine nucleotide cycle

conversion of AMP to IMP, which is reconverted to AMP during recovery

TABLE 4.2

Maximal rate of ATP production, time to reach maximal rate, and oxygen requirement of the metabolic reactions/pathways of ATP production

REACTION/PATHWAY	MAXIMAL RATE (mmol ATP/kg wet wts)	TIME	O_2 (mmol O_2/ATP)
CrP	2.4	<1.0 sec	0.0
Glucose $\leftrightarrow$ Lactate	1.3	<5.0 sec	0.0
Glucose $\leftrightarrow$ CO_2 + H_2O	0.7	3.0 min	0.167
FFA $\leftrightarrow$ CO_2 + H_2O	0.3	30.0 min	0.177

Modified from Sahlin K: Metabolic changes limiting muscle performance. In Saltin B, editor: *Biochemistry of exercise*, vol 16, Champaign, Illinois, 1986, Human Kinetics.

TABLE 4.3

Examples of activities that rely heavily on CrP, glycolysis, or mitochondrial respiration as the source for free energy to regenerate ATP in contracting skeletal muscle

ACTIVITY	DEPENDENCE*			APPROXIMATE DURATION
	CrP	GLYCOLYSIS	O_2	(HOUR:MIN:SEC)
Kicking a football	High	Low	Low	0:0:05
Weight lifting	High	Moderate	Low	0:0:05
Throwing events	High	Low	Low	0:0:10
Running up stairs	High	Low	Low	0:0:10
Pole vault	High	Moderate	Low	0:0:10
Jumping events	High	Low	Low	0:0:10
100 to 200 m run sprints	High	Moderate	Low	0:0:10 – 0:0:30
50 to 100 m swimming sprints	High	Moderate	Low	0:0:10 – 0:0:30
Weight lifting	High	Moderate	Low	0:0:30 – 0:2:00
400 to 800 m sprints	High	High	Moderate	0:1:00 – 0:3:00
Wrestling	High	High	Moderate	0:0:30 – 0:5:00
200 to 400 m swim	High	High	Moderate	0:2:00 – 0:5:00
Hill running	High	High	Moderate	0:2:00 – 0:5:00
Ice hockey	High	High	Moderate	0:2:00 – 0:8:00
1500 m run	Moderate	Moderate	High	0:3:30 – 0:5:00
5,000 to 10,000 m run	Low	Low	High	0:12:00 – 0:30:00
Marathon run	Low	Low	High	2:0:00 – 4:0:00
Triathlons	Low	Low	High	2:0:00 – 5:0:00

*Relative to the maximal potential ATP supply from that energy system. Note that no athletic/sports/exercise examples rely solely on one energy system.

Evidence exists to indicate that CrP and ADP are also involved in the shuttling of inorganic phosphate throughout the cytosol during all conditions of cellular metabolism. The source of the inorganic phosphate is the terminal phosphate of ATP formed from glycolysis and mitochondrial respiration. The term used to describe this function of CrP is the **creatine phosphate shuttle**.[13]

The presence of mitochondrial bound creatine kinase is important for the creatine phosphate shuttle to provide a rapid means of phosphate transfer from the mitochondria to the cytosol. The transfer of phosphate molecules is proposed to occur in concert with the activities of the adenylate kinase and respective ATPase enzymes.[13] For example, during muscle contraction ATP degradation would increase ADP concentrations in the region of the contractile proteins. Because of the equilibrium reactions of creatine kinase and adenylate kinase, the increased metabolic activity of the contractile proteins would increase the activity of the mitochondrial bound creatine kinase enzyme and convert ATP to ADP. Interestingly, because ADP is known to stimulate mitochondrial respiration, these equilibrium reactions provide a rapid means of communication between the contractile proteins and mitochondria. If muscle contraction is too intense for mitochondrial respiration to restore the cytosolic creatine phosphate concentration, a decrease in creatine phosphate and an increased stimulation of mitochondrial respiration will occur (see Mitochondrial Respiration). Research evidence for the function of the shuttle is presented in Chapter 10.

The phosphagen system is crucial to the muscles' ability to tolerate increases in metabolic demand. The phosphagen system not only produces ATP at a high rate, but also produces molecules that stimulate the glycogenolytic, glycolytic, and mitochondrial respiration pathways (AMP, Pi, and ADP) (see Figure 4.2). These events do not occur without potentially negative consequences. Severe decreases in CrP lead to further increases in ADP, slight decreases in ATP, production of AMP, and decreases in the cytosolic phosphorylation potential ([ATP]/[ADP]). Metabolism of AMP to IMP increases production of the ammonium ion (NH_4^+), which is removed from the muscle cell and can become toxic in blood.[47] As discussed in the following material, large increases in glycolysis eventually lead to cellular acidosis, which has the potential to impair enzymes of glycolysis, the function of myosin ATPase, and other ATP-dependent processes of muscle contraction.

Glycogenolysis

Muscle glycogen is a large molecule composed of glucose units joined together by covalent bonds (Focus Box 4.1). Figure 4.4 is an electron micrograph of the subcellular organization of a skeletal muscle fiber. Glycogen can be seen as darkly stained granules distributed throughout the fiber. The intracellular location of glycogen appears to be some-

FIGURE 4.4

An electron micrograph of skeletal muscle. The numerous small dark stained structures are glycogen granules *(G)*. The glycogen granules are distributed throughout the muscle fiber as described in the text. (From Hikida RS et al: *J Neurol Sci* 59: 185-203, 1983.)

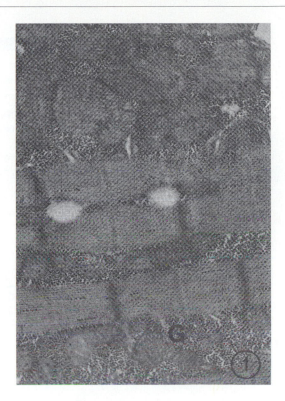

what organized.[11] Glycogen granules occur around the mitochondria beneath the sarcolemma (subsarcolemmal), presumably in support of the ATP-dependent (active transport) functions of the sarcolemma. Glycogen is also localized between myofibrils, beside Z-lines, and within the I-bands of the sarcomere.[11]

The catabolism of glycogen is termed **glycogenolysis**. Glycogenolysis requires three enzymes for optimal function. Phosphorylase (EC: 2.4.1.1) is the main enzyme and is responsible for catabolizing glucose residues from glycogen chains (see Chapter 3). Because glycogen binding to phosphorylase requires four glucose residues, the length of the glycogen chain must be greater than four residues for phosphorylase to have catalytic activity (Figure 4.5). Additional

creatine phosphate shuttle

the transfer of phosphate from mitochondrial ATP to cytosolic creatine and ADP

glycogenolytic enzymes are required to remove the remaining residues from one branch and relocate them at the end of another branch (transferase).[45] Since the transferase removes only three of the four glucose molecules, another enzyme (debranching) cleaves the alpha 1–6 bond and releases glucose. Interestingly, the majority of the increased concentration of free glucose in muscle during intense exercise is attributable to the debranching enzyme reaction.[35]

The $\Delta G^{o'}$ for the phosphorylase reaction approximates –0.5 Kcal/mol and therefore is reversible in vitro.[42] However,

---

FIGURE 4.5

The enzyme catalyzed reactions of glycogenolysis. Phosphorylase removes single glucose residues from 1-4 glu-cosidic bonds until a span of 4 residues remain. Note that phosphorylase is not the only needed enzyme. A debranching enzyme that removes a chain of three glucose residues from four that begin at a 1-6 glucosidic bond is also needed. The three residues are placed on a long chain of residues joined by the 1-4 glucosidic bond, which phosphorylase can degrade. The remaining single residue at the 1-6 bond is then released into solution without being phosphorylated.

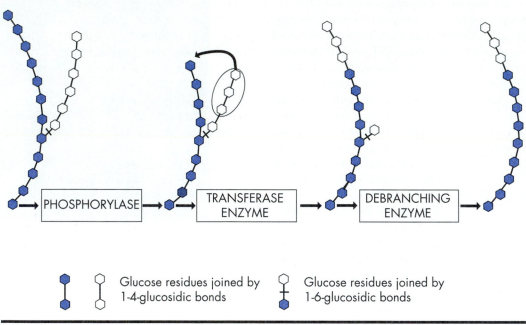

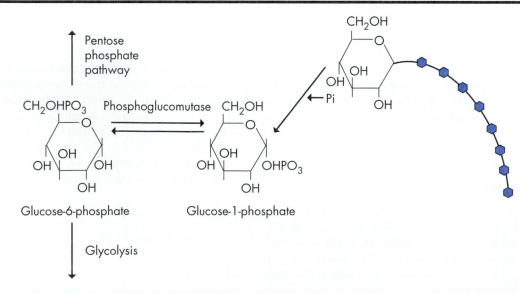

in vivo the reaction is highly exergonic as a result of the 100-fold larger concentration of Pi compared with glucose-1-phosphate and the fact that phosphorylase is believed to be located within the cell bound to protein complexes that also form part of the glycogen molecule.[33,39] The $S_{0.5}$ of glycogen for phosphorylase is estimated to be less than 1 mmol/kg wet wt, which is important because glycogen can be catabolized to release all of its stored glucose pool.[34]

The regulation of phosphorylase is detailed in Chapter 3. The covalent phosphorylation of phosphorylase-b to the phosphorylase-a structure occurs in response to increases in the intracellular second messenger cyclic AMP *(cAMP)*. cAMP is produced in response to epinephrine (a catecholamine hormone) binding to a specific receptor on the sarcolemma (see Chapters 10 and 13). cAMP activates several enzymes that eventually lead to the phosphorylation of phosphorylase and the dephosphorylation (inactivation) of the glycogen-synthesizing hormone glycogen synthase (see Chapter 3). Additional activation of phosphorylase is provided by increased concentrations of calcium. The reaction is also made more exergonic by the increasing concentrations of Pi that would occur during intense exercise from the net hydrolysis of CrP.

The importance of glycogenolysis is that it can *provide a rapid rate of production of glucose-6-phosphate* (see the Clinical Application on p. 68), which as described in the following material is the first intermediate of glycolysis.

Glycolysis

Within skeletal muscle **glycolysis** begins with either glycogenolysis or the entry of glucose into the skeletal muscle fiber. Glucose entry from the blood is facilitated by glucose binding to specialized glucose transport proteins **(GLUT proteins)** located on and below the sarcolemma. There are at least five different types of glucose transporters, and each is numbered based on the order of discovery (GLUT1 to GLUT5).[12,14,16] GLUT4 is the major transporter in skeletal muscle, and the number of GLUT4 transporters can be increased in response to insulin and exercise.[12] The exercise stimulation of glucose transporters is additive and independent of the insulin response.[12,14] GLUT1 transporters also exist in muscle and are believed to account for basal levels of glucose uptake.

The enzyme *hexokinase* (EC: 2.7.1.1) is bound to the outer mitochondrial membrane and the intracellular side of the sarcolemma[34] and catalyzes the conversion of glucose to glucose-6-phosphate coupled to the dephosphorylation of ATP. The $\Delta G^{o\prime}$ of the hexokinase reaction is -8 Kcal/mol, and when accounting for the relatively low glucose-6-phosphate concentrations in vivo, is an essentially irreversible reaction within the cell.[45] Consequently, conversion of glucose to glucose-6-phosphate (G6P) in skeletal muscle retains glucose for either glycogen synthesis or glycolysis.

Glucose-6-phosphate is broken down sequentially by nine reactions that form the central carbohydrate metabolic pathway of glycolysis (Figure 4.7). The important products of glycolysis are pyruvate, ATP, and NADH. Pyruvate can be converted to lactate in the cytosol or be incorporated into the mitochondria and catabolized to form acetyl-CoA, NADH, and carbon dioxide (CO_2). NADH is formed from NAD^+ by acquiring protons and electrons from catabolism for latter use in metabolic reactions within the mitochondria. Acetyl-CoA is an important branch point in the metabolism of both carbohydrate and lipid.

The first four reactions of glycolysis represent the first phase and involve the addition of a phosphate molecule to glucose, the conversion of the phosphorylated glucose structure to a fructose structure, and the addition of a second phosphate to the fructose structure. The phosphate additions during these reactions require the hydrolysis of ATP, and consequently, the first phase of glycolysis requires the expense of two ATP molecules. Note that when G6P molecules are produced from glycogenolysis, the ATP cost of the first phase of glycolysis is one ATP.

The main regulated enzymes of phase 1 of glycolysis are hexokinase and *phosphofructokinase* (PFK) (EC: 2.7.1.11) (Figure 4.8) (see Chapter 3). When glucose binds to hexokinase, one section of the enzyme rotates 12 degrees, enclosing the glucose molecule and developing the active site of the enzyme-substrate complex. A similar induced fit mechanism (see Chapter 3) also exists in the other kinase enzymes of glycolysis (e.g., PFK, phosphoglycerate kinase, and pyruvate kinase).[45] Hexokinase has a low $S_{0.5}$ for glucose (0.1 mmol/L), indicating that the rate of converting glucose to G6P in skeletal muscle can be high even if the vascular or intracellular concentrations of glucose are low.[34]

Glucose-6-phosphate is a substrate not only for glycolysis, but also for glycogen synthesis. To provide direction for the metabolism of G6P in glycolysis, it is understandable that a second regulatory enzyme exists. As previously stated, the second regulated enzyme is PFK (see Chapter 3). Because the PFK reaction has a large negative ΔG, essentially making the reaction irreversible in vivo, the activation of the PFK reaction would provide the thermodynamic drive for G6P catabolism in glycolysis. Remember that the ΔG values of reac-

glycogenolysis (gli-ko-jen-ol-is-is)
the removal of glucose units from glycogen, producing glucose-1-phosphate

glycolysis (gli-kol'i-sis)
reactions involving the catabolism of glucose to pyruvate

GLUT proteins
the proteins that transport glucose across the cell membrane.

Enzyme Deficiency Diseases of Catabolism

Numerous genetically determined diseases of metabolism are caused by the absence or altered regulation of key enzymes. Several of these conditions have been researched to further the understanding of the causes of accompanied limitations in exercise tolerance, the regulation of muscle or liver metabolism, and the importance of key enzymes to the optimal ability of cells to regenerate ATP.

Of the enzyme deficiency diseases known to alter glycogen catabolism (Table 4.4), the most closely studied relative to its influence on energy metabolism during exercise has been McArdle's disease.

McArdle's Disease

McArdle's disease, also known as *myophosphorylase deficiency* (MD) is a rare condition that involves the lack or defective function of skeletal muscle phosphorylase. The disease is named after B. McArdle, who in 1951 first reported a case study of the condition and its symptoms, which at that time consisted of severe muscular pain and fatigue during moderate to intense exercise, no increase in blood lactate or pyruvate during exercise, and increased catabolism of ATP to IMP and *hypoxanthine* (a muscle precursor for the formation of uric acid in the liver).[27] Subsequent muscle enzyme analysis of additional patients with similar symptoms indicated a lack of phosphorylase activity, high muscle glycogen concentrations, and the inability to produce lactate in vivo, yet the presence of an active LDH enzyme and the potential for lactate production in vitro when substrates such as glucose 6-phosphate, glucose 1-phosphate, or fructose 6-phosphate were provided.[43]

As discussed in the text, impaired muscle metabolism and exercise tolerance in individuals with MD provide compelling evidence for the importance of glycogenolysis in producing a rapid rate of ATP regeneration from both glycolysis and mitochondrial respiration.

Initial studies reported markedly lower exercise tolerance of individuals with MD, compared with control subjects.[2,27,43] Although some researchers have interpreted the negligible muscle and blood lactate concentrations as evidence for the inability of individuals with MD to produce lactate, this is not true as explained earlier, since they have a functional LDH enzyme. Lactate production is low because individuals with MD rely on glucose uptake from blood to fuel glycolysis. Blood-borne glucose does not provide a high rate of glucose-6-phosphate production, and therefore glycolytic flux is low and pyruvate production is low. Since pyruvate is the substrate for the LDH reaction, this scenario lowers the exergonic nature of the LDH reaction. Figure 4.6 illustrates the lowered blood lactate during exercise and the limited exercise tolerance (earlier fatigue) in individuals with MD compared with normal subjects. The data indicate the inability to develop metabolic acidosis because of the limited capacity for lactate production.

TABLE 4.4

Different diseases of catabolism

DISEASE	CONDITION(S)	AFFECTED ORGAN(S)
CARBOHYDRATE CATABOLISM*		
I. von Gierke's disease	Glucose-6-phosphatase deficiency	Liver
II. Pompe's disease	Alpha-1,4-glucosidase deficiency	Skeletal muscle and liver
III. Cori's disease	Amylo-1,6-glucosidase deficiency	Skeletal muscle and liver
V. McArdle's disease	Phosphorylase deficiency	Skeletal muscle
VI. Hers' disease	Liver phosphorylase deficiency	Liver
VII. Muscle phosphofructokinase deficiency		Skeletal muscle
VIII. Liver phosphorylase kinase deficiency		Liver

*Although classified as storage diseases, these specific examples directly alter catabolism of carbohydrate, which indirectly influences glycogen stores.
Modified from Stryer L: *Biochemistry,* ed 3, New York, 1988, WH Freeman.

Enzyme Deficiency Diseases of Catabolism—Cont'd

Based on the hypothesis that muscle metabolism in individuals with MD is determined by the limited flux through glycolysis, researchers have provided increased substrate either by inducing hyperglycemia and hyperinsulinemia (elevated blood glucose and insulin concentrations) during exercise or by increasing blood FFA concentrations.[31,49] These studies have shown that either alteration increases exercise tolerance in individuals with MD and decreases degradation of ATP to IMP and hypoxanthine.[50] Other researchers have shown that lactate increases during conditions of increased substrate availability.[43]

The implications of the findings from the condition of MD are that a rapid rate of glycolysis is important not only for intense exercise, but also to increase flux through mitochondrial respiration. Without muscle glycogenolysis, blood glucose uptake is insufficient to sustain even moderate-intensity steady state exercise. During moderate to intense exercise in individuals with MD, muscular fatigue and pain occur as a result of decreased creatine phosphate and the degradation of ATP to nonusable by-products. In normal muscle, the capacity to dramatically increase glycolytic flux from increased glycogenolysis delays the onset and severity of these events. Rather than an early onset of fatigue and muscular pain as in MD, individuals without MD suffer from increased acidosis.

FIGURE 4.6

The lowered blood lactate and limited exercise tolerance in individuals with McArdle's disease compared with control subjects.

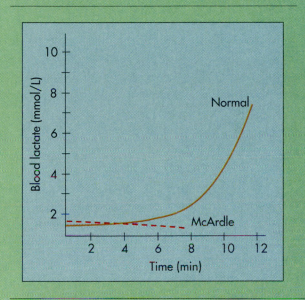

tions in a pathway can be combined to provide an overall ΔG. Conversely, despite the exergonic nature of the PFK reaction, inhibition of PFK would restrict the rate of this reaction, favoring G6P metabolism for glycogen synthesis (see Chapter 5).

During exercise, repeated intense muscle contractions increase the concentration of AMP, which binds to regulator sites on PFK and increases PFK activity for a given concentration of substrate (fructose-6-phosphate). ATP is a needed substrate for the PFK reaction, but ATP can also bind to a separate site that inhibits PFK activity. AMP increases the activity of PFK by decreasing ATP inhibition. The additional regulation mechanisms of PFK are detailed in Chapter 3. The activation of PFK during muscle contraction favors the entry of G6P into the glycolytic pathway. Despite the fact that increasing acidosis (lowered intracellular pH) enhances ATP

inhibition of PFK, it is believed that the increased concentrations of AMP overcome this detrimental effect, retain PFK activity, and provide the potential for glycolysis to continue.[34]

The second phase of glycolysis produces ATP and pyruvate and releases electrons and hydrogen ions. The first reaction of the second phase converts fructose-1,6-bisphosphate into two three-carbon molecules. Glyceraldehyde-3-phosphate is then phosphorylated and simultaneously oxidized, releasing two hydrogen ions and two electrons. The electrons and one hydrogen ion are added to nicotinamide adenine dinucleotide (NAD^+) to form NADH, with the second hydrogen ion remaining free in solution. The role of NAD^+ and NADH as coenzymes is introduced in Chapter 3. The electrons and hydrogen ions are shuttled by NADH to other reactions of metabolism (either within the mitochondria or in the cytosol). The ratio of NAD^+ to NADH is called the

FIGURE 4.7

The reactions of glycolysis can be divided into two phases. Phase 1 involves the eventual catabolism of glucose into two or three carbon molecules and is ATP costly. The second phase of glycolysis produces ATP, reduces the coenzyme NAD+, and eventually produces pyruvate. (Adapted from Lehninger AL et al: *Principles of biochemistry*, New York, 1993, Worth Publishers.)

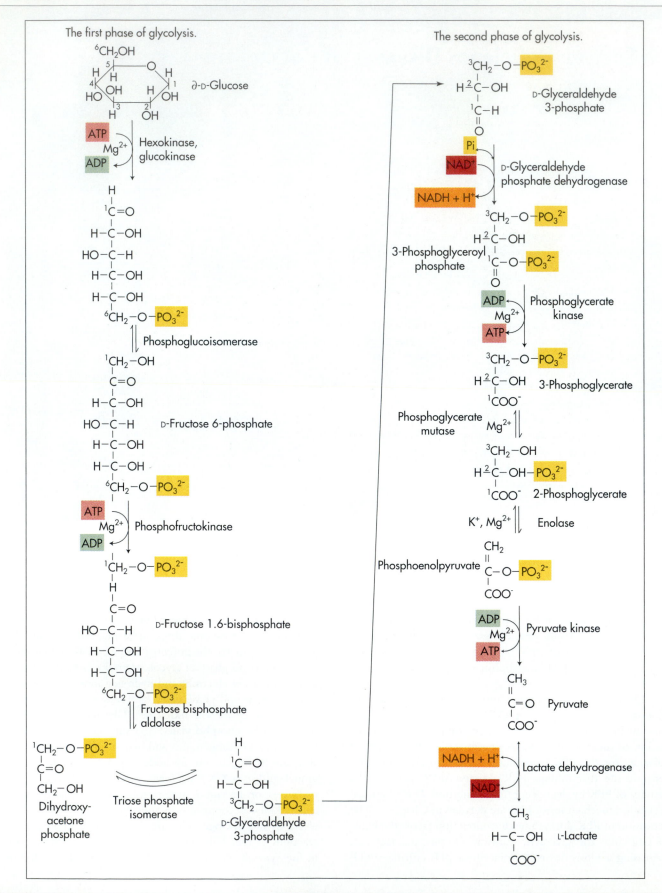

FIGURE 4.8

The regulation of the glycolytic pathway. Note that allosteric enzymes are regulated in the beginning and end of the pathway, and that pyruvate conversion to acetyl-CoA occurs during pyruvate transport through the mitochondrial membranes.

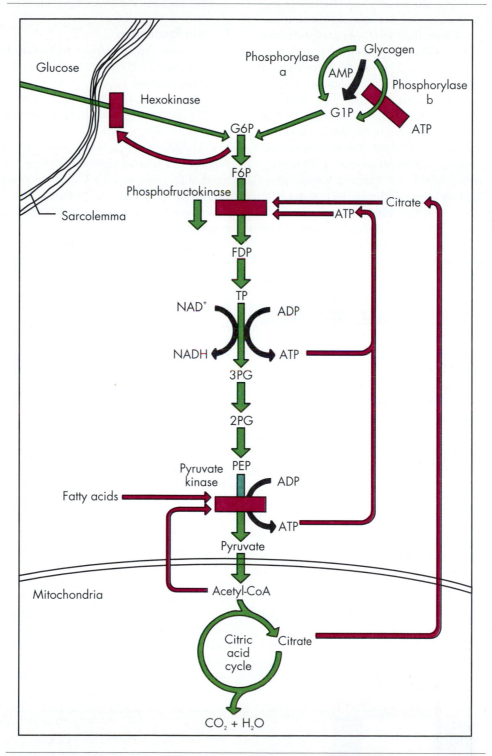

redox potential, and it is important that the cytosolic redox potential be maintained during exercise to provide NAD+ in the glyceraldehyde-3-phosphate dehydrogenase reaction and therefore to continue glycolysis.

The four remaining reactions of phase 2 result in the production of two ATP molecules. Because two three–carbon molecules are produced from fructose-1,6-bisphosphate, this total must be doubled, resulting in a net production of four ATP. Because of the ATP cost of phase 1, depending on whether glucose or glycogen was the initial substrate, the net ATP production from glycolysis is either two or three, respectively. Of the six reactions of phase 2 of glycolysis, the only one with an allosteric enzyme is the last reaction catalyzed by pyruvate kinase (EC: 2.7.1.40). The pyruvate kinase reaction is highly exergonic and therefore, like the PFK reaction, is essentially irreversible in vivo. Pyruvate kinase is activated by fructose-1,6-bisphosphate, the product of the PFK reaction, and is inhibited by ATP. Interestingly, each of the three highly exergonic reactions of glycolysis (catalyzed by hexokinase, PFK, and pyruvate kinase) are essentially irreversible in vivo and are regulated by allosteric enzymes.

The production of lactate in skeletal muscle. Lactate is the name for the deprotonated structure of lactic acid. During lactate production, pyruvate is reduced by the electrons from NADH, reforming NAD$^+$. Therefore lactate production helps to maintain the cytosolic redox potential and provides the coenzyme NAD$^+$ for the glyceraldehyde 3-phosphate dehydrogenase reaction.

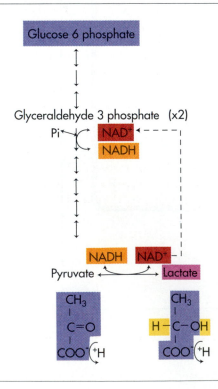

Pyruvate is recognized as the final product of glycolysis and can be reduced to lactate in the cytosol or be transported into the mitochondria and oxidized to acetyl-CoA. The production of lactate has many ramifications to muscle energy metabolism and cardiorespiratory function during exercise.

Lactate Production

Pyruvate can be reduced to **lactate** by the enzyme *lactate dehydrogenase* (LDH) (EC: 1.1.1.27), as indicated in the following equation:

$$\text{Pyruvate} + \text{NADH} + \text{H}^+ \leftrightarrow \text{Lactate} + \text{NAD}^+$$

The ΔG of the LDH reaction is close to zero, and therefore this is a near equilibrium reaction.[34] Interestingly, LDH exists as five isozymes. Each isozyme contains four subunits. LDH from myocardium contains four identical subunits (abbreviated H for "heart"), although skeletal muscle can have different proportions of the H subunit and an M (for "muscle") subunit. Controversy exists over the kinetic differences among the isozymes.[34] Preliminary findings indicated that the H-type isozyme favored lactate conversion to pyruvate, thus explaining the preference of myocardium for lactate as a substrate for catabolism and the larger production of lactate by skeletal muscle.[18] However, research has shown that under in vivo conditions there are minimal kinetic differences among the isozymes and that the equilibrium nature of the reaction governs directionality.[33] Based on the fact that enzymes do not alter directionality of chemical reactions, these later findings are most important.

The lactic acid molecule immediately releases a proton when produced at physiologic pH and is termed *lactate* (Figure 4.9). A basal level of lactate production exists in skeletal muscle, resulting in a resting muscle lactate concentration of 1 mmol/kg wet wt. This resting concentration results from a balance between lactate production, metabolism within the same muscle fiber, and its removal from the cell for metabolism in other tissues (other skeletal muscle fibers, the heart, and the liver). The production of lactate under these steady state conditions has been termed *aerobic glycolysis;* however, since glycolysis is totally anaerobic, this term is misleading and should be avoided.

Unless the proton from lactate production is buffered, lactate production results in a decrease in cellular pH. As exercise intensity increases, the rate of proton liberation eventually exceeds the buffering capacity of the cell and pH decreases, resulting in acidosis. Despite this occurrence, *lactate production is not necessarily detrimental to muscle metabolism during exercise.* The production of lactate involves the reduction of pyruvate, and the electrons and protons required for this are provided by NADH. Lactate production therefore involves the oxidation of NADH, which regenerates NAD$^+$ for the glyceraldehyde-3-phosphate dehydrogenase reaction of phase 2 of glycolysis, as previously explained. Lactate production therefore helps to maintain the *cytosolic redox potential* and to support continued glycolysis and a high rate of ATP regeneration during repeated intense muscle contractions. This is even more important when the finite store of CrP in muscle is considered. As CrP declines, continued intense exercise becomes increasingly reliant on a high rate of glycolysis to regenerate ATP. As previously explained, *lactate production retards a decrease in the cytosolic redox potential and enables glycolysis to continue.*

The metabolic conditions that cause an increase in lactate production are topics of research in exercise physiology and biochemistry. Despite evidence for lactate production during conditions of low or no oxygen (hypoxia),[19] lactate production can also occur in the presence of adequate oxygen.[3,44] Consequently, lactate production should not be viewed as evidence of hypoxia (anaerobic conditions). When the rate of pyruvate production exceeds the rate of pyruvate entry into the mitochondria, pyruvate is converted to lactate. This condition has been termed the **mass action effect**. Therefore the production of lactate is not a detrimental occurrence. Since lactate and pyruvate can be removed from the muscle for metabolism in other tissues, lactate should be viewed as a substrate of metabolism. For example, after intense exercise that results in the accumulation of muscle and blood lactate, lactate can be oxidized back to pyruvate for subsequent gluconeogenic conversion to glucose in the liver or converted to pyruvate in muscle and other tissues for further catabolism within the mitochondria for the eventual production of ATP. Table 4.5 lists the various conditions known to alter lactate production during exercise.

Finally, it should be stressed that lactate production and accumulation in skeletal muscle do not directly cause fatigue or pain. Research has frequently measured blood or muscle lactate as an indication of muscle fatigue.[5] However, lactate concentrations are used as an indirect reflection of acidosis. The production of lactate coincides with the release of a proton (H^+) and the potential for decreases in pH. It is the decrease in cellular and blood pH accompanying high rates of lactate production that has potential detriment to several enzymes of energy metabolism and muscle contraction. The problem with lactate production is the accompanying acidosis and not the lactate molecule.

Mitochondrial Respiration

During steady state exercise conditions, the majority of pyruvate is not converted to lactate but enters into the mitochondria to be further catabolized by a series of reactions that collectively yield carbon dioxide, consume oxygen, and produce large quantities of ATP. Before these reactions are discussed in detail, the function of the mitochondria and the nature of the regulation of mitochondrial function are best introduced by study of the anatomic structure and intracellular localization of mitochondria.

Mitochondria are specialized organelles that contain the enzymes for the reactions responsible for the eventual utiliza-

TABLE 4.5	
Examples of conditions known to alter skeletal muscle lactate production during exercise	
CONDITION	**EFFECTS ON LACTATE PRODUCTION**
INCREASE	**DECREASE**
Hypoxia*	Low muscle glycogen concentration
Ischemia†	Dichloroacetate ingestion‖
Blood loss‡	Hypervolemia
Carbohydrate ingestion	Blood transfusion
High muscle glycogen concentration	
Exercise hyperthermia§	

*Decrease in oxygen content of the blood.
†Decreased blood flow.
‡As in hemorrhage.
§Elevated body core temperature as a result of exercise.
‖Currently not FDA approved.

tion of oxygen (Figure 4.10). Mitochondria contain a double membrane, with the inner membrane impermeable to almost all polar molecules. The inner membrane invaginates to form many internal membrane folds *(cristae)* that penetrate the inner region *(matrix)* of the mitochondrion. The enzymes and electron transfer molecules of the electron transport chain, the protein-enzyme complex responsible for ATP synthesis, and several specialized molecule transport proteins are located on the inner membrane. The enzymes and intermediates of the TCA cycle are in solution within the matrix.

The redox potential within mitochondria is very different from that of the cytosol. Intramitochondrial concentrations of NADH are larger than in the cytosol, resulting in a redox potential that is 100 times lower. The differences are understandable since a relatively high redox potential in the cytosol favors glycolysis and the reduction of NAD^+, whereas the lower redox of the mitochondria favors mitochondrial respiration and the oxidation of NADH.[42]

redox potential
the ratio of NAD^+ to NADH

lactate (lac'tate)
product of the reduction of pyruvate

mass action effect
lactate production caused by an increased rate of glycolytic metabolism

FIGURE 4.10

The structure and shape of mitochondria. (From Thibodeau GA, Patton KT: *Anatomy & Physiology,* St. Louis, 1993, Mosby. Art by William Ober.)

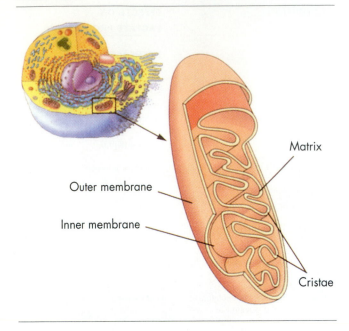

Matrix

Outer membrane

Inner membrane

Cristae

Tricarboxylic Acid Cycle

During pyruvate entry into the mitochondria it is converted to acetyl-CoA by a series of linked enzymes known collectively as pyruvate dehydrogenase. This reaction produces **acetyl-CoA**, carbon dioxide, and NADH. The acetyl-CoA formed from either carbohydrate or lipid catabolism can then enter into a catabolic pathway called the **tricarboxylic acid cycle** (TCA cycle) (Figure 4.11), which consists of nine reactions. The combined products of the TCA cycle are carbon dioxide, ATP, NADH, and FADH. All of the CO_2 produced in energy metabolism can be accounted for from pyruvate entry into the mitochondria and the TCA cycle.

The first reaction of the cycle involves the addition of acetyl-CoA to four carbon molecule—oxaloacetate. The product of this reaction is *citrate,* which is an important allosteric regulator of several enzymes in the cytosol of the muscle fiber, as discussed later in this section. The enzyme that catalyzes this reaction is *citrate synthase* (EC: 4.1.3.7) and is routinely assayed in exercise physiology and biochemistry research. For example, at given substrate and product conditions in vitro, increases in the activity of citrate synthase can occur only if there is an increased enzyme concentration.

Because citrate synthase is confined to mitochondria, measurements of increased citrate synthase activity indicate increased numbers and size of mitochondria. As discussed in Chapter 10, increased mitochondrial mass is a common chronic adaptation to endurance training.

The remaining reactions of the TCA cycle result in the production of three NADH, one FADH, one GTP, and two CO_2. The molecule GTP is guanine triphosphate and is interconvertible with ATP, so it is counted in the ATP tally of metabolism. NADH and FADH are the major products of the TCA cycle. These molecules harness electrons and protons as discussed in the section on glycolysis. The structures of NADH and FADH are provided in Chapter 2, and although they provide a similar function in enzymatic reactions, their use in mitochondrial respiration results in different amounts of ATP production.

The TCA cycle is regulated at several reactions. Citrate synthase is inhibited by ATP, and consequently conditions that are associated with adequate ATP production result in decreased conversion of acetyl-CoA and oxaloacetate to citrate. ATP and NADH inhibit isocitrate dehydrogenase (EC: 1.1.1.41), whereas increases in ADP activate the enzyme. A third site of regulation is the reaction catalyzed by alpha-ketoglutarate dehydrogenase (EC: 1.2.4.2). Consequently, even if citrate is formed, the regulation of additional reactions in the cycle when ATP and NADH concentrations are stable further decreases the entry of acetyl-CoA molecules into the cycle. Interestingly, during these conditions the citrate that is produced is more likely to leave the mitochondria where it inhibits PFK (glycolysis). These metabolic conditions would favor lipid catabolism over carbohydrate. (See Figure 4.8.)

Electron Transport Chain

The student should note that during all the catabolic pathways identified thus far, no mention has been made of oxygen or of a large production of ATP. The biochemical use of oxygen occurs in the **electron transport chain** (ETC). In the ETC the proton and electrons acquired in NADH and FADH are used to add electrons to hydrogen atoms and oxygen to form water, and generate the free energy to add a phos-

acetyl-CoA

molecule produced from carbohydrate and FFA catabolism that enters into the TCA cycle

tricarboxylic acid cycle

mitochondrial reactions involving the addition of acetyl-CoA to oxaloacetate and the eventual release of carbon dioxide, electrons, and protons during the reformation of oxaloacetate

electron transport chain

the series of electron receivers located along the inner mitochondrial membrane that sequentially receive and transfer electrons to the final electron receiver—molecular oxygen

FIGURE 4.11

The intermediates and enzymes of the tricarboxylic acid cycle (TCA cycle). The products of the cycle are CO_2, NADH, FADH, and GTP. The TCA cycle is not a closed cycle since intermediates can be used as substrates of other pathways of metabolism. Similarly, molecules (e.g., amino acids) can be converted to many of the TCA cycle intermediates and therefore integrated into catabolism.

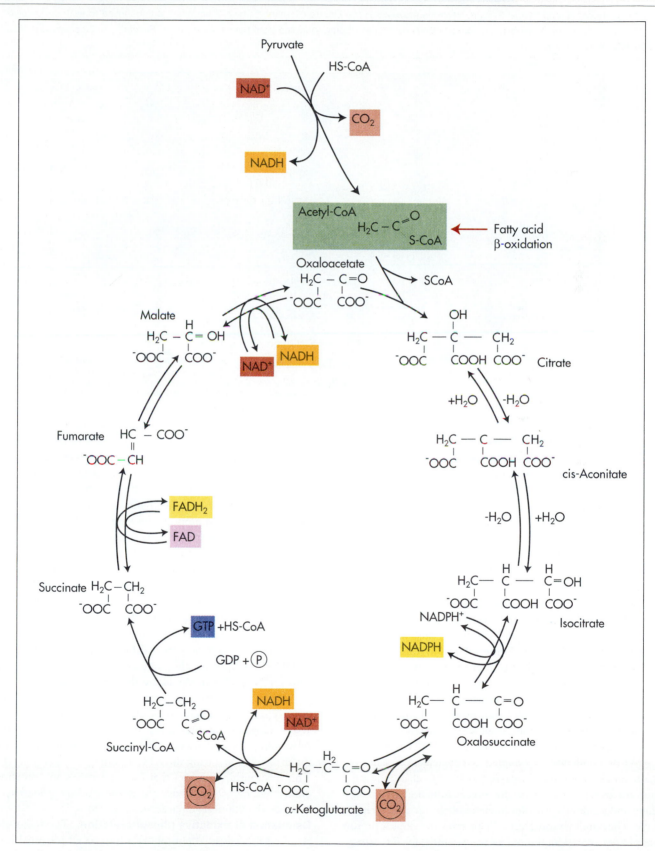

FIGURE 4.12

The change in reduction potential (E'0) as electrons move along the Electron Transport Chain. Electrons are transferred to each successive molecule because of their increasing propensity for accepting electrons. (Adapted from Lehninger AL et al: *Principles of biochemistry*, New York, 1993, Worth Publishers.)

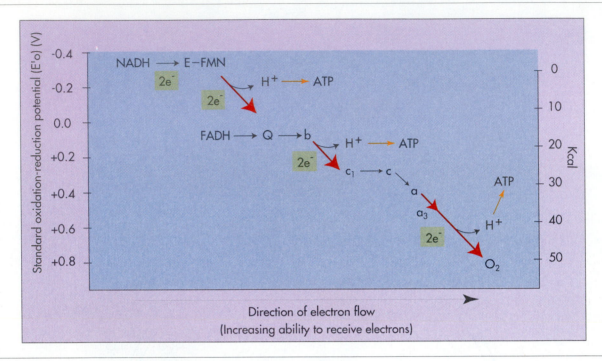

phate to ADP to form ATP. The formation of water and ATP during the ETC is termed **oxidative phosphorylation**.

Electrons are transferred unidirectionally along the electron transport chain. The unidirectionality occurs because each electron acceptor of the chain has a progressively larger affinity for electrons. In biochemical terms the measure of affinity for electrons is termed the **reduction potential**. Figure 4.12 illustrates the change in reduction potential (E'_0) for each molecular component of the electron transport chain. An increased reduction potential is indicated by a more positive E'_0. NADH donates electrons and protons to the chain at the flavine mononucleotide (FMN) complex at the start of the chain. FADH donates electrons and protons at ubiquinone (coenzyme Q) further along the chain. The last electron receiver of the electron transport chain is molecular oxygen ($1/2 O_2$), which has the largest reduction potential. Consequently, the presence of oxygen inside the mitochondria essentially drives the electron transport chain and all the reactions of the mitochondria, which ultimately depend on the function of the chain to regenerate NAD^+ and FAD^+.

ATP production is coupled to the electron transport chain. As electrons are transferred down the chain, the protons are transported across the inner mitochondrial membrane and accumulate in the intermembranous space (Figure 4.13). The unidirectional flow of protons develops a proton and pH gradient, which provides the potential for free energy to be harnessed from the controlled release of protons down the gradient. A special protein complex exists along the inner membrane that contains an ATP synthetase enzyme and allows the flow of protons down the gradient across the inner membrane. According to the chemiosmotic theory of oxidative phosphorylation proposed by Peter Mitchell in 1961, the flow of protons down the gradient provides the free energy to phosphorylate ADP to ATP.[15,28] The electrons and protons provided to the chain by each NADH results in the production of three ATP. Since FADH provides electrons and protons to coenzyme Q, which is located further along the chain than the flavin mononucleotide (FMN) prosthetic group of NADH-Q reductase, fewer protons can be transported across the membrane and only two ATP are produced for each FADH. Consequently, the generally accepted ATP equivalents for NADH and FADH are three and two, respectively.

It is apparent that the production of ATP does not result directly from the reduction of oxygen and protons to form water. However, as previously explained, a stoichiometric relationship exists between the flux of protons across the inner membrane during the ETC and the production of ATP. This relationship indicates that these processes are somehow connected, or *coupled*, hence the name *oxidative phosphorylation* (see the Clinical Application on p. 78).

Regulation of oxidative phosphorylation. The molecules required for oxidative phosphorylation are all potential can-

FIGURE 4.13

The location of the electron carrier molecules of the Electron Transport Chain across the inner mitochondrial membrane. Movement of electrons and protons occur in such a way that protons are transported within the inner-membranous space and generate a proton concentration (pH) gradient across both the inner and outer mitochondrial membranes. As explained in the text, the pH gradient is used to provide the free energy for ATP production during oxidative phosphorylation.

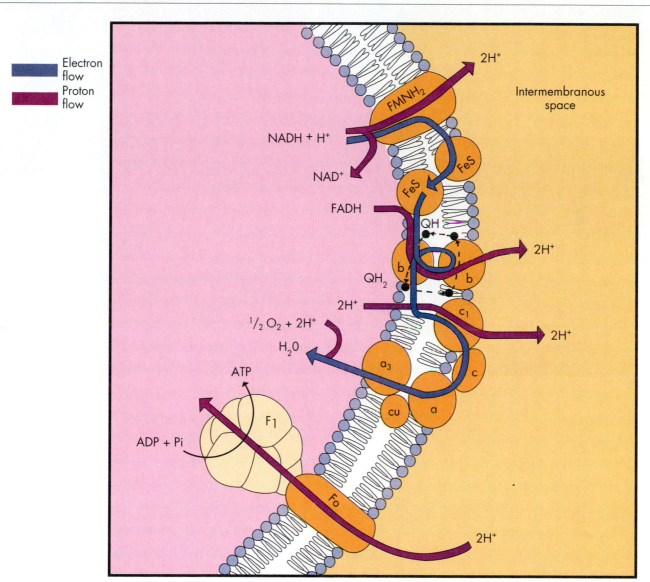

didates for controlling the rate of mitochondrial ATP production. These molecules are pyruvate, acylcarnitines, ADP, Pi, NADH, FADH, and oxygen. Investigations of in vitro mitochondrial function have shown that increases in NADH, ADP, and Pi result in increased rates of oxidative phosphorylation, but data are less convincing for in vivo conditions.[1] No single main candidate for regulation has been identified, and the consensus is that several regulators exist, with each contributing differently depending on the cellular conditions present.

oxidative phosphorylation

the production of ATP from the coupled transfer of electrons to the generation of an H⁺ gradient between the two mitochondrial membranes

reduction potential

a measure of the propensity for a molecule to receive electrons

Preventing or Uncoupling Oxidative Phosphorylation

Oxidative phosphorylation is dependent on the flow of electrons along the electron transport chain, the generation of a proton (H^+) gradient in the intermembranous space of the mitochondria, the ability to regulate the movement of H^+ down this gradient, and the harnessing of the free energy generated from the movement of the H^+ down the gradient to ADP phosphorylation to form ATP. If any one of these events is hindered, cells will generate less ATP for a given consumption of oxygen and cell function will be impaired. There are many examples of poisons that prevent electron transport, as well as molecules that prevent the coupling of the free energy of the H^+ gradient to the phosphorylation of ADP to ATP (Table 4.6).

In nature there are also instances in which the partial uncoupling of oxidative phosphorylation is a beneficial characteristic of certain tissues. Partial uncoupling of oxidative phosphorylation requires an increase in oxygen consumption for a given ATP production, and as a result of the increased metabolism accompanying this condition, also results in increased heat production. *Brown fat* is a tissue in infants and hibernating animals that has partial uncoupled oxidative phosphorylation.; This is beneficial, since the increased heat production conserves body heat in the infant and it maintains core temperature in the hibernating animal during the cold months of winter.

Poisons and "uncoupling agents" that affect oxidative phosphorylation
Figure 4.14 indicates the sites at which certain molecules are known to interfere with the process of oxidative phosphorylation. Rotenone, Amytal, Antimycin A, cyanide, carbon monoxide, and hydrogen sulfide each decrease the flow of electrons, the generation of a proton gradient, and the rate of ATP regeneration from mitochondrial respiration.[22] In contrast to the mechanism of these poisons, uncoupling agents do not interfere with the function of the electron transport chain but prevent the harnessing of the free energy of the proton gradient for use in phosphorylating ADP to ATP. This can be accomplished by either the presence of an alternate route for H^+ flux down the gradient other than the ATPase-associated F1-F0 protein or by impaired function of the F1-F0 protein.

TABLE 4.6

Poisons and "uncoupling agents" that affect oxidative phosphorylation

MOLECULE	SOURCE	MECHANISM
POISONS		
Rotenone	South American plant extract	Prevents electron transport from NADH to ubiquinone
Amytal	Barbiturate	Prevents electron transport from NADH to ubiquinone
Antimycin A	Antibiotic from *Streptomyces*	Prevents electron transfer from ubiquinone to cytochrome C
Cyanide		Prevents reduction of cytochrome a/a3 complex
Carbon monoxide	Incomplete carbon fuel combustion	Prevents reduction of molecular oxygen
Hydrogen sulfide		Prevents reduction of molecular oxygen
UNCOUPLING AGENTS		
2,4-Dinitrophenol	Laboratory	Transports protons across inner membrane, preventing the formation of the H^+ gradient

Modified from Lehninger AL: *Principles of biochemistry*, New York, 1993, Worth.

Oxidative phosphorylation can be impaired by the function of certain poisons. These molecules either hinder the process of electron transfer or the coupling between ATP regeneration and the formation of the proton gradient.

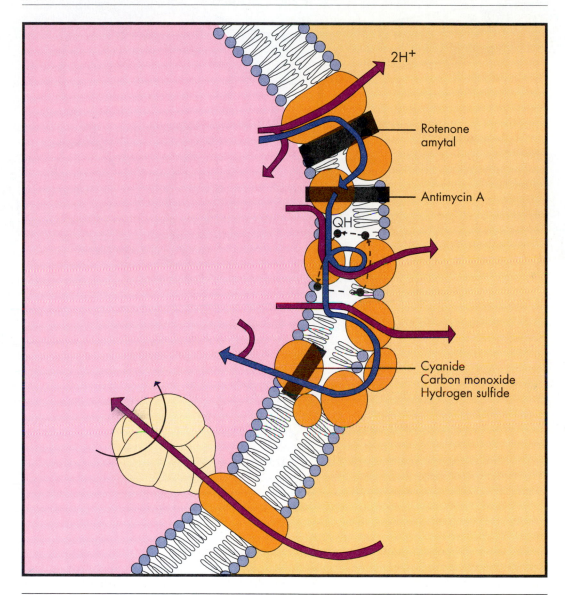

Mitochondrial Membrane Shuttles and Molecular Transport Mechanisms

Several problems exist with oxidative phosphorylation in mitochondria that are enclosed by a double membrane. If the NADH produced from glycolysis is to be used as an electron and proton donor in the ETC, there must be a means to transfer this molecule and its electrons and protons into the mitochondria. In addition, there must be a means to transfer the ADP from the cytosol into the mitochondria, as well as the ATP produced in the mitochondria to the cytosol.

Cytosolic NADH does not enter into mitochondria. Instead, the electrons and protons of NADH are added to molecules that can be transported into the mitochondria and these molecules are oxidized to release the electrons and protons to mitochondrial NAD$^+$. During cellular conditions when most of the pyruvate formed from glycolysis enters into the mitochondria, this shuttle mechanism is responsible for maintaining the cytosolic redox potential. There are two main methods of electron and proton transfer from the cytosol to mitochondria—the *glycerol-3-phosphate shuttle* and the *malate-aspartate shuttle*. Both rely indirectly on the transfer of electrons and protons from the cytosol to within the mitochondria.

The malate-aspartate shuttle involves the coupled oxidation of cytosolic NADH to NAD$^+$ and the reduction of cytosolic oxaloacetate to malate. Malate then enters the mitochondria via a transporter. Aspartate is needed in the shuttle,

FIGURE 4.15

A, The proposed roles of vascular and intracellular lipases in the mobilization of free fatty acids for muscle catabolism. Mitochondrial catabolism of lipid requires the activation of cytosolic FFA molecules by the addition of CoA.

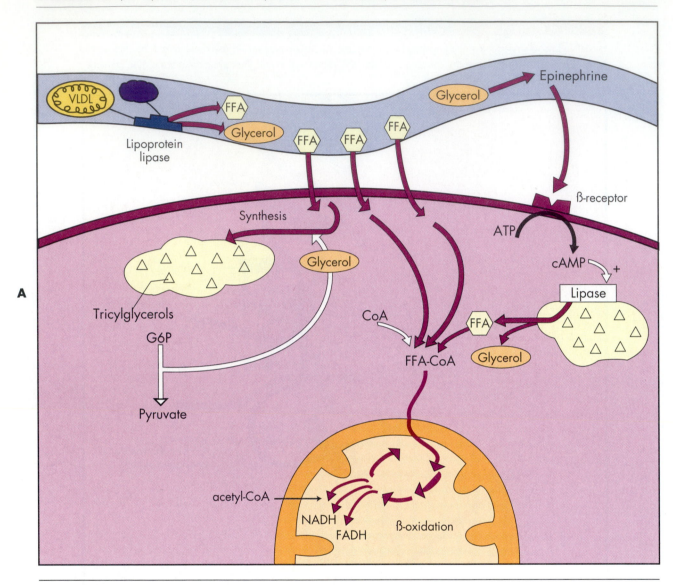

since it can leave the mitochondria and form cytosolic oxaloacetate, which is the needed reductant for the formation of malate. Once in the mitochondria, malate is oxidized to oxaloacetate, regenerating NADH and oxaloacetate.

The glycerol-3-phosphate shuttle involves the transfer of electrons from NADH to dihydroxyacetone phosphate (phase 2 of glycolysis) to form glycerol-3-phosphate. Glycerol-3-phosphate is transported into the mitochondria, where it is oxidized to form dihydroxyacetone phosphate. However, this mitochondrial reaction involves the coenzyme FAD^+ rather than NAD^+, producing FADH and an eventual two ATP rather than three.

It is stated in pure biochemistry textbooks that the malate-aspartate shuttle does not exist in skeletal muscle, but does in liver, kidney, and myocardium.[45] However, there is evidence to indicate that the malate aspartate shuttle does exist in skeletal muscle and that this enzyme-driven shuttle is more responsive to endurance training than the glycerol-3-

phosphate shuttle.[42] The student should interpret these findings to mean that both shuttles exist in skeletal muscle and that the malate-aspartate shuttle is more operable in endurance-trained muscle.

As indicated in Chapter 2, ADP and ATP are large, charged molecules. Consequently, neither molecule can diffuse through the inner mitochondrial membrane. A specific transport protein called *ADP-ATP translocase* (EC: 2.7.7.53) facilitates the movement of the adenylates between the cytosol and mitochondria. The function of the translocase requires the binding of a cytosolic ADP and a mitochondrial ATP, resulting in the coupled entry of ADP into the mitochondria and the exit of ATP. To support the electrochemical changes that occur with the transport of charged molecules from the mitochondria, many specialized transport systems exist that essentially return or remove charge to or from the mitochondria, thus requiring less ATP expenditure to maintain the mitochondrial membrane potentials.

FIGURE 4.15—Cont'd

B, The activated acyl-CoA molecule can then be transported into the mitochondria by a special carnitine shuttle mechanism. As illustrated, the shuttle requires a cytosolic and a mitochondrial enzyme. (Adapted from Lehninger AL et al: *Principles of biochemistry*, New York, 1993, Worth Publishers.)

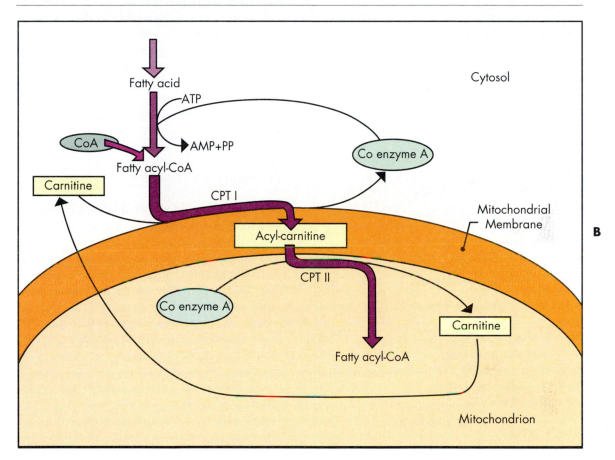

As previously discussed with the phosphagen system, creatine kinase is located on the outer mitochondrial membrane and is important for the optimal function of the creatine phosphate shuttle.

Lipolysis

Within skeletal muscle triacylglycerols are stored in lipid droplets that are easily visualized by electron microscopy (Chapters 8 and 10). Lipid catabolism begins with the breakdown of triacylglycerols **(lipolysis)** (Figure 4.15). A special intracellular lipase enzyme, *hormone-sensitive lipase* (EC: 3.1.1.3), is activated by cAMP and sequentially releases FFA molecules from the glycerol backbone of triacylglycerols.[36,37] Another lipase enzyme, *lipoprotein lipase* (EC: 3.1.1.34), is attached to the endothelial lining of blood vessels and catabolizes triacylglycerols from blood lipoprotein molecules. The FFA molecules can then be catabolized by muscle, while the remaining glycerol molecule is circulated to the liver. However, glycerol removal by the liver, heart, and kidney is a slow process, hence the use of glycerol as a marker for peripheral triacylglycerol catabolism (FFA mobilization).

The products of intramuscular lipolysis, *glycerol* and *free fatty acids,* are catabolized differently. Following intramuscular lipolysis, glycerol can be incorporated into glycolysis in the liver at the start of phase 2, although long-chain (>15 carbons) FFAs must be modified by the addition of CoA for transport into the mitochondria (Figure 4.15) where they are then catabolized in a metabolic pathway called **ß-oxidation** (Figure 4.16). The ß-oxidation pathway consists of four enzyme-catalyzed reactions that result in the removal of a two-carbon end segment, producing acetyl–CoA, NADH, FADH, and an FFA molecule that is two carbons shorter. The

lipolysis (li-pol'i-sis)

catabolism of triacylglycerol, releasing FFA and glycerol

ß-oxidation

the reactions of the oxidation of FFA molecules to acetyl-CoA

FIGURE 4.16

The reactions of β-oxidation. For every cycle, 1 acetyl-CoA, 1 NADH, and 1 FADH are produced, leaving the FFA-CoA molecule shorter by 2 carbons. (Adapted from Lehninger AL et al: *Principles of biochemistry*, New York, 1993, Worth Publishers.)

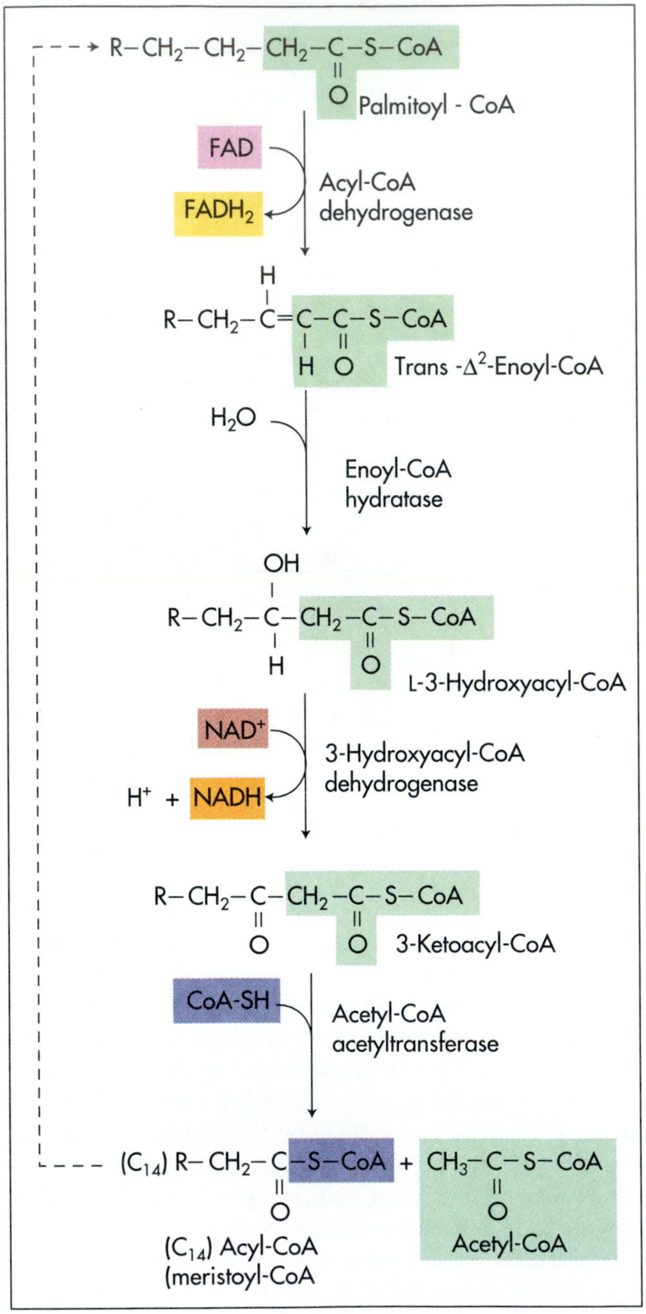

reactions are necessary to make this section of the molecule saturated, which then allows ß-oxidation to continue.

Activation of the FFA molecule is costly, since it requires that two phosphates be removed from ATP (a two ATP cost). The transport of the activated FFA into the mitochondria occurs via a **carnitine shuttle,** which involves the function of a cytosolic and a mitochondrial enzyme (Figure 4.15). During light to moderate exercise the ATP cost of FFA activation can be tolerated and the function of the mitochondrial enzyme of the carnitine shuttle and the enzymes of ß-oxidation are active. As exercise intensity and stimulation for glycogenolysis and glycolysis increase, the relative contribution of FFA catabolism decreases, with complete dependence on carbohydrate catabolism occurring at intensities above 60% to 85% VO_2max (higher for endurance-trained individuals).

Does Lipid Burn in a Carbohydrate Flame Within Skeletal Muscle?

In skeletal muscle, lipid does not burn in a carbohydrate flame. This adage implies that molecules produced from carbohydrate metabolism can enter the mitochondria and supplement TCA cycle intermediates. Unfortunately, many previous texts have indirectly promoted this adage by stating it without specific reference to a metabolically active tissue. As you will see, the adage is true for the liver. Within skeletal muscle, lipid metabolism and carbohydrate metabolism share a common means of entry into the TCA cycle, acetyl-CoA. As discussed in the section on glycogen synthesis, skeletal muscle does not have sufficient quantities of the enzymes to convert glycolytic intermediates (mainly pyruvate and phosphoenolpyruvate) into molecules that can be transported into the mitochondria to supplement TCA cycle intermediates. In fact, as indicated in the section on amino acid oxidation, a more accurate adage would be that *muscle lipid burns in an amino acid flame.*

Amino Acid Oxidation

Proteins can be catabolized to amino acids and then have the nitrogenous amino group removed *(deamination)* with the carbon skeleton incorporated into the central pathways of carbohydrate and lipid metabolism (Table 4.7). The exact location where the amino acid enters these pathways depends on the number of carbons in the molecule. The amine group from the process of deamination can be used to reform an amino acid (transamination) for storage in the free amino acid pool, be used in protein synthesis, or be released from the skeletal muscle fiber for uptake by the liver, conversion to urea, and subsequent excretion in the urine.

Figure 4.17 presents the locations at which the carbon skeletons of each amino acid can enter into catabolism. The production of acetoacetyl-CoA, a substrate of ketone body formation, can occur only in the liver and therefore does not apply to skeletal muscle metabolism. During prolonged exer-

ß-oxidation pathway can then continue, removing two carbon units with each cycle until the FFA molecule is completely catabolized. For unsaturated FFA molecules, ß-oxidation proceeds until the carbon double bond prevents further removal of two carbon units. Additional enzyme-catalyzed

TABLE 4.7		
Intermediates from energy metabolism that can be produced from amino acid oxidation in skeletal muscle and the liver		
	AMINO ACID SOURCE*	
INTERMEDIATE	**SKELETAL MUSCLE**	**LIVER**
Pyruvate	Alanine	Glycine
		Serine Cysteine
		Tryptophan
Alpha-ketoglutarate	Glutamine	Proline
	Glutamate	Histidine
		Arginine
Succinyl-CoA	Valine	Methionine
	Isoleucine	Threonine
Fumarate		Phenylalanine
		Tyrosine
Oxaloacetate		Asparagine
		Aspartate
Acetyl-CoA	Leucine	Tryrosine
	Isoleucine	Lysine
		Tryptophan

*Amino acids listed for skeletal muscle can also be catabolized in the liver.
Modified from Newsholme EA, Leech ER: *Biochemistry for the medical sciences*, Chichester, Eng, 1983, John Wiley & Sons.

cise, when muscle glycogen and blood glucose concentrations are low, the incorporation of the carbon skeletons from amino acids into the TCA cycle is important for maintaining the concentrations of the intermediates and therefore a high rate of mitochondrial respiration. The main amino acids oxidized in skeletal muscle are the branched chain amino acids isoleucine, leucine, and valine, as well as glutamine and glutamate.[34]

The deamination of amino acids is potentially harmful to cellular function. A by-product of deamination is ammonia (NH_{3+}), which is released into the circulation and becomes toxic in high concentrations. During prolonged and intermittent intense exercise, when ammonia may be produced from the purine nucleotide cycle and amino acid deamination, ammonia accumulates to small concentrations in plasma and can often be smelled in sweat. Ammonia release from skeletal muscle is reduced by the transfer of the amine group from amino acids (mainly glutamate) to pyruvate to form *alanine*. Alanine is then released into the circulation where it can be taken up by the liver and metabolized (Figures 4.18 and 4.19).

Tally of ATP Production From Catabolism

We are now ready to summarize the ATP produced from creatine phosphate, carbohydrate, lipid, and amino acid catabolism. Table 4.8 presents the sources of ATP during catabolism in skeletal muscle. Creatine phosphate provides 1 ATP per reaction, glycolysis provides 3 ATP from glycogen and 2

from glucose, one cycle of ß-oxidation provides 5 ATP, one cycle of the citric acid cycle provides 12 ATP, and the potential ATP yield from amino acid catabolism depends on the number of carbons in the molecule and therefore the location of entry into the central catabolic pathways. The net ATP yield from the catabolism of glucose is therefore 2 or 3 if pyruvate is converted to lactate and 36 when pyruvate is entered into mitochondrial respiration and the 2 cytosolic NADH enter the mitochondria via the glycerol-3-phosphate shuttle. The complete catabolism of palmitate provides 129 ATP, which accounts for the 2 ATP cost of FFA activation in the cytosol. Catabolism of valine and leucine to glutamine produces 16 molecules of ATP.[34] However, as discussed in Chapter 10, the rate of amino acid oxidation during exercise is low and increases to a maximum of only 15% of the ATP demand during prolonged (>1 hour) exercise.

Despite the comparatively larger ATP yield from palmitate than from glucose, a comparison that equates acetyl-CoA production proves interesting. Without including the ATP cost of FFA activation, the ATP yield from 2 acetyl-CoA molecules from palmitate amounts to 10, resulting from 2 NADH and 2 FADH from two cycles of ß-oxidation. The

carnitine shuttle

the enzyme-catalyzed transfer of activated long-chain free fatty acid molecules from the cytosol into the mitochondria

FIGURE 4.17

The entry points of amino acids into the main catabolic pathways of energy metabolism. The liver and skeletal muscle differ in the predominant amino acids catabolized, as indicated by color in the illustration and in Table 4.7.

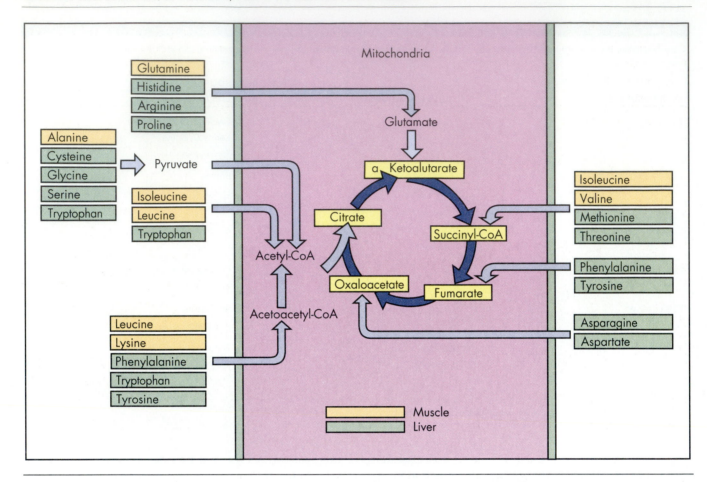

ATP yield from the production of 2 acetyl–CoA molecules from glucose equals 12 if the glycerol phosphate shuttle is operative, but equals 14 if the malate-aspartate shuttle is operative. As previously indicated, the metabolism of carbohydrate and lipid is identical after acetyl-CoA formation. Based on this ATP tally, carbohydrate metabolism produces more ATP for a given number of acetyl-CoA molecules. This would require less oxygen consumption for a given ATP production and provide the biochemical explanation for *carbohydrate having a greater caloric equivalent for 1 liter of oxygen consumed compared with lipid.* The practical implications for the difference between carbohydrate and lipid in the oxygen requirement and carbon dioxide production for a given caloric expenditure are explained in Chapter 6.

Catabolism in the Liver

Like skeletal muscle, the liver can catabolize carbohydrate, FFA, and amino acids. However, during exercise the liver functions differently from skeletal muscle. As indicated in Table 4.1, the liver is responsible primarily for blood glucose regulation, the regulation of blood lipoprotein concentrations, and the catabolism of many molecules produced in other (extrahepatic) tissues. Consequently, the liver does not experience the large increase in ATP demand that characterizes skeletal muscle during contractions. These differences result in certain enzymes being regulated differently in the liver compared with skeletal muscle, as well as the presence of additional enzymes that result in the more complex regulation of the catabolic pathways of metabolism.

Carbohydrate

Glycogenolysis

Liver glycogenolysis involves the activation of phosphorylase and therefore is similar to skeletal muscle. However, in the liver the hormone *glucagon* also induces an increase in intracellular cAMP, similar to epinephrine, which contributes to the stimulation of glycogenolysis during low blood glucose conditions. This difference is understandable given the role of the liver and glucagon in blood glucose regulation.

Glycolysis

The pathway of glycolysis in the liver is regulated differently from glycolysis in skeletal muscle. The additional enzymes operative in liver glycolysis are presented in Figure 4.20. In the liver the enzyme glucokinase (EC: 2.7.1.2) replaces hexokinase, and the additional enzyme glucose-6-phophatase (EC: 3.1.3.9) is present. Glucose-6-phosphatase is

FIGURE 4.18

The transamination and deamination of amino acids to form the TCA cycle intermediate α-ketoglutarate. These reactions produce ammonia that is circulated from the skeletal muscle to the liver, where it is incorporated into the urea cycle to form urea. (Adapted from Lehninger AL et al: *Principles of biochemistry,* New York, 1993, Worth Publishers.)

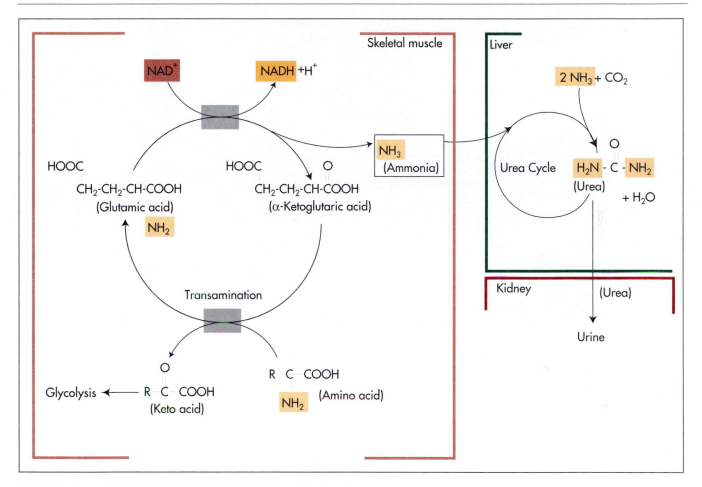

discussed in the section on gluconeogenesis. Glucokinase catalyzes an identical reaction to hexokinase, but compared with hexokinase the $S_{0.5}$ for glucose is much higher (0.1 versus 10 mmol/L). Consequently, the liver can take up and metabolize glucose to G6P only when blood glucose concentrations are high (e.g., after a meal). This initial enzymatic difference between muscle and liver enables blood glucose to be conserved for extrahepatic tissues (mainly neural, blood, adipose, and skeletal muscle tissue).

The liver contains the enzyme fructokinase (EC: 2.7.1.4), which catalyzes the addition of a phosphate to fructose, forming F6P. Because muscle contains limited amounts of this enzyme, the liver is the predominant tissue that incorporates fructose into glycolytic metabolism.

A second isozyme of phosphofructokinase (PFK_2) (EC: 2.7.1.105) is also present in the liver. PFK_2 is activated by glucose, fructose-6-phosphate (F6P), and AMP, producing the molecule fructose-2,6-bisphosphate (F2,6P). Interestingly, PFK_2 is a by-functional enzyme, since it also has reverse

(fructose-2,6-bisphosphatase) activity.[45] The phosphatase activity is inhibited by F6P and stimulated by glucagon. As indicated in Chapter 3, small concentrations of PFK_2 also exist in skeletal muscle, and F2,6P increases PFK_1 activity. Nevertheless, this stimulation is far greater in the liver.[20,21] Citrate inhibits both PFK isozymes in the liver. *Why does PFK$_2$ exist in larger concentrations in the liver?* Compared with skeletal muscle, the liver is less reliant on concentrations of creatine kinase and adenylate kinase and therefore has a lower capacity to increase concentrations of AMP, the main activator of PFK_1. F2,6P provides an alternative means of regulation for liver glycolysis.

The glucose regulation of PFK_2 is important because increased glucose availability (e.g., after a meal) requires increased liver glucose uptake and glycolysis to aid in blood glucose regulation. During low blood glucose conditions, the release of glucagon from the pancreas stimulates increased F2,6Pase activity, which decreases F2,6P and therefore decreases the stimulation of glycolysis and conserves glucose.

FIGURE 4.19

The metabolic connections between the liver, adipose tissue, and skeletal muscle. The directionality and magnitude of flow of molecules among these tissues varies depending on nutrient status and exercise intensity. The connections illustrated represent those that can exist during steady state exercise conditions.

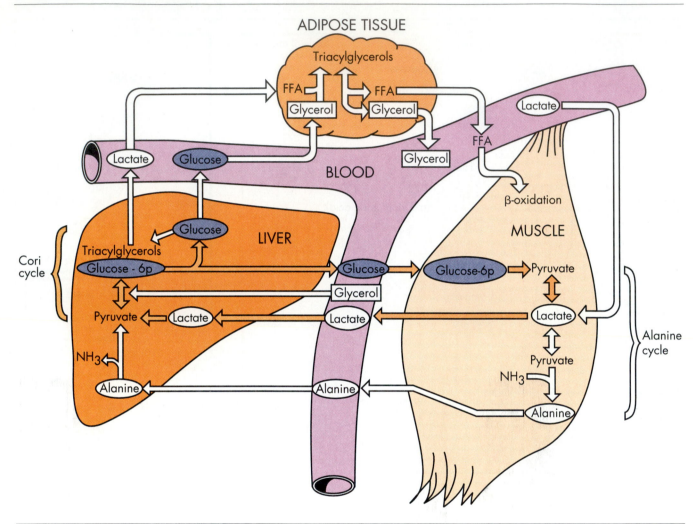

Decreased F2,6P also decreases inhibition of F1,6Pase, allowing the conversion of F1,6P to F6P.

The regulation of F1,6Pase is also important for liver glycolysis. A considerable drain on ATP would occur if both PFK$_1$ and F1,6Pase were active. F1,6Pase is inhibited by F2,6P, so that during conditions that stimulate PFK$_1$ and liver glycolysis, the reversal of the PFK$_1$ reaction is prevented. The remaining reactions of glycolysis are identical to those of skeletal muscle.

Mitochondrial Respiration

Subtle differences exist between skeletal muscle and liver metabolism in the TCA cycle (see Figure 4.20). Essentially, the presence of the enzymes phosphoenol-pyruvate carboxykinase and pyruvate carboxylase enables the conversion of phosphoenol-pyruvate and pyruvate to TCA cycle inter-

mediates in the cytosol, which can be converted to malate via malate dehydrogenase (EC: 1.1.1.37–39) and enter into the mitochondria. Hence, carbohydrate catabolism in the liver can support the TCA cycle intermediates by resupplying malate, and hence oxaloacetate. A continual supply of oxaloacetate is crucial for incorporating acetyl-CoA molecules into the TCA cycle, especially during conditions of low glucose and high lipid catabolism. The presence of these enzymes *in the liver* is the evidence for the adage, "Lipid burns in a carbohydrate flame!" Further comment is given in the sections on liver gluconeogenesis.

Lipolysis

The reactions of lipid metabolism that produce acetyl-CoA are similar in liver and skeletal muscle. The main difference in metabolic regulation occurs after acetyl-CoA forma-

TABLE 4.8

Tally of ATP production from the catabolism of creatine phophate, carbohydrate, and lipid in skeletal muscle

REACTIONS	YIELD OF HIGH-ENERGY INTERMEDIATES		
	NADH	FADH	ATP
CREATINE PHOSPHATE	**0**	**0**	**1**
ATP Tally			1
CARBOHYDRATE (GLUCOSE)*			
Glycolysis			
Phosphorylation of glucose			-1
Phosphorylation of fructose-6-phosphate			-1
Dephosphorylation of 1,3-bisphosphoglycerate	(×2)		2
Oxidation of glyceraldehyde-3-phosphate[†]	(×2)	2	4
Dephosphorylation of phosphoenolpyruvate	(×2)		2
Mitochondrial (TCA cycle and ETC)			
Pyruvate oxidation to acetyl-CoA	(×2)	2	6
Coupled phosphorylation of GTP from the oxidation of succinyl-CoA	(×2)		2
Oxidation of isocitrate, alpha-ketoglutarate, and malate	(×2)	6	18
Oxidation of succinate	(×2)	2	4
ATP Tally			36
FREE FATTY ACID (PALMITATE, 16 CARBONS)			
Cytosolic reactions			
Activation of the FFA			-2
Mitochondrial (ß-oxidation)			
Oxidation of acyl-CoA	(×7)	7	14
Oxidation of 3-hydroxyacyl-CoA	(×7)	7	21
Mitochondrial (TCA cycle and ETC)			
Acetyl-CoA	(×8)	24	72
		8	16
			8
ATP Tally			129

*The ATP cost of the first phase of glycolysis is 1 ATP if glucose-6-phosphate is produced from glycogen, which would result in either 37 or 39 ATP, depending on the NADH shuttle used.
[†]Assumes the glycero-phosphate shuttle is used.

tion. The liver has enzymes that can convert acetyl–CoA to any one of three molecules referred to as **ketone bodies** (Figure 4.19).

When blood glucose is low and therefore liver glycogen is low, minimal G6P is produced and metabolized in glycol-

ketone bodies

the product of the liver during conditions of low carbohydrate and high lipid catabolism

FIGURE 4.20

The enzymes of the liver in catabolism that differ from skeletal muscle. These differences alter the functions of glucose uptake/release, glycolysis, and acetyl-CoA production.

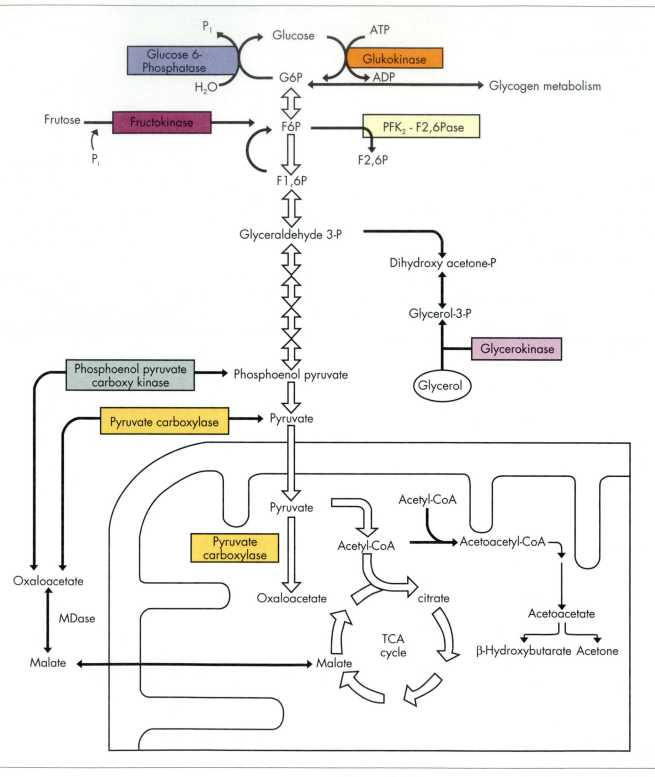

ysis. Consequently, FFA catabolism predominates via the pathway of ß-oxidation. Since several of the intermediates of the TCA cycle can be removed from the mitochondria or converted to other metabolites, mitochondrial oxaloacetate concentrations can decrease, limiting the rate at which acetyl-CoA can enter into the TCA cycle. Some of the acetyl-CoA formed from ß-oxidation must therefore be converted to other end products, namely the ketone bodies *acetoacetate, ß-hydroxybutarate,* and *acetone.* The main ketone body is acetoacetate, which is produced from two acetyl-CoA molecules via three enzyme-catalyzed reactions. Acetoacetate is converted to ß-hydroxybutarate by the enzyme ß-hydroxybutarate dehydrogenase (EC: 1.1.1.30) and can form acetone without the need for enzyme catalysis.

The ketone bodies leave the liver and are used as fuel in extrahepatic tissues. However, there is a one ATP cost for the reformation of two acetyl-CoA molecules from acetoacetate, and increases in circulating ketone bodies (ketosis) decrease blood pH, which can further impair exercise tolerance and performance by reducing the buffering capacity of the blood.

Amino Acid Oxidation

The entry of amino acids into the catabolic pathways of energy metabolism in skeletal muscle is detailed in Figure 4.17. These reactions are similar for the liver, except that small-carbon-length amino acids (e.g., glycine, alanine), which can be converted to pyruvate or phosphoenol pyruvate, can be converted to ketone bodies via acetyl-CoA.

Catabolism in Adipose Tissue

The catabolic pathways in adipose tissue are predominantly restricted to glycolysis, the purine nucleotide cycle, mitochondrial respiration, and lipolysis. Insulin is the main regulator of adipose tissue catabolism. Increased insulin inhibits adenylate cyclase activity and therefore decreases production of cAMP. To facilitate this effect, insulin increases *phosphodiesterase* (EC: 3.1.4.1) activity and cAMP degradation. The net result of these responses is to inhibit lipolysis, thus favoring glycolysis, the pentose phosphate pathway, and triacylglycerol synthesis.

The process of lipolysis is as previously described for skeletal muscle. FFA molecules are released into the circulation and, if not reesterified back to triacylglycerol, are transported in the blood bound to albumin, where they are then taken up by other tissues as a substrate for energy metabolism. As a result of the absence of the enzyme glycerokinase (EC: 2.7.1.30), adipose tissue cannot reincorporate glycerol into glycolysis and the glycerol released during lipolysis must be released into the circulation for uptake by the liver or kidney as a substrate for glycolysis.

Metabolic Connections Between Skeletal Muscle, the Liver, and Adipose Tissue

Figure 4.19 illustrates the metabolic connections among skeletal muscle, the liver, and adipose tissue during exercise conditions. Exercise increases glucose catabolism in skeletal muscle and the production of lactate. The cycle of lactate release from skeletal muscle, uptake by the liver and conversion to glucose by gluconeogenesis, and release back into the blood for eventual uptake by muscle is termed the **Cori cycle.** The similar cycle for alanine release from skeletal muscle is called the **alanine cycle.** Both the Cori and alanine cycles are more operative during exercise and times of inadequate caloric intake, when blood glucose levels need to be maintained and substrate must be continually supplied for catabolism.

Exercise-induced increases in the hormone epinephrine can stimulate triacylglycerol catabolism (lipolysis) in adipocytes, releasing free fatty acids and glycerol into the circulation. The FFA molecules can be used by skeletal muscle as a substrate for energy metabolism, whereas the glycerol is taken up by the liver and kidney for incorporation into glycolysis. Because skeletal muscle has its own supply of lipid, it is unclear how important the mobilization of adipose tissue FFA is to muscle lipid metabolism during exercise.[17,46]

Cori cycle

the release of lactate from muscle into the circulation for uptake by the liver and conversion to glucose

Alanine cycle

the release of alanine from muscle into the circulation for uptake by the liver and conversion to glucose

SUMMARY

- The design and function of metabolism in skeletal muscle are to produce ATP in rates that meet the ATP demand as well as possible. The main catabolic pathways of skeletal muscle are glycogenolysis, glycolysis, lipolysis, ß-oxidation, and cellular respiration.

- The molecules used for catabolism, referred to as *energy substrates,* consist of **glucose, fructose, glycogen, triacylglycerols, fatty acids, glycerol,** and **amino acids**.

- Skeletal muscle can produce the ATP from creatine phosphate (CrP) hydrolysis, glycolysis, and the use of oxygen in the mitochondria. The production of ATP from CrP and glycolysis does not require the presence of oxygen and has been referred to as **anaerobic metabolism**. Conversely, the ATP production from cellular respiration in mitochondria, which uses oxygen, has been termed **aerobic metabolism**. Terms that are gaining increased acceptance for qualifying the source of ATP production are the **phosphagen system, glycolytic metabolism,** and **mitochondrial respiration,** respectively.

- The CrP reaction is the most rapid means to regenerate ATP. However, the ATP production capacity of the creatine kinase reaction relies on a store of CrP, which approximates 24 mmol/kg wet wt. An additional one enzyme-catalyzed reaction exists to regenerate ATP, and the enzyme involved is called *adenylate kinase*. The adenylate kinase reaction produces the allosteric activator (AMP) of phosphorylase and phosphofructokinase, thus stimulating increased glycogenolysis and glycolysis. AMP can be converted to inosine monophosphate (IMP) during acidic conditions by the *AMP deaminase* catalyzed reaction of the **purine nucleotide cycle**.

- Evidence exists to indicate that CrP and ADP are also involved in the shuttling of inorganic phosphate throughout the cytosol during all conditions of cellular metabolism. The source of the inorganic phosphate is the terminal phosphate of ATP formed from glycolysis and mitochondrial respiration. The term used to describe this function of CrP is the **creatine phosphate shuttle**.

- The catabolism of glycogen is termed **glycogenolysis**. In vivo the phosphorylase reaction is highly exergonic and has a low $S_{0.5}$ for glycogen. The covalent modification of phosphorylase-b to the more active phosphorylase occurs via phosphorylation of the enzyme in response to increases in the intracellular second messenger cyclic AMP *(cAMP)* and calcium.

- Within skeletal muscle, **glycolysis** begins with the entry of glucose into the skeletal muscle fiber. Glucose entry is facilitated by blood glucose binding to specialized glucose transport proteins **(GLUT proteins)** located on and below the sarcolemma. The exercise stimulation of glucose transporters is additive and independent of the insulin response.

- An important regulated enzyme of glycolysis is phosphofructokinase (PFK). During exercise, repeated intense muscle contractions increase the concentration of AMP, which binds to regulator sites on PFK_1 and increases PFK_1 activity for a given concentration of substrate (fructose-6-phosphate). During the first reaction of the second phase of glycolysis, electrons and one hydrogen ion are added to nicotinamide adenine dinucleotide (NAD^+) to form NADH, with the second hydrogen ion remaining free in solution. The ratio of NAD^+ to NADH is called the **redox potential**.

- Glycolysis results in the oxidation of glucose-6-phosphate to two pyruvate molecules and the net production of two or three ATP, depending on whether glucose or glycogen was the initial substrate. Pyruvate can be converted to lactic acid by the enzyme lactate dehydrogenase (LDH). The lactic acid molecule immediately releases a proton when produced at physiologic pH and is termed **lactate.**

- Lactate production is not necessarily detrimental to muscle metabolism during exercise. The production of lactate involves the regeneration of NAD^+ and therefore helps to maintain the cytosolic redox potential and support continued glycolysis and a high rate of ATP regeneration. When the rate of pyruvate production exceeds the rate of pyruvate entry into the mitochondria, pyruvate is converted to lactate. This condition has been termed **mass action effect**.

■ During steady state exercise conditions, the majority of pyruvate is not converted to lactate but enters into the mitochondria where it is converted to **acetyl-CoA** by a series of linked enzymes known collectively as pyruvate dehydrogenase. This reaction also produces carbon dioxide and NADH. The acetyl-CoA formed from either carbohydrate or lipid catabolism can then enter into a catabolic pathway called the **tricarboxylic acid cycle** (TCA cycle), which consists of nine reactions.

■ NADH and FADH are the major products of the TCA cycle. The biochemical use of oxygen occurs in the **electron transport chain** (ETC). In the ETC, the protons and electrons acquired in NADH and FADH are used to add electrons to hydrogen atoms and oxygen to form water and generate the free energy to add a phosphate to ADP to form ATP. The formation of water and ATP during the ETC is termed **oxidative phosphorylation**. There is a unidirectional flow of electrons in the electron transport chain because each successive component of the chain has a higher affinity for electrons **(reduction potential)**.

■ **Lipolysis** refers to the breakdown of triacylglycerols to FFA molecules and glycerol. Catabolism of FFA involves their transport into the mitochondria, where they are degraded into acetyl-CoA molecules during **ß-oxidation**. The transport of the FFA into the mitochondria occurs via a **carnitine shuttle**. As exercise intensity and stimulation for glycogenolysis and glycolysis increase, the relative contribution of FFA catabolism decreases, with complete dependence on carbohydrate catabolism occurring at intensities above 60% to 85% VO_2max (higher for endurance-trained individuals).

■ In skeletal muscle lipid does not burn in a carbohydrate flame. Proteins can be catabolized to amino acids and then have the nitrogenous amino group removed (deamination) with the carbon skeleton incorporated into the central pathways of carbohydrate and lipid metabolism. Because of involvement of amino acids in supplementing the concentration of TCA cycle intermediates, a more accurate adage would be that muscle lipid burns in an amino acid flame.

■ A second isozyme of phosphofructokinase (PFK_2) (EC: 2.7.1.105) is present in the liver. PFK_2 is activated by glucose, fructose-6-phosphate (F6P), and AMP, producing the molecule fructose-2,6-bisphosphate (F2,6P), which then increases PFK_1 activity. Consequently, unless there is adequate substrate, there is minimal stimulation of liver glycolysis. Carbohydrate catabolism in the liver can support the TCA cycle intermediates by resupplying malate, and hence oxaloacetate. The presence of the enzymes that can support these reactions *in the liver* is the evidence for the adage, "Lipid burns in a carbohydrate flame."

■ The liver has enzymes that can convert acetyl-CoA to any one of three molecules referred to as **ketone bodies**. These reactions occur during conditions of minimal carbohydrate (low blood glucose) and increased reliance on lipid catabolism. The ketone bodies leave the liver and are used as fuel in extrahepatic tissues.

■ The cycle of lactate release from skeletal muscle, uptake by the liver and conversion to glucose by gluconeogenesis, and release back into the blood for eventual uptake by muscle is termed the **Cori cycle**. The similar cycle for alanine release from skeletal muscle is called the **alanine cycle**. Both the Cori and alanine cycles are more operative during exercise and times of inadequate caloric intake, when blood glucose needs to be maintained and substrate must be continually supplied for catabolism.

REVIEW QUESTIONS

1. What are the different metabolic functions of skeletal muscle, the liver, and adipose tissue during exercise?

2. How might the different rates of ATP regeneration from the catabolic reactions and pathways in skeletal muscle influence energy production during differing intensities of exercise?

3. What is the net ATP production from the different catabolic pathways of skeletal muscle?

4. What are the key allosteric enzymes of glycogenolysis and glycolysis, and how are they regulated during exercise?

5. Explain the following terms: creatine phosphate shuttle, mass action, lipolysis, carnitine shuttle, redox potential, reduction potential, oxidative phosphorylation, ketone bodies.

6. Why are the concentrations of NAD^+ and $NADH$ important to energy metabolism in the cytosol and mitochondria?

7. Why is lactate produced in skeletal muscle during exercise, and why it is wrong to view lactate as a detrimental molecule to muscle function?

8. Why is there an increasing reliance on carbohydrate catabolism during increases in exercise intensity?

9. What are the functions of the Cori and alanine cycles during exercise?

APPLICATIONS

1. There are clinical disorders of metabolism in which certain enzymes of carbohydrate catabolism are absent. Two notable examples are deficiencies in either phosphorylase (McArdle's disease) or phospho-fructokinase. How might these clinical conditions influence muscle catabolism during exercise and the person's ability to exercise?

2. The group of drugs that block the ß-receptors for epinephrine and norepinephrine (classified as ß-blockers) can alter muscle and adipocyte metabolism. How might energy metabolism be altered in a person taking ß-blocker medication in each of these tissues, and what effect would these changes have on the person's ability to exercise?

3. Type II diabetics have a decreased ability to remove glucose from the circulation in response to a given amount of circulating insulin. Why might exercise increase glucose uptake during exercise, as well as retain the body's ability for increased glucose uptake after exercise?

4. Certain poisons, such as cyanide, hinder oxidative phosphorylation. How would this interfere with muscle energy metabolism, and why can the inhalation of cyanide gas eventually cause death?

5. Agents that uncouple oxidative phosphorylation result in an increase in heat production and oxygen consumption for a given ATP regeneration. At one time, these agents were prescribed as a means to lose weight in the morbidly obese. Why would this have been done, and what dangers existed in this medical practice?

6. During a marathon, there may be times when runners must quickly increase their pace to a speed that they cannot sustain for more than two or three minutes. What pathways are supporting mitochondrial respiration in regenerating ATP under these conditions, and what metabolic reasons exist for the inability to sustain this increase in speed?

REFERENCES

1. Balaban RS: Regulation of oxidative phosphorylation in the mammalian cell, *Am J Physiol* 258(27):C377-C389, 1990.

2. Bertorini TE, Shively V, Taylor B: ATP degradation products after ischemic exercise: hereditary lack of phosphorylase or carnitine palmityltransferase, *Neurology* 35:1355-1357, 1985.

3. Carraro F, Klein S, Rosenblatt JI: Wolfe RR: Effect of dichloroacetate on lactate concentration in exercising humans, *J Appl Physiol* 66(2):591-597,1989

4. Chasiotis D: Role of cyclic AMP and inorganic phosphate in the regulation of muscle glycogenolysis during exercise, *Med Sci Sports Exerc* 20(6):545-550, 1988.

5. Chwalbinska-Moneta J, Robergs, RA, Costill DL, Fink WJ: Threshold for muscle lactate accumulation, *J Appl Physiol* 66(6):2710-2716, 1989.

6. Crabtree B, Higgins SJ, Newsholme EA: The activities of pyruvate carboxylase, phosphoenolpyruvate carboxykinase and fructose diphosphatase in muscles from vertebrates and invertebrates, *Biochem J* 130:391-396, 1972.

7. Douen AG, Ramlal T, Rastogi S et al: Exercise induces recruitment of the "insulin responsive glucose transporter," *J Biol Chem* 265(23):13427-13430, 1990.

8. Dudley GA, Terjung RJ: Influence of acidosis on AMP deaminase activity in contracting fast-twitch muscle, *Am J Physiol* 248(17):C43-C50, 1985.

9. Dudley GA, Tullson PC, Terjung RL: Influence of mitochondrial content on the sensitivity of respiratory control, *J Biol Chem* 262(19):1909-1914, 1987.

10. Fleckenstein JL, Haller RG, Lewis SF et al: Absence of exercise-induced MRI enhancement of skeletal muscle in McArdle's disease, *J Appl Physiol* 71(3):961-969, 1991.

11. Friden J, Seger J, Ekblom B: Topographical localization of muscle glycogen: an ultrahistochemical study in the human vastus lateralis, *Acta Physiol Scand* 135:381-391, 1989.

12. Fushiki T, Wells JA, Tapscott EB, Dohm GL: Changes in glucose transporters in muscle in response to exercise, *Am J Physiol* 256(19):E580-E587, 1989.

13. Gollnick PD: Metabolic regulation in skeletal muscle: influence of endurance training as exerted by mitochondrial protein concentration, *Acta Physiol Scand* 128(S556):53-66, 1986.

14. Henrikson EJ, Bourey RE, Rodnick KJ et al: Glucose transporter protein content and glucose transport capacity in rat skeletal muscle, *Am J Physiol* 259(22):E593-E598, 1990.

15. Hinkle PC, McCarry RE: How cells make ATP, *Sci Am* 238(5):104-123, 1978.

16. Houmard JA, Egan PC, Neufer PD et al: Elevated skeletal muscle glucose transporter levels in exercise-trained middle-aged men, *Am J Physiol* 261(24):E437-E443, 1991.

17. Hurley BF, Nemeth PM, Martin III WH et al: Muscle triglyceride utilization during exercise: effect of training, *J Appl Physiol* 60(2):562-567, 1986.

18. Kaplan NO, Everse J: Regulatory characteristics of lactate dehydrogenases, *Adv Enz Regul* 10:323-336, 1972.

19. Katz A, Sahlin K: Regulation of lactic acid production during exercise, *J Appl Physiol* 65(2):509-518, 1988.

20. Katz A, Spencer ME, Lillioja S et al: Basal and insulin-mediated carbohydrate metabolism in human muscle deficient in phosphofructokinase 1, *Am J Physiol* 261(24):E473-E478, 1991.

21. Kawachi M, Ono A, Nishimura T et al: Low glucose-1,6-bisphosphate and high fructose-2,6-bisphosphate concentrations in muscles of patients with glycogenolysis types VII and V, *Biochem Biophys Res Comm* 176(1):7-10, 1991.

22. Ladu MJ, Kapsas H, Palmer WK: Regulation of lipoprotein lipase in adipose and muscle tissue during fasting, *Am J Physiol* 260(29):R953-R959, 1991.

23. Lehninger AL: *Principles of biochemistry,* New York, 1993, Worth.

24. Lewis SF, Haller RG, Cook JD: Muscle fatigue in McArdle's disease studied by 31P-NMR: effect of glucose infusion, *J Appl Physiol* 59:1191-1194, 1985.

25. SF, Lewis Haller RG, The pathophysiology of McArdle's disease: clues to regulation in exercise and fatigue, *J Appl Physiol* 61:391-401, 1986.

26. Lewis SF, Haller RG: Disorders of muscle glycogenolysis/glycolysis: the consequences of substrate limited-oxidative metabolism in humans. In Taylor A, Gollnick PD, Green HJ et al, editors: *Biochemistry of exercise VII,* Champaign, Illinois, 1990, Human Kinetics.

27. McArdle B: Myopathy due to a defect in muscle glycogen breakdown, *Clin Sci Lond* 10:13-32, 1951.

28. Mayes PA: Biologic oxidation. In Murray RK, Granner DK, Mayes PA, Rodwell VW, editors: *Harper's biochemistry,* ed 22, Norwalk, Connecticut, 1990, Appleton & Lange.

29. Mayes PA: Oxidative phosphorylation and mitochondrial transport system. In Murray RK, Granner DK, Mayes PA, Rodwell VW, editors, *Harper's biochemistry,* ed 22, Norwalk, Connecticut, 1990, Appleton & Lange.

30. Mayes PA: Metabolism of glycogen. In Murray RK, Granner DK, Mayes PA, Rodwell VW: *Harper's biochemistry,* ed 22, Norwalk, Connecticut, 1990, Appleton & Lange.

31. Mineo I, Kono N, Yamada Y et al: Glucose infusion abolishes the excessive ATP degradation in working muscles of a patient with McArdle's disease, *Muscle Nerve* 13(7):618-620, 1990.

REFERENCES—Cont'd

32. Munger R, Temler E, Jallut D et al: Correlations of glycogen synthase and phosphorylase activites with glycogen concentration in human muscle biopsies: evidence for a double-feedback mechanism regulating glycogen synthesis and breakdown, *Metabolism* 42(1):36-43,1993.

33. Newsholme EA, Crabtree, J: Flux generating and regulatory steps in metabolic control, *Trends Biochem Sci* 6:53-55, 1981.

34. Newsholme EA, Leech ER: *Biochemistry for the medical sciences,* Chichester, England, 1983, John Wiley & Sons.

35. Opie LH, Newsholme EA: The activities of fructose 1,6-diphosphatase, phosphofructokinase and phosphoenolpyruvate carboxykinase in white muscle and red muscle, *Biochem J* 103:391-399, 1967.

36. Oscai LB: Type L hormone-sensitive lipase hydrolyzes endogenous triacylglycerols in muscle in exercised rats, *Med Sci Sports Exerc* 15(4):336-339, 1983.

37. Oscai LB, Palmer WK: Cellular control of triacylglycerol metabolism, *Exerc Sport Sciences Rev* 11:1-23, 1983.

38. Rodwell VW: Catabolism of the carbon skeletons of amino acids. In Murray RK, Granner DK, Mayes PA, Rodwell VW: *Harper's biochemistry,* ed 22, Norwalk, Connecticut, 1990, Appleton & Lange.

39. Ren JM, Hultman E: Regulation of glycogenolysis in human skeletal muscle, *J Appl Physiol* 67(6):2243-2248, 1989.

40. Sahlin K: Metabolic changes limiting muscle performance. In Saltin B, editor: *Biochemistry of exercise VI,* vol 16, *International Series on Sport Sciences,* Champaign, Illinois, 1986, Human Kinetics.

41. Sale EM, Denton RM: Adipose-tissue phosphofructokinase, *Biochem J* 232:897-904, 1985.

42. Schantz PG: Influence of physical training on enzyme levels of the NADH shuttles. In Schantz PG, editor: Plasticity of human skeletal muscle, *Acta Physiol Scand Suppl* 558, 1986.

43. Schmid R, Mahler R: Chronic progressive myopathy with myoglobinuria: demonstration of a glycogenolytic defect in muscle, *J Clin Invest* 38:2044-2058, 1959.

44. Stanley WC, Gertz EW, Wisneski JA et al: Systematic lactate kinetics during graded exercise in man, *Am J Appl Physiol* 249(12):E595-E602, 1985.

45. Stryer L: *Biochemistry,* ed 3, New York, 1988, WH Freeman.

46. Tarnopolsky LJ, MacDougall JD, Atkinson SA et al: Gender differences in substrate for endurance exercise, *J Appl Physiol* 68(1):302-308, 1990.

47. Terjung RL, Dudley GA, Meyer RA et al: Purine nucleotide cycle function in contracting skeletal muscle. In Saltin B, *Biochemistry of exercise VI,* vol 16, *International Series on Sport Sciences,* Champaign, Illinois, 1986, Human Kinetics.

48. Tonomi H, Fujieda K, Kajii N et al: Negative dystrophin staining in muscles of patients with complex glycerol kinase deficiency, *J Pediatr* 117:268-271, 1990.

49. Vissing J, Lewis SF, Galbo H, Haller RG: Effect of deficient muscular glycogenolysis on extramuscular fuel production in exercise, *J Appl Physiol* 72(5):1773-1779, 1992.

50. Wahren J, Felig P, Havel RJ et al: Amino acid metabolism in McArdle's syndrome, *N Eng J Med* 288:774-777,1973.

51. Winder WW, Arogyasami J, Barton RJ et al: Muscle malonyl-CoA decreases during exercise, *J Appl Physiol* 67(6):2230-2233, 1989.

RECOMMENDED READINGS

- Balaban RS: Regulation of oxidative phosphorylation in the mammalian cell, *Am J Physiol* 258(27):C377-C389, 1990.

- Chasiotis D: Role of cyclic AMP and inorganic phosphate in the regulation of muscle glycogenolysis during exercise, *Med Sci Sports Exerc* 20(6):545-550, 1988.

- Chwalbinska-Moneta J, Robergs RA, Costill DL, Fink WJ: Threshold for muscle lactate accumulation, *J Appl Physiol* 66(6):2710-2716, 1989.

- Dudley GA, Tullson PC, Terjung RL: Influence of mitochondrial content on the sensitivity of respiratory control, *J Biol Chem* 262(19):1909-9114, 1987.

- Friden J, Seger J, Ekblom B: Topographical localization of muscle glycogen: an ultrahistochemical study in the human vastus lateralis, *Acta Physiol Scand* 135:381-391, 1989.

- Hinkle PC, McCarry RE: How cells make ATP, *Sci Am* 238(5):104-123, 1978.

- Katz A, Sahlin K: Regulation of lactic acid production during exercise, *J Appl Physiol* 65(2):509-518, 1988.

- Lewis SF, Haller RG, Cook JD: Muscle fatigue in McArdle's disease studied by 31P-NMR: effect of glucose infusion, *J Appl Physiol* 59:1191-1194, 1985.

- Lewis SF, Haller RG: The pathophysiology of McArdle's disease: clues to regulation in exercise and fatigue, *J Appl Physiol* 61:391-401, 1986.

- Newsholme EA, Crabtree, J: Flux generating and regulatory steps in metabolic control, *Trends Biochem Sci* 6:53-55, 1981.

- Oscai LB: Type L hormone-sensitive lipase hydrolyzes endogenous triacylglycerols in muscle in exercised rats, *Med Sci Sports Exerc* 15(4):336-339,1983.

- Oscai LB, Palmer WK: Cellular control of triacylglycerol metabolism, *Exerc Sport Sci Rev* 11:1-23, 1983.

- Ren JM, Hultman E: Regulation of glycogenolysis in human skeletal muscle, *J Appl Physiol* 67(6):2243-2248, 1989.

- Vissing J, Lewis SF, Galbo H, Haller RG: Effect of deficient muscular glycogenolysis on extramuscular fuel production in exercise, *J Appl Physiol* 72(5):1773-1779, 1992.

CHAPTER 5

Anabolism: Skeletal Muscle, the Liver, and Adipose Tissue

OBJECTIVES

After studying this chapter you should be able to:

- Describe the cellular conditions necessary for glycogen synthesis in skeletal muscle and the liver.

- Explain the regulation of glycogen synthesis in skeletal muscle and the liver.

- Explain the enzymatic differences between the liver and skeletal muscle that permit liver gluconeogenesis.

- List the substrates used by the liver in gluconeogenesis and glycogen synthesis.

- Detail the steps involved in the synthesis of free fatty acids and triacylglycerols by the liver, their transportation to peripheral tissues, and their storage in adipocytes.

- List the main blood lipoproteins and their relative proportions of triacylglycerol and cholesterol.

- Describe the regulation and reactions of cholesterol synthesis.

- Explain the importance of triacylglycerol synthesis in skeletal muscle.

- Explain the steps involved in protein synthesis in skeletal muscle.

KEY TERMS

anabolism	translation
synthesis	gluconeogenesis
activity ratio	malonyl-CoA
fractional velocity	lipoproteins
glycogen synthetase	apoproteins
phosphatidate	pentose phosphate pathway
transamination	NADPH
transcription	ribose 5-phosphate
ribonucleic acid	cholesterol
ribosome	

The capacity for tissues of the body to synthesize molecules is essential for life. In fact, one could argue that the main role of the catabolic pathways of metabolism is to provide the free energy and reducing power necessary to synthesize molecules, thereby providing molecules for cell structure and function, and life in general. The reactions of molecular synthesis also have specific functions that support exercise, enable optimal recovery from exercise, and support chronic adaptation to exercise stress. For example, skeletal muscles need to store glucose as the branched polymer glycogen, store free fatty acids in triacylglycerols, and form proteins from amino acids. Similarly, the liver needs to reform glucose and glycogen from noncarbohydrate molecules; to produce free fatty acids, cholesterol, and proteins; and to package some of these molecules into lipoproteins, which then circulate in the blood. Adipose tissue produces free fatty acids and glycerol and stores them as triacylglycerols. The purpose of this chapter is to present the biochemical regulation of anabolism in skeletal muscle, the liver, and adipose tissue; emphasize how these functions are important for exercise; and explain how these tissues interact with each other during and following exercise for the purpose of molecular synthesis.

Anabolism

As explained in Chapter 4, **anabolism** consists of reactions that combine smaller molecules into larger molecules through the use of free energy and the electrons and protons released during catabolism. Another term used to describe the formation of molecules during anabolism is **synthesis.** It is tempting to associate the synthesis of molecules with conditions of rest, especially the recovery from exercise. However, the synthesis of amino acids, glucose and glycogen can occur during exercise in certain tissues.

During the recovery from exercise or in the days or hours before exercise competition, muscle and liver glycogen synthesis is important to optimize the body's stores of glycogen that can fuel muscle contraction or maintain blood glucose concentrations. After exercise the body has to repair damaged muscle and connective tissue, which involves protein synthesis.

Apart from increasing glycogen synthesis, the consumption of food after exercise necessitates that the liver synthesize free fatty acids, triacylglycerols, and specialized blood lipid transport proteins called *lipoproteins*. Triacylglycerols are also formed in adipose tissue and skeletal muscle. The following sections detail the biochemical processes involved in molecular synthesis in skeletal muscle, the liver, and adipose tissue.

Molecular Synthesis in Skeletal Muscle

Several important topics in skeletal muscle exercise biochemistry concern anabolic pathways. Exercise performance and duration are influenced by the magnitude of muscle glycogen stores; muscle hypertrophy is dependent on amino

---

anabolism (an-ab′o-lizm)
a part of metabolism that involves the synthesis of molecules

synthesis (sin-the′sis)
the formation of larger molecules

FIGURE 5.1

The reactions involved with glycogen synthesis. The main reaction, catalyzed by glycogen synthetase, adds a glucose residue to another, and is supported by two other enzymes. Glycogen initiator synthase catalyzes the attachment of the first glucose residue to the protein core of glycogen. Branching enzyme catalyzes the alpha, 1-6 linkages to form the branched structure of glycogen.

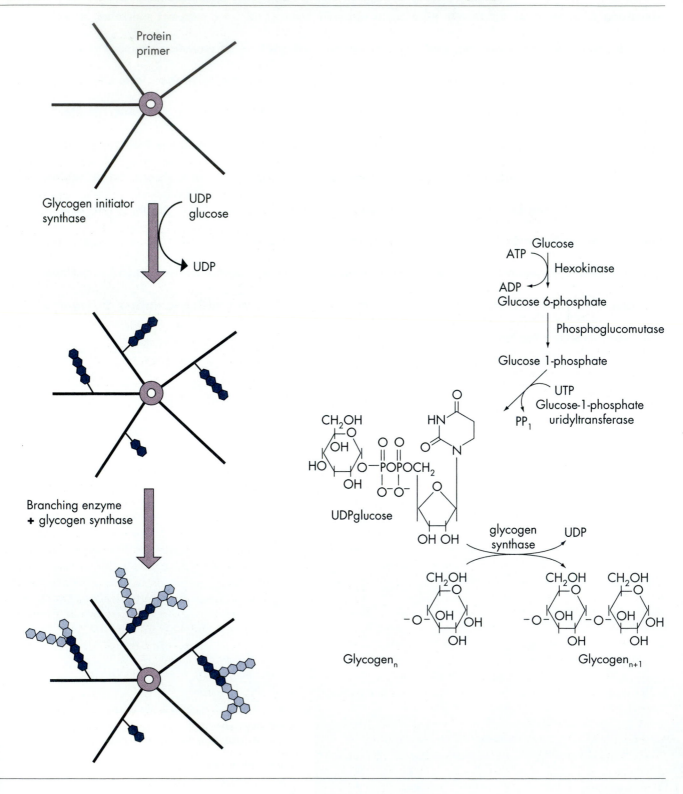

FOCUS BOX 5.1

Regulation of glycogen synthetase

Like phosphorylase, glycogen synthetase is an allosteric enzyme that is regulated by covalent phosphorylation and many metabolites. However, unlike phosphorylase, glycogen synthetase has multiple phosphorylation sites (as many as six).[6,40] Phosphorylation of glycogen synthetase decreases activity, and the sites of phosphorylation are unequal in their magnitude of influence on enzyme activity. For example, depending on the sites that are phosphorylated, glycogen synthetase can retain activity with one or two phosphate additions and lose activity with additional phosphorylation[16] (Figure 5.2). The major allosteric activator of enzyme activity is G6P. Increased concentrations of G6P activate glycogen synthetase when it is phosphorylated, yet provide little activation when unphosphorylated[38] (Figure 5.3, *A*). The inhibitors of glycogen synthetase are ATP, ADP, AMP, UDP, and Pi, with ATP being the most physiologically significant inhibitor.[38]

Despite the presence of multiple phosphorylation sites, past nomenclature has termed the unphosphorylated enzyme structure *synthetase-I*, with the "I" abbreviation indicating independence of activation by G6P. The phosphorylated structures have been termed *synthetase-D*, with the "D" abbreviation indicating dependence on G6P for activation.[40] Increased synthetase activity has been expressed by the **activity ratio** of the enzyme when the assayed activity with no G6P (denoted "I" activity) is divided by the activity with a high (usually 10 mM) G6P concentration (denoted "D" activity). A high activity ratio would indicate that the majority of the enzyme was not phosphorylated and therefore was active in vivo. However, as previously indicated, depending on the G6P concentration the I structure may not be the only active form in vivo, since several different D structures with minimal phosphorylation may exist that are activated by in vivo concentrations of G6P (0.3 mmol/kg wet wt). To account for this discrepancy, researchers have developed the measure called the **fractional velocity**, in which unlike the activity ratio, enzyme activity is measured with in vivo concentrations of G6P, as well as high concentrations of G6P.[12,21] Researchers have shown that glycogen synthesis still occurs when the activity ratio remains low but the fractional velocity is increased, which indicates activity of the D structures of the enzyme that have minor phosphorylation.[12,21]

Glycogen synthesis is also influenced by the size of the glycogen granules, which is indirectly measured by the muscle glycogen concentration.[10,23] Increased concentrations of muscle glycogen decrease the activity of the enzyme for given allosteric conditions, and vice versa. These responses are understandable, since glycogen is both a substrate and a product for the reaction and there are definite limits on the size and number of glycogen granules within a cell.

---

acid and protein synthesis; molecular adaptations to endurance and intense training can modify genetic regulation and DNA translation; and the restoration of muscle lipid stores is necessary to maintain an endogenous supply of lipid.

Glycogen Synthesis

A specific enzyme, phosphorylase, exists for the catabolism of glycogen, and the enzyme responsible for catalyzing the addition of glucose residues to glycogen is called *glycogen synthetase* (EC: 2.4.2.11) (see Chapter 3). These enzymes, and others that affect their activity, are regulated by an epinephrine-cAMP mechanism, as well as intracellular metabolic conditions that favor phosphorylase activation during contractions and synthetase activation during rest, low glycogen concentrations, and increased blood glucose and insulin concentrations.

The synthesis of glycogen is actually dependent on a series of reactions (Figure 5.1) in which G6P is converted to glucose 1-phosphate (G1P), which is activated by its addition to a nucleotide (uridine monophosphate [UMP]) to form UDP-glucose, and finally UDP is removed and the remaining glucose molecule is added to a glucose polymer chain within the large glycogen molecule. The addition of UMP to G1P is thermodynamically driven by the cleavage of two phosphate molecules (pyrophosphate) from UTP, which releases –14.6 Kcal/mol of free energy ($\Delta G^{\circ\prime}$).

As detailed in Chapter 3, the presence of allosterically regulated enzymes in the pathways of glycogenolysis, glycolysis, and glycogen synthesis determine the pathway by which G6P is metabolized. During exercise, stimulation is provided to phosphorylase and phosphofructokinase, which directs G6P metabolism into glycolysis. Conversely, during recovery, stimulation of carbohydrate catabolism is reduced and stimulation of glycogen synthesis is increased. Focus Box 5.1 details

activity ratio
in vitro ratio of glycogen synthetase activity with zero G6P divided by maximally saturating G6P concentrations

fractional velocity
similar to activity ratio, but the numerator is the glycogen synthetase activity measured with a physiologic G6P concentration

FIGURE 5.2

The decreased activity of glycogen synthetase with increasing phosphate content.

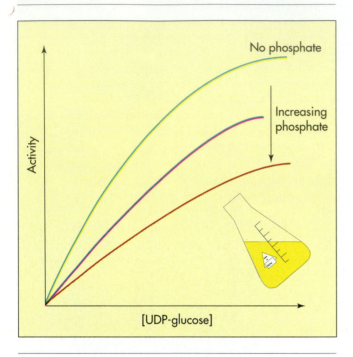

FIGURE 5.3

Increased concentrations of G6P increase the activity of glycogen synthetase. Activity is increased more when there is more phosphate content on the enzyme.

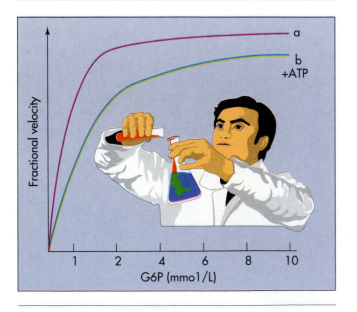

the regulation of **glycogen synthetase**, the enzyme that catalyzes the addition of glucose residues to glycogen.

Following submaximal exercise. When glycogen synthetase is activated, glycogen synthesis occurs if there is a constant supply of substrate. Substrate for glycogen synthesis in skeletal muscle can be blood glucose or intramuscular G6P. A distinction is made between the two substrates, since G6P not only is produced from the hexokinase reaction, but also can accumulate in skeletal muscle during *intense exercise* and be eventually produced from the reversal of several of the reactions of phase 1 and 2 of glycolysis.[2,31,39] During steady state exercise, or intense exercise followed by an active recovery, there is minimal metabolite accumulation, and substrate for glycogen synthesis is dependent on blood glucose as previously described.

Following intense exercise. The pathways of glycogen synthesis in skeletal muscle after exercise are presented in Figure 5.4. There is usually a slight increase in blood glucose during intense exercise as a result of the increased loss of fluid from the plasma, as well as the large increase in catecholamine-stimulated release of glucose by the liver. The importance of the hyperglycemia during intense exercise to increased muscle glycogen synthesis during recovery has not been determined.

The two irreversible reactions of glycolysis are the phosphofructokinase (PFK) reaction and the reaction catalyzed by pyruvate kinase. Although the PFK-catalyzed reaction is irreversible, the enzyme fructose 1,6–bisphosphatase (EC: 3.1.3.11) is present in skeletal muscle and provides a different catalytic mechanism for the exergonic cleavage of the phosphate at carbon–1.[2,5,35] Debate exists as to the presence in skeletal muscle of two enzymes that can bypass the pyruvate kinase reaction.[2,5,35,42] The enzymes of concern are *pyruvate carboxylase* (EC: 6.4.1.1), which catalyzes the addition of CO_2 to pyruvate to form oxaloacetate, and *phosphoenolpyruvate carboxykinase* (EC: 4.1.1.49), which catalyzes the cleavage of CO_2 from oxaloacetate and the addition of a phosphate from GTP to form phosphoenolpyruvate. As indicated in Chapter 3, reactions involving carbon dioxide addition or removal require biotin as a coenzyme.

Both pyruvate carboxylase and phosphoenolpyruvate carboxykinase are known to exist in adequate concentrations in the liver; however, it is generally believed that their concentrations in human skeletal muscle are minimal[42] despite research evidence of their existence in frog, rat, and rabbit muscle.[2,5,35] Consequently, it is widely accepted that once pyruvate is formed from glycolysis in skeletal muscle it is

glycogen synthetase

the enxyme catalyzing the addition of glucose residues from UDP-glucose to glycogen

The pathways for glycogen synthesis in skeletal muscle and the liver. The enzymes that are believed to be specific to the liver are indicated by color. The pyruvate kinase, phosphofructokinase, and hexokinase reactions are all irreversible in vivo. However, the presence of fructose bisphosphatase in skeletal muscle can bipass the PFK reaction. Consequently, skeletal muscle can not reform G6P from lactate or the TCA cycle intermediates; however, the glycolytic intermediates formed before pyruvate can be redirected to glycogen synthesis. As explained in the text, the added enzymes in the liver provide alternate pathways for lactate and pyruvate reduction to eventually reform glucose or glycogen.

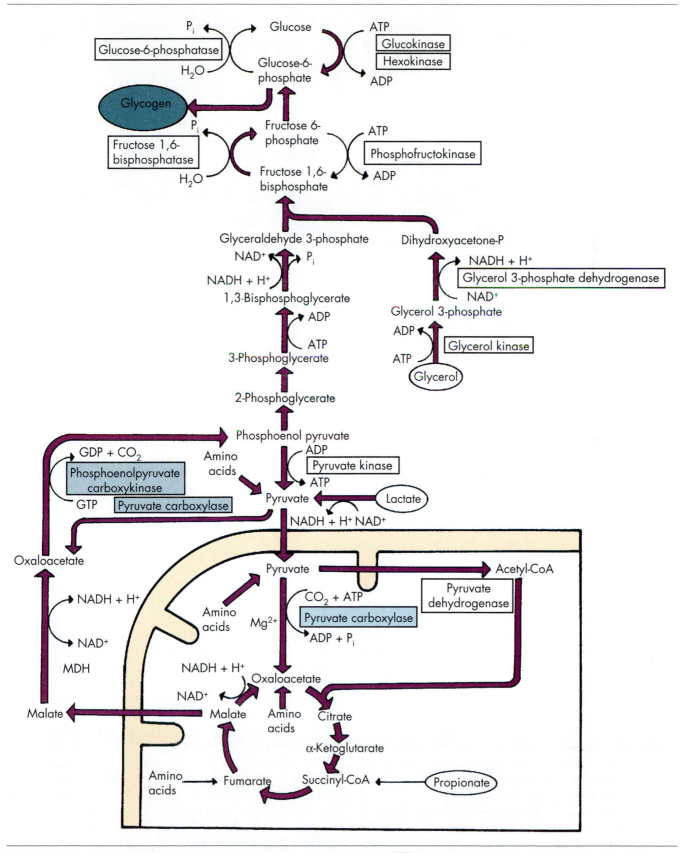

FIGURE 5.5

Triacylglycerol synthesis within skeletal muscle. The synthesis of triacylglycerols is more involved than lipolysis, since several different enzymes are required to reduce glcyerol 3-phosphate to phosphatidate and then eventually to a triacylglycerol.

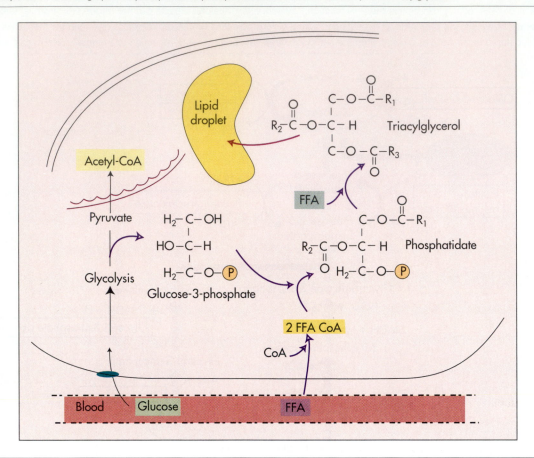

committed to either lactate or acetyl-CoA production. Because of the adequate concentrations of F1,6Pase in skeletal muscle, the intermediates before pyruvate formation can therefore be reconverted back to G6P and may be used to synthesize muscle glycogen. It has been proposed that the high rates of muscle glycogen synthesis after intense exercise are due in part to the reversal of accumulated glycolytic and glycogenolytic intermediates.[39]

Glycogen synthesis is a very efficient means of storing free energy. After G6P formation the only added energy expenditure is the two ATP cost of the pyrophosphate cleavage from GTP during the formation of UDP-glucose. This is a minimal energy cost during resting conditions, and compared with glucose glycogenolysis reduces the ATP cost of the first phase of glycolysis by one ATP.

Triacylglycerol Synthesis

The presence of lipid (triacylglycerol) droplets within skeletal muscle is discussed in Chapter 4. Because lipid is the predominant substrate catabolized during low to moderate intensities of exercise, and the majority of this lipid comes from skeletal muscle, the pathways that are responsible for these lipid stores deserve clarification.

Fatty acid synthesis does not occur at physiologically meaningful rates in skeletal muscle. The reason for this is the limited activity of the pentose phosphate pathway in skeletal muscle, which produces NADPH, the reducing coenzyme needed for several reactions in the pathway of fatty acid synthesis.[42] Although malonyl-CoA, the first molecule of fatty acid synthesis, has been shown to exist in skeletal muscle, the concentrations are too small to have metabolic significance.[46]

The question therefore arises: where do the free fatty acid (FFA) and glycerol molecules come from for muscle triacylglycerol synthesis? As illustrated in Figure 5.5, the FFA molecules are taken from the blood. The synthesis of a triacylglycerol begins with the formation of glycerol 3-phosphate, which in skeletal muscle is predominantly formed from the reduction of dihydroxyacetone phosphate (from glycolysis) and is catalyzed by glycerol 3-phosphate dehydrogenase (EC: 1.1.99.5) (Figure 5.5). Several enzymes catalyze the addition of intramuscular FFA molecules (depending on FFA length and saturation) to the glycerol 3-phosphate. The product formed after two FFA additions is called **phosphatidate** and is a branch molecule in the synthesis of triacylglycerols and phospholipids. The third FFA acid molecule is added (by a lipase) after the phosphate is removed, forming a triacylglycerol. Limited research has been completed on muscle triacylglycerol synthesis, and the regulation of these reactions is unclear. This is unfortunate, since muscle lipid is a major substrate for energy metabolism and therefore the biochemical regulation and mobilization of this energy store require further understanding.

Muscular strength is proportional to the cross-sectional area of a muscle. Based on this fact, the need for increasing muscle size by hypertrophy, and perhaps by hyperplasia (see Chapter 9), has stimulated numerous research questions. For example, there have been applied and clinical needs to understand the best training methods to produce muscle hypertrophy, the time course of the hypertrophy response, and the process of muscle wasting during detraining, immobilization, or the course of various diseases (e.g., AIDS).

The capacity of human muscle to both increase and decrease in size is phenomenal. As discussed in later chapters of this text, complex interactions among genetics, exercise training, nutrition, endocrinology, and health combine to determine the degree of hypertrophy or wasting that results from a given condition. Until the application of noninvasive methods for measuring muscle dimensions, such as the computed tomography (CT) scan, or

magnetic resonance imaging (MRI), indirect measures such as thigh girths have been used, which are obviously less valid because of the unknown contribution of the skin and subcutaneous fat to the girth measurement.

In muscle cross-sectional areas MRI has been used effectively to document changes. Figure 5.7 presents the images of the thigh for two subjects. One subject has weight trained for several years, whereas the other has not participated in regular exercise training of any sort. Muscle cross-sectional areas are obtained by digitizing the circumference of the image on a computer screen and having a program mathematically calculate the area.

Muscle hypertrophy is not a rapid process. Several weeks of training are required to induce a detectable increase in muscle mass, and large increases in muscle cross-sectional areas may take months to years of committed training.

Amino Acid and Protein Synthesis

Many of the 20 amino acid molecules of the human body are produced from intermediates of glycolysis and the TCA cycle (see Table 4.5). Ten amino acids cannot be produced from metabolism and must be provided by the diet. Therefore they are called *essential amino acids*. After the digestion and metabolism of protein into its constituent amino acids, the control of amino acid synthesis occurs via the regulated cellular metabolism of the amino acids glutamate and glutamine. For example, during cellular conditions that require an increase in amino acid synthesis, an ammonium ion (NH_4^+) is added to alpha-ketoglutarate (TCA cycle) to form glutamate via the enzyme *glutamate dehydrogenase* (EC: 1.4.1.3). This reaction requires the presence of NADPH to provide the electrons needed in this oxidation-reduction reaction. An additional amine (NH_2) can be added to glutamate, at the expense of one ATP, to form glutamine via the enzyme glutamine synthetase (EC: 6.3.1.2). Amine groups can then be transferred from glutamate and glutamine (a process termed **transamination**) to carbon skeletons to form other amino acids (Figure 5.6). Not all amino acids are produced this way. Some have more involved pathways, whereas others are produced from the modification of similarly structured amino acids.

The amino acids are joined by peptide bonds to form a chain of amino acids (polypeptide) that eventually may form a protein (Figure 5.8). The amino acid sequence of a protein is called the *primary structure,* and since many chains of proteins do not exist in a linear structure but twist into several types of formations (e.g., alpha helix of DNA), this three-dimensional arrangement is referred to as a *secondary structure.* Larger proteins can form other arrangements, in which the secondary structure twists and turns or changes structure to form the *tertiary structure* (e.g., myoglobin). Finally, some proteins are so large that they consist of multiple units of a given

tertiary structure (e.g., hemoglobin), and this arrangement is referred to as a *quaternary structure.*

Protein synthesis involves molecular events that require communication between the nucleus and cytosol of a cell. An example of the stimulation of protein synthesis is provided in Figure 5.9. Testosterone, a steroid hormone that increases protein synthesis in skeletal muscle, passes through the sarcolemma, binds to an intracellular transport protein, and is transported to the nucleus. Testosterone, like other anabolic agents, stimulates the synthesis of a sequence of nucleotides that complement a specific DNA sequence that codes for the molecules necessary for skeletal muscle hypertrophy, such as the proteins of muscle contraction, the molecules that provide structural support for the sarcomeres, membrane-bound transport proteins, and enzymes. In this process, termed **transcription**, a molecule similar to DNA is formed. This molecule, **ribonucleic acid**, has nucleotide bases that complement those of the DNA. The transcribed RNA molecule is processed to produce a messenger RNA (mRNA), which is responsible for transferring the genetic code for specific mol-

---

phosphatidate (fos-fa-ti′date)
the product formed after two FFA additions to glycerol 3-phosphate

transamination (trans-amin′a-shun)
the removal of an amino group from one amino acid and its placement on a carbon chain that forms another amino acid

transcription (trans-krip′shun)
the duplication of specific DNA regions in the form of RNA

ribonucleic acid
the nucleic acid bases that complement those of DNA

The transamination of glutamate to another amino acid, forming a TCA cycle intermediate α-ketoglutarate).

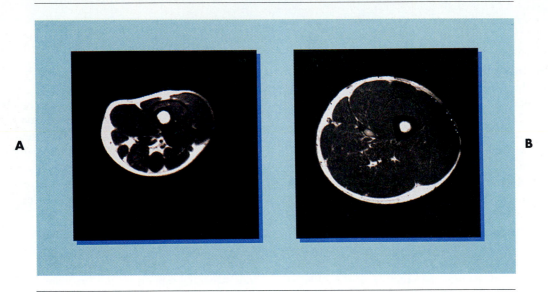

Images of the thigh obtained by MRI from **A,** an individual who has muscle wasting induced by the HIV infection and **B,** an individual trained in competitive cycling.

ecules into the cytosol. Once in the cytosol, mRNA attaches to the organelle responsible for protein synthesis, the **ribosome**. The ribosome provides the foundation from which the amino acids are connected together by peptide bonds. Many ribosomes can work together to synthesize the protein coded by an mRNA molecule.

Amino acids are transported to the mRNA-ribosome structure by another special RNA molecule, *transfer RNA* (tRNA). The tRNA molecule has a binding site *(anticodon)* for the RNA sequence that codes a specific amino acid *(codon)* and a binding site for the amino acid. Consequently, there is a specific tRNA molecule for each amino acid. In addition, specific enzymes exist that catalyze the binding of the tRNA to the mRNA and the binding of the amino acid to the tRNA.

Protein molecules are synthesized by the interactions among the ribosomes, mRNA, and tRNA–amino acid molecules. As the ribosomes move along the mRNA molecule, the protein chain is elongated by the enzymatic addition of amino acids from the specific tRNA molecules. This process

is termed **translation**. Each tRNA–amino acid attachment to the mRNA ribosome complex requires the dephosphorylation of one GTP. Like other examples within biochemistry (e.g., FFA activation), the GTP cost at this phase forms an *activated complex* that enables the formation of the peptide bond and addition of an amino acid to the chain to be a thermodynamically exergonic reaction. However, the GTP (equivalent to ATP) cost of each amino acid positioning on the ribosome mRNA complex is costly, since proteins can have more than several hundred amino acids (myoglobin = 153, Figure 5.8) that require a similarly numbered (n-1) ATP cost for synthesis.

Molecular Synthesis in the Liver

The liver functions differently from skeletal muscle during and after exercise. Like skeletal muscle, the liver synthesizes glycogen, amino acids, triacylglycerols, and proteins. However, unlike skeletal muscle, the liver produces glucose and free fatty acids and regulates the production of various

FIGURE 5.8

The formation of proteins by connecting amino acids by peptide bonds. The amino acid sequence is termed the *primary structure*. Because of interactions between charged and uncharged regions of amino acids with each other and the acqueous environment, proteins are not always linar molecules and can fold into secondary structures such as helixes (e.g., DNA) or random structures (e.g., insulin). Tertiary structures are also formed by large proteins, when several different types of secondary structures are present (e.g., myoglobin). Finally for large proteins that have multiple components (or domains), quaternary structures are formed (e.g., hemoglobin).

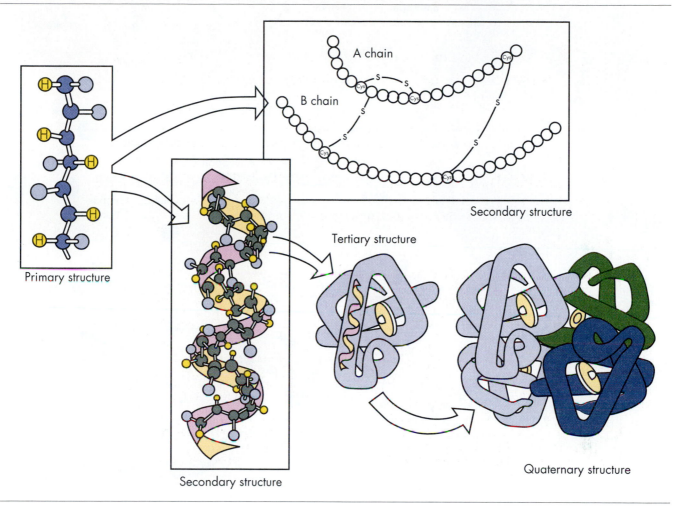

Primary structure

A chain

B chain

Secondary structure

Tertiary structure

Secondary structure

Quaternary structure

lipoprotein molecules that transport blood cholesterol, triacylglycerol, phospholipid, and protein structures to and from the extrahepatic tissues.

Gluconeogenesis

Gluconeogenesis refers to the production of glucose from noncarbohydrate precursors and is not simply the reversal of glycolysis. The enzymes glucose 6-phosphatase (G6Pase) (EC: 3.1.3.9), pyruvate carboxylase (PC), phosphoenolpyruvate carboxykinase (PEPCK), and malate dehydrogenase (MD) are additional enzymes to glycolysis important for the gluconeogenic pathway (see Chapter 4). The last three enzymes are necessary to provide alternate reactions that bypass the pyruvate kinase reaction. Pyruvate carboxylase converts pyruvate to oxaloacetate, which can be converted to phosphoenolpyruvate (PEP) by the enzyme PEPCK. Malate dehydrogenase can convert pyruvate to malate, which in turn can be converted to oxaloacetate. The PEP eventually formed from these reactions can be redirected through glycolysis to form F1,6P, which can then be reconverted to F6P by F1,6Pase, and then eventually to G6P. G6P can be converted to glucose by G6Pase, with glucose released into the circulation.

The gluconeogenic pathway is regulated by metabolites and hormones (Figure 5.10). During low glucose conditions, F2,6P production is decreased, thus decreasing activation of PFK1 and decreasing the inhibition of F1,6,Pase. Glucagon is released from the pancreas when blood glucose concentrations decrease below normal (3 to 4 mmol/L). Glucagon inhibits pyruvate kinase activity and stimulates increased liver

ribosome (ri'bo-som)
the cytosolic organelle involved in protein synthesis

translation (trans-la'shun)
the formation of amino acids from the enzymatic association among ribosomes, RNA, and tRNA

gluconeogenesis (glu'ko-ne-o-jen'e-sis)
formation of glucose from noncarbohydrates, such as amino acids or alcohol

FIGURE 5.9

Protein synthesis involves the formation of messenger RNA (mRNA), which then leaves the nucleus to attach to ribosome subunits in the cytosol. This event starts the process of joining amino acids into a protein molecule. (Courtesy Thibodeau GA, Patton KT: *Anatomy & physiology*, St. Louis, 1996, Mosby and Rolin Graphics.)

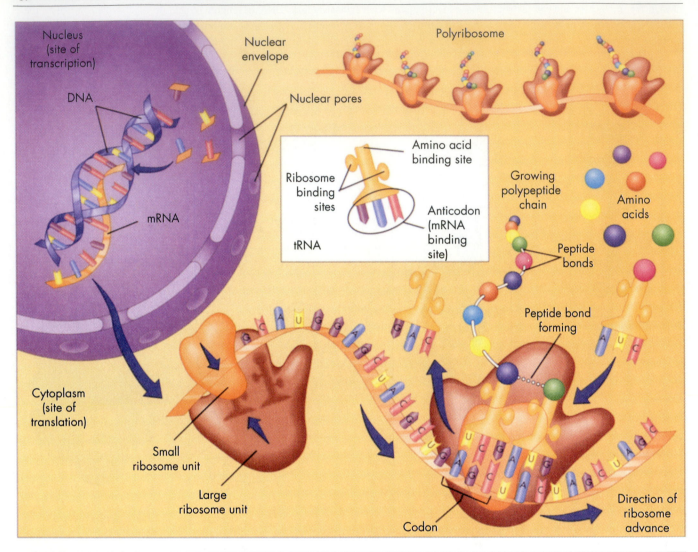

cAMP concentrations and therefore phosphorylase and glycogenolysis. The low blood glucose concentration and minimal activity of glucokinase under these conditions allow for a net production and release of glucose from the liver via the enzyme G6Pase.

Glycogen Synthesis

The main differences between liver and skeletal muscle glycogen synthesis are in the predominant substrates used. As previously mentioned, muscle glycogen synthesis occurs predominantly from glucose conversion to G6P and then to UDP-glucose. Additional G6P production can come from hexose- and triose-phosphate glycolytic intermediates before pyruvate formation. In the liver, glucose is only a substrate for glycogen synthesis in the postabsorptive state after a high carbohydrate meal, when blood glucose concentrations are elevated enough for glucokinase activity to exceed rates of the reverse reaction catalyzed by G6Pase.

Research has shown that the main substrates for liver glycogen synthesis are lactate, fructose, alanine, glutamine, and glycerol.[18,19] This phenomenon has been termed the *glucose paradox,* or the *indirect pathway,* of glycogen synthesis.[19]

Free Fatty Acid Synthesis

The acetyl-CoA formed in muscle under resting conditions is restricted from entry into the TCA cycle by the inhibition of citrate synthase, isocitrate dehydrogenase, and alpha-ketoglutarate dehydrogenase (Figure 5.11). These metabolic conditions stimulate activity of the enzyme acetyl-CoA carboxylase, which catalyzes the irreversible formation of **malonyl-CoA** in the cytosol; this is the committed step to fatty acid synthesis.

The production of malonyl-CoA involves the addition of CO_2 to acetyl-CoA, which requires the coenzyme biotin. The remaining reactions are catalyzed by a linked enzyme

malonyl-CoA

the first product of free fatty acid synthesis

FIGURE 5.10

The regulation of gluconeogenesis in the liver. The main substrates are lactate amino acids and glycerol. (+, Activation; -, inhibition.)

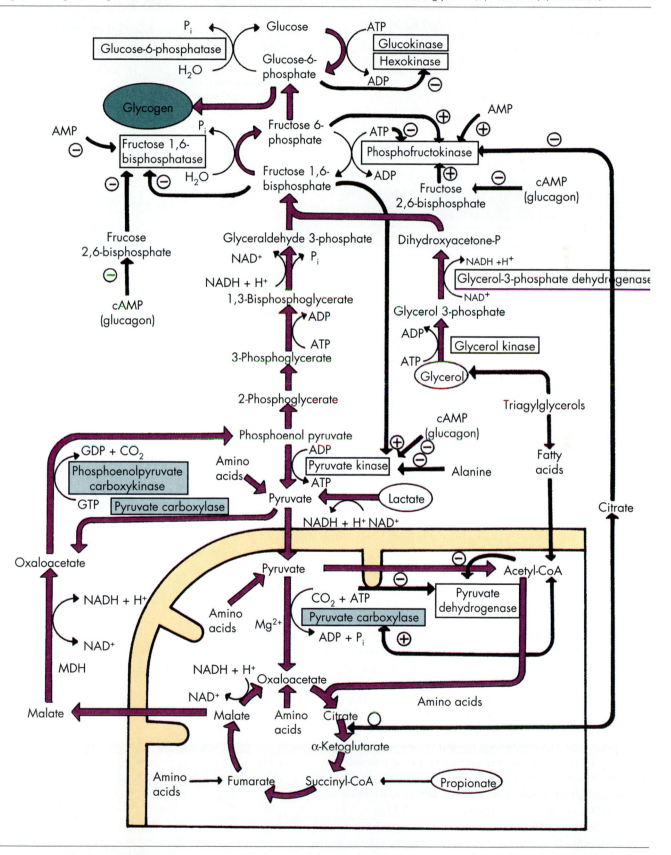

FIGURE 5.11

The regulation of free fatty acid synthesis in the liver and adipose tissue.

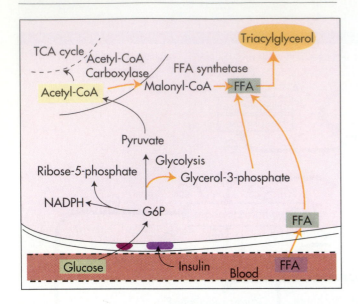

FIGURE 5.12

The reactions of the Pentose Phosphate Pathway.

complex referred to as fatty acid synthase (EC: 2.3.1.35). The fatty acid chain becomes elongated by the sequential addition of two carbon units from malonyl-CoA. Malonyl-CoA is added to the fatty acid chain by addition to a carrier protein that serves the same function as CoA during catabolism. During elongation the release of CO_2 provides the free energy that makes the reactions exergonic. The reductant (electron donor) is NADPH, which is produced from the purine nucleotide cycle (Focus Box 5.3).

Triacylglycerol Synthesis

The reactions of triacylglycerol synthesis were detailed for skeletal muscle and are identical for the liver, except that the liver has the enzyme glycerokinase (EC: 2.7.1.30), which can produce glycerol 3-phosphate from glycerol. Triacylglycerol synthesized in the liver not only is stored in lipid droplets, but also is used to form lipoprotein molecules that transport the triacylglycerol to extrahepatic tissues for metabolism (e.g., skeletal muscle) and storage (e.g., adipose tissue). Consequently, the liver forms and processes triacylglycerol for transport to extrahepatic tissues.

Lipoprotein Synthesis

Since lipid molecules are hydrophobic and cannot dissolve in aqueous solution, they must be transported in the blood bound to specific molecules. The molecules that bind to and transport lipids are **lipoproteins**. Lipoproteins are classified by their density (Table 5.1) and consist of four groups: (1) chylomicrons, formed following the intestinal absorption of triacylglycerols; (2) very low-density lipoproteins (VLDL), formed by the liver from the metabolism of chylomicrons; (3) low-density lipoproteins (LDL), the final product of VLDL catabolism, and (4) high-density lipoproteins (HDL), a product of chylomicron and VLDL metabolism by the liver.[29,30] There are differences in the relative content of the lipids contained in each lipoprotein, as indicated in Table 5.1.

FOCUS BOX 5.3

The pentose phosphate pathway provides the reducing power for molecular syntheses

The **pentose phosphate pathway** is a side branch of glycolysis, using glucose 6-phosphate as a substrate. It produces two very important molecules used in anabolism: **NADPH** and **ribose 5-phosphate**. NADPH is a modified form of NADH presented in Chapter 4 and provides reducing power and free energy for many anabolic reactions. Ribose 5-phosphate is used for the further synthesis of ribonucleic (for RNA) and deoxyribonucleic acid bases (for DNA).

The reactions of the pentose phosphate pathway are depicted in Figure 5.12. For each glucose 6-phosphate molecule conversion to ribose 5-phosphate, four reactions are involved, yielding two molecules of NADPH. In tissue such as liver, certain glands, and adipose tissue, the NADPH is used in the synthesis of free fatty acids. In the liver and adrenal cortex, NADPH is also required for the synthesis of cholesterol and the related steroid hormones estrogen, testosterone, aldosterone, and cortisol.

TABLE 5.1

Chemical constituents of lipoproteins

LIPOPROTEIN CLASS	DENSITY	TRIGLYCERIDE	CHOLESTEROL FREE	CHOLESTEROL ESTERIFIED	PHOSPHOLIPID	PROTEIN
Chylomicrons	<0.94	85	2	4	8	2
VLDL	0.94-1.006	60	6	16	18	10
IDL	1.006-1.019	30	8	22	22	18
LDL	1.119-1.063	7	10	40	20	25
HDL	1.063-1.210	5	4	15	30	50

Modified from Guton AC: *Textbook of medical physiology,* ed 8, Philadelphia, 1991, WB Saunders.
VLDL, Very low-density lipoprotein; *IDL,* intermediate-density lipoprotein; *LDL,* Low-density lipoprotein; *HDL,* high-density lipoprotein.

The lipoproteins are composed of proteins (termed *apoproteins*), triacylglycerols, phospholipid, esterified cholesterol (cholesterol esters), unesterified cholesterol (free cholesterol), and free fatty acids (FFAs) (Table 5.1). The **apoproteins** are important for the function of each lipoprotein because they can serve as cofactors, transfer lipid, and act as receptor binding sites. Many different types of apoproteins have been isolated, and several are known to be specific to certain types of lipoproteins (see the Clinical Application on p. 110 and Figure 5.13 on p. 111).

Cholesterol is an important molecule for optimal cell function. Cholesterol is found within cell membranes, and therefore every cell needs cholesterol. Almost every cell can synthesize cholesterol. The cholesterol synthesized by the body is referred to as *endogenous* cholesterol, and the cholesterol that is absorbed from the diet is termed *exogenous* cholesterol. The pathway for cholesterol synthesis is illustrated in Figure 5.14.

The role of the liver in the metabolism of lipoproteins begins with digestion (Figure 5.15). The liver produces bile and cholesterol, which are both secreted into the small intestine to aid in the digestion and absorption of lipid. The cholesterol and triacylglycerol absorbed and produced by the

lipoprotein (lip′o-pro′teen)
blood compounds containing lipid and protein

apoprotein (apo-pro′teen)
the regulatory protein constituents of lipoproteins

pentose phosphate pathway
A side branch of glycolysis resulting in the conversion of glucose 6-phosphate to NADPH and ribose 5-phosphate

NADPH
one of the main products of the pentose phosphate pathway. NADPH provides reducing power and free energy during anabolic reactions

ribose 5-phosphate
one of the main products of the pentose phosphate pathway. Ribose 5-Phosphate is a precursor of both RNA and DNA synthesis

cholesterol (ko-les′ter-ol)
a steroid lipid that is produced by almost all cells, and whose production is regulated by a receptor-mediated mechanism in both hepatic and extrahepatic tissues

Pathogenesis of Hypercholesterolemia

Cholesterol circulates in the blood packaged within specialized lipid transport proteins called lipoproteins. Almost all of the cholesterol in lipoproteins is synthesized in the liver.

When properly regulated, the total cholesterol concentration in the blood is less than 200 mg/dL.[42] Proper regulation of blood cholesterol involves the liver (hepatic) and extrahepatic tissue and the regulation of the main allosteric enzyme of cholesterol synthesis: hydroxymethylglutaryl-CoA reductase (HMG-CoA reductase).[3,4,24-26,42] This enzyme is inhibited by cholesterol and mevalonate, as well as by phosphorylation (activation) and dephosphorylation (deactivation).[42]

The regulation of HMG-CoA reductase by cholesterol via a receptor-mediated mechanism was elucidated by the research of Brown and Goldstein[3] (Figure 5.13), which resulted in their receiving the 1985 Nobel Prize for Physiology or Medicine.[4] Since then additional research findings have emphasized the importance of apoprotein function and content on lipoproteins for the normal uptake of cholesterol by hepatic and extrahepatic tissue. The main apoproteins are *apoA, apoB, apoC,* and *apoE,* and each is found on many of the lipoprotein molecules.[24] These apoproteins have different affinities for the lipoprotein receptors (Table 5-2), regulate the distribution of cholesterol between lipoproteins and cells, and function as cofactors for enzymes of lipid metabolism.[24] For example, apoA and apoC are coenzymes for the enzyme lecithin:cholesterol acyltransferase (LCAT), which attaches a free fatty acid on the cholesterol molecule, forming a cholesterol ester.

Certain individuals have defective or inadequate apoproteins, resulting in impaired removal of cholesterol from the circulation, and abnormally high cholesterol and lipoprotein concentrations (Table 5.3). These conditions are collectively termed *type III hypercholesterolemia, familial hypercholesterolemia,* and *familial defective apoB-100.*[25]

TABLE 5.2

Apoproteins associated with blood lipoproteins, the main lipoprotein receptors, and the functions of apoproteins in lipoprotein metabolism

APOPROTEINS/PHENOTYPES			TISSUE PRODUCTION	LIPOPROTEIN RECEPTOR
A	-I	Intestine/liver	HDL	
	-II	Liver	HDL	
	-III	Liver/intestine	CM	
B	-48	Intestine	All but HDL	apoB,E(LDL)
	-100	Liver	All but HDL	apoB,E(LDL)
C	-I	Liver/intestine	CM, VLDL, LDL	
	-II	Liver/intestine	CM, VLDL, LDL	
	-III	Liver/intestine	CM, VLDL, LDL	
E	-2	Liver/extrahepatic	CM, CMr, VLDL, HDL	apoE and apoB,E(LDL)
	-3	Liver/extrahepatic	CM, CMr, VLDL, HDL	apoE and apoB,E(LDL)
	-4	Liver/extrahepatic	CM, CMr, VLDL, HDL	apoE and apoB,E(LDL)

CM, Chylomicron; *CMr,* chylomicron remnant; *VLDL,* very low-density lipoproteins; *IDL,* intermediate-density lipoproteins; *LDL,* low-density lipoproteins; *HDL,* high-density lipoproteins.

Individuals with mutant forms of apoE have a decreased ability to remove cholesterol from HDL and the other intermediary lipoproteins causing elevated blood triglyceride (hypertriglyceridemia) and hypercholesterolemia: a condition termed *type II hyperlipoproteinemia.* Familial hypercholesterolemia occurs when there is a complete absence of apoB,E(LDL) receptors or their ability to bind LDLs is impaired. The extent of the inability to synthesis LDLs or their malfunction determines the extent of hyperlipoprotenemia. Individuals with defective apoB-100 do not have effective binding of LDL to the LDL receptor and therefore cannot properly inhibit the cellular synthesis of cholesterol.

TABLE 5.3

Blood lipoprotein and cholesterol concentrations (mg/dL) for normal individuals and individuals with genetic defects in lipoprotein metabolism

LIPOPROTEIN DISORDER	DEFECT	EFFECT ON LIPOPROTEIN				CHOLESTEROL	TRIGLYCERIDE
		VLDL	IDL	LDL	HDL		
Type III	ApoE mutation(s)	↑	↑	↓	↓	300-600	400-800
Familial	LDL receptor mutation(s)	↑	↑	↑	↓	350-500	100-300
ApoB-100	ApoB-100 mutation	↑	↑	↑	↓	250-300	100-300
Dietary	None	↑	↑	↑	↑	200-350	100-300

Modified from Mahley RW, Innerarity TL, Rall SC, Weisgraber KH: *J Lipid Res* 25:1277-1294, 1984; and National Cholesterol Education Program.

Since high blood cholesterol is a serious risk factor for heart and peripheral vascular disease, individuals with hypercholesterolemia are at increased risk for heart attack and stroke. Unfortunately, individuals with hypercholesterolemia have such high blood cholesterol concentrations that severe arterial blockages can develop during the teens and death often results by the age of 20.

FIGURE 5.13

The receptor mediated regulation of cholesterol synthesis as originally proposed by Brown and Goldstein. (Adapted from Brown MS, Goldstein JL: *Sci Am* 251: 58-66, 1984; and Brown MS, Goldstein JL: *Science*, 232: 34-47, 1985.)

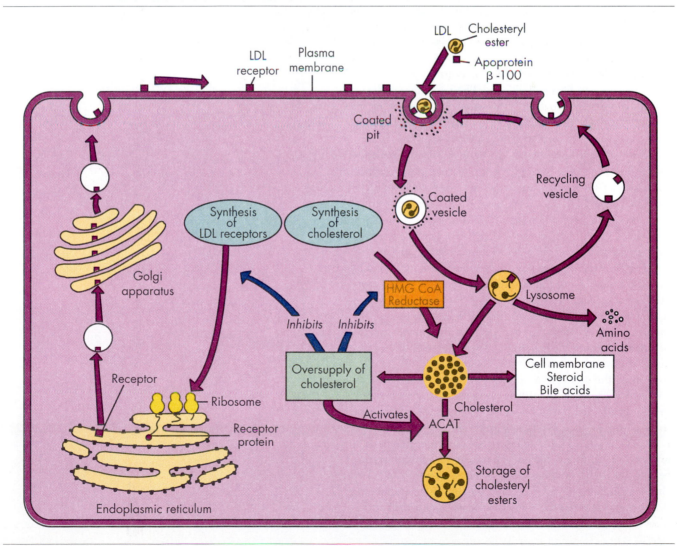

FIGURE 5.14

The condensed pathway of cholesterol synthesis. The main regulated enzyme is HMG CoA reductase.

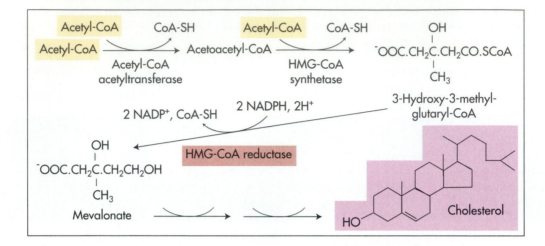

intestinal mucosa cells are packaged into chylomicrons and released into the lymph circulation. The liver then processes the chylomicrons into VLDLs, which transport triacylglycerol to the extrahepatic tissues. As previously described, the enzyme lipoprotein lipase that is bound on the inner endothelial lining of blood vessels catabolizes the circulating triacylglycerols to FFA and glycerol. The remaining remnants of VLDL are removed from circulation by the liver or are converted to LDL. The LDLs contain relatively more cholesterol than the other lipoproteins (Figure 5.16).[37]

Low-density lipoproteins are removed from circulation by the LDL receptor located on the membranes of hepatic and extrahepatic tissue. Individuals who are deficient in or have defective LDL receptors have large blood cholesterol concentrations, a condition termed *familial hypercholesterolemia* (see the Clinical Application on p. 110) These individuals have an increased risk for arterial atherosclerotic disease.

High-density lipoproteins are formed by the liver and by the addition of specific apoproteins by the liver to immature HDL produced in the small intestine. High-density lipoproteins remove free cholesterol from the circulation, esterify them, and either internalize them within their own structure or transfer them to the other lipoproteins for eventual metabolism by the liver. Consequently, having high HDL concentrations in the blood is an effective means to remove excess cholesterol from the circulation and return it to the liver for catabolism (Figure 5.15). There are two subfractions of HDL (HDL$_2$ and HDL$_3$); HDL$_2$ contains more cholesterol than HDL$_3$. It is the HDL$_2$ subfraction concentration that is inversely related to the development of atherosclerosis, because it is this subfraction that has successfully acquired cholesterol from the peripheral circulation. Exercise training is known to increase HDL$_2$ concentrations, but the mechanism for this increase remains unclear (see Chapter 27).

FIGURE 5.15

The regulation of lipoprotein molecules by the liver, intestine, and other extrahepatic tissues. (From Brown MS, Goldstein JL: *Sci Am* 251: 58-66, 1984.)

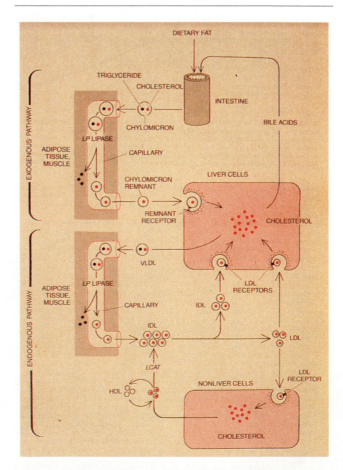

Amino Acid Synthesis

As far as exercise applications are concerned, the liver is similar to skeletal muscle with regard to the processes of amino acid synthesis. Because of the different metabolic functions of the liver and skeletal muscle, obvious differences exist in the type of proteins synthesized.

Molecular Synthesis in Adipose Tissue

The main anabolic pathway of interest within adipose tissue is triacylglycerol synthesis. This pathway has been detailed in liver and skeletal muscle metabolism. Nevertheless, the student should be aware that adipose tissue is the main store of the body's triacylglycerols, and excess carbohydrate or protein intake increases liver FFA synthesis, and that it is the majority of this lipid that ends up in adipose tissue triacylglycerol stores.

FIGURE 5.16

A diagramatic representation of a lipoprotein. Apoproteins are located on the external surface of the molecule and are important for the metabolic function of the lipoprotein. As indicated in Table 5.1, the content of cholesterol, triacylglycerols, and protein varies between lipoproteins. (From Wardlaw GM, Insel PM: *Perspectives in nutrition,* St. Louis, 1996, Mosby.)

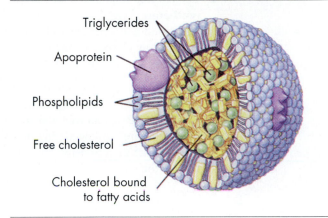

Triglycerides

Apoprotein

Phospholipids

Free cholesterol

Cholesterol bound to fatty acids

SUMMARY

- **Anabolism** consists of reactions that combine smaller molecules into larger molecules by the use of free energy and the electrons and protons released during catabolism. Another term used to describe the formation of molecules during anabolism is **synthesis**.

- The enzyme responsible for catalyzing the addition of glucose residues to glycogen is called **glycogen synthetase**. Synthetase is regulated by an epinephrine–cAMP mechanism, as well as intracellular metabolic conditions that favor phosphorylase activation during contractions and synthetase activation during rest, low glycogen concentrations, increased blood glucose and insulin levels, and increased intracellular glucose 6-phosphate (G6P) concentrations.

- The synthesis of glycogen is dependent on a series of reactions in which G6P is converted to glucose 1-phosphate (G1P), which is activated by addition to a nucleotide (uridine monophosphate) to form UDP-glucose. UDP is removed and the remaining glucose molecule is added to a glucose polymer chain within the large glycogen molecule. The in vitro assays, referred to as the **activity ratio** and **fractional velocity,** are used to detect the activity of glycogen synthetase and differ in the amount of G6P used to activate the enzyme.

- During steady state exercise, or intense exercise followed by an active recovery, there is minimal intramuscular metabolite accumulation and the substrate for glycogen synthesis is dependent on blood glucose as previously described. Because of the adequate concentrations of F1,6Pase in skeletal muscle, the intermediates before pyruvate formation can be reconverted to G6P and may be used to synthesize muscle glycogen. It has been proposed that the high rates of muscle glycogen synthesis after intense exercise are due in part to the reversal of accumulated glycolytic and glycogenolytic intermediates.

- Fatty acid synthesis does not occur at physiologically meaningful rates in skeletal muscle because of the limited activity of the **pentose phosphate pathway,** which produces **NADPH,** the reducing coenzyme needed for several reactions in the pathway of fatty acid synthesis, as well as **ribose 5-phosphate,** an intermediate used in the synthesis of nucleotide bases.

- The synthesis of a triacylglycerol in skeletal muscle begins with FFA uptake from the blood. The intracellular FFA is combined with glycerol 3-phosphate. The product formed after two FFA additions is called **phosphatidate** and is a branch molecule in the synthesis of triacylglycerols and phospholipids. The third FFA acid molecule is added (by a lipase) after the phosphate is removed, forming a triacylglycerol.

- Many of the 20 amino acid molecules of the human body are produced from intermediates of glycolysis and the TCA cycle. Ten amino acids cannot be produced from metabolism and must be provided by the diet, and therefore are termed *essential amino acids.* Amine groups can be transferred from amino acids and used to form other amino acids, a process termed **transamination.** Not all amino acids are produced this way. Some have more involved pathways, whereas others are produced from the modification of similarly structured amino acids.

- Testosterone, like other anabolic agents, stimulates the **transcription** of specific DNA sequences that code for cellular proteins. The process of transcription involves the formation of a molecule similar to DNA but has nucleotide bases that complement those of the DNA. This molecule is a **ribonucleic acid** (RNA), referred to as *messenger RNA* (mRNA), and is responsible for transferring the genetic code for specific molecules into the cytosol. Once in the cytosol, the mRNA is attached to the organelle responsible for protein synthesis, the **ribosome.** The ribosome provides the foundation from which the amino acids are connected together by peptide bonds. Many ribosomes can work together to synthesize the protein coded by an mRNA molecule.

- Protein molecules are synthesized by the interactions among the ribosomes, mRNA, and tRMA–amino acid molecules. Because the ribosomes move along the mRNA molecule, the protein chain is elongated by the enzymatic addition of amino acids from the specific tRNA molecules, a process termed **translation.** Each tRNA–amino acid attachment to the mRNA ribosome complex requires the dephosphorylation of one GTP.

■ **Gluconeogenesis** refers to the production of glucose from noncarbohydrate precursors, occurs in the liver, and is not simply the reversal of glycolysis. The enzymes glucose 6-phosphatase (G6Pase), pyruvate carboxylase (PC), phosphoenolpyruvate carboxykinase (PEPCK), and malate dehydrogenase (MD) are additional enzymes to glycolysis important for the gluconeogenic pathway.

■ The gluconeogenic pathway is regulated by metabolites and hormones. During low-glucose conditions, F2,6P production is decreased, thus decreasing activation of PFK1 and the inhibition of F1,6Pase. Glucagon is released from the pancreas when blood glucose concentrations decrease below normal (3 to 4 mmol/L). Glucagon inhibits pyruvate kinase activity and stimulates increased liver cAMP concentrations and therefore phosphorylase and glycogenolysis. The low blood glucose concentration and minimal activity of glucokinase under these conditions allow for a net production and release of glucose from the liver via the enzyme G6Pase.

■ In the liver, glucose is only a substrate for glycogen synthesis in the postabsorptive state after a high carbohydrate meal, when blood glucose concentrations are elevated enough for glucokinase activity to exceed rates of the reverse reaction catalyzed by G6Pase. The main substrates for liver glycogen synthesis are lactate, fructose, alanine, glutamine, and glycerol. This phenomenon has been termed the *glucose paradox,* or the "indirect pathway" of glycogen synthesis.[27]

■ The entry of acetyl-CoA into the TCA cycle in the liver is restricted by the inhibition of citrate synthase, isocitrate dehydrogenase, and alpha-ketoglutarate dehydrogenase. These conditions stimulate activity of the enzyme acetyl-CoA carboxylase, which catalyzes the irreversible formation of **malonyl-CoA** in the cytosol; this is the committed step to fatty acid synthesis.

■ The production of malonyl-CoA involves the addition of CO_2 to acetyl-CoA. The remaining reactions are catalyzed by a linked enzyme complex referred to as fatty acid synthase (EC: 2.3.1.35). The fatty acid chain becomes elongated by the sequential addition of two carbon units from malonyl-CoA. Malonyl-CoA is added to the fatty acid chain by addition to a carrier protein that serves the same function as CoA during catabolism. During elongation the release of CO_2 provides the free energy that makes the reactions exergonic. The reductant (electron donor) is NADPH.

■ The molecules that bind to and transport lipids are **lipoproteins.** Lipoproteins are classified by their density and consist of four groups: (1) chylomicrons, formed following the intestinal absorption of triacylglycerols; (2) very low-density lipoproteins (VLDLs), formed by the liver from the metabolism of chylomicrons; (3) low-density lipoproteins (LDLs), the final product of VLDL catabolism; and (4) high-density lipoproteins (HDLs), a product of chylomicron and VLDL metabolism by the liver.

■ The lipoproteins are composed of proteins **(apoproteins),** triacylglycerols, phospholipid, esterified **cholesterol** (cholesteryl esters), unesterified cholesterol (free cholesterol), and free fatty acids (FFAs). The cholesterol and triacylglycerol absorbed and produced by the intestinal mucosa cells are packaged into chylomicrons and released into the lymph circulation. The liver then processes the chylomicrons into VLDLs, which transport triacylglycerol to the extrahepatic tissues. The enzyme lipoprotein lipase that is bound on the inner endothelial lining of blood vessels catabolizes the circulating triacylglycerols to FFA and glycerol. The remaining remnants of VLDL are removed from circulation by the liver, or converted to LDLs. The LDLs contain relatively more cholesterol than the other lipoproteins.

■ Low-density lipoproteins are removed from circulation by the LDL receptor located on the membranes of extrahepatic tissue. Individuals who are deficient or have defective LDL receptors have large blood cholesterol concentrations, and this condition is termed *familial hypercholesterolemia.* These individuals are exposed to increased risk for arterial atherosclerotic disease.

■ High-density lipoproteins are formed by the liver and by the addition of specific apoproteins by the liver to immature HDLs produced in the small intestine. High-density lipoproteins remove free cholesterol from the circulation, esterify them, and either internalize them within their own structure or transfer them to the other lipoproteins for eventual metabolism by the liver. There are two subfractions of HDL (HDL_2 and HDL_3); HDL_2 contains more cholesterol than HDL_3. It is the HDL_2 subfraction concentration that is inversely related to the development of atherosclerosis, because it is this subfraction that has successfully acquired cholesterol from the peripheral circulation. Exercise training is known to increase HDL_2 concentrations, but the mechanism for this increase is unclear.

REVIEW QUESTIONS

1. Which metabolites activate and inhibit the enzyme glycogen synthetase?

2. How does the regulation of glycogen synthesis differ in skeletal muscle and the liver?

3. Can glycolysis be reversed in skeletal muscle? Explain.

4. What are the enzymes and their reactions that enable the liver to synthesize glucose from pyruvate, lactate, and amino acids?

5. Under what conditions do the liver and adipose tissue convert acetyl-CoA to malonyl-CoA?

6. Why is it accepted that skeletal muscle does not synthesize free fatty acids?

7. If skeletal muscle does not synthesize free fatty acids, where are they synthesized, and how can skeletal muscle have an endogenous store of triacylglycerols?

8. What does the term esterification mean?

9. Why are the amino acids glutamate and glutamine important in the synthesis of many amino acids?

10. What are the differences between transcription and translation?

11. What are the functions of mRNA, tRNA, ribosomes, and GTP during protein synthesis?

12. What are the different classes of lipoproteins, and how do they differ in lipid and protein composition?

13. What is the role of the LDL receptor in the regulation of blood cholesterol?

14. What are the roles of the liver in the regulation of blood lipoprotein concentrations?

15. What are the functions of apoproteins in the metabolism of lipoproteins?

APPLICATIONS

1. Individuals with type I or II diabetes have an impaired capacity for glucose uptake by skeletal muscle. How would this influence their ability to synthesize muscle glycogen and their muscles' dependence on FFA metabolism?

2. Would the need for carbohydrate ingestion after exercise be similar for individuals who participate in intense exercise and those who participate in steady state exercise? Why?

3. Skeletal muscle sources of FFA are the predominant source of lipid used in energy catabolism during exercise. However, exercise training can eventually decrease adipose tissue stores of fat. What interactions between muscle and adipose FFA metabolism must exist to explain these facts?

4. Recent research has indicated that the RDA for protein (0.8 g/kg/day) needs to be increased for athletes. What functions of skeletal muscle in well-trained athletes would require increased amino acid and protein synthesis?

5. There are enormous individual differences in the role of diet in influencing fasting blood lipoprotein and cholesterol concentrations. Based on the regulation of blood lipoproteins, what are the best explanations for these differences?

REFERENCES

1. Bak JF, Pedersen O: Exercise-induced activation of glycogen synthase in human skeletal muscle, *AM J Physiol* 258(21):E957-E963, 1990.

2. Bendall JR, Taylor AA: The Meyerhof quotient and the synthesis of glycogen from lactate in frog and rabbit muscle, *Biochem J* 118:887-893, 1970.

3. Brown MS, Goldstein JL: How LDL receptors influence cholesterol and atherosclerosis, *Sci Am* 251:58-66, 1984.

4. Brown MS, Goldstein JL: A receptor-mediated pathway for cholesterol homeostasis, *Science* 232:34-47, 1985.

5. Crabtree B, Higgins SJ, Newsholme EA: The activities of pyruvate carboxylase, phosphoenolpyruvate carboxykinase and fructose diphosphatase in muscles from vertebrates and invertebrates, *Biochem J* 130:391-396, 1972.

6. DePaoli-Roach AA, Roach PJ, Larner J: Multiple phosphorylation of rabbit skeletal muscle glycogen synthase, *J Biol Chem* 254(23):12062-12068, 1979.

7. Douen AG, Ramlal T, Rastogi S et al: Exercise induces recruitment of the "Insulin responsive glucose transporter," *J Biol Chem* 265(23):13427-13430, 1990.

8. Friden J, Seger J, Ekblom B: Topographical localization of muscle glycogen: an ultrahistochemical study in the human vastus lateralis, *Acta Physiol Scand* 135:381-391, 1989.

9. Fushiki T, Wells JAS, Tapscott EB, Dohm GL: Changes in glucose transporters in muscle in response to exercise, *Am J Physiol* 256(19):E580-E587, 1989.

10. Goldsmith E, Sprang S, Fletterick R: Structure of maltoheptose by difference Fourier methods and a model for glycogen, *J Mol Biol* 156:411-427, 1982.

11. Grannar DK: Protein synthesis and the genetic code. In Murray RK, Granner DK, Mayes PA, Rodwell VW, editors: *Harper's biochemistry*, ed 22, Norwalk, Conn, 1990, Appleton & Lange.

12. Guinovart JJ, Salavert A, Massague J et al: Glycogen synthase: a new activity ratio assay expressing a high sensitivity to the phosphorylation state, *FEBS Lett* 106(2):284-288, 1979.

13. Guyton AC: *Textbook of medical physiology*, ed 8, Philadelphia, WB Saunders.

14. Henrikson EJ, Bourey RE, Rodnick KJ et al: Glucose transporter protein content and glucose transport capacity in rat skeletal muscle, *Am J Physiol* 259(22):E593-E598, 1990.

15. Houmard JA, Egan PC, Neufer PD et al: Elevated skeletal muscle glucose transporter levels in exercise-trained middle-aged men, *Am J Physiol* 261(24):E437-E443, 1991.

16. Huang K, Huang FL: Phosphorylation of rabbit skeletal muscle glycogen synthase by cyclic AMP-dependent protein kinase and dephosphorylation of the synthase by phosphatase, *J Biol Chem* 255(7):3141:3147, 1980.

17. Huang K, Lee S, Huang FL: Phosphorylation of rabbit skeletal muscle glycogen synthesis I by a cyclic AMP–independent synthase kinase, *J Biol Chem* 254(9):9867-9870, 1980.

18. Johnson JL, Bagby GJ: Gluconeogenic pathway in liver and muscle glycogen synthesis after exercise, *J Appl Physiol* 64(4):1591-1599, 1988.

19. Katz J, McGarry JD: The glucose paradox: is glucose a substrate for liver metabolism? *J Clin Invest* 74:1901-1909, 1984.

20. Kochan RG, Lamb DR, Lutz SA et al: Glycogen synthase activation in human skeletal muscle: effects of diet and exercise, *Am J Physiol* 236(6):E660-E666, 1979.

21. Kochan RG, Lamb DR, Reinman EM, Schlender KK: Modified assays to detect activation of glycogen synthase following exercise, *Am J Physiol* 240(3):E197-E202, 1981.

22. Ladu MJ, Kapsas H, Palmer WK: Regulation of lipoprotein lipase in adipose and muscle tissue during fasting, *Am J Physiol* 260(29):R953-R959, 1991.

23. Larner J, Takeda Y, Hizukuri S: The influence of the chain size and molecular weight on the kinetic constants for the span glucose to polysaccharide for rabbit muscle glycogen synthase, *Mol Cell Biochem* 12(3):131-136, 1976.

24. Mahley RW, Innerarity TL, Rall SC, Weisgraber KH: Plasma lipoproteins: apolipoprotein structure and function, *J Lipid Res* 25:1277-1294, 1984.

25. Mahley RW, Weisgraber KH, Innerarity TL, Rall Jr. SC: Genetic defects in lipoprotein metabolism: evaluation of atherogenic lipoproteins caused by impaired catabolism, *JAMA* 265(1):78-83, 1991.

26. Mahley RW: Apolipoprotein E: cholesterol transport protein with expanding role in cell biology, *Science* 240:622-630, 1988.

27. Mayes PA: Metabolism of glycogen. In Murray RK, Granner DK, Mayes PA, Rodwell VW, editors, *Harper's biochemistry*, ed 22, Norwalk, Conn, 1990, Appleton & Lange.

28. Mayes PA: Gluconeogenesis and control of blood glucose. In Murray RK, Granner DK, Mayes PA, Rodwell VW, editors, *Harper's biochemistry*, ed 22, Norwalk, Conn, 1990, Appleton & Lange.

29. Mayes PA: Lipid transport and storage. In Murray RK, Granner DK, Mayes PA, Rodwell VW, editors, *Harper's biochemistry*, ed 22, Norwalk, Conn, 1990, Appleton & Lange.

REFERENCES—Cont'd

30. Mayes PA: Cholesterol synthesis, transport, and excretion. In Murray RK, Granner DK, Mayes PA, Rodwell VW, editors, *Harper's biochemistry,* ed 22, Norwalk, Conn, 1990, Appleton & Lange.

31. McLane JA, Holloszy JO: Glycogen synthesis from lactate in three types of skeletal muscle, *J Biol Chem* 254(14):6548-6553, 1979.

32. Munger R, Temler E, Jallut D et al: Correlations of glycogen synthase and phosphorylase activities with glycogen concentration in human muscle biopsies: evidence for a double-feedback mechanism regulating glycogen synthesis and breakdown, *Metabolism* 42(1):36-43, 1993.

33. Newgard CB, Hirsch LJ, Foster DW, McGarry JD: Studies on the mechanism by which exogenous glucose is converted into liver glycogen in the rat, *J Biol Chem* 258(13):8046-8052, 1983.

34. Newsholme EA, Leech ER: *Biochemistry for the medical sciences,* Chichester, England, 1983, John Wiley & Sons.

35. Opie LH, Newsholme EA: The activities of fructose 1,6-diphosphatase, phosphofructokinase and phosphoenolpyruvate carboxykinase in white muscle and red muscle, *Biochem J* 103:391-399, 1967.

36. Oscai LB: Type L hormone-sensitive lipase hydrolyzes endogenous triacylglycerols in muscle in exercised rats, *Med Sci Sports Exerc* 15(4):336-339, 1983.

37. Oscai LB, Palmer WK: Cellular control of triacylglycerol metabolism, *Exerc Sport Sciences Rev* 11:1-23, 1983.

38. Piras R, Staneloni R: In vivo regulation of rat muscle glycogen synthetase activity, *Biochemistry* 8(5):2153-2160, 1969.

39. Robergs RA: Nutritional and exercise determinants of post-exercise muscle glycogen synthesis, *Int J Sports Nutr* 1:307-337, 1991.

40. Roach PJ, Takeda Y, Larner J: Rabbit skeletal muscle glycogen synthase. I. Relationship between phosphorylation state and kinetic properties, *J Biol Chem* 251(7):1913-1919, 1976.

41. Sale EM, Denton RM: Adipose-tissue phosphofructokinase, *Biochem J* 232:897-904, 1985.

42. Stryer L: *Biochemistry,* ed 3, New York, 1988, WH Freeman.

43. The National Institutes of Health: *Detection, evaluation, and treatment of high blood cholesterol in adults,* NIH Pub No 93-3095, Bethesda, Maryland, 1993, National Institutes of Health.

44. Watson JD, Hopkins NH, Roberts JW et al: *Molecular biology of the gene,* ed 4, Menlo Park, Calif, 1987, Benjamin Cummings.

45. Winder WW, Arogyasami J, Barton RJ et al: Muscle malanyl-CoA decreases during exercise, *J Appl Physiol* 67(6):2230-2233, 1989.

46. Yan Z, Spencer MK, Bechtel PJ, Katz A: Regulation of glycogen synthase in human muscle during isometric contraction and recovery, *Acta Physiol Scand* 147:77-83, 1993.

47. Yeagle PL: *The membranes of cells,* ed 2, San Diego, 1993, Academic Press.

RECOMMENDED READINGS

- Bak JF, Pedersen O: Exercise-induced activation of glycogen synthase in human skeletal muscle, *Am J Physiol* 258(21):E957–E963, 1990.

- Friden J, Seger J, Ekblom B: Topographical localization of muscle glycogen: an ultrahistochemical study in the human vastus lateralis, *Acta Physiol Scand* 135:381–391, 1989.

- Goldsmith E, Sprang S, Fletterick R: Structure of maltoheptose by difference Fourier methods and a model for glycogen, *J Mol Biol* 156:411–427, 1982.

- Johnson JL, Bagby GJ: Gluconeogenic pathway in liver and muscle glycogen synthesis after exercise, *J Appl Physiol* 64(4):1591–1599, 1988.

- Katz J, McGarry JD: The glucose paradox: is glucose a substrate for liver metabolism? *J Clin Invest* 74:1901–1909, 1984.

- Kochan RG, Lamb DR, Lutz SA et al: Glycogen synthase activation in human skeletal muscle: effects of diet and exercise, *Am J Physiol* 236(6):E660–E666, 1979.

- Kochan RG, Lamb DR, Reinman EM, Schlender KK: Modified assays to detect activation of glycogen synthase following exercise, *Am J Physiol* 240(3):E197–E202, 1981.

- Ladu MJ, Kapsas H, Palmer WK: Regulation of lipoprotein lipase in adipose and muscle tissue during fasting, *Am J Physiol* 260(29):R953–R959, 1991.

- McLane JA, Holloszy JO: Glycogen synthesis from lactate in three types of skeletal muscle, *J Biol Chem* 254(14):6548–6553, 1979.

- Oscai LB, Palmer WK: Cellular control of triacylglycerol metabolism, *Exerc Sport Sciences Rev* 11:1–23, 1983.

- Piras R, Staneloni R: In vivo regulation of rat muscle glycogen synthetase activity, *Biochemistry* 8(5):2153–2160, 1969.

- Robergs RA: Nutritional and exercise determinants of post-exercise muscle glycogen synthesis, *Int J Sports Nutr* 1:307–337, 1991.

- Roach PJ, Takeda Y, Larner J: Rabbit skeletal muscle glycogen synthase. I. Relationship between phosphorylation state and kinetic properties, *J Biol Chem* 251(7):1913–1919, 1976.

CHAPTER 6

Ergometry and Calorimetry

OBJECTIVES

After studying this chapter you should be able to:

- Define ergometry and provide examples of its application to exercise.

- Calculate work and power for bench step, cycle, and treadmill ergometry examples.

- Use conversion factors to equate work, energy, and power expressed in different units.

- Explain the differences between direct and indirect calorimetry.

- Calculate oxygen consumption, carbon dioxide production, and energy expenditure for given exercise and measured data examples.

- List the caloric equivalents (per unit weight and also relative to oxygen consumption) for pure fat and pure carbohydrate catabolism.

- State the assumptions and limitations of the nonprotein respiratory exchange ratio (RER) values.

- Explain why an increase in protein catabolism during exercise can affect calculations of caloric expenditure and the contributions of fat and carbohydrate to energy metabolism.

- Identify the modern methods available for indirect calorimetry data measurement and computation during exercise.

- Describe the importance of indirect calorimetry to the calculation of oxygen consumption and how this measure is important in the study and research of exercise physiology.

KEY TERMS

ergometry

ergometer

work

power

calorimetry

calorimeter

respiratory quotient

respiratory exchange ratio

Haldane transformation

economy

efficiency

The ability to externally regulate and quantify exercise intensity has been invaluable to the scientific study of exercise physiology. For example, the introduction of the stationary cycle enabled the quantification of work and power output during cycle exercise. Similarly, the development of equipment and techniques allowing the measurement of *oxygen consumption* provided an indirect means to quantify the metabolic intensity of steady state exercise and to calculate changes in energy expenditure with changes in exercise intensity. When controlling exercise intensity, metabolic responses can be compared between differing individuals (male versus female, young versus old, etc.), or for the same individual exposed to differing circumstances (pretraining to posttraining, low versus high altitude, etc.). Conversely, studying how differing exercise intensities affect the human body has resulted in advances in our understanding of the body at all the levels of function: molecular, cellular, tissue, organ, system, and the integrated whole.

Knowing how to quantify exercise intensity is a fundamental component of knowledge in the exercise sciences. Consequently, the purpose of this chapter is to explain the methods available for quantifying exercise intensity for various modes of exercise and to present the methods used to measure, or indirectly calculate, the energy expenditure of the body. The importance of the concepts of energy, work, and power during exercise in the science of exercise physiology cannot be overemphasized.

Ergometry

The science of **ergometry** concerns the measurement of work. Work (W) is accomplished during the application of force against gravity (F) over a distance (D), and hence is expressed as follows:

6-1
$$W = F \times D$$

Like the science of thermodynamics, ergometry was originally applied to mechanical systems. However, since the body is based on lever systems, which can produce mechanical work during dynamic muscle contraction, ergometry also has application to human movement. A device that can be used to calculate work is called an **ergometer**.

One of the earliest ergometers was a bench step (Figure 6.1, *A*). To measure work and power, subjects stepped up and down on a bench, thus raising their body weight against gravity. When a person steps on a bench of a known height at a constant rate the amount of work performed is equal to:

Force	= Body weight = 70 kg
Distance	= Step height × Rate = 0.25 m/step
	× 30 steps/min × 30 min
	= 225 m
Work	= 70 kg × 225 m
	= 15,750 kgm

6-2

Power	= Work/Time (min)
	= 15,750 kgm/30
	= 525 kgm/min

ergometry (er-gom′e-tree)
the science of the measurement of work and power

ergometer (er-gom′e-ter)
a device used to measure work

Appendix A at the end of the text provides conversions between different scientific units. The internationally recognized unit of work is the joule (J), and the recognized unit for power is J/sec (or J/min).[23] These units are extremely small, so they are often expressed in increments of 1000 as kilojoules (kJ). Unfortunately, the scientific literature in many countries uses alternate units; energy is still often expressed as kilocalories (Kcal), and power is expressed as watts (W). This is especially true for the United States. An understanding of the relationships between Kcal and kJ, and watts and kJ/sec is advantageous for the understanding of research findings published in internationally circulated journals.

Using the scientific conversions of Appendix A (1 watt = 6.118 kgm/min = 0.060 kJ/min, 1 kgm = 0.0023 Kcal, and 1 cal = 4.1860 kJ), the bench stepping exercise involved an average power output of 85.8 watts (5.1480 kJ/min), and a total mechanical energy cost of 36.23 Kcal or 151.66 kJ. This energy value is not the biologic energy expended for this activity, but the energy derived from the mechanical work produced. Because the body is not 100% efficient in converting chemical energy to mechanical energy, *the biologic energy expenditure by the body during exercise is always greater than the mechanical energy produced*. The concept of efficiency is explained, and values are calculated, in a later section of this chapter.

The distinction between work and power is important during exercise. Almost any individual can perform a given amount of work if allowed enough time. However, not all individuals can perform a similar quantity of work in a given time interval. Consequently, exercise intensity is quantified in units of power, which enables comparisons to be made within and among individuals. Individuals who can sustain high power outputs during prolonged exercise without becoming fatigued have high cardiorespiratory endurance fitness. Conversely, individuals who can generate high maximal power values during very short bursts of exercise have high muscle power and are suited to sprint and other intense short-term exercises.

Cycle Ergometry

The development of the *cycle ergometer* enabled the calculation of work and power during cycle exercise. A modern example of a cycle ergometer and the principles that it uses to quantify work and power are illustrated in Figure 6.1, *B*.

The application of friction via a belt around the front flywheel is quantified by the force required to move a pendulum attached to the belt. The distance moved by the pendulum is calibrated and generally labeled in 0.5 kg units on a scale fixed behind the pendulum. A person pedaling the bike spins the front flywheel and the product of the distance traversed by the circumference of the flywheel and the frictional force applied to the belt is equal to work and is expressed as kilogram meters (kgm). Bikes can differ in the circumferential distance traversed with one crank revolution.

The Body Guard and Monark ergometers traverse 6 m per crank revolution, and the Tunturi traverses 3 m per crank revolution.

For a Monark ergometer, **work** and **power** can then be calculated as follows:

6-3   Work = Cadence (rpm) × Load (kg) × 6 (m)
× Duration (minutes)

For example, a person riding at 60 rpm against a 2 kg load for 30 minutes performs work equal to:

$$\text{Work (kgm)} = 60 \times 2 \times 6 \times 30$$
$$= 21{,}600$$

When expressing power relative to work performed in a minute (kgm per minute, kgm/min), the previous example computes to:

$$
\begin{aligned}
\text{Power (kgm/min)} &= 21{,}600/30 \\
&= 720 \\
\text{Power (watts)} &= 720/6.118 \\
&= 118 \\
\text{Power (kJ/min)} &= 118 \times 0.060 \\
&= 7.08
\end{aligned}
$$

Many different types of cycle ergometers are used in research and fitness facilities. A popular cycle ergometer used in well-equipped research laboratories is the *constant load ergometer* (Figure 6.1, *C*). The constant load ergometer has an electronic resistance mechanism that applies resistance, varying with cadence, to a flywheel. The ability to apply variable resistance enables the subject to vary cadence within a range specified by the bike manufacturer. Consequently, unlike the traditional cycle ergometer, the bike automatically maintains a given power output (usually set as watts) across a wide range of cadence. This is advantageous in a research setting, since less time and effort by the researchers are required to ensure the correct cadence for a given exercise intensity, which decreases the likelihood of experimental error.

Another type of cycle ergometer is the isokinetic ergometer. This cycle provides the user with the option to set a given cadence and then measures the force applied to the crank shafts during cycling. These forces are used to calculate both power and work. With advances in computer and video technology, the isokinetic ergometer is becoming popular in many fitness facilities because of additional options, such as

work (wer′k)
the product of an applied force exerted over a known distance against gravity

power (pow′er)
the application of force relative to time

FIGURE 6.1

Common ergometers used during exercise. **A,** The step test. **B,** The cycle ergometer. During cycle ergometry resistance is usually applied via a friction belt surrounding the front flywheel. This friction system is calibrated with the frictional resistance, or load, and measured in kilograms. **C,** The constant load cycle ergometer. Electrical resistance is applied to a copper flywheel, and the resistance is automatically adjusted with increases or decreases in cadence to maintain a constant power output. **D,** The treadmill. The movement of the treadmill belt at given velocities is used to generate known walking or running speeds. Walking or running up hill can also be mimicked by increasing the inclination of the treadmill. **E,** Arm ergometer, which is based on the principles used in cycle ergometry. *(B through E, Courtesy Quinton Instrument Co., Bothell, Washington.)*

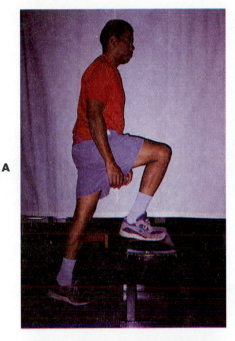

A

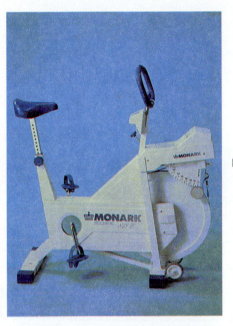

B

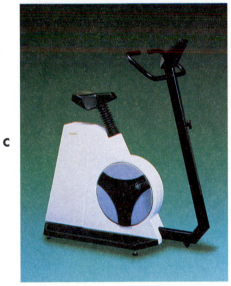

C

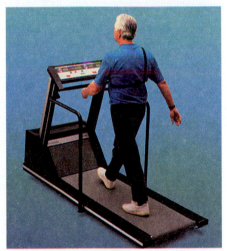

D

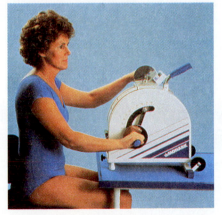

E

FIGURE 6.2

A, The inclination of a treadmill is measured as a percent grade (% grade), which is defined as the vertical rise per 100 units of horizontal translation. It is easily calculated as the tangent of the angle multiplied by 100. However, in reality measuring the angle is not easy or accurate. Consequently, measuring the vertical height (rise) of a triangle (y) and dividing it by the horizontal length of the triangle (x) yields the grade expressed as a fraction. The inverse tangent of this value is the angle. **B,** Suspension of a weight from the subject provides a force exerted against gravity, thus allowing the calculation of work during treadmill exercise. **C,** Instead of a weight, subjects can also be connected to a strain gauge positioned at the rear of a special low resistance free-spinning treadmill. During walking or running, the subject's attempts at forward movement spins the treadmill belt and force is exerted by the body on the strain gauge.

$\sin \sigma = (\text{rise} / \text{hypotenuse})$
where,
$\sigma = \text{angle} (°)$
hypotenuse = belt distance that forms a
        rignt angled triangle
if rise = 8 cm and belt distance = 58 cm,
then $\sin \sigma = (8 / 58) = 0.1379$
        $\sigma = \text{inverse sine } 0.1379$
          $= 7.9°$
percent grade = $\sin \sigma \times 100$
          $= 0.1379 \times 100 = 13.8$

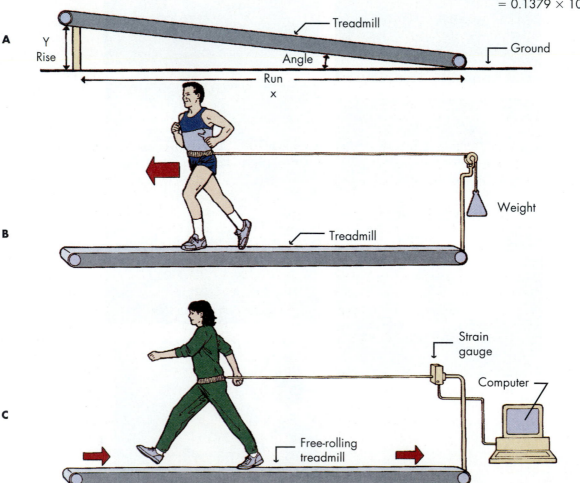

video-tape integration, competitive racing programs, and specific terrain-imitating circuits. Similar ergometers also exist for rowing and cross-country skiing.

Both constant load and isokinetic ergometers have faults. The traditional cycle ergometer can be calibrated manually, but constant load and isokinetic ergometers need to be returned to the manufacturer for recalibration. Each ergometer should be routinely checked for correct calibration.

Treadmill Ergometry

Compared with cycling, it is more difficult to apply principles of ergometry to treadmill running or walking. Level walking or running does not directly involve a translation of force against gravity. Although the body's center of gravity is moved vertically during a stride, this height is hard to quantify, differs among individuals, and is therefore hard to control. The easiest solution to this problem is to have the subject walk or run on a treadmill set at an incline (Figure 6.1, *D*). The larger the angle, the steeper the grade, and vertical distance (against gravity) can be calculated from the application of simple trigonometry (Figure 6.2, *A*). The accepted unit of treadmill grade is percent grade (% grade) and represents the relative expression of the vertical distance divided by the horizontal distance during treadmill walking or running. The conversions between %grade and angle (degree) for various % grades are presented in Table 6.1

Another method used to alleviate the problem is to attach the subject to a weight and pulley so that the weight is suspended against gravity by the subject's maintained position on the treadmill (Figure 6.2, *B*). Work and power can then be calculated in the units of kgm and kgm/min, as for cycle ergometry.

Researchers from Loughborough University in England developed a previously described method[22] to quantify work and power during sprint running on a treadmill (Figure 6.2, *C*).[8] Subjects are connected to a strain gauge, and the faster they run on the treadmill, the greater is the force they apply to the strain gauge. This equipment has been beneficial in furthering understanding of the energetics and physiologic demands of sprint running.

Swimming Ergometry

Of all the popular exercise modes, swimming has proved the most resistant to application of the principles of ergometry. The main method to gauge and quantitate exercise intensity during swimming is based on a simple pulley and suspended weight system (Figure 6.3, *A*). Maintaining the suspended weight in the same position requires effort that can be expressed as a force (weight against gravity), exerted continuously over time. Although there is no true distance component, and therefore calculations of power and work cannot be performed, this method enables researchers to perform

tests with increments of intensity, similar to the principles of a treadmill or cycle ergometer incremental exercise test.

Another swimming method more suitable for ergometry is the swimming power test developed by David Costill[11] (Figure 6.3, *B*). A belt is placed around the waist of a swimmer, and a wire that is connected to a modified isokinetic device is attached to the belt. The swimmer then swims as hard as possible. The isokinetic device maintains a constant velocity, and the strain exerted on the wire is measured as a force. This test provides data of maximal power generation during swimming and has been used to correlate swimming power and performance in competitive swimmers, as well as to monitor the effects of training programs and skill coaching on in-water power development. Similar systems have been developed for assessing velocity changes during the varied propulsive phases of the different strokes.[10,13]

Additional systems have also been developed. Waterproof strain gauges[14] have been placed on the subject's hands to measure force application in the water and, when combined with high-speed cinematography, allow calculations of power and propulsion.[13]

Finally, swimming research can be conducted with a flume (Figure 6.3, *C*). A swimming flume is a small swimming pool fitted with electronically controlled water circulation devices that generate known water velocities within the

TABLE 6.1

Conversion between angle and %grade of a treadmill

% GRADE	TANGENT Ø	Ø (DEGREES)
1	0.01	0.57
2	0.02	1.15
3	0.03	1.72
4	0.04	2.29
5	0.05	2.86
6	0.06	3.43
7	0.07	4.00
8	0.08	4.57
9	0.09	5.14
10	0.10	5.70
12	0.12	6.28
14	0.14	7.97
16	0.16	9.09
18	0.18	10.20
20	0.20	11.31

FIGURE 6.3

Methods used to quantify exercise intensity, or measure power and velocity, during swimming. **A,** The suspended weight method. **B,** The use of an isokinetic system enables the measurement of power developed by the swimmer in the water. Connecting the wire device suitable for velocity measurement provides information of changes in speed. **C,** The swimming flume. (B, Adapted from Costill DL et al: *J Swim Res* 2(1): 16-19, 1986.)

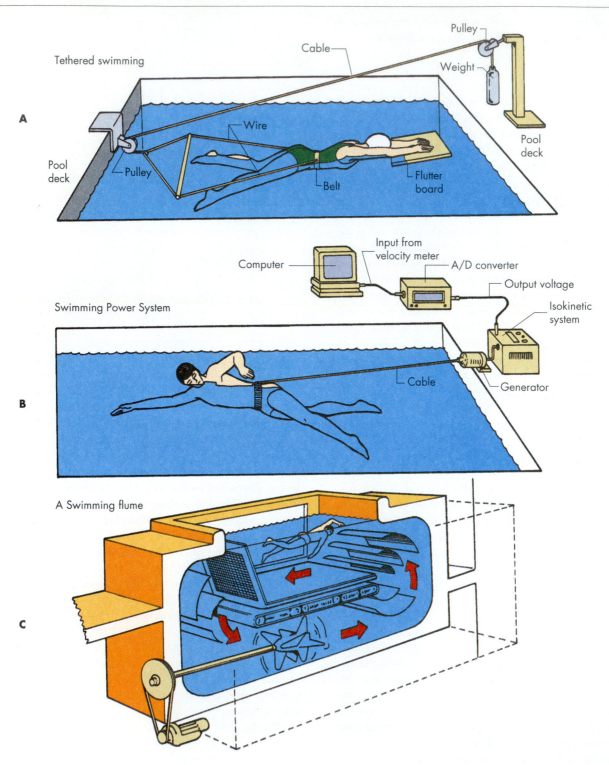

pool. Swimmers must swim against the water velocity to maintain their position in the flume, thereby swimming at a known speed. Indirect calorimetry procedures can be performed with the swimmer in the water and swimming at various velocities. As explained in Chapter 10, research of this description has determined the variation in energy cost of different swimming strokes, as well as differences between individuals with differing swimming techniques for a given stroke. Obviously the ability to measure the effectiveness of different stroke technique changes is important for improvement in swimming technique of both elite and recreational swimmers. For these and other reasons swimming flumes have been installed at the International Center For Aquatics Research, U.S. Olympic Training Center, Colorado Springs, and at the Institute for Exercise and Environmental Medicine, Dallas. Many European countries also have swimming flumes to improve the technique of their elite athletes.

Calorimetry

Many chemical reactions occur to support the body's basic needs for function and survival. The sum of all these reactions is referred to as *metabolism*. Recalling the first law of thermodynamics from Chapter 2, energy is neither created or destroyed, but simply changes form. The forms of energy that concern the body are heat, light, and chemical energy, and the products of changes in energy are work, mechanical work, and entropy. It is difficult to measure and quantify changes in entropy, light, and the chemical energy of the body. However, mechanical work can be measured as previously described in the section on ergometry and, as will be explained, changes in heat are suited to measurement and the calculation of energy expenditure in both animals and humans.

Another important meaning of the first law of thermodynamics is that energy release from the combustion of chemicals is a constant. The quantity of heat release, free energy, and entropy from the breakdown of glucose to water and carbon dioxide is the same regardless of how the breakdown occurs.

$$C_6H_{12}O_6 + 6O_2 \leftrightarrow 6CO_2 + G\ H_2O + Energy;\ \Delta G$$
$$= -648\ Kcal/mol$$

Glucose $CO_2/O_2 = 6/6 = 1.0$

$$C_{16}H_{32}O_2 + 23O_2 \leftrightarrow 16CO_2 + 16\ H_2O + Energy;$$
$$\Delta G = -2340\ Kcal/mol$$

Palmitate $CO_2/O_2 = 16/23 = 0.69$

For example, the catabolism of glucose yields 648 Kcal/mol (3.72 Kcal/g) of energy if the catabolism occurs via the numerous reactions of the body, or if the glucose molecule is combusted in a flame.[21,24] For palmitate, the body's predominant free fatty acid molecule, the heat release from its

FIGURE 6.4

The divisions of calorimetry.

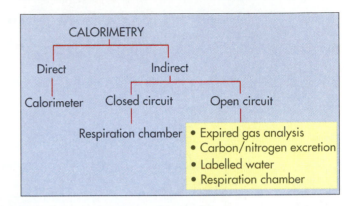

complete catabolism or combustion amounts to 2340 Kcal/mol (9.3 Kcal/g).[21,24] Because heat is a major by-product of the chemical reactions in the body, the heat production from reactions is proportional to the number or rate of the reactions. Therefore the amount of heat generated by the body is a reflection of the metabolic rate.

The science that quantifies the heat release from metabolism is termed **calorimetry** (Figure 6.4). Calorimetric methods that directly measure heat dissipation from the body are termed *direct calorimetry*.[28] When heat dissipation is calculated from other measurements, these methods are termed *indirect calorimetry*. Indirect calorimetry can be subdivided into *open-* and *closed-circuit* systems. Closed-circuit indirect calorimetry involves the recirculation of inhaled and exhaled air, thus necessitating the removal of carbon dioxide and the replenishment of oxygen. Open-circuit indirect calorimetry can involve the inhalation of atmospheric air and the sampling and measurement of exhaled air for respiratory gas analysis. Other forms of indirect open-circuit calorimetry exist, such as measuring total carbon and nitrogen exchange and measuring the exchange of labeled water within the body. Before we elaborate on direct and indirect calorimetry, the historical development of the science of calorimetry is explained.

History of Calorimetry

Table 6.2 is a time line identifying the dates of important scientific discoveries that influenced the development of calorimetry. As indicated, calorimetry dates back to the eighteenth century. The initial findings of the importance of air for life and the release of heat during combustion were identified by scientists such as Crawford and Antoine-Laurent

calorimetry (kal'o-ri-met'ri)

the measurement of body metabolism from heat release from the body

TABLE 6.2

Time line for important scientific developments in calorimetry

NAME	DEVELOPMENT	DATE	DEVELOPMENT	NAME
		1688	Air known to be necessary for life and combustion	Mayow
Crawford, Lavoisier	First direct animal calorimetry research	1770s		
		1785	Discovery of hydrogen	Cavendish
		1790	Observation that exercise increased V_{O_2}	Lavoisier
Despret, Dulong	First combined calorimeters and respirometers	1820-1840		
		1837	Discovery that blood contains oxygen	Magnus
Mayer	First law of thermodynamics formulated	1842		
Joule	Mechanical equivalent of heat determined	1842		
		1849	First description of a closed-circuit respirometer	Renault, Reiset
Pettenkofer, Voit	First open-circuit respirometer built	1862		
Pettenkofer, Voit	First experiments on the affects of exercise on metabolism	1860s	Heat value of certain foodstuffs and urea determined from bomb calorimetry	Frankland
		1866	Proportions of carbon, notrogen, and oxygen in metabolism were determined	Pettenkofer, Voit
		1866	Animal experimental results supported a nitrogen equilibrium	Voit
Rubner	Dietary thermogenesis shown to be larger for protein than fat or carbohydrate	1885		
Haldane	Development of an open-circuit respiratory apparatus	1892		
Atwater, Rosa	First description of the Atwater-Rosa respiration calorimeter	1897		
		1901	Gram caloric value of carbohydrate, fat, and protein catabolism determined in animals (4.1, 9.3, and 4.1 kcal/g, respectively)	Rubner
Rubner, Atwater	Validation of indirect respiratory methods of calorimetry	1902-1903		
Rubner	Basal metabolism known to be proportional to body surface area	1902		
		1903	Rubner's findings replicated in humans	Atwater, Benedict
Tissot	Development of Tissot tank for expired air collection	1904		
		1905	Development of the Douglas bag for expired air collection	Douglas

TABLE 6.2—Cont'd

Time line for important scientific developments in calorimetry

NAME	DEVELOPMENT	DATE	DEVELOPMENT	NAME
Atwater, Benedict	Refinement of the Atwater-Rosa respiration closed-circuit calorimeter	1905		
		1906	Development of a portable, back-mounted open-circuit calorimetry apparatus	?
Shaffer	First experimental human evidence for no increase in protein metabolism during exercise	1908		
Loewy	Caloric equivalents for protein catabolism determined in body, urine, and feces; Value for protein RER calculated	1911	Oxygen and carbon dioxide requirement of one gram of urinary nitrogen calculated (8.49 and 9.35 g, respectively)	Loewy
		1913	Mechanical efficiency calculated to be 33% for stationary cycling	Benedict, Cathcart
		1914	Basal Vo_2 shown to increase with increased body temperatures	Krogh
Du Bois	Developement of the height-weight formula for calculating body surface area	1916		
Lusk	Publication of the nonprotein RER and caloric equivalent table	1924		
Michaelis	Nomogram for determining the caloric equivalent for Vo_2 from the nonprotein RER, amount of urinary nitrogen, and Vo_2	1926		
Michaelis	Application of electronic gas analyzers and temperature gradient instrumentation	post WWII		
		1952	Development of the Max Planck respirometer	Muller
Lifson	Validation of the doubly labeled body water technique	1955		
		1958	Development of the pneumotachograph	Wolff

Lavoisier. It was Lavoisier who theorized that a component of air, which he called "oxygen," supported life and combustion. Lavoisier also theorized that the heat released during combustion and metabolism resulted from the process of oxidation of carbon and the formation of carbon dioxide. Unfortunately, Lavoisier's premature death in 1794 prevented him from proving his theories and little development occurred in the science of calorimetry until 1822.

In 1822 the Academie de Sciences in Paris announced "The Determination of the Source of Animal Heat" as the topic of a prize study.[26] This award prompted the development of several direct calorimeters combined with the closed-circuit measurement of oxygen consumption and carbon dioxide production *(respiration calorimeters)* (Figure 6.5).

Although the initial research with these devices did not support an association between heat release estimates from gas analysis and direct calorimetric measurements, the subsequent formulation of the first law of thermodynamics in 1842 provided sound reasoning that the total heat release from metabolism should be accounted for if all of the products of metabolism could be quantified and the heat release associated with each known.

In 1842 work was also being performed on the nitrogen balance of the body. Liebig had demonstrated that protein contains nitrogen, that measuring urine nitrogen is an indirect means to measure protein catabolism, and that the nitrogen lost in the urine accounts for a large proportion of the nitrogen consumed in food.[26]

FIGURE 6.5

An illustration of the Atwater-Benedict respiration calorimeter, which was developed during the early 1900s. The walls of the chamber are insulated. Direct calorimetry measurements were made from the chamber from the simple measurement of the change in temperature of water as it was circulated through the chamber. Indirect calorimetry measurements were made from the circulation of air through the chamber, requiring oxygen replenishment to replace that used, and the removal of the carbon dioxide produced by soda lime. Carbon dioxide production was then measured chemically by the change in the weight and composition of the soda lime per unit time. (Adapted from McLean JA, Tobin G: *Animal and human calorimetry,* New York, 1987, Cambridge University Press.)

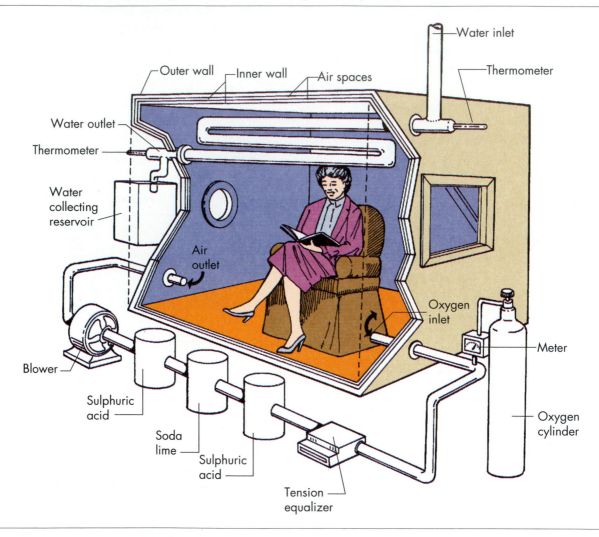

Renault and Reiset built the first closed-circuit respirometer and reported their findings in 1849. These scientists experimented with different species of animals and demonstrated that the ratio of carbon dioxide production and oxygen consumption varies with the type of food ingested. These findings sparked the inquiry of several German researchers and resulted in the development of the first open-circuit respirometer by Pettenkofer.[26] Pettenkofer and Voit used this chamber to measure carbon dioxide production and excretion of carbon and of nitrogen. From these data oxygen consumption was calculated, and results indicated that

metabolism could be accounted for by the oxidation of three food-stuffs: carbohydrate, fat, and protein. Furthermore, the data proved that nitrogen excretion could be accounted for by the nitrogen content of urine and feces, and therefore that the body could be in a state of nitrogen equilibrium. When nitrogen excretion was greater than ingestion, the body was in a state of protein catabolism. When nitrogen excretion was less than ingestion, the body was in a state of protein synthesis.

In 1860 Bischoff and Voit completed calculations on the caloric and respiratory gas exchange involved in the combustion of certain foods and pure nutrients. The calorimeter used

FIGURE 6.6

A typical bomb calorimeter. The calorimeter consists of a heavy insulated metal shell, a capsule for the sample to be combusted, a water bath pressurized with at least 20 atmospheres of oxygen, a thermometer to measure water temperature, and an electric fuse to ignite the food sample. The number of calories used to combust the food is determined by the increase in water temperature. Analyzing the air for decreases in oxygen and increases in carbon dioxide, enable calculations of oxygen consumption and carbon dioxide production. (Adapted from Bursztein S et al: *Energy metabolism, indirect calorimetry, and nutrition,* Baltimore, 1989, Williams & Wilkins.)

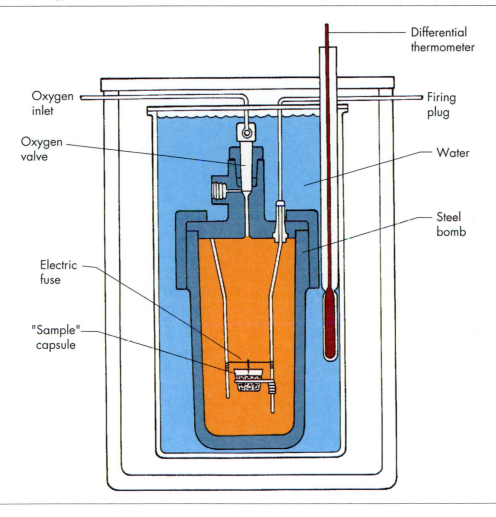

to combust food was called a *bomb calorimeter.* Bomb calorimetry was an important advancement to understanding the energy value of foods. A typical bomb calorimeter is shown in Figure 6.6. When a food source is ignited in an oxygen-rich environment, the heat release is measured via the increase in temperature of circulating water, and measurements of oxygen consumption and carbon dioxide are also made. Consequently, if a given quantity of pure carbohydrate, fat, or protein is combusted, given amounts of oxygen consumption, carbon dioxide production, and heat release can be measured. These values are listed in Table 6.3.

Researchers knew that the products of carbohydrate and fat catabolism were similar for the body and combustion; however, for nitrogen catabolism the products of metabolism were different from those of combustion. Catabolism of protein in the body yielded carbon dioxide, water, urea, nitrogen waste in feces, and additional carbon compounds in urine and feces (e.g., creatinine). Consequently, the excreted nitrogen and carbon compounds accompanying protein metabolism represented a loss in potential heat release, which had to be subtracted from known bomb calorimetry caloric equivalents for protein.

Rubner determined the caloric value of protein combustion in a bomb calorimeter, measured the energy release of dried urine and feces, and calculated the difference in energy release from protein between bomb calorimetry and

TABLE 6.3

Heat release* and caloric equivalants for oxygen† for the main macronutrients of catabolism

FOOD	RUBNER'S Kcal/gm	Kcal/g BOMB Cal	Kcal/g BODY	RQ	Kcal/L O_2
MIXED CARBOHYDRATE	4.1	4.1	4.0	1.0	5.05
Glycogen		4.2		1.0	5.05
Glucose		3.7		1.0	4.98
Fructose		3.7		1.0	5.00
Glycerol		4.3		0.86	5.06
MIXED FAT	9.3	9.3	8.9	0.70	4.73
Palmitate (C 16:0)		9.3		0.70	4.65
Stearate (C 18:0)		9.5		0.69	4.65
Triacylglycerol (C 18:0)		9.6		0.70	4.67
Medium chain length					
Triacylglycerols		8.4		0.74	4.69
MIXED PROTEIN	4.1	5.7	4.3	0.81	4.46
Alanine		4.4		0.83	4.62
Aspartate		2.69		1.17	4.60
Glutamate		3.58		1.0	4.58
Isoleucine		6.89		0.73	4.64
ALCOHOL		7.1	7.0	0.82	4.86
MIXED DIET				0.84	4.83

*Data compiled from Lusk,[26] Livesey and Elia,[24] Bursztein et al,[5] and Fox et al.[19]
†RQ = VCO_2 / VO_2; Kcal / LO_2 = caloric equivalent for oxygen.

metabolism. In 1901 Rubner published caloric equivalent values for different types of carbohydrate, fat, and protein molecules that are metabolized in the body (see Table 6.3).[26]

Assuming percentage contributions of these molecules to total metabolism, Rubner deduced that the appropriate average values to use for carbohydrate, fat, and protein were 4.1, 9.3, and 4.1 Kcal/g, respectively. Rubner's findings were replicated in human subjects by Atwater and Benedict in 1903 with a more sophisticated closed–circuit respiration calorimeter[1,26] (see Figure 6.6). It is ironic that Atwater, an American, has received historical recognition for these values when the pioneering original work was published by Rubner, a German, before the experiments of Atwater and Benedict had begun.

Knowledge of the caloric equivalents for excreted nitrogen and carbon and metabolized carbohydrate, fat, and protein enabled researchers to discern their contributions to heat release. The data for metabolic heat release and the respiratory gas requirements of protein catabolism were based on Rub-

ner's and Lowey's documentation that 1 g of urinary nitrogen represented 25.98 Kcal of energy from protein catabolism, which would require 8.49 and 9.35 g of oxygen consumption and carbon dioxide production, respectively. Lusk[26] removed the caloric release, oxygen consumption, and carbon dioxide production because of basal protein catabolism from total body metabolism. The remainder of oxygen consumption, carbon dioxide production, and heat release was then attributable to carbohydrate and fat metabolism. Because carbohydrate and lipid catabolism differ in oxygen consumption and carbon dioxide production, the ratio of the volume of carbon dioxide production and oxygen consumption (respiratory quotient [RQ]) was used to indicate the predominance of carbohydrate or fat as the substrate for catabolism.

Data from Lusk, published in 1928, are presented in Table 6.4 and represent oxygen consumption, carbon dioxide production, and caloric equivalents for different mixtures of carbohydrate and fat during metabolism. As a result of the subtraction of protein from this data set, it is often referred to

TABLE 6.4

Caloric equivalents for the range of nonprotein respiratory quotient (RQ) values (caloric values from carbohydrate and fat are also listed for each RQ value)

RQ	Kcal/L O_2	% Kcals CHO	Kcal/L O_2 CHO	% Kcals FAT	Kcal/L O_2 FAT
1.00	5.047	100.00	5.047	0.0	0.000
0.99	5.035	96.80	4.874	3.18	0.160
0.98	5.022	93.60	4.701	6.37	0.230
0.97	5.010	90.40	4.529	9.58	0.480
0.96	4.998	87.20	4.358	12.80	0.640
0.95	4.985	84.00	4.187	16.00	0.798
0.94	4.973	80.70	4.013	19.30	0.960
0.93	4.961	77.40	3.840	22.60	1.121
.092	4.948	74.10	3.666	25.90	1.281
0.91	4.936	70.80	3.495	29.20	1.441
0.90	4.924	67.50	3.324	32.50	1.600
0.89	4.911	64.20	3.153	35.80	1.758
0.88	4.899	60.80	2.979	39.20	1.920
0.87	4.887	57.50	2.810	42.50	2.077
0.86	4.875	54.10	2.637	45.90	2.238
0.85	4.862	50.70	2.465	49.30	2.397
0.84	4.850	47.20	2.289	52.80	2.561
0.83	4.838	43.80	2.119	56.20	2.719
0.82	4.825	40.30	1.944	59.70	2.880
0.81	4.813	36.90	1.776	63.10	3.037
0.80	4.801	33.40	1.603	66.60	3.197
0.79	4.788	29.90	1.432	70.10	3.356
0.78	4.776	26.30	1.256	73.70	3.520
0.77	4.764	22.30	1.062	77.20	3.678
0.76	4.751	19.20	0.912	80.80	3.839
0.75	4.739	15.60	0.739	84.40	4.000
0.74	4.727	12.00	0.567	88.00	4.160
0.73	4.714	8.40	0.396	91.60	4.318
0.72	4.702	4.76	0.224	95.20	4.476
0.71	4.690	1.10	0.052	98.90	4.638
0.707	4.686	0.0	0.000	100.00	4.686

To convert Kcal to kJ, multiply by 4.184.
*Modified from Lusk G: *The elements of the science of nutrition,* ed 4, Philadelphia, 1928, WB Saunders.

FIGURE 6.7

A nomogram for altering the caloric equivalents of oxygen for catabolism at nonprotein RQ values for given relative increases in urinary nitrogen. (Adapted from Michaelis AM: *J Biol Chem* 59: 51-58, 1924.)

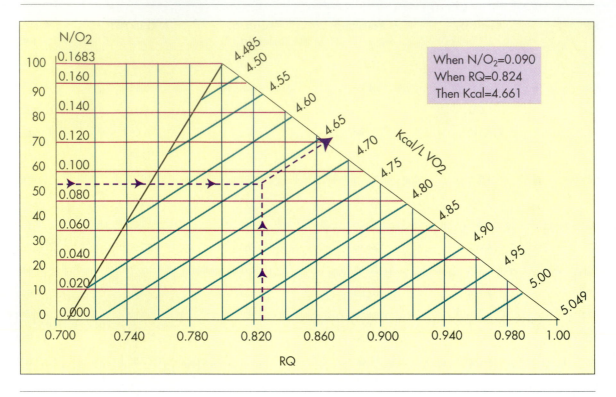

as *nonprotein* data. As early as 1866 Pettenkofer and Voit demonstrated that moderate amounts of exercise did not increase protein metabolism and therefore that increased energy was provided by the metabolism of carbohydrate and fat.[26] These findings were supported by more elaborate research by Atwater in 1904,[1] and again by Shaffer in 1908.[32] However, research has also been completed that contradicted these findings. Campbell and Webster[7] reported that a man who expended 100,000 kgm of work on a cycle ergometer increased urinary nitrogen from 8.01 g/day to 10.25 g/day. Additional research involving more intense and shorter duration exercise also indicated an increase in protein catabolism.[26] Ironically, the implications of these early findings were overshadowed by the many studies in humans and animals that verified the predominance of carbohydrate and fat catabolism during exercise.[26]

As explained in Chapter 10, an increase in protein catabolism during exercise was reevaluated in the 1970s and sophisticated techniques proved that prolonged exercise can increase protein catabolism. Nevertheless, the nonprotein RQ and caloric equivalents are still used today for computing caloric expenditure during many, but not all, rest and exercise conditions.

Knowledge of the caloric equivalents for excreted nitrogen and carbon and metabolized carbohydrate, fat, and protein enables researchers to discern their contributions to heat release. Figure 6.7 presents a nomogram, developed by Michaelis in 1924,[29] to determine the contribution of protein, carbohydrate, and fat catabolism to caloric expenditure. From this nomogram it is clear that for a given nonprotein RQ an increase in protein catabolism lowers the caloric equivalent for oxygen consumption and the contribution of carbohydrate and fat catabolism to energy production.

The validation of indirect (respiration) methods of calorimetry enabled application of indirect open–circuit gas analysis calorimetry to varied metabolic conditions. Researchers measured basal energy requirements under different environmental conditions and established the relationships between metabolic rate and body temperature, body surface area, and the intensity of exercise.[6,7,26,27] Interestingly, research completed as early as 1910 demonstrated the superiority of carbohydrate as the main dietary component to fuel the muscles during exercise.[26]

The recent history of calorimetry witnessed the development of more sophisticated instrumentation and alternate methods of both direct and indirect calorimetry. For indirect calorimetry, expired gas collection bags (Douglas bags), portable gas collection and analysis units, improved electronic gas volume and gas analyzer instrumentation, and computerization of data collection have enabled greater use of this technique during varied conditions (Figure 6.8). Direct calorimeters are currently used in many metabolic and nutri-

FIGURE 6.8

Common methods used to collect and sample expired gases during indirect gas analysis calorimetry. **A,** The use of a Douglas bag, gas analyzers, and a gas flow meter to obtain measurements required in calorimetry. The air collected in the Douglas bag is saturated with water vapor and at room temperature. A small volume of this collected air is pumped through gas analyzers to determine the fraction of oxygen and carbon dioxide. The volume of collected air is then measured via a flow meter. The expired volume must be converted to standard conditions before being used in the calculations of Focus Box 6.1 (See Appendix B). **B,** A simple, portable, time-averaged system for indirect calorimetry. Expired gas flow is measured via a pneumotach, expired air is sampled from a mixing bag and pumped to oxygen and carbon dioxide electronic analyzers, and data is acquired, processed, and calculations completed by a computer. **C,** An advanced breath-by-breath system. Rapidly responding analyzers and powerful computerization enable calculations to made every breath. (C, Courtesy Medical Graphics Corp., St. Paul Minnesota.)

A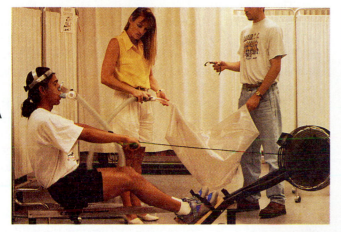

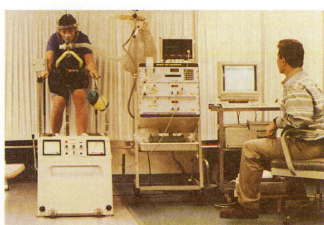 B

C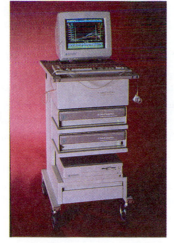

tion divisions of hospitals to research metabolic abnormalities in patients, and the validation of alternative indirect methods such as doubly labeled body water has enabled research of long-term metabolism without the expense and confinement of large direct calorimeters. Nevertheless, the science of direct and indirect calorimetry still relies on classic work by such researchers as Rubner, Voit, and Atwater, which testifies to the quality of their work especially since the equipment they used was more labor intensive, tedious, and open to error than today's scientific equipment and methodology.

Direct Calorimetry

As noted in previous description of the historical development of calorimetry, the direct **calorimeter** was the first tool used to measure caloric expenditure in animals and humans. Direct calorimeters are expensive pieces of equip-

calorimeter (kal'o-rim'eter)
an instrument that measures heat release from the body

ment. In addition, they are more suited to measuring basal metabolic demands than those of exercise for several reasons: (1) exercise performed in a direct calorimeter causes added heat production from friction developed by the ergometer and the subject; (2) during exercise the body stores heat, as evidenced by this rise in core temperature; and (3) the method is not suited to providing data in small time intervals, which is necessary to measure the rapidity of the changes in metabolic rate during changes in exercise intensity.

Today direct calorimetry is used to study basal metabolic rate, daily energy expenditure, and the influence of altered environmental or physiologic conditions on these values. For example, direct calorimeters large enough to allow people to live inside for several days have been used to determine the factors that influence basal and daily metabolic rate.[3]

Indirect Calorimetry

The fact that a known amount of oxygen is required to combust gram equivalents of carbohydrate, fat, and protein is extremely important. If oxygen consumption can be measured and quantified, the proportion of carbohydrate, fat, or protein used during metabolism and heat release (caloric expenditure) can be calculated. The most common procedure for this is *indirect gas analysis calorimetry*. As previously stated, indirect gas analysis calorimetry can be performed via an open- or closed-circuit system.

Open-Circuit Indirect Calorimetry

Although the mathematic calculations of open-circuit indirect calorimetry have remained unchanged since the respiration calorimetry work of Rubner and Atwater, the equipment that was originally used differs considerably from today's computerized systems. The principles, equations, and assumptions of indirect calorimetry are presented in Focus Box 6.1.

When concerned with exercise, the predominant application of indirect calorimetry is the measurement of oxygen consumption, which can be used to assess the metabolic intensity of exercise. Also, the ratio between carbon dioxide production and oxygen consumption is used to indicate the contribution of fat and carbohydrate substrates to energy production. However, as discussed in the section on energy production, several factors can invalidate the accurate use of indirect calorimetric calculations for determining the contribution of fat and carbohydrate to energy production.

Respiratory quotient and the respiratory exchange ratio. The ratio between carbon dioxide production and oxygen consumption is traditionally called the **respiratory quotient (RQ)**. This measure is calculated the same way as the **respiratory exchange ratio (RER)**, but the conditions of production of carbon dioxide differ. The RQ is used to indicate cellular respiration and therefore the VO_2 and VCO_2 resulting from the catabolism of food. The RER is used when VO_2 and VCO_2 are measured from ventilated air resulting from

external respiration at the lung. When sampling air from the lung, the ratio of VCO_2/VO_2 can be modified by increased exhalation of CO_2 that is unrelated to the cellular production of CO_2 from the catabolic pathways of carbohydrate, fat, or protein. *When calculated or measured gas volumes relate solely to cellular respiration, the term RQ should be used. When measured gas volumes can be influenced by additional sources of CO_2, the term RER should be used.* These rules are adhered to in this text.

<u>6-4</u> $$RER = VCO_2 / VO_2$$

The energy released from catabolism for every liter of oxygen consumed at different nonprotein RQ values is listed in Table 6.4. The RQ values theoretically reflect carbohydrate and lipid catabolism, with an RQ value of 1.0 reflecting pure carbohydrate catabolism and an RQ value of 0.71 reflecting pure lipid catabolism.

The RQ is important because when carbon dioxide production is occurring only from cellular metabolism, and assuming that no change in protein (amino acid) catabolism occurs during exercise, the RQ value can be used to accurately reflect the proportion of fat and carbohydrate catabolized for energy during exercise, which allows calculations of energy expenditure during exercise.

For many metabolic and exercise conditions the RER is often assumed to be equal to the RQ. Therefore the RER is used to calculate contributions of either fat or carbohydrate to catabolism and to calculate caloric expenditure. However, the assumption of equality between RQ and RER cannot be made under certain conditions. These conditions and their interpretations include the following:

1. *Metabolic acidosis:* Within the cell the production of carbon dioxide cannot exceed the consumption of oxygen, and the maximal value of 1.0 for VCO_2/VO_2 occurs from the metabolism of pure carbohydrate. During metabolic conditions that increase acid production (intense exercise, ketosis, etc.), the added carbon dioxide produced from the buffering of acid in the body increases VCO_2 independent of oxygen consumption (VO_2), and therefore RER values can exceed 1.0. Consequently during exercise the RER value can also be used as an indirect measure of exercise intensity. During exercise, if the RER increases to above 1.0, it can be concluded that acid production (presumably lactate) is increasing. If the RER continues to increase above 1.0 during exercise, fatigue is imminent unless the exercise intensity is decreased. Basal conditions of acidosis, such as during ketosis, raise the RER and cause an incorrect assumption of an increased contribution of carbohydrate to catabolism.

2. *Non–steady state conditions:* When a person has increased his or her exercise intensity, it takes time for the VO_2 to increase to a level that accounts for the ATP produced during metabolism. During these times the ATP is produced from alternative sources,

FOCUS BOX 6.1

Principles, equations, and assumptions of indirect gas analysis calorimetry

Principles

The fundamental principle of indirect calorimetry is that the volume of oxygen consumed by the body equals the difference between the volumes of inspired (V_IO_2) and expired oxygen (V_EO_2)

6-5, A
$$VO_2 = V_IO_2 - V_EO_2$$

The variables V_IO_2 and V_EO_2 can be further partitioned, with equation (6.5, A) expressed differently as:

6-5, B
$$VO_2 = V_IF_IO_2 - V_EF_EO_2$$

where
F_IO_2 = fraction of oxygen in inspired air
F_EO_2 = fraction of oxygen in expired air

To solve the dilemma of needing to measure both inspired and expired volumes of air when using equation (6.5, B), the fact that nitrogen is physiologically inert, and therefore that on average inspired nitrogen must equal expired nitrogen, is used to solve for V_I.

6-5, C
$$V_IN_2 = V_EN_2$$

6-5, D and, $\quad V_IF_IN_2 = V_EF_EN_2$

6-5, E thus, $\quad V_I = V_EF_EN_2 / F_IN_2$

6-5, F $\quad V_I = V_E (F_EN_2 / F_IN_2)$

The gas fractions in atmospheric air are as follows:

Gas	Fraction
Oxygen	0.2093
Nitrogen	0.7903
Carbon dioxide	0.0003
Argon, helium, etc.	0.0001
Total	**1.0**

If the rare gas component of air is neglected, the F_EN_2 can be rewritten as $[1-(F_ECO_2 + F_EO_2)]$, and equation (6.5, F) can be rewritten as:

6-5, G
$$V_I = V_E \times \frac{[1 - (F_ECO_2 + F_EO_2)]}{0.7903}$$

Equating V_I by assuming inspired nitrogen equals expired nitrogen is called the **Haldane transformation.**[25] Although data also exist to refute its accuracy,[9,15] replicated studies have been performed that have all documented the similarity of inspired and expired nitrogen volumes.[18,25,33,35] Consequently the Haldane transformation and resulting indirect calorimetry equations for calculating oxygen consumption, carbon dioxide production, and energy expenditure are widely accepted by educators and scientists.

Incorporating equation (6.5, G) into equation (6.5, B) provides the final equation to calculate oxygen consumption:

6-5, H $\quad VO_2 = (V_E \times \dfrac{[1 - (F_ECO_2 + F_EO_2)]}{0.7903} \times F_IO_2) - V_E \times F_EO_2$

Carbon dioxide production

Carbon dioxide production is equal to the carbon dioxide expired minus the carbon dioxide inspired.

6-5, I
$$VCO_2 = V_EF_ECO_2 - V_IF_ICO_2$$

Solving for this equation is relatively easy compared with calculating oxygen consumption. Assuming that oxygen consumption is calculated first, V_I is then already calculated, and all that is needed is to incorporate V_I, V_E (measured), F_ICO_2 (0.0003), and F_ECO_2 (measured) into equation (6.5, I). Because of the small value of F_ICO_2, a ventilation even as large as 150 L/min would yield a value of only 0.045 L/min for inspired carbon dioxide. Consequently, seemingly accurate values can be obtained by simply equating $VCO_2 = V_EF_ECO_2$. Nevertheless, it is recommended that the student complete the calculation with equation (6.5, I) to uphold the principle of the measurement.

namely creatine phosphate hydrolysis and glycolysis. Calculating VO$_2$ during non–steady state conditions would give a lower metabolic intensity than if the person were at steady state. In addition, a higher RER may be calculated, and together these values would yield incorrect calculations of energy expenditure and the contribution of fat and carbohydrate to steady state catabolism. If the exercise intensity is not too high, approximately 3 minutes are required for the attainment of steady state.

3. *Hyperventilation:* Excessive exhalation increases the volume of carbon dioxide exhaled from the lung. If

respiratory quotient
the ratio of carbon dioxide production to oxygen consumption during metabolism

respiratory exchange ratio
the ratio of carbon dioxide production to oxygen consumption, as measured from expired gas analysis indirect calorimetry

Haldane transformation
the use of equal inspired and expired nitrogen volumes to solve for either inspired or expired ventilatory volumes

this phenomenon occurs without similar increases in VO_2 a higher VCO_2 results from indirect gas analysis calorimetry, yielding an inflated RER value.

4. *Excess postexercise VO_2:* After exercise, VO_2 declines but remains above pre-exercise values for several minutes, whereas VCO_2 decreases rapidly. Consequently the RER may decline below resting values for several minutes.

The previously mentioned circumstances that can alter RER values must be understood when performing research or interpreting exercise responses. These circumstances could cause error in calculations of the contribution of foodstuffs to catabolism and, as explained, in the calculations of energy expenditure.

Energy Expenditure

The calculation of energy expenditure using the non-protein data of Lusk (see Table 6.4) is a simple process involving the multiplication of oxygen consumption (L/min), time (minutes), and the caloric equivalent for the respective RER of the exercise (Kcal/LO_2).

6-6   Kcal = VO_2 (L/min) × RER caloric equivalent (Kcal/L)
× Time (minutes) (6-6).

For example, when exercise is performed for 30 minutes requiring a VO_2 of 1.5 L/min, with an average RER of 0.9 (see Table 6.4), caloric expenditure can be calculated as:

$$Kcal = 1.5 \times 4.924 \times 30$$
$$= 221.6$$

Based on Table 6.4, the contribution of fat and carbohydrate to the energy expenditure can be calculated. For example, from the previous calculation of VO_2, RER, and Kcal:

% Kcal from fat = [(1-RQ)/(1-0.7)] × 100
% Kcal from carbohydrate (CHO) = 100 − (% Kcal from fat)

With a reported RQ=0.9, 33.3% of the Kcal are derived from fat, while 66.7% of the Kcal are derived from carbohydrates.

Kcals from fat = 0.33 × (221.6 Kcal/30 min) = 2.46 Kcal/min
Kcals from CHO = 0.667 × (221.6 Kcal/30 min) = 4.93 Kcal/min

Assume caloric densities of 4 Kcal/g for CHO and 9 Kcal/g for fat.

fat usage = (2.46 Kcal/min) / (9 Kcal/g) = 0.27 g fat/min
CHO usage = (4.93 Kcal/min) / (4 Kcal/g) = 1.23 g CHO/min

If dietary, disease, or exercise conditions exist that are accompanied by increased protein catabolism, calculations of energy expenditure using the nonprotein RER data of Lusk

may be inaccurate. However, even as early as the 1920s it was understood that the error inherent in increased protein catabolism was negligible. For example, using the data of Michaelis[29] (see Figure 6.7), a 10% increase in urinary nitrogen with an RER of 0.9 lowers the caloric equivalent for oxygen from 4.925 to 4.90 Kcal/L O_2, resulting in a 1% error in caloric expenditure for a VO_2 of 2.0 L/min. Recent nutrition research by Livesey and Elia[24] has supported this fact. However, although the errors are negligible when computing caloric expenditure during conditions of increased protein catabolism, approximating contributions of fat or carbohydrate to energy expenditure can have errors as large as 60% under these conditions.[24] Metabolic conditions that increase protein catabolism are starvation, diabetes mellitus, prolonged exercise during restricted carbohydrate nutrition, and excess protein ingestion.

Table 6.3 presented known heat release and caloric equivalents for the combustion of certain carbohydrates, fats, and amino acids. The caloric release during food combustion has high variability within and between food categories, and high variability also exists for the measures of RQ and Kcal/L O_2. The lower values for the caloric release during combustion in the body compared to the bomb calorimeter are due to relative inefficiencies of digestion. The respective adjustments for carbohydrate, fat, and protein for the inefficiency of digestion are -2%, -5%, and -25% (-8% digestion and -17% loss in urine).[18]

Systems Used In Indirect Calorimetry

Remarkable research involving indirect calorimetry was completed by such scientists as Rubner, Atwater, and Zuntz during the late 1890s and early 1900s. In those days, without the convenience of electronic gas analyzers, gas mass spectrometers, and computerization, scientists analyzed gas fractions and calculated oxygen consumption by tedious manual methods. As illustrated in Figure 6.5, respiration calorimeter studies of basal metabolism required that carbon dioxide be chemically removed from air and measured as a change in weight of the reactants. Oxygen was provided at a rate that equaled its consumption, and therefore oxygen consumption was relatively easy to measure.[5,26,28] However, the need to measure respiratory gases during different exercise intensities required that methods be devised for sampling gases at known intervals. Expired air samples were obtained in special airtight glass syringes and later analyzed chemically in either a Scholander or a Haldane apparatus (Figure 6.9). Expired gas volumes were measured from timed gas samples collected in large meteorologic balloons or Douglas bags (see Figure 6.8, *A*).

Within the last 20 years the sophistication of the equipment used in indirect calorimetry has increased remarkably. Today, data are obtained, processed, and calculated within seconds, enabling the monitoring of changes during very small time intervals. Figure 6.8, *B* and *C* illustrate some of the

FIGURE 6.9

A diagram of the Haldane apparatus, used to chemically quantify the fraction of oxygen and carbon dioxide in air samples. This device is in stark contrast to the sophisticated computer interfaced electronics of today's indirect calorimetry equipment. (Figure 6.8). *A*, Thermobarometer; *B*, measuring burette; *C*, mercury reservoir; *D*, absorption chamber; *E*, absorption chamber; *F*, KOH reservoir; *G*, 1,2,4-benzenetriol reservoir. (From McLean JA, Tobin G: *Animal and human calorimetry*, New York, 1987, Cambridge University Press. Reprinted with the permission of Cambridge University Press.)

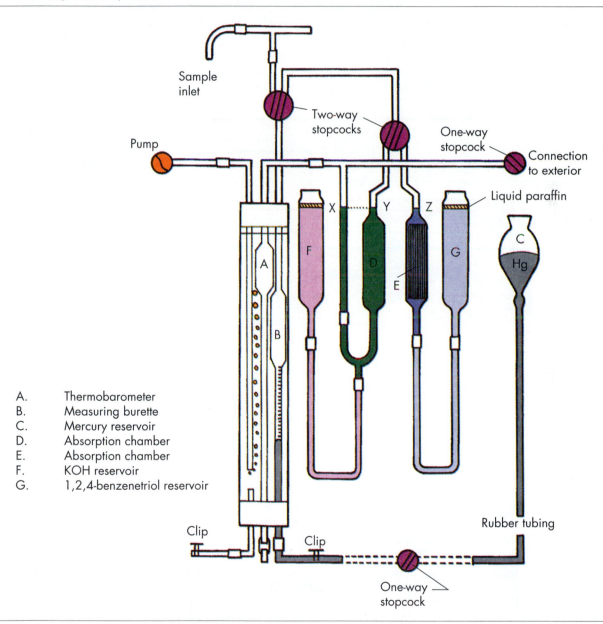

A. Thermobarometer
B. Measuring burette
C. Mercury reservoir
D. Absorption chamber
E. Absorption chamber
F. KOH reservoir
G. 1,2,4-benzenetriol reservoir

advances in equipment since the time of the Scholander apparatus. Ventilation measurement is now performed by advanced electronics less than one tenth the size of the original volume meters, and the response times of the electronic analyzers for oxygen and carbon dioxide are now as short as 100 ms. When these improvements are combined with computer software and hardware advances that enable the handling of information at high speed, the automation of indirect calorimetry data collection is now a common feature of many advanced research and clinical exercise testing laboratories.

Time-Averaged and Breath-By-Breath Calculations of Oxygen Consumption

Today's computerized sophistication with indirect calorimetry has enabled the production of several different systems.[20] The basic designs of computerized indirect calorimetry systems are illustrated in Figure 6.10. For the

FIGURE 6.10

Schematics of time-averaged and breath-by-breath indirect calorimetry systems. **A,** A typical time-averaged system. Ventilation is measured on the inspired side via a large capacity low resistance flow meter. Expired air is directed to a mixing chamber, from which air is pumped to electronic oxygen and carbon dioxide analyzers. The flow meter and analyzers are electronically connected to an analog to digital (A-D) converter, and digital signals are received by a computer that runs software enabling the calculations of indirect calorimetry to be made and printed or displayed on a screen. **B,** The breath-by-breath system is configured differently. Expired air samples are obtained from tubing connected to the mouthpiece and are pumped to rapidly responding analyzers. Expired air flow rate is measured by a pneumotach, or a low resistance impeller, with the exhaust air returned to the room. Electronic connections to a powerful high capacity computer enables calculations to be performed and the display of data on the screen in tabular or graphic form while the test is conducted.

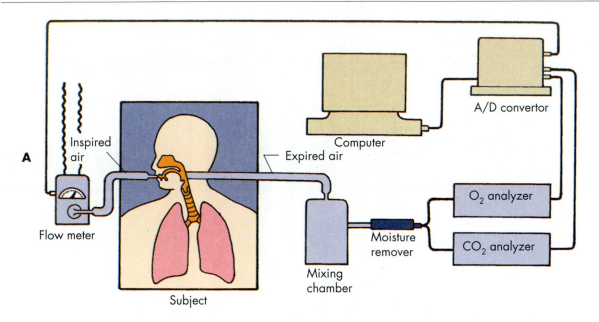

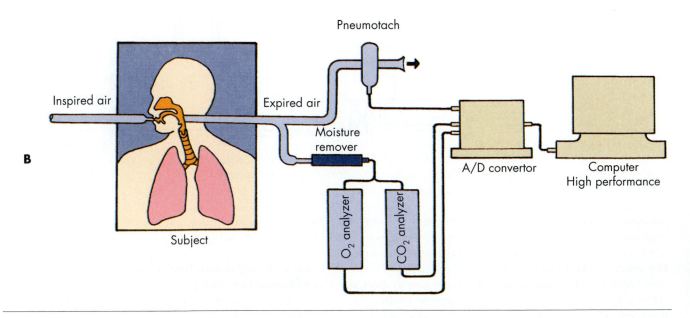

FIGURE 6.11

Oxygen consumption (VO_2) data obtained from time-averaged and breath-by-breath indirect calorimetry systems during exercise. Although the changes in VO_2 appear similar from both systems, the rate of change in VO_2 is more rapid from the breath-by-breath system. However, the numerous data points of the breath-by-breath system also reveal the variability inherent in calculating VO_2 every breath.

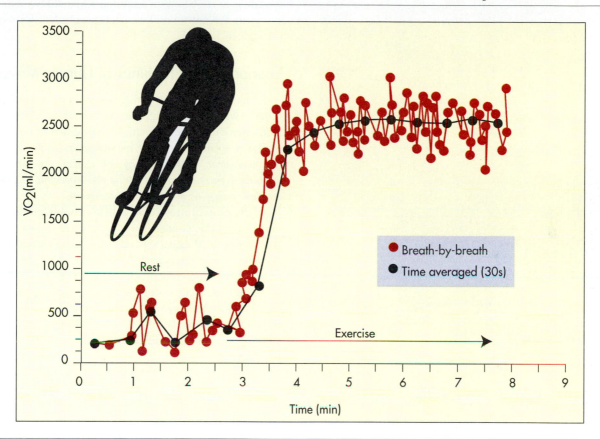

time–averaged system (see Figures 6.8 and 6.10), the subject breathes room air through a volume-measuring device and expired air is directed to flow into a mixing chamber. Air from the mixing chamber is continuously pumped to and through separate oxygen and carbon dioxide analyzers. Electrical signals from the volume measurement and gas analyzers are diverted to a computer where they are first converted from electrical current (analog) to digital signal via an analog to digital (A–D) converter. For example, for ventilation and gas fraction measurement, electronic accessory equipment is connected to the equipment so that a change in the measurement condition of the instrument exerts a proportional change in electrical voltage output. This voltage change is converted to computer language by the A–D converter.[5,34]

Time-averaged systems are able to calculate indirect calorimetry values, such as VO_2, VCO_2, RER, caloric expenditure, and other respiratory parameters in intervals of time restricted by software and hardware capacities. For example, if the ventilation meter and gas analyzers have slow response

times and the computer processor has small memory and slow processing speed, data may be calculated in intervals of 15 or 30 seconds.

Some indirect calorimetry systems have rapidly responding analyzers and advanced computerization that enable the calculation of parameters with every breath. These systems are appropriately called breath-by-breath systems (see Figures 6.8, *C* and 6.10, *B*). The circuitry of a breath-by-breath system is a little different from that of time-averaged systems. Expired air is sampled close to the mouth, avoiding the need for a mixing chamber, and ventilation is measured by sophisticated devices such as a pneumotach or a low-mass impeller, rather than the traditional volume meter (Figure 6.11, *B*). Time-averaged and breath-by-breath data for a given exercise condition are graphed in Figure 6.12. The breath-by-breath system clearly reveals the improved ability to detect the rapidity of change in VO_2 and is therefore the system of choice for research of the kinetics of gas exchange during changes in metabolic conditions.

FIGURE 6.12

The change in oxygen consumption (VO$_2$) for 2 subjects when running at different velocities on a level treadmill.

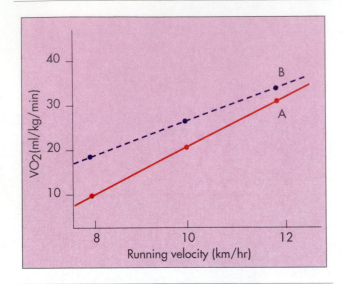

Ventilated Hood Systems

A major difficulty when using expired gas analysis is the presence of a valve apparatus within the subject's mouth, or a mask firmly pressed against the subject's face. These conditions can influence the frequency and depth of breathing, causing potential for hyperventilation and increased movement to invalidate gas analysis estimations of basal caloric expenditure. These difficulties are not significant during exercise. To solve for these problems during basal conditions, hoods have been developed for placement over the head of the subject and can be either a closed- or open-circuit system.[5] For the preferred open-circuit system, air is pumped through the hood at a high rate (e.g., 75 L/min), which ensures that all expired air is collected, mixed, and sampled for gas content.[5,28,34] These ventilated systems require precise flow rates because the flow rate is used to solve for exhaled gas volumes based on a simple dilution of the high carbon dioxide and enrichment of the low oxygen in exhaled air relative to environmental air.

Closed-Circuit Indirect Calorimetry

As previously mentioned, the respirometers used in the late nineteenth century and early twentieth century were based on a closed-circuit system (see Figure 6.5). Air was recirculated through the chamber, with oxygen added at a rate matching VO$_2$, and carbon dioxide was removed. The nitrogen content of the air remained stable because of the physiologically inert nature of gaseous nitrogen.

Today closed-circuit indirect calorimetry systems are rarely used. However, an example of a closed-circuit system that is used for purposes other than calorimetry is the *spirometer* (see Chapter 18). Unless the CO$_2$ produced from metabolism can be measured, closed-circuit systems may accurately provide only data concerning VO$_2$. Estimations of energy expenditure are based on assuming a mixed RQ value (0.83) and using the corresponding caloric equivalent for oxygen to calculate VO$_2$.

Economy and Efficiency of Human Movement

The words *economy* and *efficiency* are often used synonymously when describing exercise conditions. This is incorrect, since these terms pertain to very different conditions of the body. **Economy** of movement refers to *the energy cost of that movement*.[4,12] **Efficiency** of movement refers to *the mechanical energy produced during the movement relative to the metabolic energy used to cause the movement*.

Economy of movement is best exemplified during running and in this context has been termed *running economy*.[12] Another term used to describe this energy demand is *submaximal oxygen consumption*.[4] Figure 6.12 presents data for two different individuals running on a treadmill. Subject A has better running economy because for a given running speed subject A consumes less oxygen relative to body weight than subject B. Researchers have explained differences in running economy by different running techniques (biomechanics).

The concept of efficiency, and some difficulties inherent in calculating efficiency, is best illustrated using subjects A and B of Figure 6.12 as an example. These two runners have differing submaximal oxygen consumptions (differing economy), and the increase in VO$_2$ for a given intensity is also different between the two individuals. To compute the efficiency of movement for an individual, the change in energy output during ergometry is expressed relative to the change in the chemical energy used during the movement. In this instance, subject B requires a smaller increase in VO$_2$ for a given increase in intensity. If all else were equal (i.e., mechanics), this would mean that subject B was more efficient.

6-7   Efficiency = Δ energy generation/Δ energy of metabolism

However, this definition poses problems when trying to compute efficiency of running. As previously described, the calculation of mechanical work during level treadmill walk-

economy (e-kon'o-mi)

the concept pertaining to the oxygen consumption required to perform a given task

efficiency (e-fish'en-si)

when applied to exercise; the ratio (expressed as percentage) between the mechanical energy produced during exercise and the energy cost of the exercise

ing or running requires a modification in method, such as running or walking up a grade, measuring the horizontal force applied by the subject to a strain gauge, or the vertical force from a suspended weight attached to the subject. Unless one of these modifications is accomplished, the term *efficiency* has little meaning to level running, walking, or cross-country skiing.

For a change in exercise intensity during cycle ergometry from 100 to 250 watts, a subject increases energy generation each minute from 1.4333 Kcal to 3.5832 Kcal. If the subject's steady state VO_2 during the two cycle intensities was 1.6 L/min and 3.1 L/min, respectively, with an RER of 0.83, efficiency can be calculated as:

6-8   Efficiency = Δ mechanical energy production /
Δ metabolic energy cost

$$= (3.5832\text{-}1.4333 \text{ Kcal/min})$$
$$(14.9978\text{-}7.7408 \text{ Kcal})$$
$$= 2.1499 \text{ Kcal/min}/7.2570 \text{ Kcal/min}$$
$$= 8.9995 \text{ kJ/min}/30.3778 \text{ kJ/min}$$
$$= 0.2962$$
$$= 29.62\%$$

Generally, efficiency during exercise is very similar among individuals as a result of the constant efficiency of our metabolic pathways. For example, the standard free energy change of glycolysis is equal to -47.0 Kcal/mol glucose, and the production of two ATP in muscle from glucose during glycolysis is equal to -14.6 Kcal/mol glucose. The ratio of the two is equal to 0.361, or 36%. This value is slightly higher than the normal range of total body efficiency during exercise of 25% to 30%.[18]

SUMMARY

- The science of **ergometry** concerns the measurement of work. A device that can be used to measure work is called an **ergometer**. Examples of ergometers used for exercise and research are the bench step, cycle, treadmill, and rowing apparatus.

- Ergometry enables the calculation of **work**, **power**, and external energy production during exercise. The general components of these calculations are a resistance or load, a distance the load is moved against gravity and over time, and the duration (repetition) of the movement. The preferred unit to express energy is the kJ, which equals 4.186 Kcal. Power is expressed as kJ/min, where 1 kJ/min equals 16.667 watts.

- Exercise intensity is quantified in units of power. Individuals who can sustain high power outputs during prolonged exercise without becoming fatigued have high cardiorespiratory endurance fitness. Individuals who can generate high maximal power during very short bursts of exercise are suited to explosive exercises such as sprinting or weight lifting.

- The direct measurement of heat dissipation is termed *direct calorimetry*. When heat dissipation is calculated from other measurements, these methods are termed *indirect calorimetry*. Indirect calorimetry can also be subdivided into open- and closed-circuit systems.

- The direct **calorimeter** was the first tool used to measure caloric expenditure in animals and humans. With the validation of indirect calorimetry, and therefore less expensive methods of calorimetry, attention became focused away from direct methods.

- The most common method of indirect calorimetry involves the collection and measurement of expired gases, allowing the computation of oxygen consumption (VO_2) and carbon dioxide production (VCO_2). These calculations are based on the **Haldane transformation**, which is derived from the fact that nitrogen is physiologically inert. The ratio of VCO_2 to VO_2 is termed the **respiratory quotient** (RQ) and when measured under conditions of ventilatory gas exchange is termed the **respiratory exchange ratio** (RER). The RQ is important because when carbon dioxide production is solely from cellular metabolism, and assuming that no change in protein (amino acid) catabolism occurs during exercise, the RQ value can be used to calculate energy expenditure more accurately.

- The following conditions alter VCO_2 disproportionately to VO_2 and invalidate use of RER values in energy expenditure calculations: metabolic acidosis, non–steady state exercise conditions, hyperventilation, and excess postexercise VO_2.

- Electronic gas analyzers and computer sophistication have enabled the production of several different indirect calorimetry systems. Time-averaged systems are able to calculate indirect calorimetry values, such as VO_2, VCO_2, RER, caloric expenditure, and other respiratory parameters, in intervals of time restricted by software and hardware capacities. If these measurement instruments have rapid response times with high accuracy, data can be calculated in time intervals less than 1 second.

- Other indirect methods of measuring caloric expenditure are determining carbon and nitrogen excretion from the body and assessing the exchange of isotopes in water during basal metabolism. These methods are suited to long-term basal energy expenditure conditions, whereas gas analysis indirect calorimetry remains the method of choice to compute changes in caloric expenditure during exercise.

- **Economy** of movement refers to the energy cost of that movement. **Efficiency** of movement refers to the mechanical energy production of the movement relative to the metabolic energy used to cause the movement and approximates 30% during exercise.

REVIEW QUESTIONS

1. Define the terms *ergometry, economy, efficiency,* and *calorimetry.*

2. Calculate work and power for the following exercise examples:

   A. An 84 kg person bench stepping a 15 cm bench, 20 times per minute, for 15 minutes.

   B. A person riding a cycle ergometer with a 6 m per revolution fly wheel, for 35 minutes, at a load setting of 2.0 kg and a cadence of 70 rpm.

   C. A person riding the aforementioned cycle ergometer for 2 minutes at a load of 5.0 kg at 95 rpm.

   D. Between examples B and C above, which example would be more likely to be maintained at a metabolic steady state? Why?

3. What are the difficulties of applying principles of ergometry to treadmill walking or running and swimming?

4. What are the differences between direct and indirect calorimetry?

5. What are the differences between open- and closed-circuit indirect calorimetry?

6. Calculate V_ESTPD, V_ISTPD, VO_2, RER, and energy expenditure for the examples provided in Appendix B.

7. How were nonprotein caloric equivalent and RQ data derived?

8. What does an increase in protein catabolism during exercise influence more, total energy expenditure or the relative contribution of fat and carbohydrate catabolism? Why?

9. What is the difference between the respiratory quotient (RQ) and the respiratory exchange ratio (RER)?

10. Under what conditions does the RER not equal the RQ?

11. What are the components of a modern computerized system for indirect gas analysis calorimetry?

12. How do modern systems for indirect gas analysis calorimetry differ from methods used before electronic gas analyzers and computerization?

13. Why are special expired gas sampling methods required when performing measurements of basal metabolic rate? What are some examples of these systems?

APPLICATIONS

1. You tested one highly trained endurance runner and one novice runner for VO_2 during three different speeds of running. Would you expect them to have the same VO_2 for each of the speeds? Explain.

2. The measure of economy has many clinical applications. For example, individuals who wear a knee brace are likely to be less economical while running or walking, and individuals who wear artificial limbs have been shown to have an increased oxygen cost (lower economy) for given walking speeds. What are other examples of clinical scenarios in which economy of motion might be an important measure of both disability and improvement of a disability following rehabilitation?

3. Why is the measure of VO_2 max a widely used statistic in exercise science research?

REFERENCES

1. Atwater WO: Coefficients of digestibility and availability of the nutrients of food, *Proc Am Physiol Soc* :30, 1904.

2. Ballor DL, Katch VL, Becque MD, Marks CR: Resistance weight training during caloric restriction enhances lean body weight maintenance, *Am J Clin Nutr* 47:19-25, 1988.

3. Bisdee JT, James WPT, Shaw MA: Changes in energy expenditure during the menstrual cycle, *Br J Nutr* 61:187-199, 1989.

4. Bransford DR, Howley ET: Oxygen cost of running in trained and untrained men and women, *Med Sci Sports Exerc* 9:41-44, 1977.

5. Bursztein S, Elwyn DH, Askanazi J, Kinney JM: *Energy metabolism, indirect calorimetry, and nutrition,* Baltimore, 1989, Williams & Wilkins.

6. Campbell JA, Hargood-Ash D, Hill L: Effect of cooling power of the atmosphere on body metabolism, *J Physiol Lond* 52:259-264, 1922.

7. Campbell JA, Webster TA: Day and night urine during complete rest, laboratory routine, light muscular work and oxygen administration, *Biochem J* 15:660-664, 1921.

8. Cheetham ME, Boobis LH, Brooks S, Williams C: Human muscle metabolism during sprint running, *J Appl Physiol* 61(1):54-60, 1986.

9. Cissik J, Johnson R: Myth of nitrogen equality in respiration: its history and implications, *Aerospace Med* 43:755-758, 1972.

10. Costill DL, Lee G, D'Aquisto LJ: Video-assisted analysis of swimming technique, *J Swim Res* 3(2):5-9, 1987.

11. Costill DL, Rayfield F, Kirwan J, Thomas R: A computer based system for the measurement of force and power during front crawl swimming, *J Swim Res* 2(1):16-19, 1986.

12. Daniels JT: A physiologist's view of running economy, *Med Sci Sports Exerc* 17(3):332-338, 1985.

13. D'Aquisto LJ, Costill DL, Gehlsen GM et al: Breastroke economy, skill, and performance: study of breastroke mechanics using a computer based "velocity-video" system, *J Swim Res* 4(2):9-13, 1988.

14. deGroot G: Fundamental mechanics applied to swimming: technique and propelling efficiency. In Ungerechts BE, Reischle K, editors: *Swimming science V: international series on sport sciences* 18:17-30, 1986.

15. Dudka L, Inglis H, Johnson R et al: Inequality of inspired and expired gaseous nitrogen in man, *Nature* 232:265-267, 1971.

16. Dupuis R, Adrian M, Yoneda Y, Jack M: Forces acting on the hand during swimming and their relationships to muscular, spatial, and temporal factors. In Terauds J, Bedingfield EW, editors: *Swimming III: international series on sport sciences* 8:110-117, 1978.

17. Elia M, Livesey G: Theory and validity of indirect calorimetry during net lipid synthesis, *Am J Clin Nutr* 47:591-601, 1988.

18. Fox EL, Bowers R: Steady-state equality of respiratory gaseous N_2 in resting man, *J Appl Physiol* 35(1):143-144, 1973.

19. Fox EL, Bowers RW, Foss ML: *The physiological basis for exercise and sport,* ed 5, Madison, Wis, 1993, Brown & Benchmark.

20. Jones NL: Evaluation of a microprocessor-controlled exercise testing system, *J Appl Physiol* 57:1312-1318, 1984.

21. Kleiber M: *The fire of life: an introduction to animal energetics,* Melbourne, Fla, 1975, Robert E Kreiger Publishing.

22. Lakomy HKA: An ergometer for measuring the power generated during sprinting, *J Physiol Lond* 354:33P, 1984 (abstract).

23. Lippert H, Lehmann HP: *SI units in medicine: an introduction to the international system of units with conversion tables and normal ranges,* Baltimore, 1978, Urban & Schwarzenberg.

24. Livesey G, Elia M: Estimation of energy expenditure, net carbohydrate utilization, and net fat oxidation and synthesis by indirect calorimetry: evaluation of errors with special reference to the detailed composition of fuels, *Am J Clin Nutr* 47:608-628, 1988.

25. Luft U, Myhre L, Loeppky J: Validity of Haldane calculation for estimating respiratory gas exchange, *J Appl Physiol* 35(4):546-551, 1973.

26. Lusk G: *The elements of the science of nutrition,* ed 4, Philadelphia, 1928, WB Saunders.

27. Lusk G, DuBois EF: On the constancy of the basal metabolism, *J Physiol Lond* 54:213-216, 1924.

28. McLean JA, Tobin G: *Animal and human calorimetry,* New York, 1987, Cambridge University Press.

29. Michaelis AM: Clinical calorimetry—36th paper. A graphic method for determining certain numerical factors in metabolism, *J Biol Chem* 59:51-58, 1924.

30. Morgan DW, Martin PE, Krahenbuhl GS, Baldini FD: Variability in running economy and mechanics among trained male runners, *Med Sci Sports Exerc* 23(3):378-383, 1991.

31. Passmore R, Durnin JVGA: Human energy expenditure, *Physiol Rev* 35:801-840, 1955.

32. Shaffer P: Diminished muscular activity and protein metabolism, *Am J Physiol* 22:445-456, 1908.

REFERENCES—Cont'd

33. Wagner J, Horvath S, Dahms T, Reed S: Validation of open-circuit method for the determination of oxygen consumption, *J Appl Physiol* 34(6):859-863, 1973.

34. Weissman C, Damask MC, Askanazi J et al: Evaluation of a non-invasive method for the measurement of metabolic rate in humans, *Clin Sci* 69:135-141, 1985.

35. Wilmore J, Costill DL: Adequacy of the Haldane transformation in the computation of exercise V_{O_2} in man WJ, *J Appl Physiol* 35(1):85-89, 1973.

36. Wong WW, Cochran WJ, Klish WJ et al: In vivo isotope-fractionation factors and the measurement of deuterium- and oxygen-18-dilution spaces from plasma, urine, saliva, respiratory water, and carbon dioxide, *Am J Clin Nutr* 47:1-6, 1988.

37. Young DS: Implementation of SI units for clinical laboratory data: style specifications and conversion tables, *Ann Intern Med* 106:114-120, 1987.

RECOMMENDED READINGS

▪ Bursztein S, Elwyn DH, Askanazi J, Kinney JM: *Energy metabolism, indirect calorimetry, and nutrition,* Baltimore, 1989, Williams & Wilkins.

▪ Daniels JT: A physiologist's view of running economy, *Med Sci Sports Exerc* 17(3):332-338, 1985.

▪ Livesey G, Elia M: Estimation of energy expenditure, net carbohydrate utilization, and net fat oxidation and synthesis by indirect calorimetry: evaluation of errors with special reference to the detailed composition of fuels, *Am J Clin Nutr* 47:608-628. 1988.

▪ Lusk G: *The elements of the science of nutrition,* ed 4 Philadelphia, 1928, WB Saunders.

▪ McLean JA, Tobin G: *Animal and human calorimetry,* New York, 1987, Cambridge University Press.

Muscle Contraction

KEY TERMS

fibers	t-tubule
excitability	triad
contractility	sarcoplasmic reticulum
extensibility	contraction cycling
elasticity	concentric
striated	eccentric
motor unit	isometric
myofibrils	isokinetic
sarcomere	summation
sarcolemma	tetanus
myosin	intrinsic rhythmicity
actin	calveoli
tropomyosin	calmodulin
troponin	

The previous chapter introduced the body's abilities to respond to stimuli that perturb homeostasis (e.g., exercise) and develop altered function that can result in a steady state condition. Because exercise is a stress that is caused by repeated or sustained muscle contractions, knowledge of muscle function and the molecular events of muscle contraction provides a foundation for a comprehensive understanding of exercise physiology. The scientific study of exercise is biased toward treating movement and skeletal muscle contraction synonymously. However, movement is not confined to the total body, and therefore to skeletal muscle. Just as muscle contraction causes the movement of our limbs, muscle also causes the movement of some of our organs. Organs within the body, such as the heart, stomach, lungs, eyes, and blood vessels, move. The regulated function of all muscle is crucial to life and to the body's ability to adapt to exercise. The purpose of this chapter is to identify the different types of muscle, to detail their mechanisms and regulation of contraction, and to explain how their different contraction characteristics support their specific functions during exercise.

Types of Muscle in the Human Body

Three types of muscle are located in the human body: skeletal muscle, cardiac muscle, and smooth muscle. The individual cells in each muscle type are referred to as muscle **fibers**. All three types of muscle have the properties of **excitability, contractility, extensibility,** and **elasticity**.

General functions of the types of muscle are also similar. Muscles cause movement, which refers not only to total body exercise, but also to the dynamic functions of many of our internal hollow organs and structures, such as the heart, stomach, and blood vessels. In the process of muscle contraction, which can cause movement, muscles produce heat. Heat is the product of the chemical reactions that cause and support contraction and accounts for almost two thirds of the energy release during these reactions. Because muscle accounts for more than 40% of the body mass in most individuals, muscle is the tissue most responsible for maintaining and increasing body temperature. This is especially true when we are cold, since shivering involves the involuntary contraction of skeletal muscle and can result in a sevenfold increase in basal metabolic rate and heat production.[1,9,18]

---

fibers (**fi** 'bers)
muscle cells

excitability (**ex-si**' ta-**bil**' i-ti)
the ability to respond to a stimulus (e.g., a neurotransmitter or hormone) by the generation and conduction of a reversal in membrane potential (action potential)

contractility (**kon**-trak' **til** i-ti)
the ability of muscle to contract and generate tension, at the expense of metabolic energy, when an adequate stimulus is received

extensibility (**ex-ten**'si-**bil**-i-ti)
the ability of muscle to be stretched

elasticity (e-**las**' **tis**' i-ti)
the ability of muscle to resume its resting length after being either stretched or contracted

Examples of body functions dependent on muscle contraction are listed in Table 7.1.

<table>
<tr><td colspan="2">TABLE 7.1</td></tr>
<tr><td colspan="2">Body functions involving the contraction of one or more of the three types of muscle</td></tr>
<tr><td>FUNCTION</td><td>PREDOMINANT MUSCLE TYPE</td></tr>
<tr><td>Body movement</td><td>Skeletal</td></tr>
<tr><td>Speech</td><td>Skeletal</td></tr>
<tr><td>Eye movement</td><td>Skeletal</td></tr>
<tr><td>Stomach movement</td><td>Smooth</td></tr>
<tr><td>Urination and defecation</td><td>Smooth</td></tr>
<tr><td>Heart pumping</td><td>Cardiac</td></tr>
<tr><td>Shivering</td><td>Skeletal</td></tr>
<tr><td>Sweat extrusion</td><td>Smooth</td></tr>
<tr><td>Breathing</td><td>Skeletal</td></tr>
<tr><td>Blood vessel constriction</td><td>Smooth</td></tr>
</table>

A Simple Comparison Among Skeletal, Cardiac, and Smooth Muscle

The three types of muscle each have a different cellular organization and appearance (Table 7.2). Skeletal muscle and cardiac muscle *(myocardium)* are composed of intracellular proteins arranged in discrete units that give the muscle a striated appearance. Hence both are termed **striated** muscle. Skeletal muscle and myocardium differ in the size and arrangement of the cells *(fibers)* and the neurologic innervation of the fibers. Skeletal muscle fibers are aligned linearly, can be very long, and are grouped into functional units that are each innervated by a common nerve *(motor units)*. Myocardial fibers are shorter, do not need neural innervation to contract, are more randomly aligned yet connect to each other end to end, and are able to conduct action potentials to one another. Smooth muscle fibers are not striated and consist of contractile proteins that are aligned with intracellular filaments having differing orientations. The inability to microscopically visualize the arrangement of contractile proteins in smooth muscle has resulted in the categorization name of *smooth* rather than striated muscle. There are diverse arrangements among multiple smooth muscle fibers within

striated (stri-ate′ed)

pertaining to the highly organized dark and light stained pattern of skeletal muscle fibers, as seen through microscopy

<table>
<tr><td colspan="4">TABLE 7.2</td></tr>
<tr><td colspan="4">Comparison between skeletal, cardiac, and smooth muscle</td></tr>
<tr><td>CHARACTERISTIC</td><td>SKELETAL</td><td>CARDIAC</td><td>SMOOTH</td></tr>
<tr><td>Anatomic location</td><td>Attaches to bones or skin</td><td>Attaches to fibrous walls of the heart</td><td>In or surrounding walls of blood vessels and organs</td></tr>
<tr><td>Multicellular arrangement</td><td>Cells (fibers) grouped into fascicles, which comprise a whole muscle</td><td>Atrial and ventricular fibers separated by a connective tissue sheath
Single fibers connected a fibrous skeleton</td><td>Single cells within a connective tissue matrix</td></tr>
<tr><td>Cellular morphology</td><td>Single, long, cylindric, striated, and multinucleated</td><td>Branching cells, uninucleated or binucleated, and striated</td><td>Single, uninucleated, and nonstriated</td></tr>
</table>

TABLE 7.2—Cont'd

Comparison between skeletal, cardiac, and smooth muscle

CHARACTERISTIC	SKELETAL	CARDIAC	SMOOTH
Subcellular morphology	Myofibrils with sarcomeres	Myofibrils with sarcomeres, filaments	Dispersed actin and myosin
	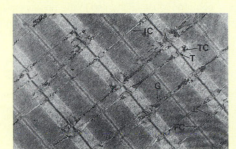	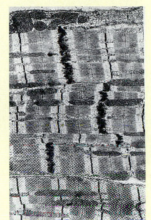	
Presence/location of t-tubules	Yes, at A-I junctions	Yes, at Z lines	No
Sarcoplasmic reticulum	Elaborate	Elaborate	Rudimentary
Gap junctions	No	Yes, at intercollated discs	Yes, in single unit muscle
Nerve-muscle interaction	Yes, neuromuscular junctions	No	Yes, in multiunit muscle
Regulation of contraction	Voluntary nervous system	Involuntary nervous system, intrinsic rhymicity, and hormones	Involuntary nervous system, hormones, local chemicals, stretch
Source(s) of calcium	Sarcoplasmic reticulum	Sarcoplasmic reticulum and extracellular fluid	Sarcoplasmic reticulum and extracellular fluid
Contraction mechanisms	Actin and myosin	Actin and myosin	Calmodulin and myosin
Autorhythmicity	No	Yes	Yes, single unit muscle
Type of contraction	Motor units	Atrial and ventricular syncytium	Singular or multi-unit
Speed of contraction	Heterogenous slow to fast	Homogenous slow	Homogenous very slow
Stretch response	Contraction	Contraction	Relaxation
Metabolism	Heterogenous oxidative to glycolytic	Homogenous oxidative	Homogenous mainly oxidative

(*Photos left*, From Gottfried S: *Human biology*, St Louis, 1994, Mosby. Photos by Richard Gross/Biological Photography. *Photos above*, From Fawcett DW: *A textbook of histology*, New York, 1994, Chapman & Hall.)

the body, and it is difficult to generalize as can be done for skeletal and cardiac muscle. The detailed functions of each type of muscle are provided in the specific sections that follow.

Specific Structure and Function of Muscle

Skeletal Muscle

An understanding of the general function of skeletal muscle is a first step in learning its structure. Skeletal muscle functions to contract and cause either body movement or the stability of body posture. Skeletal muscle contraction must be able to be performed with a decrease or increase in muscle length. In performing these functions, skeletal muscle is required to contract and generate tension throughout the length of the muscle. Depending on the muscle and movement, skeletal muscle must also be able to develop a wide range of tensions, with the ability to alter tension in small increments. These general requirements necessitate a structure that can have a large change in length and can be structurally and functionally organized to contract and generate both minutely small and extremely large forces.

Structure

Not all skeletal muscles are similar in anatomic appearance. For example, muscles that are frequently analyzed for changes in energy metabolism during exercise are the vastus lateralis, medial gastrocnemius, soleus, biceps brachii, medial deltoid, tibialis anterior, and the forearm flexors. The anatomic arrangements of bone, muscle, and tendon for these muscles are presented in Figure 7.1. Depending on the muscle, muscle fibers are aligned differently with respect to the tendon. In addition, the neural and metabolic characteristics of these muscles may differ, resulting in different functional properties (see Chapter 8).

Skeletal muscle is surrounded by a sheath of connective tissue known as *fascia,* which serves to protect each muscle from movement over hard structures (e.g., bones, ligaments, tendons) and over or beside other muscles. Three other layers of connective tissue exist within skeletal muscle. Between the fascia and the muscle itself is the *epimysium;* the *perimysium* separates discrete bundles of muscle fibers (fascicles); and the *endomysium* separates individual muscle fibers (Figure 7.2).

One nerve (termed an *alpha motor nerve*) diverges and innervates many muscle fibers, and this structural and functional unit of muscle contraction is called a **motor unit.** Consequently, contraction of a skeletal muscle results from the combined contraction of many motor units. Motor units within skeletal muscle can differ in the ease of recruitment, conduction velocity of the nerve, contractile force generation, the duration of contraction, and specific metabolic capacities. The detailed physiology and research of neuromuscular function are presented in Chapter 8.

FIGURE 7.1

The anatomic location of the major muscles studied in research of muscle metabolism or recruitment during exercise. Traditionally, muscle biopsy has been performed on the vastus lateralis (cycling), medial gastrocnemius (running), soleus (running), medial deltoid (swimming), and biceps and triceps (weight lifting). The forearm flexor muscles, gastrocnemius, and tibialis anterior have been common muscles studied in the noninvasive methods of proton and phosphorous magnetic resonance imaging and spectroscopy.

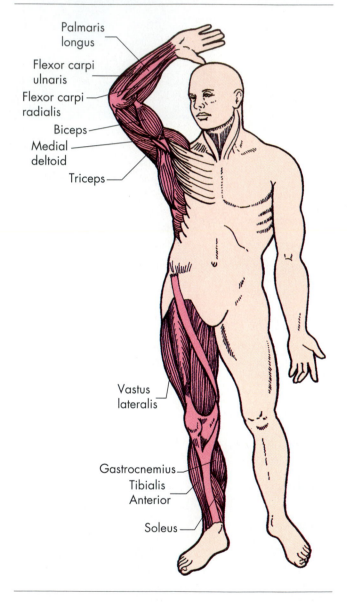

When viewed in transverse section (Figure 7.3, *A*), the striated appearance of skeletal muscle fibers results from the organized arrangement of proteins. The main proteins of skeletal muscle are *myosin, actin, tropomyosin,* and *troponin.* Myosin and actin are involved in the process of muscle contraction, whereas troponin and tropomyosin are involved in the regulation of muscle contraction. These and other proteins involved in muscle contraction are presented in Table 7.3.

FIGURE 7.2

The fascia and anatomic divisions of skeletal muscle.

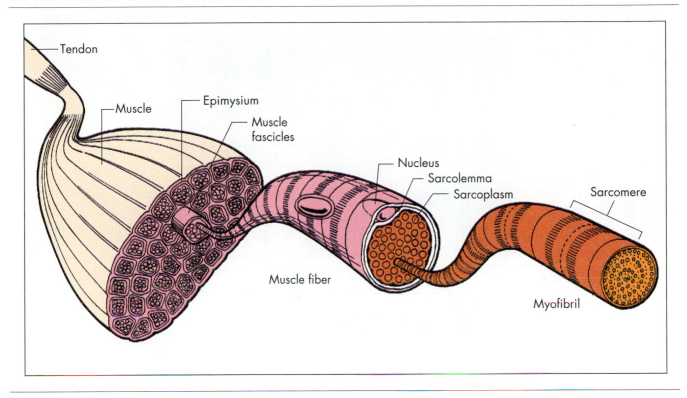

Striated muscle proteins are organized into subcellular structures called **myofibrils,** which extend along the length of the muscle fiber. The myofibrils are aligned beside each other resulting in a similar three-dimensional pattern of the contractile proteins within the entire fiber. Within a myofibril the contractile proteins are arranged in units called **sarcomeres** (Figure 7.3, *B*). The sarcomere is bordered by proteins that form the Z-lines. F-actin molecules extend from each Z-line toward the middle of the sarcomere. The myosin molecules do not extend to each Z-line but are maintained in the central region of the sarcomere by proteins that form the M-line. When viewed three-dimensionally, each myosin molecule is associated with six different F-actin molecules in a hexagonal structure.

The different visual regions of the sarcomere have been named (Figure 7.3, *C*). The darkly stained region indicating the region of myosin is termed the *A-band*. Located centrally within the A-band is a less darkly stained region where no actin is associated with the myosin, termed the *H-zone*. On either side of the Z-lines is an unstained region that is composed solely of actin molecules, termed the *I-band*.

The cellular structure of skeletal muscle is even more complex and highly organized than illustrated in Figure 7.3. Skeletal muscle fibers have multiple nuclei, many mitochondria, glycogen granules, droplets of triacylglycerol, ribosomes, t-tubules, Golgi and sarcoplasmic reticulum membranous networks, calcium stores, and of course the proteins required

for muscle contraction (Figure 7.4). The nuclei are located beneath the sarcolemma, the mitochondria and lipid droplets are located between myofibrils and immediately beneath the sarcolemma, glycogen granules are dispersed throughout the cytosol and are even found between the contractile proteins of the sarcomere,[4] and the t-tubule and sarcoplasmic reticulum membranes are diffusely located within the myofibrils and throughout the cytosol. In addition, a large number of enzymes that catalyze the reactions of metabolism exist in cytosolic solution and within the mitochondria. These intracellular structures are housed within a specialized excitable cell membrane **(sarcolemma)** containing specific proteins

motor unit
an alpha motor nerve and the muscle fibers that it innervates

myofibrils (mi'o-fi'brils)
the longitudinal anatomic unit within skeletal and cardiac muscle fibers that contains the contractile proteins

sarcomere (sar'ko-mere)
the smallest contractile unit of skeletal muscle, consisting of the contractile proteins between the two Z-lines

sarcolemma (sar'ko-lem'ah)
the cell membrane of a muscle fiber

FIGURE 7.3

The organization of the contractile proteins in skeletal muscle as viewed through an electron microscope. **A,** The relationship between the contractile proteins and myofibrils of skeletal muscle fibers. **B,** The regions of a sarcomere are more clearly identified in this hand-drawn illustration. During contraction, the I band decreases in length, the H-zone disappears, and the A band retains its length. **C,** When viewed at a higher magnification, the arrangement between the contractile proteins and membranes of the sarcomere are apparent. (**B,** From Berne RM, Levy MN: *Physiology,* ed 3, St. Louis, 1993, Mosby, and Squire JM: *The structural basis of muscular contraction,* New York, 1981, Plenum Press.)

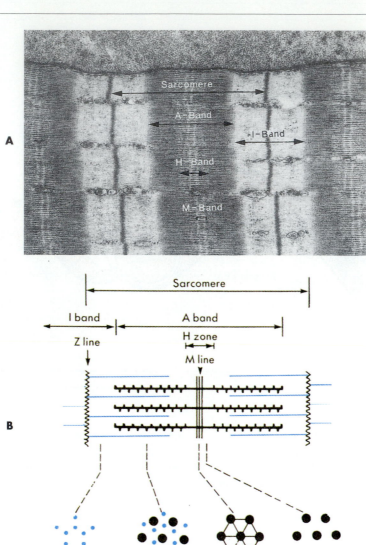

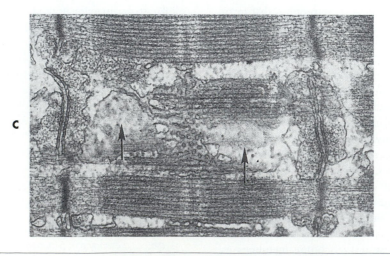

TABLE 7.3

Proteins associated with the myofibrillar structure of striated muscle and the process of muscle contraction

PROTEIN	STRUCTURE	LOCATION	FUNCTIONS
G-actin	Globular protein	Actin polymer	Forms F-actin polymer
F-actin	Polymer of G-actin in helical chain	Sarcomere thin filament	Contractile protein interacts with myosin
Myosin	Rodlike; multi-subunit protein	Sarcomere thick filament	Contractile protein; interacts with F-actin
Troponin-I*	Globular	F-actin	Blocks actin-myosin binding site in relaxed state
Troponin-T*	Globular	F-actin	Binds to tropomyosin
Troponin-C*	Globular	F-actin	Binds calcium; when bound, troponins and tropomyosin move
Tropomyosin	Double helical coil	Positioned at regular intervals on F-actin	Associated with troponins and F-actin; covers actin-myosin binding site in relaxed state
M-protein	Thin filament	M-line of sarcomere	Structure and stability of sarcomere
Alpha-actinin	Thin filament	Z-line	Structure and stability of sarcomere
Titin	Longitudinal filament	Parallel and connected to actin and myosin	Elastic connections between actin, myosin, and Z-lines
Nebulin	Longitudinal filament	Parallel and connected to actin and myosin	Elastic connections between actin, myosin, and Z-lines

*The troponin molecules are grouped and function as a single molecule.

required for the transport of molecules and electrolytes into and from the fiber.

The contractile proteins of the myofibrils differ in structure and function (Figure 7.5). **Myosin** is the largest of the proteins, is a two-stranded helical structure, and occurs in two forms (light and heavy) that are composed of six different noncovalently bound polypeptides. For example, exposure of myosin to denaturing agents separates one pair of long *heavy chains* and two pairs of short *light chains*. In vivo the two heavy chains contain a hinged region, a linear end region, and two globular heads *(S1 units)* at one end. The two pairs of light chains are associated noncovalently with S1 units.[3,23,27,29] In skeletal muscle there are two types of light chains, termed *essential* and *regulatory,* and a pair of each are associated with the S1 units of one myosin molecule.[1,3,18] The regulatory light chain can be phosphorylated, whereas the essential light chains cannot. Furthermore, the enzyme myosin ATPase, as well as an ATP binding site and a site for ATP hydrolysis, is located in the S1 heads. The activity of myosin ATPase is believed to be influenced by the myosin light chains.[14,29,30]

In vivo many myosin molecules aggregate to form a large structure called *meromyosin,* in which the hinge region and S1 units of multiple myosin molecules are angled away from the central region of the molecule.[7] The darkly stained molecule that is visualized by electron microscopy in Figures 7.3 and 7.4 is meromyosin.

Actin is a globular protein (G-actin), but in vivo it aggregates to form a two-stranded helical structure (F-actin) (Figure 7.5). Associated with F-actin is a rod-shaped mole-

myosin (mi'o-sin)
the largest of the contractile proteins of skeletal muscle

actin (ac'tin)
a contractile protein of skeletal muscle

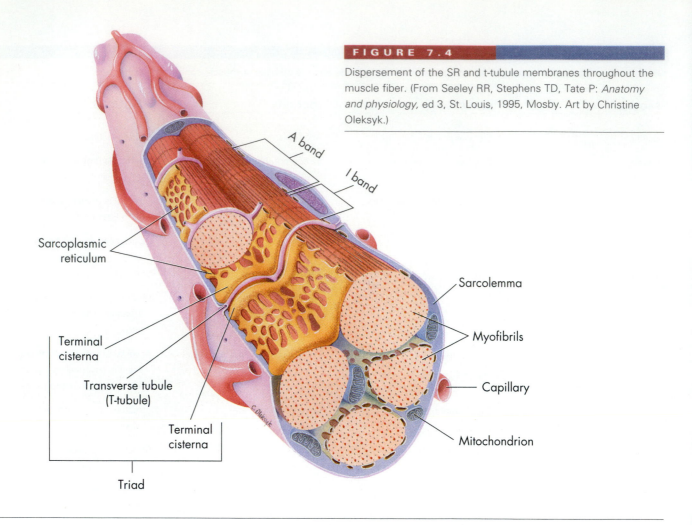

FIGURE 7.4

Dispersement of the SR and t-tubule membranes throughout the muscle fiber. (From Seeley RR, Stephens TD, Tate P: *Anatomy and physiology*, ed 3, St. Louis, 1995, Mosby. Art by Christine Oleksyk.)

cule called **tropomyosin,** which exists as multiple strands that each associate with six or seven G-actin molecules along the length of the F-actin.[1,11,12] At the end of each tropomyosin molecule is bound a **troponin** molecule, which, as discussed later, is involved in the regulation of skeletal muscle contraction.

Other proteins that add to the structure of the sarcomere have also been isolated. Of these, titin and nebulin have been the most important in the process of muscle contraction. Wang[26] has proposed that titin and nebulin assist the "sliding" of actin and myosin during the actual contraction process. Because titin and nebulin are highly elastic proteins, their presence may explain how the associations between actin, myosin, and the Z-lines are maintained throughout the entire range of sarcomere relaxation and contraction.

Contraction and Regulation

The electrochemical and molecular events during muscle contraction are listed in sequential order in Focus Box 7.1 and illustrated in Figure 7.6. When an action potential is transmitted to and propagated along the sarcolemma, the depolarization is internalized within the fiber by the **t-tubule** network. When the wave of depolarization reaches the junction of the t-tubule and sarcoplasmic reticulum **(triad)**, calcium is released from the **sarcoplasmic reticulum** and increases the concentration of free calcium within the fiber. The mechanism of calcium release is believed to be regulated by an inositol triphosphate-calmodulin second messenger system.[1,15,17]

---

tropomyosin (tro′po-my′osin)
a contractile protein of striated muscle

troponin (tro′po′nin)
the regulatory calcium binding contractile protein of striated muscle

t-tubules (t tu′buls)
transverse tubule system connecting the sarcolemma to the sarcoplasmic reticulum in skeletal and cardiac muscle

triad (tri′ad)
junction between a t-tubule and the sarcoplasmic reticulum

sarcoplasmic reticulum (sar′ko-plas-mik re-tik′u-lum)
extensive intracellular membrane compartment that stores calcium

FIGURE 7.5

The molecular structure of the contractile proteins of skeletal and cardiac muscle. Filamentous actin (F actin) is composed of separate units of G actin. Troponin and tropomyosin are located along the F-actin filament. Myosin is a more complex molecule than actin. Myosin can be enzymatically cleaved at two sites. The long tail is termed *light meromyosin* (LMM), and the remaining hinge and two head structure is termed *heavy meromyosin* (HMM). HMM can be further divided into two S1 units, with each S1 unit having two light chains. One of the light chains from each S1 head is a regulatory light chain. The enzyme myosin ATPase is also located on each S1 unit.

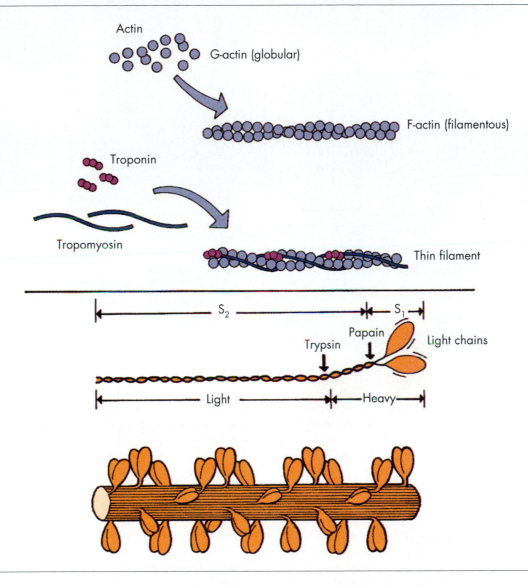

The binding of the calcium ions to the troponin molecules induces a conformational shift in the actin–troponin–tropomyosin association. This shift in three-dimensional molecular structure exposes a site that enables the noncovalent association of actin and the S1 units of myosin. The position of the myosin S1 units before calcium release from the SR is often illustrated as a vertical structure. Research performed as early as 1971 indicates that this vertically aligned position requires the expenditure of free energy,[15] and consequently, that the S1 units are in an unstable or strained position. As will be explained, the hydrolysis of ATP provides the free energy for the S1 units of myosin to be in the vertical (strained) position.

The binding of the S1 units to actin enables the release of the ADP and Pi molecules, which strengthens the actin-myosin complex.[20] During this event the S1 units return to

FOCUS BOX 7.1

Sequence of events during contraction in striated muscle

When striated muscle is relaxed, ADP and Pi are bound to the S1 unit of myosin, the myosin head is in the vertical "strained" position, the intracellular calcium concentration is low, and therefore actin-myosin binding and contraction are negligible.

1. The depolarization is received at the sarcolemma and is propagated down the t-tubule network to the sarcoplasmic reticulum (SR).

2. Depolarization of the SR in the region of the triad initiates the release of calcium from the SR and an increase in intracellular calcium.

3. Increased intracellular calcium increases calcium binding to troponin.

4. The troponin-calcium complex causes a structural change in the position of troponin and tropomyosin on the F-actin polymer, enabling actin to bind to the S1 units of myosin.

5. Actin-myosin binding enables the S1 units to move immediately to their "relaxed" position, thus causing the movement of the attached actin toward the central region of the sarcomere. During this process, ADP and Pi are released from each S1 unit. This constitutes muscle contraction.

6. Since actin is connected to the Z-lines, actin movement results in the shortening of each sarcomere within the fibers of the stimulated motor unit, resulting in muscle contraction.

7. Provided ATP is continually replenished at the myosin-actin sites of the sarcomere, ATP molecules once again bind to the myosin S1 units, which causes the release of the S1 units from actin. During the release of actin and myosin, ATP is hydrolyzed to ADP and Pi, causing the S1 units to change conformation to a vertical strained position. The ATP hydrolysis is believed to provide the free energy needed to move the S1 units to the strained position.

8. If the increased intracellular calcium concentration is maintained (because of continued neural stimulation), the myosin S1 units continue the cyclical attachment and detachment to actin, termed *contraction cycling*.

9. Relaxation occurs when the action potentials are not received by the neuromuscular junction and calcium is actively "pumped" back into the SR.

---

their unstrained or "favored" position, causing shortening of the sarcomere. The myosin and actin association is broken by the binding of ATP to the myosin S1 heads and the release of ADP. The hydrolysis of ATP then provides the free energy to move the S1 units of myosin to their strained position. The presence of ADP and Pi on the S1 units retains the S1 units in this position until calcium ions bind to troponin. Consequently, if free calcium is still present within the myofibrillar apparatus and calcium remains bound to troponin, as soon as the S1 units are returned to their strained position the contraction process occurs again. The continued cycling of the S1 units, which requires the presence of calcium and the continual production and hydrolysis of ATP, is termed **contraction cycling.** Contraction cycling accounts for the ability of skeletal muscle to generate force despite no (isometric) or minimal changes in length and for the ATP and metabolic demands of these contractions. The summation of contraction cycling and sarcomere shortening within a myofibril, muscle fiber, and motor unit results in the shortening of muscle during dynamic muscle contraction.

Because muscle contraction and relaxation are dependent on the molecular interaction between calcium and troponin, troponin is an important regulatory protein for muscle contraction. However, other proteins exist that regulate

the velocity of contraction cycling. The myosin light chains function by affecting the rate of movement of the S1 heads during contraction.[30] The regulatory light chains become phosphorylated when the intracellular calcium concentration increases, and phosphorylation increases the rate at which the S1 unit can move between the strained and unstrained positions.

Function

Types of contractions. Skeletal muscle can contract in a variety of ways. Contractions causing a change in muscle length are called *isotonic* contractions. When the muscle shortens, the isotonic contraction is referred to as a **concentric** contraction. When the muscle lengthens during con-

---

contraction cycling
the repeated cycling of actin and myosin binding, movement, and release during contraction

concentric (kon-sen′trik)
in reference to skeletal muscle contraction; a contraction involving the shortening of muscle

FIGURE 7.6

The sequence of events during skeletal and cardiac muscle contraction. The depolarization of the sarcolemma is propagated down the t-tubules and causes calcium release from the SR. As long as calcium is not pumped back into the SR, the sequence of events from **B** to **F** continues, and represents contraction cycling. Removal of calcium from the cytosol by the ATP dependent pumps prevents the binding between the myosin S1 units and actin. Caption B without calcium would therefore represents muscle in a relaxed state. (From Seeley RR, Stephens TD, and Tate P: *Anatomy and physiology*, ed 3, St. Louis, 1995, Mosby. Art by Barbara Cousins.)

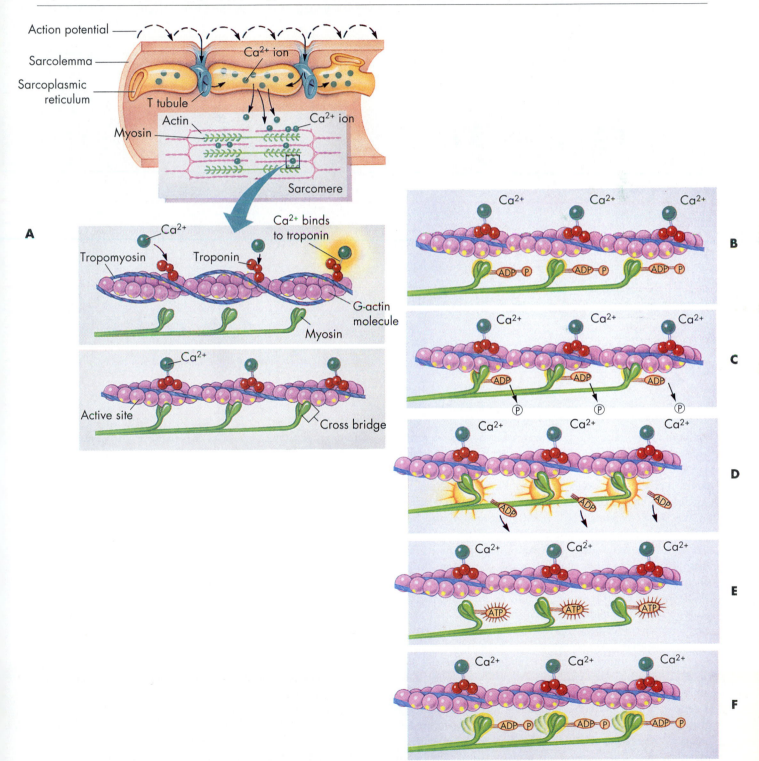

FIGURE 7.7

The different types of skeletal muscle contraction. Concentric contractions occur with a rapid increase in *external force* application. However, because of the influence of joint angle on force development, *contractile tension* varies during a full joint range of motion contraction. During eccentric contractions the *external force* profile is similar to that of concentric contractions; however, muscle tension development is greatest when the force of gravity is perpendicular to the lever arm. Greater forces can be developed during eccentric contractions than for concentric contractions. Isokinetic contractions performed with maximal effort produce a variable force. Force production is less for the start and end of a contraction, where musculo-skeletal mechanics (joint angles) limit force generation. (Adapted from Thorstensson A, Grimby G, Karlsson J: *J Appl Physiol* 40(1):12-16, 1976)

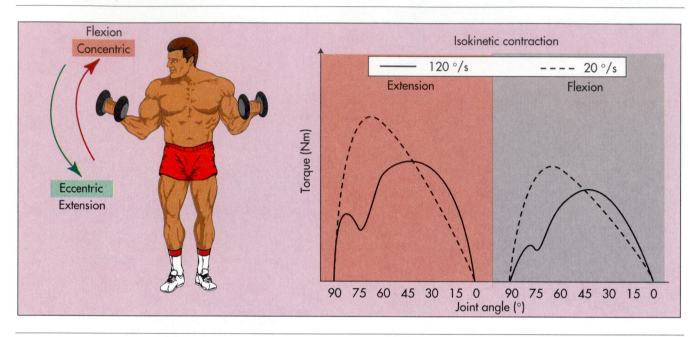

traction, the isotonic contraction is referred to as **eccentric.** However, by definition a *contraction* involves muscle shortening. For this reason many researchers now refer to an eccentric contraction as an *eccentric* action. Nevertheless, since the American College of Sports Medicine recommends that use of the word *contraction* be retained because of the broad acceptance and use of its nonspecific meaning,[22] it is used in this text. Eccentric muscle contractions can generate greater force than concentric actions[28] because of combined effects of gravity assistance (when performed with gravity), stored elastic energy, and the passive tension of the contractile proteins and musculotendinous junctions (Figure 7.7, *A*). Muscle contractions causing no change in muscle length are called **isometric** actions.

How can muscle contract and lengthen at the same time? An eccentric contraction involves the movement of a limb against resistance while the muscle is lengthening. Most eccentric contractions are performed against the force of gravity, but eccentric contractions are also performed by antagonistic muscles during deceleration, so the reference to gravity is not all-inclusive. Thus muscles contracting eccentrically function to oppose either the force of gravity or the

force of antagonistic muscles in a manner that allows a controlled and slowed movement of the limb. To do this the muscle(s) must contract, which involves myosin and actin interaction and contraction cycling. Unlike concentric contractions, this contraction cycling does not have to completely overcome the gravitational and load force, but to partially retard it. The muscle is able to lengthen because relatively limited actin-myosin interaction and contraction cycling occur. This explains the reduced metabolic demand generated during eccentric contractions compared with concentric contractions.[28]

A third type of contraction (muscle action) is **isokinetic.** Isokinetic contractions are a special type of concentric contraction in which the velocity of muscle shortening remains constant (hence the term *isokinetic*). These contractions require specialized and expensive equipment that instantaneously modifies resistance in proportion to the force generated at specific joint angles (Figure 7.7). The result of this is to provide maximal resistance when musculoskeletal mechanics allow maximal force production, and vice versa. Data from research using isokinetic systems are presented in Chapter 9.

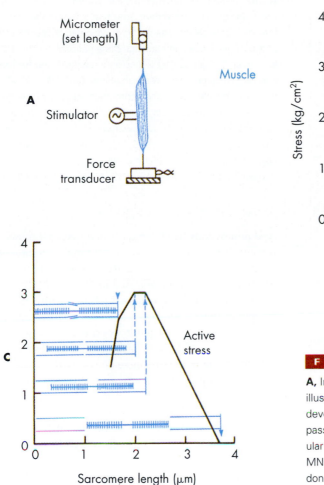

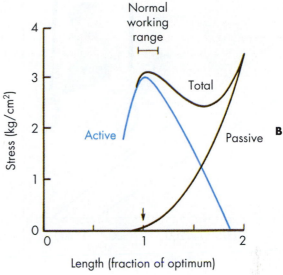

FIGURE 7.8

A, In vitro research of muscle contraction has produced curves illustrating the relationship between muscle length and tension development. **B,** Active tension is the tension remaining after the passive tension component is removed, **C,** and reflects the molecular interaction between actin and myosin. (From Berne RM, Levy MN: *Physiology*, ed 3, St. Louis, 1993, Mosby; and data from Gordon AM et al: *J Physiol* [London], 184:170, 1966.)

Length-tension relationship. For a given muscle the force of a maximal concentric contraction depends on the length of the muscle.[1] When a muscle is removed from the body, with one end connected to a micrometer and the other end connected to a force transducer, stimulation of the muscle causes contraction without shortening (isometric), and the development of tension on the force transducer (Figure 7.8, *A*). By stimulating the muscle and recording the resulting forces for various muscle lengths, the data can be graphed as a length-tension curve (Figure 7.8, *B*). However, since simply stretching the muscle generates passive tension, this passive component must be subtracted from the total tension measured, resulting in the active tension.

Muscle length influences tension development because excessive stretch and inadequate length decrease actin and myosin interaction (Figure 7.8, *C*). These facts have direct application to exercise, because warm-up and flexibility preparation before an event optimize the length-tension relationship of skeletal muscle, allow increased force production and power generation, and improve performance.

Force-velocity and power-velocity relationships. Skeletal muscle tension development is also known to vary with the velocity of the contraction. Greatest tension development occurs in zero velocity (isometric) contractions. As contraction velocity increases, maximal tension development decreases (Figure 7.9, *A*). The force-velocity curve can differ between muscles and between individuals who differ in fiber

eccentric (e-sen′trik)
in reference to skeletal muscle contraction; a contraction involving the lengthening of muscle

isometric (i-so-met′rik)
in reference to skeletal muscle contraction; a contraction involving no change in the length of muscle

isokinetic (i-so-ki-net′ik)
in reference to skeletal muscle contraction; a contraction involving a constant velocity

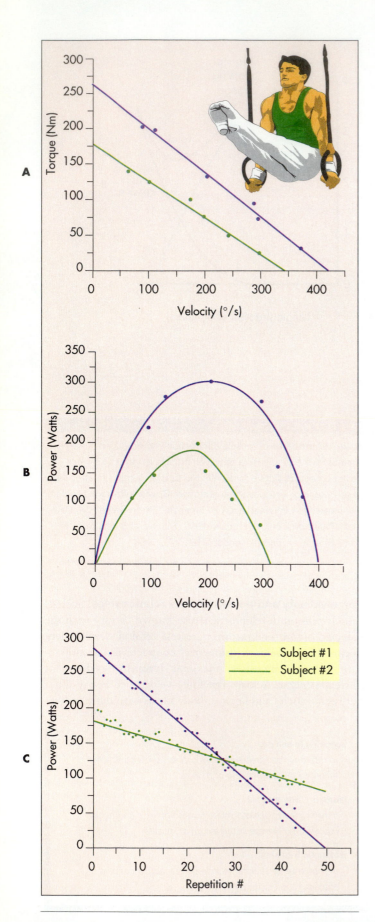

FIGURE 7.9

A, The relationship between muscle contraction force and contraction velocity. Data are shown from two subjects that have different maximal force capabilities of the quadriceps. Subject 1 is an untrained individual, and subject 2 is a national competitive triathlete. Even though subject 2 was endurance trained for prolonged exercise, subject 1 had greater maximal force. **B,** The relationship between muscle power and contraction velocity of the quadriceps for the same two subjects. Subject 1 had greater power, with both subjects having the optimal power-velocity relationship at velocities between 150 to 200 °/s. **C,** The decrease in power during multiple contractions of skeletal muscle in the same two subjects. Subject 1 had far greater endurance (less decrease in power).

type proportions (see Chapter 9). The skeletal muscle power-velocity curve reveals that an optimal velocity exists for developing power. This velocity can differ between people and muscle groups, as indicated in Figure 7.9, *B*.

During repeated maximal effort contractions, muscle fatigues. Fatigue is illustrated as an exponential decay in force generation with subsequent contractions (Figure 7.9, *C*). Interestingly, muscle with greater force generation capabilities, or muscle trained to increase strength, exhibits increases in maximal force generation with similar relative decreases in muscle force.

Summation and tetanus. The skeletal muscle twitch response is extremely long compared with the action potential (Figure 7. 10). As previously explained, skeletal muscle contraction results from the combined contraction of many motor units. The long contraction time and short stimulation time provide opportunity for additional neural stimulation before the complete relaxation of the muscle or motor unit. In these circumstances the force of the total muscle or motor unit twitch can increase with increased stimulation frequency and is called **summation**. As stimulation frequency increases, twitch tension also increases until a smooth maximal tension is reached, which is called **tetanus**. Tetanus is not a normal occurrence during voluntary muscle contraction but is an experimental condition that exemplifies the ability of skeletal muscle to respond to high-frequency stimulation. Furthermore, during abnormal muscle function, such as during cramp, the resulting tetanus response can often exceed the maximal voluntary force of contraction.

Resting muscle tone. At rest a small amount of muscle motor unit contraction occurs to maintain firmness or *tone* of skeletal muscle. The resting muscle tone is known to be caused by neural stimulation, since neurally isolated muscles are flaccid. In addition, when afferent nerves from muscle are cut, preventing feedback from muscles to the central nervous system, muscle tone is lost.[1] This fact illustrates that resting muscle tone is caused by afferent nerve feedback from mus-

FIGURE 7.10

A, Time course of the action potential and muscle twitch from skeletal muscle. When additional neural stimulation is received during the twitch response, tension development increases (summation). If the rate of neural stimulation increases, the summation of tension can increase to cause a plateau in tension development (tetanus). **B,** For the myocardium, the action potential is elongated due to the influx of calcium ions during depolarization. The duration of both the cardiac muscle depolarization and twitch shorten in response to increased sympathetic neural and hormonal stimulation.

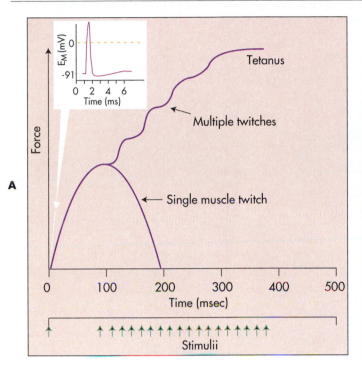

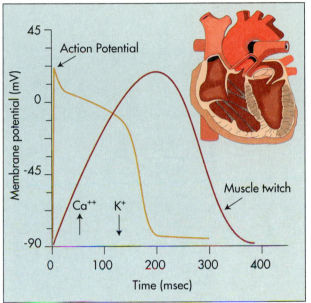

cle to the spinal cord, which then stimulates efferent fibers that innervate a small number of skeletal muscle motor units.[1]

Cardiac Muscle

The purpose of cardiac muscle contraction is not to cause musculoskeletal movement, but to generate pressure within the blood–filled atrial and ventricular chambers of the heart and propel blood down a pressure gradient. These very different functions of skeletal and cardiac muscle necessitate different structural, contractile, and regulatory characteristics.

Structure

Cardiac muscle is striated, like skeletal muscle, and therefore has contractile proteins arranged into sarcomeres. However, this is where the similarity to skeletal muscle ends. The myocardial fibers are connected end to end and project at different angles from one another, resulting in a network of short fibers that collectively span the heart (Figure 7.11). The general angulation of these fibers changes with increasing depth within the wall of myocardium, and, as explained in Chapter 11, this improves the heart's function as a pump.

The myocardial fibers are not functionally arranged into motor units, so the heart does not have multiple nerves initiating contraction. The depolarization of cardiac muscle therefore requires the propagation of the action potential from fiber to fiber. This propagation is aided by specialized membranes called *intercalated discs,* which transmit the action potential rapidly between myocardial fibers via *gap junctions* (see Figure 7.11, *A*). The intercalated discs and the electrical separation of the atrial and ventricular myocardium result in two separate regions of the heart (atrial and ventricular) for the spread of the depolarization and collective contraction of the myocardium (termed a *syncytium*). Consequently the heart has both an atrial and a ventricular syncytium.

summation (sum-a′shun)
the increase in muscle force during contraction caused by the frequent stimulation of the same or multiple motor units

tetanus (tet′a-nus)
sustained maximal contraction of a muscle

FIGURE 7.11

Electron micrographs of cardiac muscle fibers. **A,** The anatomic arrangement of the fibers in cardiac muscles is less linear than skeletal muscle, and fibers are shorter and connect end to end at differing angles. **B,** When viewed with higher magnification, the organization of contractile proteins into sarcomers and myofibrils is apparent, as are the many mitochondria, t-tubules, and intercollated discs. **C,** In the heart, cardiac fibers are layered, with the general orientation of the fibers differing between the layers. The layered and angulated arrangement of cardiac fibers (myocardium) is suited to their function of constricting the three dimensional volume of the heart to eject blood. (A, From Fawcett DW: *A textbook of histology,* ed 12, New York, 1994, Chapman Hall; B, From Berne MN: *Physiology,* ed 3, St. Louis, 1993, Mosby; C, From Thibideau GA Patton KT: *Anatomy and physiology,* St Louis, 1996, Mosby. Art by Rusty Jones.)

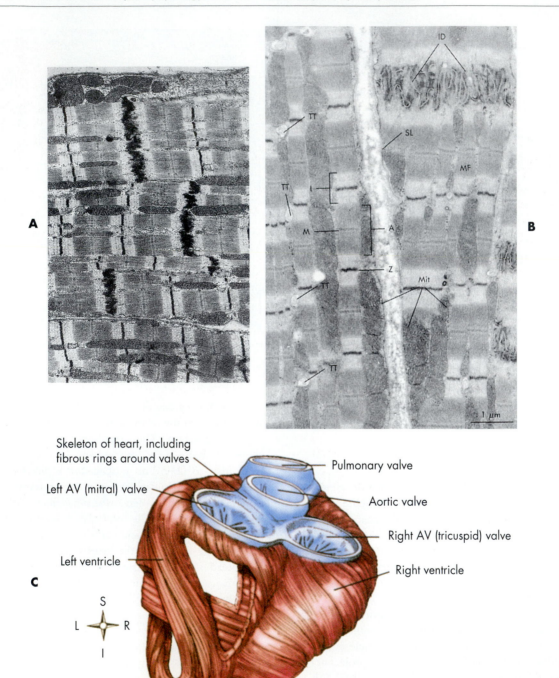

FIGURE 7.12

The direct neural, hormonal, and intrinsic regulation of myocardial contraction. Parasympathetic nerves innervate the SA node and atrial myocardium. Sympathetic nerves innervate both the SA and AV nodes, and also the ventricular myocardium to cause an increase in heart rate and ventricular contractility. An increased venous return increases myocardial end diastolic stretch, thus increasing the force of myocardial contraction. (From Seeley RR, Stephens TD, and Tate P: *Anatomy and physiology*, ed 3, St. Louis, 1995, Mosby. Art by Christine Oleksyk.)

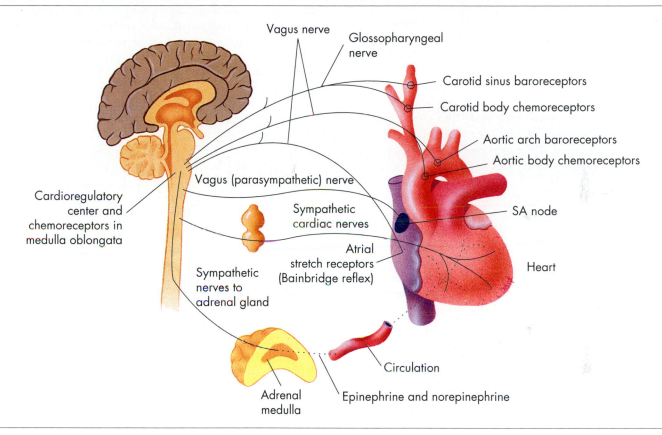

Myocardial fibers also possess an intrinsic ability to depolarize and initiate a contraction. This so-called **intrinsic rhythmicity** allows myocardial fibers to initiate a heartbeat and thereby to serve as additional pacemakers to the sinoatrial and atrioventricular nodes.

Because of the lack of motor units in cardiac muscle, the myocardium is a homogenous fiber type, consisting of many mitochondria, an extensive capillary supply, and metabolic capacities that favor ATP production by oxidative phosphorylation. Since the heart is continually contracting throughout a lifetime and must increase contractile force and frequency during exercise, this aerobic metabolic bias is understandable.

Contraction and Regulation

Cardiac muscle is striated and therefore has a cellular contraction mechanism similar to that of skeletal muscle. As illustrated in Figure 7.11, *A*, a cardiac muscle fiber consists of myofibrils, with sarcomeres and myosin and actin alignment similar to skeletal muscle. However, the light chains associated with cardiac muscle myosin differ from those of skeletal muscle.[2,14,27] The sequence of events during contraction (see Table 7.3) is identical for skeletal and cardiac muscle. However, the electrical characteristics of contraction are very different, as is the regulation of muscle contraction.

The myocardial fiber has a longer action potential than skeletal muscle, with a very different shape. (See Figure 7.10.) The length and shape of the myocardial action potential are caused primarily by the proteins that form ion channels allowing specific electrolytes to pass through the cell membrane. The ion channels are slower to open and close in cardiac muscle. In addition, an added channel for calcium is opened during depolarization, allowing calcium ions to move

intrinsic rhythmicity (in'trin-sik rith-miss i'ti)
the ability of a tissue to develop its own depolarization, usually at some consistent rate

from their relatively high extracellular concentration (2.4 mEq/L) to the extremely low intracellular concentration (0.0001 mEq/L) (Figure 7.10, B).[9] The influx of additional positive charge (Ca^{2+}) delays the repolarization of the membrane, prolonging the action potential and muscle contraction.

The regulation of cardiac muscle contraction has neural, hormonal, and intrinsic components (Figure 7.12). Nerves from the parasympathetic and sympathetic divisions of the autonomic nervous system innervate the heart to influence both the rate of contraction (heart rate) and the force and velocity of contraction *(contractility)* (Figure 7.13). Parasympathetic nerves innervate both the sinoatrial (SA) and atrioventricular (AV) nodes and result in a decreased heart rate. Sympathetic nerves innervate each node and the ventricular myocardium, resulting in an increased heart rate and increased contractility. Circulating catecholamines (epinephrine and norepinephrine) also increase heart rate and myocardial contractility.

Intrinsic regulation of the heart implies that the cardiac muscle itself responds to certain stimuli to either enhance or decrease contractile function. Cardiac muscle can do this because of the relationship between myocardial fiber length and tension. For cardiac muscle the length of the fibers is influenced by the filling of the chambers of the heart during diastole. Using the left ventricle as an example, the greater the ventricular filling, the greater the stretch and the greater the force of contraction (Figure 7.14). This response is called the *Frank-Starling mechanism* (see Chapter 11).

Function

The structural and electrochemical uniqueness of cardiac muscle has important functional consequences. The relatively long duration of the action potential prolongs the duration of the cardiac muscle twitch. In addition, the prolonged action potential prevents the rapid generation of successive action potentials and the possibility for twitch summation and the development of tetanus. Because cardiac muscle has no motor unit organization, contracts synchronously, and has no summation effect causing increased twitch tension, factors that increase myocardial contractility provide the only means to regulate myocardial contraction. As discussed in Chapter 11, each of the factors that increase myocardial contractility is involved in the body's acute response to exercise and allows the heart to function better as a demand pump.

Smooth Muscle

The function of smooth muscle is not necessarily to contract and cause a linear change in muscle length, like that of cardiac and skeletal muscle. Smooth muscle contracts to change the internal diameter of hollow organs and to maintain the shape of organs against force that can be constant or highly variable. Furthermore, smooth muscle must be able to maintain contraction for long periods (e.g., blood vessel diameter) and also to contract forcefully and intermittently

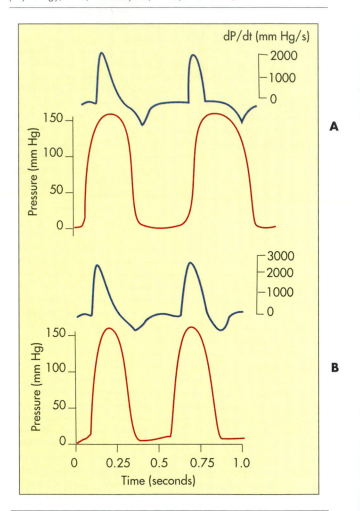

FIGURE 7.13

Cardiac muscle responds to hormonal stimulation by increasing the force of contraction (contractility) for a given stretch stimulus. Since measuring the force of myocardial contraction normally requires invasive measurements, an indirect method is to measure the rate of change in ventricular pressure over time (dP/dT). **A,** The change in ventricular pressure and dP/dT from a normal heart without sympathetic stimulation. **B,** When stimulated (isoproterenol), the rate of contraction increases (more frequent and shorter duration ventricular pressure waves) and the dP/dT curve increases in magnitude. (From Sodeman WA, Sodeman TM, editors: *Pathologic physiology,* ed 6, Philadelphia, 1979, Saunders.)

(e.g., peristalsis). As with cardiac and skeletal muscle, the structure and molecular characteristics of smooth muscle contraction are suited to its specific functions.

Structure

The simple cellular appearance of a smooth muscle fiber is illustrated in Figure 7.15. The fiber is elongated and can be connected to other smooth muscle fibers at varied regions of

FIGURE 7.14

Increasing the volume of blood in each chamber of the heart increases the stretch (length) of the myocardium, which like skeletal muscle, increases the force of the contraction (Starling's Law). In the healthy heart, an increased force of contraction results in increased cardiac function. This intrinsic response exists for differing extrinsic conditions that effect contractility (e.g., catecholamine stimulation). (Adapted from Underhill SL et al: *Cardiac nursing*, Philadelphia, 1982, JB Lippincott.)

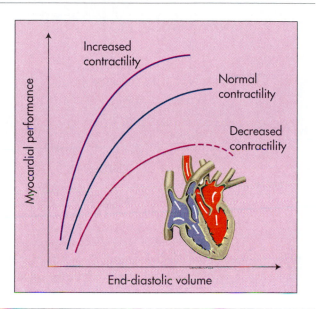

FIGURE 7.15

The cellular structure and cell–cell connections between smooth muscle fibers. (From Berne RM, Levy MN: *Physiology,* ed 3, St. Louis, 1993, Mosby.)

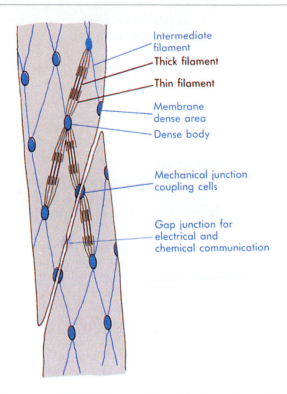

its cell membrane. These cell-to-cell connections are important for structural integrity within the smooth muscle mass and for the spread of depolarization during stimulation. The junctions that provide low resistance to the spread of depolarization are termed *gap junctions*. Figure 7.15 reveals that at the site of gap junctions exist numerous saclike invaginations called **calveoli** that are believed to be involved in the transmission of the depolarization between adjacent fibers.[5] Consequently, smooth muscle fibers connected by gap junctions contract as a multicellular unit, similar to the syncytium of the myocardium. However, in certain anatomic regions of the body, smooth muscle functions as isolated cellular units and therefore requires separate cellular stimulation.

Smooth muscle fibers do not have t-tubules. Rather, the sarcoplasmic reticulum is connected to the calveoli, from which it becomes depolarized during stimulation and releases calcium as in cardiac and skeletal muscle. The smooth muscle sarcoplasmic reticulum can be as extensive as in cardiac and skeletal muscle.[1] The smooth muscle sarcolemma also has calcium channels that allow calcium to enter directly from the extracellular compartment during depolarization. As will be explained, the extracellular pool of calcium is very important for the contractile mechanisms of smooth muscle.

The cytoskeletal and contractile filaments of smooth muscle are not aligned in a routine fashion, hence the inability to visualize them through electron microscopy. However, the inability to visualize these proteins does not mean smooth muscle lacks an organized array of contractile proteins. The fact that smooth muscle contraction is successful and can cause movement of hollow organs is a testament to an effective intracellular structure and contractile mechanism.

As a result of the need to contract in a three-dimensional manner, smooth muscle does not operate by a longitudinal system involving Z-lines and sarcomeres. Rather, smooth muscle fibers have dense bodies to which are attached actin filaments that are involved in contraction and the structural integrity of the fiber (see Figure 7.15). These dense bodies and their proteins are aligned within and between smooth muscle fibers, providing cellular connec-

calveoli (kal-ve′ol′i)

small circular invaginations located on sarcolemma of smooth muscle that transmit the depolarization to sarcoplasmic reticulum

tions that make a functional unit of a mass of many separate smooth muscle fibers.

The contractile proteins of smooth muscle are similar to those of striated muscle, except that smooth muscle does not contain troponin. Smooth muscle myosin is similar to striated muscle myosin, since in both myosin subfragments exist and the S1 unit has light chains that are essential for contractile activity.

The content of contractile proteins is very different between smooth and striated muscle. The smooth muscle cellular content of actin and tropomyosin is approximately double that of striated muscle, whereas the myosin content is one fourth that of striated muscle.[1]

Contraction and Regulation

The previous anatomic and molecular description of smooth muscle implies that the molecular mechanism of muscle contraction must differ from that of skeletal muscle. Because of the lack of troponin, the intracellular regulation of smooth muscle contraction is dependent on changes in the intracellular calcium concentration. An increase in intracellular calcium increases calcium binding to **calmodulin**, which in turn activates the enzyme myosin kinase. As detailed in Figure 7.16, myosin kinase catalyzes the phosphorylation of myosin regulatory light chains. The phosphate additions to the light chains are essential for the activation of myosin and actin and the resulting contraction of smooth muscle. The removal of calcium inhibits myosin kinase activity and activates myosin phosphatase, which catalyzes the removal of the phosphate from myosin light chains. However, as explained in the following material, unlike skeletal and cardiac muscle, the decrease in intracellular calcium may not necessarily result in complete smooth muscle relaxation.[1,8,10,17,19]

A fast and slow cycle of contraction exists in smooth muscle (Figures 7.16 and 7.17). The fast cycle is very ATP costly, since ATP is required in myosin phosphorylation and in detachment of the actin and myosin complex. This fast cycle predominates during phasic smooth muscle contractions, as exemplified by peristaltic contractions along the esophagus or gastric movement. The slow cycle, or *latch mechanism,* predominates when intracellular calcium concentrations are slightly raised, providing a slow rate of myosin phosphorylation. A proportion of the phosphorylated myosin that is in the contracted state is dephosphorylated by myosin phosphatase, and because this process is relatively slow, results in continued contraction with no added ATP cost. The result of the slow phase of contraction is that smooth muscle contractile tension is maintained without contraction cycling, hence the term *latch mechanism.* The slow phase of contraction typifies smooth muscle contractions during blood vessel and sphincter constriction.

The stimulation of smooth muscle contraction can occur from the neural release of a neurotransmitter or by circulating hormones. Unlike skeletal muscle, smooth muscle does not have specialized neuromuscular junctions. Enlarged regions along the axon (varicosities) release the vesicles that

FIGURE 7.16

The molecular sequence of events during smooth muscle contraction. The phosphorylation of the myosin regulatory light chain is essential for actin and myosin interaction and muscle contraction. The continued presence of calcium and the phosphorylated light chain of myosin results in crossbridge cycling and the expenditure of ATP in a similar manner to skeletal and cardiac muscle contraction. (From Berne RM, Levy MN: *Physiology,* ed 3, St. Louis, 1993, Mosby.)

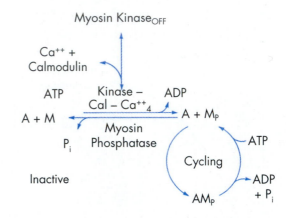

contain the transmitter. The transmitter then diffuses to the smooth muscle membrane where there is little specialization of the sarcolemma. If the smooth muscle mass is not connected by gap junctions (multiunit), each fiber must receive the neurotransmitter for eventual contraction. However, if the gap junctions connect fibers, and therefore propagate an action potential or respond to an intracellular second messenger, there is less need for multiple receptors on each fiber.

Function

From the previous description of the molecular events of contraction, phasic smooth muscle contraction and force generation are more dependent on the intracellular calcium activation of myosin kinase activity than are tonic contractions. In tonically contracting smooth muscle, force generation continues despite a decline in intracellular calcium and the rate of crossbridge cycling.

Compared with skeletal muscle, the velocity of smooth muscle contraction is extremely slow. However, the degree of myosin regulatory light chain phosphorylation is proportional to the velocity of smooth muscle contraction. Interestingly, the added ATP cost of phasic contraction in smooth muscle decreases its efficiency to one half that of skeletal muscle, whereas the tonic contraction of smooth muscle requires 300 times less ATP than skeletal muscle for a given tension development.

calmodulin (cal′mod-u′lin)

an intracellular protein that binds four calcium ions, and when bound to calcium can activate specific enzymes within the cell

FIGURE 7.17

The fast (phasic) and slow (tonic) mechanisms of smooth muscle contraction. (Adapted from Berne RM, Levy MN: *Physiology,* ed 3, St. Louis, 1993, Mosby.

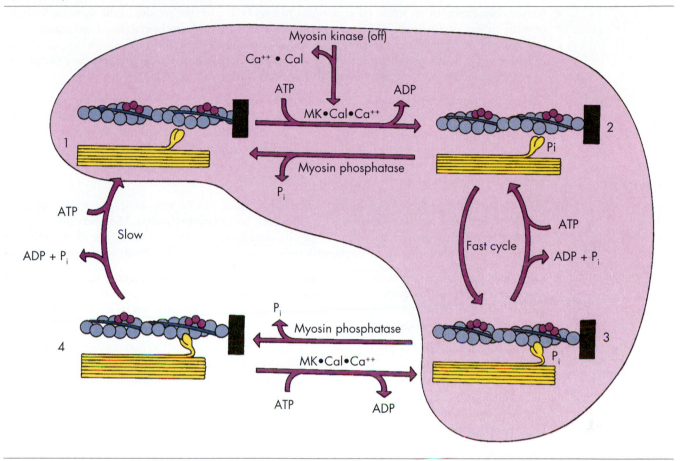

SUMMARY

- Muscles cause movement, which refers not only to total body exercise, but also to the dynamic functions of many of our internal organs. Skeletal muscle causes or resists musculoskeletal movement, cardiac muscle causes heart constriction and blood flow, and smooth muscle constricts or maintains the dimensions of many of the body's hollow organs. The cells, or **fibers,** of all three types of muscle have the properties of **excitability, contractility, extensibility**, and **elasticity.**

- Skeletal muscle and cardiac muscle (myocardium) are termed *striated muscle* because of the visual microscopic organization of the contractile proteins **actin** and **myosin.** Additional proteins, such as **troponin** and **tropomyosin,** are also present and involved in the regulation of contraction. Within striated muscle fibers, these proteins are organized into **sarcomeres** and **myofibrils.** Smooth muscle also contains actin and myosin, but the arrangement and proportions of these proteins are different and they cannot be visualized by microscopy.

- Skeletal muscle fibers are aligned linearly, are multinucleated, can be very long, and are grouped into functional units that are each innervated by a common nerve **(motor units)**. The fibers from different motor units can differ in mechanical and metabolic characteristics. A depolarization spreads from the **sarcolemma** via **t-tubules** to the **sarcoplasmic reticulum**–tubule junction **(triad)** within the sarcomeres.

- Continued stimulation of muscle results in sustained contraction, and this process is explained by **contraction cycling.** Whole muscle contractions are categorized as concentric, eccentric, isometric, or isokinetic. Increased frequencies of muscle stimulation can cause the **summation** of tension and can result in the condition of **tetanus**.

- Skeletal muscle contractions causing a change in muscle length are called *isotonic* contractions. When the muscle shortens, the isotonic contraction is referred to as a **concentric** contraction. When the muscle lengthens during contraction, the isotonic contraction is referred to as **eccentric.** Muscle contractions causing no change in muscle length are called **isometric** actions. A third type of contraction (muscle action) is **isokinetic.** Isokinetic contractions are a special type of concentric contraction in which the velocity of muscle shortening remains constant (hence the term *isokinetic*).

- Myocardial fibers are relatively short, possess **intrinsic rhythmicity**, are randomly aligned with one another, and are of a homogenous metabolic fiber type. The anatomic arrangement of myocardial fibers and their neural regulation during contraction differ from skeletal muscle. Cardiac muscle action potential is long and of similar duration to the cardiac muscle twitch as a result of an influx of calcium. The involvement of calcium in the process of myocardial depolarization also improves the velocity and force of contraction, termed *contractility.*

- Smooth muscle fiber is elongated and has dense bodies dispersed throughout it to which are attached protein filaments involved in contraction and the structural integrity of the fiber. Smooth muscle fibers can be connected to other fibers through gap junctions, and saclike invaginations called *calveoli* transmit electrical stimulation to the sarcoplasmic reticulum where calcium is released. Like cardiac muscle, smooth muscle depolarization also causes an influx of calcium. Smooth muscle fibers do not have t-tubules or the protein troponin; however, another protein, **calmodulin,** functions like troponin during contraction. The increase in intracellular calcium during depolarization results in the phosphorylation of myosin light chains, which is essential for smooth muscle contraction. Although the complete removal of excess calcium causes smooth muscle relaxation, decreases in calcium can be associated with sustained contraction and tension development. The sustained contraction results from the slow detachment of the actin and myosin complex *(latch mechanism)* when the phosphates are removed from the myosin light chains.

REVIEW QUESTIONS

1. What are the different functions of skeletal, cardiac, and smooth muscle?

2. How do the anatomic, molecular, and regulatory aspects of muscle contraction for skeletal, myocardial, and smooth muscle enable them to exert their functions?

3. Detail and list in sequence the molecular events of skeletal and cardiac muscle contraction.

4. Explain the differences among concentric, eccentric, and isokinetic muscle contractions.

5. How does the influx of calcium during cardiac muscle depolarization affect the action potential and the duration of the contraction? Compare the cardiac action potential and contractile response to those of skeletal muscle.

6. How does the velocity of skeletal muscle contraction affect force and power development?

7. What are the functional implications of the length-tension relationship for skeletal and cardiac muscle?

8. What are the differences between multi-unit and single unit smooth muscle?

9. What is the "latch mechanism" of smooth muscle contraction?

APPLICATIONS

1. The condition of heart failure often develops because of a chronic overstretch of the ventricular myocardium. Based on the length-tension relationship, explain how this condition might affect the function of the heart.

2. During episodes of skeletal muscle cramp, relief is often promoted by immediate massage and the stretching of the muscle. Explain why these immediate treatment modalities might be effective.

3. Explain the reasons that electrolyte (Na^+, K^+, Ca^{2+}) imbalances in blood can impair the ability of muscle to respond appropriately to neural stimulation.

4. During exercise, skeletal muscle must contract and relax in very short time intervals. What demands does this place on the cellular regulation of muscle contraction?

5. If the latch mechanism of smooth muscle contraction did not exist, what might the ramifications be to the regulation and energetic demands of blood vessels and blood flow through these vessels?

REFERENCES

1. Berne RM, Levy MN: *Physiology,* ed 3, St Louis, 1993, Mosby.

2. Canale ED, Campbell GR, Smolich JJ, Campbell JH: *Cardiac muscle,* New York, 1986, Springer-Verlag.

3. Collins JH: Myosin light chains and troponin C: structural and evolutionary relationships revealed by amino acid sequence comparisons, *J Muscle Res Cell Motil* 12(1):3-25, 1991.

4. Friden J: Topographical localization of muscle glycogen: an ultrahistochemical study in the human vastus lateralis, *Acta Physiol Scand* 135(3):381-392, 1989.

5. Gabella G: General aspects of fine structure of smooth muscles. In Motta PM, editor: *Ultrastructure of smooth muscle,* Boston, 1990, Kluwer Academic.

6. Geneser F: *Textbook of histology,* Philadelphia, 1986, Lea & Febiger.

7. Goldfine SM, Einheber S, Fischman DA: Cell-free incorporation of newly synthesized myosin subunits into thick myofilaments, *J Muscle Res Cell Motil* 12:161-170, 1991.

8. Golenhofen K: Spontaneous activity and functional classification of mammalian smooth muscle. In Bulbring E, Shuba MF, editors: *Physiology of smooth muscle,* New York, 1978, Raven Press.

9. Guyton AC: *Textbook of medical physiology,* ed 8, Philadelphia, 1991, WB Saunders.

10. Haraki H, Hori M, Sato K et al: Regulation of smooth muscle contraction by the myosin light chain phosphorylation-dependent and –independent mechanisms. In Frank GB, Bianchi CP, ter Keurs HED: *Excitation-contraction coupling in skeletal, cardiac, and smooth muscle,* New York, 1992, Plenum Press.

11. Huxley HE: Molecular basis of contraction in cross-striated muscle. In Bourke GH, editor: *The structure and function of muscle,* vol 1, part 1, New York, 1972, Academic Press.

12. Ishikawa H, Sawada H, Yamada E: Surface and internal morphology of skeletal muscle. In Peachey LD, Adrian RH, Geiger SR, editors: *Handbook of physiology,* section 10, *Skeletal muscle,* Bethesda, Md, 1983, American Physiological Society.

13. Katz A: *Physiology of the heart,* New York, 1977, Raven Press.

14. Lowey S, Risby D: Light chains from fast and slow muscle myosins, *Nature* 234:81-85, 1971.

15. Lymn RW, Taylor EW: Mechanism of adenosine triphosphate hydrolysis by actomyosin, *Biochemistry* 10(25):4617-4624, 1971.

16. Marieb EN: *Human anatomy and physiology,* Redwood City, California, 1995, Benjamin Cummings Publishing.

17. Marston SB: What is latch? New ideas about tonic contraction in smooth muscle, *J Muscle Res Cell Motil* 10:97-100, 1989.

18. Mornet D, Bonet A, Audemard E, Bonicel J: Functional sequences of the myosin head, *J Muscle Res Cell Motil* 10:10-24, 1989.

19. Onishi H, Maita T, Matsuda G, Fujiwara K: Interaction between the heavy and the regulatory light chains in smooth muscle myosin subfragment 1, *Biochemistry* 31:1201-1210, 1992.

20. Pate E, Cooke R: A model of crossbridge action: the effects of ATP, ADP and Pi, *J Muscle Res Cell Motil* 10:181-196, 1989.

21. Peachey LD, Franzini-Armstrong C: Structure and function of membrane systems of skeletal muscle cells. In Peachey LD, Adrian RH, Geiger SR, editors: *Handbook of physiology,* section 10, *Skeletal muscle,* Bethesda, Md, 1983, American Physiological Society.

22. Raven PB, *Med Sci Sports Exer* 23(7):777-778, 1991.

23. Schmalbruch H: *Skeletal muscle,* New York, 1985, Springer-Verlag.

24. Sedeen M: In touch with the world. In National Geographic Society: *The incredible machine,* Washington DC, 1986, National Geographic Society.

25. Underhill SL, Woods SL, Sivarajan ES, Halpenny CJ: *Cardiac nursing,* Philadelphia, 1982, JB Lippincott.

26. Wang K: Sarcomere-associate cytoskeletal lattices in striated muscle. In Shay JW, editor: *Cell muscle motility,* vol 6, New York, 1985, Plenum Publishing.

27. Weeds AG, Pope B: Chemical studies on light chains from cardiac and skeletal muscle myosins, *Nature* 234:85-88, 1971.

28. Westing SH, Segar Y: Eccentric and concentric torque-velocity characteristics, torque output comparisons and gravity effect torque corrections for quadriceps and hamstring muscles in females, *Int J Sports Med* 10:175-180, 1989.

29. Winkelmann DA, Baker TS, Rayment I: Three dimensional structure of myosin subfragment-1 from electron microscopy of sectioned crystals, *J Cell Biol* 114(4):701-713, 1991.

30. Young OA: A possible role for myosin light chain 1 slow of bovine muscle, *J Muscle Res Cell Motility* 10:403-412, 1989.

RECOMMENDED READINGS

▪ Gabella G: General aspects of fine structure of smooth muscles. In Motta PM, editor: *Ultrastructure of smooth muscle,* Boston, 1990, Kluwer Academic.

▪ Guyton AC: *Textbook of medical physiology,* ed 8, Philadelphia, 1991, WB Saunders.

▪ Haraki H, Hori M, Sato K et al: Regulation of smooth muscle contraction by the myosin light chain phosphorylation-dependent and –independent mechanisms. In Frank GB, Bianchi CP, ter Keurs HED: *Excitation-contraction coupling in skeletal, cardiac, and smooth muscle,* New York, 1992, Plenum Press.

▪ Ishikawa H, Sawada H, Yamada E: Surface and internal morphology of skeletal muscle. In Peachey LD, Adrian RH, Geiger SR, editors: *Handbook of physiology,* section 10, *Skeletal muscle,* Bethesda, Md, 1983, American Physiological Society.

▪ Peachey LD, Franzini-Armstrong C: Structure and function of membrane systems of skeletal muscle cells. In Peachey LD, Adrian RH, Geiger SR, editors: *Handbook of physiology,* section 10, *Skeletal muscle,* Bethesda, Md, 1983, American Physiological Society.

CHAPTER 8

Neuromuscular Function and the Control of Movement

OBJECTIVES

After studying this chapter you should be able to:

- Define and provide examples of different neurotransmitters, and associate their presence to functions of the body.

- Explain the importance of sensory receptors to the control of muscle contraction.

- Identify the functions of the autonomic nervous system that contribute to the body's physiologic response to exercise.

- Identify complex anatomy and related functions of the muscle spindle.

- Explain the terms *proprioception* and *kinesthesis,* and how neuromuscular interactions enable these capacities.

- Describe the neural sequence of events that occurs during the instigation and execution of movement.

- Describe the morphology and function of the neuromuscular junction.

- Define and explain the function of motor units and the neural, contractile, and metabolic differences between motor units.

- Identify the order of motor unit recruitment, and explain how this recruitment order can influence muscle energy metabolism and exercise performance.

KEY TERMS

synapse

neurotransmitter

axon hillock

ganglia

receptor

sensory receptor

neural adaptation

muscle spindle

alpha-gamma coactivation

kinesthesis

proprioception

somatosensory cortex

neuromuscular junction

muscle biopsy

fiber type

*N*erve function and the integrated control of nerve function enable us to consciously and subconsciously control our bodies and to be aware of our body parts. Specific components of the nervous system deal with conscious and subconscious control of movement, as well as regulate body functions that support movement. The autonomic nervous system provides the subconscious regulation of muscles used to breathe, determines the tone of smooth muscle surrounding arterioles and veins in certain tissue beds, and influences hormones released during exercise. During exercise the integration between nerves originating in the motor cortex of the brain and skeletal muscle fibers allows the voluntary control of muscle contraction. As explained in this chapter, nerves also dictate the strength and intensity of muscle contraction and therefore the intensity of exercise. Consequently, to understand the metabolic responses to exercise the student must understand how the nervous system and skeletal muscle interact to cause muscle contraction and movement. The purpose of this chapter is to detail the important interactions that exist between nerves and skeletal muscle and to document the heterogeneous neural and muscle metabolic properties of the human neuromuscular system.

Divisions of the Nervous System

*T*he nervous system can be divided into anatomic and functional divisions. Anatomically, the nervous system comprises the central and peripheral systems (Figure 8.1), where the central system comprises the brain and spinal cord and the peripheral system comprises sensory and motor nerves. The functional divisions of the nervous system are the involuntary and voluntary control divisions. However, since brain, spinal cord, and motor pathways do not function as discrete entities, have both voluntary and involuntary functions, and combine to give certain functions, further differentiation according to function is more complex than the anatomic classification.

The major functions of the nervous system are listed in Figure 8.2. Generally the central nervous system (CNS) functions on three levels: the cortical or higher brain level, the lower brain level, and the spinal cord level. Simple reflex movements (e.g., blinking of the eye, stretch reflex, gastrointestinal movements) are controlled within the spinal cord, while the majority of the remaining subconscious functions of the body, such as ventilation, blood pressure regulation, and emotion, are controlled in the lower brain. The midbrain is responsible for receiving and processing neural signals from the many specialized centers within the CNS and relays the processed nerve signals to the higher brain (or cortical level), which is responsible for memory, complex movement patterns, the awareness of peripheral stimuli, and the sending of movement patterns to the $A\alpha$ motor nerves.

The Synapse

*T*he previous description of the functions of the nervous system indicates that many nerves must connect with one another. For example, nerves of the cortical

FIGURE 8.1

The anatomic divisions of the nervous system. (From Thibodeau GA, Patton KT: *Anatomy and physiology*, ed 3, St. Louis, 1996, Mosby.)

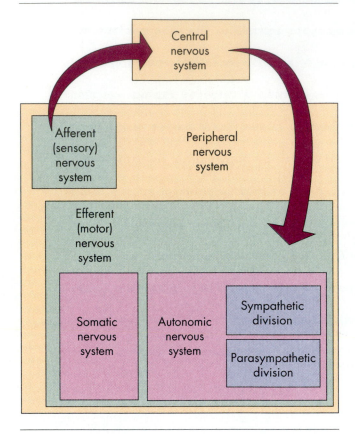

region of the presynaptic membrane, voltage-gated calcium channels open and calcium diffuses down its concentration gradient into the presynaptic nerve region, increasing the concentration of intracellular free calcium. This increased calcium concentration is believed to result in the migration of *acetylcholine*-containing vesicles to the presynaptic membrane, where acetylcholine is released via the process of *exocytosis.* Acetylcholine is an example of a **neurotransmitter.** The acetylcholine diffuses across the short (<300 angstroms = <0.03 µm) synaptic cleft, where it binds to specialized acetylcholine receptors. The binding of acetylcholine to the receptors opens special Na^+ channels (acetylcholine-gated Na^+ channels). If enough acetylcholine is released from the presynaptic membrane and binds to the receptors of the postsynaptic membrane, sufficient Na^+ channels open and the postsynaptic membrane depolarizes.

Whether the depolarization of a postsynaptic membrane is sufficient to cause an action potential depends on the location of the synapse in the nervous system, the level of neuronal excitation, and the spatial summation of other nerve synaptic transmissions, which may have excitatory or inhibitory effects on the postsynaptic membrane.

The location of the synapse is important, since this influences the number of nerves that synapse on another nerve and therefore have influence on the postsynaptic membrane potential. A suitable example of the importance of synapses is the neural connections to the Aα motor nerve (see Figure 8.4). The Aα motor nerve is located within the spinal cord and may have more than 100 synapses. When there is a general excitation of the somatic nervous system, 20 to 40 of the excitatory synapses may be active and their separate influences on the postsynaptic membrane are summed *(spatial summation),* which may cause a further increase in the postsynaptic membrane potential from –65 to –45 mV. Increases in the postsynaptic membrane potential are referred to as *excitatory postsynaptic potentials.* Of course, if the synapses that are active are inhibitory in nature, the neurotransmitter they release causes an increase in the permeability of the membrane to K^+, resulting in a more negative postsynaptic membrane potential and the less likely event of an action potential being developed.

The summation of the inhibitory and excitatory nerves acting on the soma through the dendrites determines whether the membrane of the soma depolarizes sufficiently to reach threshold. Because the Na^+ channels on the membrane of the soma are not voltage gated, an action potential cannot originate here. In the region where the axon leaves the soma, called the **axon hillock,** a large density of voltage-gated Na^+ channels is present in the nerve membrane. When the summed depolarization exceeds the given threshold potential for the nerve, the voltage-gated Na^+ channels of the axon hillock open and an action potential is propagated along the axon. For the Aα motor nerve, this results in the contraction of all the muscle fibers *innervated* by the nerve (see section on motor units).

region of the brain connect to many other locations within the cortical level and also to nerves within the lower brain and spinal cord levels. Similarly, the afferent nerves from the periphery connect to nerves located within the spinal cord, and the Aα motor nerves leave the spinal cord from connections to nerves from the spinal cord and also nerves from the lower and cortical levels of the brain. For the effective transmission of the action potential from one nerve to another, these junctions must function very effectively.

The junction site between two different nerves is called a **synapse** (Figures 8.3 and 8.4). Almost all the synapses of the body function by releasing a chemical substance from the *presynaptic membrane* that diffuses across the space between nerves, or *synaptic cleft,* where the chemical binds to special receptors on the *postsynaptic membrane*. All synapses function unidirectionally.

Synaptic Transmission

The biochemical and electrochemical events of synaptic transmission for a typical stimulatory synapse are depicted in Figure 8.3. When the action potential reaches the terminal

FIGURE 8.2

The major functions of the nervous system localized to the regions of control. The three levels of function of the central nervous system are illustrated, as are the peripheral functions of the autonomic and sensory nerves (involuntary control) and voluntary motor nerves.

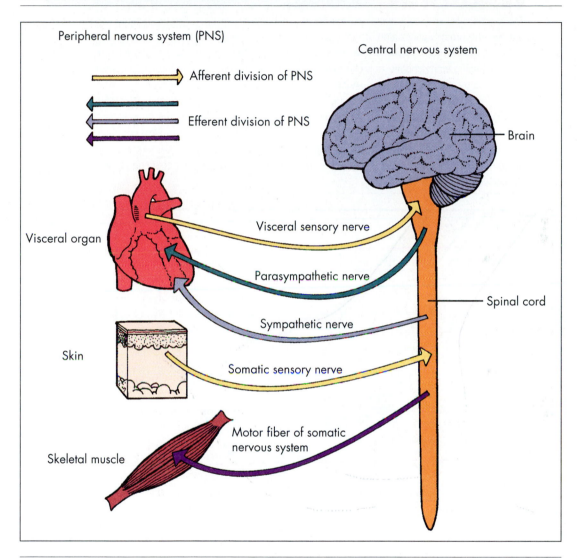

Acetylcholine:
Not the Only Neurotransmitter

As mentioned, there are stimulatory and inhibitory synapses, and almost all synapses are located within the central nervous system. Table 8.1 lists some of the known neurotransmitters and their location within the nervous system. The neurotransmitters of interest for the function of the nervous system during exercise are mainly acetylcholine and norepinephrine (Figure 8.5); however, additional neurotransmitters in the CNS are essential for our cognition of movement and emotional responses to exercise. Acetylcholine is the neurotransmitter for the conduction of the action potential to skeletal muscle fibers, for a small number of synapses

synapse (sin'aps)

the junction between two nerves

neurotransmitter (nu'ro-**trans**-mit'er)

a chemical released at a synapse in response to the depolarization of the presynaptic membrane

axon hillock

the region of a cell body near the axon that is responsible for the development of an action potential

FIGURE 8.3

The biochemical and electrochemical events of synaptic transmission. The propagated depolarization reaches the presynaptic region of the axon and opens voltage-gated calcium channels. Calcium enters the presynaptic region of the axon. The increase in free calcium causes the migration of vesicles containing acetylcholine to move to and to bind with the presynaptic membrane. Acetylcholine is released by the process of exocytosis. Acetylcholine diffuses across the synaptic cleft, where it binds to acetylcholine receptors or is degraded to acetate and choline by acetylcholinesterase. Binding of acetylcholine molecules to a sufficient number of receptors causes the depolarization of the sarcolemma of the skeletal muscle fiber, leading to the cellular events of muscle contraction. Once bound, acetylcholine is also degraded into acetate and choline by acetylcholinesterase, and the sarcolemma membrane potential is restored to resting values, ready to once again be receptive to neuromuscular stimulation.

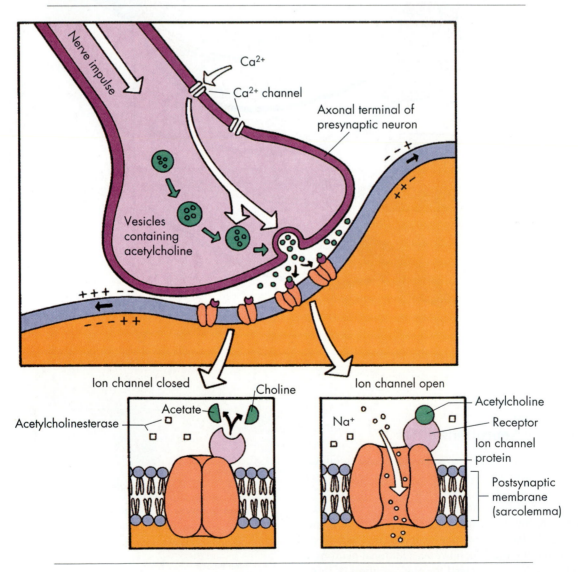

FIGURE 8.4

The stimulatory and inhibitory synapses on the soma of a typical Aα motor nerve within the spinal cord. The inhibitory nerves are orange, whereas the stimulatory nerves are green. The enlarged region shows the Axon of Hillock, where voltage-gated Na+ channels are present and convert an above threshold membrane potential of the soma to an action potential that is propagated along the nerve axon.

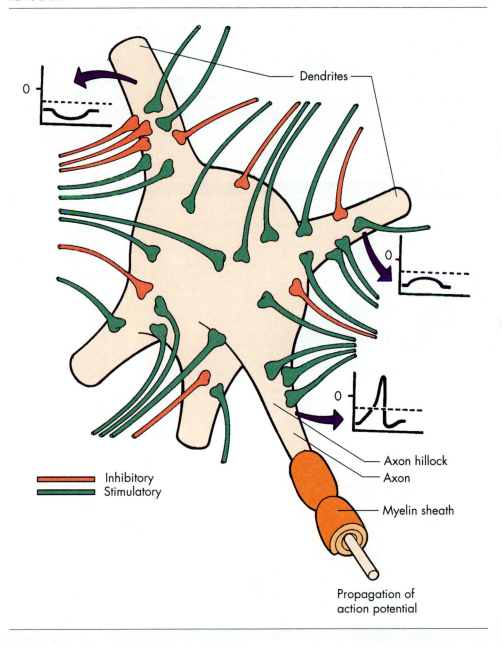

Dendrites

Inhibitory
Stimulatory

Axon hillock
Axon

Myelin sheath

Propagation of
action potential

TABLE 8.1

Examples of the fast-acting* neurotransmitters of the nervous system, and the main regions of the nervous system in which they are released

NEUROTRANSMITTER	LOCATIONS
Acetylcholine	Motor cortex, basal ganglia, Aα motor nerves, some nerves of the autonomic nervous system
Norepinephrine	Brain stem, hypothalamus, most postganglionic nerves of the sympathetic nervous system
Epinephrine	Adrenal medulla
Dopamine	Basal ganglia
Serotonin	Brain stem, spinal cord, hypothalamus
γ -Aminobutyric acid (GABA)	Brain stem, spinal cord, cerebellum, cortex

*The nervous system also uses slow-acting neurotransmitters, or neuropeptides, that are synthesized in the soma of a nerve and not the presynaptic region of the nerve.

FIGURE 8.5

The nerves, neurotransmitters, and receptors of the sympathetic and parasympathetic divisions of the autonomic nervous system. (From Thibodeau GA, Patton KT: *Anatomy and physiology,* ed 3, St. Louis, 1996, Mosby.)

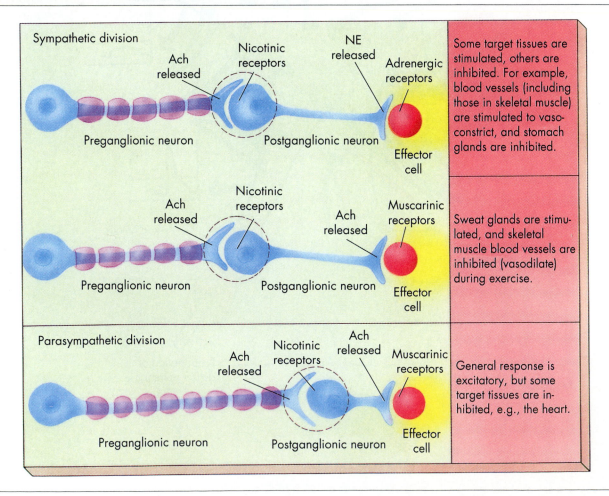

FIGURE 8.6

The organs and tissues innervated by the parasympathetic and sympathetic divisions of the autonomic nervous system. (From Thibodeau GA, Patton KT: *Anatomy and physiology,* ed 3, 1996, Mosby. Art by Barbara Cousins.)

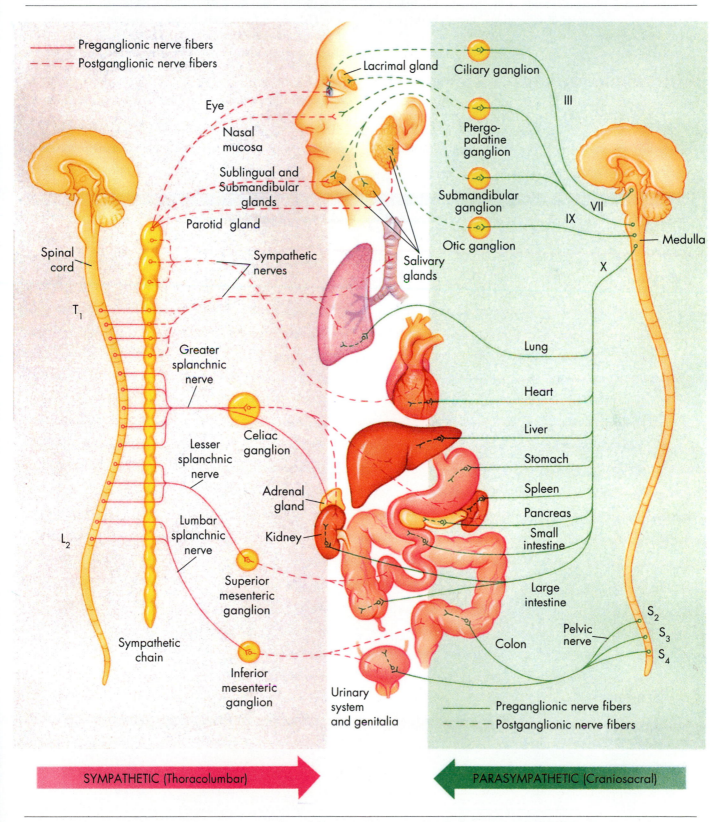

Preganglionic nerve fibers
Postganglionic nerve fibers

Lacrimal gland
Ciliary ganglion
III
Eye
Nasal mucosa
Ptergo-palatine ganglion
Sublingual and Submandibular glands
Submandibular ganglion
VII
IX
Parotid gland
Otic ganglion
Medulla
Spinal cord
Sympathetic nerves
Salivary glands
X
T_1
Greater splanchnic nerve
Lung
Heart
Liver
Stomach
Spleen
Pancreas
Small intestine
Lesser splanchnic nerve
Celiac ganglion
Adrenal gland
Lumbar splanchnic nerve
Kidney
L_2
Superior mesenteric ganglion
Large intestine
S_2
Pelvic nerve
S_3
S_4
Sympathetic chain
Colon
Inferior mesenteric ganglion
Urinary system and genitalia
Preganglionic nerve fibers
Postganglionic nerve fibers

SYMPATHETIC (Thoracolumbar)   PARASYMPATHETIC (Craniosacral)

from sympathetic nerves of the autonomic nervous system, and for all the *preganglionic* synapses of the sympathetic (e.g., sweat gland) and parasympathetic nerves of the autonomic nervous system. Norepinephrine is the neurotransmitter for the *postganglionic* synapses of sympathetic nerves of the autonomic nervous system.

Autonomic Nervous System

*A*s the name suggests, the autonomic nervous system functions without voluntary control. However, emotions such as excitement, fear, depression, and anxiety cause alterations in the function of the autonomic nervous system. The autonomic nervous system can be functionally and anatomically divided into the *sympathetic* division and the *parasympathetic* division.

The nerves from both divisions innervate organs such as the heart and smooth muscle of the lungs, blood vessels, sweat glands, and bladder. Control of these organs by reciprocal changes in the activity of sympathetic and parasympathetic nerves results in the control of body functions or conditions such as temperature, blood pressure, hydration, urination, and heart rate (Figure 8.6).

The functions altered by the sympathetic and parasympathetic divisions of the nervous system that are pertinent to

TABLE 8.2

Important functions altered by the sympathetic and parasympathetic nervous system during exercise

TISSUE	ACTIVITY	RECEPTOR	RESPONSE
SYMPATHETIC			
Heart	↑	β1	↑ Heart Rate
Myocardium	↑	β1	↑ Contractility
Myocardial blood vessels	↑	β2	Vasodilation
	↓	α	Vasoconstriction
Lungs	↑	β2	↓ Airway resistance
Skeletal muscle	↑	β2	↑ Glycogenolysis
Skeletal muscle blood vessels	↑	β	Vasodilation
	↑	Nicotinic	Vasodilation
	↑	α	Vasoconstriction
Cutaneous blood vessels	↑	α	Vasoconstriction
Adipose	↑	β1	↑ Lipolysis
Liver	↑	β2	↑ Glycogenolysis
Abdominal viscera blood vessels	↑	α	Vasoconstriction
Sweat glands	↑	Nicotinic	↑ Sweating
Iris	↑	α	Dilation
Intestinal tract lumen	↑	β2	↓ Tone
PARASYMPATHETIC			
Heart	↓	Muscarinic	↑ Heart rate
Myocardial blood vessels	↓	Muscarinic	↓ Vasodilation
Atrial myocardium	↓	Muscarinic	↑ Contractility
Intestinal tract lumen	↓	Muscarinic	↓ Tone

Modified from Guyton AC: *Textbook of medical physiology,* ed 8, Philadelphia, 1991, WB Saunders.

exercise conditions are listed in Table 8.2. Although it is tempting to use the words *sympathetic* and *excitatory* synonymously, this is inaccurate because some sympathetic nerves cause smooth muscle relaxation in certain vascular beds (e.g., bronchioles of the lung) and some parasympathetic nerves cause smooth muscle contraction (e.g., bladder, certain glands). However, it is clear from Table 8.2 that sympathetic stimulation induces changes that improve the body's response to exercise, whereas parasympathetic stimulation generally opposes these functions.

Sympathetic and Parasympathetic Divisions

Figure 8.6 illustrates the anatomic arrangement and the organs influenced by the sympathetic and parasympathetic divi-sions of the autonomic nervous system. Regions of the midbrain and lower brain influence the activity of the autonomic nervous system. For example, neural stimulation from the hypothalamus can alter the regulation of the heart, peripheral vasculature, body temperature, and gastrointestinal activity.[24]

For the sympathetic division, two nerves are responsible for stimulating a peripheral organ. The first nerve, called a *preganglionic nerve,* leaves the spinal cord through an anterior root and enters within the sympathetic chain of **ganglia** located external to the spinal cord, where it either synapses with a peripheral nerve or leaves the sympathetic chain to synapse with a peripherally located ganglion (e.g., adrenal medulla, anal sphincter). The synapse of the preganglionic nerve to the second nerve, called a *postganglionic nerve,* is outlined in Figure 8.5. As previously described, the neurotransmitter acting at the preganglionic synapses is acetylcholine. Norepinephrine is the neurotransmitter released in all postganglionic synapses, except for sweat glands and certain blood vessels, which release acetylcholine.

A unique component of the sympathetic nervous system is the preganglionic nerve that extends to the adrenal medulla where it synapses with special nervelike cells that secrete epinephrine and norepinephrine into the circulation. Approximately 85% of the neural secretion by the adrenal medulla is epinephrine, with the remainder norepinephrine.[24] Together, epinephrine and norepinephrine are referred to as *catecholamines.* This source of the catecholamine hormones extends the function of the sympathetic system from neural to hormonal, making the norepinephrine available to all cells of the body that possess the appropriate receptors. Similarly, epinephrine also becomes available to all cells of the body, and because of the similar structure of norepinephrine and epinephrine, epinephrine can also bind to norepinephrine receptors and elicit a cellular response.

For the parasympathetic division, two nerves are also involved in the innervation of peripheral organs. However, unlike the sympathetic neural arrangement, the preganglionic nerve extends directly from the CNS to the peripheral organ, within which lies the postganglionic nerve. The parasympa-

thetic nerves leave the lower brain or sacral level of the spinal cord and innervate the peripheral organs illustrated in Figure 8.6. More than 75% of all parasympathetic nerves leave the CNS at the level of the lower brain via cranial nerves III, VII, IX, and X.[24]

The importance of the parasympathetic and sympathetic divisions of the autonomic nervous system is revealed by the decreased neuromuscular and cardiorespiratory function experienced by individuals with spinal cord injury, as explained in the Clinical Application on p. 184.

Importance of Membrane Receptors

*F*or nerves to conduct an action potential across a synapse and to have an effect on an organ, the receptive membrane must have a **receptor** on which the neurotransmitter binds. The presence of the receptor and the type of receptor determine the cellular response to the neurotransmitter.

There are two receptors for acetylcholine, and their names are derived from foreign molecules that are known to bind to them and elicit a biologic response: muscarine poison from toadstools activates the *muscarinic receptor,* and nicotine activates the *nicotinic receptor.* There are also two main types of norepinephrine receptors, called *alpha* (α) *and beta* (β) *receptors.* Both the α and β receptors have two subdivisions (α1 and 2, β1 and 2), with the β1 and β2 subdivisions having more distinct separation of function. Binding of norepinephrine to β2 receptors causes vasodilation of the coronary arteries, whereas binding of norepinephrine to α receptors on coronary arteries and the arterioles of skeletal muscle causes vasoconstriction. Similarly, the membranes of smooth muscle surrounding the bronchioles of the lung contain β2 receptors and dilate when bound to norepinephrine, whereas the β1 receptors of the heart induce increased Na^+ permeability of certain membranes (e.g., the sinoatrial node) and improvements in myocardial metabolism and contractile function.

The catecholamine system has further complexity, since norepinephrine and epinephrine have differing affinity for the α and β receptors. Norepinephrine exerts its main cellular response via the α receptors, whereas epinephrine is equally effective for both α and β receptors. This difference is important when comparing the systemic release of the catecholamines from the adrenal medulla during exercise with

ganglia (gang-gli-ah)
an aggregation of nerve cell bodies located in the peripheral nervous system

receptor (re-sep'tor)
a protein located within a membrane that is able to bind another molecule

Neuromuscular Implications of Spinal Cord Injury

Spinal cord injury (SCI) is classified by the level of the spinal cord that is injured and by the completeness of the injury. Based on the level of injury, individuals with SCI are grouped as either *paraplegic*, when the injury is lower than the seventh cervical vertebra, or *quadriplegic*, when the injury is above this level. Complete injuries involve the complete severance of the spinal cord. Complete injuries result in the loss of voluntary and involuntary neural control of not only muscles, but all organs that rely on sympathetic neural inner-

vation from the spinal cord below the level of injury (see Figure 8.6). In addition, afferent feedback to the spinal cord from these organs is detrimentally affected. Although the public's general impression is that paraplegics and quadriplegics have no voluntary use of their muscles below their level of injury, this is not always true. Incomplete spinal cord injuries also exist. For example, an individual with an incomplete SCI at a cervical vertebra is classified as a quadriplegic, yet may be able to walk with the assistance of a cane.

TABLE 8.3

Impaired autonomic nervous system regulation of bodily functions caused by complete spinal cord injury*

SPINAL LEVEL	ORGANS SUPPLIED	IMPAIRED BODILY FUNCTION
SYMPATHETIC		
T11-L2	Large intestine, ureter, bladder	Loss of voluntary control of urination and defecation
T10-L2	Lower limbs	Loss of sweat gland stimulation
T9-T10	Small intestine	Decreased vasoconstriction, inability to regulate blood flow
T7-T9	Liver	Decreased vasoconstriction, inability to regulate blood flow
T6-T10	Stomach, spleen, pancreas	Poor blood glucose regulation
T5-T9	Adrenal glands	Impaired catecholamine responses to stress
T2-T5	Upper limbs	Loss of sweat gland stimulation
T2-T4	Bronchi and lungs	Increased airway resistance
T1-T5	Head, neck, and heart	Sympathetic innervation of heart decreased heart rate and contractility
PARASYMPATHETIC		
S2-S4	Large intestine, bladder	Loss of voluntary control of urination and defecation

*The higher the injury, the more diverse the impairment.

Neuromuscular Implications of Spinal Cord Injury—Cont'd

Bodily Functions Impaired By Complete Spinal Cord Injury

Based on the material presented in Figure 8.9, physiologic functions impaired or totally lost from spinal cord injury are listed in Table 8.3. Because the parasympathetic second, seventh, ninth, and tenth cranial nerves leave the spinal cord at the medullary level, the parasympathetic functions of the spinal cord are minimally affected by SCI. However, since parasympathetic regulation of the bowel and bladder leaves the spinal cord at the sacral level, almost all complete SCIs results in impaired control of the bowel and bladder.

The ability of individuals with SCI to exercise depends greatly on the level of injury (see Table 8.3). Injuries high in the thoracic vertebrae can result in decreased stimulation of central cardiovascular function that limits maximal abilities to consume oxygen. The inability to dilate the airways increases the work of breathing at high ventilation rates, and the inability to constrict the blood vessels of the splanchnic region decreases the fraction of the cardiac output that is directed toward the contracting muscle. In addition, if exercise is performed in a vertical position, or if the paralyzed limbs are placed below the heart, blood pooling can occur in the venous circulation, further decreasing venous return and blood flow to contracting muscle. Loss of sympathetic innervation to sweat glands and the cutaneous circulation, as well as the adrenal gland, decreases heat dissipation by radiation and evaporative cooling, causing increased risk for heat injury. However, the decreased sweat response decreases the risk for exercise-induced dehydration.

More information on how individuals with SCI respond to exercise is presented in Clinical Applications in Chapters 13 and 15.

---

norepinephrine release from nerve synapses. The systemic release of both epinephrine and norepinephrine decreases the tissue specificity of neural innervation and causes a widespread sympathetic stimulation to the body. In this context the type and density of the receptors on cells dictate the cellular response.

Synthesis and Degradation of Neurotransmitters

Norepinephrine is synthesized from the amino acid tyrosine, with epinephrine formed by the addition of a methyl group (CH_3) to norepinephrine.[10] When secreted by a nerve, norepinephrine is (1) rapidly reabsorbed by the nerve endings (50% to 80%), (2) circulated away from the synapse, taken up by other tissues, and broken down by the enzyme *catechol-O-methyl transferase*, and a small amount is broken down within the synapse by the enzyme *monoamine oxidase*.[24] Consequently, after norepinephrine is released from nerves it has a short half-life (less than 5 seconds). However, the epinephrine and norepinephrine secreted into the circulation from the adrenal medulla remain active for up to 30 seconds, with their removal accounted for by uptake by tissues and enzymatic destruction by catechol-O-methyl transferase.

Acetylcholine is formed in an enzyme-catalyzed reaction from the substrates acetyl-CoA and choline. When released into the synapse, acetylcholine is rapidly broken down by the enzyme *acetylcholinesterase* to acetate and choline. Acetate is circulated away from the synapse, whereas the majority of choline is reabsorbed by the presynaptic membrane for further synthesis of acetylcholine.

Nerve-Muscle Interactions

*N*erve-muscle interactions, or *neuromuscular* functions, comprise both efferent and afferent nerves; peripheral smooth, cardiac, and skeletal muscles; and specialized regions of the CNS. As discussed in Chapter 7, efferent nerves interact with skeletal muscle to cause muscle contraction; however, a complete understanding of neuromuscular function requires knowledge of sensory, as well as motor, functions of the neuromuscular system.

Sensory Functions

During rest and exercise conditions, neural functions of our bodies are continually operating to provide feedback to the CNS of the conditions experienced by our internal organs and more peripheral tissues. The neural information is derived from specialized **sensory receptors** that convert a

sensory receptor
a specialized region of an afferent nerve that is receptive to a specific stimulus that can result in the change in receptor membrane potential and the eventual generation of an action potential

biochemical (e.g., retina of the eye), physical (e.g., temperature), or mechanical (joint movement) stimulus into an action potential that is propagated to the CNS. The main sensory receptors that function during exercise are listed in Table 8.4. Of these, the receptors of importance to neuromuscular function are the muscle spindle, Golgi tendon organ, and joint receptors. The role of the muscle receptors that influence cardiovascular function is discussed in Chapter 11.

General Function of Sensory Receptors

The function of receptors and their afferent nerves is to "inform" the CNS of changes in local conditions. To do this effectively, there must be a means to detect these changes and to relay neural information of the magnitude of these changes.

Receptor Potential. A given receptor has a specialized structure that enables a specific sensory stimulus (modality) to alter the membrane potential. The depolarization of the receptor membrane is called a *receptor potential*. As with the postsynaptic membrane, or the soma of a nerve, if the receptor potential exceeds a *threshold* value, an action potential is generated and propagated toward the CNS.

The magnitude of the stimulus to a receptor is relayed to the CNS by the rate of action potentials leaving the receptor. The greater the stimulus strength, the larger the receptor potential, and if above threshold the greater the rate of action potentials leaving the receptor. However, depending on the receptor, the initial frequency of action potentials may not be retained even if the stimulus is continued. The decrease in the

---

TABLE 8.4

Sensory receptors of the body most pertinent to exercise

RECEPTOR	FUNCTION DURING EXERCISE
MECHANORECEPTORS	
Muscle spindle	Smooth muscle contractions, kinesthesis
Golgi tendon organ	Prevention of muscle injury
Pacinian corpuscles	Pressure sensation
Joint receptors	↑ Ventilation rate
Free nerve endings?	↑ Blood pressure and heart rate
Cochlea	Sound
Vestibular apparatus	Equilibrium and balance
Baroreceptors	Blood pressure and blood volume regulation
Atrial stretch receptors	Blood pressure and blood volume regulation
THERMORECEPTORS	
Cold receptors	Thermoregulation
Warm receptors	Thermoregulation
ELECTROMAGNETIC RECEPTORS	
Rod and cone cells	Vision
CHEMORECEPTORS	
Aortic and carotid bodies	Blood O_2 and CO_2 concentrations, ventilatory regulation
Osmoreceptors	Blood osmolality
	Fluid balance, kidney function, and blood volume regulation
CNS blood CO_2 sensors	Ventilatory regulation, blood acid-base regulation
Glucose receptors	Blood glucose regulation, carbohydrate metabolism

Modified from Guyton AC: *Textbook of medical physiology*, ed 8, Philadelphia, 1991, WB Saunders.

FIGURE 8.7

The skeletal muscle spindle. The muscle spindle is located in parallel to the extrafusal fibers of a muscle. The spindle consists of several smaller, and relatively more specialized intrafusal fibers that are encapsulated in a connective tissue sheath. As explained in the text, the differentiation between afferent and efferent nerve association among the intrafusal fibers is integral to the multiple functions of the spindle.

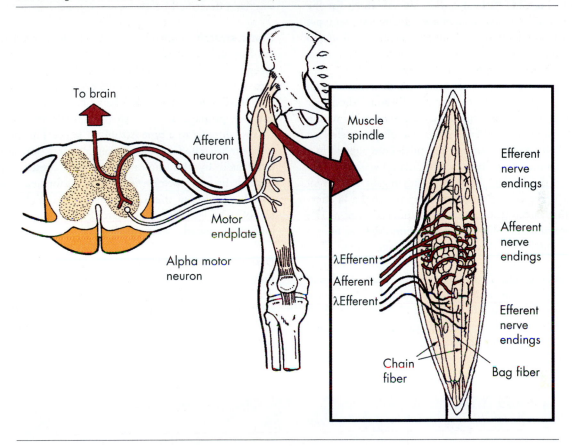

frequency of action potentials from a receptor when a stimulus is retained is termed **neural adaptation.**

Not all receptors exhibit the same degree of neural adaptation. Joint receptors and muscle spindles have minimal adaptation, whereas the hair receptor and pacinian corpuscle receptors of the skin adapt rapidly. These differences are understandable, for the rapid adaptation of skin receptors allows us to be unaware of the clothes on our bodies, or the surface of our bodies when we sit or lean against a chair. Conversely, since the function of the muscle spindle and joint receptor is to provide essential information of body movement and posture, providing "body awareness," it is to our benefit that these receptors adapt minimally.

Muscle Spindle

During exercise, when many muscles are contracting during very complex movements, the complex interactions that must exist between nerves and muscle are easy to over-

look. In fact, the contraction of skeletal muscle is only one of several neuromuscular interactions during movement. During muscle contraction and the movement of the body, there is continual feedback by afferent nerves that originate in receptors within skeletal muscle. The main skeletal muscle receptor of interest is the **muscle spindle,** which continually allows neural information about muscle stretch, muscle length, and the rate of change in muscle length to be relayed

neural adaptation

the decrease in discharge frequency of action potentials that leave a sensory receptor

muscle spindle

the sensory receptor within skeletal muscle that is sensitive to static and dynamic changes in muscle length back to the CNS. These functions are a result of the anatomic arrangement between afferent and efferent nerves and the components of the muscle spindle (Figure 8.7).

The muscle spindle contains specialized muscle fibers, which are collectively termed *intrafusal fibers*. These fibers run parallel to the normal skeletal muscle fibers, which for the sake of clarity are termed *extrafusal fibers*. There are two types of intrafusal fibers, which are termed *nuclear bag* and *nuclear chain* fibers, and the typical spindle has several of each type, with the chain fiber being more numerous.[9,19,24,29]

The nuclear bag and chain fibers get their name from their anatomic appearance. Nuclear bag fibers are the larger of the two and have multiple nuclei clustered centrally within the fiber. Nuclear chain fibers also have multiple nuclei, yet because of their smaller diameter the nuclei are aligned in a single line, resembling a chain in the central region of the fiber. The intrafusal fibers also differ with regard to efferent and afferent nerve connections. The bag fiber has a Ia afferent nerve that encapsulates the central nuclear region. The multiple encapsulation of the Ia nerve around the bag fiber is termed an *annulospiral ending* (actually the origin of the afferent nerve). The chain fibers also have annulospiral Ia afferent nerve connections and, in addition, have group II afferent connections *(flower spray endings)* located distal and proximal to the central region of the fiber. The Ia afferent nerves have a greater conduction velocity than the group II afferents and therefore relay information faster to the CNS. Both the bag and chain fibers have γ efferent nerves innervating the distal and proximal ends of each fiber, which are where the contractile proteins are located.

Functions of the spindle. The muscle spindle is sensitive to static stretch, dynamic stretch, and to changes in muscle length, as described below.

Static stretch. During static stretch the central regions of the bag and chain fibers are forcefully elongated and cause receptor potentials in the annulospiral and flower spray endings of the type Ia afferents of the bag and chain fibers and in type II afferent nerves of the chain fibers. These action potentials are propagated back to the spinal cord, where they synapse directly to a type Aα motor nerve. This nerve innervates the stretched muscle, causing a contraction of the fibers innervated by the motor nerve. This stretch response is termed the *static stretch reflex*, as it is performed at the spinal cord level without the involvement of the higher level centers of the CNS. The static stretch reflex is maintained for as long as the muscle is stretched.

Dynamic stretch. The neuromuscular response to dynamic stretch is slightly different from the static stretch reflex. A sudden stretch of a skeletal muscle induces a receptor potential solely in the type Ia annulospiral endings from the bag and chain fibers. The ensuing reflex is rapid, causing a forceful contraction of the stretched muscle, and is completed in a fraction of a second.

FOCUS BOX 8.1

Proprioception and kinesthesis: functions for everyday life and athletic success

Our abilities to be aware of our body parts and their movement in three-dimensional space enable us to perform miraculous functions in everyday life. The simple task of typing on a computer keyboard while watching the screen involves simultaneous finite movement patterns and cerebral processing. For example, the trained proprioceptive and kinesthetic responses between the fingers and brain enable the correct keys to be touched in the correct sequence. During this remarkable skill, cognitive effort is directed toward the thought processes forming the words and sentences typed. Of course, many other examples can be found in day-to-day life, such as merely walking and running, scratching your back, or loosening shoelaces that have been tied too tightly.

The realm of athletics and sports also demands well-developed capacities for proprioception and kinesthesis. Within the realm, activities exist that demand more from these capacities. The skills of the gymnast demand exemplary body awareness to enable the completion of difficult maneuvers in short periods of time. Similarly, the ballerina, dancer, or figure skater must not only perform difficult maneuvers but do so with controlled grace to express the aesthetics of his or her movements.

The quarterback in American football must throw the ball at the right speed, accuracy, and timing to complete a pass to a receiver. The cricket batsman must swing the bat correctly to hit the ball down and through an opening between fielders, the golfer must control the backswing without moving his or her head to ensure correct alignment of the club during the downswing for successful contact with the ball, and the baseball batter must make optimal contact with a ball with less that 1 second of visual information of ball position and speed.

Another example of proprioception and kinesthesis at work is the practice of *mental rehearsal*, often used by skilled performers before competitive participation. Athletes who mentally rehearse before performance mimic movements that their bodies would make in competition, in slow motion. Such warming up of the body's neuromuscular system is thought to improve neuromuscular function during the event (see Chapter 18).

Changes in muscle length. During muscle contraction and relaxation there is a repeated increase and decrease in the length of the extrafusal fibers. If the muscle spindle is to remain effective in responding to changes in muscle length, at differing initial lengths, the spindle must also change length in concert with the extrafusal fibers. This does happen and represents a very important additional function of the γ efferent nerves. When Aα nerves are stimulated, γ nerves are also stimulated so that the change in length of the intrafusal fibers matches that of the extrafusal fibers. This process is called **alpha-gamma coactivation** and allows the spindle to be at near optimal sensitivity regardless of the changing length of the extrafusal muscle fibers.

How does alpha-gamma coactivation assist muscle contraction? The best example is to imagine a muscle contracting against a large resistance. Simultaneous alpha-gamma stimulation of the intrafusal and extrafusal fibers allows a slowed contraction of the extrafusal fibers (as does occur during muscle contraction against resistance) to cause stretch on the spindle, resulting in a reflex additional increase in Aα motor nerve stimulation and subsequent increased strength of muscle contraction. In addition, dynamic muscle contractions stimulate in Ia afferent nerves. Alpha-gamma coactivation therefore also enables continual afferent feedback from the contracting muscle that informs the CNS of muscle length almost continually during a contraction. This dynamic sense has been termed **kinesthesis,** whereas the term **proprioception** is used to describe the general state of body awareness in the resting state. Our abilities of proprioception and kinesthesis are used in daily activities, as well as in exercise and athletic performance (Focus Box 8.1).

Other Muscle Receptors

As well as the muscle spindle, other receptors exist that connect to afferent nerves and the CNS. As the name implies, the *Golgi tendon organs* are located in the tendons of skeletal muscle. They are receptive to tension generated in the tendon during excessively strong muscle contractions, and action potentials are directed to the spinal cord by type Ib afferent nerves, where they synapse on an inhibitory interneuron, which then inhibits the respective Aα motor nerve(s).

Research has documented the existence of other muscle afferents that are probably special mechanoreceptors or receptors sensitive to metabolites from metabolism, or both. Muscle contraction is known to elicit increases in cardiovascular parameters, such as heart rate and blood pressure, and to increase ventilation.[33,34] These afferent nerves are believed to be type III and IV nerves and therefore to have a slower conduction velocity compared with the Ia and Ib nerves of the spindle and Golgi tendon organ.[24] These added receptors provide evidence for the role of nerves in orchestrating extremely rapid multisystemic responses to muscle contraction, and therefore partially explain how the body can rapidly adapt to exercise stress.

Ascending Afferent Nerve Pathways Within the CNS

The pathways in which the afferent nerves return to the higher levels of the CNS are anatomically distinct and exist as two sensory pathways referred to as (1) the *dorsal column–lemniscal system,* and (2) the *anterolateral system.*

The dorsal column–lemniscal system consists of myelinated type I and II nerves from the mechanoreceptors of the periphery. These nerves send information of sensations that have a high degree of spatial and intensity resolution (mechanoreceptors of the skin, joints, and skeletal muscle) to a specialized cortical region of the brain concerned with integrating the sensory information, the *somatosensory cortex.* In fact, there is already some spatial organization of these afferent nerves within the spinal cord, and as a result of the crossing of the nerves to the opposite side within the medulla, the left side of the body is neurally connected to the right side of the lower and cortical regions of the brain. Some nerves of this pathway diverge many times and enter other lower brain regions such as the cerebellum, the importance of which is apparent in the sections that follow.

The anterolateral system of ascending afferent nerves provides information from receptors for pain, heat and cold, itch, and tickle stimuli and represents sensory signals that have a low degree of spatial and intensity resolution. These nerves are predominantly type II and IV afferents and form two relatively distinct anterior and lateral pathways that both cross within the spinal cord. Thus, as with the dorsal column lemniscal pathway, the left side of the body is represented by the right side of the somatosensory cortex.

Somatosensory Cortex

The **somatosensory cortex** is located posterior to the central gyrus and consists of several layers of specialized nerves. The sensory afferent nerves project to a spatial region of the somatosensory cortex that is specific to the anatomic origin of the action potentials. As the afferent nerves cross the spinal cord in the ascending pathways, each side of the

---

alpha-gamma coactivation
the interaction between alpha and gamma motor nerves and type I and II afferent nerves of skeletal muscle and muscle spindles that results in smooth and controlled dynamic muscle contractions

kinesthesis (kin'es-the'sis)
the sense of awareness of moving body parts

proprioception (pro'pri-o-sep'shun)
the sense of awareness of body part positions in space

somatosensory cortex
the three-dimensional region of the cerebral cortex responsible for receiving afferent nerves from peripheral receptors

somatosensory cortex receives nerves from the opposite side of the body.

Clearly, a larger area of the cortex exists for anatomic regions of the body that have high spatial sensitivity, with the tongue, lips, face, fingers, and feet having the largest representation relative to real anatomic size. Because of the spatial discrimination within the somatosensory cortex, we are able to recognize the type of stimulation and the anatomic location of the source of stimulation.

Voluntary Motor Functions

The origin of most movement is not skeletal muscle, the Aα motor nerve, or specific synapses of the spinal cord. Complex movement patterns, like the muscle contractions performed during exercise, have their origin in structures of the midbrain and lower brain (Figure 8.8). Neural connections between the motor cortex and specific nerve nuclei and structures such as the cerebellum refine the pattern of action potentials that leave the motor cortex, resulting in controlled muscle contractions and movement. Simple motor patterns may not require input from the motor cortex and may be initiated from the cerebellum and certain nuclei of the lower brain. The neural events involved in movement are outlined in their order of function in the following sections.

FIGURE 8.8

The anatomic and functional association between the neuromuscular components involved in body movement. (From Thibodeau GA, Patton KT: *Anatomy and physiology*, ed 3, St. Louis, 1996, Mosby.)

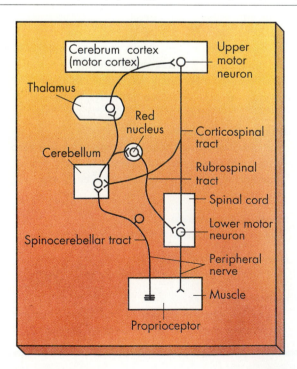

Initiating Movement

Figure 8.9 illustrates the anatomic location of the neural components involved in skeletal muscle contraction. The primary motor cortex is located anterior to the central gyrus of the cortex, and more anterior to this are the premotor area and the supplemental motor area. As with the somatosensory cortex, the premotor area and primary motor cortex are organized according to anatomic locations, with regions requiring more discrete movement control having the largest three-dimensional area. For example, more than 50% of the primary motor cortex concerns the muscles of the hands and face.[24] Cortical regions also exist for specialized motor functions that are distinct from the motor cortex. The regions are known to involve head rotation, eye movements, speech, and fine hand movements.

The nerves that leave the motor cortex group together at the level of the lower brain and pass down the spinal cord in the *corticospinal tract* (or *pyramidal tract*). These nerves can pass directly into this tract, or indirectly via the cerebellum and nuclei such as the *basal ganglia* and *red nucleus* (Figure 8.8). Every time action potentials travel down the nerves of the corticospinal tract, these additional regions of the brain receive neural input. The nerves of the corticospinal tract cross in the medulla, so that the right side of the motor cortex controls movement in the left side of the body, and vice versa.

Nerve connections to the cerebellum, basal ganglia, and red nucleus are important for the refinement of the patterns of action potentials that leave the motor cortex. The cerebellum is essential for coordinating and correcting rapid motor patterns, for preparing future motor patterns, and for storing correct movement sequences.[24] To perform these functions, the cerebellum has a complex arrangement of nerves that is too involved to discuss in this text. Neural output from the cerebellum is responsible for exciting agonist muscles and inhibiting antagonist muscles. For example, during running the cerebellum is responsible for the timing of quadriceps contraction and hamstring relaxation during knee extension and for the opposite stimulation during knee flexion. As the cerebellum receives afferent input from peripheral mechanoreceptors, it immediately adjusts errors to make the completion of the motor pattern smoother. In addition, when we learn new motor patterns, part of this learning occurs in the cerebellum. Yet, as we are all aware, this learning may take several weeks of practice and may not progress as well for some individuals as for others.

The basal ganglia are several nuclei within the mid brain and lower brain that receive nerves from the motor cortex and primarily return nerves back to the cortex. Skilled movements and movements requiring cognitive input, such as throwing, kicking, shoveling, and writing, require the presence of the basal ganglia. The main nucleus of the basal ganglia, the caudate nucleus, receives input from numerous regions of the brain and combines these inputs to "inform" the motor cortex of appropriate movement patterns or of the appropriate speed at which movement patterns should occur.

The red nucleus is responsible for assisting the motor cortex in causing refined movement of the distal muscles of the body, such as the forearms and lower leg. The red nucleus has a spatial arrangement similar to the motor cortex.

As illustrated in Figure 8.8, all the components of the motor control regions of the brain operate together in a complex manner that results in the controlled and precisely orchestrated series of action potentials that are propagated to the appropriate Aα motor nerves of the spinal cord. Many nerves innervate the soma of an Aα motor nerve, since efferent nerves from the different components of the motor control system of the brain can synapse either directly or indirectly on the Aα nerve. In addition, afferent nerves function to invoke inhibition or excitation of the Aα motor nerve, as was discussed with the muscle spindle and Golgi tendon organs, thus providing important refinement at the level of the spinal cord.

The distribution of Aα motor nerves down the spinal cord is somewhat organized into a *segmental distribution* (Figure 8.9). The Aα motor nerves leave the spinal cord at a ver-tebral level that reflects the anatomic position of the skeletal muscle.[11,13] For example, the Aα motor nerves from the motor units of the muscles of the shoulder girdle, abdominal muscles, and muscles from the upper and lower leg leave the spinal cord at various levels of the cervical, thoracic, and sacral vertebrae, respectively.

This relative order of the spinal level of the Aα motor nerves adds to the spatial order of the motor cortex and somatosensory cortex and is important for understanding the neuromuscular impairment resulting from injury to select levels of the spinal cord. An individual with a complete spinal cord lesion above the fifth thoracic vertebra would not have abdominal neural innervation or complete intercostal muscle innervation. Because these muscles aid in the increased depth of breathing, the person would experience poor tolerance to moderate or intense exercise intensities. Furthermore, the impaired arm motor function of individuals with spinal cord lesions above seventh cervical vertebra is explained by the loss or incomplete innervation of the muscles of the shoulder girdle, upper arm, and forearm.

FIGURE 8.9

The vertebral organization of the Aα motor nerves relative to the location of the skeletal muscles they innervate. (From Thibodeau GA, Patton KT: *Anatomy and physiology*, ed 3, St. Louis, 1996, Mosby, and Network Graphics.)

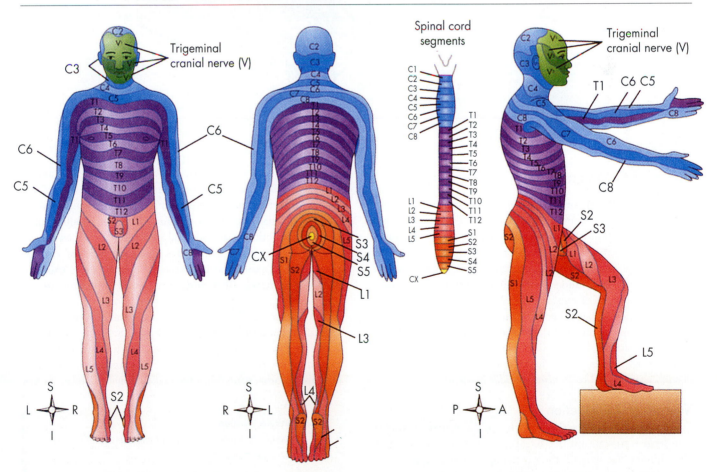

FIGURE 8.10

The motor nerve and muscle fiber components of the motor unit.

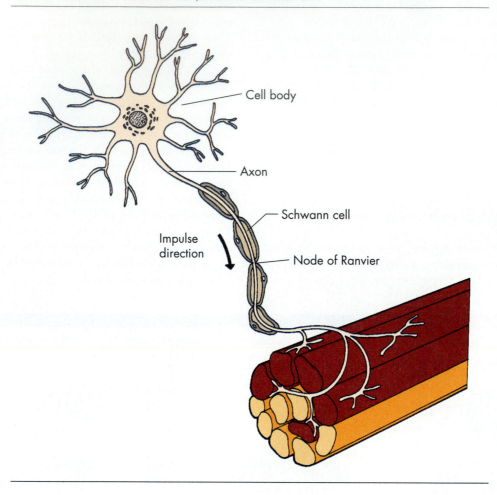

Cell body

Axon

Schwann cell

Impulse direction

Node of Ranvier

Instigating Movement

The stimulation of the Aα motor nerves results in the propagation of action potentials to the skeletal muscle fibers of the muscles required to contract during the given movement. For one muscle, hundreds of separate Aα nerves may be stimulated, and for a given Aα motor nerve, divergence of the main axon into hundreds of branches results in the innervation of hundreds of muscle fibers. The muscle fibers and the Aα motor nerve that innervates them compose a *motor unit* (Figure 8.10). The divergence of the Aα motor nerve results in the formation of many junctions between the nerve and skeletal muscle fibers. These junctions are special synapses and as such are referred to as *neuromuscular junctions.*

Neuromuscular Junction

As for the synapse, the function of the **neuromuscular junction** is to transmit the action potential across a synaptic cleft. Unlike the synapse, the postsynaptic membrane is not a nerve but the sarcolemma of a skeletal muscle fiber.

Electron micrographs of tissue preparations containing many neuromuscular junctions are presented in Figure 8.11. A few important features are prominent. Some muscle fibers have more than one neuromuscular junction. Each neuromuscular junction is an enlarged structure that extends over an area far greater that the cross-sectional area of the Aα motor nerve axon, and an extensive invagination exists in the skeletal muscle fiber under the neural extensions of the junction.

An enlarged illustration of the cross section of a neuromuscular junction is presented in Figure 8.12. Acetylcholine is released from vesicles via calcium-mediated exocytosis, as explained for the nerve synapse. The postsynaptic region of the sarcolemma, sometimes termed the *motor endplate,* is not

neuromuscular junction

the connection between a branch of an alpha motor nerve and a skeletal muscle fiber

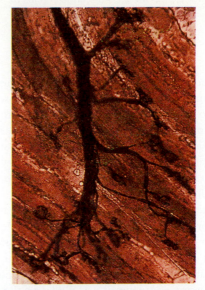

A

FIGURE 8.11

Electron micrographs of neuromuscular junctions. **A,** A scanning electronmicrograph of a motor nerve and its divergence to numerous muscle fibers. It is clear that several of the muscle fibers have more than one neuromuscular junction. **B,** A scanning electron micrograph of a motor nerve axon and its neuromuscular junction. The neuromuscular junction is an enlarged end region of the nerve axon that extends in many directions across the surface of the muscle fiber. **C,** When the axon and neural components of the neuromuscular junction are removed, invaginations can be seen in the muscle fiber, within which are further clefts and folds. (*A,* From Thibideau GA, Patton KT: *Anatomy and Physiology,* St. Louis, 1992, Mosby. *B,* From Desaki J, Vehara Y: *J Neurocytol* 10:101-110, 1981. *C,* From Peachey LD et al: *Handbook of physiology,* Bethesda, Maryland, 1983, American physiology society.)

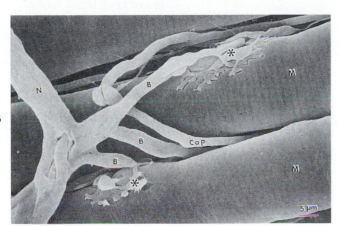

B

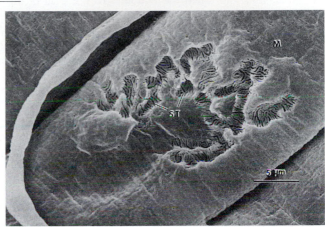

C

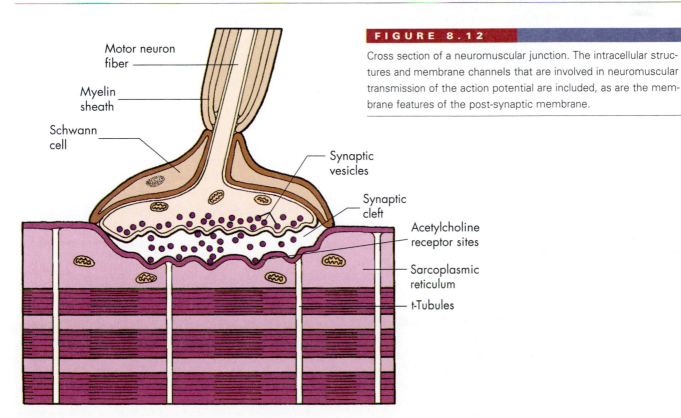

Motor neuron fiber

Myelin sheath

Schwann cell

Synaptic vesicles

Synaptic cleft

Acetylcholine receptor sites

Sarcoplasmic reticulum

t-Tubules

FIGURE 8.12

Cross section of a neuromuscular junction. The intracellular structures and membrane channels that are involved in neuromuscular transmission of the action potential are included, as are the membrane features of the post-synaptic membrane.

only a large invagination, but within it exist numerous other invaginations that serve to increase the cross-sectional area exposed to the release of acetylcholine. As with the postsynaptic membrane of a nerve synapse, the region of the sarcolemma at the neuromuscular junction contains acetylcholine-gated Na^+ channels and the enzyme acetylcholinesterase, which rapidly catalyzes the degradation of acetylcholine into acetate and choline.

The action potential that is received at the neuromuscular junction is always sufficient to release adequate acetylcholine to depolarize the motor endplate above threshold. This event stimulates the voltage-gated Na^+ channels to open and instigate the propagation of the action potential across the sarcolemma and down the t-tubules to the triad of the sarcoplasmic reticulum. The biochemical and molecular structure sequence of events involved in muscle contraction then follows (see Chapter 7).

Motor Units and Muscle Fiber Types

Research of neuromuscular function was first conducted using samples from animals. The earliest animal models used to research nerve function and muscle contraction were the triceps surae and gastrocnemius muscles of the cat.[7,9,10,25,26] This research showed that differences existed in the morphology and function between the nerves of certain motor units and that the metabolic characteristics of muscle fibers innervated by different nerves were also different. These findings were replicated in the rat hindlimb model.[15] The complete classification of a motor unit requires data of nerve and muscle morphology and physiology, and differences in these characteristics have resulted in a motor unit classification based on nerve recruitment order and conduction velocity, muscle contraction velocity and force, and muscle fiber metabolic capacities (Table 8.5). Motor units exist in human muscle that are fast twitch (FT) and slow twitch (ST). Within the fast twitch category are two subdivisions that differ in oxidative capacity.

Nerve and Recruitment Characteristics

As previously explained, the origin of a motor unit is the soma of the Aα motor nerve that is located in the spinal cord. The spinal cord and higher order nerves of the central nervous system synapse on cell bodies of the Aα motor nerves (motor neuron pool) of the motor units of the respective muscles used during the movement. Generally, the soma of the SO motor unit requires less supraspinal excitation to reach threshold and propagate an action potential than do the somas of the FOG and FG motor units (see Figure 8.13). It is believed that this difference is due to a combination of the smaller size of the soma and nerve axon and the less inhibitory synapses of the SO than of the FOG and FG motor units.[8,27]

The earlier attainment of a threshold membrane potential of the soma of the nerve of an SO motor unit than of

TABLE 8.5

Classification nomenclature of mammalian skeletal muscle motor units*

CLASSIFICATION METHOD	NOMENCLATURE
Visual	Red
	White
Contractile velocity†	Slow twitch
	Fast twitch
Contractile velocity‡ and metabolism	I, slow twitch
	IIab, fast twitch intermediate
	IIa, fast twitch fatigue resistant
	IIb, fast twitch fatigable
Contractile velocity§ and metabolism	S, slow twitch
	F (int), fast twitch intermediate
	FR, fast twitch fatigue resistant
	FF, fast twitch fatigable
Contractile velocity and metabolism‖	Slow twitch oxidative (SO)
	Fast twitch oxidative glycolytic (FOG)
	Fast twitch glycolytic (FG)

Modified from Burke RE: Motor units: anatomy; physiology and functional organization. In Brooks VB, editor: *Handbook of physiology: the nervous system,* vol II, Bethesda, Maryland, 1981, American Physiological Society.
*A more complex classification, resulting in additional subdivisions, can be found in Pette D, Straron RS: *Rev Physiol Biochem Pharmacol,* 116:2-76, 1990.
†Modified from Henneman E, Somjen G, Carpenter DO: *J Neurophysiol* 28:599-620, 1965.
‡Modified from Brook MH, Kaiser K: *J Histochem Cytochem* 18:670-672, 1970.
§Burke RE, Levine DN, Tsairis P, Zajac FE: *J Physiol London* 234:723-748, 1973.
‖Peter JB, Barnard RJ, Edgerton VR et al: *Biochemistry* 11:2627-2633, 1972.

FOG and FG motor units results in a recruitment order of motor units. SO motor units are recruited first during incremental exercise, followed by a progressive increase in FOG and FG motor unit recruitment as exercise intensity increases. This pattern of recruitment, termed the *size principle,* causes SO motor units to be recruited predominantly during low to moderate exercise intensities, and each of SO, FOG, and FG motor units to be recruited during exercise requiring intense contractions against high resistance or fast muscle contractions.* During contractions of increased velocity the size principle is still retained, but the difference in recruitment order between the different types of motor units is less pronounced.[19] As discussed in Chapter 9, this recruitment order results in a recruitment profile of motor units from those with low contraction tension, slow velocity, and high fatigue resistance to those with high contraction strength, fast velocity, and low fatigue resistance.[15]

Apart from the soma and recruitment order, the Aα motor nerves of different motor units differ in size, conduc-

*References 15, 19, 25, 26, 27, and 47.

FIGURE 8.13

The different neural, stimulatory, contractile, and metabolic differences among the three main types of motor units of human skeletal muscle. *SO*, Slow twitch oxidative; *FOG*, fast twitch oxidative glycolytic; *FG*, fast twitch glycolytic. (Adapted from Edington DW, Edgerton VR: Muscle fibertype population of human leg muscles, *Histochem J* 7:259-266, 1975.

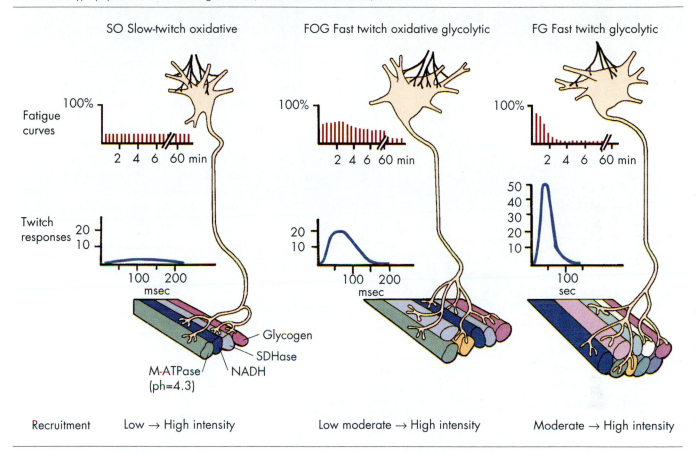

tion velocity, and stimulation characteristics (Figure 8.13). The area dimensions of the soma and cross-sectional area of the axon of the Aα motor nerve are larger in FG than in SO motor units.[8,15,27,47] In addition, the Aα motor nerve has a higher conduction velocity in FG than SO motor units, and SO motor units are stimulated more consistently than the rapid and intermittent manner of FG motor units.[27] However, because of considerable overlap between motor units for these characteristics, Burke[8] has commented that motor units cannot be classified based on nerve characteristics alone.

The contribution of human motor unit recruitment to muscle function has been indirectly studied using *electromyography* (EMG) (Focus Box 8.2). The signal obtained from EMG is proportional to electrical activity, which in turn is proportional to the number of muscle fibers and therefore the number of motor units stimulated to contract.[3] EMG has revealed the increase in electrical activity that occurs with muscle contractions that develop increased tension, as well as the different electrical activity and recruitment for concentric, eccentric, and isokinetic muscle contractions.

Neuromuscular Junction Characteristics

Henneman[27] has shown that the divergence of the Aα motor nerve is proportional to axon diameter, and therefore that the number of neuromuscular junctions and muscle fibers within a motor unit is larger for fast twitch than slow twitch motor units. There are generally more SO motor units within a muscle than FG motor units, but the variability in fiber numbers is large and little information exists on fiber number differences in human muscle.[48] There appear to be no differences in the morphology and function of the neuromuscular junction between the different motor units.

Muscle Characteristics

The muscle fibers of a motor unit have biochemical and contractile capacities that influence how the motor unit is suited to different types of exercise and exercise intensities.

Contractile force and velocity. The contractile force of muscle within the different motor units increases in progression from SO to FOG to FG motor units (see Figure 8.13), whereas the duration of the contraction decreases in the pro-

FOCUS BOX 8.2

Application of electromyography to muscle contraction during exercise

What is Electromyography?

Electromyography (EMG) is the study of muscle function from the detection of electrical activity emanating from the depolarization of nerves and muscle membranes that accompanies contraction.[3] The electrical activity is detected by the placement of one or more electrodes close to the contracting muscle(s) of interest. The electrodes can be either needle or surface. Needle electrodes are inserted into a muscle belly or a specific nerve, and surface electrodes are placed on the skin over the anatomic locations of interest (Figure 8.14).

Electromyography Signal

An example of the signal that can be obtained from EMG of skeletal muscle contraction is presented in Figure 8.15. The observed unprocessed signal is the composite of all neural and muscle membrane depolarizations and as such consists of signals from Aα motor nerves of the recruited motor units, muscle receptors, and afferent nerves. Understandably, the EMG signal can be very complex. The raw signal can be processed by adding the squared deviations from the baseline signal, and this signal processing when expressed relative to the duration of the signal is referred to as *integrated EMG*. Another method of analysis is to record the frequency of individual spikes in the EMG signal. Increased frequency of EMG signals is interpreted to indicate increased conduction velocities (and/or increased FT recruitment), whereas a decrease in frequency has been interpreted to represent muscle fatigue.[3] In addition, the ability of skeletal muscle to increase force application after exercise training despite no increase in EMG signal has been used to indicate a neural component to training adaptation, such as an increased synchronization of motor unit firing.[20,39]

Electromyography Evidence of Motor Unit Recruitment

The use of the EMG to detect changes in motor unit recruitment has been based on an increase in signal amplitude and an increase in integrated EMG signal (Figure 8.16). Both parameters increase in an exponential manner as the muscle contraction force increases; however, this methodology is not very sensitive and the ability to distinguish the recruitment of separate motor units is not possible from EMG.

Other Uses of Electromyography In Exercise-Related Research

The most beneficial use of EMG has been in documenting the activity of specific muscles during specific movement patterns. Thus EMG has shown whether certain muscles contribute to movement, at what time within a movement muscles contract, and based on signal processing relative to muscle size, which muscles contribute the most to certain movements. This use of EMG is probably the most scientifically valid and reliable, and it is common to read of the use of EMG in research that requires additional proof to support biochemical findings of increased metabolism in specific muscles during certain exercises.

FIGURE 8.14

Photograph of an EMG with surface electrodes attached to a subject.

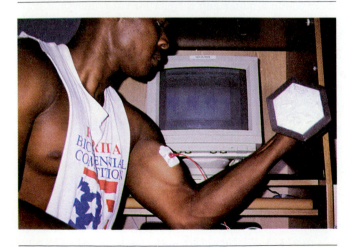

FIGURE 8.15

Raw signal obtained from EMG during concentric and eccentric muscle contractions of the biceps brachii.

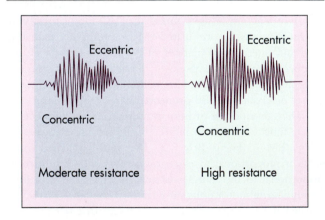

gression from SO to FOG to FG motor units. The force of contraction of a motor unit is determined by the size and number of the muscle fibers within a motor unit. As previously described, FT motor units generally contain more muscle fibers that ST motor units.

Contractile velocity of motor units is determined by the conduction velocity of the Aα motor nerves and the type of myosin proteins and myosin ATPase enzyme within the muscle fibers. As discussed in Chapter 7, skeletal muscle myosin is a complex molecule that consists of heavy (rod and S1 units) and light chain components and different isozymes of the enzyme myosin ATPase.[44,45] The myosin heavy and light chains and ATPase isozymes are known to result from separate genes, and their expression is therefore determined by the controls of gene translation, which are believed to be differentiated within the first year of life.[8] Specific isozymes of the myosin light chains are known to be present in FT compared to ST muscle fibers, as are isozymes of the enzyme myosin ATPase. These differences result in faster contraction times in FT compared to ST motor units, but the contribution from other determinants to contractile velocity, such as neuromuscular transmission, t-tubule and sarcoplasmic reticulum density, and calcium pump characteristics is unknown.[47]

Muscle fiber biochemical and enzymatic capacities. Skeletal muscle fibers from SO motor units have a high oxidative capacity. In other words, they possess relatively high concentrations of myoglobin, high mitochondrial membrane density, and therefore relatively high concentrations of the enzymes of the TCA cycle, β-oxidation, and electron trans-

port chain. The added myoglobin and mitochondria of SO muscle compared with FG muscle are the reasons for the "red" appearance and "white" appearance of the respective muscle types. Muscle fibers from FOG motor units have moderate concentrations of these molecules and enzymes, and muscle from FG motor units have the lowest concentrations (Figure 8.13). However, the differentiation of muscle fibers based on metabolic capacities is far less sensitive than that of histochemical staining based in the different pH stability of myosin ATPase and has been interpreted as evidence of a metabolic continuum that exists within and between muscle fibers of different motor units (see Focus Box 8.3).[8,9,22,47]

These metabolic differences make SO motor units more suited to prolonged exercise and the muscle catabolism of lipid and carbohydrate via mitochondrial respiration. Conversely, the low mitochondrial density of the skeletal muscle fibers from FG motor units makes these muscle fibers reliant on glycolytic catabolism and therefore the production of lactate and the development of acidosis. Muscle fibers from SO motor units are therefore termed *fatigue resistant,* while muscle fibers from FG motor units are *fatigable.*

Researchers have documented the metabolic differences between muscle fibers from different motor units by several methods. An increasingly common but laborious technique is to isolate individual muscle fibers from a biopsy sample, determine their fiber type by an enzymatic assay, pool the fibers into different fiber type populations, and assay the muscle samples for the activity of additional enzymes of either glycolysis, β-oxidation, the TCA cycle, or the electron transport chain.[12,30] Researchers can also analyze whole muscle biopsy samples, and based on additional myosin ATPase fiber typing, compare enzyme activities between samples that have differing percentages of ST and FT muscle fibers. Yet another method is to histochemically assay sections of muscle biopsy samples for specific enzyme activities.

Based on single fiber research, muscle fibers from the different motor units are shown to have distinctive enzymatic capacities best discriminated by the activity of mitochondrial enzymes or by ratios of activities from enzymes of glycolytic versus mitochondrial pathways.[45] When histochemical methods are used to detect differences in the quantity of NADH in muscle fibers, SO fibers stain darkest and a progressive decrease in stain intensity occurs for the FOG and FG fibers. Nevertheless, histochemical methods have revealed that fast twitch muscle fibers do have mitochondria and therefore the ability to increase oxygen consumption during contraction, and that there is considerable diversity in metabolic capacities for fibers that stain similarly from myosin ATPase activity. The perception that fast twitch muscle fibers are devoid of any potential for oxidative phosphorylation is incorrect.

Because of the connections among lactate production, acidosis, and muscle fatigue, the difference between fiber types for capacities for lactate production and removal has been widely researched. Glycolytic enzyme activity is higher in FT muscle fibers than in ST fibers, and FT fibers have con-

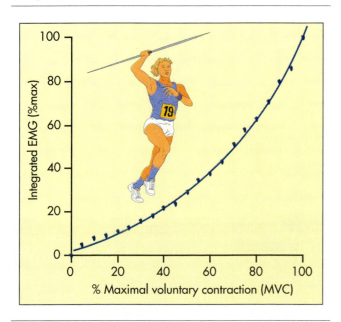

FOCUS BOX 8.3

Applications of muscle biopsy to exercise physiology

Muscle Biopsy Procedure

Human muscle biopsy is an invasive procedure that enables the removal of a small piece of muscle tissue from the human body. It is performed by first injecting a local anesthetic into the skin and underlying connective tissue where the biopsy is to be performed. Once the anesthetic has taken effect, a small incision (usually 1 cm long) is made through the skin and down through the fascia sheath covering the muscle. The biopsy needle (Figure 8.17) is then forced into the opening. When in place, the center plunge and guillotine are raised, and to increase the size of the biopsy sample, suction is generated within the needle to force muscle into the window of the needle.[18] The guillotine is then forcefully lowered, cutting the muscle. The needle is withdrawn with the muscle specimen inside.

How Are Muscle Biopsy Specimens Processed and Analyzed?

When the muscle specimen is removed from the needle, it can be processed in several ways. For biochemical assay the muscle specimen is frozen in liquid nitrogen as rapidly as possible.

Some researchers place the needle, with the muscle inside, immediately into liquid nitrogen to prevent the added delay in removing the muscle from the needle. If the specimen is to be used for histologic preparations, the rapidity of freezing is less important (see the following discussion).

Freeze drying versus wet weight

When frozen, the muscle specimen can be stored as is, or the water content of the tissue can be removed by vacuum sublimation (freeze drying). If the muscle is left frozen in its raw form, it contains a large amount of water, which dilutes the concentration of metabolites. Conversely, freeze drying enables the water to be removed, increasing the concentration of metabolites and thereby improving the ability to detect metabolites by enzymatic assays. The drawback to freeze drying is that metabolites are not in their true in vivo concentration; however, dividing metabolite concentrations expressed relative to muscle dry weight (i.e., mmol/kg dry wt) by 4.11 gives a concentration close to wet weight values (depending on the change in tissue hydration).[28]

FIGURE 8.17

Biopsy needle, identifying the inner guilotene, window for muscle sampling, and attached suction device. The needle can come in several different sizes, with the size of the standard needle approximating the diameter and length of a lead pencil.

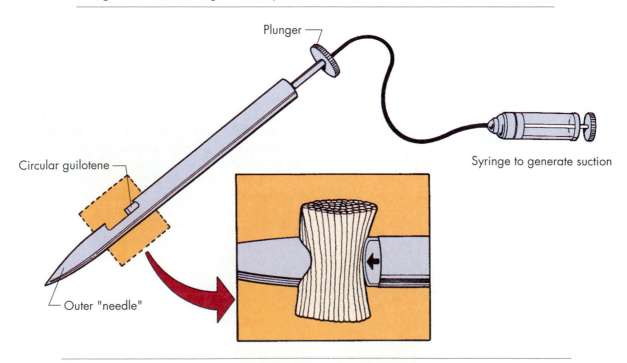

Plunger

Circular guilotene

Outer "needle"

Syringe to generate suction

FOCUS BOX 8.3

Applications of muscle biopsy to exercise physiology—Cont'd

Enzymatic biochemistry

Muscle metabolites and enzyme activities are most frequently determined by first homogenizing the muscle in a solution containing buffers and electrolytes. For the assay of metabolites a sample of this homogenate is added to test tubes containing appropriate enzymes, substrates, and enzyme activators to induce reactions that eventually increase the concentration of a suitable end product that can be measured via an indirect technique (usually NAD^+ or NADH, which can be measured by spectrophotometry or fluorometry).

Histology

For histologic preparation, the muscle specimen must be cleaned of excess blood and connective tissue and mounted within a special paste on a small platform (usually cork). The mounted specimen is then frozen slowly in an organic solvent (e.g., isopentane) to prevent damage to the specimen that occurs during rapid freezing. It is then stored in liquid nitrogen for later histologic preparation.

Microscopically thin slices of frozen tissue are obtained in a *cryostat.* Serial sections of the tissue are then placed in solutions containing chemicals that specifically favor a given reaction or selectively denature enzymes in given muscle fiber types. For example, the periodic acid–Schiff (PAS) stain produces a pink color, with the color intensity proportional to muscle carbohydrate (glycogen) (Figure 8.18).

The histochemical procedures used to stain for myosin ATPase activity are outlined in Focus Box 8.4. The myosin ATPase stain, if it involves a preincubation of the sections in an acid medium of pH 4.3, denatures the enzyme in fast twitch muscle fibers and allows the following incubation and reactions to deposit cobalt in the slow twitch fibers whose myosin ATPase is still active (Figure 8.19). This stains slow twitch fibers black and leaves fast twitch fibers unstained (white) when viewed by light microscopy. A preincubation in a solution of pH 10.3 denatures the myosin ATPase from slow twitch muscle fibers, allowing subsequent incubations to stain the fast twitch muscle fibers, which have active myosin ATPase. Consequently, when preincubated at pH 10.3, fast twitch fibers stain black and slow twitch fibers remain unstained. If the preincubation is at a moderately low pH (pH 4.6), some muscle fibers that are classified as fast twitch by either the 4.3 or 10.3 preincubation procedures retain some myosin ATPase activity. These fibers reveal a slight stain from the incubation and reactions that follow and have been classified as fast twitch oxidative (IIa or FOG) fibers.

FIGURE 8.18

Sections of skeletal muscle stained for carbohydrate content by the Periodic Acid Schiff stain. **A,** Before prolonged submaximal exercise; **B,** after prolonged submaximal exercise.

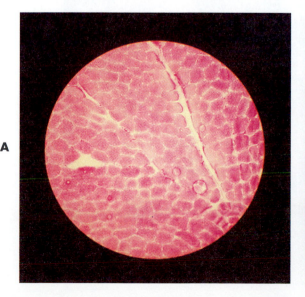

A

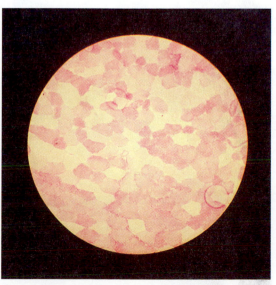

B

FIGURE 8.19

Myosin ATPase staining of serial sections of skeletal muscle preincubated at different pH values and for different preincubation durations. Reference fibers are denoted *1, 2,* and *3*. Slow twitch fibers are denoted *S*. **A,** Staining after preincubation at pH=10.3. Slow twitch (ST) fibers are unstained, whereas fast twitch (FT) fibers are stained black. **B,** Staining for NADH tetrazolium reductase (NADH TR). Stain intensity is proportional to mitochondrial density. **C** to **H,** Staining after preincubation as pH=4.34 for durations of 0.25, 1.0, 1.5, 2.0, 3.0, and 5.0 min. Note that after 5 min of incubation in an acidic medium (pH=4.34), myosin ATPase staining is the reverse of that at a pH of 10.3. Muscle fibers that stain dark for NADH TR and as fast twitch from myosin ATPase staining have been termed fast twitch oxidative fibers (FOG) ____= 100 um. (From Gollnick, P.D., et al: Differentiation of fiber types in skeletal muscle from the sequential inactivation of myofibrillar actomyosin during acid preincubation. *Histochem* 77:543-555, 1983.)

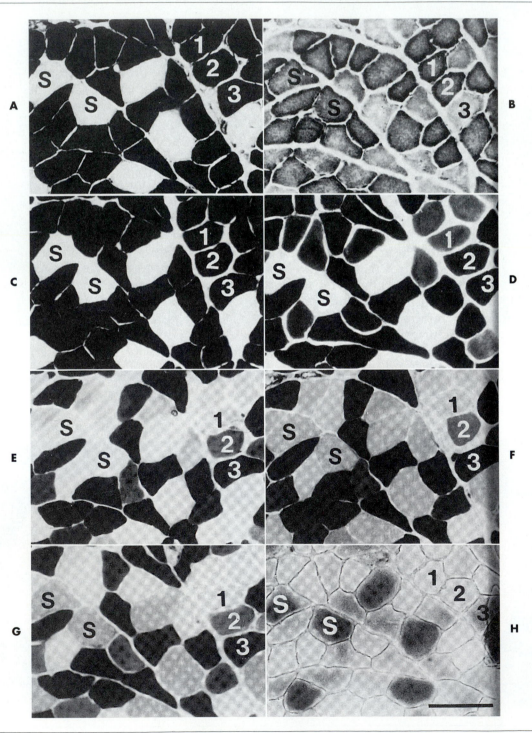

FOCUS BOX 8.4

Procedures for staining muscle sections for myosin ATPase activity

1. Muscle biopsy specimens are sectioned in a cryostat, producing serial sections of muscle.

2. Serial sections of muscle are placed on a cover slip.

3. The cover slips with their muscle sections are placed into an incubation (Columbia) jar.

4. A preincubation solution is added to the jar. Depending on the staining required, this will be a solution approximating a pH of either 4.34, 4.6, or 10.3. (See Fig. 8.20.) Typically, serial sections are placed on multiple cover slips, and in multiple staining jars, so that preincubation of serial sections can occur at each pH.

5. The sections are incubated in their respective solution for 5 minutes. The solution is then discarded, and the sections are rinsed in distilled water.

6. An alkaline incubation solution containing ATP is added, and the sections are incubated for 45 min. The solution is then discarded, and the sections are rinsed in distilled water.

7. The sections are incubated in a 1% calcium chloride solution. The solution is then discarded, and the sections are rinsed in distilled water.

8. The sections are incubated in a 2% cobalt chloride solution for 3 minutes. The solution is then discarded, and the sections are rinsed in distilled water.

9. The sections are incubated in a 1% ammonium sulphide solution for 1 minute. The solution is then discarded, and the sections are rinsed in distilled water. The sections can air dry or dehydrate in ascending alcohol and clear xylene solutions.

The aforementioned staining procedure is based on the following biochemical conditions and reactions. The preincubation at specified pH values denatures the myosin ATPase enzyme from specific fiber types. The ATP and calcium incubation solution provides substrate for the ATPase enzyme that remains active in certain fiber types. The free phosphate reacts with the calcium to form calcium phosphate, which under alkaline conditions is deposited on the muscle fiber. Exposure to cobalt chloride fosters the exchange of cobalt with the calcium deposits. Finally, the exposure of the cobalt containing fibers to ammonium sulphide forms cobaltous sulphide, an insoluble black compound that completes the staining procedure.

The muscle section shown resulted from staining after a preincubation pH of 4.6. Note the multiple shades of gray, as well as the black and unstained fibers.

---

siderably lower capacities for mitochondrial respiration. In addition, FT fibers have an isozyme of lactate dehydrogenase that has a lower $S_{0.5}$ for pyruvate than does ST muscle. These differences favor increased lactate production for a given activity of glycolysis.

Despite the lower activity of lactate dehydrogenase in ST muscle fibers, the ST isozyme is kinetically more suited to oxidizing lactate to pyruvate, and thus aiding in lactate removal from the circulating blood and its incorporation into the carbohydrate catabolic pathways.[41]

Muscle glycogen stores. Muscle glycogen stores have been reported to be higher in FT than ST muscle fibers before exercise.[35,46,49,52] However, because of the recruitment order of motor units and the bias to ST muscle metabolism that exists in daily locomotion requirements, this finding may be more a result of an activity-related lowering of muscle glycogen in ST muscle fibers than a difference in glycogen storage.

FIGURE 8.20

Staining muscle fibers for myosin ATPase activity.

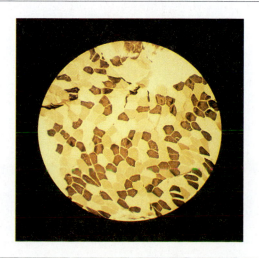

This interpretation is understandable given the predominance of carbohydrate catabolism in skeletal muscle during both prolonged intense exercise and short-term intense exercise (see Chapter 9).

Capillary density. Research on animal muscle capillarization has revealed that within a muscle of homogenous fiber type, greater capillary density is evident in slow twitch compared to fast twitch muscle. Because human muscle is heterogenous in fiber type, a similar investigation can not be completed. Nevertheless, Anderson[1] studied the capillarization of human muscle relative to the area occupied by either of the fiber types. Greatest capillary density occurred around SO muscle fibers, and there was no difference in capillary density between FG and FOG muscle fibers. Consequently, even in human muscle with a heterogenous distribution of fiber types there appear to be more capillaries surrounding SO muscle fibers.

Fiber Type Proportions

The differences in biochemical capacities and myosin ATPase pH stability between the muscle fibers of differing motor units have enabled histochemical methods to become those predominantly used to determine motor unit proportions in human **muscle biopsy** samples (see Focus Box 8.3) from skeletal muscle. However, because the myosin ATPase histochemical procedure involves only the muscle fiber component of the motor unit, the term **fiber type** has often replaced the more correct expression of SO, FOG, and FG *motor unit* proportions. This is unfortunate, since evidence exists to indicate that muscle fibers have a greater potential for diversity than do the neural components of the entire motor unit. For example, at least eight different muscle fiber types based on the myosin ATPase stain have been shown,[22] and as discussed in Chapter 9, exercise training can alter the genetic function of skeletal muscle fibers, resulting in the

---

FIGURE 8.21

The mean and range of human SO fiber type proportions in different muscles obtained from autopsy whole muscle specimens.

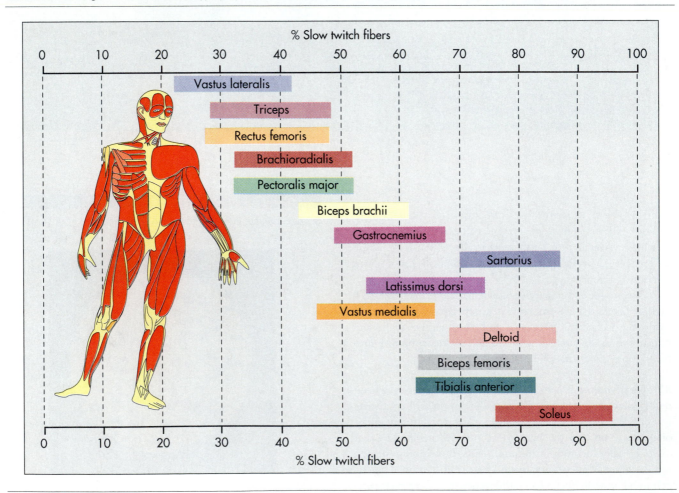

transcription of myosin light chains that typically occur in other fiber type subcategories.[45] Consequently, changes in fiber type proportions may not reflect actual motor unit changes, and it remains unclear whether fiber type changes are more important than nerve changes for the function of motor units during exercise.

Methodologic Concerns

The estimation of fiber type proportions is a common method in exercise physiology and biochemistry research. Because of the heterogeneous and unequal three-dimensional spatial distribution of motor units within a given human skeletal muscle, one muscle biopsy may not provide a fiber type proportion representative of the entire muscle. Although numerous researchers since the 1970s have published data on muscle fiber types determined from one biopsy sample, which contains approximately 300 to 600 fibers,[16,36] recent research involving biopsies from the human vastus lateralis muscle indicate that as many as three separate biopsy samples (> 1200 fibers) are required to decrease sampling error and the error in calculating fiber type proportions to less than ±10%.[16,36] Nevertheless, research studies using single muscle biopsies for the estimation of muscle fiber type proportions continue to be published.

Fiber Type Proportions of Different Muscles

The fiber type proportion of skeletal muscle varies not only within a muscle, but also between muscles and between individuals.[32] Figure 8.21 illustrates the mean and variation in SO fiber type proportions in various muscles determined from human autopsy samples of entire muscles. Muscles ranged from predominantly slow twitch (tibialis anterior, soleus) to fast twitch (orbicularis oculi). More evenly proportioned muscles were the biceps brachii, medial gastrocnemius, latissimus dorsi, and vastus lateralis. Nevertheless, the variability in fiber type proportions for the potentially evenly proportioned muscles is large, indicating the genetic variability in fiber type proportions in specific muscles.

> **muscle biopsy**
> *the procedure of removing a sample of skeletal muscle from an individual*
>
> **fiber type**
> *a categorization of muscle fibers based on their enzymatic and metabolic characteristics*

SUMMARY

- Anatomically, the nervous system comprises the central system, composed of the brain and spinal cord, and the peripheral system, composed of sensory and motor nerves. The functional divisions of the nervous system can be divided into voluntary and involuntary control divisions, with the latter comprising the parasympathetic and sympathetic divisions of the autonomic nervous system.

- The junction site between two different nerves is called a **synapse.** Almost all the synapses of the body function by releasing a chemical substance, termed **neurotransmitter,** from the *presynaptic membrane* that diffuses across the space between nerves, or *synaptic cleft,* where the chemical binds to special **receptors** on the *postsynaptic membrane.* All synapses function unidirectionally. Whether the depolarization of a postsynaptic membrane is sufficient to cause an action potential depends on (1) the location of the synapse in the nervous system, (2) the level of neuronal excitation, and (3) the spatial summation of other nerve synaptic transmissions, which may have excitatory or inhibitory effects on the postsynaptic membrane.

- When the summed depolarization exceeds the given threshold potential for the nerve, the voltage-gated Na^+ channels of the **axon hillock** open and an action potential is propagated along the axon.

- Acetylcholine is the neurotransmitter for the conduction of the action potential to skeletal muscle fibers, for a small number of synapses from sympathetic nerves of the autonomic nervous system, and for all the *preganglionic* synapses of the sympathetic and parasympathetic nerves of the autonomic nervous system. Norepinephrine is the neurotransmitter for the *postganglionic* synapses of sympathetic nerves of the autonomic nervous system.

- The autonomic nervous system can be functionally and anatomically divided into two divisions: the *sympathetic* division and the *parasympathetic* division. The **ganglia** of the sympathetic division are outside the spinal cord. Control of organ function by reciprocal changes in the activity of sympathetic and parasympathetic nerves results in the control of body functions or conditions such as temperature, blood pressure, hydration, urination, and heart rate.

■ The neural information derived from specialized **sensory receptors** results in the conversion of a biochemical (e.g., retina of the eye), physical (e.g., temperature), or mechanical (joint movement) stimulus into an action potential that is propagated to the CNS. The magnitude of the stimulus to a receptor is relayed to the CNS by the rate of action potentials leaving the receptor. The greater the stimulus strength, the larger the *receptor potential* and, if above threshold, the greater the rate of action potentials leaving the receptor. The decrease in the frequency of action potentials from a receptor when a stimulus is retained is termed **neural adaptation.**

■ The main skeletal muscle receptor of interest is the **muscle spindle,** which continually allows neural information to be relayed back to the CNS of muscle stretch, muscle length, and the rate of change in muscle length. The interaction of afferent and efferent functions of the muscle spindle enables highly controlled muscle contractions, and this process is termed **alpha-gamma coactivation.** In addition, this process enables afferent information to be returned to the brain to provide awareness of body part movement and spatial position, which are conditions termed **proprioception** and **kinesthesis,** respectively. Afferent information from peripheral sensory receptors returns to the **somatosensory cortex** of the brain.

■ The distribution of motor nerves down the spinal cord is somewhat organized into a segmental distribution. The motor nerves leave the spinal cord at a vertebral level that reflects the anatomic position of the skeletal muscle. For example, the motor nerves from the motor units of the muscles of the shoulder girdle, abdominal muscles, and muscles from the upper and lower leg leave the spinal cord at various levels of the cervical, thoracic, and sacral vertebrae, respectively.

■ The muscle fibers and the motor nerve that innervates them comprise a *motor unit.* The divergence of the motor nerve results in the formation of many junctions between the nerve and skeletal muscle fibers. The postsynaptic region of the sarcolemma, sometimes termed the *motor endplate* or **neuromuscular junction,** is a large invagination, and within it exist numerous other invaginations that serve to increase the cross-sectional area exposed to the release of acetylcholine.

■ The complete classification of a motor unit requires data of nerve and muscle morphology and physiology, and differences in these characteristics have resulted in a motor unit classification based on nerve recruitment order and conduction velocity, muscle contraction velocity and force, and muscle fiber metabolic capacities. Motor units exist in human muscle that are fast twitch and slow twitch. Within the fast twitch category are two subdivisions that differ in oxidative capacity. Muscle motor unit proportions can also be determined from metabolic and contractile characteristics from muscle samples obtained from **muscle biopsy,** and these divisions of muscle fiber metabolic capacities are more correctly termed **fiber types.**

■ Generally the soma of the SO motor unit requires less supraspinal excitation to reach threshold and propagate an action potential than do the somas of the FOG and FG motor units. The earlier attainment of a threshold membrane potential of the relatively small SO motor nerve results in a recruitment order of motor units. This pattern of recruitment has been termed the *size principle.* This recruitment order results in a recruitment profile of motor units from those with low contraction tension, slow velocity, and high fatigue resistance to those with high contraction strength, fast velocity, and low fatigue resistance.

REVIEW QUESTIONS

1. How is an action potential transmitted across a synapse?

2. How can the nervous system be divided based on both structure and function?

3. What are the functional benefits of having different types of receptors and neurotransmitters?

4. What are the roles of the motor cortex, cerebellum, and spinal cord in determining a motor pattern for movement?

5. What are the functions of the muscle spindle?

6. What is a motor unit, and how do motor units differ within and between different muscles of the body?

7. What is a fiber type, and how are fiber types determined in research?

8. Using an individual with a lower level spinal cord injury as an example, why is the autonomic nervous system important for optimal function of the body during exercise?

9. What is electromyography, and how has it been used in exercise-related research?

APPLICATIONS

1. The muscle contraction and movement impairments that accompany spinal cord injury are obvious repercussions of the condition. However, many other neuromuscular and neural issues affect body functions. What are these impaired functions?

2. Would individuals who have different proportions of motor units in their muscles have different genetically determined potential for either endurance or sprint activities? Explain.

3. Imagine that you are blindfolded and must retie your shoelace. List and explain the neuromuscular processing that is involved in this act.

REFERENCES

1. Anderson P: Capillary density in skeletal muscle of man, *Acta Physiol Scand* 95:203-205, 1975.

2. Baldwin KM, Klinkerfuss GH, Terjung RL et al: Respiratory capacity of white, red and intermediate muscle: adaptive response to exercise, *Am J Physiol* 222:373-378, 1972.

3. Basmajian JV, DeLuca CJ: *Muscles alive: their functions revealed by electromyography,* ed 5, Baltimore, Maryland, 1985, Williams & Wilkins.

4. Bell DG, Jacobs I: Muscle fiber-specific glycogen utilization in strength-trained males and females, *Med Sci Sports Exerc* 21(6):649-654, 1989.

5. Bradford HF: *Chemical neurobiology: an introduction to neurochemistry,* New York, 1986, WH Freeman.

6. Brooke MH, Kaiser K: Three "myosin adenosine triphosphatase" systems: the nature of their pH lability and sulfhydryl dependence, *J Histochem Cytochem* 18:670-672, 1970.

7. Burke RE: Firing patterns of gastrocnemius motor units in the decerebrate cat, *J Physiol* 196:631-654, 1968.

8. Burke RE: Motor units: anatomy, physiology and functional organization. In Brooks VB, editor: *Handbook of physiology: the nervous system,* vol II, Bethesda, Maryland, 1981, American Physiological Society.

9. Burke RE, Edgerton VR: Motor unit properties and selective involvement in movement, *Exerc Sport Sci Rev* 3:31-81, 1975.

10. Burke RE, Levine DN, Tsairis P, Zajac FE: Physiological types and histochemical profiles in motor units of the cat gastrocnemius, *J Physiol London* 234:723-748, 1973.

11. Carpenter MB, Sutin J: *Human neuroanatomy,* ed 8, Baltimore, Maryland, 1983, Williams & Wilkins.

12. Chi MM-Y, Hintz CS, Coyle EF et al: Effects of detraining on enzymes of energy metabolism in individual human muscle fibers, *Am J Physiol* 244:C276-C287, 1983.

13. Chusid JG: *Correlative neuroanatomy and functional neurology,* ed 19, Los Altos, California, 1985, Lange Medical.

14. Edgerton VR, Smith JL, Simpson DR: Muscle fiber type populations in human leg muscles, *Histochem J* 7:259-266, 1975.

15. Edstrom L, Grimby L: Effect of exercise on the motor unit, *Muscle Nerve* 9:104-126, 1986.

16. Elder GCB, Bradbury K, Roberts R: Variability of fiber type distributions within human muscles, *J Appl Physiol* 53(6):1473-1480, 1982.

17. Essen B, Jansson E, Henriksson J et al: Metabolic characteristics of fiber types in human skeletal muscle, *Acta Physiol Scand* 95:153-165, 1975.

18. Evans WJ, Phinney SJ, Young VR: Suction applied to muscle biopsy maximizes sample size, *Med Sci Sports Exerc* 14:101-102, 1982.

19. Freund HJ: Motor unit and muscle activity in voluntary motor control, *Physiol Rev* 63:387-436, 1983.

20. Garfinkel S, Cafarelli E: Relative changes in maximal force, EMG, and muscle cross-sectional area after isometric training, *Med Sci Sports Exerc* 24(11):1220-1227, 1992.

21. Gollnick PD, Armstrong RB, Saubert CW et al: Enzyme activity and fiber composition in skeletal muscle of untrained and trained men, *J Appl Physiol* 33(3):312-319, 1972.

22. Gollnick PD, Hodgson RD: The identification of fiber types in human skeletal muscle: a continual dilemma, *Exerc Sport Sci Rev* 14:81-104, 1986.

23. Gollnick PD, Reidy M, Quintinskie JJ, Bertocci LA: Differences in metabolic potential of skeletal muscle fibers and their significance for metabolic control, *J Exp Biol* 115:91-199, 1985.

24. Guyton AC: *Textbook of medical physiology,* ed 8, Philadelphia, 1991, WB Saunders.

25. Henneman E, Somjen G, Carpenter DO: Excitability and inhibitability of motor neurons of different sizes, *J Neurophysiol* 28:599-620, 1965.

26. Henneman E, Somjen G, Carpenter DO: Functional significance of cell size in spinal motor neurons, *J Neurophysiol* 28:560-580, 1965.

27. Henneman E, Mendell LM: Functional organization of motorneurone pool and its inputs. In Brooks VB editor: *Handbook of physiology: The nervous system,* vol II, Bethesda, Maryland, 1981, American Physiological Society.

28. Hultman E, Sahlin K: Acid-base balance during exercise, *Exerc Sport Sci Rev* 7:41-128, 1980.

29. Hunt CC: Mammalian muscle spindle: peripheral mechanisms, *Physiol Rev* 70(3):643-662, 1991.

30. Ivy JL, Chi MM-Y, Hintz CS et al: Progressive metabolite changes in individual human muscle fibers with increasing work rates, *Am J Physiol* 252(21):C630-C639, 1987.

31. Ivy JL, Withers RT, Van Handel PJ et al: Muscle respiratory capacity and fiber type as determinants of the lactate threshold, *J Appl Physiol* 48(3):523-527, 1980.

32. Johnson MA, Polgar J, Weightman D, Appleton D: Data on the distribution of fibre types in thirty-six human muscles: an autopsy study, *J Neurol Sci* 18:111-129, 1973.

33. Kaufman MP, Waldrop TG, Rybicki KJ et al: Effects of static and rhythmic twitch contractions on the discharge of group III and IV muscle afferents, *Cardiovasc Res* 18:663-668, 1984.

REFERENCES—Cont'd

34. Kniffki KD, Mense S, Schmidt RF: Muscle receptors with fine afferent fibers which may evoke circulatory reflexes. *Circ Res* 48(b)(SuppI):I25-I25, 1981.

35. Lesmes GR, Benham DW, Costill DL, Fink WJ: Glycogen utilization in fast and slow twitch muscle fibers during maximal isokinetic exercise, *Ann Sports Med* 1:105-108, 1983.

36. Lexel J, Taylor C, Sjostrom M: Analysis of sampling errors in biopsy techniques using data from whole muscle cross sections, *J Appl Physiol* 59(4):1228-1235, 1985.

37. Lowry CV, Kimmey JS, Felder S et al: Enzyme patterns in single human muscle fibers, *J Biol Chem* 253:8269-8277, 1978.

38. Minneman KP: Adrenergic receptor molecules. In Schulster D, Levitzki A: *Cellular receptors for hormones and neurotransmitters,* Chichester, England, 1981, John Wiley.

39. Narici M, Roi G, Landoni L et al: Changes in force, cross-sectional area, and neural activation during strength training and detraining of the human quadriceps, *Eur J Appl Physiol* 59:310-319, 1989.

40. Nemeth P, Hofer HW, Pette D: Metabolic heterogeneity of muscle fibers classified by myosin ATPase, *Histochemistry* 163:191-201, 1979.

41. Newsholme E, Leech ER: *Biochemistry for the medical sciences,* Chichester, England, 1983, John Wiley & Sons.

42. Nicoll R, Malenka R, Kauer J: Functional comparison of neurotransmitter receptor subtypes in mammalian central nervous system, *Physiol Rev* 70:513-565, 1990.

43. Peter JB, Barnard RJ, Edgerton VR et al: Metabolic profiles of three types of skeletal muscle in guinea pigs and rabbits, *Biochemistry* 11:2627-2633, 1972.

44. Pette D: Activity-induced fast to slow transitions in mammalian muscle, *Med Sci Sports Exerc* 16(6):517-528, 1984.

45. Pette D, Straron RS: Cellular and molecular diversities of mammalian skeletal muscle fibers, *Rev Physiol Biochem Pharmacol* 116:2-76, 1990.

46. Robergs RA, Pearson DR, Costill DL et al: Muscle glycogenolysis during differing intensities of weight-resistance exercise, *J Appl Physiol* 70(4):1700-1706, 1991.

47. Saltin B, Gollnick PD: Skeletal muscle adaptability: significance for metabolism and performance. In *Handbook of physiology,* Section 10: *Skeletal muscle,* Bethesda, Maryland, 1983, American Physiological Society.

48. Saltin B, Henriksson J, Nygaard E, Anderson, P: Fiber types and metabolic potentials of skeletal muscles in sedentary man and endurance runners, *Ann NY Acad Sci* 301:3-29, 1977.

49. Secher NH, Jenssen NE: Glycogen depletion patterns in type I, IIA, and IIB muscle fibers during maximal voluntary static and dynamic exercise, *Acta Physiol Scand Suppl* 440:174, 1976.

50. Stephens JA, Usherwood TP: The mechanical properties of human motor units with special reference to their fatigability and recruitment threshold, *Brain Res* 125:91-97, 1977.

51. Tesch PA, Thorsson A, Kaiser P: Muscle capillary supply and fiber type characteristics in weight and power lifters, *J Appl Physiol* 56(1):35-38, 1984.

52. Vollestad NK, Blom PCS, Gronnerod O: Resynthesis of glycogen in different muscle fiber types after prolonged exhaustive exercise in man, *Acta Physiol Scand* 137:15-21, 1989.

53. Wastek GJ, Yamamura HI: Acetylcholine receptors. In Yamamura HI, Enna ST, editors: *Neurotransmitter receptors,* Part 2, Receptors and recognition, Series B, vol 10, New York, 1981, Chapman & Hall.

RECOMMENDED READINGS

▪ Brooke MH, Kaiser K: Three "myosin adenosine triphosphatase" systems: the nature of their pH lability and sulfhydryl dependence, *J Histochem Cytochem* 18:670–672, 1970.

▪ Burke RE: Motor units: anatomy, physiology and functional organization. In Brooks VB, editor: *Handbook of physiology: the nervous system,* vol II, Bethesda, Maryland, 1981, American Physiological Society.

▪ Gollnick PD, Hodgson RD: The identification of fiber types in human skeletal muscle: a continual dilemma, *Exerc Sport Sci Rev* 14:81-104, 1986.

▪ Henneman E, Mendell LM: Functional organization of motorneurone pool and its inputs. In Brooks VB editor: *Handbook of physiology: The nervous system,* vol II, Bethesda, Maryland, 1981, American Physiological Society.

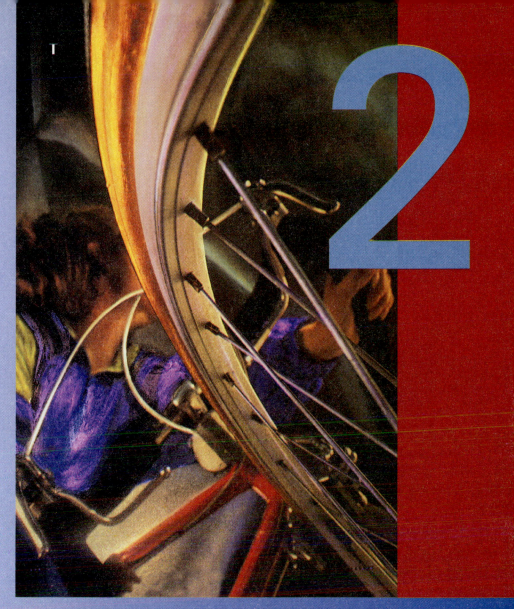

2

Systemic

Responses

to Exercise

CHAPTER 9

Neuromuscular Adaptations to Exercise

OBJECTIVES

After studying this chapter you should be able to:

- Explain how the recruitment of specific motor units during exercise can influence muscle energy metabolism.

- Explain why certain fiber type proportions may be beneficial or detrimental to specific exercise intensities, sports, and athletic events.

- Describe the potential changes in muscle fiber type proportions after endurance, strength, or power training.

- Identify the alteration in fiber type proportions that occurs during periods of extreme disuse like bed rest, limb immobilization, or deinnervation.

KEY TERMS

resistance exercise

torque

hypertrophy

hyperplasia

artificial electrical stimulation

deinnervation

As explained in Chapter 8, muscle contraction occurs by the regulated recruitment of motor units. Because the muscle fibers in different motor units possess different metabolic capacities, and since motor unit recruitment occurs in progressive order from slow twitch to fast twitch, motor unit recruitment during exercise can influence muscle energy metabolism and blood acid-base balance. Therefore knowledge of motor unit recruitment, and thus the contributions of different muscle fibers to the metabolic demands of exercise, aids in understanding many of the body's metabolic adaptations to exercise. Similarly, the body's responses to training may be further understood by knowing differences in how muscle fibers adapt to certain exercise-induced stresses and why certain individuals excel in specific events while others cannot. The purpose of this chapter is to present research findings of the acute adaptations of muscle motor unit and fiber type function during different exercise conditions, during recovery from exercise, and after different types of exercise training.

Metabolic Contribution of Muscle Fiber Types During Exercise

The dissimilar metabolic capacities of muscle fibers from different motor units, combined with the recruitment transition of slow to fast twitch motor units during increases in exercise intensity, emphasize the need to interpret metabolic changes during and following exercise relative to the specific contributions from specific types of muscle fiber. The following sections are structured to present research of fiber type–specific contributions to muscle metabolism relative to the intensity of exercise and specific metabolic pathways.

Steady State Exercise and Intense Exercise

Glycogenolysis

During exercise at intensities that can be sustained for periods in excess of 30 minutes, research using serial muscle sections stained by the PAS and myosin ATPase methods has revealed greater use of glycogen from SO compared to FG and FOG muscle fibers.[61,83] Figure 9.1 indicates that after 60 minutes of cycling at 43% VO_2max, muscle biopsy specimens sectioned and stained by the PAS procedure revealed that SO muscle fibers contributed 80% of the change in muscle glycogen, with the remainder a result of FOG fiber recruitment. The FOG contribution to glycogen breakdown increased at 61% VO_2max, and at 91% VO_2max glycogen breakdown continued to occur in SO and FOG fibers, as well as in FG fibers.[83] In similar research on muscle glycogen changes during an active recovery at 40% VO_2max, muscle glycogen increased in FOG and FG muscle fibers that were presumably not recruited during the low-intensity exercise.[61] Collectively this evidence is used to indirectly indicate preferential recruitment of SO motor units during low-intensity long-duration exercise.

The previous evidence does not mean that fast twitch motor units are never recruited during low-intensity exer-

FIGURE 9.1

The changing contribution of glycogenolysis in SO, FOG, and FG muscle fibers during increasing exercise intensity. (From references 7, 34, 61, 65, 83 to 85.)

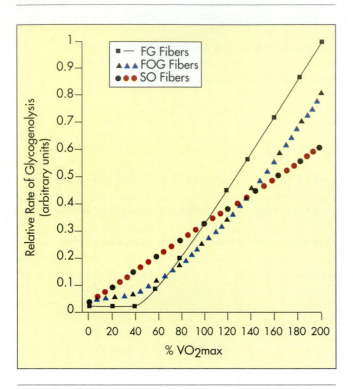

accumulation is due to production or uptake of lactate from the fast twitch muscle fibers.[43]

Weight Lifting Exercises

Minimal research on fiber type–specific glycogen depletion has occurred during weight lifting or **resistance exercise.** Nevertheless, data indicate that glycogenolysis occurs simultaneously and equally in slow and fast twitch fibers during maximal single leg isokinetic leg extension exercise at 180 degrees/sec.[7] This result is to be expected for such moderate speed muscle contraction because of the intensity-dependent recruitment of motor unit types. However, animal research has shown that rapid muscle contraction can preferentially recruit fast twitch motor units.[12,14] Whether this is true for human voluntary exercise remains unclear.

Fiber Type Determinants of Exercise Performance

The metabolic and contractile differences between slow and fast twitch motor units can not only alter metabolic response to exercise, but can also influence exercise performance. For elite athletes, whose muscle metabolic capacities are highly developed, motor unit proportions can set genetic limitations to the magnitude of adaptations obtainable from training.

Long-Term Endurance Exercise

A summary of research of human muscle fiber type proportions in elite athletes from different activities is presented in Figure 9.2. Based on this compilation of cross-sectional data, elite athletes involved in long-term activities, such as distance running, cycling, or swimming have predominantly SO muscle fibers in the muscles that contribute most to their respective exercise. Conversely, FG and FOG muscle fibers predominate in athletes who excel in activities more reliant on muscle strength and power. The data from Figure 9.2 are derived from genetically favored individuals and should not be interpreted as evidence for muscle fiber type changes that are specific to the intensity and duration of exercise training (see Training Adaptations).

Experimental evidence exists to provide a mechanistic association between fiber type proportions and exercise performance. For example, a high SO proportion in muscle causes a high mitochondrial capacity, a high capacity for oxygen consumption,[44] a high lactate threshold (see Chapter 10), and superior distance running and cycling performance.[20,44]

Short-Term Intense Exercise

A high FT proportion in muscle is accompanied by the continued ability to generate power at increasing contraction

cise. As muscle glycogen is depleted from SO muscle fibers and exercise is continued, FOG and FG motor units are recruited to allow for continued activity.[85] However, the level of motor skill often diminishes during these conditions because of the larger number of muscle fibers of the FOG and FG motor units and therefore the decrease in refinement of contractile strength. In addition, as explained in Chapter 10, decreases in muscle glycogen are associated with decreases in liver glycogen and blood glucose, which are conditions that invoke additional metabolic adaptations that decrease the ability to maintain a high steady state exercise intensity.

Muscle Lactate Accumulation

As discussed in Chapter 10, increased muscle lactate production causing lactate accumulation in muscle or blood occurs at intensities that are not at steady state. Consequently, during prolonged steady state exercise, where slow twitch motor unit recruitment predominates, minimal lactate is produced. However, as exercise intensity increases above the lactate threshold (see Chapters 4 and 10), lactate production increases. Part of the cause for increased lactate production is the recruitment of fast twitch glycolytic motor units. Single muscle fiber research has shown that lactate accumulation is larger in fast twitch than slow twitch muscle. However, it is uncertain how much of the slow twitch muscle fiber lactate

FIGURE 9.2

The proportions of ST and FT muscle fibers in elite athletes from different events. The more long-term the activity, the greater is the proportion of ST muscle fibers in select muscles of the athletes. (Data from Bergh U et al: Maximal oxygen uptake and muscle fiber types in trained and untrained humans, *Med Sci Sports* 10:151, 1978.)

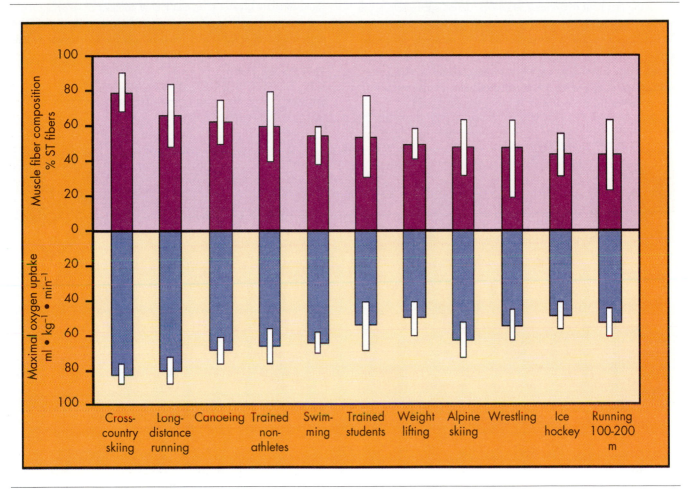

velocities[40,82] and superior performance in explosive activities.[19,22,40] It has often been accepted that such a bias toward FT proportions favors all types of intense exercise; however, some contradictory research exists. Colliander et al[19] investigated performance during three bouts of intense single leg knee extensions performed at 180 degrees/sec, with the bouts separated by 1 minute of recovery. Individuals with high FT fiber type proportions generated greater **torque** than those with predominantly ST proportions during the first bout of contractions (Figure 9.3), but torque was no different between groups for bouts two and three. Individuals with greater ST fiber type proportions in the vastus lateralis muscle had greater metabolic recovery between bouts. The results indicated that when multiple bouts of intense exercise are to be performed, ST muscle fibers are important for allowing recovery between bouts. Conversely, individuals with greater FT fiber proportions will probably perform bet-

ter if they are provided more recovery time between successive bouts of intense exercise.

Weight Lifting Exercise

Research using isokinetic exercise equipment has provided added evidence for the potential for varied fiber type

resistance exercise
muscle contractions performed against a resistance, typically in the form of external loads like those used in weight lifting

torque (tork)
force applied to a lever system that causes rotational movement

The difference in torque generation among individuals having different FT and ST fiber type proportions in their vastus lateralis muscles. Individuals with high FT proportions generated greater torque during the first bout of exercise. However, during successive bouts of exercise separated by 1 min of recovery, individuals with more ST fiber type proportions demonstrated better recovery, yet overall torque was not different between the two divergent groups of individuals. (Data from Collainder EB et al: Skeletal muscle fiber composition and performance during repeated bouts of maximal, concentric contractions, *Eur J Appl Physiol* 58:81-86, 1988.)

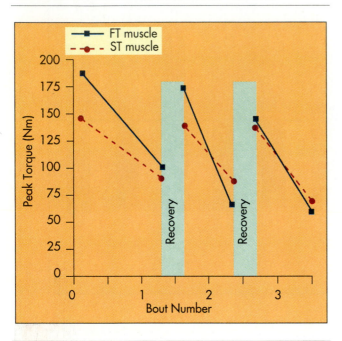

The difference in torque generation at different contraction velocities for an individual with different FT and ST muscle fiber type proportions. Individuals having higher FT muscle fiber proportions could generate greater torque at higher contraction velocities. However, torque generation was similar for isometric contractions. (Data from Gregor RJ et al: Torque-velocity relationships and muscle fiber composition in elite female athletes, *J Appl Physiol* 47(2):388-392, 1979.)

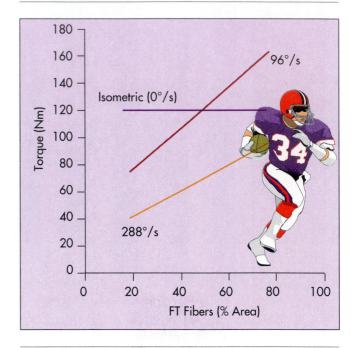

proportions to influence strength and endurance exercise performance.[40,82] In this research design, muscle fiber type proportions determined from myosin ATPase staining for individuals are compared with the abilities of these individuals to contract their muscles to generate torque at different velocities of contraction. Figure 9.4 indicates that individuals with high FT fiber type proportions in the vastus lateralis can produce greater torque at contraction velocities between 90 and 300 degrees/sec.[40] These results are similar for trained males and females.[40,82] Interestingly, at low contraction velocities and isometric contractions, where force generation is greatest (see Chapter 3), there is no difference in force generation between individuals with high ST or high FT fiber type proportions.[40]

These results suggest that individuals involved in powerful single contraction events would benefit by having a greater FT fiber type proportion in their active muscles. Conversely, for pure strength development, the fiber type proportion is less influential in determining performance.

Metabolism in Muscle Fiber Types During the Recovery From Exercise

Recovery of muscle involves the replenishment of energy stores, such as creatine phosphate, glycogen, and lipid, and the removal or further metabolism of waste products, such as lactate, protons, carbon dioxide, and ammonia. Consequently, muscle recovery is an energy-dependent process and is dependent on an intact circulation for recovery of creatine phosphate, restoration of normal concentrations of glycolytic intermediates, decreases in acidosis, and glycogen storage. The greater mitochondrial mass of SO fibers favors recovery in these muscle fibers. Although an active recovery at low exercise intensities has been shown to decrease muscle glycogen synthesis,[83] an active recovery is known to improve the metabolic recovery from exercise (see Chapter 10).

Training Adaptations

The following sections focus on how exercise training affects the additional characteristics of muscle fibers that are important in distinguishing their classification into SO, FOG, or FG fiber types. These characteristics are central nervous system activation and neuromuscular function, fiber size and number, myosin ATPase and myosin isozyme content, and capillary density. Specific comment and reference to different exercise intensities are provided in each section.

Central Nervous System Activation and Neuromuscular Function

The recruitment of motor units is known to be important for determining the strength of a muscle contraction. During intense exercise involving the recruitment of ST and FT motor units, the ability to voluntarily increase the number of motor units recruited or alter the asynchronous nature of the recruitment can increase muscular strength. Since drastic changes in fiber type proportions are unobtainable through training muscle by voluntary contractions, increased recruitment and summation are the main ways to improve strength without muscle hypertrophy.

Coyle et al[22] and Caiozzo et al[16] reported evidence for altered neuromuscular involvement during muscle contraction after resistance training. Training specifically at fast or slow contraction velocities resulted in different abilities to generate torque, without alterations in muscle fiber type proportions. Training at fast contraction velocities caused specific improvements only at high velocities. Conversely, training at a slower velocity produced improvements across all speeds. These differences indicated that neural activation differed, which may reflect an improved ability to recruit motor units after resistance training.[16] Coyle's findings differed slightly from Caiozzo's but confirmed the possibility of neural involvement in improved strength and power of muscle contractions after strength training.

Increasing evidence from animal research supports morphologic alterations of the neuromuscular junction (NMJ) in response to increased activity.[23] In rats the combination of maturation and endurance training increases the size and complexity of the NMJ.[66] Similar evidence exists that exercise training increases acetylcholine stores in the presynaptic terminal, alters isozymes of acetylcholinesterase and the acetylcholine receptor, and delays the occurrence of NMJ fatigue during chronic stimulation.[23] Although this research has not been applied to human models, it indicates that the neural component of adaptation to exercise may be important to more completely understand increased exercise tolerance and performance after training.

Fiber Size and Number

The increase in size, or more specifically the cross-sectional area, of muscle fibers is termed **hypertrophy.** In endurance-trained individuals the SO muscle fibers can be larger than either the FOG or FG muscle fibers,[34] with considerable variation in size within a fiber type in the same muscle.[13] These findings indicate some degree of selective hypertrophy of muscle fibers from different motor units and are presumably a result of an increased mitochondrial and membranous mass and increased muscle filaments within the fibers.

During more intense exercise, such as sprinting or weight lifting, muscle hypertrophy is greater than that for endurance activities.[18,24] The fiber type hypertrophy is not as distinct for endurance exercise, since all motor unit types are recruited in these activities.[52]

Animal research has indicated the potential for muscle fibers to split and form new fibers during intense training.[4] Although there are various animal models, those involving voluntary exercise, and therefore most similar to human exercise, have repeatedly reported increases in muscle fiber numbers from 5% to 15% after long-term resistance training (> 10 weeks).[38,77] The increase in the number of muscle fibers is termed **hyperplasia.** It is unclear whether hyperplasia occurs from the splitting of existing fibers or the generation of new fibers.

Although there is no experimental evidence for hyperplasia in human muscle following training for long-term muscular endurance, Antonio and Gonyea[4] have meticulously detailed the large body of indirect evidence for hyperplasia. When entire muscles have been obtained post mortem, comparison between left and right tibialis anterior muscles from previously healthy men revealed a 10% difference in fiber numbers.[74] Research that has compared muscle fiber areas between hypertrophied trained athletes and sedentary control subjects has revealed no difference in fiber areas, yet large differences in muscle size.[2,47,79] However, a similar body of research has shown the muscle fiber hypertrophy can account for differences in muscle cross-sectional area between trained and untrained individuals.[41,53,63,72]

The generally accepted interpretation of the findings is that muscle fiber hypertrophy accounts for the largest increases in muscle cross-sectional area, with a possible small contribution from hyperplasia.

Myosin ATPase and Myosin Isozyme Content

Animal research has clearly documented the importance of neural activation and muscle contraction as determinants of the altered expression of myosin and myosin ATPase in skeletal muscle fiber types. Both *nerve cross-reinnervation* and

hypertrophy (hi-per'tro-fi)
the increase in size of skeletal muscle resulting from the increased size of individual muscle fibers

hyperplasia (hi'per-pla'zi-ah)
the increase in muscle fiber number in skeletal muscle

artificial electrical stimulation of motor nerves have been shown to reverse the metabolic and contractile profiles of muscle fibers.[26,29,39] Connecting muscle fibers to an opposite motor nerve or stimulating a nerve in the opposite frequency and intensity converts the muscle fibers to reflect the muscle normally innervated by the nerve and stimulation profile.[26,39,67] However, these interventions are extreme and do not represent voluntary activation of human motor units in patterns that reflect low-intensity or high-intensity muscle contractions.

In humans, exercise training for improvement in long-term muscular endurance, strength, or power lifting causes changes in the genetic expression of myosin ATPase, certain structural components of the myosin molecule (heavy and light chains), and the contractile function of myosin in select populations of muscle fibers.[1] These changes result in altered contractile function that favors the specific demand of training. However, in human voluntary exercise training these changes do not alter the basic proportions of slow and fast twitch muscle fibers. Rather, endurance training increases the

CLINICAL APPLICATION

Regenerating Paralyzed Muscle By Artificial Electrical Stimulation

Artificial Electrical Stimulation

Artificial electrical stimulation (AES) of skeletal muscle involves the placement of surface or needle electrodes on or in muscles of interest and the stimulation of these muscles with a small electric current at predetermined intervals. This stimulation results in the synchronous contraction of all motor unit types, with the number of motor units recruited dependent on the strength (voltage) of the stimulation.

Artificial electrical stimulation has been used in both animal and human experimental research. Several studies have exploited the near maximal motor unit recruitment potential of AES in human muscle biochemistry research to document extreme muscle metabolic adaptations to intense contractions and to verify the potential of AES to induce muscle metabolic adaptations even in human muscle with normal neuromuscular function.[31] However, a more specific application has been to train previously paralyzed muscle to reverse the atrophy that accompanies paralysis. Researchers from Wayne State University in the United States have enabled individuals with complete spinal cord injury to perform cycle ergometry or walking by providing computer-controlled AES to several muscles. For example, correctly programmed AES to the quadriceps, hamstring, and gluteal muscles can result in movement of the lower legs similar to voluntary cycling. Such use of AES has been termed *computerized functional electrical stimulation (CFES)* (Figure 9.5), and has enabled many individuals with complete spinal cord injury to once again experience the movement pattern of riding a bike.

Human Paralyzed Muscle Training by Electrical Stimulation

Individuals with complete spinal cord injury resulting in the paralysis of the muscles of the lower limbs experience incredible wasting of these muscles during the initial years after injury. The known denervated muscle fibers decrease in number and size and when histologically prepared resemble diseased muscle, similar to dystrophic muscle (usually a large cross-sectional area with consistent staining). Paralyzed muscle also experiences an increase in fast twitch fiber type expression.[56] Collectively these alterations decrease the contractile function and endurance of the muscle, as indicated by the minimal endurance and strength capabilities of paralyzed muscle when exposed to AES.[46]

Artificial electrical stimulation and CFES have been shown to increase the endurance capacity of paralyzed muscle.[46] When AES is used as a means of exercise training, there is an increase in slow twitch muscle fiber type expression toward normal values and associated increases in mitochondrial enzyme activity.[56] In addition, if multiple muscles are stimulated and therefore the muscle mass stimulated is large, there is a considerable production of lactate that can raise systemic blood lactate concentrations above 4 mmol/L even for extremely small exercise intensities.[46]

Initial application of AES to paralyzed muscle causes muscle fatigue and contractile failure within as little as 1 minute, with the fatigue probably a result of neuromuscular or intramuscular electrochemical impairment.

Individuals with spinal cord injury who have been exposed to AES in a training program experienced remarkable increases in muscular endurance.

FIGURE 9.5

An individual with spinal cord injury receiving computerized functional electrical stimulation (CFES) that enables her to perform cycle ergometry. (Courtesy, Therapeutic Technologies, Inc., Dayton, Ohio.)

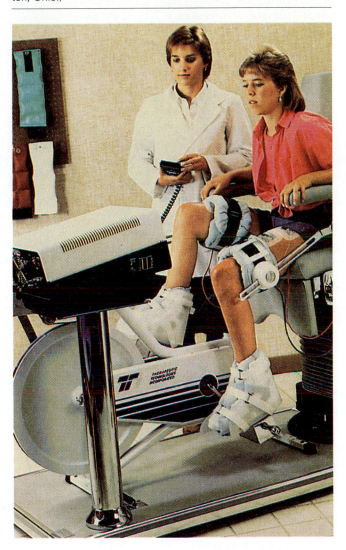

proportion of FT muscle that stains as FOG fibers, whereas strength training increases the proportion of muscle fibers that stain as FG fibers (see Chapter 8).[1,5,52,55,57]

Capillary Density

Exercise training for long-term muscular endurance also increases the number of capillaries per cross-sectional area of muscle. As previously mentioned, Anderson[3] documented a selective increase in capillary density around SO muscle fibers in human muscle samples that have a heterogenous distribution of fiber types. Exercise training for long-term endurance further increases capillary density, providing more potential for blood flow to and from the contracting muscle fibers. Since these new capillaries cannot be associated with only SO muscle fibers, this adaptation also provides a more oxygen-rich microenvironment to certain FG and FOG fibers, further supporting the potential for increased capacities for mitochondrial respiration in these fibers.

Disuse Atrophy

During detraining, muscle mitochondrial metabolic capacities are lost at a fast rate and those of glycolysis remain unchanged or increase slightly.[17] However, alteration in fiber type proportions requires more severe disuse, like that of forced bed rest, immobilization of a limb (e.g., limb casts),[52] or **deinnervation** (e.g., spinal cord injury).[56] Generally there is a shift in fiber type from SO to FOG to FG; however, the shift is not consistent in all muscles affected by the intervention.[67,68,75] Increased activity, even artificial electrical stimulation of the immobilized muscle(s), can reverse this atrophy response.[56]

artificial electrical stimulation

the application of needle or surface electrodes that provide small electrical stimulations to skeletal muscle, resulting in muscle contraction

deinnervation (de-in'er-va'shun)

the complete removal of neural connections to skeletal muscle

SUMMARY

■ Research based on the changing content of glycogen within specific muscle fibers is used to indirectly indicate preferential recruitment of SO motor units during low-intensity long-duration exercise. As muscle glycogen is depleted from SO muscle fibers and exercise is continued, FOG and FG motor units are recruited to allow for continued activity.

■ Single muscle fiber research has shown that lactate accumulation is larger in fast twitch than slow twitch muscle. However, it is uncertain how much of the slow twitch muscle fiber lactate accumulation is due to production or uptake of lactate from the fast twitch muscle fibers.

■ Minimal research of fiber type–specific glycogen depletion has focussed on weight lifting or **resistance exercise.** Nevertheless, data indicate that glycogenolysis occurs simultaneously and equally in slow and fast twitch fibers during maximal single leg isokinetic leg extension exercise at 180 degrees/sec. Animal research has shown that rapid muscle contraction can preferentially recruit fast twitch motor units, but whether this is true for human voluntary exercise remains unclear.

■ Based on a compilation of cross-sectional data, elite athletes involved in long-term activities, such as distance running, cycling, or swimming, have predominantly SO muscle fibers in the muscles that contribute most to their respective exercise. Conversely, a high FT proportion in muscle is accompanied by the continued ability to generate **torque** at increasing contraction velocities and superior performance in explosive activities.

■ Muscle recovery is an energy-dependent process and is dependent on an intact circulation for recovery of creatine phosphate, restoration of normal concentrations of glycolytic intermediates, decreases in acidosis, and glycogen storage. The greater mitochondrial mass of SO fibers favors recovery in these muscle fibers.

■ The increase in size, or more specifically the cross-sectional area, of muscle fibers is termed **hypertrophy.** In endurance-trained individuals, the SO muscle fibers can be larger than either the FOG or FG muscle fibers, with considerable variation in size within a fiber type in the same muscle. During more intense exercise, such as sprinting or weight lifting, muscle hypertrophy is greater than for endurance activities. The fiber type hypertrophy is not as distinct for endurance exercise because all motor unit types are recruited in these activities.

■ Animal research has indicated the potential for muscle fibers to split and form new fibers during intense training. The increase in the number of muscle fibers is termed **hyperplasia.** It is unclear whether hyperplasia occurs from the splitting of existing fibers or the generation of new fibers. Although there is no experimental evidence for hyperplasia in human muscle following training for long-term muscular endurance, research that has compared muscle fiber areas between hypertrophied trained athletes and sedentary controls has revealed no difference in fiber areas, yet large differences in muscle cross-sectional area. Many scientists believe that this is indirect evidence of hyperplasia.

■ Both nerve cross-reinnervation and **artificial electrical stimulation** of motor nerves have been shown to reverse the metabolic and contractile profiles of muscle fibers. Connecting muscle fibers to an opposite motor nerve, or stimulating a nerve in the opposite frequency and intensity, converts the muscle fibers to reflect the muscle normally innervated by the nerve and stimulation profile. In humans, endurance training increases the proportion of FT muscle that stains as FOG fibers, whereas strength training increases the proportion of muscle fibers that stain as FG fibers (see Chapter 8).

■ Exercise training for long-term endurance further increases capillary density, thus providing more potential for blood flow to and from the contracting muscle fibers. Since these new capillaries cannot be totally associated with only SO muscle fibers, this adaptation also provides a more oxygen-rich microenvironment to certain FG and FOG fibers, thus further supporting the potential for increased capacities for mitochondrial respiration in these fibers.

SUMMARY—Cont'd

■ During detraining, muscle mitochondrial metabolic capacities are lost at a fast rate and those of glycolysis remain unchanged or increase slightly. However, alteration in fiber type proportions requires more severe disuse, like that of forced bed rest, immobilization of a limb (e.g., limb casts), or **deinnervation** (e.g., spinal cord injury). Generally there is a shift in fiber type from SO to FOG to FG, but the shift is not consistent in all muscles that are affected by the intervention. Increased activity, even by artificial electrical stimulation of the immobilized muscle(s), can reverse this atrophy response.

REVIEW QUESTIONS

1. Why can the fiber type proportion of a muscle influence muscle energy metabolism?

2. How might the preferential decrease in muscle glycogen from SO muscle fibers influence performance during exercise lasting in excess of 2 hours?

3. What might the benefit be for lactate production by FG muscle, and its uptake and metabolism in SO muscle during exercise?

4. Why do you think human exercise research has not verified the isolated recruitment of FT muscle fibers during intense rapid muscle contractions?

5. Can extremes in fiber type proportions influence an individual's potential for success in given types of exercise or sports competition? Explain.

6. What evidence is there to support the trainability of the neural and neuromuscular components of the motor unit pool of skeletal muscles?

7. What are the changes in muscle fiber type proportions that can be expected from training for either endurance or muscular power?

8. When muscles increase in cross-sectional area after resistance training, is the increase a result of hypertrophy or hyperplasia?

9. What muscle fiber changes occur during severe disuse, like immobilization of a limb or deinnervation?

APPLICATIONS

1. Individuals who are in rehabilitation from injury often experience severe wasting of skeletal muscle. Are there ways to minimize this wasting during the rehabilitation, and if so, what would the benefits of this be for the individual?

2. Try to explain why muscle that is experiencing disuse atrophy increases in FT fiber type proportion rather than ST proportion.

3. Individuals with spinal cord injury can receive artificial electrical stimulation to their paralyzed muscles and, when used in training, experience muscle hypertrophy. Apart from the aesthetic implications of this change, what other benefits may come from increasing the muscle mass of their lower limbs? What are some potential problems that may arise?

4. When using isokinetic equipment to test or train muscles, is the speed of contraction an important variable for determining outcome? Explain.

REFERENCES

1. Abernethy PJ, Jurimae J, Logan PA et al: Acute and chronic response of skeletal muscle to resistance exercise, *Sports Med* 17(1):22-38, 1994.

2. Alway SE, Grumbt WH, Stray-Gundersen J, Gonyea WJ: Effects of resistance training on elbow flexors of highly competitive bodybuilders, *J Appl Physiol* 72(4):1512-1521, 1992.

3. Anderson P: Capillary density in skeletal muscle of man, *Acta Physiol Scand* 95:203-205, 1975.

4. Antonio JA, Gonyea WJ: Skeletal muscle fiber hyperplasia, *Med Sci Sports Exerc* 25(12):1333-1345, 1993.

5. Baldwin KM, Klinkerfuss GH, Terjung RL et al: Respiratory capacity of white, red, and intermediate muscle: adaptive response to exercise, *Am J Physiol* 222:373-378, 1972.

6. Basmajian JV, Deluca CJ: *Muscles alive: their functions revealed by electromyography,* ed 5, Baltimore, 1985, Williams & Wilkins.

7. Bell DG, Jacobs I: Muscle fiber-specific glycogen utilization in strength-trained males and females, *Med Sci Sports Exerc* 21(6):649-654, 1989.

8. Berridge MJ: The molecular basis of communication within the cell. In *The molecules of life,* 1985, New York, Scientific American, WH Freeman.

9. Bradford HF: Chemical neurobiology: an introduction to neurochemistry, New York, 1986, WH Freeman.

10. Brooke MH, Kaiser K: Three "myosin adenosine triphosphatase" systems: the nature of their pH lability and sulfhydryl dependence, *J Histochem Cytochem* 18:670-672, 1970.

11. Brown AM, Birnbaumer L: Ionic channels and their regulation by G protein subunits, *Annu Rev Physiol* 52:197-214, 1990.

12. Burke RE: Firing patterns of gastrocnemius motor units in the decerebrate cat, *J Physiol* 196:631-654, 1968.

13. Burke RE: Motor units: anatomy, physiology and functional organization. In Brooks VB, editor: *Handbook of physiology: the nervous system,* vol II, Bethesda, Md, 1981, American Physiological Society.

14 Burke RE, Edgerton VR: Motor unit properties and selective involvement in movement, *Exerc Sport Sci Rev* 3:31-81, 1975.

15. Burke RE, Levine DN, Tsairis P, Zajac FE: Physiological types and histochemical profiles in motor units of the cat gastrocnemius, *J Physiol London* 234:723-748, 1973.

16. Caiozzo VJ, Perrine JJ, Edgerton VR: Training-induced alterations of the in vivo force-velocity relationship of human muscle, *J Appl Physiol* 51(3):750-754, 1981.

17. Chi MM-Y, Hintz CS, Coyle EF et al: Effects of detraining on enzymes of energy metabolism in individual human muscle fibers, *Am J Physiol* 244:C276-C287, 1983.

18. Clarke DH: Adaptations in strength and muscular endurance resulting from exercise, *Exerc Sports Sci Rev* 1:73-102, 1973.

19. Colliander EB, Dudley GA, Tesch PA: Skeletal muscle fiber composition and performance during repeated bouts of maximal, concentric contractions, *Eur J Appl Physiol* 58:81-86, 1988.

20. Costill DL, Fink WJ, Pollock ML: Muscle fiber composition and enzyme activities of elite distance runners, *Med Sci Sports Exerc* 8(2):96-100, 1976.

21. Costill DL, Jansson E, Gollnick PD, Saltin B: Glycogen utilization in leg muscles of men during level and uphill running, *Acta Physiol Scand* 91:475-481, 1974.

22. Coyle EF, Feiring DC, Rotkis TC et al: Specificity of power improvements through slow and fast isokinetic training, *J Appl Physiol* 51(6):1437-1442, 1981.

23. Deschenes MR, Cocault J, Kraemer WJ, Maresh CM: The neuromuscular junction: muscle fiber type differences, plasticity and adaptability to increased and decreased activity, *Sports Med* 17(6):358-372, 1994.

24. Dons B, Bollerup K, Bonde-Peterses F, Hancke S: The effect of weight lifting exercise related to muscle fiber composition and muscle cross-sectional area in humans, *Eur J Appl Physiol* 40:95-106, 1979.

25. Edgerton VR, Smith JL, Simpson DR: Muscle fiber type populations in human leg muscles, *Histochem J* 7:259-266, 1975.

26. Edstrom L, Grimby L: Effect of exercise on the motor unit, *Muscle Nerve* 9:104-126, 1986.

27. Essen B, Jansson E, Henriksson J: Metabolic characteristics of fiber types in human skeletal muscle, *Acta Physiol Scand* 95:153-165, 1975.

28. Evans WJ, Phinney SJ, Young VR: Suction applied to muscle biopsy maximizes sample size, *Med Sci Sports Exerc* 14:101-102, 1982.

29. Freund HJ: Motor unit and muscle activity in voluntary motor control, *Physiol Rev* 63:387-436, 1983.

30. Garfinkel S, Cafarelli E: Relative changes in maximal force, EMG, and muscle cross-sectional area after isometric training, *Med Sci Sports Exerc* 24(11):1220-1227, 1992.

31. Gauthier JM, Theriault R, Theriault G et al: Electrical stimulation-induced changes in skeletal muscle enzymes of men and women, *Med Sci Sports Exerc* 24(11):1252-1256, 1992.

32. Giddings CJ, Gonyea WJ: Morphological observations supporting muscle fiber hyperplasia following weight-lifting exercise in cats, *Anatom Rec* 233:178-195, 1992.

REFERENCES—Cont'd

33. Gollnick PD: Metabolism of substrates: energy substrate metabolism during exercise and as modified by training, *Fed Pro* 44:353-357, 1985.

34. Gollnick PD, Armstrong RB, Saubert CW et al: Enzyme activity and fiber composition in skeletal muscle of untrained and trained men, *J Appl Physiol* 33(3):312-319, 1972.

35. Gollnick PD, Hodgson RD: The identification of fiber types in human skeletal muscle: a continual dilemma, *Exerc Sport Sci Rev* 14:81-104, 1986.

36. Gollnick PD, Piehl K, Saltin B: Selective glycogen depletion pattern in human skeletal muscle fibers after exercise of varying intensity and at varying pedal rates, *J Physiol* 241:45-57, 1974.

37. Gollnick PD, Reidy M, Quintinskie JJ, Bertocci LA: Differences in metabolic potential of skeletal muscle fibers and their significance for metabolic control, *J Exp Biol* 115:91-199, 1985.

38. Gonyea WJ, Sale DG, Gonyea FB, Mikesky A: Exercise-induced increases in muscle fiber number, *Eur J Appl Physiol* 55:137-141, 1986.

39. Gordon T, Pattullo M: Plasticity of muscle fiber and motor unit types, *Exer Sport Sci Rev* 21:331-362, 1993.

40. Gregor RJ, Edgerton VR, Perrine JJ et al: Torque-velocity relationships and muscle fiber composition in elite female athletes, *J Appl Physiol* 47(2):388-392, 1979.

41. Haggmark T, Jansson E, Svane B: Cross-sectional area of the thigh muscle in man measured by computed tomography *Scand J Clin Lab Invest* 38:355-360, 1978.

42. Henneman E, Mendell LM: Functional organization of motorneurone pool and its inputs. In Brooks VB, editor: *Handbook of physiology: the nervous system,* vol II, Bethesda, Md, 1981, American Physiological Society.

43. Ivy JL, Chi MM-Y, Hintz CS et al: Progressive metabolite changes in individual human muscle fibers with increasing work rates, *Am J Physiol* 252(21):C630-C639, 1987.

44. Ivy JL, Withers RT, Van Handel PJ et al: Muscle respiratory capacity and fiber type as determinants of the lactate threshold, *J Appl Physiol* 48(3):523-527, 1980.

45. Kaufman MP, Waldrop TG, Rybicki KJ et al: Effects of static and rhythmic twitch contractions on the discharge of group III and IV muscle afferents, *Cardiovasc Res* 18:663-668, 1984.

46. Kraus J, Robergs RA, DePaepe JL et al: Cardiorespiratory effects of computerized functional electrical stimulation (CFES) and hybrid training in individuals with spinal cord injury, *Med Sci Sports Exerc* 25(9):1054-1061, 1993.

47. Larsson L, Tesch PA: Motor unit fiber density in extremely hypertrophied skeletal muscles in man, *Eur J Appl Physiol* 55:130-136, 1986.

48. Lesmes GR, Benham DW, Costill DL, Fink WJ: Glycogen utilization in fast and slow twitch muscle fibers during maximal isokinetic exercise, *Ann Sports Med* 1:105-108, 1983.

49. Lowey S: Cardiac and skeletal muscle polymorphism, *Med Sci Sports Exerc* 18(3):284-291, 1986.

50. Lowry CV, Kimmey JS, Felder S et al: Enzyme patterns in single human muscle fibers, *J Biol Chem* 253:8269-8277, 1978.

51. MacDougall JD, Elder GCB, Sale DG et al: Effects of strength training and immobilization on human muscle fibers, *Eur J Appl Physiol* 43:25-34, 1980.

52. MacDougall JD, Sale DG, Elder GCB, Sutton JR: Muscle ultrastructural characteristics of elite power lifters and body builders, *Eur J Appl Physiol* 48:117-126, 1982.

53. MacDougall JD, Sale DG, Elway SE, Sutton JR: Muscle fiber number in biceps brachii in body builders and control subjects, *J Appl Physiol* 57:1399-1403, 1984.

54. MacDougall JD, Sale DG, Moroz JR et al: Mitochondrial volume density in human skeletal muscle following heavy resistance training, *Med Sci Sports Exerc* 11:164-166, 1979.

55. MacDougall JD, Ward GR, Sale DG, Sutton JR: Biochemical adaptation of human skeletal muscle to heavy resistance training and immobilization, *J Appl Physiol* 43:700-703, 1977.

56. Martin TP, Stein RB, Hoeppner PH, Reid DC: Influence of electrical stimulation on the morphological and metabolic properties of paralyzed muscle, *J Appl Physiol* 72(4):1401-1406, 1992.

57. Mikesky AE, Giddings CJ, Mathews W, Gonyea WJ: Changes in muscle fiber size and composition in response to heavy-resistance exercise, *Med Sci Sports Exerc* 23(9):1042-1049, 1992.

58. Moritani T, DeVries HA: Neural factors versus hypertrophy in the time course of muscle strength gain, *Am J Phys Med* 58:115-130, 1979.

59. Muscacchia XJ, Steffen JM, Fell RD: Disuse atrophy of skeletal muscle: animal models, *Exerc Sport Sci Rev* 16:61-88, 1988.

60. Narici M, Roi G, Landoni L et al: Changes in force, cross-sectional area, and neural activation during strength training and detraining of the human quadriceps, *Eur J Appl Physiol* 59:310-319, 1989.

61. Nordheim K, Vollestad NK: Glycogen and lactate metabolism during low-intensity exercise in man, *Acta Physiol Scand* 139:475-484, 1990.

62. Pette D: Activity-induced fast to slow transitions in mammalian muscle, *Med Sci Sports Exerc* 16(6):517-528, 1984.

REFERENCES—Cont'd

63. Prince FP, Hikida RS, Hagerman FC: Human muscle fiber types in power lifters, distance runners and untrained subjects, *Pflugers Arch* 363:19-26, 1976.

64. Reidy M, Matoba H, Vollestad NK et al: Influence of exercise on the fiber composition of skeletal muscle, *Histochemistry* 80:553-557, 1984.

65. Robergs RA, Pearson DR, Costill DL et al: Muscle glycogenolysis during differing intensities of weight-resistance exercise, *J Appl Physiol* 70(4):1700-1706, 1991.

66. Rosenheimer J: Effects of chronic stress and exercise on age-related changes in endplate architecture, *J Neurophysiol* 53:1582-1589, 1985.

67. Roy RR, Baldwin KM, Edgerton VR: The plasticity of skeletal muscle: effects of neuromuscular activity, *Exerc Sport Sci Rev* 19:269-312, 1991.

68. Sale DG: Influence of exercise and training on motor unit activation, *Exerc Sport Sci Rev* 15:95-151, 1987.

69. Saltin B, Gollnick PD: Skeletal muscle adaptability: significance for metabolism and performance. In *Handbook of physiology: skeletal muscle,* Section 10, Bethesda, Md, 1983, American Physiological Society.

70. Saltin B, Henriksson J, Nygaard E, Anderson P: Fiber types and metabolic potentials of skeletal muscles in sedentary man and endurance runners, *Ann N Y Acad Sci* 301:3-29, 1977.

71. Sargeant AJ, Davies CT, Edwards RHT et al: Functional and structural changes after disuse of human muscle, *Clin Sci Mol Med* 52:337-342, 1977.

72. Schantz P, Randall Fox E, Norgen P, Tyden A; The relationship between muscle fiber area and the muscle cross-sectional area of the thigh in subjects with large differences in thigh girth, *Acta Physiol Scand* 113:537-539, 1981.

73. Secher NH, Jenssen NE: Glycogen depletion patterns in type I, IIA, and IIB muscle fibers during maximal voluntary static and dynamic exercise, *Acta Physiol Scand Suppl* 440:174 (abstract 287), 1976.

74. Sjostrom M, Lexell J, Eriksson A, Taylor CC: Evidence of fiber hyperplasia in human skeletal muscles from healthy young men, *Eur J Appl Physiol* 62:301-304, 1992.

75. Staron RS, Malicky ES, Leonardi MJ et al: Muscle hypertrophy and fast fiber type conversions in heavy resistance-trained women, *Eur J Appl Physiol* 60:71-79, 1989.

76. Stephens JA, Usherwood TP: The mechanical properties of human motor units with special reference to the fatigability and recruitment threshold, *Brain Res* 125:91-97, 1977.

77. Tamaki T, Uchiyama S, Nakano S: A weight-lifting exercise model for inducing hypertrophy in the hindlimb muscle of rats, *Med Sci Sports Exerc* 24:881-886, 1992.

78. Terjung RL, Baldwin KM, Winder WW, Holloszy JO: Glycogen repletion in different types of skeletal muscles and liver after exhaustive exercise, *Eur J Appl Physiol* 55:362-366, 1986.

79. Tesch PA, Larsson L: Muscle hypertrophy in body builders, *Eur J Appl Physiol* 49:301-306, 1984.

80. Tesch PA, Thorsson A, Fujitsuka N: Creatine phosphate in fiber types of skeletal muscle before and after exhaustive exercise, *J Appl Physiol* 66(4):1756-1759, 1989.

81. Tesch PA, Thorsson A, Kaiser P: Muscle capillary supply and fiber type characteristics in weight and power lifters, *J Appl Physiol* 56(1):35-38, 1984.

82. Thorstensson A, Grimby G, Karlsson J: Force-velocity relations and fiber composition in human knee extensor muscles, *J Appl Physiol* 40(1):12-16, 1976.

83. Vollestad NK, Blom PCS: Effect of varying exercise intensity on glycogen depletion in human muscle fibers, *Acta Physiol Scand* 125:395-405, 1985.

84. Vollestad NK, Blom PCS, Gronnerod O: Resynthesis of glycogen in different muscle fiber types after prolonged exhaustive exercise in man, *Acta Physiol Scand* 137:15-21, 1989.

85. Vollestad NK, Vaage O, Hermansen L: Muscle glycogen depletion pattern in type I and subgroups of type II fibers during prolonged severe exercise, *Acta Physiol Scand* 122:433-440, 1984.

RECOMMENDED READINGS

- Abernethy PJ, Jurimae J, Logan PA et al: Acute and chronic response of skeletal muscle to resistance exercise, *Sports Med* 17(1):22-38, 1994.

- Alway SE, Grumbt WH, Stray-Gundersen J, Gonyea WJ: Effects of resistance training on elbow flexors of highly competitive bodybuilders, *J Appl Physiol* 72(4):1512-1521, 1992.

- Antonio JA, Gonyea WJ: Skeletal muscle fiber hyperplasia, *Med Sci Sports Exerc* 25(12):1333-1345, 1993.

- Brooke MH, Kaiser K: Three "myosin adenosine triphosphatase" systems: the nature of their pH lability and sulfhydryl dependence, *J Histochem Cytochem* 18:670-672, 1970.

- Burke RE: Motor units: anatomy, physiology and functional organization. In Brooks VB, editor: *Handbook of physiology, the nervous system,* vol II, Bethesda, Md, 1981, American Physiological Society.

- Gollnick PD, Hodgson RD: The identification of fiber types in human skeletal muscle: a continual dilemma, *Exerc Sport Sci Rev* 14:81-104, 1986.

- Henneman E, Mendell LM: Functional organization of motorneurone pool and its inputs. In Brooks VB, editor: *Handbook of physiology: the nervous system,* vol II, Bethesda, Md, 1981, American Physiological Society.

- Mikesky AE, Giddings CJ, Mathews W, Gonyea WJ: Changes in muscle fiber size and composition in response to heavy-resistance exercise, *Med Sci Sports Exerc* 23(9):1042-1049, 1992.

- Saltin B, Gollnick PD: Skeletal muscle adaptability: significance for metabolism and performance. In *Handbook of physiology: skeletal muscle,* Bethesda, Md, 1983, American Physiological Society.

- Vollestad NK, Blom PCS: Effect of varying exercise intensity on glycogen depletion in human muscle fibers, *Acta Physiol Scand* 125:395-405, 1985.

CHAPTER 10

Muscle Metabolic Adaptations to Exercise

During the muscle contractions that accompany exercise there is a sudden increase in ATP utilization and the stimulation of metabolic *adaptations* that enable the muscle fibers to increase the regeneration of ATP. From the content of Chapter 6, the main pathways stimulated to increase ATP regeneration are the creatine kinase and adenylate kinase reactions, glycolysis, and mitochondrial respiration. The immediate *(acute)* metabolic adaptations that occur in skeletal muscle during exercise are classic examples of the responsiveness of skeletal muscle to metabolic stress. Apart from the acute changes in muscle metabolism, we know that skeletal muscle can undergo long-term *(chronic)* structural and functional changes when exposed to exercise performed repeatedly over several weeks or months. This chapter presents information that reveals the acute changes that occur in muscle metabolism to meet the muscles' needs to increase the regeneration of ATP, and the chronic adaptations that improve the muscles' abilities to regenerate ATP during exercise.

Importance of Exercise Intensity and Duration

The metabolic response of skeletal muscle is determined by the intensity of muscle contractions and therefore the intensity of the exercise. Since exercise of high intensity can be performed only for several seconds, and in the opposite extreme, low-intensity exercise can be maintained in excess of 1 hour, exercise intensity also determines exercise duration. There are several biochemical pathways from which muscle can regenerate ATP. The most immediate and fastest way to regenerate ATP is to use the muscle store of creatine phosphate (see Chapter 4). Glycolysis yields the next highest rate of ATP regeneration, followed by mitochondrial respiration. As a result of the time and rate dependence of each main pathway in ATP regeneration, it has been common to illustrate each metabolic pathway's relative contribution to ATP regeneration across increasing durations of exercise (Figure 10.1).

Figure 10.1 shows the connection between exercise duration (intensity) and the predominance of a certain pathway. Figure 10.1 applies to maximal exercise performed to fatigue, so that if fatigue occurred at 30 seconds, most of the ATP would have been regenerated from creatine phosphate hydrolysis. Exercise causing fatigue after 2 minutes would rely mainly on ATP from glycolysis, whereas exercise performed in excess of 3 minutes would rely more on ATP from mitochondrial respiration. The illustration should not be interpreted to indicate that creatine phosphate is used only in the first 30 seconds of exercise and that glycolysis then follows,

adaptation (ad-ap-**ta**'shun)
change in function or structure in response to changing conditions

acute (a-**kut**)
immediate

chronic (**kron**'ik)
long term

FIGURE 10.1

The relationships between exercise duration and the contribution of the creatine phosphate, glycolytic, and mitochondrial respiration pathways of ATP regeneration.

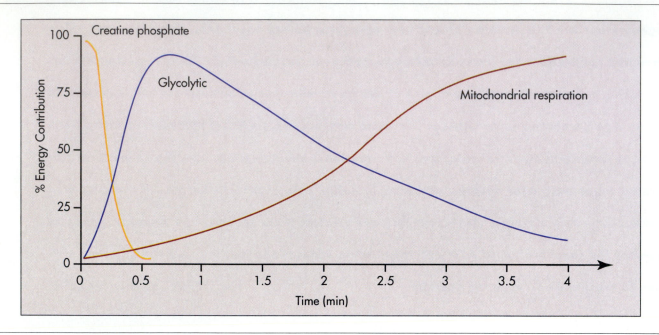

with mitochondrial respiration being important only after 3 minutes. Experimental evidence is presented in this chapter to indicate that creatine phosphate plays a role even during long-duration exercise, that glycogenolysis and glycolysis are stimulated almost immediately after muscle contraction begins, and that creatine phosphate hydrolysis and increased glycolysis also occur whenever exercise exceeds an individually specific intensity.

Acute Adaptations

*A*cute metabolic adaptations to exercise occur during the stress of exercise and also during the recovery after exercise. During exercise, catabolic reactions are stimulated to release the free energy required to regenerate the ATP that is used to fuel muscle contraction. During the recovery after exercise, both catabolic and anabolic reactions occur to replenish the energy stores used during exercise. The acute metabolic responses to exercise enable the muscles to meet or attempt to meet the ATP demand. During the recovery the ability of skeletal muscle to replenish energy and substrate stores as rapidly as possible prepares the muscle to better tolerate successive bouts of exercise. For these reasons the following sections are organized to describe acute adaptations to exercise relative to when they occur, the intensity of the exercise, and the type of metabolic pathway involved.

Adaptations During Exercise

Incremental Exercise

Incremental exercise involves the increase in exercise intensity over time. Other names for this type of exercise are *progressive* or *graded.* Incremental exercise protocols can be either *continuous,* in which successive increases in intensity occur without rest periods, or *intermittent,* in which a rest period is provided between increments. In addition, incremental protocols can be *maximal,* requiring the subject to exercise against increasing intensities until volitional fatigue, or *submaximal,* in which exercise is terminated at a predetermined intensity before volitional fatigue. Incremental exercise protocols can also vary in the duration of each specific intensity *(stage)* and the magnitude of the increment. If steady state is to be attained at each stage, stage durations must be at least 3 minutes in duration; however, the time requirement for this can be prohibitive. Depending on the purposes of the test, short-duration small increment stages are often used. In fact, *ramp protocols* exist that continuously increase intensity over time (speed and grade on a treadmill and resistance on a cycle ergometer).

Maximal oxygen consumption. Maximal oxygen consumption (VO$_2$max) is the maximal rate at which the body can consume oxygen during exercise. It is detected as a plateau in VO$_2$ despite further increases in intensity and as an RER that exceeds 1.1.[35,59] As you will discover, and as indicated by the RER requirement, the test of maximal oxygen

FIGURE 10.2

During incremental exercise, VO_2 increases in a manner that is dependent on the type of protocol used. The linear increase in VO_2 during cycle ergometry using a ramp protol (see text). During a 50 Watt incremental protocol, with 3 min stage durations, VO_2 increases to near steady state values at each stage during the early part of the test, revealing a "staircase" effect. During the last half of the test, the intensity increment and absolute intensity are too great for a steady state to be attained, and VO_2 increases more linearly to VO_2max.

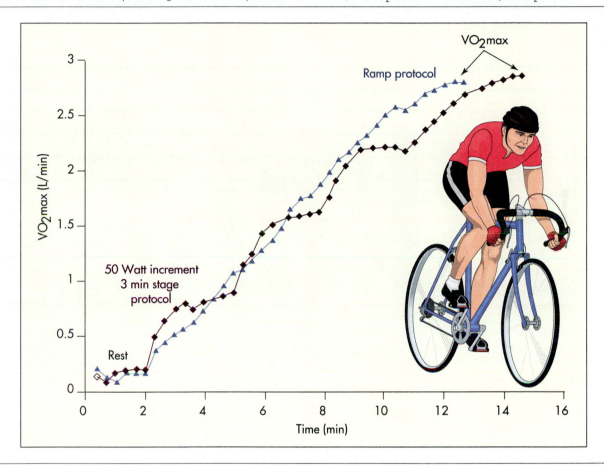

consumption is an example of both low- and high-intensity exercise; however, it is an important measurement that must be understood before a discussion of energy metabolism during both steady state and intense exercise conditions.

Figure 10.2 presents the change in VO_2 during two different protocols (A, ramp; B, 50-watt increment 3-minute stages) for the same individual using breath-by-breath indirect calorimetry. The ramp protocol increased VO_2 in a smooth linear manner to the plateau at VO_2max; however, during the initial stages the 3-minute stage protocol induced a "staircase" effect in the increase in VO_2. This effect makes it difficult to plot and interpret changes in metabolism over time during incremental protocols; however, it provides steady state VO_2 values for the lower exercise intensities, which may be useful for computing economy. Furthermore, despite the staircase effect, a line drawn through the VO_2 val-

ues at the end of each 3-minute stage would show a linear increase in VO_2 with an increase in intensity. As explained in subsequent sections, ramp protocols, or those involving small frequent increases in intensity (e.g., 20 watts every minute), provide more data points corresponding to the linear increase in VO_2 and therefore increase the temporal resolution of the metabolic response to incremental exercise.

incremental exercise

exercise performed at intensities that progressively increase over time

maximal oxygen consumption (VO_2max)

the maximal rate of oxygen consumption by the body

FIGURE 10.3

The variation in VO_2max for individuals that range in functional capacity from the chronically ill, to elite cross country skiers. These differences are not totally explained by training, as the genetic determinants of VO_2max include motor unit and central cardiovascular capacities that provide a foundation of genetic potential that will determine the magnitude of training improvement. (Adapted from Saltin B, Åstrand P: Maximal oxygen uptake in athletes, *J Appl Physiol* 25:353, 1967.)

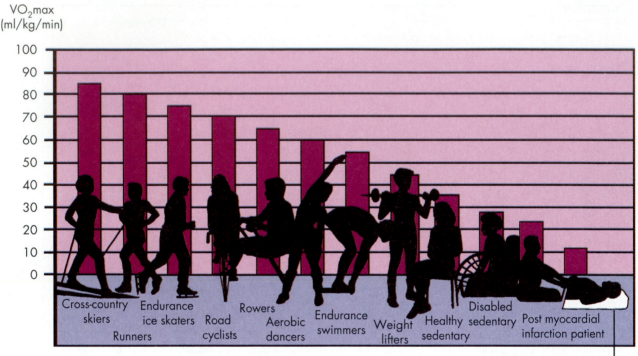

Individual variation in VO_2max. VO_2max values can be expressed as an absolute volume of oxygen per unit time (L/min) or relative to body mass (ml/kg/min). Typically, the absolute expression is used for exercise modes in which body weight is externally supported, and the relative expression is used for exercise modes in which body weight is supported by the individual and therefore contributes to the intensity of the exercise.

VO_2max values range from those of persons with extremely low capacities, such as chronically ill individuals (<20 ml/kg/min), to those of well-trained and elite endurance athletes (>80 ml/kg/min) (Figure 10.3). The factors that combine to influence VO_2max are a high proportion of slow twitch motor units, high central and peripheral cardiovascular capacities, and the quality and duration of training. Having more slow twitch muscle fibers increases the oxidative capacity of the muscle.[71] As discussed in Chapter 8, muscle motor unit proportions are genetically determined, and therefore a person's abilities to respond to endurance training and increase VO_2max have important genetic constraints.

VO_2max during different exercise modes. VO_2max is known to differ depending on the type of exercise and the type and extent of training performed by the individual. Figure 10.4 provides a comparison among VO_2max values obtained from treadmill run, step test, cycle ergometry, arm ergometry, and swimming incremental protocols. Generally, VO_2max is largest during running and stepping and lowest during arm ergometry. The reason for these differences is believed to be muscle mass, since a larger muscle mass is exercised during running and a relatively small muscle mass is exercised during arm ergometry.[35] However, when cycling and treadmill running are compared, VO_2max values have been shown to be largest in the trained exercise mode, with cycling VO_2max equal to or larger than treadmill VO_2max in well-trained cyclists.[43] This training specificity has also been demonstrated in well-trained swimmers, who can attain or exceed treadmill run VO_2max values during swimming or arm ergometry protocols.[50]

Percent of VO_2max: a relative measure of exercise intensity. The measurement of VO_2max not only is important in itself, but also serves as a value for the relative expression of exercise intensity. Because the increase in VO_2 is a linear function of exercise intensity, exercise intensities below VO_2max can be expressed as a percentage of VO_2max (%VO_2max), which allows a comparison of metabolic responses at the

FIGURE 10.4

A comparison between VO_2max obtained for a given individual during different exercise modes. The VO_2max values are expressed relative to treadmill run VO_2max, which represents the zero value of the y-axis. The changes for relatively untrained individuals is provided, with values for individuals highly trained in one exercise mode also provided.

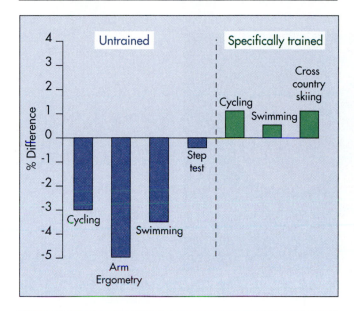

same relative intensity among individuals who may have very different VO_2max values. In addition, the linear relationship between intensity and VO_2 enables synonymous use of the expressions *%VO_2max* and *% workload at VO_2max*. Exercise intensities above VO_2max can also be expressed as a %VO_2max, with these values exceeding 100%. Workloads above 100%VO_2max have been incorrectly termed *supramaximal,* which has caused some confusion because a supramaximal load would theoretically be one that could not be performed! The expression of exercise intensities relative to VO_2max or the % workload at VO_2max is common in exercise-related research.

Creatine Phosphate

The previous description and graphic representation of a maximal exercise test indicated the development of metabolic acidosis, as evidenced by an RER exceeding unity, and the fact that the test is terminated by volitional fatigue. Obviously muscle creatine phosphate stores must be used to supplement ATP regeneration from mitochondrial respiration during the later stages of the test. The changing metabolic conditions during an incremental exercise test are presented in Figure 10.5, and the increasing reliance on creatine phosphate is shown to occur above intensities corresponding to 60% of the maximal incremental workload.

Application of *phosphorus magnetic resonance spectroscopy* (^{31}P MRS) (Focus Box 10.1) to exercise has improved our

understanding of the role of creatine phosphate in energy metabolism during exercise. Figure 10.6, *B*, presents successive ^{31}P MRS spectrum obtained during forearm incremental exercise to fatigue. In Figure 10.6, *C*, the data are analyzed and graphed as a change in Pi/CrP and the muscle hydrogen ion concentration (10^{-pH}) ([H^+]) with increases in intensity. As exercise intensity increased, Pi/CrP increased linearly with a low slope, indicating minimal reductions in CrP concentrations. After a given intensity of exercise, Pi/CrP increased abruptly and corresponded with increases in muscle acidosis (increased [H^+]). Obviously there is a region of exercise intensity in which muscle metabolism reverts from use of minimal muscle CrP to an increase in metabolic acidosis and the need to use CrP. For the forearm, this intensity corresponds to approximately 60% of the intensity attained at fatigue during incremental exercise, although this value can vary among individuals.[9,97] A low initial slope of Pi/CrP before the abrupt increase has been interpreted as an indicator of increasing muscle mitochondrial respiration.[1,9,27]

Glycogenolysis and Glycolysis

The previously described changes in RER and muscle CrP during incremental exercise, and the associated increase in muscle acidosis, indicate that increased glycogenolysis and glycolysis must also occur with an increase in intensity. Furthermore, at intensities greater than 60% of the maximum, lactate production must also increase to account for the change in muscle acidosis. Increased glycogenolysis and glycolysis during incremental exercise have been measured indi-

Text continues on p. 235.

FIGURE 10.5

The changing metabolic conditions, and primary sources of ATP regeneration, during an incremental exercise test to VO_2max.

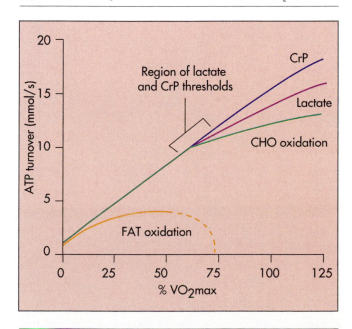

FIGURE 10.6

Data from a test using ¹H MRS and ³¹P MRS. **A,** A ¹H relaxation time image of the exercised muscles used during forearm wrist-flexion exercise. **B,** A stack plot of individual ³¹P spectrum obtained from the flexor carpi radialis during an incremental exercise protocol. **C,** Data from the ³¹P MRS spectrum that have been plotted as a change in Pi/CrP with increasing exercise intensity. The initial slope of this plot is interpreted to represent the CrP involvement in the creatine phosphate shuttle and general ATP demands of muscle contraction and membrane function. The steep increase in Pi/CrP represents the need to use CrP to supplement ATP regeneration when the rate of ATP demand exceeds the rate of ATP supply from mitochondrial respiration. The steep increase in Pi/CrP coincides with the development of intramuscular acidosis.

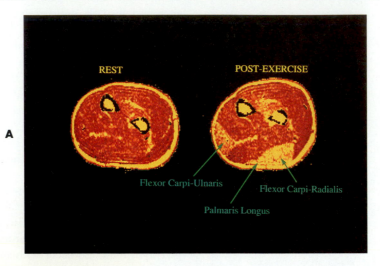

A

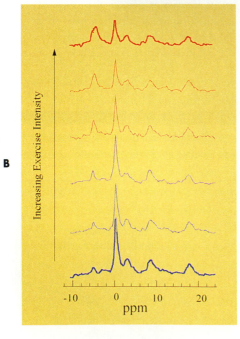

B

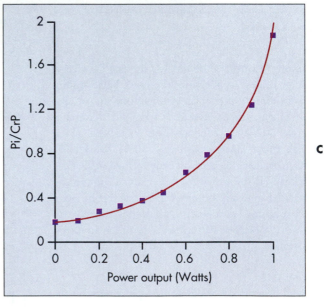

C

FOCUS BOX 10.1

Applications of magnetic resonance to exercise physiology

What is magnetic resonance?

Some atomic nuclei (e.g., of hydrogen and phosphorus atoms) have magnetic properties that make them directional, like an arrow or compass needle rather than a ball. Nuclear magnetic resonance (hereafter called **magnetic resonance [MR]**) detects the *precession* of these nuclei about a magnetic field applied by a large magnet. Precession refers to a motion similar to the spinning of a top about the earth's gravitational field (Figure 10.7). The nuclei precess at a frequency that is directly proportional to the strength of the magnetic field.

Since atoms reside in many different chemical environments, they have different neighboring atoms, some of which are magnetic and create their own magnetic fields like bar magnets. Therefore atomic nuclei feel slightly different magnetic field strengths depending on their chemical environment. Thus these nuclei have different precession frequencies from one another. The difference in precession between different nuclei, and between the same nuclei in different chemical environments, provides one of the applications of MR—to *noninvasively* analyze the distribution of chemically inequivalent atoms.

The nuclei most suited to study in biologic MR are listed in Table 10.1. The differences among them for natural abundance, relative tissue concentration, and MR sensitivity, coupled with their

FIGURE 10.7

The model of how a nucleus will precess in a magnetic field when forced out of alignment. The maximal radius of rotation is obtained when the nucleus is "tipped" at a 90° angle, and this also provides the maximal radiofrequency (rf) signal emitted from the nucleus.

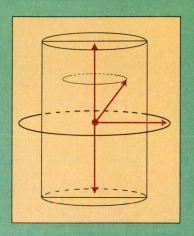

biologic relevance, determine the usefulness of the nuclei for MR studies. For example, ¹H (proton) is the most commonly

TABLE 10.1

Properties of nuclei used in biologic magnetic resonance

NUCLEI	NATURAL ABUNDANCE	TISSUE* CONCENTRATION	SENSITIVITY†	MR TECHNIQUE	APPLICATION
Hydrogen (^{1}H)	99.9%	99	1.0	Imaging Spectroscopy	Metabolism Anatomy Fat distribution
Deuterium (^{2}H)	0.015%	Trace	0.001	Spectroscopy	Body water
Sodium (^{23}Na)	100%	0.08	0.093	Imaging	Anatomy
Phosphorus (^{31}P)	100%	0.075	0.066	Imaging Spectroscopy	Metabolism
Flourine (^{19}F)	100%	4×10^{-6}	0.083	Contrast imaging	Anatomy
Carbon (^{13}C)	1.1%	Trace	0.016	Contrast imaging Spectroscopy	Metabolism

Modified from American Hospital Association: *Hospital Technology Series* 4(3-4):1-235, 1985.
*Relative to total hydrogen = 100. †For the same number of nuclei at constant field strength.

magnetic resonance (MR)
the ability of objects to precess when forced out of alignment in a magnetic field

used MR nucleus because of its high natural abundance, high concentration in tissues, and great MR sensitivity. Another important property, omitted to save space, is the precession frequency of different nuclei in a given magnetic field. For example, in a magnetic field of 1.9 Tesla the precession frequency of ^{1}H is 80.34 MHz (million cycles/second, comparable to FM radio broadcast frequencies), and for phosphorus it is 32.5 MHz.

The strength of a magnetic field is measured in units called *Tesla.* One Tesla equals 10,000 Gauss. When expressed relative to the earth's magnetic field, which equals 0.5 Gauss, a 1.9 Tesla magnet has a magnetism 38,000 times that of the earth. The magnetic field is generated by the conduction of an electric current (approximating 100 amperes) by bobbins of superconducting wires that surround the core of the magnet. These wires are bathed in cryogenic liquid helium (at a temperature of 269° C or 4° K), surrounded in turn by a vacuum and liquid nitrogen (-196° C or 77° K). Magnets used for MR applications come in all sizes (Figure 10.8), from the clinical MR imagers in hospitals that can image the whole body to high field strength instruments used by chemists that can accept only samples in 5-mm diameter tubes.

The details of how nuclear precessions are detected are not germane to the basic understanding of the relation of MR data to physiology. Brief operational descriptions are included here, but MR texts should be consulted for the complex and interesting implications of how the data are obtained in the myriad of different MR experiments.

For any MR experiment the desired sample (e.g., test tube, small animal, human forearm or leg) is placed into a suitable magnet and is subjected to radiofrequency magnetic fields (in addition to the field of the magnet itself) that excite the nuclei so that they yield a detectable MR signal. The detected signal is recorded and analyzed in a computer. One of the beauties of MR is that neither the field of the magnet nor the auxiliary radiofrequency field (analogous to radio waves that make TV and radio work) has known harmful effects on living tissue (unlike x-rays).

Most MR experiments work better at the strongest magnetic field strength possible. However, there are trade-offs in the strength of the magnetic field and the size of the magnet that generates it. The clinical machines used for human subjects usually have field strengths of up to 1.5 Tesla, whereas small sample instruments can have field strengths of 11 Tesla (six times stronger than a 1.9 Tesla magnet).

What is MR spectroscopy?

It was pointed out in the previous section that MR can noninvasively yield the distribution of chemically inequivalent atoms. This is the basis of **magnetic resonance spectroscopy (MRS).** In effect, researchers can obtain spectra (histograms proportional to concentrations) of specific atoms in different chemical sites of the same molecule (e.g., ATP) or different molecules (e.g., creatine phosphate versus inorganic phosphate).

Modern MRS experiments are performed with pulses of radio wave excitation (as opposed to the continuous radio waves used in the past). The signal elicited from these radio waves is a mixture from all pertinent nuclei precessing at different frequencies. For example, in ^{31}P MRS of skeletal muscle the signals from ^{31}P in adenosine triphosphate, creatine phosphate, and inorganic phosphate are combined. A mathematic operation called *Fourier transform* (FT) is used to separate the signal contributions from the nuclei precessing at slightly different frequencies. The result of the FT is the spectrum.

Because the spectrum is a distribution in precession frequency, the independent variable (x axis) has the units of frequency, usually in Hertz (Hz). However, because the difference in precession frequencies between nuclei in different chemical sites is proportional to the strength of the magnet, data from different magnets are best compared relative to fractions of the field strength (parts per million [ppm]).

Examples of common superconducting magnets used in MRS and MRI. **A,** A 1.9 Tesla superconducting magnet used for ^{31}P MRS studies of forearm or calf muscle. **B,** A 1.5 Tesla whole body magnet used for ^{1}H MRI and ^{1}H MRS.

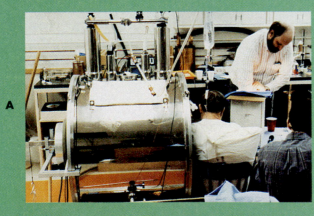

A

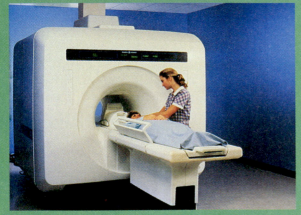

B

Examples from ^{31}P MRS

For living tissue like muscle, the phosphorus atoms detected by ^{31}P MRS are within inorganic phosphate (Pi), creatine phosphate (CrP), and the three phosphate groups of adenosine triphosphate (ATP). Figure 10.9, *A*, presents a typical unprocessed ^{31}P MRS signal (*free induction decay* [FID]) of a human forearm. This FID represents the average decay in the precession frequencies from the phosphorus nuclei. When the FID is Fourier transformed, it is typical for CrP to be aligned to zero ppm, with Pi located between 3.5 to 5 ppm away from CrP, and the three phosphate groups of ATP are positioned on the other side of CrP in the order of gamma (γ), alpha (α), and beta (β) phosphorus groups, respectively (Figure 10.9, *B*). As muscle pH decreases, the free Pi in the cell becomes more protonated.[67] This protonation alters the frequency emitted by these phosphorus nuclei and decreases the ppm difference between Pi and CrP (σ) (Figure 10.9, *B*). The ppm difference between Pi and CrP is used in a modified Henderson-Hasselbach acid-base equation (see Chapter 12) to calculate pH.*

FIGURE　10.9

The radiofrequency data received from the surface coil during ^{31}P MRS of the forearm. **A,** The raw radiofrequency signals from rest and high-intensity exercise. Each signal is referred to as a free induction decay (FID). **B,** After FID has been fourier transformed, it is converted to a spectrum revealing the intensity of signal of separate ^{31}P containing molecules and the signal frequency difference between each molecule.

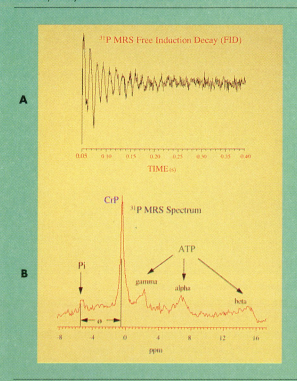

*References 2,7,9,16,24,85,92,115.

$$pH = 6.75 + \log\,[(\sigma - 3.27)/(5.69 - \sigma)]$$

The area under each peak obtained from MRS is proportional to concentration; however, in human muscle it is impossible to use an internal standard from which a known concentration equals a given area under a peak. Researchers using ^{31}P MRS with in vivo models do one of two things to combat this problem. The area under the curve of the alpha ATP peak is used as a standard that represents the known intramuscular concentration of 5 to 8 mmol/kg wet wt.[7] The concentrations represented by the area under the curves of CrP and Pi are then calculated. A more common strategy is to express the changes in CrP and Pi as a ratio of Pi/CrP,[96] or CrP/(Pi + CrP).[7,27] These ratios provide a measure of the relative change in CrP and Pi and prevent errors resulting from changes in specific peaks caused by movement artifact.

The applied difficulty with ^{31}P MRS is the long relaxation time of phosphorus nuclei, which for a 1.9 Tesla magnetic field takes approximately 2.5 seconds. To ensure complete relaxation of the nuclei in different chemical environments, researchers normally wait for five times the relaxation time. The chemical reactions involving CrP hydrolysis and phosphorylation are rapid, and the muscle CrP concentration can change significantly in a few seconds. Also, unless the magnetic field strength is large, the signal from phosphorus nuclei is small (Table 10.1) and requires the accumulation of several FIDs. Together these characteristics of ^{31}P MRS decrease the time resolution of the method, and prevent ^{31}P MRS from being applied to high-intensity exercise conditions when CrP metabolism is rapid.

Other Biologic Applications of MRS: ^{1}H and ^{13}C MRS
Magnetic resonance imaging

Proton MRS is the most commonly performed spectroscopy study, but not always in physiologic applications. This is because the proton spectrum is very narrow compared with the ^{31}P spectrum and has many more molecules of interest in living tissue and therefore more peaks; it is difficult to resolve each peak with acceptable accuracy.

The most favorable human organ for ^{1}H MRS is the brain. Figure 10, *A*, is a spectrum from H$^+$ MRS of the human brain at 1.5 Tesla, with the main peaks indicated. Figure 10, *B*, is a H$^+$ MRS spectrum of human muscle, identifying muscle lipid, creatine, and carnitine.[20,122] After exercise a new peak is present, which may be mobilized free fatty acid molecules (Figure 10.10, *C*). With sophisticated analyses of ^{1}H MRS data, a lactate peak can also be identified.

---

magnetic resonance spectroscopy (MRS)

the detection of differing radio frequency sound waves from precessing objects in a magnetic field, and the processing of these signals allowing the graphic illustration and quantification of the different signals and their respective intensities

FIGURE 10.10

Examples of ¹H MRS of human tissue. The human gastrocnemius muscle at **A,** rest, **B,** 10 minutes after 60 min of running exercise at 50% VO₂max, and **C,** after 60 min of recovery from the running exercise. The new peak from the skeletal muscle spectrum revealed after exercise is believed to represent increased intramuscular free fatty acids. **D,** The human brain, with the identification of the chemicals represented by specific peaks.

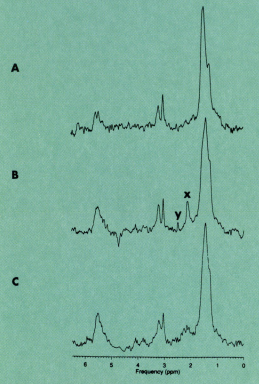

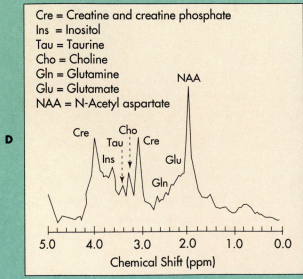

Cre = Creatine and creatine phosphate
Ins = Inositol
Tau = Taurine
Cho = Choline
Gln = Glutamine
Glu = Glutamate
NAA = N-Acetyl aspartate

One percent of all carbon atoms in nature have an extra neutron, resulting in an atomic mass of 13 instead of 12. This isotope, ¹³C, yields valuable MR spectra, but because of its low abundance requires either a high field strength apparatus or isotope enrichment of the sample being analyzed (e.g., ingestion of ¹³C in food for researching muscle glycogen). In fact, muscle glycogen measured by biochemical assay from biopsy samples and by natural abundance ¹³C MRS has produced amazingly similar concentrations,[130] thus indicating the potential of ¹³C MRS to further increase our understanding of glycogen metabolism.

Other Biologic Applications of MR: Proton Imaging

The magnetic resonance of proton nuclei in a magnetic field is the basis for the process of **magnetic resonance imaging (MRI).** MRI is used in clinical settings as a diagnostic tool for the anatomic location of internal structures of the body, thus aiding detection of injury, incorrect structure, or abnormal growths. The proton is a good nuclei to investigate with MR techniques, since it is abundant in water, fat, and to a lesser degree membranous tissue. These differences in proton content, and therefore signal intensity, provide a means to distinguish between different tissues in the body. Tissues rich in protons, such as fat, bone marrow, or the watery medium of blood, appear bright on MRI, whereas tissues low in protons appear dark (e.g., bone). The different proton signal from connective tissue and skeletal muscle enables the cross-sectional area of muscle to be quantified, as well as regional estimations of body fat content.

Proton T₂-weighted imaging

Researchers have been able to detect increased muscle metabolic activity by developing images that reflect changes in the *relaxation characteristics* of the proton nuclei(T₂).[40,41,74] For example, Figure 10.6, *A,* (see p. 230) presents rest and postexercise images that reveal the exercised muscles of the quadriceps appeared lighter in contrast to the remaining muscles because of a prolonged relaxation time of protons. Changes in muscle that may alter the relaxation of the proton nuclei include water movement between different compartments of tissue, resulting in an increased interstitial water content.[42]

magnetic resonance imaging (MRI)
the detection of different radio frequencies of precessing objects in a magnetic field and the processing of this informa-tion to provide a visual two-dimensional picture of the anatomic distribution of these frequencies

rectly via measurement of changes in blood or muscle lactate. As with muscle Pi/CrP, blood and muscle lactate concentrations increase abruptly at a certain exercise intensity, which has been termed the **lactate threshold.**

Lactate thresholds. The lactate threshold has been studied mainly during cycle ergometry and treadmill running. When increased lactate concentrations are measured from blood, the measurement is termed the *blood lactate threshold*. When increasing lactate concentrations are measured in muscle, the measurement is termed the *muscle lactate threshold*.[26,53,77]

Blood lactate threshold. Figure 10.11, *A*, presents a typical graph of blood lactate concentrations from venous blood during incremental exercise. In this example, at an exercise intensity approximating 70% VO₂max, blood lactate concentrations begin to increase abruptly. This particular intensity can be expressed as a VO₂, Watts (if cycling), or running speed (if treadmill running). Research indicates that the intensity at the lactate threshold represents the maximal intensity at which steady state exercise can be maintained.[86,138] Consequently, studies that have correlated running velocity at the lactate threshold to long distance running have reported correlations exceeding 0.9 for running distances from 5 km to the marathon (46 km).[86] The higher the intensity at the lactate threshold, the higher the intensity that can be sustained in endurance exercise.

The difficulty in measuring the lactate threshold occurs in the method selected to detect the exact intensity at which it occurs.[12,65,139,142] Obviously, visual methods of detection are open to experimenter error. For this and other reasons there has been considerable debate as to the scientific validity of the lactate threshold concept. Additional methlogic concerns over the lactate threshold have been that (1) blood lactate may increase in an exponential rather than a threshold manner,[21,65] (2) blood lactate concentrations differ in different blood compartments (capillary, venous, arterial),[111] (3) blood lactate and the lactate threshold can be altered by changing the carbohydrate content of the diet,[143] and (4) blood lactate results from lactate appearance and disappearance from the blood, and therefore using blood lactate as a reflection of lactate production is invalid.[19,28,29,126]

Techniques used to decrease the visual error in detecting the lactate threshold have been based on converting the data to logarithmic values. One or both of the lactate and intensity axes can be expressed on a logarithmic scale, or the data converted to log values (see Figure 10.11, *B*).[12] The reasoning for this is that if there are different exponential associations between blood lactate and intensity below compared with above the lactate threshold, converting data to a log form would produce data that fit a linear function below the threshold, and data that fit a different linear function above the threshold. From Figure 10.12, *B,* it is clear that the data can be fitted with two separate linear regression lines, and the intersection of the two lines used as the lactate threshold.

The change in blood lactate concentrations during an incremental exercise test. **A,** The identification of the lactate threshold from visual detection of the abrupt increase in blood lactate. **B,** The detection of the lactate threshold by converting lactate and VO₂ to log values. The lactate threshold represents the intensity at which two regression lines intersect. Note that after endurance training, the lactate threshold occurs at a higher exercise intensity, even when expressed as %VO₂max.

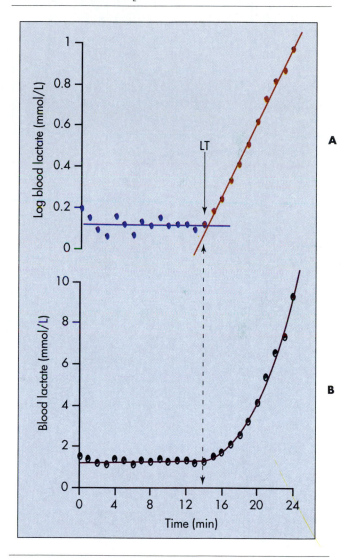

However, from these two methods it is clear that a slightly different time is detected for the lactate threshold, and the argument that a specific threshold intensity does not validly represent the data may have merit.[65]

lactate threshold
the term used to denote the intensity of exercise when there is an abrupt increase in lactate accumulation in blood or muscle

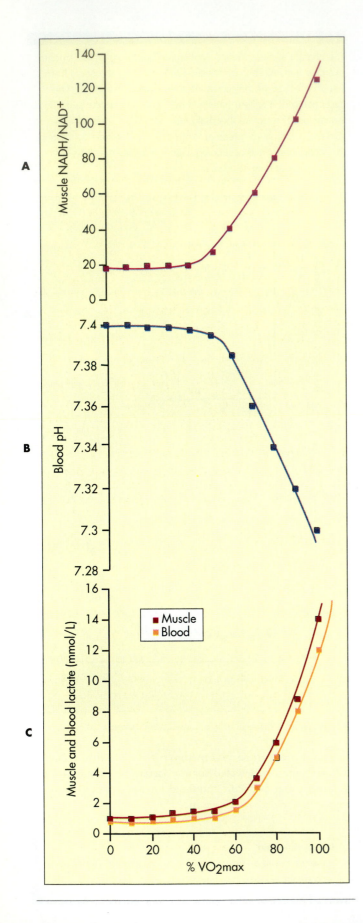

FIGURE 10.12

A combination figure revealing the temporal relationship between changes in **A,** muscle NADH, **B,** muscle lactate, and **C,** blood pH during an incremental exercise test.

Muscle lactate threshold. We know that a similar lactate threshold occurs in muscle. As early as 1972, data existed that demonstrated that during low-intensity exercise muscle lactate remained close to rest concentrations (1 mmol/kg wet wt), and after a given intensity, muscle lactate then increased abruptly.[76] Despite these early findings, more recent research has indicated that muscle lactate production may increase linearly with exercise intensity.[52] However, these findings have not been reproduced, whereas those of a threshold increase in muscle lactate accumulation have been reproduced.[26] In addition, a temporal connection between the blood and muscle lactate thresholds and decreases in blood pH has been shown[26] (Figure 10.12).

What may cause a blood and muscle lactate threshold? Several explanations have been proposed for a lactate threshold:

    (1) Decreased removal of lactate from the circulation
    (2) Increased recruitment of fast twitch glycolytic motor units
    (3) Imbalance between the rate of glycolysis and mitochondrial respiration
    (4) Decreased redox potential (increased NADH relative to NAD^+)
    (5) Hypoxia (lowered blood oxygen content)
    (6) Ischemia (lowered blood flow to skeletal muscle)

Decreased lactate removal. Research using radioactive isotopes has demonstrated that lactate production increases even during low-intensity exercise, and that as exercise intensity increases beyond a certain point the removal of lactate from the circulation does not increase at the same rate (Figure 10.13).[126] However, these data do not provide a mechanism for the further increase in lactate production during incremental exercise.

Increased Fast Twitch Glycolytic Motor Unit Recruitment. The delayed recruitment of fast twitch glycolytic (FG) motor units during incremental exercise influences lactate production. Muscle fibers from FG motor units have a high glycolytic capacity and a low oxidative capacity. Therefore recruiting FG motor units biases metabolism away from mitochondrial respiration to glycolysis. The inevitable result is an increase in lactate production.

    The fiber type proportion determinants of the lactate threshold have also been revealed from comparing the intensity of the lactate threshold with the proportion of slow twitch fiber types in muscle and with muscle oxidative

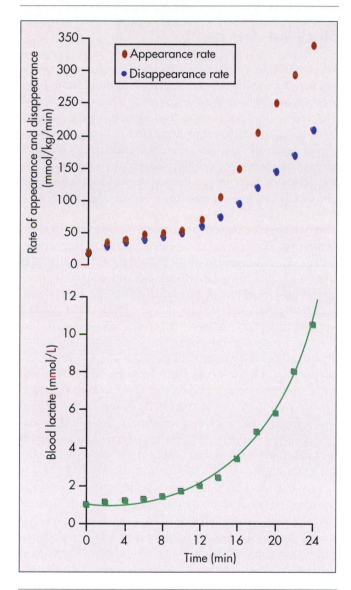

FIGURE 10.13

The change in lactate appearance and disappearance during a cycle ergometry incremental exercise test. (Adapted from Stanley WC et al: Systemic lactate kinetics during graded exercise in man, *Am J Physiol* 249(12):E595-E602, 1985.)

may exceed the ability of all pyruvate molecules to enter into the mitochondria and be converted to acetyl-CoA. Biochemical support for this hypothesis is that administration of dichloroacetate to humans decreases blood lactate concentrations at rest, during exercise, and during the recovery from exercise.[23] Because dichloroacetate stimulates pyruvate dehydrogenase, the lower lactate concentrations with dichloroacetate would indicate that there is some limitation to pyruvate conversion to acetyl-CoA within the mitochondria during exercise. Nevertheless, in this study there was no change in the exercise intensity at the lactate threshold, and pyruvate may have still been converted to lactate to prevent decreases in glycolysis because of an accumulation of pyruvate and decreasing concentration of cytosolic NAD^+.

Decreased cytosolic redox. The lactate dehydrogenase reaction converts pyruvate to lactate and vice versa. Apart from pyruvate, an important substrate for this reaction is NADH, which provides the electrons and protons necessary to reduce pyruvate to lactate. Consequently, the production of lactate also regenerates NAD^+, which is a coenzyme for the glyceraldehyde 3-phosphate dehydrogenase reaction of glycolysis. Figure 10.12 illustrates that lactate concentrations in muscle do not increase, despite increases in pyruvate, until there is an increase in cytosolic NADH. The increase in muscle NADH during exercise is known to occur in both slow and fast twitch fibers.[106] Lactate production can be viewed as a result of a decreased capacity for exchange of NAD^+ and NADH between the mitochondria and cytosol, as would occur when mitochondrial NADH increases.

Is there an anaerobic threshold? The name **anaerobic threshold** was first reported in 1964 by Wasserman.[136] At that time the sudden increase in blood lactate was interpreted to indicate increased lactate production. The concept of an anaerobic threshold was based on experimental research that documented increased lactate production during conditions of low blood oxygen partial pressures *(hypoxia)* or low blood flow conditions *(ischemia)*. At that time Wasserman and McIlroy thought it logical for increased lactate production during incremental exercise to be interpreted as evidence for a lack of oxygen in the contracting muscles. However, there was no experimental evidence for the development of hypoxia within muscle during incremental exercise, and because of methodologic constraints, even today we are still unable to measure intracellular partial pressures of oxygen.

capacity.[70] The oxidative potential of the muscle, and therefore the genetic and training determinants of this capacity, are important determinants of the exercise intensity at the lactate threshold.

Mass action. The argument that lactate production increases because of a greater rate of glycolysis than mitochondrial respiration has been termed the *mass action* effect. As a result of the large potential increases in glycogenolysis and glycolysis during exercise, pyruvate can be produced at high rates that

anaerobic threshold

the term used to denote the intensity of exercise when there is an abrupt increase in creatine phosphate hydrolysis and glycolysis, resulting in increased lactate production and the decrease in muscle creatine phosphate

Despite our inability to measure intracellular pressures of oxygen, several indirect measures may indicate reduced cellular oxygen content. Each of these measures is based on the fact that if there is a lack of oxygen in muscle, the rate of electron transport would be slowed, which would slow the rate of the TCA cycle. These events would increase the concentration of NADH in both the mitochondria and cytosol and would decrease the concentration of NAD^+. Consequently, the NAD^+/NADH, or *redox potential,* would be a reflection of the oxygen availability in muscle. Since most of the NAD^+ and NADH is found in the mitochondria,[79,114,116] a total muscle measure of NAD^+/NADH reflects the mitochondrial redox potential. Rather than measure actual NAD^+ or NADH concentrations, researchers have measured substrate and product concentrations for equilibrium reactions involving NAD^+ or NADH coenzymes. Presumably, the relationship between substrates and products would also reflect NAD^+/NADH (e.g., the lactate dehydrogenase reaction lactate/pyruvate).[7,79,80] A decrease in the muscle redox potential has been observed during incremental exercise[116] (see Figure 10.13, D). The muscle redox potential increased (increased NAD^+) during low-intensity exercise (<45% VO_2max) and then decreased well below resting values for intensities greater than 75% VO_2max.[116]

Despite this evidence, in vitro research with isolated mitochondria has shown that oxygen does not limit mitochondrial respiration until oxygen partial pressures are as low as 0.3 mm Hg.[79,80] The main argument against this impressive finding is that in vivo muscle function and metabolism are different from those in isolated mitochondria. In vivo there is a need for oxygen diffusion from blood to myoglobin, oxygen diffusion from myoglobin to the mitochondria, and additional reactions that can add or remove TCA cycle intermediates. The differences between isolated mitochondria and in vivo conditions could only increase the critical pressure of oxygen that limits mitochondrial respiration. In addition, blood flow to contracting skeletal muscle is known to decrease during muscle contraction,[110,135] and be unequally distributed within a given muscle.[69] The combination of temporal and regional disparity in blood flow (oxygen provision) to oxygen demand may cause some regions of muscle to become hypoxic, even though average muscle partial pressures of oxygen (PO_2) values are above a so-called critical value.[110] No definitive statement that a muscle becomes deficient in oxygen during submaximal exercise can be made; however, evidence that oxygen limitation affects muscle metabolism is mounting.

The lactate threshold has also been estimated from gas exchange parameters determined from indirect gas analysis calorimetry. The term *ventilatory threshold* reflects the measurement's dependence on ventilation. Because the ventilatory threshold involves acute ventilatory responses to incremental exercise, it is explained in Chapter 12.

All of the previous explanations of the lactate threshold may be involved in determining when blood or muscle lactate may increase abruptly. A lack of oxygen causes the mito-

chondrial redox, cytosolic redox, and mass action scenarios to develop. The increase in fast twitch motor unit recruitment exacerbates the aforementioned conditions. The actual mechanisms causing the lactate threshold remain a challenging research topic, but the importance of the lactate threshold to endurance performance is clear.

Steady State Exercise

As explained in Chapter 2, *steady state* exercise is attained when all the ATP demand from muscle contraction is met by oxidative phosphorylation. Therefore during steady state exercise, oxygen consumption has reached a plateau and *metabolic acidosis* does not develop. The metabolic issues of interest involve how steady state is attained, how glycogenolysis, glycolysis, lipolysis, β-oxidation, and amino acid oxidation contribute substrates to mitochondrial respiration, and how the contribution of these substrates may change with different steady state exercise intensities and durations.

Oxygen kinetics during transitions to increased exercise intensity. The increment in intensity causing an increase in VO_2 until steady state can be isolated and studied (Figure 10.14). For low to moderate intensities, small increases in intensity result in an exponential increase in VO_2 until steady state is reached. The time to reach steady state is approximately 3 minutes[53-55,60,64,139]; however, this time varies depending on the magnitude of the increment and the fitness of the individual.[54,60] The larger the increment, the longer the time to steady state, although individuals with high cardiorespiratory endurance have a shorter time to steady state (see Figure 10.14). Presumably the oxygen cost of recovering from the use of these immediate sources of ATP regeneration occurs during the steady state exercise and also during the recovery from the exercise (see section on EPOC).

As a result of the time delay in attaining steady state, ATP must be regenerated by creatine phosphate hydrolysis and glycolysis to enable continued muscle contraction. The energy provided by creatine phosphate and glycolysis that supplements mitochondrial respiration is called the **oxygen deficit.** Since endurance training can decrease the time to steady state, it also decreases the oxygen deficit.[54,60] Performing a warm-up can also decrease the oxygen deficit. Presumably a *warm-up* increases the body's ability to respond to exercise by increasing blood flow, muscle temperature, and stimulation of mitochondrial respiration.[111]

What stimulates the increase in mitochondrial respiration? After exercise is started, biochemical events must develop that stimulate the mitochondria to increase metabolic rate. This stimulation must occur rapidly to prevent a large oxygen deficit, but this need is complicated by the compartmentalization of the mitochondria by a double membrane. Metabolic signals must exist within the cytosol that communicate the increased ATP demand of muscle contraction to within the mitochondria.

FIGURE 10.14

The change in VO_2 during the transition from rest to submaximal exercise, revealing **A,** the exponential increase in VO_2 and the detection of the time to steady state. The difference between the integrated differences between measured VO_2 and the steady state VO_2 represents the oxygen deficit. For a given increment in intensity, the oxygen deficit will be less in an individual trained for long-term endurance. **B,** The oxygen deficit increases for larger increments in exercise intensity. For a given increment in exercise intensity, the oxygen deficit will be less in an individual trained for long-term endurance.

A 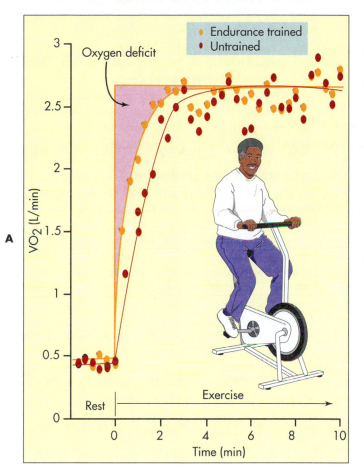 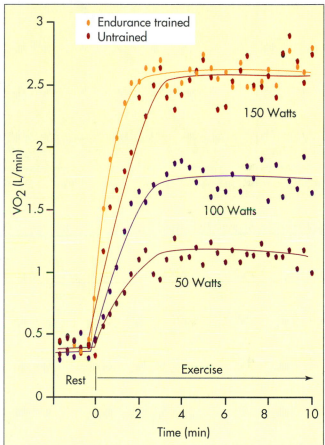 **B**

In vitro research has shown that increasing the concentrations of ADP and Pi stimulates increased mitochondrial respiration.[8] However, increases in VO_2 occur in vivo during submaximal exercise without increases in either ADP or Pi. Obviously, additional regulation must exist. For mitochondrial oxygen consumption to increase, there must be a simultaneous increase in mitochondrial concentrations of NADH, supplied through either glycolysis or the TCA cycle. The shuttling of cytosolic NADH into the mitochondria (as NADH or FADH) would be a responsive system because of the near-immediate stimulation of glycolysis during muscle contraction. However, an increased TCA cycle activity is also a recognized response to muscle contraction. A possible agent for increasing mitochondrial enzyme activity is calcium, which increases in concentration within the cytosol during muscle contraction. Calcium is a known activator of mitochondrial dehydrogenase enzymes, of which the pyruvate dehydrogenase complex is an important example.[8]

Sahlin et al[115] measured TCA cycle intermediates before and during continuous exercise to fatigue at 75% VO_2max. There was almost a tenfold increase in TCA cycle intermediates after the first 5 minutes of exercise, followed by a gradual decline to concentrations that were five times that of rest at fatigue (75 minutes). The tenfold increase in TCA cycle intermediates within 5 minutes of exercise is remarkable. More intermediates within the TCA cycle would increase the maximal rate of pyruvate entry into the mitochondria because the increased concentrations of oxaloacetate would combine with acetyl-CoA to form citrate. How can the TCA

oxygen deficit

the difference between oxygen consumption and the oxygen demand of exercise during non–steady state exercise conditions

The change in **A,** RER, **B,** VO₂ and VCO₂ during an incremental exercise test.

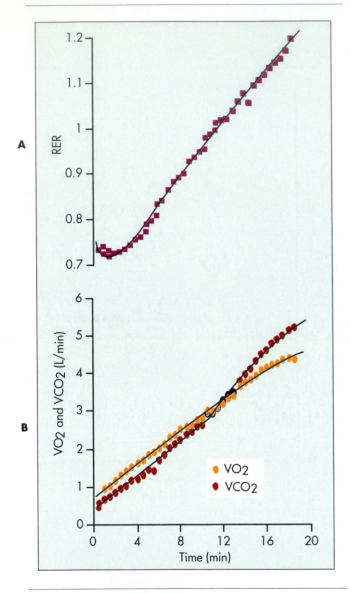

approximately 3 minutes, prolonged exercise at a given sub-maximal intensity causes a slight increase in VO₂, known as **oxygen drift.** Westerlind et al[138] demonstrated that the oxygen drift was significantly greater (approximately 18 to 22 ml/kg/min) during 30 minutes of downhill running at 40% VO₂max compared with level running at the same intensity, for which no drift was reported. However, in studies that evaluated VO₂ for longer periods and at higher submaximal steady state exercise intensities (>60% VO₂max), an upward drift in VO₂ has been reported.[30,53] It seems that a combination of increased muscle temperature and circulating catecholamine hormones contributes to the oxygen drift during level running. Apparently the larger oxygen drift during downhill running is not caused by muscle damage but results from the greater increases in muscle temperature during negative work.[138]

Carbohydrate and lipid catabolism. The metabolic data obtained from indirect calorimetry for steady state exercise at different intensities are graphed in Figure 10.15. The increasing VO₂, VCO₂, and RER values at steady state for increases in exercise intensity indicate that VO₂ increases linearly with an increase in intensity, VCO₂ increases linearly but at a slightly larger rate, and RER increases linearly. The difference between the VO₂ and VCO₂ response is explained by RER. An increase in RER indicates an increasing reliance on carbohydrate catabolism, which involves an increase in CO₂ production. For example, at rest, when lipid catabolism predominates, RER approximates 0.7 and indicates that VCO₂ is less than VO₂. During exercise the increase in RER toward unity indicates an increase in VCO₂ relative to VO₂. Consequently, exercise performed at a low intensity, when RER is closest to 0.7, involves lipid as the predominant substrate.

Other measurements have been used to document the contribution of lipid and carbohydrate to muscle energy metabolism. Researchers have measured muscle *glycogen* and *triglyceride* stores,[22,68] and the blood metabolites *lactate, free fatty acid* (FFA), and *glycerol* can be used to indirectly assess carbohydrate and lipid contributions to metabolism.[22,68,108] For example, increasing blood lactate concentrations during exercise are often interpreted to indicate increased muscle glycogenolysis and carbohydrate catabolism. Similarly, increasing serum free fatty acid and glycerol concentrations are interpreted to reflect increased mobilization of free fatty acids from triglycerides within lipoproteins or adipose tissue. However, care should be taken when interpreting blood metabolite concentrations, since increased free fatty acids and glycerol may not necessarily reflect increased free fatty acid uptake by muscle, and increasing blood lactate may be influenced by decreased lactate removal from the circulation.[19]

cycle intermediates increase in concentration? There must be sites other than pyruvate at which carbohydrates or amino acids can enter into the TCA cycle. As explained in Chapter 5, the minimal amount of pyruvate carboxylase in skeletal muscle favors the use of amino acids for increasing TCA cycle intermediates.

The regulation of mitochondrial respiration appears to be a multifaceted phenomenon. This is probably a good thing, since having many regulators allows a more sensitive response to conditions that require increased oxygen consumption and ATP regeneration.

Drift in VO₂ during prolonged exercise. Although exercise at a submaximal intensity results in a steady state VO₂ after

oxygen drift
the increase in oxygen consumption during presumably "steady state" exercise when it is performed for extended periods

FIGURE 10.16

The change in **A,** muscle glycogen, **B,** ratings of perceived exertion (RPE) during prolonged submaximal exercise, and **C,** blood glucose. The association between decreases in muscle glycogen and blood glucose, and the increase in RPE may indicate the role of hypoglycemia in the mechanism of fatigue during prolonged exercise (see Chapter 24).

Where does the lipid come from that fuels muscle contraction during low-intensity steady state exercise? Traditionally, lipid catabolism was thought to involve the mobilization of free fatty acids from triglycerides stored in plasma lipoproteins or adipose tissue. These free fatty acids were assumed to enter into muscle fibers from the capillary circulation and be used in β-oxidation. These interpretations were based on animal and human research revealing that free fatty acid uptake into skeletal muscle increased in proportion to the concentration of free fatty acids in blood.[31,108] However, several studies have indicated that circulating free fatty acids are not the only or major source of lipid during muscle lipid catabolism. Carlson et al[22] found that more than 60% of lipid used during submaximal exercise comes from lipid stores within the contracting skeletal muscle. In addition, Hurley et al[68] demonstrated that after endurance training, when lipid catabolism increases for a given exercise intensity, circulating FFA and glycerol concentrations decrease and the use of muscle triglycerides increases. These data indicate that during submaximal exercise the main source of lipid for metabolism is not blood or adipose tissue, but intramuscular stores of lipid (see Chapters 4 and 5).

The enzyme responsible for lipolysis is *lipoprotein lipase* (LPL), which exists in two possible forms. One form is located attached to the inner lumen of capillaries and the other is located intracellularly (see Figure 4.15). Both forms are thought to have tissue-specific regulation. For example, research using rats has shown that total muscle LPL activity (vascular and intracellular) increases in response to exercise, while that of adipose tissue decreases.[84] These findings support the human experimental evidence of Hurley et al,[68] since with the decreased activity of adipose tissue, FFA from blood triglycerides perfusing contracting muscle or intramuscular triglyceride stores is the remaining source of free fatty acids used during exercise.

Not all steady state exercise relies predominantly on lipid as a fuel. O'Brien et al[100] mimicked the marathon run inside a laboratory using a treadmill and demonstrated that RER averaged 0.99 for fast runners (<165 minutes duration at 73.3% VO$_2$max). Interestingly, both muscle glycogen and blood glucose were substrates for muscle catabolism. The muscle, liver, and blood stores of carbohydrate are therefore important to more intense steady state exercise, as indicated in Figure 10.5.

The rate of muscle glycogenolysis during steady state and intense exercise depends on exercise intensity. The lower the exercise intensity, the longer the time until muscle glyco-

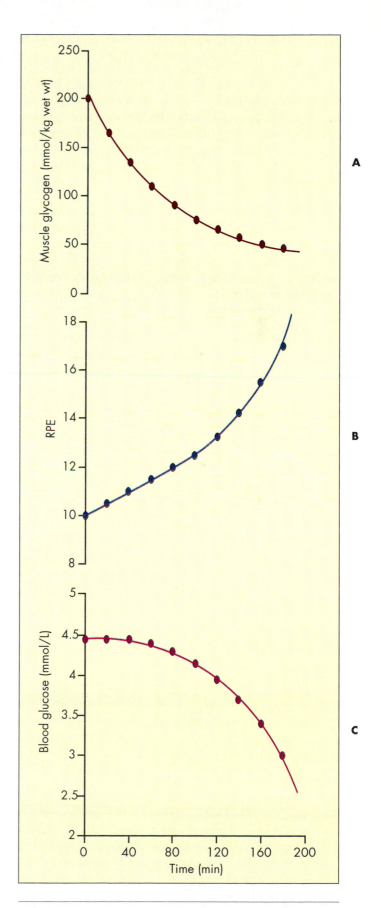

gen depletion. For the near maximal steady state intensities (60% to 80% VO$_2$max), muscle glycogen stores would become low after more than 2 hours. As muscle glycogen concentrations become low, glycogenolysis and glycolysis lessen, the concentrations of the TCA cycle intermediates decrease,[115] reliance on lipid catabolism increases,[47] the rate of mitochondrial respiration decreases, blood glucose concentrations decrease, and an individual's perceived effort increases (Figure 10.16). Low muscle glycogen concentrations are therefore associated with decreases in exercise performance and a metabolic shift away from carbohydrate catabolism. As explained in Chapter 22, it is during these metabolic conditions that carbohydrate supplementation during exercise is beneficial.

Amino acid and ketone body catabolism during submaximal exercise. The depletion of muscle and liver glycogen during prolonged exercise requires that additional substrates be used to fuel muscle contraction. The main additional source of carbohydrate is blood glucose, and like muscle the liver has a finite store of glycogen. As liver glycogen stores become low, the liver is forced to produce glucose from sources other than glycogen. Consequently, liver gluconeogenesis increases, with the molecules lactate and amino acids as the main substrates. Similarly, in skeletal muscle the decreasing TCA cycle intermediates must be replaced if mitochondrial respiration is to be maintained at a relatively high rate. The main additional substrates for supplementing muscle TCA cycle intermediates are muscle and blood amino acids.

An increased *free amino acid pool* during exercise can result from increased muscle or liver protein degradation, decreased protein synthesis, or both[37,88,140,141] (Figure 10.17). These amino acids can be oxidized for catabolism or conversion to other molecules, or can be converted to glucose by liver gluconeogenesis. The indirect evidence for an increase in **amino acid oxidation** during long-term steady state exercise is the increase in blood and muscle *ammonia* (NH$_3$).[88] Ammonia is formed from the deamination of amino acids that are oxidized in the catabolic pathways or from the conversion of AMP to IMP (inosine monophosphate). Because there is minimal production of AMP during steady state exercise, as well as minimal activity of the enzyme AMP deaminase (activated by decreased pH) that catalyzes this reaction, ammonia

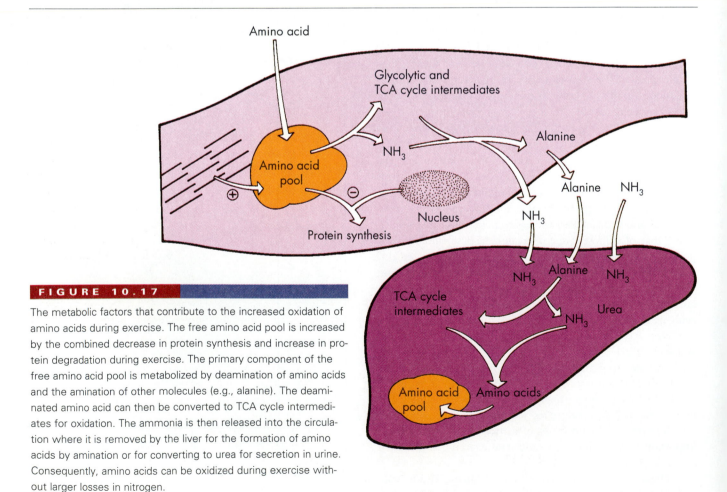

The metabolic factors that contribute to the increased oxidation of amino acids during exercise. The free amino acid pool is increased by the combined decrease in protein synthesis and increase in protein degradation during exercise. The primary component of the free amino acid pool is metabolized by deamination of amino acids and the amination of other molecules (e.g., alanine). The deaminated amino acid can then be converted to TCA cycle intermediates for oxidation. The ammonia is then released into the circulation where it is removed by the liver for the formation of amino acids by amination or for converting to urea for secretion in urine. Consequently, amino acids can be oxidized during exercise without larger losses in nitrogen.

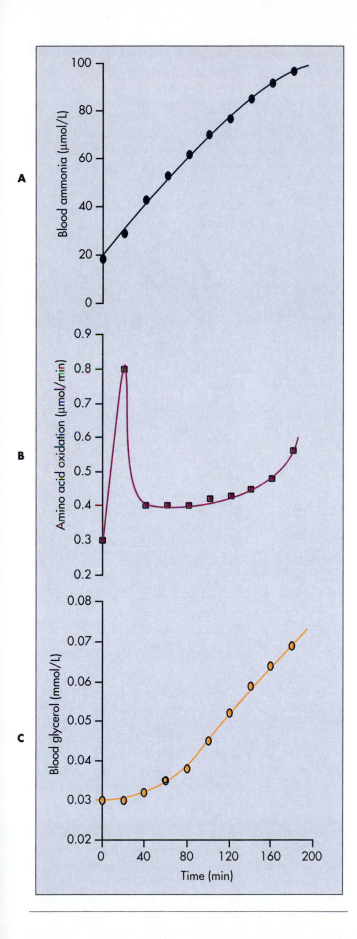

FIGURE 10.18

The change in **A,** blood ammonia, **B,** amino acid oxidation, and **C,** blood glycerol during prolonged exercise.

is produced predominantly from amino acid oxidation during steady state exercise.[88,141]

Other evidence used to indicate increased amino acid oxidation during prolonged exercise is increased *urinary nitrogen excretion* during the recovery after exercise, the urinary excretion of specific amino acid derivatives that can be produced only from muscle proteins (e.g., 3-methyl histidine),[37] and the formation of carbon dioxide from radioactive or natural isotope–labeled amino acids fed to subjects before or during exercise.[140]

The changes in blood ammonia and muscle amino acid concentrations and amino acid oxidation during prolonged exercise are presented in Figure 10.18. The main amino acids oxidized during exercise are the branched–chain amino acids (valine, isoleucine, leucine).[88] Research has been focused on the oxidation of the essential amino acid leucine.[37] As indicated in Chapter 6, amino acids can be converted to pyruvate, phosphoenol pyruvate, and several TCA cycle intermediates, where further oxidation can occur. Dohm[37] has calculated from his research with rats that leucine oxidation can account for up to 25% of the energy used during prolonged exercise; however, evidence in human subjects indicates that leucine oxidation may not represent total body amino acid catabolism.[139,140] Nevertheless, findings clearly show that amino acid catabolism increases during long-term exercise and may contribute as much as 10% of the energy expenditure. The catabolized amino acids come from muscle proteins, intramuscular amino acid stores, and the amination of molecules within the liver or muscle to form nonessential amino acids that are used by other tissues (e.g., the alanine cycle). Therefore amino acid catabolism during exercise is important for three reasons: (1) to provide free energy for muscle contraction during exercise, (2) to increase concentrations of TCA cycle intermediates, and therefore support carbohydrate and lipid catabolism, and (3) to serve as gluconeogenic precursors for the liver.

Prolonged exercise during low muscle and liver carbohydrate conditions also increases the production of **ketone bodies** in the liver. The ketone bodies are then released and

amino acid oxidation

the catabolism of amino acids involving the removal of the amine group and subsequent oxidation of the remaining carbon chain in the TCA cycle

ketone bodies

the molecules produced by the liver from acetyl-CoA derived from β-oxidation when TCA cycle activity is compromised from a lack of carbohydrate are used by more active tissues (skeletal muscle, heart, kidney) as a form of carbohydrate. The main ketone body from the liver, β-*hydroxybutarate* (βHB) is released from the liver during exercise (or starvation) and circulated to the active skeletal muscle where it is taken up, converted to two acetyl–CoA molecules, and used in mitochondrial respiration. Interestingly, in severe cases of ketosis, such as diabetes, the increased blood concentration of βHB can induce acidosis. However, it is unclear whether the increased acid production by βHB during prolonged exercise contributes to the increased perception of fatigue.

Creatine phosphate. As illustrated in Figure 10.15 some creatine phosphate is used at the start of exercise and during the initial period of adjustment to increases in intensity. However, recent research indicates that creatine phosphate may also be important for the exchange of phosphate molecules throughout the cytosol during steady state exercise, as discussed in the creatine phosphate shuttle concept of Chapter 4. The evidence for this interpretation is that creatine kinase enzymes are bound to the mitochondrial membrane and that a slight linear increase in Pi/CrP occurs during increasing exercise intensity (see Figure 10.6, *C*), when the absolute intensity is still relatively low and before the abrupt increase in Pi/CrP.[24,27] This suggests that creatine phosphate is used even during steady state metabolic conditions.

Intense Exercise

Intense exercise can be defined as *any intensity that exceeds an individual's capability to maintain a steady state condition.* Consequently, ATP regeneration must be met by creatine phosphate hydrolysis and by glycolysis terminating in the production of lactate and the eventual development of acidosis. The extent and rate of change in creatine phosphate stores, glycolytic rate, and development of *metabolic acidosis* during exercise have been heavily researched topics. Intense exercise can be performed in many ways, such as the intense *powerful* exercises of sprint running, cycling, swimming, skating, and skiing and the more *strength*-dependent exercise of *weight lifting.*

Intense powerful exercises

Mitochondrial respiration. The easiest way to assess increases in mitochondrial respiration is to measure increases in oxygen consumption. Generally exercise physiologists do this by measuring total body changes in VO_2 during exercise using indirect gas analysis calorimetry as outlined in Chapter 7.

During intense exercise the increase in mitochondrial respiration occurs quickly. For example, during 30 seconds of maximal cycling, the contribution of ATP from mitochondrial respiration to muscle contraction is estimated to be between 25% and 40%.[92,94,95] Figure 10.19 presents the different curves obtained from the breath-by-breath measurement of VO_2 when changing from unloaded cycling to different absolute exercise intensities for 5 minutes. The larger the intensity, the more rapid the increase in VO_2. However,

FIGURE 10.19

The increase in VO_2 determined by breath-by-breath indirect gas analysis calorimetry during an increment from rest to a steady state intensity and during large increments from rest to nonsteady state intensities. The rate of change in the VO_2 response to the nonsteady state conditions were larger than that for steady state. However, no difference existed between the rates of VO_2 increase during the three nonsteady state intensities. Obviously, the oxygen deficit is larger for increments in intensity to nonsteady state conditions.

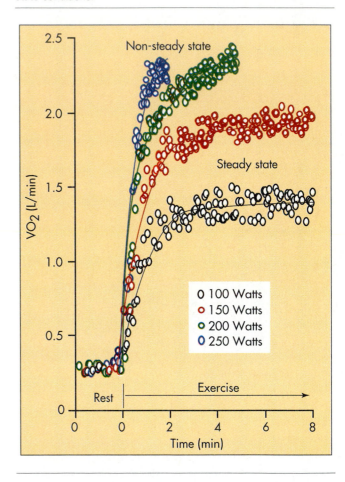

since these curves reveal a gradual increase in VO_2 over time, other energy sources must be supplying the ATP needed to supplement the delayed increase in ATP from mitochondrial respiration, as explained by the oxygen deficit concept. For a given individual, the greater the exercise intensity, the larger is the oxygen deficit, and therefore the greater the reliance on creatine phosphate and glycolysis for ATP regeneration.

Creatine phosphate. Figure 10.20 illustrates results from muscle biopsy research (see Focus Box 8.1) that measured the decrease in muscle creatine phosphate at different intervals of a 100 meter sprint.[61] The resting muscle creatine phosphate store was 22 mmol/kg wet wt, and decreased during a warm up to 11mmol/kg wet wt. During the sprinting the decrease

FIGURE 10.20

The decrease in muscle creatine phosphate and increase in blood lactate during different segments of the 100m sprint.

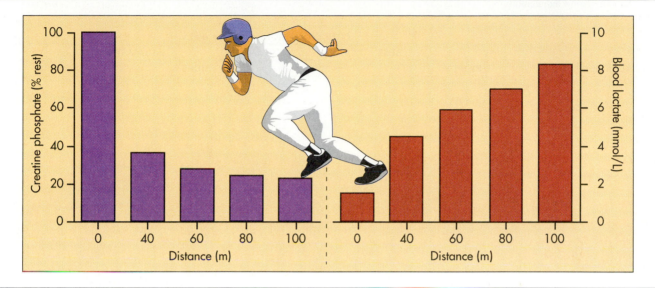

in creatine phosphate was largest during the first 40 meters and then decreased in small decrements in each remaining 20 meter segment. Interestingly, speed increased exponentially to 60 meters and then gradually and consistently decreased to 100 meters. Although muscle biopsy research can be applied to field settings, such as the one described, the time delay in having the subjects stop exercising, positioning them for the biopsy, performing the biopsy, and freezing the muscle sample can be as long as 20 seconds, during which considerable creatine phosphate may be re-formed.

Research has also demonstrated that creatine phosphate content is higher in fast twitch than in slow twitch muscle fibers, resulting in a greater decrease in creatine phosphate from fast twitch muscle during intense exercise.[132] As described in Chapter 8, the metabolic and recruitment pattern differences between fast and slow twitch motor units are important determinants of changes in muscle energy metabolism or total body indirect measures of metabolism (e.g., blood lactate and pH, ventilation).

During intense exercise ^{31}P MRS has also revealed that muscle ATP concentrations remain stable and ADP concentrations increase. The concentrations of ADP in skeletal muscle are too small to detect by ^{31}P MRS but can be calculated by using the creatine kinase equilibrium equation (see Chapter 4). ADP concentrations can also be calculated after intense exercise. Table 10.2 presents measurements of muscle creatine phosphate (CrP), inorganic phosphate (Pi), ATP, ADP, pH, and hydrogen ion (H^+) concentrations at rest and after intense exercise to fatigue determined by biochemical assay from muscle biopsy and by ^{31}P MRS. The concentrations of several important glycolytic intermediates are also listed.

Intense exercise to fatigue almost completely depletes muscle creatine phosphate, causes reciprocal increases in inorganic phosphate, and lowers cellular pH from 7.0 to approximately 6.1.[9,14,96] Interestingly, lower muscle pH values can be detected by ^{31}P MRS than by methods using muscle biopsy samples. Similarly, muscle ADP concentration changes are more extreme when detected by ^{31}P MRS than by biochemical analyses from muscle biopsy specimens. This fact is important due to the role of ADP in stimulating mitochondrial respiration and reveals how the muscle damage and the time lag in obtaining the muscle biopsy and freezing the specimen may alter the biochemical conditions within the muscle fibers. Nevertheless, it is apparent that muscle biopsy enables the measurement of many more different metabolites in skeletal muscle than have been provided by ^{31}P MRS.

Glycogenolysis. The larger the exercise intensity, the greater the decrease in muscle glycogen for a given time. The maximal rate of skeletal muscle glycogenolysis during voluntary exercise, based on the decrease in muscle glycogen, has been measured during maximal isokinetic cycling[92] and approximates 0.65 mmol glucosyl units/kg/sec wet wt. The rate of glycogenolysis during repeated contractions of isolated muscle during weight-resistive exercise and during sprint running is also close to this rate.[25,112] However, researchers have also calculated the maximal rate of glycogenolysis by summing concentrations of intramuscular metabolites and glycolytic intermediates. When blood flow in a leg is blocked by a tourniquet, no oxygen delivery is possible. After a small equilibration period, negligible mitochondrial respiration could occur. In these circumstances, during exercise muscle

TABLE 10.2

Concentrations of phosphate metabolites, pH, adenine nucleotides, and several glycolytic intermediates in skeletal muscle at rest and after intense exercise to exhaustion

| | CONCENTRATION (mmol/kg wet wt) | | | |
| | REST | | EXHAUSTION | |
MEASUREMENT	BIOPSY	^{31}P MRS	BIOPSY	^{31}P MRS
ATP	8.0	8.0	6.0	6.0
ADP	0.05	0.05	0.07	0.5
AMP	0.05	—	0.15	—
IMP	0.05	—	1.0	—
CrP	26	4	2.0	1.0
Cr	10.0	—	28.0	—
Pi	5.0	4.0	28.0	30.0
pH	7.0	7.0	6.4	6.1
[H+] (x 10^{-7})	1.0	1.0	4.0	8.0
Glucose	0.5	—	1.5	—
G6P	0.4	—	2.0	—
F6P	0.08	—	2.0	—
F16P	0.03	—	0.08	—
Lactate	1.0	—	30.0	—

Data modified from 1, 9, 25, 57, 71, 87, 96, 123, 124, 131, and 145.
For specific molecules, concentrations obtained from muscle biopsy biochemical assay and ^{31}P MRS methodologies are presented.

glycogenolysis increases muscle concentrations of lactate and glycolytic intermediates.

$$\text{Glycogenolysis} = [\Delta([G1P] + [G6P] + [F6P])] + [\Delta([La] + [Glyc3P])/2]$$

Based on this method the maximal rate of glycogenolysis has been calculated as 1.7 mmol glucosyl units/kg/sec wet wt,[123] which is considerably higher than the glycogen-based calculation. The difference is due to the known decrease in glycogenolysis over time[94,123] or during successive bouts of intense exercise.[92] For example, muscle glycogenolysis has been shown to decrease from 1.7 to 0.7 mmol glucosyl units/kg/sec wet wt within 32 muscle contractions, with a further decrease to 0.2 mmol glucosyl units/kg/sec wet wt after 64 contractions.[123] Calculations of glycogenolysis based on decreases in muscle glycogen are performed over a relatively large time frame and represent an average value. Consequently, muscle glycogenolysis is highest during the initial period or bout of intense exercise and decreases over time in an exponential decay.

Is intense exercise performance impaired when muscle glycogen levels are low? It appears that muscle glycogen concentrations as low as 50 mmol/kg wet wt do not impair muscle contraction during intense exercise.[14] However, researchers have not answered this question when muscle glycogen concentrations are very low (<20 mmol/kg wet wt). If the time-averaged maximal rate of glycogenolysis (0.6 mmol glucosyl units/kg/sec wet wt) occurred during 1 minute of intense exercise when only 20 mmol/kg wet wt of glycogen was available in the muscle, the muscle would deplete all glycogen in 33 seconds. Obviously, muscle glycogen is important for intense exercise, but generally the short time to fatigue and the progressively decreasing rates of glycogenolysis during intense exercise decrease the need for large preexercise muscle glycogen stores.

Glycolysis. During intense exercise the glycolytic pathway converts glucose 6-phosphate to pyruvate. A large proportion of the pyruvate is then converted to lactate rather than transported into the mitochondria. The reason for increased lactate production during intense exercise is a controversial topic in exercise physiology and biochemistry. This section presents research data that have quantified the increase in glycolytic rate during intense exercise and that have associated lactate production with the development of metabolic acidosis.

Increased glycolytic rate. Since blood glucose and glucose 6-phosphate are substrates of glycolysis and because the end product of glycolysis (pyruvate) can either be converted to lactate or enter into the mitochondria, the rate of glycolysis is difficult to measure. Nevertheless, as with the rate of glycogenolysis, researchers have quantified the glycolytic rate by summing metabolites and glycolytic intermediates[123]:

$$\text{Glycolysis} = \Delta \ ([\text{La}] + [\text{Glycerol 3-phosphate}]/2)$$

Based on this principle researchers have measured increases in muscle lactate and glycolytic intermediates after intense exercise and have calculated a maximal glycolytic rate of 1.3 mmol glucosyl units/kg wet wt.[120] As with glycogenolysis, this rate decreases over time.

What stimulates an increase in glycolysis?

Table 10.2 indicates that AMP concentrations increase in skeletal muscle during intense exercise. AMP is an activator of phosphorylase and phosphofructokinase (PFK), the important allosteric enzymes that increase the rate of glycogenolysis (and therefore glucose 6-phosphate [G6P] production) and of the fructose 6-phosphate (F6P) to fructose 1,6-bisphosphate (F1,6P) reactions, respectively (see Chapters 3 and 4). The remaining reactions of glycolysis are either close to equilibrium or highly exergonic, so that increasing G6P production and activating PFK essentially activate the entire glycolytic pathway.

Alanine production. The release of amino acids from skeletal muscle increases during intense exercise.[137] Based on radioactive labeling research, it has been deduced that the primary source of the alanine is the amination of pyruvate formed from glycolysis and that the capacity for alanine formation was greater in more oxidative muscle fibers than in pure fast twitch fibers.[137]

These findings are important because they show that amino acid involvement in energy metabolism is not confined to prolonged exercise during low-carbohydrate nutrition states. In addition, the removal of pyruvate from muscle as alanine prevents further increases in acidosis by providing a pathway for pyruvate other than lactate formation.

Lactate production and acidosis. Figure 10.12 presents the change in blood pH that occurs during incremental exercise and compares this change to muscle lactate concentrations. Both muscle and blood **acidosis** are characteristics of high-intensity exercise. As explained in Chapter 4, the production of lactic acid from the oxidation of pyruvate occurs at a pH that, even during intense exercise (pH = 6.1 to 6.4), greatly exceeds the pK of lactic acid (pH = 3.7). Consequently, a pro-

ton is immediately released from the carboxylic acid group, resulting in the molecule lactate. The released proton is free to bind to other proteins, be buffered by the intracellular phosphate buffer system, or leave the muscle cell to be buffered by blood bicarbonate, plasma proteins, or hemoglobin (see the section on buffering capacity within chronic adaptation).

Lactate and protons leave the muscle fiber by a similar mechanism. Roth and Brooks[113] have presented the kinetics of a lactate transporter and have shown that it is a saturated transport process. It is believed that protons leave the muscle in combination with the lactate transporter via facilitated transport,[126] which accounts for similar changes in blood lactate and acidosis during intense exercise.

Muscle biopsy research has measured muscle pH as low as 6.4[66]; however, ^{31}P MRS has measured muscle pH as low as 6.1,[9,14,16] which represents an eightfold increase in muscle [H$^+$] compared with rest. Blood pH does not vary across the range evident in muscle. During intense exercise to volitional fatigue, venous blood pH has been reported to decrease to 7.15, which represents almost a doubling of (H$^+$) above the normal resting blood pH of 7.4. In arterial blood, pH changes are not as large and pH may decrease to 7.24.[107] As explained in Chapter 12, the blood and lungs combine to be a powerful buffer of acidosis.

Can muscle acidosis impair muscle energy metabolism? Since enzyme function can be negatively affected by acidosis, research has evaluated whether increased muscle acidosis can have a measurable effect on the glycolytic rate. As previously stated, the main regulatory enzyme of glycolysis is PFK, and in vitro research has indicated that it can be inhibited by low pH.[107] Researchers indirectly assess pH inhibition of PFK by measuring the concentrations of fructose 6-phosphate (F6P) and fructose 1,6-bisphosphate (F1,6P). An increase in the ratio F6P/F1,6P indicates that there is a rate limitation at the PFK reaction, which has been interpreted to be a result of in vivo pH inhibition of PFK.[25,123,124] A decreasing cellular pH can also affect other enzymes, such as the ATPases that are associated with muscle contraction, calcium pumps, and the Na$^+$K$^+$ pump, but the magnitude of pH inhibition of these enzymes in vivo has not been determined.

What is the anaerobic capacity of skeletal muscle? This is an important question, since being able to measure an individual's **anaerobic capacity** would provide a value that could reflect his or her suitability for intense exercise.

---

acidosis (as′i-**do**′sis)
the decrease in pH (increase in free hydrogen ion concentration)

anaerobic capacity
the maximal amount of ATP able to be regenerated from creatine phosphate hydrolysis and glycolysis during intense exercise

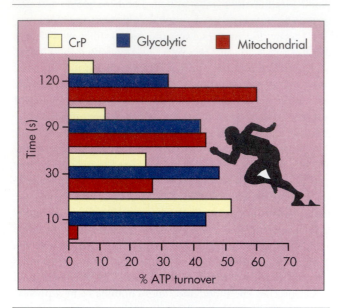

FIGURE 10.21

The different rates of ATP regeneration from mitochondrial respiration, creatine phosphate, and glycolysis during short-term intense exercise. (Adapted from references 9, 25, 61, 71, 92, 95, 122.)

Researchers have attempted to calculate the energy released from anaerobic pathways during intense muscle contraction.[94,95,122,123] Figure 10.21 presents the rates and contribution to ATP production from creatine phosphate, glycolysis, and mitochondrial respiration at different times during intense exercise. As with muscle glycogenolysis, the rates of creatine phosphate hydrolysis, glycolysis, and lactate production exhibit exponential decays. However, the contribution of anaerobic ATP regeneration to total ATP turnover can continue for approximately 2 minutes of intense exercise. Despite this fact, muscle fatigue can reduce muscle tension to values less than 50% of the initial force application in less than 1 minute. The topic of muscle fatigue, and the research that has attempted to elucidate the mechanisms causing muscle fatigue, is presented in Chapter 24.

Medbo et al[94,95] have published several articles on how measuring the total oxygen deficit during a bout of exercise can be used as a measure of the capacity of the anaerobic sources of ATP regeneration. When the ATP provision from accumulated muscle lactate and decreases in creatine phosphate was calculated and compared with the ATP provision calculated from accumulating the oxygen deficit, the correlation obtained was 0.94. Comparable findings have also been reported for the oxygen deficit calculated from regional (blood flow × arterial-venous oxygen content) versus indirect gas analysis calorimetry determinations.[10] These findings demonstrate the importance of the oxygen deficit, since it provides an indirect means to quantify the ability of skeletal muscle to regenerate ATP from sources other than mitochondrial respiration. The ability to generate a large oxygen deficit during intense exercise should correspond to an increased capacity to perform intense exercise; however, this has yet to be proved by research.

Adaptations During the Recovery After Exercise

Muscle recovery occurs after exercise and is characterized by the continued removal of waste products and by-products of metabolism (lactate, H^+, CO_2) and the restoration of endogenous substrates used during exercise (creatine phosphate, glycogen, lipid). Depending on the exercise duration and intensity, and the conditions of the recovery (active versus passive, nutrition), these processes may take from minutes to several days. Since the long-term recovery of energy substrates in muscle is determined mainly by exercise nutrition, a detailed discussion of the exercise and nutritional determinants of postexercise muscle glycogen resynthesis is presented in Chapter 17. The remainder of the material pertinent to understanding muscle recovery after exercise is organized by the intensity of exercise, metabolic pathways, and when appropriate, whether the recovery is passive or active.

Steady State Exercise

As previously explained, during steady state exercise muscle metabolism depends predominantly on a combination of fat and carbohydrate catabolism. Creatine phosphate stores are not taxed, and glycolysis occurs at a rate that does not induce metabolic acidosis. Therefore recovery primarily concerns the effects of the intensity of exercise and the type of recovery on mitochondrial respiration and the restoration of endogenous stores of glycogen and triacylglycerols.

Mitochondrial respiration. After exercise during a passive recovery the body's VO_2 decreases in an exponential manner, with an initial fast component followed by a slow component (Figure 10.22, *A*). Consequently, the body has an elevated VO_2 after exercise. In 1922 A.V. Hill proposed that the elevated VO_2 after exercise was an oxygen debt, which existed to pay back the oxygen deficit occurring during exercise. Hill's interpretation was based on the oxygen cost of replenishing creatine phosphate and for the oxidation of lactate to glycogen, glucose, or TCA cycle intermediates. However, we now know that several factors contribute to the retained elevation in VO_2 after exercise:

(1) Replenishment of creatine phosphate and metabolism of lactate
(2) Muscle glycogen and protein metabolism
(3) Reoxygenation of venous blood
(4) Increased body temperature
(5) Increased heart rate
(6) Increased ventilation rate
(7) Increased circulating concentrations of catecholamine hormones

Each of the aforementioned factors would increase metabolic rate and therefore increase VO_2. Researchers have

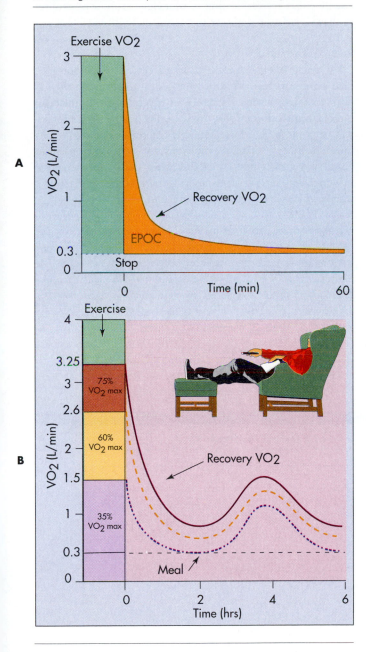

A, The continued elevation of VO_2 (EPOC) during the recovery from exercise. **B,** EPOC is increased when exercise intensity is above 60% VO_2max and performed for longer durations. The ingestion of a meal raises EPOC, but by a magnitude no different to food ingestion when prior exercise had not been performed.

abbreviated the excess postexercise oxygen consumption as **EPOC**.[5,6,46]

The intensity and duration of exercise determine the relative contribution of each factor to the size of EPOC (Figure 10.22, *B*). For example, 20, 40, and 80 minutes of cycling at 70% VO_2max retained a 12-hour EPOC that amounted to 24, 33 and 69 kcal, respectively.[6] Conversely, studies that required lower intensities of exercise (35% to 55% VO_2max) demonstrated an EPOC that lasted less than 1 hour.[15,101,102] In an attempt to determine the influence of exercise intensity and duration on EPOC, Gore and Withers[51] tested nine highly trained (mean VO_2max = 63 ml/kg/min) male subjects by treadmill running at several intensities for several exercise durations. The thermic effect of a meal was also investigated. EPOC lasted for less than 1 hour for exercise intensities less than 50% VO_2max, regardless of duration. No added thermic effects of digestion occurred following a meal for these intensities. However, for intensities and durations in excess of 50% VO_2max and 20 minutes, EPOC remained elevated beyond 2 hours. Exercise sessions of two durations at 70% VO_2max produced a larger EPOC than one session alone. No increased dietary thermogenesis was evident for these higher intensities of exercise and more prolonged exercise durations.

Reproducible values for the maximal EPOC range between 15 and 21 L O_2. Assuming a caloric equivalent of 4.74 kcal/L O_2, this amounts to an added expenditure of between 70 and 100 kcal. Findings of larger values for EPOC have been reported for cycle ergometry and less endurance-trained individuals.[90] However, it is unclear how endurance training status, time of day, and exercise mode combine to influence EPOC.

Glycogen synthesis. The ability of exercised skeletal muscle to resynthesize glycogen after steady state exercise depends on diet, the presence of muscle damage, and whether the recovery is active or passive. The dietary contribution to postexercise muscle glycogen synthesis is discussed in Chapter 17.

Passive recovery. During steady state exercise muscle glycogen can be decreased to low levels if exercise is performed long enough. During the recovery, if adequate carbohydrate is ingested (0.7 g/kg body wt/hr), the maximal rate of synthesis approximates 7 to 10 mmol/kg wet wt/hr, with minimal synthesis occurring without carbohydrate ingestion.[109]

This rate of glycogen resynthesis may be lowered if the exercise bout induced muscle damage, as is common when running downhill for extended periods, especially in those unaccustomed to downhill running.[33,38,109,138] However, the impaired muscle glycogen synthesis accompanying muscle damage is not apparent until after 12 hours of recovery.[33,38] It is believed that glycogen synthesis is lowered during muscle damage because of the infiltration of macrophages and leukocytes into the damaged region. (See Chapter 15.) Because white blood cells rely solely on blood glucose as a substrate for catabolism, the white blood cells compete with the exercised muscle for blood glucose, resulting in decreased glucose availability to muscle. It is because of the simple competition for glucose that raising the carbohydrate content of the diet and further increasing the blood glucose response to the ingested food can increase muscle glycogen synthesis toward normal rates.[109]

Active recovery. During an active recovery a metabolic load is still placed on the muscles and the resynthesis of glycogen is impaired.[17,18] Consequently, muscle glycogen concentrations continue to decrease.

Triacylglycerol synthesis. Previous descriptions of lipid metabolism in skeletal muscle have indicated the limited knowledge we have of the regulation, rates, and timing of triacylglycerol lipolysis during exercise. The same is true for muscle triacylglycerol synthesis after exercise and the source of free fatty acids used to fuel muscle metabolism during the recovery. Based on research that has documented muscle tria-

cylglycerol hydrolysis as the major source of free fatty acids metabolized during exercise, there must be reactions within skeletal muscle that influence the free fatty acid concentrations in muscle and the increase or further decrease in the muscle triacylglycerol stores. The mobilized free fatty acids, whether from muscle stores or the blood, must be used during exercise by either reesterification to triacylglycerols or catabolism in the β-oxidation pathway of the mitochondria.

Intense Exercise

During intense exercise to volitional fatigue, blood glucose concentrations become elevated, muscle blood flow is near maximal, several substrates of glycolysis accumulate in muscle, muscle lactate may increase from 1 to 30 mmol/kg wet wt,* and blood lactate may increase from 1 to 25 mmol/L.[13,36,44,131] These conditions are very different from blood and muscle conditions following steady state exercise, in which blood flow is less and no metabolites or glycolytic intermediates have accumulated in muscle or blood.

Mitochondrial respiration. As a result of the large oxygen deficit generated during intense exercise, the larger concentrations of circulating catecholamine hormones, and the higher VO$_2$, EPOC is more elevated during the initial recovery following intense exercise than steady state exercise. These issues are illustrated in Figure 10.22.

---

*References 57,66,71,76,95,112,123,124.

FIGURE 10.23

The influence of the intensity of exercise on the kinetics of blood lactate during a passive and active recovery.

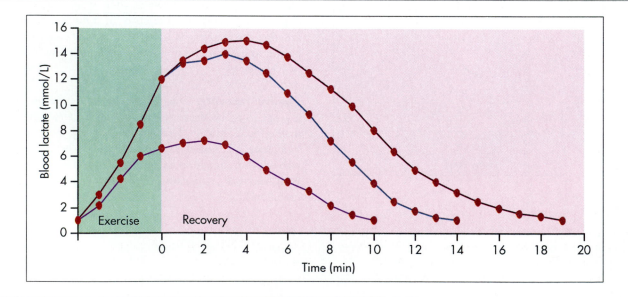

Glycolysis and glycogen synthesis. The perturbed intramuscular environment after intense exercise necessitates the continued flux of intermediates through glycolysis and mitochondrial respiration to normalize muscle concentrations of creatine phosphate and to regenerate electrolyte concentration gradients within the muscle fibers and across the sarcolemma. The balance between continued catabolic metabolism and anabolic metabolism depends on the type of recovery.

Passive recovery. Research on the role of glycogen synthesis during the passive recovery after intense exercise has produced varied results. In those studies with sound methodology, glycogen synthesis has been reported at rates between 12 to 15 mmol/kg wet wt/hr, even without carbohydrate ingestion. This high rate of glycogen synthesis is believed to be evidence for lactate reconversion to pyruvate, with a subsequent reversal of glycolysis producing glucose 6-phosphate, which can then be diverted to glycogen storage.[17,109] Nevertheless, this is a controversial topic, since research has not documented adequate activity of the enzymes phosphoenolpyruvate carboxykinase or pyruvate carboxylase in skeletal muscle.[109] As explained in Chapter 5, these enzymes are necessary to avoid the essentially irreversible pyruvate kinase reaction in the conversion of pyruvate to phosphoenolpyruvate. In addition, lactate is known to be removed from skeletal muscle by a transport mechanism,[113] and this process is known to be effective from the rapid increase in blood lactate during the initial minutes of recovery. However, studies that have used radioactive isotopes have documented that lactate carbons do end as muscle glycogen, as well as carbon dioxide, amino acids, and presumably glycolytic intermediates.[125,126] The high rate of glycogen synthesis after intense exercise is difficult to explain without accounting for endogenous glycogen precursors within skeletal muscle.

Lactate removal and oxidation. When concerned with lactate removal into the circulation, the intensity of exercise and therefore the muscle lactate concentration combine to influence the kinetics of the blood lactate response during a passive recovery.[44] The greater the increase in muscle lactate, the longer the time to peak blood lactate concentrations and the more prolonged the decrease in blood lactate concentrations to normal resting values (Figure 10.23). These data support a saturable lactate transporter on the sarcolemma of skeletal muscle or an inhibition of the transporter with the increasing acidosis of larger muscle lactate concentrations.

Active recovery

Glycogen synthesis. During an active recovery after intense exercise, the accumulated intermediates of glycolysis and muscle lactate are converted to pyruvate and used in mitochondrial respiration. Obviously an active recovery removes the potential glycogen precursor molecules that have accumulated in skeletal muscle, lowering the rate of synthe-

FIGURE 10.24

A, The recovery of forearm muscle acidosis following forearm wrist flexion exercise to fatigue. **B,** The recovery of creatine phosphate is known to be influenced by muscle acidosis, as recovery is more rapid during near normal muscle pH conditions. (Adapted from Arnold DL et al: *J Mag Reson Med* 1(3):307-315, 1984.)

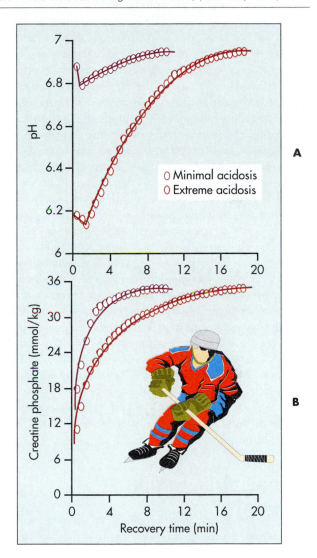

○ Minimal acidosis
○ Extreme acidosis

Recovery time (min)

sis. Glycogen synthesis during the subsequent passive recovery would therefore be as described for steady state exercise.

Lactate removal. The influence of the type of recovery on blood lactate concentrations has been studied.[13,36] Performing exercise between 35% and 50% VO₂max during the recovery from fatiguing exercise increased the removal of lactate from blood. Although it is tempting to interpret these data as evidence for improved recovery when submaximal exercise is performed, such an interpretation is premature. Lactate is not a molecule that impairs muscle function. The biochemical and physiologic detriment of lactate production is the stoichiometric production of hydrogen ions, which, unless buffered, lower pH. The issues of concern are how muscle and blood acidosis are recovered from and what factors positively and negatively affect these processes.

Acidosis and creatine phosphate. The multiple data acquisitions and increased temporal resolution provided by ^{31}P MRS have increased our understanding of the recovery from muscle acidosis and the recovery of creatine phosphate stores. Muscle acidosis and creatine phosphate recovery need to be discussed together because of the involvement of a free proton in the creatine kinase reaction (see Chapter 6). The greater and more prolonged the acidosis, the longer the time required for complete recovery of creatine phosphate.[7]

Figure 10.24, *A,* presents the recovery curve of forearm muscle acidosis, and Figure 10.24, *B,* presents the recovery curves of creatine phosphate during minimal and extreme muscle acidosis. Muscle creatine phosphate recovery reveals a dual exponential curve having a fast and slow component.[7,24,82,133] The fast component of CrP recovery is complete within less than 2 minutes and represents approximately 80% to 90% of complete CrP recovery. The complete recovery of CrP requires a prolonged period that extends beyond the normalization of muscle pH[133] and may be related to the energy requirements of cellular recovery from exercise.

The recovery from muscle acidosis is influenced by the exchange of intracellular protons and other positive and negatively charged molecules and ions between the intracellular and extracellular compartments.[83] The recovery from extreme muscle acidosis requires approximately 5 minutes during a passive recovery; however, little is known of the influence of exercise duration and the severity of muscle acidosis on the kinetics of recovery from acidosis.

Chronic Adaptations

*T*he physiologic health benefits of exercise and the improved performance that occurs following training result in part from chronic adaptations of muscle to repeated exercise stress. Chronic muscle adaptations to exercise are specific to the type of exercise performed. Therefore, as with other subjects of this chapter, the intensity and duration of exercise dictate which metabolic pathways adapt and the extent of their adaptation. However, because training for prolonged exercise often involves intense intervals, and many athletes who compete in high-intensity events also complete endurance training, chronic adaptations are categorized by metabolic pathways and whether the exercise training is predominantly long term or short term. The chronic training adaptations discussed in this chapter assume that correct training is performed. Discussion of the different training strategies used by athletes is found in Chapter 16.

Long-Term Muscular Endurance

Muscular endurance can be defined as the ability of muscle to contract repeatedly over time. Muscular endurance has just as much meaning for short-duration as long-duration exercise. Consequently, the term *endurance exercise* has little meaning unless a time frame is clarified. *Long-term muscle endurance* refers to the ability of skeletal muscle to repeatedly contract for periods in excess of 5 minutes. Based on Figure 10.1, exercise times in excess of 5 minutes rely heavily on ATP regeneration from mitochondrial respiration.

The chronic skeletal muscle adaptations to training for long-term muscular endurance are summarized in Table 10.3. The subdivisions used in the table are also used to divide the subsequent discussion of research findings.

During muscle contraction, oxygen must be supplied to and used by the contracting muscle fibers. When oxygen is released from hemoglobin at the tissue level, it must be transferred from the capillary to within the muscle fiber and then to within mitochondria. This requirement has raised the question of whether endurance training for long-term endurance increases stores of muscle myoglobin. Despite convincing evidence from animal research, endurance training research with human subjects has not shown an increase in myoglobin concentrations.[72,73,98] It is unclear why myoglobin does not increase in human muscle, especially when activities of the enzymes of mitochondrial respiration increase dramatically, and a potential mechanism of the lactate threshold may be intramuscular anaerobiosis.[79,80,130]

Mitochondrial Respiration

Perhaps the most important chronic adaptation increasing long-term muscular endurance is an increase in the number and size of mitochondria. Research that has documented more mitochondria has usually been based on an increased density of mitochondria seen by electron microscopy. Because electron microscopy provides a two-dimensional evaluation, it is unclear whether the mitochondria increase in number or size after endurance training, revealing more sections of what might be a continuous mitochondrial matrix. In either case the adaptation provides a greater mitochondrial surface area exposed to the cytosol, and a greater mitochondrial volume within which are located the enzymes and intermediates of mitochondrial respiration.

Importance of Mitochondrial Membrane Surface Area

An increase in the surface area of mitochondrial membranes increases the capacity for the exchange of metabolites between the cytosol and mitochondria. As already explained, the metabolites of importance to stimulating mitochondrial respiration are pyruvate, NADH, ADP, Pi, and oxygen. This increased capacity increases the sensitivity for mitochondria to be stimulated by a given metabolic stress.[39] Consequently, it is not surprising that the oxygen deficit developed during

TABLE 10.3

Chronic skeletal muscle metabolic adaptations resulting from exercise training for long-term muscular endurance

METABOLIC PATHWAY	ADAPTATION	CONSEQUENCE
Mitochondrial respiration	↑ Number and size of mitochondria	↑ Rate of mitochondrial respiration
		↑ Capacity to oxidize carbohydrate
		↑ Sensitivity to stimulation
		↓ Oxygen deficit
	↑ Activity of TCA cycle enzymes	↑ Capacity to oxidize acetyl-CoA
	↑ Activity of β-oxidation enzymes	↑ Capacity to oxidize lipid
		↑ Sparing of muscle glycogen
Glycogen	↑ Concentration	↑ Time to exhaustion at steady state
Glycolysis	↑ Activity of phosphorylase	↑ Capacity of glycogenolysis
	↑ Activity of phosphofructokinase	↑ Capacity of glycolysis
	↑ Lactate threshold	↑ Maximal steady state intensity
	↑ Lactate removal	↑ Capacity to normalize blood lactate
Creatine phosphate	↑ Threshold	↑ Maximal steady state intensity
Buffering capacity	No change	

Data modified from 11, 32, 42, 48, 49, 50, 54, 56, 58, 59, 60, 62, 63, 68, 73, 76, 98, and 108.

the transition from rest to steady state exercise decreases after endurance training (see Figure 10.14).

Importance of Mitochondrial Volume

The increased volume of mitochondria provides a greater concentration of mitochondrial enzymes, which includes enzymes of the TCA cycle, β-oxidation, the electron transport chain coupled to ADP phosphorylation, and also cellular concentrations of the iron-containing electron transfer molecules of the electron transport chain. Since enzyme concentration is proportional to enzyme activity, it is no surprise that research has shown large increases in mitochondrial enzyme activity after chronic training for long-term muscular endurance.

Figure 10.25 illustrates the increases in the activity of important TCA cycle enzymes after several weeks of training for long-term muscular endurance. Increases in mitochondrial volume also increase the activity of the enzymes of lipolysis, mitochondrial transport (NADH shuttles), and β-oxidation. The functional importance of these adaptations is to increase the ability to catabolize both fat and carbohydrate during exercise. An increased capacity to catabolize carbohydrate in mitochondrial respiration results in an increased maximal rate of ATP regeneration from oxidative phosphorylation and an increased maximal steady state intensity. During submaximal exercise an increased capacity to catabolize lipid would spare muscle and liver glycogen and conserve the body's carbohydrate stores.

Hurley et al[68] studied nine subjects for 12 weeks by having them train six times per week at intensities between 75% to 100% VO_2max and durations of exercise between 5 to 40 minutes. After training, the subjects could perform a given bout of exercise using less muscle glycogen and more muscle triglyceride compared with pretraining. As discussed in the following material, the aforementioned muscle metabolic responses to endurance training can be explained by improvements in one or both of VO_2max and the lactate threshold.

VO_2max

An increased mitochondrial volume would also provide skeletal muscle with the ability to increase maximal oxygen consumption. However, cardiovascular adaptations are also involved in increasing VO_2max after training, and muscle adaptations should not be viewed as the sole determinants of VO_2max (see Chapters 11 and 24).

The extent of improvement in VO_2max depends on the value of VO_2max before training. Figure 10.26 illustrates that for individuals with high VO_2max values, the extent of improvement possible by training for long-term endurance may be less that 5%. The largest training response reported for VO_2max has been 57%, which was accomplished by individ-

muscular endurance
the ability of muscle to contract repeatedly over time

The increase in key enzymes of the mitochondrial oxidation of carbohydrate and lipid after training for long-term muscular endurance.

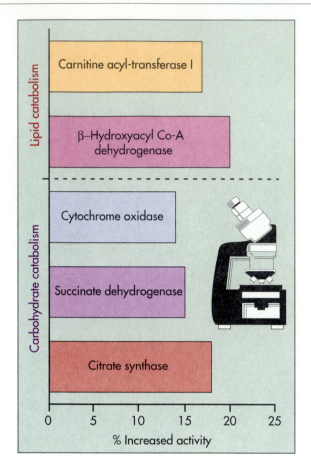

The relationship between the improvement in VO_2max and the initial VO_2max before training. For a given individual, the larger the initial VO_2max, the less the improvement for a given training program.

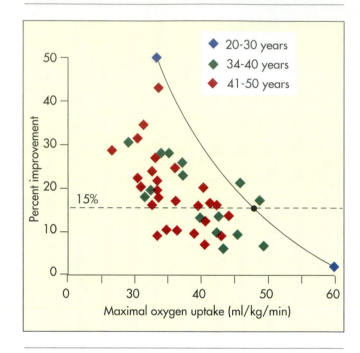

Improvements in metabolic thresholds. The combination of an increased mitochondrial volume and mass results in increases in the blood and muscle lactate thresholds and the muscle creatine phosphate threshold. Coggan et al[27] reported a high negative correlation (-0.63) between muscle mitochondrial enzyme activity (citrate synthase) and the slope of the increase in Pi/CrP, which indicates that an increased mitochondrial capacity must also increase the rate of ATP demand necessary to tax muscle creatine phosphate stores.

Findings similar to those for creatine phosphate metabolism during incremental exercise have been obtained for the lactate thresholds. In fact, long-term endurance training has been shown to increase the lactate threshold without increasing VO_2max, suggesting that the mechanisms for adaptation of these capacities are different.[35] An increased lactate threshold would allow a person to exercise at a higher intensity, while still being at steady state (see Figure 10.11). Consequently, a runner, cyclist, cross country skier, or swimmer would be able to maintain a faster pace longer, resulting in a decreased finishing time and improved performance.

Running economy. As explained in Chapter 6, running economy refers to the oxygen consumption during a given intensity of steady state exercise. Good running economy relates to a relatively low VO_2 for a given running pace. Although no study has demonstrated improvements in run-

uals who had sustained a myocardial infarction, who then trained for and completed a marathon.[81] Although Figure 10.27 indicates that training improvement in VO_2max decreases as an exponential decay of the initial VO_2max value, some evidence to disprove this exists. When training intensity was kept constant relative to VO_2max, subjects demonstrated a linear increase in VO_2max during 10 weeks of training. VO_2max values increased on average from 38 to 55 ml/kg/min, a 45% increase. Obviously there would eventually be a plateau in VO_2max improvement, but it appears that the type and quality of training are also important. Discussion of the influence of different training strategies on metabolic capacities and exercise performance is presented in Chapter 16.

The ability to improve VO_2max should not be confused with submaximal oxygen consumption. After long-term endurance training a person's VO_2 for a given exercise intensity remains unchanged unless there are improvements in economy.

ning economy after training, the duration of training for these studies has been relatively short (<15 weeks). Comparisons among well-trained long distance runners, well-trained middle-distance runners, and untrained individuals indicate large differences between running economy and suggest that long-term training may be necessary to induce decreases in submaximal oxygen consumption (improved economy).[34] The determinants of improved running economy are believed to be biomechanical rather than biochemical or physiologic.[34]

Joyner[75] combined the importance of the lactate threshold, VO₂max, and running economy in the development of a model to predict optimal race performance in the marathon. By optimizing VO₂max (85 ml/kg/min) and lactate threshold (85% VO₂max) and using an estimate of running economy corrected for air resistance and oxygen drift, he calculated an optimal average marathon running pace of 21.46 km/hr. These estimates could lead to a new world record marathon time of 1:57:58 (hr:min:sec) (the current record is 2:06:50) and emphasize the applied importance of muscle adaptations to training. Time will tell if the genetically gifted human body can adapt to training to attain this "optimal" marathon time.

Glycogen

Experimental evidence exists to support a long-term endurance training–associated increase in muscle glycogen concentrations. For example, Piehl et al[105] measured muscle glycogen concentrations in contralateral trained and untrained legs (cycling) of four subjects. Resting muscle glycogen concentrations were higher in the trained than in the untrained leg (119 versus 81 mmol/kg wet wt). Similar findings have been reported for runners and swimmers.[32,50] However, the muscle glycogen concentrations reported for trained subjects in these studies are relatively low (<150 mmol/kg wet wt), since resting muscle glycogen concentrations can exceed 200 mmol/kg wet wt in well-trained long- or short-term endurance- and strength–trained individuals.

Glycogenolysis and Glycolysis

Long-term endurance training increases the activities of the two main regulated enzymes of the glycogenolytic and glycolytic pathways: phosphorylase (PHOS) and phosphofructokinase (PFK) (Figure 10.27).[32,50,72] The increased activity of these enzymes is not as great as for the enzymes of the mitochondria; nevertheless, when combined with the larger store of muscle glycogen they reflect an increased capacity for glycolysis to produce pyruvate for subsequent mitochondrial respiration.

Creatine Phosphate and Buffering Capacity

Long-term endurance exercise predominantly uses skeletal muscle creatine phosphate for the shuttling of phosphate molecules from the mitochondria to the contractile proteins. Data presented on the acute adaptations of creatine phosphate during incremental exercise indicated that crea-

FIGURE 10.27

The increase in enzyme activity from glycogenolysis and glycolysis resulting from training for long-term and short-term muscle endurance. *PHOS*, Phosphorylase; *PFK*, phosphofructokinase; *CS*, citrate synthase.

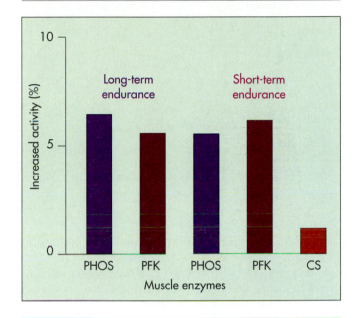

tine phosphate stores do not decrease at exercise intensities corresponding to less than 60% VO₂max. These intensities do not provide a stimulus for improvement and therefore chronic adaptation.

The temporal connection between muscle acidosis and creatine phosphate hydrolysis is presented in Figure 10.25. As discussed in the section on acidosis during short-term intense exercise, muscle buffering capacity of endurance-trained individuals is no greater than that of untrained individuals.

Short-Term Muscular Endurance

For exercise that is terminated because of muscular fatigue (see Chapter 22), the intensity must have been too high to maintain a steady state condition. Endurance is more dependent on the nonmitochondrial sources of ATP regeneration, as well as the ability to retard or tolerate acidosis (Table 10.4). Consequently, the chronic adaptations to intense exercise are very different from those that have been documented for long-term less intense exercise conditions.

Weight Lifting Exercises

Compared with intense dynamic exercise, such as sprint running and cycling, limited research has been completed on the adaptations of skeletal muscle to weight lifting or resis-

TABLE 10.4

Chronic skeletal muscle metabolic adaptations resulting from exercise training for short-term muscular strength and power

METABOLIC PATHWAY	ADAPTATION	CONSEQUENCE
Mitochondrial respiration	↑ Small	No importance to intense exercise
Glycogen	↑ Concentration	↑ Store of substrate to fuel glycolysis
Glycolysis	↑ Phosphorylase ↑ PFK	↑ Rate of glycogenolysis and glycolysis ↑ Rate of glycolysis
ATP	↑ Small	↑ Tolerance of intense exercise
Creatine phosphate	↑ Small	↑ Capacity to rapidly regenerate ATP
Buffering capacity	↑ Capacity	Delays fatigue from acidosis ↑ ATP capacity of glycolysis

Data modified from 72, 76, 86, 99, and 117.

tance-type exercises. During heavy resistance exercise, muscle fatigue can occur in as little as 30 seconds. Despite this short time there is adequate stimulation of glycogenolysis and glycolysis to induce a moderate intramuscular lactate accumulation and lactate acidosis. However, the intramuscular accumulation of lactate and the degree of acidosis are significantly less than when performing intense exercise for periods in excess of 1 to 2 minutes.[25,67,92,124]

Mitochondrial Respiration

During intense exercise, exercise duration is limited by the development of muscle acidosis and the depletion of creatine phosphate, resulting in exercise durations less than 2 to 3 minutes. These time frames are inadequate for the development of large metabolic adaptations in mitochondrial respiration. However, a study of strength-trained individuals has reported small increases in citrate synthase activity,[72] although it is unclear how this change influences the development of muscle fatigue.

Glycogenolysis and Glycolysis

As for long-term endurance training, short-term endurance training stimulates increased resting concentrations of muscle glycogen. In addition, the enzymes phosphorylase and phosphofructokinase increase to levels comparable to those with long-term endurance training (Figure 10.27).

Creatine Phosphate and ATP

Studies evaluating chronic adaptations to weight training have reported significant (but small) increases in resting muscle concentrations of creatine phosphate and ATP.[86] However, similar results have not been found for sprint training.[72,99] A larger store of creatine phosphate would theoretically provide added potential for a high rate of ATP regeneration during the initial seconds of intense exercise. However, because the

increase in creatine phosphate is only minor, it is doubtful that this adaptation is physiologically meaningful.

Buffering Capacity

The term **buffering capacity** refers to the ability to bind free protons and therefore resist increases in the free hydrogen ion concentration ([H^+]). Since the negative logarithm of the free [H^+] represents the pH unit (pH = $-\log[H^+]$), an increased buffering capacity retards decreases in pH. The physiology of acid-base buffering is presented in Chapter 12.

As previously described, during intense exercise, muscle contraction increases lactate production with a stoichiometric increase in H^+ production. Hultman and Sahlin[67] have proposed that 94% of the H^+ release during exercise comes from lactic acid. Given the potential large increases in lactate production in skeletal muscle, a large exercised muscle mass could result in an H^+ release that would decrease the pH of an unbuffered solution to less than 1.5.[103] Based on the data in Table 10.5, this obviously does not happen, and the reason is the buffering capacity of muscle and blood.

The potential buffers in muscle and blood comprise molecules that can receive a proton, and this buffering system is referred to as *physicochemical buffering*. Table 10.5 presents the molecules within muscle, with their pK values, that are potential buffers of protons. The pK value represents the pH at which half the number of the molecules in question would have a proton attached. At this pH the molecule is better able to receive added protons and therefore buffer a solution. Of these molecules, the phosphate (HPO_4^{2-}), bicarbonate (HCO_3^-), carnosine, and protein (amino acid) components

buffering capacity

the capacity to remove free hydrogen ions from solution

TABLE 10.5

Potential physicochemical buffers within skeletal muscle

SUBSTANCE	pK	CELLULAR CONCENTRATION OR RANGE*
Bicarbonate	10.2	5.0
ATP	6.97	5.0-8.0
Carnosine	6.80	4.5
Pi	6.78	4.0-30.0
Glyceraldehyde 3-phosphate	6.75	1.0-5.0
ADP	6.75	0.01
Dihydroxyacetone phosphate	6.45	1.0-3.0
Glycerol 1-phosphate	6.44	0.05-4.0
Fructose 1,6-phosphate	6.31	0.03-0.08
AMP	6.2-6.4	0.05-0.15
Glucose 1-phosphate	6.13	0.01-0.03
Glucose 6-phosphate	6.11	0.03-3.0
Fructose 6-phosphate	6.11	0.08-2.0
Histidine	6.0[†]	35-42
Creatine phosphate	4.50	3.0-26.0

Data modified from references 1, 9, 25, 57, 67, 71, 87, 96, 123, 124, 136, and 145.
*Units of mmol/kg wet wt.
[†]Average of carboxylic acid and amine groups.

FIGURE 10.28

The influence of training for short-term muscular endurance on muscle buffer capacity. (Data from Hultman EH, Sahlin K: Acid-base balance during exercise, *Exerc Sport Sci Rev* 7:41-128, 1980.)

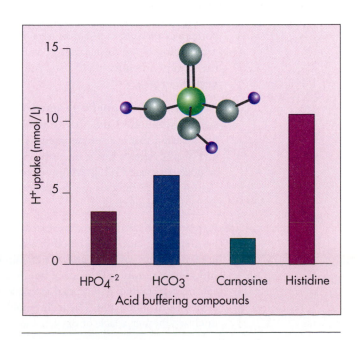

are the major contributors to physicochemical buffering. The most powerful intracellular buffers are proteins, followed by bicarbonate, phosphate, and carnosine molecules.

Research on the influence of training on muscle buffer capacity in human subjects is limited, primarily because valid measurement of muscle buffer capacity is difficult to obtain. Typically, researchers perform muscle biopsy, homogenize the muscle in a buffer solution, and either titrate the sample or determine the pH of the homogenate by automated methods. In either case the influence of homogenizing the muscle on the final [H^+] is unknown.

A summary of research based on the biopsy and titration method is presented in Figure 10.28. It is clear that training for short-term endurance increases the muscle buffer capacity, whereas long-term endurance training results in a muscle buffer capacity no different from that of untrained control subjects.[93,103] In addition, Parkhouse[103] demonstrated that the increased buffer capacity of short-term endurance–trained athletes was associated with increased concentrations of carnosine. Carnosine is a histidine-containing dipeptide that because of its histidine content (see Table 10.5) and relatively unknown function within muscle was hypothesized to be important as a buffer. Consequently, the improved muscle buffer capacity associated with training may be a result of increased amino acid and protein contributions to physicochemical buffering.

Conclusion

From the data presented for chronic muscle adaptations to short-term endurance exercise, the improvement in muscle buffer capacity represents the main adaptation. This is in contrast to the myriad of adaptations associated with the increase in mitochondrial density after training for long-term muscular endurance. Consequently, the muscle fibers' abilities to respond to prolonged exercise are superior to those for short-term exhaustive exercise. This difference raises the question of what stimulates the increased mitochondrial density. If the stimulus were a lack of oxygen, this would be more severe during short-term intense exercise. The questions concerning the cellular stimuli to training adaptations are the focus of current and future research involving applications of molecular biology and biochemistry to muscle function during exercise and training.

SUMMARY

■ Repeated muscle contractions stimulate alterations, or **adaptations,** in metabolism. Immediate **(acute)** and long-term **(chronic)** metabolic adaptations can occur that increase the potential for ATP regeneration within skeletal muscle. The acute and chronic adaptations of skeletal muscle are determined by the intensity of muscle contractions and therefore the intensity of the exercise. The exercise intensity in turn determines the maximal exercise duration and which muscle metabolic pathways are predominantly stressed during exercise.

■ When **incremental exercise** is performed, resulting in a gradual increase in exercise intensity, the **maximal oxygen consumption (VO$_2$max)** attained during exercise can be measured. It is detected as a plateau in VO$_2$ despite further increases in intensity and as an RER that exceeds 1.1. VO$_2$max values range from those of persons with extremely low capacities, such as chronically ill individuals (<20 ml/kg/min) to those of well-trained and elite endurance athletes (>80 ml/kg/min). The factors that combine to influence VO$_2$max are a high proportion of slow twitch motor units, high central and peripheral cardiovascular capacities, and quality and duration of training. Exercise intensities relative to VO$_2$max, the exercise intensity at VO$_2$max, and the %workload at VO$_2$max are common measurements in exercise-related research.

■ Application of **magnetic resonance (MR)** to exercise physiology has improved the understanding of muscle metabolism and activity patterns. Phosphorus **magnetic resonance spectroscopy** (^{31}P MRS) has revealed that as exercise intensity increases, Pi/CrP remains stable, indicating little if any decrease in CrP stores. After a given intensity, Pi/CrP increases abruptly and corresponds with increases in muscle acidosis (increased [H$^+$]). **Magnetic resonance imaging (MRI)** has been used to identify which muscles, or parts of muscles, are used during specific types of muscle contraction, as well as to document fluid shifts within muscles.

■ Researchers have measured increased glycogenolysis and glycolysis during incremental exercise indirectly by measuring changes in blood or muscle lactate. As with muscle Pi/CrP, blood and muscle lactate concentrations increase abruptly at a certain exercise intensity, which has been termed the **lactate threshold.** The intensity at the lactate threshold represents the maximal intensity at which steady state exercise can be maintained. A temporal connection exists between the blood and muscle lactate thresholds and decreases in blood pH. These thresholds were once termed the **anaerobic threshold;** however, it is unclear whether a lack of oxygen causes these events.

- The possible causes of the lactate threshold are (1) the decreased removal of lactate from the circulation, (2) an increased recruitment of fast twitch motor units, (3) an imbalance between the rate of glycolysis and mitochondrial respiration *(mass action),* (4) a decreased *redox potential* (increased NADH relative to NAD^+), and (5) a lack of oxygen.

- Steady state exercise is attained when all the ATP demand from muscle contraction is met by oxidative phosphorylation. When exercise intensity increases by a small magnitude, VO_2 increases until steady state is reached. The energy provided by creatine phosphate and glycolysis that supplements mitochondrial respiration during transitions between increasing exercise intensity is called the **oxygen deficit.** As steady state exercise is continued, there is a slight continual increase in oxygen consumption, termed **oxygen drift.**

- The predominant energy substrate used during steady state exercise is dependent on exercise intensity. The lower the intensity of steady state exercise, the greater is the contribution from lipid. In trained individuals the majority of lipid used during steady state exercise comes from intramuscular stores of triacylglycerols. As exercise intensity increases toward the lactate threshold, carbohydrate predominates as the energy source, and the main source of carbohydrate is muscle glycogen.

- As muscle glycogen concentrations become low there is a decrease in continued glycogenolysis and glycolysis, the concentrations of the TCA cycle intermediates decrease, there is increased reliance on lipid catabolism, the rate of mitochondrial respiration decreases, blood glucose concentrations decrease, **amino acid oxidation** increases, and an individual's perception of effort increases. During prolonged exercise when blood glucose decreases, the liver increases the production of **ketone bodies,** which are released and used by peripheral tissues as a form of carbohydrate.

- The increase in amino acid catabolism during long-term exercise may contribute as much as 10% of the energy expenditure and is important for three reasons: (1) to provide free energy for muscle contraction during exercise, (2) to increase concentrations of TCA cycle intermediates and therefore support carbohydrate and lipid catabolism, and (3) to serve as gluconeogenic precursors for the liver.

- Intense exercise can be defined as any intensity that exceeds an individual's capabilities to maintain a steady state condition. Consequently, ATP regeneration must be met by creatine phosphate hydrolysis and by glycolysis terminating in the production of lactate and the eventual development of acidosis. During intense exercise the increase in mitochondrial respiration occurs quickly. The larger the intensity, the more rapid the increase in VO_2. However, the greater the exercise intensity, the larger the oxygen deficit and therefore the greater the initial reliance on creatine phosphate and glycolysis for ATP regeneration.

- Intense exercise to fatigue almost completely depletes total muscle creatine phosphate, causes reciprocal increases in inorganic phosphate, and lowers cellular pH from 7.0 to approximately 6.1, resulting in severe **acidosis.** Lower muscle pH values can be detected by ^{31}P MRS and from methods using muscle biopsy samples.

- The maximal rate of skeletal muscle glycogenolysis during voluntary exercise has been calculated from the accumulation of glycolytic intermediates and lactate and equals 1.7 mmol glucosyl units/kg/sec wet wt. This rate rapidly decreases during a 2 minute time frame. The maximal rate of glycolysis approximates 1.3 mmol glucosyl units/kg/sec wet wt. As with glycogenolysis, this rate decreases over time. The muscles' capacity to regenerate ATP from creatine phosphate and glycolysis represents the **anaerobic capacity.**

- After exercise during a passive recovery, the body's VO_2 decreases in an exponential manner, with an initial fast component followed by a slow component. Researchers have abbreviated the excess postexercise oxygen consumption as **EPOC.** The intensity and duration of exercise determine the size of EPOC. Reproducible values for the maximal EPOC range between 15 to 21 L O_2. Assuming a caloric equivalent of 4.74 kcal/L O_2, this amounts to an added expenditure of between 70 and 100 kcal.

SUMMARY—Cont'd

■ During steady state exercise, muscle glycogen can be decreased to low levels if exercise is performed long enough. During the recovery, if adequate carbohydrate is ingested (0.7 gm CHO/kg body wt/hr), the maximal rate of synthesis approximates 7 to 10 mmol/kg wet wt. Minimal synthesis occurs if no carbohydrate is ingested. This rate of glycogen resynthesis may be lowered if the exercise bout induced muscle damage, as is common when running downhill for extended periods of time, especially in those unaccustomed to downhill running. During an active recovery a metabolic load is still placed on the muscles and the resynthesis of glycogen is impaired.

■ During intense exercise to volitional fatigue, blood glucose concentrations are elevated, muscle blood flow is near maximal, several substrates of glycolysis have accumulated in muscle, muscle lactate may increase from 1 to 25 mmol/kg wet wt, and blood lactate may increase from 1 to 20 mmol/L. These conditions are very different from blood and muscle conditions following steady state exercise and are associated with glycogen synthesis rates between 12 to 15 mmol/kg wet wt/hr, even without carbohydrate ingestion. The high rate of glycogen synthesis after intense exercise is difficult to explain without accounting for endogenous glycogen precursors of skeletal muscle.

■ Performing exercise between 35% to 50% VO_2max during the recovery from fatiguing exercise increases the removal of lactate from muscle and blood. However, it is unclear how an active recovery decreases muscle acidosis. The increased temporal resolution provided by ^{31}P MRS has increased our understanding of the recovery from muscle acidosis and the recovery of creatine phosphate stores. Muscle creatine phosphate recovery reveals a dual exponential curve, having a fast (<2 minutes) and a slow component (5 to 10 minutes). The recovery from extreme muscle acidosis requires approximately 5 minutes during a passive recovery. The recovery of creatine phosphate is faster during conditions of minimal muscle acidosis; however, the complete recovery of CrP requires time that extends beyond the normalization of muscle pH.

■ The chronic skeletal muscle adaptations to training for long-term **muscular endurance** include increased mitochondrial mass and oxidative capacity, increased glycogenolytic and glycolytic enzyme activity, and increased stores of glycogen. These adaptations decrease the oxygen deficit, increase VO_2max, and increase the creatine phosphate and lactate metabolic thresholds. The chronic skeletal muscle metabolic adaptations resulting from exercise training for short-term muscular endurance include a small increase in muscle oxidative capacity, increased glycogen stores, increased activity of glycolytic enzymes, small increases in muscle ATP and creatine phosphate stores, and an increased muscle **buffer capacity.**

REVIEW QUESTIONS

1. Why does the exercise intensity determine which pathway predominates in ATP regeneration?

2. Why is the incremental exercise test important in understanding the metabolic responses to exercise?

3. Try to determine why it is necessary for the body to generate a large oxygen deficit to attain its highest rate of oxygen consumption. If this question sounds paradoxical, you are right, but try nevertheless!

4. What factors combine to determine the magnitude of the oxygen deficit during a transition of an increased exercise intensity?

5. How have researchers used the method of ^{31}P MRS to evaluate the oxidative potential of skeletal muscle?

6. List the muscle adaptations resulting from training for long-term and short-term muscular endurance. Why do you think muscle is so limited in its chronic adaptability to intense training?

REVIEW QUESTIONS—Cont'd

7. Develop an argument, based on experimental evidence, for an oxygen limitation to muscle causing the lactate threshold. Then develop an opposing argument that is based on experimental evidence. What is your opinion?

8. Explain why muscle pH affects the recovery of creatine phosphate.

9. Explain the factors that contribute to the excess postexercise oxygen consumption (EPOC).

10. What exercise conditions increase and prolong EPOC? Does EPOC represent a significant amount of added caloric expenditure?

11. What muscle adaptations may explain why muscle buffer capacity increases after training for short-term muscular endurance?

12. Explain how the relative contributions of energy substrates used to fuel muscle contraction are forced to change during prolonged exercise lasting more than 2 hours.

APPLICATIONS

1. Individuals with impaired cardiovascular or respiratory function cannot perform incremental exercise that results in a large oxygen deficit. Is this fact likely to prevent the attainment of a true VO_2max? If so, what should this VO_2 measure be called?

2. Individuals with McArdle's disease (see Chapter 4) cannot degrade glycogen and increase glycolytic activity in skeletal muscle. How might their ^{31}P MRS spectrum be abnormal after exercise to volitional fatigue?

3. Some clinical physiologists believe that measuring VO_2max is not as suitable for equating exercise intensities and metabolic responses to exercise between individuals as is the percent of the lactate threshold. Would there be a difference, and if so, which do you think would be the better measure?

4. Many individuals with atherosclerotic artery disease develop stenoses in peripheral arteries such as the femoral artery. This event decreases blood flow to the lower limbs and compromises oxygen delivery to the extent that even mild exercise (e.g., walking) is accompanied by severe pain. How would this condition, termed *claudication,* affect the metabolic capacities of the skeletal muscle involved in walking or running?

5. For the exercise condition of progressing from seated rest to immediately cycling at 50 watts, how and why would the oxygen deficit be different from normal for individuals that (1) are endurance trained, (2) suffer from chronic obstructive pulmonary disease, (3) suffer from heart failure, (4) have claudication of the lower limbs?

6. Individuals with diabetes can develop ketosis caused by the overproduction of ketone bodies by the liver, which in turn lowers blood pH. How would this condition influence exercise performance?

REFERENCES

1. Achten E, Van Cauteren M, Willem R et al: ^{31}P-NMR spectroscopy and the metabolic properties of different muscle fibers, *J Appl Physiol* 68(2):644-649, 1990.

2. Adams GR, Foley JM, Meyer RA: Muscle buffer capacity estimated from pH changes during rest-to-work transitions, *J Appl Physiol* 69(3):968-972, 1990.

3. American Hospital Association: NMR—issues for 1985 and beyond, *Hosp Tech Series* 4(3-4):1-235, 1985.

4. Armon Y, Cooper DM, Flores R et al: Oxygen uptake dynamics during high-intensity exercise in children and adults, *J Appl Physiol* 70(2):841-848, 1991.

5. Bahr R, Sejerste OM: Effect of feeding and fasting on excess postexercise oxygen consumption, *J Appl Physiol* 71(6):2088-2093, 1991.

6. Bahr R, Ingnes I, Vaage O et al: Effect of duration of exercise on excess postexercise O_2 consumption, *J Appl Physiol* 62(2):485-490, 1987.

7. Baker AJ, Kostov KG, Miller RG, Weiner MW: Slow force recovery after long-duration exercise: metabolic and activation factors in muscle fatigue, *J Appl Physiol* 74(5):2294-2300, 1993.

8. Balaban RS: Regulation of oxidative phosphorylation in the mammalian cell, *Am J Physiol* 258(27):C377-C389, 1990.

9. Bangsbo J, Johansen L, Quistorff B, Saltin B: NMR and analytic biochemical evaluation of CrP and nucleotides in the human calf during muscle contraction, *J Appl Physiol* 74(4):2034-2039, 1993.

10. Bangsbo J, Gollnick PD, Graham TE et al: Anaerobic energy production and O_2 deficit-debt relationship during exhaustive exercise in humans, *J Physiol* 422:539-559, 1990.

11. Bassett DR, Merrill PW, Nagel FJ et al: Rate of decline in blood lactate after cycling exercise in endurance-trained and un-trained subjects, *J Appl Physiol* 70(4):1816-1820, 1991.

12. Beaver WL, Wasserman K, Whipp BJ: Improved detection of lactate threshold during exercise using a log-log transformation, *J Appl Physiol* 59(6):1936-2940, 1985.

13. Belcastro AN, Bonen A: Lactic acid removal rates during controlled and uncontrolled recovery exercise, *J Appl Physiol* 39(6):932-936, 1975.

14. Bertocci LA, Fleckenstein JL, Antonio J: Human muscle fatigue after glycogen depletion: a ^{31}P magnetic resonance study, *J Appl Physiol* 73(1):75-81, 1992.

15. Bielinski R, Schutz Y, Jequier J: Energy metabolism during the postexercise recovery in man, *Am J Clin Nutr* 42:69-82, 1985.

16. Binzoni T, Ferretti G, Schenker K, Cerretelli P: Phosphocreatine hydrolysis by ^{31}P-NMR at the onset of constant-load exercise in humans, *J Appl Physiol* 73(4):1644-1649, 1992.

17. Bonen A, McDermott JC, Hutber CA: Carbohydrate metabolism in skeletal muscle: an update of current concepts, *Int J Sports Med* 10:385-401, 1989.

18. Bonen A, Ness GW, Belcastro AN, Kirby RL: Mild exercise impedes glycogen repletion in muscle, *J Appl Physiol* 58(5):1622-1629, 1985.

19. Brooks GA: Lactate production under fully aerobic condition: the lactate shuttle during rest and exercise, *Fed Proc* 45:2924-2929, 1986.

20. Bruhn H, Frahm J, Gyngell ML et al: Localized proton NMR spectroscopy using stimulated echoes: applications to human skeletal muscle in vivo, *Mag Res Med* 17:82-94, 1991.

21. Campbell ME, Hughson RL, Green HJ: Continuous increase in blood lactate concentration during different ramp exercise protocols, *J Appl Physiol* 66(3):1104-1107, 1989.

22. Carlson LA, Ekelund L, Froberg SO: Concentration of triglycerides, phospholipids and glycogen in skeletal muscle and of free fatty acids and β-hydroxybutyric acid in blood in man in response to exercise, *Eur J Clin Invest* 1:248-254, 1971.

23. Carraro F, Klein S, Rosenblatt JI, Wolfe RR: Effect of dichloracetate on lactate concentration in exercising humans, *J Appl Physiol* 66(20):591-597, 1990.

24. Chance B, Sapega A, Sokolow D et al: Fatigue in retrospect and prospect: ^{31}P NMR studies of exercise performance. In Knuttgen HG, Vogel JA, Poortmans J: *Biochemistry of exercise: international series on sport sciences,* vol 13, Champaign, Ill, 1982, Human Kinetic.

25. Cheetham ME, Boobis LH, Brooks S, Williams C: Human muscle metabolism during sprint running, *J Appl Physiol* 61(1):54-60, 1986.

26. Chwalbinska-Moneta J, Robergs RA, Costill DL, Fink W: Threshold for muscle lactate accumulation during progressive exercise, *J Appl Physiol* 66(60):2710-2716, 1989.

27. Coggan AR, Abduljalil AM, Swanson SC et al: Muscle metabolism during exercise in young and older untrained and endurance-trained men, *J Appl Physiol* 75(5):2125-2133, 1993.

28. Connett RJ, Gayeski TEJ, Honig CR: Lactate accumulation in fully aerobic, working, dog gracilis muscle, *Am J Physiol* 246(15):H120-H128, 1984.

29. Connett RJ, Gayeski TEJ, Honig CR: Energy sources in fully aerobic rest work conditions: a new role for glycolysis, *Am J Physiol* 248(17):H922-H929, 1985.

30. Costill DL: Metabolic responses during distance running, *J Appl Physiol* 28(3):251-255, 1970.

31. Costill DL, Fink WJ, Getchell H et al: Lipid metabolism in skeletal muscle of endurance-trained males and females, *J Appl Physiol* 47(4):787-791, 1979.

REFERENCES—Cont'd

32. Costill DL, Fink WJ, Hargreaves M et al: Metabolic characteristics of skeletal muscle detraining from competitive swimming, *Med Sci Sports Exerc* 17(3):339-343, 1985.

33. Costill DL, Pascoe DD, Fink WJ et al: Impaired muscle glycogen resynthesis after eccentric exercise, *J Appl Physiol* 69(1):46-50, 1990.

34. Daniels JT: A physiologist's view of running economy, *Med Sci Sports Exerc* 17(3):332-338, 1985.

35. Davis JA, Vodak P, Wilmore JH et al: Anaerobic threshold and maximal aerobic power for three modes of exercise, *J Appl Physiol* 41(4):544-550, 1976.

36. Dodd S, Powers SK, Callender T, Brooks E: Blood lactate disappearance at various intensities of recovery exercise, *J Appl Physiol* 57(5):1462-1465, 1984.

37. Dohm LG, Kasperek GJ, Tapscott EB, Barakat HA: Protein metabolism during endurance exercise, *Fed Proc* 44:348-352, 1985.

38. Doyle JA, Sherman WM: Eccentric exercise and glycogen synthesis, *Med Sci Sports Exerc* 24(4):S98, 1991(abstract 587).

39. Dudley GA, Tullson PC, Terjung RL: Influence of mitochondrial content on the sensitivity of respiratory control, *J Biol Chem* 262(19):9109-9114, 1987.

40. Fisher MJ, Meyer RA, Adams GR et al: Direct relationship between proton T2 and exercise intensity in skeletal muscle MR images, *Invest Radiol* 25:480-485, 1990.

41. Fleckenstein JL, Watumull D, McIntire DD et al: Muscle proton T2 relaxation times and work during repetitive voluntary exercise, *J Appl Physiol* 74(6):2855-2859, 1993.

42. Flynn MG, Costill DL, Kirwan JP et al: Muscle fiber composition and respiratory capacity in triathletes, *Int J Sports Med* 8(6):383-386, 1987.

43. Forster J, Morris AS, Shearer JD et al: Glucose uptake and flux through phosphofructokinase in wounded rat skeletal muscle, *Am J Physiol* 256(19):E788-E797, 1989.

44. Freund H, Oyono-Enguelle S, Heitz A et al: Work rate-dependent lactate kinetics after exercise in humans, *J Appl Physiol* 61(3):932-939, 1986.

45. Fullerton GD, Potter JL, Dornbluth NC: NMR relaxation of protons in tissues and other macromolecular water solutions, *Mag Res Imag* 1:209-228, 1982.

46. Gaesser G, Brooks G: Metabolic bases of post-exercise oxygen consumption: a review, *Med Sci Sports Exerc* 16:29-43, 1984.

47. Gollnick PD: Metabolism of substrates: energy substrate metabolism during exercise and as modified by training, *Fed Proc* 44:353-357, 1985.

48. Gollnick PD, Piehl K, Saltin B: Selective glycogen depletion pattern in human muscle fibers after exercise of varying intensity and at varying pedal rates, *J Physiol (Lond)* 241:45-57, 1974

49. Gollnick PD, Armstrong RB, Saubert IV CW et al: Enzyme activity and fiber composition in skeletal muscle of untrained and trained men, *J Appl Physiol* 33(3):312-319, 1972.

50. Gollnick PD, Armstrong RB, Saltin B et al: Effect of training on enzyme activity and fiber composition of human skeletal muscle, *J Appl Physiol* 34(1):107-111, 1973.

51. Gore CJ, Withers RT: Effects of exercise intensity and duration on postexercise metabolism, *J Appl Physiol* 68(6):2362-2368, 1990.

52. Green HJ, Hughson RL, Orr GW, Ranney DA: Anaerobic threshold, blood lactate, and muscle metabolites in progressive exercise, *J Appl Physiol* 54(4):1032-1038, 1983.

53. Hagberg HA, Mullin JP, Nagle FJ: Oxygen consumption during constant-load exercise, *J Appl Physiol* 45(3):381-384, 1978.

54. Hagberg JM, Hickson RC, Ehsani AA, Holloszy JO: Faster adjustment to and recovery from submaximal exercise in the trained state, *J Appl Physiol* 48:218-224, 1980.

55. Haouzi P, Fukuba Y, Casaburi R et al: O2 uptake kinetics above and below the lactic acidosis threshold during sinusoidal exercise, *J Appl Physiol* 75(4):1683-1690, 1993.

56. Harms EH, Hickson RC: Skeletal muscle mitochondria and myoglobin, endurance, and intensity of training, *J Appl Physiol* 54(3):798-802, 1983.

57. Harris RC, Hultman E, Sahlin K: Glycolytic intermediates in human skeletal muscle after isometric contraction, *Pflugers Arch* 389:277-282, 1989.

58. Henriksson J, Reitman JS: Time course of changes in human skeletal muscle succinate dehydrogenase and cytochrome oxidase activities and maximal oxygen uptake with physical activity and inactivity, *Acta Physiol Scand* 99:91-97, 1977.

59. Hickson RC, Bomze HA, Holloszy JO: Linear increase in aerobic power induced by a strenuous program of endurance exercise, *J Appl Physiol* 42(3):372-376, 1977.

60. Hickson RC, Bomze HA, Holloszy J: Faster adjustment of O2 uptake to the energy requirement of exercise in the trained state, *J Appl Physiol* 44(6):877-881, 1978.

61. Hirvonen J, Rehunen S, Rusko H, Harkonen M: Breakdown of high-energy phosphate compounds and lactate accumulation during short supramaximal exercise, *Eur J Appl Physiol* 56:253-259, 1987.

62. Holloszy JO, Coyle EF: Adaptations of skeletal muscle to endurance training and their metabolic consequences, *J Appl Physiol* 56(4):831-838, 1984.

63. Holloszy JO, Oscai LB, Don IJ, Mole PA: Mitochondrial citric acid cycle and related enzymes: adaptive response to exercise, *Biochem Biophys Res Comm* 40(6):1368-1373, 1970.

REFERENCES—Cont'd

64. Hughson RL, Cochrane JE, Butler GC: Faster O_2 uptake kinetics at the onset of supine exercise with and without lower body negative pressure, *J Appl Physiol* 75(5):1962-1967, 1993.

65. Hughson RL, Weisiger KD, Swanson GD: Blood lactate concentration increases as a continuous function in progressive exercise, *J Appl Physiol* 62(5):1975-1981, 1987.

66. Hultman EH: Carbohydrate metabolism during hard exercise and in the recovery period after exercise, *Acta Physiol Scand* 128(suppl 556):75-82, 1986.

67. Hultman EH, Sahlin K: Acid-base balance during exercise, *Exerc Sport Sci Rev* 7:41-128, 1980.

68. Hurley BF, Nemeth PM, Martin III WH et al: Muscle triglyceride utilization during exercise: effect of training, *J Appl Physiol* 60(2):562-567, 1986.

69. Iversen PO, Standa M, Nicolaysen G: Marked regional heterogeneity in blood flow within a single skeletal muscle at rest and during exercise hyperemia in the rabbit, *Acta physiol Scand* 136:17-28, 1989.

70. Ivy JL, Withers RT, Van Handel PJ et al: Muscle respiratory capacity and fiber type as determinants of the lactate threshold, *J Appl Physiol* 48(3):523-527, 1980.

71. Jacobs I: Lactate in human skeletal muscle after 10 and 30 seconds of supramaximal exercise, *J Appl Physiol* 55(20):365-367, 1983.

72. Jacobs I, Esbjornsson M, Sylven C et al: Sprint training effects on muscle myoglobin, enzymes, fiber types, and blood lactate, *Med Sci Sports Exerc* 19(4):368-374, 1987.

73. Jansson E, Sylven C, Sjodin B: Myoglobin concentration and training in humans. In Knuttgen HG, Vogel JA, Poortmans J: *Biochemistry of exercise: international series on sport sciences,* vol 13, Champaign, Ill, 1982, Human Kinetic.

74. Jenesen JAL, van Dobbenburgh JO, van Echteld CJA et al: Experimental design of ^{31}P MRS assessment of human forearm muscle function: restrictions imposed by functional anatomy, *Mag Res Med* 30:634-640, 1993.

75. Joyner MJ: Modeling: optimal marathon performance on the basis of physiological factors, *J Appl Physiol* 70(2):683-687, 1991.

76. Karlsson J, Nordesjo L, Jorfeldt L, Saltin B: Muscle lactate, ATP, and CP levels after physical training in man, *J Appl Physiol* 33(2):199-203, 1972.

77. Katz A, Broberg S, Sahlin K, Wahren J: Muscle ammonia and amino acid metabolism during dynamic exercise in man, *Clin Physiol* 6:365-379, 1986.

78. Katz A, Sahlin K: Effects of decreased oxygen availability on NADH and lactate contents in human skeletal muscle during exercise, *Acta Physiol Scand* 131:119-128, 1987.

79. Katz A, Sahlin K: Regulation of lactic acid production during exercise, *J Appl Physiol* 65(2):509-518, 1988.

80. Katz A, Sahlin K: Role of oxygen in regulation of glycolysis and lactate production in human skeletal muscle, *Exerc Sport Sci Rev* 18:1-28, 1990.

81. Kavanagh T, Shephard R, Pandit V: Marathon running after myocardial infarction, *JAMA* 229:1602-1605, 1974.

82. Kemp GJ, Taylor DJ, Thompson CH et al: Quantitative analysis by ^{31}P magnetic resonance spectroscopy of abnormal mitochondrial oxidation in skeletal muscle during recovery from exercise, *NMR Biomed* 6:302-310, 1993.

83. Kowalchuk JM, Heigenhauser GJF, Lindinger MI et al: Role of lungs and inactive muscle in acid-base control after maximal exercise, *J Appl Physiol* 65(5):2090-2096, 1988.

84. Ladu MJ, Kapsas H, Palmer WK: Regulation of lipoprotein lipase in muscle and adipose tissue during exercise, *J Appl Physiol* 71(2):404-409, 1991.

85. LaFontaine TP, Londeree BR, Spath WK: The maximal steady state versus selected running events, *Med Sci Sports Exerc* 13(3):190-192, 1981.

86. MacDougall JD, Ward GR, Sale DG, Sutton JR: Biochemical adaptation of human skeletal muscle to heavy resistance exercise training and immobilization, *J Appl Physiol* 43(4):700-703, 1977.

87. MacDougall JD, Ward GR, Sale DG, Sutton JR: Muscle glycogen repletion after high intensity intermittent exercise, *J Appl Physiol* 42(2):129-132, 1977.

88. MacLean DA, Spriet LL, Hultman E, Graham TE: Plasma and muscle amino acid and ammonia responses during prolonged exercise in humans, *J Appl Physiol* 70(5):2095-2103, 1991.

89. Madden A, Leach MO, Sharp JC et al: A quantitative analysis of the accuracy of in vivo pH measurements with ^{31}P NMR spectroscopy: assessment of pH measurement methodology, *NMR Biomed* 4(1):1-11, 1991.

90. Maelum S, Grandmontagne M, Newsholme EA, Sejersted OM: Magnitude and duration of excess post exercise oxygen consumption in young healthy subjects, *Metabolism* 35(5):425-429, 1986.

91. McCain DC: ^{31}P nuclear spin relaxation. In Burt CT, editor: *Phosphorus NMR in biology,* Boca Raton, Fla, 1987, CRC Press.

92. McCartney N, Spriet LL, Heigenhauser GJF et al: Muscle power and metabolism in maximal intermittent cycling, *J Appl Physiol* 60(4):1164-1169, 1986.

93. McKenzie DC, Parkhouse WS, Rhodes EC et al: Skeletal muscle buffering capacity in elite athletes. In Knuttgen HG, Vogel JA, Poortmans J: *Biochemistry of exercise: international series on sport sciences,* vol 13, Champaign, Ill, 1982, Human Kinetic.

REFERENCES—Cont'd

94. Medbo JI, Tabata I: Anaerobic energy release in working muscle during 30 sec to 3 min of exhausting exercise, *J Appl Physiol* 75(4):1654-1660, 1993.

95. Medbo JI, Mohn A, Tabata I et al: Anaerobic capacity determined by maximal accumulated O_2 deficit, *J Appl Physiol* 64(1):50-60, 1988.

96. Minotti JR, Johnson EC, Hudson TL et al: Forearm metabolic asymmetry detected by ^{31}P-NMR during submaximal exercise, *J Appl Physiol* 67(1):324-329, 1989.

97. Mondon CE, Dolka CB, Tobey T, Reaven GM: Causes of the triglyceride-lowering effect of exercise training in rats, *J Appl Physiol* 57(5):1466-1471, 1984.

98. Nemeth PM, Chi NM, Hintz CS, Lowry OH: Myoglobin content of normal and trained human muscle fibers. In Knuttgen HG, Vogel JA, Poortmans J: *Biochemistry of exercise: international series on sport sciences,* vol 13, Champaign, Ill, 1982, Human Kinetic.

99. Nevill ME, Boobis LH, Brooks S, Williams C: Effect of training on muscle metabolism during treadmill sprinting, *J Appl Physiol* 67(6):2376-2382, 1989.

100. O'Brien MJ, Viguie CA, Mazzeo RS, Brooks GA: Carbohydrate dependence during marathon running, *Med Sci Sports Exerc* 25(9):1009-1017, 1993.

101. Pacy PJ, Barton N, Webster JD, Garrow JS: The energy cost of aerobic exercise in fed and fasted normal subjects, *Am J Clin Nutr* 42:764-768, 1985.

102. Pacy PJ, Webster JD, Isaacs G et al: The effect of aerobic exercise on subsequent 24 hour resting metabolic rate in normal male subjects, *Proc Nutr Soc* 46:4A, 1987(abstract).

103. Parkhouse WS, McKenzie DC, Hochochka PW et al: The relationship between carnosine levels, buffering capacity, fiber type and anaerobic capacity in elite athletes. In Knuttgen HG, Vogel JA, Poortmans J: *Biochemistry of exercise: international series on sport sciences,* vol 13, Champaign, Ill, 1982, Human Kinetic.

104. Pascoe DD, Costill DL, Fink WJ et al: Glycogen resynthesis in skeletal muscle following resistive exercise, *Med Sci Sports Exerc* 25(3):249-354, 1993.

105. Piehl K, Adolfsson S, Nazar K: Glycogen storage and glycogen synthase activity in trained and untrained muscle of man, *Acta Physiol Scand* 90:779-788, 1974.

106. Ren JM, Henriksson J, Katz A, Sahlin K: NADH content in type I and type II human muscle fibers after dynamic exercise, *Biochem J* 25:183-187, 1988.

107. Renaud JM, Allard Y, Mainwood GW: Is the change in intracellular pH during fatigue large enough to be the main cause of fatigue? *Can J Physiol Pharmacol* 64:764-767, 1986.

108. Rennie MJ, Winder WW, Holloszy JO: A sparing effect of increased plasma free fatty acids on muscle and liver glycogen content in the exercising rat, *Biochem J* 156:647-655, 1976.

109. Robergs RA: Nutritional and exercise determinants of post exercise muscle glycogen synthesis, *Int J Sports Nutr* 1(4):307-337, 1991.

110. Robergs RA, Icenogle MV, Hudson TL, Greene ER: Brachial artery blood flow during twist flexion exercise, *Med Sci Sports Exerc,* 24 (5) (abstract 988) 1992.

111. Robergs RA, Pascoe DD, Costill DL et al: Effects of warmup on muscle glycogenolysis during intense exercise, *Med Sci Sports Exerc* 23(1):37-43, 1991.

112. Robergs RA, Pearson DR, Costill DL et al: Muscle glycogenolysis during differing intensities of weight-resistance exercise, *J Appl Physiol* 70(4):1700-1706, 1991.

113. Roth DA, Brooks GA: Facilitated lactate transport across muscle membranes, *Med Sci Sports Exerc* 21(2):S35, 1989(abstract).

114. Sahlin K: NADH in human skeletal muscle during short-term intense exercise, *Pfluegers Arch* 403:1983-1986, 1985.

115. Sahlin K, Katz A, Broberg S: Tricarboxylic acid cycle intermediates in human muscle during prolonged exercise, *Am J Physiol* 259(28):C834-C841, 1990.

116. Sahlin K, Katz A, Henriksson J: Redox state and lactate accumulation in human skeletal muscle during dynamic exercise, *Biochem J* 245:551-556, 1987.

117. Sale DG, Jacobs I, MacDougall JD, Garner S: Comparison of two regimens of concurrent strength and endurance training, *Med Sci Sports Exerc* 22(3):348-356, 1990.

118. Saltin B, Nazar K, Costill DL et al: The nature of the training response: peripheral and central adaptations to one legged cycling, *Acta Physiol Scand* 96:289-305, 1976.

119. Sapega AA, Sokolow DP, Graham TJ, Chance B: Phosphorus nuclear magnetic resonance: a non-invasive technique for the study of muscle bioenergetics during exercise, *Med Sci Sports Exerc* 19(4):410-420, 1987.

120. Schick F, Eismann B, Jung W et al: Comparison of localized proton NMR signals of skeletal muscle and fat tissue in vivo: two lipid compartments in muscle tissue, *Mag Res Med* 29:158-167, 1993.

121. Shearer JD, Amarai JF, Caldwell MD: Glucose metabolism of injured skeletal muscle: contribution of inflammatory cells, *Circ Shock* 25:131-138, 1988.

122. Spriet LL, Sonderland K, Bergstrom M, Hultman E: Anaerobic energy release in skeletal muscle during electrical stimulation, *J Appl Physiol* 62(2):611-615, 1987.

123. Spriet LL, Soderlund K, Bergstrom M, Hultman E: Skeletal muscle glycogenolysis, glycolysis, and pH during electrical stimulation in men, *J Appl Physiol* 62(2):616-621, 1987.

124. Spriet LL, Lindinger ML, McKelvie RS et al: Muscle glycogenolysis and H^+ concentration during maximal intermittent cycling, *J Appl Physiol* 66(1):8-13, 1988.

REFERENCES—Cont'd

125. Stainsby WN, Brooks GA: Control of lactic acid metabolism in contracting muscles and during exercise, *Exerc Sport Sci Rev* 18:29-64, 1990.

126. Stanley WC, Gertz EW, Wisneski JA et al: Systematic lactate kinetics during graded exercise in man, *Am J Physiol* 249(12):E595-E602, 1985.

127. Stromme SB, Ingjer F, Meen HD: Assessment of maximal aerobic power in specifically trained athletes, *J Appl Physiol* 42(6):833-837, 1977.

128. Tanokura M, Yamada K: Changes in intracellular pH and inorganic phosphate concentrations during and after muscle contraction as studied by time-resolved ³¹P-NMR, *FEBS Lett* 171(2):165-168, 1984.

129. Taylor R, Price TB, Rothman DL et al: Validation of ¹³C NMR measurement of human skeletal muscle glycogen by direct biochemical assay of needle biopsy samples, *Mag Res Med* 27:13-20, 1992.

130. Terrados N, Jansson E, Sylven C, Kaijser L: Is hypoxia a stimulus for synthesis of oxidative enzymes and myoglobin? *J Appl Physiol* 68(6):2369-2372, 1990.

131. Tesch PA, Collainder EB, Kaiser P: Muscle metabolism during intense, heavy resistance exercise, *Eur J Appl Physiol* 55:362-366, 1986.

132. Tesch PA, Thorsson A, Fujitsuka N: Creatine phosphate in fiber types of skeletal muscle before and after exhaustive exercise, *J Appl Physiol* 66(40):1756-1759, 1989.

133. Tonokura M, Yamada K: Changes in intracellular pH and inorganic phosphate concentration during and after muscle contraction as studied by time-resolved ³¹P=NMR, *Fed Eur Biochem Soc* 171(2):165-168, 1984.

134. Vollestad NK, Sejersted OM, Biochemical correlates of fatigue: a brief review, *Eur J Appl Physiol* 57:336-347, 1988.

135. Walloe L, Wesche J: Time course and magnitude of blood flow changes in the human quadriceps muscles during and following rhythmic exercise, *J Physiol* 405:257-273, 1988.

136. Wasserman K, Beaver WL, Whipp BJ: Mechanisms and patterns of blood lactate increase during exercise in man, *Med Sci Sports Exerc* 18(30):344-352, 1986.

137. Weicker H, Bert H, Rettenmeier A et al: Alanine formation during maximal short-term exercise. In Knuttgen HG, Vogel JA, Poortmans J: *Biochemistry of exercise: international series on sport sciences,* vol 13, Champaign, Ill, 1982, Human Kinetics.

138. Westerlind KC, Byrnes WC, Mazzeo RS: A comparison of the oxygen drift in downhill vs. level running, *J Appl Physiol* 72(20):796-800, 1992.

139. Whipp BJ, Wasserman K: Oxygen uptake kinetics for various intensities of constant-load work, *J Appl Physiol* 33(3):351-356, 1972.

140. Wolfe RR: Does exercise stimulate protein breakdown in humans?: isotopic approaches to the problem, *Med Sci Sports Exerc* 19(15):S172-S178, 1987.

141. Wolfe RR, Wolfe MH, Nadel ER, Shaw JHF: Isotopic determination of amino-acid-urea interactions in exercise in humans, *J Appl Physiol* 56(1):221-229, 1984.

142. Yeh MP, Garfner RM, Adams TD et al: "Anaerobic threshold": problems of determination and validation, *J Appl Physiol* 55(4):1178-1186, 1983.

143. Yoshida T: Effect of dietary modifications on the anaerobic threshold, *Sports Med* 3(3):4-8, 1986.

144. Zachwieja JJ, Costill DL, Pascoe DD et al: Influence of muscle glycogen depletion on the rate of resynthesis, *Med Sci Sports Exerc* 23(1):44-48, 1990.

145. Zanconato S, Buchthal S, Barstow TJ, Cooper DM: ³¹P-magnetic resonance spectroscopy of leg muscle metabolism during exercise in children and adults, *J Appl Physiol* 74(5):2214-2218, 1993.

RECOMMENDED READINGS

■ Baker AJ, Kostov KG, Miller RG, Weiner MW: Slow force recovery after long-duration exercise: metabolic and activation factors in muscle fatigue, *J Appl Physiol* 74(5):2294-2300, 1993.

■ Balaban RS: Regulation of oxidative phosphorylation in the mammalian cell, *Am J Physiol* 258(27):C377-C389, 1990.

■ Bangsbo J, Gollnick PD, Graham TE et al: Anaerobic energy production and O_2 deficit-debt relationship during exhaustive exercise in humans, *J Physiol Lon* 422:539-559, 1990.

■ Bangsbo J, Johansen L, Quistorff B, Saltin B: NMR and analytic biochemical evaluation of CrP and nucleotides in the human calf during muscle contraction, *J Appl Physiol* 74(4):2034-2039, 1993.

■ Beaver WL, Wasserman K, Whipp BJ: Improved detection of lactate threshold during exercise using a log-log transformation, *J Appl Physiol* 59(6):1936-2940, 1985.

■ Bonen A, McDermott JC, Hutber CA: Carbohydrate metabolism in skeletal muscle: an update of current concepts, *Int J Sports Med* 10:385-401, 1989.

■ Chance B, Sapega A, Sokolow D et al: Fatigue in retrospect and prospect: ^{31}P NMR studies of exercise performance. In Knuttgen HG, Vogel JA, Poortmans J: *Biochemistry of exercise: international series on sport sciences,* vol 13, Champaign, Ill, 1982, Human Kinetics.

■ Gollnick PD, Metabolism of substrates: energy substrate metabolism during exercise and as modified by training, *Fed Proc* 44:353-357 , 1985.

■ Gore CJ, Withers RT: Effects of exercise intensity and duration on postexercise metabolism, *J Appl Physiol* 68(6):2362-2368, 1990.

■ Holloszy JO, Coyle EF: Adaptations of skeletal muscle to endurance training and their metabolic consequences, *J Appl Physiol* 56(4):831-838, 1984.

■ Hughson RL, Weisiger KD, Swanson GD: Blood lactate concentration increases as a continuous function in progressive exercise, *J Appl Physiol* 62(5):1975-1981, 1987.

■ Jenesen JAL, van Dobbenburgh JO, van Echteld CJA et al: Experimental design of ^{31}P MRS assessment of human forearm muscle function: restrictions imposed by functional anatomy, *Mag Res Med* 30:634-640, 1993.

■ Joyner MJ: Modeling: optimal marathon performance on the basis of physiological factors, *J Appl Physiol* 70(2):683-687, 1991.

■ Medbo JI, Tabata I: Anaerobic energy release in working muscle during 30 sec to 3 min of exhausting exercise, *J Appl Physiol* 75(4):1654-1660, 1993.

■ Robergs RA: Nutritional and exercise determinants of post exercise muscle glycogen synthesis, *Int J Sports Nutr* 1(4):307-337, 1991.

■ Sapega AA, Sokolow DP, Graham TJ, Chance B: Phosphorus nuclear magnetic resonance: a non-invasive technique for the study of muscle bioenergetics during exercise, *Med Sci Sports Exerc* 19(4):410-420, 1987.

■ Stromme SB, Ingjer F, Meen HD: Assessment of maximal aerobic power in specifically trained athletes, *J Appl Physiol* 42(6):833-837, 1977.

■ Yeh MP, Garfner RM, Adams TD et al: "Anaerobic threshold": problems of determination and validation, *J Appl Physiol* 55(4):1178-1186, 1983.

CHAPTER 11

Cardiovascular Function and Adaptation to Exercise

OBJECTIVES

After studying this chapter you should be able to:

- Describe the structural and functional differences between the pulmonary and systemic circulations.

- Identify the diverse functions of blood.

- Describe the process of erythropoiesis and how iron is transported in the blood.

- Identify approximate volumes of blood and plasma and their relationships to fitness and body mass.

- Describe the circulation of blood through the heart.

- Describe the changes in ventricular volumes and pressures for the right and left sides of the heart during the cardiac cycle.

- Identify the physical laws that govern fluid flow through vessels.

- Describe the structural and functional differences among the different types of blood vessels.

- Explain the regulation of blood vessels.

- Describe the chronotropic and inotropic regulation of the heart.

- Explain how cardiovascular function changes during different exercise conditions.

- Explain how cardiovascular function changes in response to endurance training.

KEY TERMS

cardiovascular system	stroke volume
blood	ejection fraction
hematocrit	cardiac output
erythrocytes	compliance
transferrin	vasoconstriction
ferritin	vasodilation
polycythemia	hemodynamics
anemia	muscle pump
osmolality	precapillary sphincter
pulmonary circulation	chronotropic
systemic circulation	inotropic
cardiac cycle	hemoconcentration
preload	hemolysis
intercalated discs	hyperemia
afterload	autoregulation

Despite the almost immediate neuromuscular and metabolic responses to muscle contraction, continued contractions for extended periods of time require an increased delivery of oxygen. This oxygen originates in atmospheric air and must be transferred to blood to be circulated to the contracting skeletal muscles. The cardiovascular system provides the means to transport the oxygen, metabolic nutrients, and waste products throughout the body. In addition, cardiovascular function is required for optimal regulation of body temperature and blood pressure during both rest and exercise conditions. The purpose of this chapter is to briefly outline the components of the cardiovascular system, explain the regulation of cardiovascular function during exercise, and detail the acute and chronic exercise adaptations to cardiovascular function.

Components of the Cardiovascular System

The cardiovascular system is composed of blood, the heart, and the vasculature within which blood is pumped throughout the body. The heart is a biologic pump that generates the pressure that drives blood throughout the vasculature, and therefore life depends on its continual effective function. Anatomic and functional aspects of the heart are referred to as *cardiac,* whereas anatomic and functional aspects of the circulation of blood around the body are referred to as *vascular,* hence the term *cardiovascular.* The heart, blood, and blood vessels of the body constitute the **cardiovascular system** (or *circulatory system*), which consists of the *pulmonary circulation* of the lungs and the *systemic circulation* to the remainder of the body. Within the systemic circulation are local circulation beds, such as that of the head and brain (*cranial* circulation), liver (*hepatic* circulation), kidney (*renal* circulation), abdominal viscera and intestinal tract (*splanchnic* circulation), skin (*cutaneous* circulation), and *skeletal muscle* circulation. The combined function of the cardiovascular system and lungs is referred to as *cardiorespiratory* function.

Blood

Blood is the liquid medium that circulates within the vascular system. Blood can be divided into cellular and non-

---

cardiovascular system
the heart and blood vessels of the body

blood
the fluid medium that contains cells that function to transport oxygen and carbon dioxide, cells involved in immunity, certain proteins involved in blood clotting and the transport of nutrients, and electrolytes necessary for optimal cell function

The cellular and liquid components of blood, as they appear after centrifugation. (From Thibodeau GA, Patton KT: *Anatomy and physiology*, ed 3, St. Louis, 1996, Mosby. Art by Rolin Graphics.)

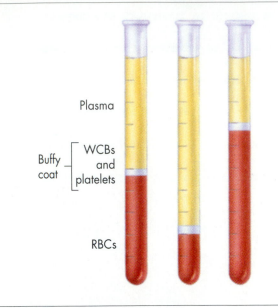

Plasma

Buffy coat { WCBs and platelets

RBCs

TABLE 11.1

Main functions of the cellular and liquid components of blood

COMPONENT	FUNCTIONS
Cellular	Transport of oxygen and carbon dioxide
	Blood clotting
	Acid-base buffering
	Immune functions
	Tissue repair and destruction
Liquid	Blood clotting
	Circulation of cellular components and their contents
	Heat transfer and thermoregulation
	Water exchange and transport
	Circulation of hormones
	Acid-base buffering
	Circulation of metabolites, nutrients, and waste products

cellular components, as illustrated in Figure 11.1. The general functions of the cellular and liquid components of blood are presented in Table 11.1.

Blood serves many functions, and although the transport of blood gases is crucial to life, other functions of blood can be equally important during rest (e.g., immune functions) and certain exercise conditions (e.g., thermoregulation, water exchange).

Cellular Components

The cell content of blood constitutes approximately 45% of the total blood volume, and this measure is termed **hematocrit.** Hematocrit is lower in females than males and varies with hydration status. Total blood volume approximates 5 L for the average individual, but is greater for larger, more endurance-trained and altitude-acclimated individuals. As discussed in later sections, the finite store of blood in the body and the potentially large muscle mass that can be recruited during exercise can severely challenge the functional capacity of the cardiovascular system.

Blood consists of several types of cells, which all emanate from stem cells located in bone marrow (Figure 11.2). The original stem cell can differentiate into precursors of white blood cells *(leukocytes)*, red blood cells **(erythrocytes),** or cell fragments known as *platelets.* During the synthesis of erythrocytes *(erythropoiesis)*, the stem cell is differentiated into nucleated cells that synthesize hemoglobin. These cells are released into the circulation when they have lost their nuclei and are then termed *reticulocytes.* The reticulocyte has remnants of

RNA and continues to synthesize hemoglobin. The differentiation of the stem cell to a reticulocyte requires 2 days, and development of the reticulocyte to a mature erythrocyte may take an additional 2 days.[11,37] The stimulation of erythropoiesis is under the control of the hormone *erythropoietin,* as discussed in Chapter 13.

The shape of the erythrocyte resembles a biconcave disk and in humans is approximately 8 μm in diameter and 2 μm thick at the perimeter.[11] Molecules of hemoglobin are located on the membrane surface of erythrocytes and function by transporting oxygen and carbon dioxide and by buffering protons (see Chapter 12). Since erythrocytes have an average life span of 120 days, *erythropoiesis* is a continual process that occurs in the bone marrow and spleen. The iron from hemoglobin of the destroyed erythrocytes is recycled by the liver, and along with the nutritional intake of iron, is transported in the blood bound to **transferrin** (iron-binding globulin). Iron can be stored in plasma and certain tissues (heart, liver, spleen) as **ferritin,** which is a complex of water-

hematocrit (he-mat'-o-krit)
the ratio of the volume of blood cells and formed elements of blood to total blood volume; usually expressed as a percentage

erythrocyte (e-rith'ro-syt)
red blood cell

transferrin (trans-fer'in)
an iron transporting β-globulin of the blood

ferritin (fer'-itin)
an iron protein complex, found mainly in the liver, small intestine, and spleen, but also present in blood

FIGURE 11.2

A simplified illustration of the heomatopoeitic system showing the formation of erythrocytes, leukocytes, and platelets. All blood cells and cellular components have a common precursor cell. Subsequent differentiation commits to certain blood cell types. The hormone that stimulates the differentiation of the progenator cell to erythrocytes is erythropoietin. (From Thibodeau GA, Patton KT: *Anatomy and physiology,* ed 3, St. Louis, 1996, Mosby. Art by Kathryn A. Born.)

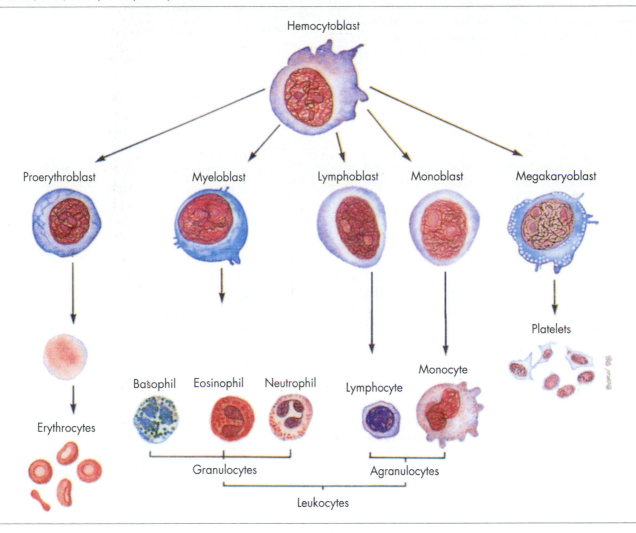

soluble protein and reduced iron (ferrous hydroxide). An increased production of erythrocytes can result in elevated red blood cell counts, and this condition is termed **polycythemia.** Conversely, an inadequate iron intake, excessive bleeding, or exaggerated erythrocyte destruction can result in a lowered red blood cell count, or **anemia.** As discussed in Chapters 17 and 23, despite the body's abilities to store iron, iron intake can be a nutritional concern for many athletes.

Liquid Component

The liquid component of blood is termed *plasma.* Plasma is the medium within which the blood cells, metabolites,

hormones, and nutrients are circulated around the body, body heat and water are distributed, and certain reactions occur. When blood is drawn from the body, the clotting process

polycythemia (pol'i-**si-the'**mi-ah)
　above normal increase in the erythrocyte content of the blood

anemia (a-**ne'**mi-ah)
　abnormally low erythrocyte content, hemoglobin concentration, or hematocrit of the blood

forms fibrinogen and the remaining fluid component of blood is termed *serum*.

Since plasma represents 55% of total blood volume (1.0 − 0.45 [hematocrit] = 0.55), it approximates a volume of 3 L. Plasma volume can be measured by injecting a substance that is known to remain in the vascular compartment. The total blood volume is then calculated from simple dilution equations, and plasma volume is obtained after adjustment for hematocrit. Plasma volume varies in proportion with lean body mass, more so than with either total body mass or even fitness,[107] and for healthy young men (age range 18 to 35) can be estimated from the following equation:

11.1   men:*   PV = 0.042 (LBM) + 0.567

Plasma contains many soluble molecules and electrolytes, which are summarized in Table 11.2. The presence of electrolytes and proteins in plasma generates an osmotic force to attract and retain water within the vasculature. This osmotic force is best reflected by the number of particles in solution, which is termed **osmolality.** As indicated in Table 11.2, sodium has the largest concentration and is the main electrolyte that influences osmolality. Changes in osmolality are detected by several specialized cells in the central nervous system and also in peripheral tissues such as the kidney; these changes are important for the processes involved in the control of hydration and kidney function (see Chapter 13).

The Heart

The heart is a muscular organ that is required to contract without voluntary control. You can estimate for yourself the number of times the heart must beat in a lifetime, assuming an average heart rate of 100 beats per minute (bpm) and an average life span of 75 years! What is all the more amazing about the heart is that it can be regulated to rapidly increase its rate of beating (heart rate) from what could be resting values of less than 50 bpm to maximal values that could reach 200 bpm. In addition, while pumping blood the healthy heart can generate average circulation pressures that increase from 90 to over 140 mm Hg without signs or symptoms of impaired function. The ability to generate pressure is crucial for the function of the heart and the function of the rest of the body, for as explained in later sections, the blood circulates throughout the body down a pressure gradient in which pressures are largest where blood leaves the heart and lowest where blood returns to the heart.

The microanatomy, electrophysiology, and metabolic characteristics of the myocardium are presented in Chapter 7. As described in that chapter, the pumping function of the heart is influenced by the unique qualities of myocardial fibers

TABLE 11.2	
Electrolyte and protein constituents of plasma	
CONSTITUENT*	**CONCENTRATIONS**
ELECTROLYTES (mEq/L)†	
Cations	
Sodium	135-145
Potassium	3.5-5.0
Calcium	2.2-2.5
Magnesium	1.5-2.0
Anions	
Chloride	95-107
Bicarbonate	22-16
Lactate	1.0-1.8
Sulfate	1.0
Phosphate	2.0
PROTEINS	
Albumin (g/L)	34-50
Total globulin (g/L)	22-44
Transferrin (mg/L)	2500
Ferritin (µg/L)	15-300
Total protein (g/L)	60-80
OSMOLALITY	
(mOsm/kg H_2O)	290-300

*In addition, metabolites exist bound to certain protein molecules (e.g., cholesterol, steroid hormones) or in solution (e.g., glucose, lactate). See Appendix B.
†mEq/L, mmol/L × charge (e.g., 1 mmol/L Ca^{2+} = 2 mEq/L).

and their properties of excitability and contraction. Readers need to remember these facts when studying the function of the heart in the operation of the cardiovascular system.

The heart is illustrated in Figure 11.3 to reveal the flow of blood through the four chambers. Blood returns to the right atrium of the heart via veins called the superior and inferior venae cavae, passes into the right ventricle through the tricuspid valve, and is pumped by the right ventricle through the pulmonary valve into the **pulmonary circulation** where it returns to the left atrium. The blood then passes through the mitral valve into the left ventricle, where it is pumped through an artery, the aorta, to the circulation of the remainder of the body, or **systemic circulation.** As indicated, the heart functions as a double pump, and the special one-way valves exist to prevent backflow of blood and

---

*PV, plasma volume; LBM, lean body mass. Modified from Sawka MN: Exerc Sports Sci Rev 14:175-211, 1986.

FIGURE 11.3

Blood flow through the valves and chambers of the heart to the pulmonary and systemic circulations. (From Thibodeau GA, Patton KT: *Anatomy and physiology,* ed 3, St. Louis, 1996, Mosby. Art by Christine Oleksyk.)

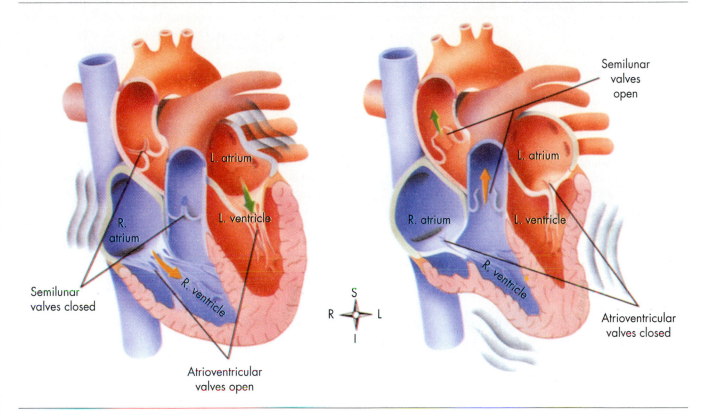

the decreased effectiveness of the pump. One pump, the right side of the heart, receives blood from the systemic circulation and pumps it through the pulmonary circulation of the lungs. The other pump, the left side of the heart, receives blood from the pulmonary circulation and pumps it through the systemic circulation. The right and left sides of the heart contract and pump blood together, resulting in a closed loop circulation (see Figure 11.3). Because the pump is a closed loop, the volume of blood pumped by the right and left sides of the heart must be equal or a backlog of blood will occur in either the pulmonary or the systemic circulation and cause serious impairment to pulmonary and cellular respiration.

Cardiac cycle

The previous description of blood flow through the heart and vasculature is referred to as the **cardiac cycle** and is illustrated in Figure 11.4. Note that the volumes and pressures of this diagram are shown specifically for the left side of the heart. During the cardiac cycle the volumes and pressures of blood in the atria and ventricles change in an organized and repeatable fashion, as do the blood pressures within the systemic and pulmonary circulations.

At rest, right atrial blood pressure is between 0 and 4 mm Hg and central venous blood pressure is only slightly

higher. During inspiration the enlargement of the thoracic cavity reduces not only pleural and alveolar pressure, but also the pressure exerted on the vasculature within the thoracic cavity. This serves to lower the pressure gradient between the inferior and superior venae cavae and the right atrium. Conversely, the increased thoracic pressures obtained during expiration increase the pressure gradient between the veins and right atrium, thus acting to pump blood to the right side of the heart. This phenomenon, termed the *ventilatory pump,* accounts for a noticeable (<5 bpm) slower heart rate during expiration than during inspiration.[82]

osmolality (oz′mo-lal′i-ti)
the number of particles per kilogram of solvent

pulmonary circulation
the vasculature that connects the heart to the lungs

systemic circulation
the vasculature of the body other than the pulmonary circulation

cardiac cycle
the events in a functional heart that occur between successive heart beats

FIGURE 11.4

The changes in pressures and volumes corresponding to phases of the cardiac cycle for the left side of the heart. (From Thibodeau GA, Patton KT: *Anatomy and physiology*, ed 3, St. Louis, 1996, Mosby.)

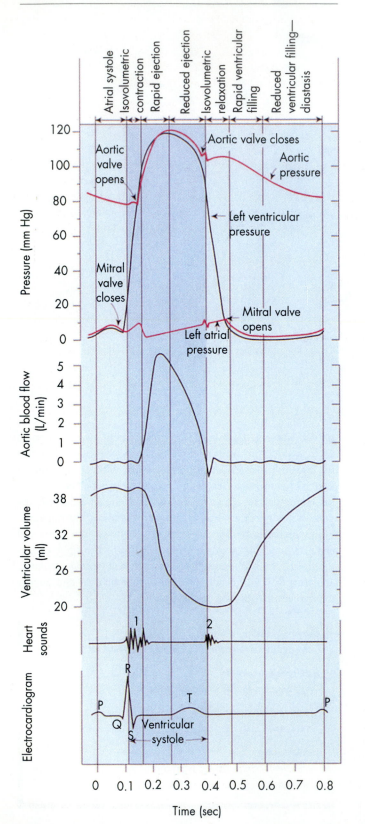

During the phase of the cardiac cycle when the myocardium is relaxed, termed *diastole,* blood flows passively into the right and left atrium and then into the respective ventricles. During this *passive filling* phase the atrial pressures do not increase, since minimal blood accumulates in these chambers at this stage. The discharge of an action potential from the sinoatrial (SA) node then starts the electromechanical events of the cardiac cycle. The action potential spreads throughout the right and left atrial myocardium, causing contraction of the myocardium. This atrial contraction, termed *atrial systole* (or *atrial kick*) contributes an extra 30% of total ventricular filling. The volume of blood in each ventricle, referred to as *end-diastolic volume* (EDV), exerts a stretch on the ventricular myocardium. This stretch can be interpreted as a load and is known as **preload** in clinical cardiology and cardiac rehabilitation. The greater the EDV and the greater the stretch, the faster the resultant ventricular myocardial contraction. This relationship is known as the *Frank-Starling law* of the heart.

In the average heart the EDV may approximate 120 ml, but as discussed in later sections, genetically gifted individuals may have a large heart and an end-diastolic volume exceeding 180 ml. Endurance training is also known to increase EDV.

The action potential that is propagated throughout the atrial myocardium is directed to the atrioventricular (AV) node via specialized neural tissue. Within the AV node are numerous nonmyelinated nerves that delay the propagation of the action potential by up to 0.1 second. This delay allows for the time required to complete the atrial kick and resultant increased ventricular filling. The action potential is then directed through the bundle of His to where the neural tissue branches into a right, left anterior, and left posterior branch, or *bundle branch*. These branches extend inferiorly toward the apex of the heart, where they diverge to spread the action potential to the apical myocardium. The neural tissue of the diverging bundle branches is referred to as the *Purkinje fibers* and is important for causing the contraction of the ventricular myocardium to occur in an inferior to superior direction.

The action potentials spread rapidly throughout the ventricular myocardium because of the diffuse presence of specialized low-resistance conducting tissue, termed **intercalated discs.** Blood is ejected from the ventricles during ventricular contraction, or *ventricular systole.* Ejection actually occurs when the ventricular myocardium generates ventricular pressures that exceed arterial pressures, which causes a short time interval in which contraction is occurring but no blood is ejected (*isovolumetric contraction*). For the right ventricle the pulmonary arterial pressure before ventricular systole (or *end diastole*) approximates 8 mm Hg, whereas the end diastolic pressure of the aorta artery approximates 80 mm Hg. These end diastolic pressures are also termed the **afterload.** Thus the left ventricle must generate more pressure than the right ventricle, causing it to perform more work for a given volume of blood pumped, which accounts for the larger myocardial mass surrounding the left compared with the right ventricle.

During ventricular systole not all blood is ejected from each ventricle. The volume of blood pumped from each ventricle per beat is termed **stroke volume,** and when expressed relative to the EDV is known as the **ejection fraction.** The ejection fraction for a healthy heart at rest approximates 0.6, or 60%. As discussed in later sections, the ejection fraction can increase to 80% during exercise. The product of stroke volume (SV) and heart rate (HR) quantifies the volume of blood pumped by the heart per unit time and is referred to as **cardiac output** (Q).

11.2 $$Q \text{ (ml/min)} = SV \text{ (ml)} \times HR \text{ (b/min)}$$

At rest the normal value for cardiac output approximates 5 L/min, but output may increase to greater than 35 L/min during the exercise intensities at or close to VO_2max.

Once the ventricular pressures return below the respective artery pressures and the momentum of ejected blood is overcome, the one-way valves of each ventricle close, the ventricular myocardium relaxes *(ventricular diastole),* and passive filling from the atrium occurs. The cardiac cycle is then complete and is repeated over and over again.

A useful application of cardiac output and arterial and central venous concentrations of oxygen is in the calculation of oxygen consumption using the Fick equation:

11.3 $$VO_2 \text{ (ml/min)} = Q \text{ (L/min)} \times \Delta a\text{-}VO_2 \text{ (ml/L)}$$

Where Δa-VO_2 equals the difference between the concentration of oxygen in arterial and mixed venous blood and represents the volume of oxygen consumed by the cells of the body for every liter of blood circulated in the body.

The tremendous increase in VO_2 during exercise is explained by the increase in both cardiac output and the increase in oxygen extraction from the blood. Muscle metabolic aspects of oxygen extraction are discussed in Chapter 10. Endurance training increases both components, and the application of the Fick equation to calculating VO_2 is testament to the importance of cardiovascular function to VO_2 and submaximal and maximal exercise performance.

The Vasculature

The flow of blood through almost all the circulatory beds within the body proceeds in the order of arteries, arterioles, capillaries, venules, and veins. However, there are a few exceptions to this rule in tissues such as the pituitary gland and liver, where one capillary bed is connected to another by an intermediate vein. Each of these special circulation beds is referred to as a *portal circulation.*

The artery has the thickest wall and the greatest ability to stretch and then recoil to its original dimension, a property termed *elasticity.* Conversely, arteries have a limited ability to be distended and increase their vascular volume, a property termed **compliance.** Arterioles possess properties similar to those of arteries but in addition can be surrounded circumferentially by layers of smooth muscle fibers. The contraction of this smooth muscle is regulated by nerves, hormones from the circulation, local metabolites, and perhaps even local pressure and electrical changes that result in either the constriction or the relaxation of the muscle.[*] Contraction of smooth muscle surrounding an arteriole decreases the diameter of the lumen, increases resistance to blood flow, and thereby decreases flow, a process termed **vasoconstriction.** Conversely, smooth muscle relaxation around an arteriole increases the diameter, decreases resistance, and increases blood flow, a process termed **vasodilation.**

Capillaries are the smallest diameter blood vessels and possess a wall composed of a single cell layer. The cells of the capillary wall are not tightly connected, and pores exist that allow the movement of fluid into and from the vascular compartment, as well as certain white blood cells and small pro-

---

[*]References 4, 11, 37, 51, 60, and 98.

preload
the load to which a muscle is subjected before shortening. Preload is usually explained as the stretch induced on the myocardium by the filling of the ventricles of the heart

intercalated discs
low resistance, high-conduction velocity tissue dispersed through the myocardium, causing a rapid depolarization of the myocardium when stimulated

afterload
the blood pressure exposed to the aortic valve immediately before ventricular contraction

stroke volume
the volume of blood ejected from the ventricle with each beat

ejection fraction
the volume of blood pumped by the heart per beat, expressed relative to the end diastolic volume of the ventricle

cardiac output
the blood volume pumped by the heart each minute

compliance (kom-pli'ans)
the measure of the ease at which a structure can increase its volume capacitance; the reciprocal of elasticity

vasoconstriction (vas'o-kon-strik'shun)
narrowing of the lumen diameter of blood vessels

vasodilation (vas'o-di-la'shun)
widening of the lumen diameter of blood vessels

FIGURE 11.5

The changes in systemic blood pressure, vascular cross-sectional area, and blood flow velocity in the progression from arteries to veins.

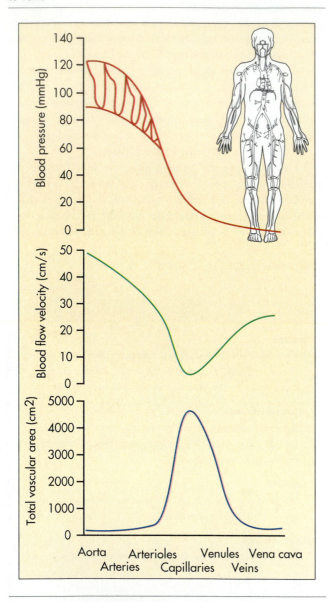

flows from the left ventricle through the arteries to the veins and right atrium. The variation in blood pressure is largest in the left ventricle, and because of the elastic properties and recoil of the arteries during ventricular diastole, systemic diastolic pressure remains well above zero (80 mm Hg). The pressure change in the vasculature is largest as blood flows through the arterioles, and for this reason arterioles are the pressure-regulating vessels of the body. Decreasing smooth muscle tone (contraction) around the arterioles would decrease this pressure differential by lowering arterial systemic blood pressure, while increasing smooth muscle tone would increase vasoconstriction, raise systemic blood pressure, and increase this pressure differential (see Focus Box 11.1). Blood pressure continues to decline as blood flows through the capillaries and veins and, as previously described, approximates zero within the right atrium.

The changes in blood pressure throughout the systemic circulation are explained by the changes in vascular cross-sectional area and blood flow velocity. The divergence of the vascular system increases in the progression from arteries to capillaries, followed by convergence of the venules and veins into the inferior and superior venae cavae. As explained in Focus Box 11.1, the increase in vascular cross-sectional area resulting from the large increase in the number of blood vessels reduces pressure, and a given blood flow can be received and directed to the venules at a lower velocity. A longer capillary transit time in the peripheral circulation favors the equilibration of gas partial pressures between the blood and cells of the respective tissue bed.

The low-pressure venous circulation presents a problem to the circulation of blood back to the heart, especially for the vasculature exposed to hydrostatic pressures when positioned below heart level, as is the case for the lower limbs during most forms of exercise. Two aspects of the venous circulation assist venous blood flow against gravity back to the heart. As previously indicated, veins possess one-way valves that prevent backflow away from the heart. However, these valves do little propelling blood toward the heart. This aspect is aided by the contraction of muscles, which increase intramuscular and extravascular pressures, serving to squeeze the blood-filled veins. Because of the one-way valves, the only direction that blood can flow is toward the heart. This mechanism has been termed the **muscle pump.**

The Microvasculature

Recent research has identified the importance of the microvasculature to the regulation of skeletal muscle blood flow and metabolism during exercise.[16,63,64,123] Consequently, the factors that regulate smooth muscle tone surrounding the arterioles and capillaries warrant special attention.

teins and metabolites. In certain regions of the circulatory bed, smooth muscle may also be present around the junctions between arterioles and capillaries, as discussed in the section on the microcirculation. The walls of venules and veins are not as thick as those of the arteries or arterioles and do not have high elasticity, but they do have high compliance. Veins are also surrounded by smooth muscle, which because of the compliance of the venous circulation, functions to regulate the cross-sectional dimensions of the veins and therefore the volume of blood that is in the venous circulation.

Figure 11.5 illustrates the changes in blood pressure, vasculature cross-sectional area, and blood flow velocity as blood

muscle pump

the action of contracting muscles that forces venous blood flow against gravity toward the heart

FOCUS BOX 11.1

Hemodynamics of circulation throughout the human body

The rhythmic contraction of the heart and the changing pressures of the cardiac cycle cause the flow of blood within the vasculature to be pulsatile. The vasculature of the body diverges and converges, causing numerous branches and changing vessel diameters, and the cellular components of blood make it a suspension of varied viscosity rather than a true fluid. These facts make the physical modeling of the cardiovascular system a difficult, if not impossible, process. Nevertheless, the application of several physical principles and equations to cardiovascular function is useful in appreciating the physical constraints the body must overcome to effectively circulate blood. The branch of physics that concerns the dynamics of fluid flow is termed *hydrodynamics*, and when the fluid is blood, the subdiscipline is termed **hemodynamics.**

Types of Blood Flow

Most laws of hemodynamics assume that blood flow is *laminar*. Laminar flow is characterized by the fluid having a uniform velocity throughout the radial dimensions of the vessel (Figure 11.6). In contrast, *turbulent* flow is characterized by irregular directioned fluid flow throughout the lumen of the vessel, often resulting in sections that have reversed flow (vortices). The main consequence of the two different flows within the cardiovascular system is that turbulent flow requires the generation of larger pressures for a given flow rate, which would increase the work of the heart. *Reynold's number* (N_R) is used to determine when a given fluid in a given vessel will develop turbulence. For $N_R < 2000$ flow is laminar, but for $N_R > 3000$ flow is turbulent.[11,37]

11.4, A $\qquad\qquad N_R = \rho D \, v / \eta$

Where ρ, fluid density; D, vessel diameter; v, mean velocity; η, viscosity.

From the equation, fluid flows more easily become turbulent for fluids with low viscosity flowing through vessels with large diameters at a high velocity. The turbulent flow of blood in the cardiovascular system is exploited in various measurements. For example, the measurement of blood pressure by auscultation is dependent on the audible detection of sound resulting from turbulent flow within the brachial artery. Similarly, the sounds generated from turbulent flow through the valves of the heart are exaggerated when there are valve abnormalities, such as

---

hemodynamics (he'mo-di-nam'iks)

the study of the dynamics of the blood circulation

FIGURE 11.6

The difference between laminar and turbulant fluid flow within a vessel. (From Berne RM, Levy MN: *Physiology*, ed 3, St. Louis, 1993, Mosby.)

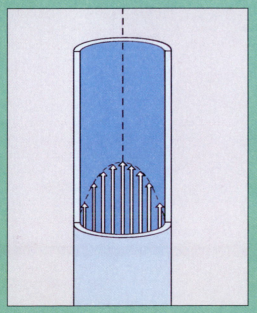
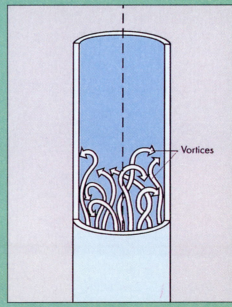

stenoses or regurgitation, and these sounds are used in conjunction with Doppler flowmetry to diagnose valvular abnormalities.

Blood Flow and Pressure

The law that applies to the laminar flow of fluid through cylindric tubes is Poiseuille's law (Figure 11.7).

11.4, B $Q = \pi(Pi - Po) r^4 / 8\eta l$

Where Q, flow; $(Pi - Po)$, pressure difference at two ends of a vessel; r, radius; η, viscosity; l, length of the vessel.

The greater the pressure gradient, the larger the radius, and the lower the viscosity and length of the vessel, the greater the flow. For the human cardiovascular system, the important relationships in this law are for the radius and length of the vessel. For the systemic circulation, where arteries are longer, a greater pressure difference is required to maintain a given flow. When the radius is decreased, such as during vasoconstriction, this has a large influence on decreasing flow because of the fourth power function. These facts partially explain the larger systemic blood pressures compared with the pulmonary blood pressures.

Importance of vascular resistance

Ohm's law, which was devised to explain the relationships between electrical resistance (R), voltage changes(V_{ab}), and current flow (I) (R = V_{ab}/I), can be applied to the cardiovascular system by rearranging Poiseuille's law.

11.4, C $R = [(Pi - Po) / Q] = 8\eta l / \pi r^4$

Thus, when the assumptions of Poiseuille's law apply, for a given blood flow the resistance along a vessel is increased by larger changes in pressure. Interestingly, this relationship can be applied to the total systemic arterial circulation, where Q represents cardiac output, MAP represents mean arterial blood pressure, and PVR represents peripheral vascular resistance.

FIGURE 11.7

The geometric features of a straight vessel, and their relationship to resistance and flow as described by Poiseuille's law.

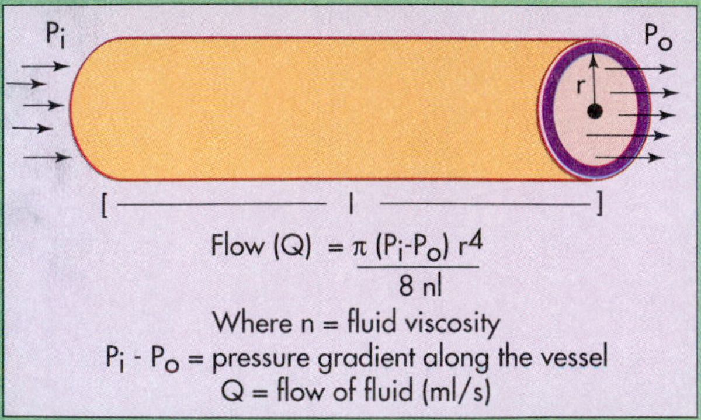

$$\text{Flow (Q)} = \frac{\pi (P_i - P_o) r^4}{8 nl}$$

Where n = fluid viscosity

$P_i - P_o$ = pressure gradient along the vessel

Q = flow of fluid (ml/s)

11.4, D $PVR = MAP / Q \text{ or } Q = MAP / PVR$

The important implications for the latter expression of the equation concern the change in mean arterial pressure during increases in cardiac output, such as those that occur during exercise. Because cardiac output can increase from 5 to over 30 L/min, and MAP may increase from 90 to approximately 140 mm Hg, PVR must decrease from 0.018 to 0.0047 mm Hg/ml/min to maintain proportionality. If PVR did not decrease during exercise, then to maintain the increase in cardiac output, mean arterial pressure would have to increase to over 540 mm Hg! Obviously, the regulation of the microvasculature and mean arterial pressures is an important acute adaptation to exercise.

Series and parallel resistances

As with Ohm's law, a model of electronic circuitry can be applied to understanding the operation of resistance circuits within the cardiovascular system. As discussed in the text, the circulatory system progresses from arteries to arterioles to capillaries to venules to veins. Similarly, during this progression there is a change in the number of vessels and total cross-sectional areas represented by the vessels (see Figure 11.7). If this increase in vessel number and cross-sectional area did not occur and each microvascular bed were connected end to end, it would reflect vascular beds or resistances arranged *in series* (Figure 11.8).

As indicated in Figure 11.8, the total resistance of these in series resistances equals the sum of the individual resistances. Clearly, the cardiovascular system could not function this way, since a phenomenally large pressure would result for even resting blood flow, let alone the demands resulting from increased blood flow during exercise.

A model more typical of the body is when multiple vascular beds (resistances) are formed from one vessel, and this arrangement is termed *in parallel* resistances. In this situation the total resistance equals the sum of the reciprocals of the individual resistances, which is obviously far less than in series resistances.

The cardiovascular system is a special example of in parallel resistances. The divergence from arteries to arterioles results in an increase in the number of vessels; however, as explained in the text, the arterioles are the sites of the largest resistance and therefore the largest changes in pressure in the cardiovascular system. In this example the divergence of the arteries is insufficient to overcome the resistances of the smaller diameter arterioles. For a given vessel that diverges into vessels having a quarter the diameter of the original vessel, four times the total cross-sectional area is needed to match the resistance of the single large vessel. Thus, when viewing Figure 11.5, the tremendous increase in cross-sectional area (increased number of vessels) from the arterioles to the capillaries is sufficient to overcome the increased resistance from divergence to smaller diameter vessels.

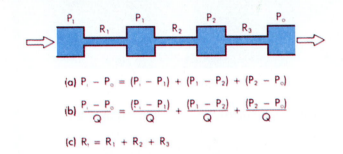

FIGURE 11.8

Comparison between in-series and in-parallel resistance circuits, and how they effect vascular resistance. (From Berne RM, Levy MN: *Physiology*, ed 3, St. Louis, 1993, Mosby.)

(a) $P_i - P_o = (P_i - P_1) + (P_1 - P_2) + (P_2 - P_o)$

(b) $\dfrac{P_i - P_o}{Q} = \dfrac{(P_i - P_1)}{Q} + \dfrac{(P_1 - P_2)}{Q} + \dfrac{(P_2 - P_o)}{Q}$

(c) $R_t = R_1 + R_2 + R_3$

(a) $Q_1 = Q_1 + Q_2 + Q_3$

(b) $\dfrac{Q_1}{P_i - P_o} = \dfrac{Q_1}{(P_1 - P_o)} + \dfrac{Q_2}{(P_1 - P_o)} + \dfrac{Q_3}{(P_1 - P_o)}$

(c) $\dfrac{1}{R_t} = \dfrac{1}{R_1} + \dfrac{1}{R_2} + \dfrac{1}{R_3}$

FIGURE 11.9

The role of skeletal muscle and vascular endothelium in the local regulation of blood flow.

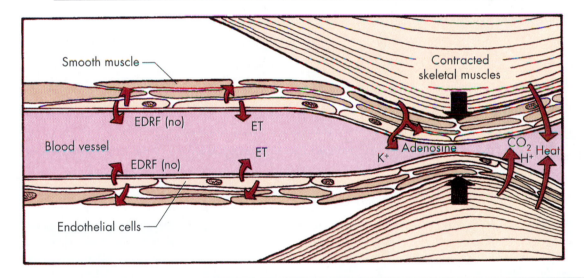

Figure 11.9 presents the relationships between the endothelial lining of the lumen of arterioles, capillaries, and veins within skeletal muscle, and the smooth muscle that often surrounds these vessels. The endothelium can produce and release several molecules that influence smooth muscle tone, stimulate immune function, influence blood clotting, and for the capillaries possibly induce vascular regeneration after damage and the formation of new capillaries.[47,119] Endothelium–derived relaxing factor (EDRF), now known as *nitrous oxide,* is a potent vasodilator, whereas endothelin is a potent vasoconstrictor of the peripheral vasculature.[62,93,123] The muscle fibers also release metabolites and electrolytes that are known to have vasodilator functions, such as potassium, adenosine, and protons (decreased pH), and vasodilation is also supported by decreases in the arterial partial pressure of oxygen (PaO$_2$) and increases in the arterial partial pressure

of carbon dioxide (PaCO$_2$) and temperature. These local controls of circulation within skeletal muscle are important for regulating the contraction or relaxation of smooth muscle that surrounds certain capillaries **(precapillary sphincters).** When the smooth muscle of these capillaries is stimulated to relax, the diameter of the capillary is increased and blood is permitted to flow into the capillary network. This event decreases resistance to blood flow, thereby increasing blood flow. (See Focus Box 11.2.)

precapillary sphincter

region of smooth muscle that surrounds blood vessels before the capillary bed

FOCUS BOX 11.2

Methods used to measure cardiac output, cardiac dimensions, and peripheral blood flow in humans

The measurement of blood flow in humans has been conducted by numerous methods both invasive and noninvasive. These methods are listed in Table 11.3.

TABLE 11.3

Main methods used to measure cardiac output, cardiac dimensions, and blood flow* in humans

METHOD	INVASIVENESS	TEMPORAL RESOLUTION	WHEN MEASURED
CARDIAC OUTPUT			
CO_2 rebreathing	Noninvasive	Averaged over several minutes	During exercise
Doppler flowmetry	Noninvasive	Every cardiac cycle (beat-to-beat)	During exercise
CARDIAC DIMENSIONS			
Echocardiography	Noninvasive	Usually at end-systole and diastole	At rest
PERIPHERAL ARTERIAL BLOOD FLOW			
Dye dilution	Invasive	Averaged over several seconds	During immediate recovery
Thermal dilution	Invasive	Averaged over several seconds	During immediate recovery
Doppler flowmetry[†]	Noninvasive	Every cardiac cycle (beat-to-beat)	During exercise
Venous occlusion plethysmography	Noninvasive	Averaged over several seconds	During immediate recovery
MUSCLE BLOOD FLOW			
Xenon clearance	Invasive	Averaged over several seconds	During immediate recovery

*All blood flow measures are normally expressed as a volume flow per minute (ml/min)
[†]Doppler flowmetry is the only method that resolves blood flow to the cardiac cycle.

As discussed in the text, research has mainly employed echocardiography as the method to evaluate cardiac dimensions and function. However, a number of methods have been used to measure blood flow in peripheral arteries of limbs. Of these methods, Doppler flowmetry is proving to be the most valid and informative, since the invasiveness of dye dilution, thermal dilution, or Xenon clearance has the risk of interfering with normal blood flow profiles. Furthermore, the method of venous occlusion plethysmography has been shown to interfere with arterial blood flow,[4,42] and as it measures flow during the recovery after contractions, provides exaggerated blood flow information because of the known hyperemia that occurs between dynamic muscle contractions.[94,125,126] As a result of these facts, only information that focuses on the function of echocardiography and Doppler flowmetry is presented in this focus box.

Echocardiography

During the echocardiographic evaluation of cardiac anatomy and function. The subject is usually in a modified supine position and two-dimensional images of the heart are displayed on a computer screen. These images are stored on video cassette for later evaluation. Echocardiography is based on the principle that very high-frequency sound waves (ultrasound > 20,000 Hz [cycles/s]) directed by a transducer to penetrate the body are reflected back to the transducer by structures within the body.[49] The returning sound-wave patterns are processed to show differences in sound waves, which provide the two-dimensional image on the screen.

Doppler Flowmetry

Doppler flowmetry is similar to echocardiography in that it uses high-frequency nonaudible sound waves; however, it differs in that the frequency of the sound waves that are reflected back to the instrument is processed to determine both a velocity of flow and the direction of flow. Thus, when the sound waves are directed to an artery or vein, blood flow velocity and direction can be measured. Blood flow velocity can be calculated from the Doppler equation.

FIGURE 11.10

Doppler flowmetry is based on the principle that a moving object will change the wavelength of sound that is directed towards the object. The best example of this principle is the change in pitch of a train whistle when the train is approaching or leaving a station. Sound from an object traveling away from a person will cause the sound to be of a lower pitch, or wavelength. Conversely, sound coming from an object moving towards a person will cause the sound to be at a higher pitch, or a higher wavelength. Doppler flowmetry applies this same principle to detect the changing frequency of sound as it rebounds off moving blood vessels. The direction of the change in frequency depends on which way the blood is flowing relative to the Doppler crystal used to direct the high frequency sound wave.

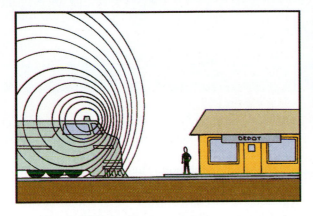
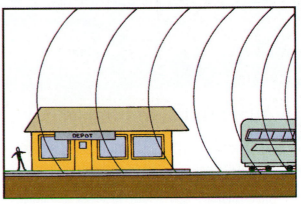

Compressed wavelength—increased frequency   Elongated wavelength—decreased frequency

FIGURE 11.11

When Doppler flowmetry is used to measure blood flow from the heart, or in a peripheral blood vessel, a measure of artery diameter is needed, and the Doppler equation is modified to convert blood flow velocity into a volume of blood flow per unit time. **A,** An image of an artery. **B,** An example of a Doppler blood velocity spectrum. Forward flow is represented by the signal above the x-axis, and reverse flow is represented by signal below the x-axis. Apart from detecting blood flow direction, Doppler flowmetry is also advantageous in that blood flow is resolved to each cardiac cycle.

A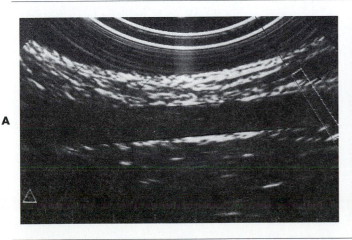
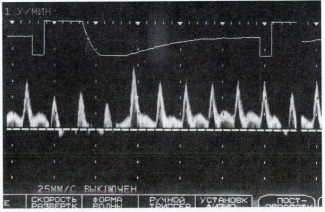 B

$$V = (fr - fo) \times (c/2fo) \times (cos \: ø)^*$$

where ø is the symbol for the angle (°). *fr*, Frequency of reflected sound beam; *fo*, frequency of transmitted sound beam (MH$_3$); *c*, speed of sound (1540 m/s).

The velocity calculation is converted to a blood flow volume by measuring the diameter of the vessel by conventional echocardiography and using this value in a modified form of the Doppler equation. The ability to detect blood flow direction is based on the change in sound wave frequency that occurs when objects are moving (see Figure 11.10). The resulting data reveal shaded peaks that represent a range of change in frequency and signal

intensity (Figure 11.11). Generally, the area under the curve generated by these velocity spectra is used as a measure of average frequency change. It is this average frequency shift that is used in the Doppler equation.

The raw signal from the Doppler system is presented in Figure 11.11 for the brachial artery of the forearm. It is clear that Doppler flowmetry can distinguish between blood flow bursts that correspond to each cardiac cycle, and that within a given cardiac cycle, reverse flow (below baseline) can be detected and quantified.

*See Tchakovsky ME, Shoemaker JK, Hughson RL: *J Appl Physiol* 79(3):713-719, 1995.

Acute Adaptations to Exercise

Considerable material has already been presented on the transition from rest to exercise. There is an instantaneous increase in ventilation and VO$_2$, and these facts alone indicate that similar increases in cardiac function and pulmonary and systemic blood flow must also occur. For example, an increased ventilation would be futile if it occurred without increases in pulmonary blood flow, since a greater mismatch between ventilation and blood flow would result (see Chapter 12). Similarly, an increase in VO$_2$ by exercising muscles could not occur or be sustained without an increase in blood flow, which supplies the added oxygen for metabolism.

The immediate response of the cardiovascular system to exercise is discussed relative to changes in heart (cardiac) function, changes in blood, and changes in peripheral blood flow and is classified according to the type of exercise performed.

Cardiac Function

The heart must respond rapidly to exercise stress. Not only is there a need for increasing the rate at which blood is pumped by the heart, but the heart must increase systemic blood pressures to assist the increasing flow of blood within the closed and finite vascular volume of the body. For the healthy heart, these demands are handled surprisingly well because of the sensitivity and effectiveness of the numerous factors that control heart function.

Regulation of the Cardiac Cycle

There are two main types of regulation of heart function: regulation that affects heart rate, known as **chronotropic** regulation, and regulation that affects the velocity of myocardial contraction *(contractility),* known as **inotropic** regulation. The start of exercise stimulates both chronotropic and inotropic regulation, resulting not only in increased heart rates, but also in improved abilities of the myocardium and heart to function as a pump. The importance of the neuroen-

docrine regulation of cardiac function is emphasized in individuals after heart transplantation (Clinical Application, p. 283).

Chronotropic regulation. The frequency of heart contractions (heart rate) is controlled by the neural and hormonal regulation of specialized neural tissue within the heart itself (see Chapter 7). The SA node is composed of neural tissue that can be permeated by sodium, resulting in regular intervals of depolarization that produce action potentials, repolarization, and depolarization once again. Parasympathetic innervation causes this neural tissue to become hyperpolarized, thus delaying the occurrence of the threshold potential required to propagate an action potential and causing a slower rate of discharge and slower heart rate. Conversely, sympathetic stimulation from neural secretion of norepinephrine or hormonal stimulation by circulating norepinephrine and epinephrine increases the leakiness of the membranes to sodium, decreasing the time to reach a threshold potential and increasing the rate of action potential discharge. Sympathetic stimulation also increases the excitability of the nerves within the AV node, resulting in a lesser delay in the propagation of the action potential through the AV node and to the ventricular myocardium.

Two additional neural reflexes can alter heart rate by influencing the balance between parasympathetic and sympathetic regulation of the heart. When venous return increases, there is a slight stretch on the right atrial wall, which stimulates pressure receptors that then return action potentials to the cardiovascular control region within the medulla. An increase in sympathetic stimulation of the heart occurs, so that cardiac output can increase and almost instantaneously propel this blood through the lungs and systemic circulation and prevent an increased blood volume in the venous circulation. When the blood pressure in the systemic circulation increases above normal values, pressure receptors in the carotid and aortic arteries return action potentials to the cardiac control center that stimulate increased parasympathetic stimulation of the heart. A lowered heart rate and cardiac output result, which in turn lower systemic blood pressure and

Clinical Examples of Altered Cardiovascular Regulation: Heart Transplantation and Spinal Cord Injury

Heart Transplantation

Individuals who consent to open heart surgery for the implantation of a new heart do so to prolong life, but are then forced to a life with risk of infection and cardiovascular compromise. Implantation of a new heart necessitates the dissection of the efferent nerves that innervate the SA node, the AV node, and the ventricular myocardium and any afferent nerves that leave the heart. The denervation of the heart leaves circulating catecholamines to provide chronotropic and inotropic regulation during rest and exercise.

Cardiac function at rest

At rest, the posttransplant heart has a relatively high resting rate resulting from the absence of vagal tone at the SA node. Ventricular filling, end-diastolic volume, ejection fraction, stroke volume, and cardiac output are at the low end of normal ranges.[121]

Cardiac function during exercise

Studies of heart transplant patients during exercise have indicated a delayed increase in heart rate, a blunted increase in heart rate for a given exercise intensity, and blunted stroke volume and cardiac output responses. Oxygen consumption is normal because of an increased Δa-VO_2. There is a prolonged elevation of heart rate during recovery from exercise.[121]

Since almost all of the heart rate response to exercise is removed during β-blockade, the circulatory catecholamine response to exercise is important for exercise tolerance after heart transplantation. Despite a stable heart rate response during β-blockade, cardiac output increases and reflects the role of venous return and stroke volume increases in determining cardiac output in this population.[121] Blood pressure responses to dynamic exercise are also blunted after heart transplant, but the rise in systemic blood pressure during isometric exercise is similar to normal innervated hearts.

Spinal Cord Injury

Unlike heart transplantation and the accompanied denervation of the heart, spinal cord injury (SCI) below the cervical level retains both parasympathetic and sympathetic innervation of the SA and AV nodes and myocardium. However, the higher the level of injury in the thoracic vertebrae, the greater the impairment to the sympathetic innervation of the adrenal gland and vasculature of the gut and lower limbs. These ailments result in decreased circulating concentrations of epinephrine and norepinephrine (see Chapter 8) and the reduced ability to regulate the smooth muscle of the peripheral vascular system. Not surprisingly, regulation of blood pressure both at rest and during upper body exercise is detrimentally affected by spinal cord injury.[114] It is not uncommon for individuals with thoracic level SCI to experience syncope after exercise in the vertical position because of venous pooling of blood in their paralyzed lower body musculature.

The heart rate response to upper body exercise is blunted in individuals with SCI compared with uninjured persons[114] and venous return and cardiac output are significantly lower. As for the heart transplant patient, exercise tolerance is more dependent on an increasing Δa-VO_2 and muscular fatigue has an earlier onset, which decreases exercise tolerance. The importance of central cardiovascular dynamics to exercise in individuals with SCI has been verified by application of artificial electrical stimulation of paralyzed leg muscle during upper body exercise. This form of hybrid exercise increases venous return, maximal heart rate, and maximal cardiac output and improves exercise tolerance in this population.

Heart transplantation and spinal cord injury are two examples of altered cardiovascular function that provide further insight to the importance of cardiovascular function to optimal exercise tolerance.

---

reduce the stretch (pressure) on the walls of the aorta and carotid arteries (see Focus Box 11.1).

Inotropic regulation. Inotropic regulation concerns changes in the velocity of contraction. Figure 11.12 presents the relationship between EDV and contractile force. This relationship, first reported by Frank in 1895 on frog myocardium and

chronotropic (kron′o-trop′ik)
pertaining to the rate of myocardial contraction (heart rate)

inotropic (in-o-trop′ik)
pertaining to the contractility of the myocardium

FIGURE 11.12

The relationship between end diastolic volume (EDV), the velocity of myocardial contraction, and contractility. Increasing EDV (increasing venous return) causes an increase in myocardial contraction velocity. Stimulation by catecholamines generates a different curve for EDV and contraction velocity, thereby increasing contractility.

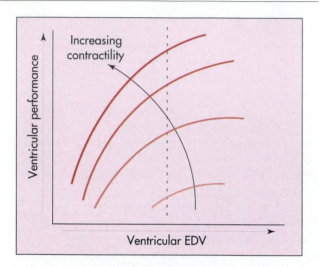

refined and quantified by Starling in 1914, is termed the *Frank-Starling law*.[11] This curve can be altered by increasing catecholamine stimulation to the myocardium, which results in the raising of the curve and therefore increases the velocity of contraction for a given EDV. An increase in myocardial contraction velocity for a given EDV is referred to as increased *contractility*.

During catecholamine-induced increases in contractility (Figure 11.12) the epinephrine and norepinephrine bind to β_1 receptors on the sarcolemma of the myocardial fibers and cause an increase in cAMP, which in turn eventually increases lipolysis, the phosphorylation of myosin light chains, and the increased cycling velocity of the myosin-actin contraction mechanism.[11] In addition, stimulatory G proteins simultaneously increase the conductance of calcium across the membrane, which further aids myocardial contraction velocity and force[11] (see Chapter 7).

Changes in Cardiac Function During Exercise

Not all exercise elicits the same cardiac response. Dynamic exercise induces increases in heart rate, stroke volume, cardiac output, and blood pressure that differ from isometric exercise. Similarly, dynamic upper body exercise, which involves a smaller muscle mass than the dynamic exercise of the larger muscles of the legs, also elicits a slightly different cardiac response.

Dynamic lower body exercise

Heart rate. The onset of exercise is associated with near simultaneous sympathetic stimulation of the SA node, AV

node, and ventricular myocardium. In addition, the contraction of skeletal muscle induces an increase in venous return, and these factors combine to increase heart rate and myocardial contractility.

Figure 11.13, *A*, presents the increases in heart rate, stroke volume, cardiac output, and oxygen consumption during several submaximal steady state exercise intensities during cycle ergometry. The rapidity of the increases in heart rate is obvious, as is the rapid decrease in heart rate after exercise is terminated. When the data for heart rate and time are plotted during a ramp protocol, it is clear that heart rate does not increase linearly with intensity (Figure 11.14). However, over a given range of submaximal exercise intensities the heart rate response is close to linear and can be used to estimate the exercise intensity. The wide individual variation in the slope of the heart rate response, as well as the nonlinearly, results in considerable error in predicting VO_2max from heart rates (see Chapter 19).

Recently, mathematic transformations have been applied to heart rates during different conditions. Interestingly, when a Fourier transformation is applied to resting steady state heart rates, which expresses heart rates based on the variability rather than rate, the normal beat to beat variability results in the appearance of three peaks in a frequency (Hz) spectrum (Figure 11.15). The lowest frequency peak (~ 0.03 Hz) reflects sympathetic stimulation of the SA node, whereas the highest frequency peak (~ 0.3 Hz) reflects parasympathetic stimulation of the SA node. The midpeak is influenced by both parasympathetic and sympathetic stimulation.[52,115] This is an exciting technique to evaluate competing parasympathetic and sympathetic stimulation of the heart. Application of the frequency analysis of heart rate variability during exercise has shown that the sympathetic frequency curve is decreased and the parasympathetic curve is completely removed,[52] indicating the decreased involvement of neural regulation of heart rate during exercise. Presumably, humoral regulation of the heart rate predominates during exercise.[52]

Stroke volume and cardiac output. The increasing venous return and sympathetic myocardial stimulation induce an increased end-diastolic volume, which for a given ejection fraction increases stroke volume (Figure 11.16). In addition, because of the increased contractility of the ventricular myocardium, there is an increased ejection fraction of the

FIGURE 11.13

The changes in **A,** oxygen consumption (VO_2), **B,** heart rate, **C,** stroke volume, and **D,** cardiac output during several intermittent steady state exercise intensities. The sudden increases and decreases in heart rate reflect its intricate regulation.

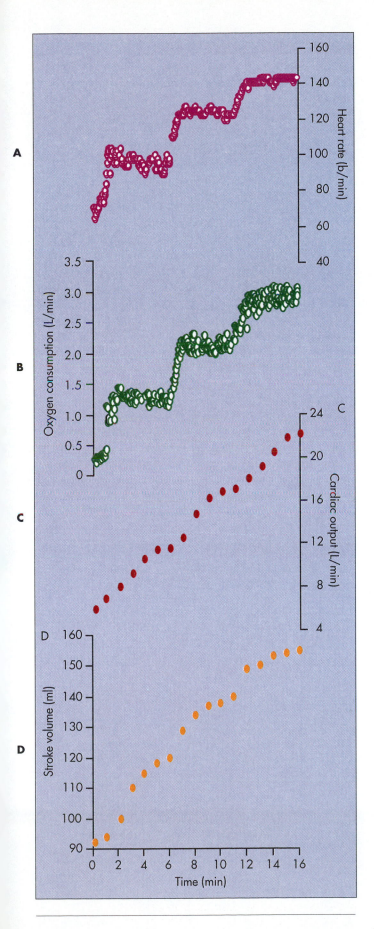

FIGURE 11.14

Although it has been generally accepted that heart rate increases linearly with exercise intensity, when heart rate is plotted against time during a ramp protocol, the relationship is curvilinear, with only a small portion of the curve resembling a linear function.

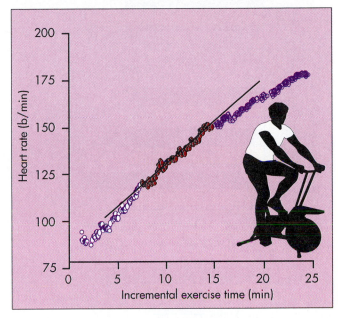

FIGURE 11.15

The frequency power spectrum of resting heart variability. The three peaks in the order from lowest to highest frequency represent variability that is due to sympathetic stimulation, both sympathetic and parasympathetic stimulation, and parasympathetic stimulation, respectively.

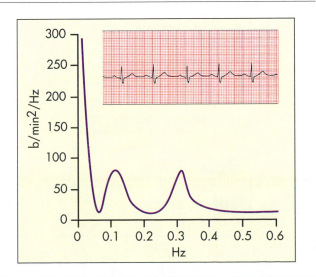

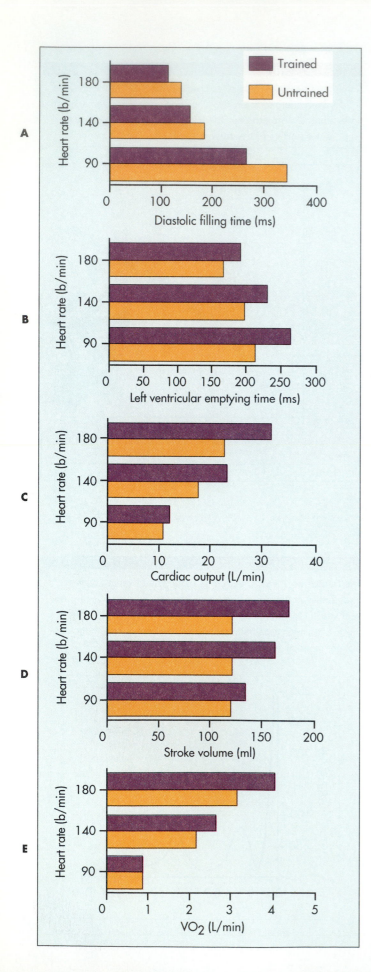

FIGURE 11.16

The changes in **A,** diastolic filling, **B,** left ventricular emptying, **C,** stroke volume, **D,** cardiac output, and **E,** oxygen consumption (VO_2) at given heart rates for untrained and endurance-trained individuals. (Adapted from Gledhill ND, et al: Endurance athletes' stroke volume does not plateau: major advantage is diastolic function, *Med Sci Sports Exerc* 26(9):1116-1121, 1994.)

heart during exercise, which further increases stroke volume. As indicated in Figure 11.17, stroke volume increases as exercise intensity increases from rest to approximately 50% VO_2max in relatively untrained individuals, and thereafter plateaus. In trained individuals, stroke volume continues to increase to VO_2max, which coincides with significant increases in maximal cardiac output and VO_2max.[35] These responses are typical only for exercise performed in the vertical position. Research conducted on individuals exercising in a recumbent or supine position has shown that maximal stroke volumes are attained at the onset of exercise,[15,71] presumably resulting from the lack of hydrostatic pressures that resist venous return to the heart.

The importance of an increased myocardial contractility for increasing or maintaining stroke volumes cannot be overemphasized. For example, Figure 11.18 compares the durations of diastolic filling and left ventricular ejection for differing heart rates for untrained and endurance-trained individuals. At increasing heart rates there is less time for diastolic filling and ventricular ejection, with the duration of dias-

FIGURE 11.17

The different increase in stroke volume for trained and untrained individuals during increases in relative exercise intensity.

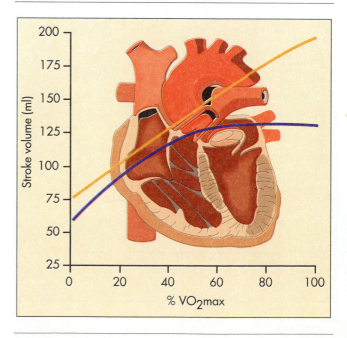

FIGURE 11.18

The decreasing durations of diastole and systole during increasing heart rate, like those that accompany exercise. (Adapted from Gledhill ND, et al: Endurance athletes' stroke volume does not plateau: major advantage is diastolic function, *Med Sci Sports Exerc* 26 (9):1116-1121, 1994.)

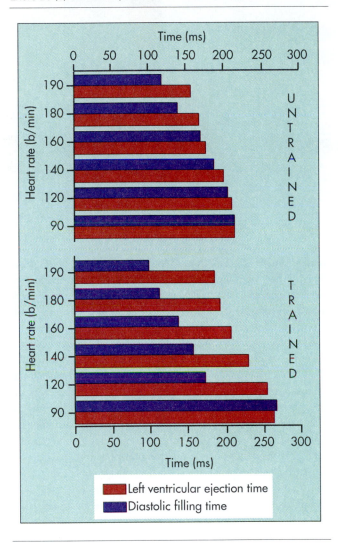

tolic filling being less than ventricular ejection. Endurance-trained individuals have an even shorter diastolic filling time, which is accounted for by a longer ventricular ejection period because of their greater stroke volume. This means that the heart must receive blood flow at a higher rate during exercise to ensure faster filling, which in turn means that the ventricular myocardium must generate pressures faster to eject larger volumes of blood from the ventricles in less time.

The increased heart rates and stroke volumes that accompany exercise result in an increase in cardiac output. This increase, relative to exercise intensity, is also linear and plateaus at intensities that correspond to maximal heart rate and VO$_2$max.

Blood pressure. Based on the hemodynamic information presented in Focus Box 11.1, peripheral vascular resistance must decrease when cardiac output increases to avoid large increases in systemic blood pressure. Although this does occur during exercise, mean blood pressure still rises with an increase in exercise intensity.

Figure 11.19 presents the change in systolic, diastolic, and mean blood pressures during an incremental exercise test. Mean blood pressure is not the average of systolic (SBP) and diastolic blood pressures (DBP), since the durations of systole and diastole differ. At rest, mean arterial blood pressure (MAP) is estimated from the calculation:

11.5 $$MAP = DBP + [(SBP - DBP) / 3]$$

This calculation is based on the duration of diastole being approximately three times that of systole. However, as indicated in Figure 11.18, this time relationship changes with increases in heart rate. During exercise, systolic and mean pressures increase, while diastolic pressure remains close to or slightly less than resting values (<80 mm Hg). This information indicates that during conditions of increasing cardiac output, ejection of blood from the left ventricle exceeds the compliant properties of the arterial vasculature, yet the reduced peripheral vascular resistance maintains a low diastolic pressure despite the reduced interval between successive ejections from the left ventricle.

Research on pulmonary blood pressures during exercise indicates that there is only a minimal increase in mean pres-

FIGURE 11.19

The change in systolic, diastolic, and mean blood pressures during an incremental cycle ergometer test. Note the steady diastolic blood pressure. The increases in mean blood pressure are therefore a result of the increase in systolic blood pressure.

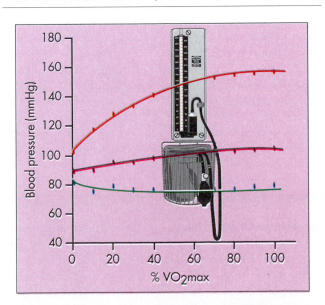

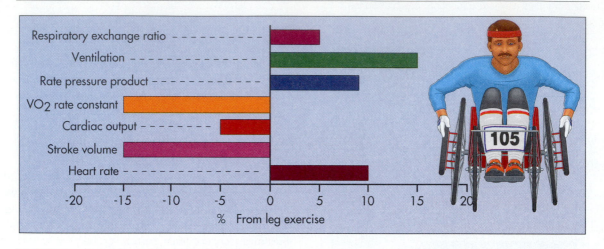

FIGURE 11.20

Differences between the cardiovascular responses to upper body and lower body exercise requiring a similar submaximal VO$_2$. (Data from Pendergast DR: Cardiovascular, respiratory, and metabolic responses to upper body exercise, *Med Sci Sports Exerc* 21(5):S121-S125, 1989.)

sure (approximately 10 mm Hg) during even intense exercise. This is understandable given the proximity of the pulmonary vasculature to the heart, the large divergence and capillary network, and therefore the low resistance to flow that would exist even at high flow rates.

Upper body exercise. The cardiovascular responses to upper body dynamic exercise invoke a different heart rate, stroke volume, and blood pressure response compared with lower body dynamic exercise (see Figure 11.20). For a given submaximal steady state VO$_2$, heart rate, ventilation, and systemic blood pressures are higher during arm ergometry than during lower body exercise.[73,75,87] Cardiac output is similar and understandably stroke volume is lower. The higher blood pressures are because of the small muscle mass involved in arm exercise and the large lower body vasculature that remains undilated and provides resistance to peripheral circulation.[84] For a given submaximal exercise intensity expressed relative to heart rate, muscle blood flow is similar between upper and lower body exercise;[73] however, the VO$_2$ is lower because of a lower extraction of oxygen as indicated by the Δa-VO$_2$.[87]

For maximal exercise, upper body exercise has a 30% lower cardiac output, a slightly lower maximal heart rate, 30% to 40% lower stroke volumes, and ventilations that are 80% of lower body maximal values. Despite these differences, systemic blood pressures are similar.

Isometric exercise. Muscle blood flow, systemic blood pressures, and central cardiac function also differ between dynamic and static, or isometric, exercise. Sustained isometric contractions are characterized by increased vascular resistance within the exercised muscle mass. Furthermore, there is a

greater muscle afferent nerve feedback to the cardiovascular center of the medulla, providing added stimulation for blood flow redistribution, which in turn further increases peripheral vascular resistance. Sustained contraction at 20% maximal voluntary contraction (MVC) induced a rapid increase in both systolic and diastolic blood pressures, whereas the blood pressure response during dynamic exercise was dampened.[10]

When isometric exercise is performed, additional increases in blood pressure may also occur if the person attempts to exhale against a closed trachea. This maneuver is similar to a clinical procedure known as the *Valsalva maneuver,* in which subjects exhale at greatly increased airway pressures. The result is to increase thoracic pressures because of added muscular contraction of the muscles of expiration against a near constant lung volume. These pressures raise systemic diastolic blood pressure, lower stroke volumes, and make the heart work harder for a given cardiac output.

The intramuscular pressures of isometric contractions cause blood flow to be almost completely occluded at 30% MVC. Consequently, this form of exercise is very fatiguing for the local muscles, and after the contraction, dramatic *hyperemia* occurs because of the effects of the local regulators of blood flow on the local arteriolar and capillary vasculature.

Blood

A known acute effect of exercise on blood is to cause a release of fluid from the vascular compartment, which decreases the volume of plasma and blood. This fluid loss from the plasma decreases plasma volume and causes the hematocrit and plasma metabolite concentrations to increase, which is termed **hemoconcentration.** In fact, a significant hemoconcentration occurs when a person moves from a

FIGURE 11.21

A, The increased hemoconcentration during changes in posture and exercise intensity. Hemoconcentration can be detected by measuring changes in serum protein, blood hemoglobin and hematocrit, or measuring or estimating changes in plasma volume. **B,** The changes in plasma volume, hematocrit, and hemoglobin concentration during endurance exercise training. The increased expansion of the plasma volume can decrease hematocrit and hemoglobin, even though total red cell and total hemoglobin masses also increase with training.

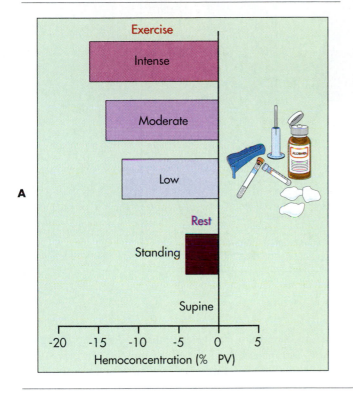

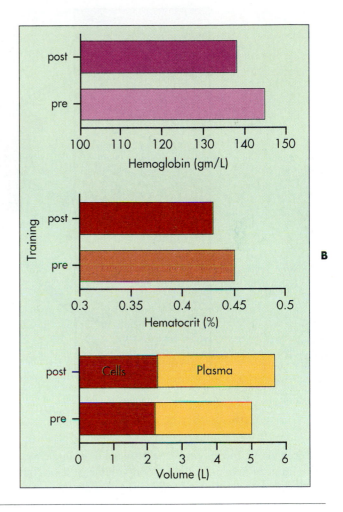

supine to a vertical position. Furthermore, the added hemoconcentration of exercise is predominantly confined to the transition from rest to exercise.[15,33,43,69,77] This response is followed by a more gradual hemoconcentration that occurs with increases in exercise intensity (Figure 11.21), and these changes are larger during the larger blood pressures associated with resistance exercise than during more prolonged dynamic exercise.

As discussed in Chapter 29, prolonged exercise involving sweating increases fluid loss from the body, and the degree of hemoconcentration can be measured by either directly measuring plasma volume or estimating relative changes in plasma volume from hemoglobin and hematocrit measurements.[24]

Apart from the hemoconcentration of exercise, additional acute changes occur in blood. Blood viscosity increases above what would be expected for hemoconcentration effects, which indicates that plasma viscosity also increases.[69] In addition, during prolonged exercise there is a destruction

of erythrocytes, termed **hemolysis,** which increases plasma hemoglobin concentrations. However, even during exercise that lasts for several hours the number of erythrocytes that are destroyed is negligible and does not significantly decrease oxygen transport capacities of the blood.[116]

Peripheral Blood Flow

The finite blood volume of the body and limited increase in cardiac output present potential limitations to

hemoconcentration (he'mo-kon'sen-tra'shun)
increased hematocrit resulting from the loss of plasma volume

hemolysis (he-mol'i-sis)
destruction of red blood cells causing the release of hemoglobin into solution

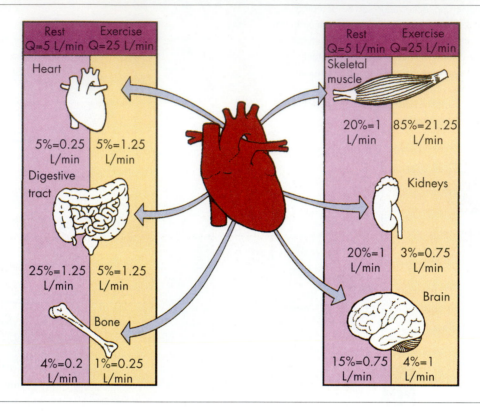

FIGURE 11.22

The distribution of cardiac output to the main tissues of the body during rest and exercise conditions.

increased blood flow to peripheral tissues. For example, a cardiac output of 5 L/min and a blood volume of 5 L require the complete recirculation of the entire blood volume every minute. During exercise, cardiac output may increase to 30 L/min, and the blood volume must be recirculated six times per minute. When compared with the potential twentyfold increase in demand for oxygen during exercise, the sevenfold potential increase in blood flow appears meager.

We can tolerate the increased metabolic demand of intense exercise because the systemic circulation is regulated to redistribute blood flow to the more metabolically active skeletal muscle tissue. In addition, the acute metabolic adaptations that occur in skeletal muscle result in an increased extraction of oxygen from the capillary blood, causing an increased Δa-VO$_2$.

Blood Flow Redistribution

Figure 11.22 compares the relative contribution of the cardiac output with the main tissue beds of the body during rest and exercise conditions. During exercise the vasoconstriction of arterioles supplying the brain, gut, and kidney reduces the percent of the cardiac output that perfuses these tissues. The result is that an increasing percentage of total blood flow is directed to the working skeletal muscle. Con-

sequently, blood flow to skeletal muscle (assuming 20 kg of muscle) can increase from 50 ml/kg muscle/min, representing 15% to 20% of cardiac output at rest, to over 1000 ml/kg/min, which represents 80% of maximal cardiac output. Furthermore, during exercise maximal muscle blood flow to a smaller muscle mass has been measured at over 2000 ml/kg/min.[6]

The redistribution of blood flow is regulated by both neural and local controls of vascular vasoconstriction. The arterioles supplying the splanchnic, renal, and cranial circulations constrict from α-adrenergic stimulation, whereas skeletal muscle blood flow increases by a general β-adrenergic stimulation, as well as local mediators such as potassium, adenosine, lowered PaO$_2$, increased PaCO$_2$ and temperature and as yet unknown substances released from the vascular endothelium.[147,75,98,102] Discussion of blood flow to the cutaneous circulation is provided in a subsequent section.

Peripheral Artery and Skeletal Muscle Blood Flow

As with cardiac output, blood flow in peripheral arteries and muscle increases linearly with increases in exercise intensity (Figure 11.23, *A*). However, this response should not be interpreted to indicate a uniform flow to skeletal muscle or uniform perfusion of the entire skeletal muscle mass. Animal

A, The linear increase in peripheral blood flow during increases in exercise. **B,** However, when blood flow is measured by Doppler flowmetry during dynamic wrist flexion exercise, an uneven blood flow to skeletal muscle is evident. Beat to beat variation in the volume of blood pumped to contracting muscle is dependent on the phase of the contraction cycle: rest, concentric contraction, eccentric contraction. It is clear that as exercise intensity increases, the amount of blood able to flow to the muscle is dramatically reduced during the concentric phase of the contraction because of an increase in intramuscular pressure. Conversely, during the recovery phases there is an exaggerated increase in blood flow, or hyperemia.

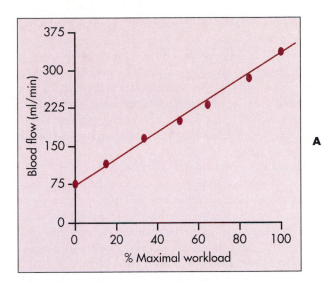

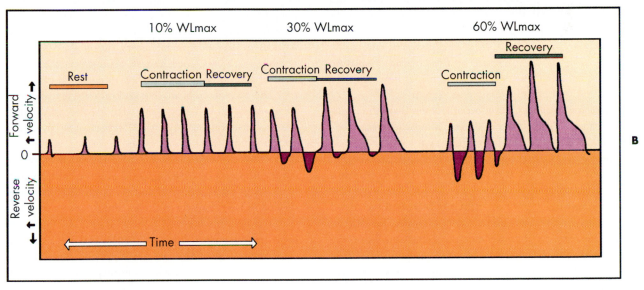

research has identified a marked blood flow heterogeneity in contracting skeletal muscle, resulting in regions that are over-perfused and underperfused.[46] This inequality can result in regions of the muscle that do not receive adequate oxygenation and may compromise muscle metabolism. As a result of methodologic constraints, it is unclear whether this nonuniform perfusion occurs in human muscle.

Variation in blood flow during contractions has been documented in humans. Walloe et al[125] reported that intense muscle contractions compress the vasculature within the muscle, causing a reduction in blood flow immediately followed by increased flow, termed **hyperemia,** during muscle relaxation. Similar findings have been reported from dynamic exercise of the forearm musculature[94] (see Figure 11.23, *B*), and show that blood flow to muscle is influenced by the contracting muscle. During the concentric contraction phase, blood flow is impeded by the intramuscular pressures of contraction. This impedance occurs as early as 20% of the maxi-

mal incremental workload, becomes more severe as exercise intensity increases, and causes reverse flow at higher intensities. Despite this response, average blood flow still increases with workload because of the hyperemia that occurs during muscle relaxation. The influence of this temporal pattern of blood flow to muscle metabolism has not been determined.

Increased Oxygen Extraction

As indicated in Chapters 10 and 12, under resting conditions blood flow from the central arterial to central venous circulation causes a reduction in the partial pressure of oxy-

hyperemia (hi-per-e'mi-ah)
increased blood flow above normal; usually expressed relative to a particular tissue

gen in the blood from 100 mm Hg to 40 mm Hg. Use of the oxyhemoglobin dissociation curve reveals that such a pressure difference would amount to a 50 ml/L change in oxygen content (200 to 150 ml O_2/L blood), which is the arterial to mixed venous difference in oxygen content (Δa-$\dot{v}O_2$). During maximal exercise the Δa-$\dot{v}O_2$ is used to reflect the added uptake of oxygen by the skeletal muscle and can increase to over 150 ml/L during running and cycling in highly trained endurance athletes.

The use of central blood volume measures of the concentration of arterial oxygen (CaO_2) and mixed venous oxygen ($C\dot{v}O_2$) can be misleading. For example, the previously identified central blood volume values for Δa-$\dot{v}O_2$ indicate that the body is unable to extract all the oxygen from the blood. This is not true for the localized microvasculature, where muscle PO_2 values have been estimated to be as low as 2 mm Hg.[67,109,117] If equilibration between capillary and tissue PO_2 is assumed, these values indicate an almost complete uptake of oxygen from the capillary circulation. Why is there such a high value for $C\dot{v}O_2$? The answer is due to the combination of blood returning to the central vasculature from nonactive tissues, as well as to the spatial heterogeneity in blood flow within the exercised muscle mass.[46,88]

The near complete extraction of oxygen from the capillary circulation within muscle during intense exercise provides further evidence of the high capacity of the muscle fibers for oxygen extraction. Central circulation and oxygen provision to the muscles are the limiting factors to maximal oxygen consumption. In fact, research that has artificially increased blood flow[8,9,13,14] or artificially increased red blood cell numbers in the circulation (erythrocythemia) has shown that the capacity to increase oxygen extraction from the blood increases,[116] which is why blood doping and injections of erythropoietin to stimulate polycythemia work and are banned in athletic events (see Chapters 18 and 22).

Cutaneous Circulation

The adjustments to skin (cutaneous) blood flow during exercise in a cool environment (see Chapter 26 for exercise in a hot environment) are integral components of the body's ability to dissipate heat to the surroundings. Unlike the splanchnic, renal, and portal circulations that vasoconstrict during exercise, the start of exercise initially induces an adrenergic vasoconstriction of the skin, which is followed by a sympathetic cholinergic vasodilation.[54,55,56] This response is characteristic of dynamic exercise, since static exercise is known to immediately induce a vasodilation of the skin.[57] During dynamic exercise the vasodilation occurs after the core temperature of the body, and therefore arterial blood temperature, increases.[57] This response is believed to be controlled by the hypothalamus, as well as the release of metabolites from the active muscle mass.[57]

Skin blood flow is also known to depend on exercise intensity.[57,87] During incremental exercise, skin blood flow decreases as exercise intensity increases above approximately 80% VO_2max. This response is interpreted to result from the

increasing circulating catecholamines in the blood at high exercise intensities[57] and from increasing systemic blood pressures that further stimulate the baroreceptors, causing an inhibition of the cholinergic vasodilator response.[54,55,56] The net functional result of this changing skin blood flow is to redistribute blood flow to favor the skeletal muscle.

Is There a Blood Flow Limitation to Contracting Skeletal Muscle?

The reduction in skin blood flow during increasing exercise intensities raises the question of whether the body's blood flow redistribution is adequate to maximally perfuse skeletal muscle. Numerous research findings using animal and human models support this interpretation.

Increasing the rate of perfusion (blood flow) through in vitro muscle preparations is known to increase VO_2 and decrease muscle fatigue during intense intermittent muscle contractions.[8,9,13,14] Furthermore, in humans, isolation of exercise to a muscle group (single leg extension exercise) induces greater peripheral artery blood flow than exercise involving the same muscle mass with simultaneous contractions of additional muscle, such as two-legged cycle ergometry.[6] These results indicate that skeletal muscle tissue is capable of receiving more blood flow than can be provided during exercise involving a large muscle mass. The overwhelming interpretation of the previously described research is that blood flow through skeletal muscle is limited more by limitations imposed by a finite blood volume and limitations to increases in cardiac output and its maximal redistribution to skeletal muscle than the muscles' abilities to extract oxygen.

The reason for blood flow limitation during exercise of large muscle masses has been explained by a sympathetic vasoconstriction of the arteries supplying the active skeletal muscle.[4,27,51,70,85] However, additional factors such as the hemodynamic changes caused by blood vessel compression during intense muscle contractions also compromise blood flow. For example, Walloe et al[125] demonstrated that dynamic contractions of the quadriceps muscles when performed at 10% to 30% of the maximal voluntary contraction (MVC) can occlude blood flow in the femoral artery. Roberts et al[94] extended these findings to show that dynamic contractions of the wrist extensor muscles of the forearm can impair brachial artery blood flow at intensities as low as 5% MVC (or 50% of the maximal incremental workload). Consequently, blood flow to skeletal muscle is not only pulsatile because of the cardiac cycle, but also during exercise the pulsatile flow is exaggerated by changing intramuscular pressures and compression of blood vessels during a contraction cycle (see Figure 11.23, B).

A Summary of Cardiovascular Adaptation to Exercise

Figure 11.24 summarizes the acute responses of the cardiovascular system to exercise. Once again the Fick equation is used to differentiate the components responsible for

FIGURE 11.24

A summary of the acute cardiovascular adaptations that combine to increase oxygen consumption during exercise.

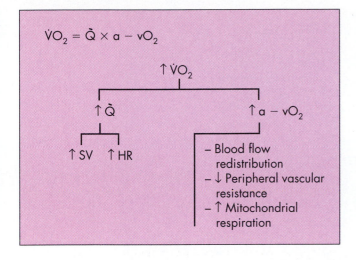

FIGURE 11.25

Data from a cross-sectional evaluation of elite athletes, indicating that the cardiac mass index (CMI) was larger in athletes involved in more endurance type activities.

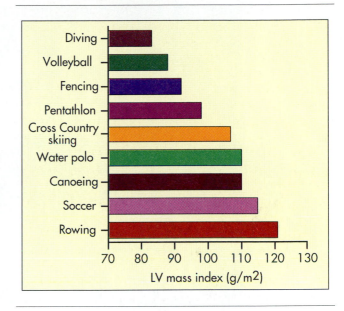

increasing VO_2 at the systemic level, as well as the peripheral level of function.

Systemic function of the cardiovascular system is based on the neural and humoral regulation of heart rate and ventricular contractility. In the periphery, blood flow is determined not only by the increase in cardiac output, but also by redistribution of cardiac output and the local regulators of blood flow (**autoregulation**). The combined effects of local and central regulation of cardiovascular function are crucial for the body to increase tolerance of exercise stress.

Chronic Adaptations to Exercise

Prolonged and repeated exposures to exercise cause structural and functional changes in the cardiovascular system. The extent of these changes is dependent on the type and quality of exercise training and is known to differ between training for long-term endurance and training for short-term muscular endurance, strength, and power. The following description of chronic training adaptations is organized principally by the type of exercise training and by the component of the cardiovascular system.

Comment must also be made on the influence of genetics to cardiovascular capacities and adaptability. Research that compares two or more groups that differ in training status (cross-sectional studies) is biased by potential genetic differences that have caused individuals to select certain exercise modes and intensities. Conversely, research that measures changes in cardiovascular parameters in individuals exposed to training (experimental) is more likely to focus on training-induced adaptation. However, these training studies are relatively short term, lasting for several weeks or months rather than several years, and therefore the full potential of cardio-

vascular adaptation to exercise alone remains unclear. Where appropriate, clarification is given as to whether research findings are from cross-sectional or experimental studies.

Adaptations from Training for Long-Term Endurance

Cardiac Structure and Function

Data from cross-sectional evaluations of cardiac dimensions and capacities indicate that heart dimensions and end-diastolic volumes are greater in endurance athletes than athletes involved in activities of a short duration[86] (Figure 11.25). This information has developed the notion of an *athletic heart* that is larger than the heart of a sedentary individual. Endurance training has also been shown to elicit increases in cardiac mass and function in previously sedentary individuals.[21] The end-diastolic volume of the left ventricle (LVEDV) increases after 9 weeks of endurance training in males, and similar responses have been shown in females.[103] These adaptations occur rapidly; increased measures of ventricular dimensions have been reported after as little as 1 week of endurance training, whereas myocardial mass responds more slowly.[26] As discussed in the following mater-

autoregulation (aw'to-**reg**-u-la'shun)
the ability of a tissue bed to retain near normal blood flow despite changes in systemic blood pressure

FIGURE 11.26

A summary of the chronic adaptations of the cardiovascular system after exposure to training for long-term endurance. Adaptations are related to their effects during both maximal and submaximal exercise.

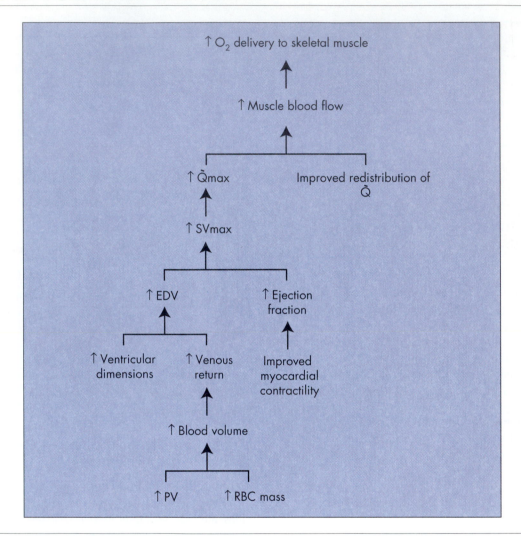

ial, the rapidity of the increase in cardiac dimensions is due primarily to a rapid increase in plasma and blood volume.[33,43]

The larger LVEDV after endurance training is associated with an increased stroke volume and decreased heart rate for a given submaximal exercise intensity. Contradictory information exists as to whether these stroke volume and heart rate responses are cause-and-effect.[18] For example, at rest the lower heart rate is also accompanied by increased parasympathetic innervation of the heart and reductions in resting and exercise heart rates have been documented without increases in stroke volume.[18] It is logical to interpret the research findings as evidence for combined increases in stroke volume and parasympathetic innervation as the causes of the lower heart rates after training.

Blood

Endurance training increases the volume of plasma in blood. Simultaneous increases in red blood cell counts and hemoglobin also occur, but their concentration relative to the volume of blood decreases because of the diluting effect of the relatively larger increases in plasma volume (see Figure 11.21, *B*).

The increase in plasma volume is known to occur without a large training stimulus. For example, Gillen et al[33] reported that just one session of intense intermittent cycle ergometry exercise performed at 85% VO_2max induced a 10% increase in plasma volume after 24 hours. This chronic increase was predominantly a result of an increase in plasma albumin. The time course of further change in plasma volume during a training program is unknown; however, maximal training-induced increases in plasma volume have been reported between 300 and 800 ml.[22,33,43]

The benefits of an increased plasma volume have been documented in studies that have artificially increased plasma volume by either saline infusion or an increase in the osmolality of blood (e.g., dextran infusion), thereby retaining more fluid in the vascular space. These studies have shown that an increased plasma volume increases venous return to the heart, increases ventricular preload, and thereby increases stroke volume for a given exercise intensity.[22,43] The increased plasma volume also has thermoregulatory benefits, as detailed in Chapter 26.

During detraining the loss of plasma volume is also rapid and accounts for the swift reversal of central cardiac function improvements (increased stroke volume and maximal cardiac output) that accompany the endurance-trained state.[22,26]

Skeletal Muscle Circulation

In Chapter 9, comment was given to the increase in capillary density that occurs after endurance training. Anderson and Henriksson[5] performed histologic studies and muscle biopsy tissue sectioning before and after training and revealed a 20% increase in capillary density that was consistent between the different fiber types and occurred in combination with a 16% increase in VO_2max and a 40% increase in select mitochondrial enzyme activities. Increased capillary density would increase maximal muscle blood flow capacities, decrease perfusion heterogeneity, and prolong the *capillary transit time*. The latter two responses are probably the more meaningful, since increased oxygen extraction is known to occur after training even when maximal cardiac output is not increased.[18]

A Summary of the Benefit of Cardiovascular Adaptations to Endurance Training

The chronic cardiovascular adaptations to endurance training benefit both maximal and submaximal exercise performance (Figure 11.26). Maximal exercise performance results from an improvement in VO_2max, whereas submaximal improvement results from a combined lowering of the relative intensity of given absolute intensities, as well as the raising of the lactate threshold as explained in Chapter 8.

SUMMARY

■ Anatomic and functional aspects of the heart are referred to as **cardiac,** whereas anatomic and functional aspects of the circulation of blood through the body are referred to as **vascular,** hence the term *cardiovascular.* The heart, blood, and blood vessels of the body constitute the **cardiovascular system.**

■ **Blood** is the liquid medium that circulates within the vascular system. Blood can be divided into cellular and noncellular components and functions to transport gases, aid immune function, transfer heat, and distribute water, nutrients, and wastes throughout the body. The cell content of blood constitutes approximately 45% of the total blood volume, and this measure is termed **hematocrit.** Blood cells are all derived from a stem cell, that differentiates into precursors of white blood cells *(leukocytes),* red blood cells **(erythrocytes),** or cell fragments known as *platelets.*

■ Molecules of hemoglobin are located on the membrane surface of erythrocytes and function by transporting oxygen and carbon dioxide and buffering protons. Erythrocytes have an average life span of 120 days. The iron from hemoglobin of the destroyed erythrocytes is recycled by the liver, and along with the nutritional intake of iron, is transported in the blood bound to **transferrin** (iron-binding globulin). Iron can be stored in plasma and certain tissues (heart, liver, spleen) as **ferritin,** which is a complex of water-soluble protein and reduced iron (ferrous hydroxide). An increased production of erythrocytes can result in elevated red blood cell counts, a condition termed **polycythemia.** Conversely, an inadequate iron intake, excessive bleeding, or exaggerated erythrocyte destruction can result in a lowered red blood cell count, or **anemia.**

■ The liquid component of blood is termed *plasma.* When blood is drawn from the body, the clotting process forms fibrinogen and the remaining fluid component of blood is termed *serum.* Since plasma represents 55% of total blood volume (1.0−0.45 [hematocrit] = 0.55), it approximates a volume of 3 L. Plasma contains many molecules and electrolytes. The number of molecules per kg of plasma is termed **osmolality,** and approximates 300 mOsm/kg H_2O.

■ The healthy heart can generate average circulation pressures that increase from 90 to over 140 mm Hg without signs or symptoms of impaired function. Blood returns to the right atrium of the heart via the superior and inferior venae cavae, passes into the right ventricle through the tricuspid valve, and is pumped by the right ventricle through the pulmonary valve into the **pulmonary circulation** where it returns to the left atrium. The blood then passes through the mitral valve into the left ventricle, where it is pumped through the aorta to the circulation of the remainder of body, or **systemic circulation.** The right and left sides of the heart contract and pump blood together, resulting in a closed loop circulation.

■ The movement of blood through the heart and vasculature is referred to as the **cardiac cycle.** During the phase of the cardiac cycle when the myocardium is relaxed, termed *diastole,* blood flows passively into the right and left atria and then into the respective ventricles. The atrial contraction, termed *atrial systole* (or *atrial kick*), contributes an extra 30% of total ventricular filling. The volume of blood in each ventricle is referred to as *end-diastolic volume* (EDV) and exerts a stretch on the ventricular myocardium. This stretch can be interpreted as a load and is known as **preload** in clinical cardiology and cardiac rehabilitation. The greater the EDV and the greater the stretch, the faster the resultant ventricular myocardial contraction. This is denoted as the *Frank-Starling law* of the heart. The velocity of myocardial contraction for a given EDV, termed *contractility,* increases with increased sympathetic stimulation.

■ Action potentials spread rapidly throughout the ventricular myocardium because of the diffuse presence of specialized low-resistance conducting tissue, termed **intercalated discs.** Blood is ejected from the ventricles during ventricular contraction, or *ventricular systole.* Ejection actually occurs when the ventricular myocardium generates ventricular pressures that exceed arterial pressures, which causes a short time interval where contraction is occurring but no blood is ejected *(isovolumetric contraction).* For the right ventricle the pulmonary arterial pressure before ventricular systole (or *end diastole*) approximates 8 mm Hg, whereas the end diastolic pressure of the aorta artery approximates 80 mm Hg. These end diastolic pressures are also termed the **afterload.**

SUMMARY—Cont'd

■ During ventricular systole, not all blood is ejected from each ventricle. The volume of blood pumped from each ventricle per beat is termed **stroke volume** and when expressed relative to the EDV is known as the **ejection fraction.** The ejection fraction for a healthy heart at rest approximates 0.6, or 60%. The product of stroke volume and heart rate quantifies the volume of blood pumped by the heart per unit time and is referred to as **cardiac output** (Q). A useful application of cardiac output and arterial and central venous concentrations of oxygen is in the calculation of oxygen consumption using the Fick equation: VO_2 ml/min $= Q$(L/min) $\times \Delta a - \dot{v}O_2$ (ml/L)

■ The branch of physics that concerns the dynamics of fluid flow is termed *hydrodynamics,* and when the fluid is blood the subdiscipline is termed **hemodynamics.** The law that applies to the laminar flow of fluid through cylindrical tubes is Poiseuille's law: $Q = \pi(Pi - Po)\ r^4/8\eta l$. The greater the pressure gradient, the larger the radius, and the lower the viscosity and length of the vessel, the greater the flow. For the systemic circulation, where arteries are longer, a greater pressure difference is required to maintain a given flow. When the radius is decreased, such as during vasoconstriction, this has a large influence on decreasing flow because of the fourth power function. These facts partially explain the larger systemic blood pressures compared with the pulmonary blood pressures.

■ Ohm's law, which was devised to explain the relationships between electrical resistance, voltage changes, and current flow ($R = V_{ab}/I$), can be applied to the cardiovascular system by rearranging Poiseuille's law: $R = [(Pi - Po)\ /\ Q] = 8\eta l\ /\ \pi r^4$. Thus, when the assumptions of Poiseuille's law apply, for a given blood flow the resistance along a vessel is increased by larger changes in pressure. Interestingly, this relationship can be applied to the total systemic arterial circulation, where *Q* represents cardiac output, *MAP* represents mean arterial blood pressure, and *PVR* represents peripheral vascular resistance: PVR = MAP/Q or Q = MAP/PVR.

■ For a given vessel that diverges into vessels having one-fourth the diameter of the original vessel, four times the total cross-sectional area is needed to match the resistance of the single large vessel. Thus the tremendous increase in cross-sectional area (increased number of vessels) from the arterioles to the capillaries is sufficient to overcome the increased resistance from divergence to smaller diameter vessels.

■ The artery has the thickest wall and the greatest ability to stretch and then recoil to its original dimension, a property termed *elasticity.* Conversely, arteries have a limited ability to be distended and increase their vascular volume, a property termed **compliance.** Arterioles possess properties similar to arteries but in addition can be surrounded circumferentially by layers of smooth muscle fibers. Contraction of smooth muscle surrounding an arteriole decreases the diameter of the lumen, increases resistance to blood flow, and thereby decreases flow, a process termed **vasoconstriction.** Conversely, smooth muscle relaxation around an arteriole increases the diameter, decreases resistance, and increases blood flow, a process termed **vasodilation.**

■ Capillaries are the smallest diameter blood vessels and possess a wall composed of a single cell layer. Some arteriole to capillary junctions are also surrounded by a layer of smooth muscle and function to regulate blood flow through a capillary bed: such structures are termed **precapillary sphincters.** The walls of venules and veins are not as thick as those of the arteries or arterioles and do not have high elasticity, but do have high compliance. Veins are also surrounded by smooth muscle, which because of the *compliance* of the venous circulation, functions to regulate the cross-sectional dimensions of the veins and therefore the volume of blood in the venous circulation. Venous blood volume is also increased by contracting skeletal muscle that functions as a **muscle pump** to propel blood in veins through the one-way valves back to the heart.

■ There are two main types of regulation of heart function: regulation that affects heart rate, known as **chronotropic** regulation, and regulation that affects the velocity of myocardial contraction *(contractility),* known as **inotropic** regulation. The start of exercise stimulates both chronotropic and inotropic regulation, resulting not only in increased heart rates, but also in improved abilities of the myocardium and heart to function as a pump. Inotropic regulation concerns changes in the velocity of contraction, or *contractility.* Increased contractility results from the sympathetic neural and hormonal stimulation of the ventricular myocardium.

SUMMARY—Cont'd

■ Not all exercise elicits the same cardiac response. Dynamic exercise induces increases in heart rate, stroke volume, cardiac output, and blood pressures that differ from isometric exercise. Similarly, dynamic upper body exercise, which involves a smaller muscle mass than the dynamic exercise of the larger muscles of the legs, also elicits a slightly different cardiac response. The onset of exercise is associated with near simultaneous sympathetic stimulation of the SA node, AV node, and ventricular myocardium. In addition, the contraction of skeletal muscle induces an increase in venous return, and these factors combine to increase heart rate and myocardial contractility.

■ The increasing venous return and sympathetic myocardial stimulation during exercise induce an increased end diastolic volume, which for a given ejection fraction increases stroke volume. Stroke volume increases as exercise intensity increases from rest to approximately 50% VO_2max in relatively untrained individuals, and thereafter plateaus. In trained individuals, stroke volume continues to increase to VO_2max. These responses are typical only for exercise performed in the vertical position. Research conducted on individuals exercising in a recumbent or supine position has shown that maximal stroke volumes are attained at the onset of exercise, presumably because of the lack of hydrostatic pressures that resist venous return to the heart.

■ Mean blood pressure is not the average of systolic and diastolic blood pressures, since the durations of systole and diastole differ. At rest, mean arterial blood pressure (MAP) is estimated from the calculation $MAP = DBP + [(SBP - DBP)/3]$. This calculation is based on the duration of diastole being approximately three times that of systole. During exercise, systolic and mean pressures increase, whereas diastolic pressure remains close to or slightly less than resting values (<80 mm Hg).

■ The cardiovascular responses to upper body dynamic exercise invoke a different heart rate, stroke volume, and blood pressure response compared with lower body dynamic exercise. For a given submaximal steady state VO_2, heart rate, ventilation, and systemic blood pressures are higher during arm ergometry than lower body exercise. Cardiac output is similar, and understandably stroke volume is lower. For maximal exercise, upper body exercise has a 30% lower cardiac output, a slightly lower maximal heart rate, 30% to 40% lower stroke volumes, and ventilations that are 80% of lower body maximal values. Despite these differences, systemic blood pressures are similar.

■ Sustained isometric contractions are characterized by increased vascular resistance within the exercised muscle mass. When isometric exercise is performed, additional increases in blood pressure may also occur if the person attempts to exhale against a closed trachea. The result of this is to increase thoracic pressures because of the added muscular contraction of the muscles of expiration against a near constant lung volume, which in turn raises systemic diastolic blood pressure, lowers stroke volumes, and makes the heart work harder for a given cardiac output.

■ A known acute effect of exercise on blood is to cause a release of fluid from the vascular compartment, which decreases the volume of plasma and blood. This fluid loss from the plasma decreases plasma volume and causes the hematocrit and plasma metabolite concentrations to increase, which is termed **hemoconcentration.** During prolonged exercise there is also a destruction of erythrocytes, termed **hemolysis.**

■ We can tolerate the increased metabolic demand of intense exercise because the systemic circulation is regulated to redistribute blood flow to the more metabolically active skeletal muscle tissue. In addition, the acute metabolic adaptations that occur in skeletal muscle result in an increased extraction of oxygen from the capillary blood, causing an increased Δa-$\dot{v}O_2$.

■ The redistribution of blood flow is regulated by both neural and local controls of vascular vasoconstriction. The arterioles supplying the splanchnic, renal, and cranial circulations consist from α-adrenergic stimulation, whereas skeletal muscle blood flow increases **(hyperemia)** by a general β-adrenergic stimulation as well as local mediators such as potassium, adenosine, lowered PaO_2, increased $PaCO_2$ and temperature and as yet unknown substances released from the vascular endothelium. The ability of tissues to regulate their own blood flow is termed **autoregulation.**

SUMMARY—Cont'd

■ As with cardiac output, peripheral artery and muscle blood flow increases linearly with increases in exercise intensity. However, animal research has identified a marked blood flow heterogeneity in contracting skeletal muscle, resulting in regions that are overperfused and underperfused, and variation in blood flow during contractions has also been documented in humans.

■ Heart dimensions and end-diastolic volumes are greater in endurance athletes than in athletes involved in activities of a short duration. This information has led to the notion of an *athletic heart* that is larger than the heart of a sedentary individual. Endurance training has also been shown to elicit increases in cardiac mass and function in previously sedentary individuals. The larger LVEDV after endurance training is associated with an increased stroke volume and decreased heart rate for a given submaximal exercise intensity. Contradictory information exists as to whether these stroke volume and heart rate responses are cause-and-effect.

■ Endurance training increases the volume of plasma in blood. Simultaneous increases in red blood cell counts and hemoglobin also occur, but their concentration relative to the volume of blood decreases because of the diluting effect of the relatively larger increases in plasma volume. This chronic increase is due predominantly to an increase in plasma albumin. The time course of further change in plasma volume during a training program is unknown; however, maximal training-induced increases in plasma volume have been reported between 300 and 800 ml.

REVIEW QUESTIONS

1. Why is the work of the myocardium less for the right ventricle than the left ventricle?

2. What are normal values for blood volume, plasma volume, hemoglobin concentration, and hematocrit? How do these values change with endurance training?

3. What has recent research revealed about the functions of the endothelial lining of blood vessels?

4. Explain the techniques of echocardiography and Doppler flowmetry. How are these techniques used in exercise-related research?

5. Explain the regulation of heart function based on chronotropic and inotropic regulation.

6. How do heart rate, stroke volume, and cardiac output change during incremental exercise to VO_2max? Are responses different after endurance training? If so, how?

7. Explain the different cardiovascular responses between exercise performed with the upper body, compared with lower body exercise.

8. Why is the body's ability to redistribute blood flow (cardiac output) important for exercise tolerance?

9. Is blood flow to skeletal muscle constant during all types of exercise and exercise intensities? What implications might these blood flow profiles have on muscle energy metabolism?

10. Is there a blood flow limitation to contracting skeletal muscle in humans during increasing exercise intensities to VO_2max?

11. List all the improvements in cardiovascular function after endurance training, and organize these to reveal potential cause-effect relationships to VO_2max.

APPLICATIONS

1. Heart failure is characterized by a dramatic decrease in myocardial contractility for a given end-diastolic volume. What symptoms might this central cardiovascular failure have on muscle metabolism during exercise?

2. How would β_1-blockade affect heart function at rest and during exercise?

3. How could echocardiography be used to determine whether heart function has improved after endurance training?

4. Why is the catecholamine response to exercise more important for individuals who have undergone heart transplantation?

5. Explain the importance of the sympathetic regulation of blood vessel tone during exercise for regulating blood flow redistribution and maximizing muscle blood flow.

6. What is a cardiovascular problem for individuals with spinal cord injury, especially during exercise in the vertical position? How could the impact of this problem be decreased?

7. How could the chronic adaptations of the central cardiovascular system help individuals recovering from myocardial infarct?

REFERENCES

1. Adams KF Jr, McAllister SM, El-Ashmawy H et al: Interrelationships between left ventricular volume and output during exercise in healthy subjects, *J Appl Physiol* 73(5):2097-2104, 1992.

2. Adams TD, Yanowitz FG, Fisher AG et al: Heritability of cardiac size: an echocardiographic and electrocardiographic study of monozygotic and dizygotic twins, *Circulation* 71(1):39-44, 1985.

3. Ahlborg G, Jensen-Urstad M: Arm blood flow at rest and during arm exercise, *J Appl Physiol* 70(2):928-933, 1991.

4. Anderson EA, Mark AL: Flow-mediated reflex changes in large peripheral artery tone in humans, *Circulation* 79:93-100, 1989.

5. Anderson P, Henriksson J: Capillary supply of the quadriceps femoris muscle of man: adaptive response to exercise, *J Physiol* 270:677-690, 1977.

6. Anderson P, Saltin B: Maximal perfusion of skeletal muscle in man, *J Physiol* 366:233-249, 1985.

7. Balaban EP, Cox JV, Snell P et al: The frequency of anemia and iron deficiency in the runner, *Med Sci Sports Exerc* 21(6):643-648, 1989.

8. Barklay JK: A delivery-independent blood flow effect on skeletal muscle fatigue, *J Appl Physiol* 61(3):1084-1090, 1986.

9. Barklay JK, Stainsby WN: The role of blood flow in limiting maximal metabolic rate in muscle, *Med Sci Sports Exerc* 7(2):116-119, 1975.

10. Beglund B, Birgegard G, Hemmingsson P: Serum erythropoietin in cross-country skiers, *Med Sci Sports Exerc* 20(2):208-209, 1988.

11. Berne RM, Levy MN: *Physiology*, ed 3, St. Louis, 1993, Mosby.

12. Bers D: Calcium regulation in cardiac muscle, *Med Sci Sports Exerc* 23(10):1157-1162, 1991.

13. Brechue WF, Ameredes BT, Andrew GM, Stainsby WN: Blood flow elevation increases VO_2 maximum during repetitive tetanic contraction of dog muscle in situ, *J Appl Physiol* 74(4):1499-1503, 1993.

14. Brechue WF, Barklay JK, O'Drobinak DM, Stainsby WN: Difference between VO_2 maxima of twitch and tetanic contractions are related to blood flow, *J Appl Physiol* 71(1):131-135, 1991.

15. Burge CM, Carey MF, Payne WR: Rowing performance, fluid balance, and metabolic function following dehydration and rehydration, *Med Sci Sports Exerc* 25(12):1358-1364, 1993.

16. Burton HW, Barclay JK: Metabolic factors from exercising muscle and the proliferation of endothelial cells, *Med Sci Sports Exerc* 18(4):390-395, 1986.

17. Celsing F, Nystrom J, Pihlsted P et al: Effect of long term anemia and retransfusion on central circulation during exercise, *J Appl Physiol* 61(4):1358-1362, 1986.

REFERENCES—Cont'd

18. Clausen JP: Effect of physical training on cardiovascular adjustments to exercise in man, *Physiol Rev* 57(4):779-815, 1977.

19. Clausen JP, Lassen NA: Muscle blood flow during exercise in normal man studied by the [133]Xenon clearance method, *Cardiovascular Res* 5:245-254, 1971.

20. Cowley A: Long-term control of arterial blood pressure, *Physiol Rev* 72:231-300, 1992.

21. Cox ML, Bennett III JB, Dudley GA: Exercise training-induced alterations of cardiac morphology, *J Appl Physiol* 61(3):926-931, 1986.

22. Coyle EF, Hemmert MK, Coggan AR: Effects of detraining on cardiovascular responses to exercise: role of blood volume, *J Appl Physiol* 60(1):95-99, 1986.

23. Cullinane EM, Sady SP, Vadeboncoeur L et al: Cardiac size and VO_2max do not decrease after short-term exercise cessation, *Med Sci Sports Exerc* 18(4):420-424, 1986.

24. Dill DM, Costill DL: Calculation of percentage changes in volumes of blood, plasma, and red cells in dehydration, *J Appl Physiol* 37(2):247-248, 1974.

25. Dodd SL, Powers SK, Brooks E, Crawford MP: Effects of reduced O_2 delivery with anemia, hypoxia, or ischemia on peak VO_2 and force in skeletal muscle, *J Appl Physiol* 74(1):186-191, 1993.

26. Ehsani AA, Hagberg JM, Hickson RC: Rapid changes in left ventricular dimensions and mass in response to physical conditioning and deconditioning, *Am J Cardiol* 42:52-56, 1978.

27. Eldridge F, Millhorn DE, Kiley JP, Woldrup TG: Stimulation by central command locomotion, respiration, and circulation during exercise, *Respir Physiol* 59:313-337, 1985.

28. Eldrige MW, Alverson DC, Howard EA, Berman W: Pulsed Doppler ultrasound: principles and instrumentation. In Berman W, editor: *Pulsed Doppler ultrasound in clinical pediatrics,* New York, 1983, Futura.

29. Franklin BA: Aerobic exercise training programs for the upper body, *Med Sci Sports Exerc* 21(50):S141-S148, 1989.

30. Friedman DB, Peel C, Mitchell JH: Cardiovascular responses to voluntary and nonvoluntary static exercise in humans, *J Appl Physiol* 73(50):1982-1985, 1992.

31. Gaebelein CJ, Senay LC, Jr: Influence of exercise type, hydration, and heat on plasma volume shifts in men, *J Appl Physiol* 49(1):119-123, 1980.

32. Gangelhoff J, Cordain L, Tucker A, Sockler J: Metabolic and heart rate responses to submaximal arm lever and arm crank ergometry, *Arch Phys Med Rehab* 69:101-105, 1988.

33. Gillen CM, Lee R, Mack GW et al: Plasma volume expansion in humans after a single intense exercise protocol, *J Appl Physiol* 71(5):1914-1920, 1991.

34. Gledhill N: Blood doping and related issues: a brief review, *Med Sci Sports Exerc* 14(3):180-183, 1982.

35. Gledhill N, Cox D, Jamnik R: Endurance athlete's stroke volume does not plateau: major advantage is diastolic function, *Med Sci Sports Exerc* 26(9):1116-1121, 1994.

36. Gordon NF, Van Rensburg JP, Van Den Heever DP et al: Effect of dual β-blockade and calcium antagonism on endurance performance, *Med Sci Sports Exerc* 19(1):1-6, 1987.

37. Guyton AC: *Textbook of medical physiology,* ed 8, Philadelphia, 1991, WB Saunders.

38. Hainsworth R: Reflexes from the heart, *Physiol Rev* 71:617-658, 1991.

39. Hammond MD, Gale GE, Kapitan KS et al: Pulmonary gas exchange in humans during exercise at sea level, *J Appl Physiol* 60(5):1590-1598, 1986.

40. Hawley JA, Dennis SC, Laidler BJ et al: High rates of exogenous carbohydrate oxidation from starch ingested during prolonged exercise, *J Appl Physiol* 71(5):1801-1806, 1991.

41. Herd J: Physiological response to stress, *Physiol Rev* 71:305-330, 1991.

42. Hiatt WR, Huang SY, Regensteiner JG et al: Venous occlusion plethysmography reduces arterial diameter and flow velocity, *J Appl Physiol* 66(5):2239-2244, 1989.

43. Hopper MK, Coggan AR, Coyle EF: Exercise stroke volume relative to plasma-volume expansion, *J Appl Physiol* 64(1):404-408, 1988.

44. Hsieh SS, Freedson PS, Mroz MC, Stewart PM: Exercise intensity and erythrocyte 2,3-diphosphoglycerate concentration, *Med Sci Sports Exerc* 18(1):82-86, 1986.

45. Hughson RL: Failure of impedance plethysmography to follow exercise-induced changes in limb blood flow, *Clin Sci* 75:41-46, 1988.

46. Iversen PO, Standa M, Nicolaysen G: Marked regional heterogeneity in blood flow within a single skeletal muscle at rest and during exercise hyperaemia in the rabbit, *Acta Physiol Scand* 136:17-28, 1989.

47. Jaffee EA: Cell biology of endothelial cells, *Human Pathol* 18:234-239, 1987.

48. Jansson E, Sylven C, Arvidsson I, Eriksson E: Increase in myoglobin content and decrease in oxidative enzyme activities by leg muscle immobilization in man, *Acta Physiol Scand* 132:515-517, 1988.

REFERENCES—Cont'd

49. Jawad IA: *Practical guide to echocardiography and cardiac Doppler ultrasound,* Boston, 1990, Little, Brown.

50. Joyner MJ, Freund BJ, Jilka SM et al: Effects of β-blockade on exercise capacity of trained and untrained men: a hemodynamic comparison, *J Appl Physiol* 60(4):1429-1434, 1986.

51. Joyner MJ, Lennon RL, Wedel DJ et al: Blood flow to contracting muscles: influence of increased sympathetic activity, *J Appl Physiol* 68(4):1453-1457, 1990.

52. Kamath MV, Fallen EL, McKelvie R: Effects of steady state exercise on the power spectrum of heart rate variability, *Med Sci Sports Exerc* 23(4):428-434, 1991.

53. Kanstrup IL, Marving J, Hoilund-Carlsen PF: Acute plasma expansion: left ventricular hemodynamics and endocrine function during exercise, *J Appl Physiol* 73(50):1791-1796, 1992.

54. Kellog DL Jr, Johnson LM, Kosiba WA: Selective abolition of adrenergic vasoconstrictor responses in the skin by local iontophoresis of bretylium, *Am J Physiol* 257(26):H1599-H1606, 1989.

55. Kellog DL Jr, Johnson LM, Kosiba WA: Baroreflex control of the cutaneous active vasodilator system in humans, *Circ Res* 66:1420-1426, 1990.

56. Kellog DL Jr, Johnson LM, Kosiba WA: Competition between the cutaneous active vasoconstrictor and vasodilator systems during exercise in man, *Am J Physiol* 261(30):H1184-H1189, 1991.

57. Kenney WL, Johnson JM: Control of skin blood flow during exercise, *Med Sci Sports Exerc* 24(3):303-312, 1992.

58. Kenno KA, Durstine JL, Shepherd RE: Distribution of cyclic AMP phosphodiesterase in adipose tissue from trained rats, *J Appl Physiol* 61(4):1546-1551, 1986.

59. Keyser RE, Andres FF, Wojta DM, Gullett SL: Variations in cardiovascular response accompanying differences in arm-cranking rate, *Arch Phys Med Rehab* 69:941-945, 1988.

60. Kiens B, Saltin B, Walloe L, Wesche J: Temporal relationship between blood flow changes and release of ions and metabolites from muscles upon single weak contractions, *Acta Physiol Scand* 136:551-559, 1989.

61. Klauson K, Secher NH, Clausen JP et al: Central and regional circulatory adaptations to one-leg training, *J Appl Physiol* 52(4):976-983, 1982.

62. Lawlor MR, Thomas DP, Michele JJ et al: Effects of chronic β-adrenergic blockade on hemodynamic and metabolic responses to endurance training, *Med Sci Sports Exerc* 17(3):393-400, 1985.

63. Lerman A, Hildebrand FL Jr, Aarhus LL, Burnett JC Jr: Endothelin has biological actions at pathophysiological concentrations, *Circulation* 83:1808-1814, 1991.

64. Lerman A, Hildebrand FL Jr, Margulies MB et al: Endothelin: a new cardiovascular regulatory peptide, *Mayo Clin Proc* 65:1441-1455, 1990.

65. Levensen JA, Peronneau PA, Simon A, Safar ME: Pulsed Doppler: determination of diameter, blood flow velocity, and volume flow of brachial artery in man, *Cardiovascular Res* 15:164-170, 1981.

66. Loftin M, Boileau RA, Massey BH, Lohman TG: Effect of arm training on central and peripheral circulatory function, *Med Sci Sports Exerc* 20(2):136-141, 1988.

67. Lundgren F, Bennegard K, Elander A et al: Substrate exchange in human limb muscle during exercise at reduced flow, *Am J Physiol* 255(24):H1156-H1164, 1988.

68. Mackie BG, Terjung RL: Blood flow to different skeletal muscle fiber types during contraction, *Am J Physiol* 245(14):H265-H275, 1983.

69. Martin DG, Ferguson EW, Wigutoff S et al: Blood viscosity responses to maximal exercise in endurance-trained and sedentary female subjects, *J Appl Physiol* 59(2):348-352, 1985.

70. Martin WH III, Spina RJ, Korte E, Ogawa T: Effects of chronic and acute exercise on cardiovascular β-adrenergic response, *J Appl Physiol* 71(4):1523-1528, 1991.

71. McCartney N, McKelvie RS, Marin J et al: Weight-training-induced attenuation of the circulatory response of older males to weight lifting, *J Appl Physiol* 74(3):1056-1060, 1993.

72. McCloskey D, Mitchell J: Reflex cardiovascular and respiratory responses originating in exercising muscle, *J Physiol* 224:173-186, 1972.

73. Miles DS, Cox MH, Bomze JP: Cardiovascular responses to upper body exercise in normals and cardiac patients, *Med Sci Sports Exerc* 21(5):S126-S131, 1989.

74. Miles DS, Sawka MN, Hanpeter DE et al: Central hemodynamics during progressive upper and lower-body exercise and recovery, *J Appl Physiol* 57(2):366-370, 1984.

75. Mitchell J: Neural control of the circulation during exercise, *Med Sci Sports Exerc* 22(2):141-154, 1990.

76. Montain SJ, Coyle EF: Fluid ingestion during exercise increases skin blood flow independent of increases in blood volume, *J Appl Physiol* 73(3):903-910, 1992.

77. Montain SJ, Coyle EF: Influence of graded dehydration on hyperthermia and cardiovascular drift during exercise, *J Appl Physiol* 73(4):1340-1350, 1992.

78. Montner P, Chick T, Reidesel M et al: Glycerol hyperhydration and endurance exercise, *Med Sci Sports Exerc* 24(5):S157, 1992 (abstract 940).

79. Morganroth J, Maron BJ, Henry WL, Epstein SE: Comparative left ventricular dimensions in trained athletes, *Ann Intern Med* 82:521-524, 1975.

REFERENCES—Cont'd

80. Nakamura T, Moriyasu F, Ban N et al: Quantitative measurement of abdominal arterial blood flow using image-directed Doppler ultrasonography: superior mesenteric, splenic, and common hepatic arterial blood flow in normal adults, *J Clin Ultrasound* 17:261-268, 1989.

81. Newhouse IJ, Clement DB, Taunton JE, McKenzie DC: The effects of prelatent/latent iron deficiency on physical work capacity, *Med Sci Sports Exerc* 21(3):263-268, 1989.

82. Novac V, Noval P, De Champlain J et al: Influence of respiration on heart rate and blood pressure fluctuations, *J Appl Physiol* 74(2):617-626, 1993.

83. Parker BM, Londeree BR, Cupp GV, Dubiel JP: The non-invasive cardiac evaluation of long distance runners, *Chest* 73:376-381, 1978.

84. Paulson W, Boughner DR, Ko P et al: Left ventricular function in marathon runners: echocardiographic assessment, *J Appl Physiol* 51(4):881-886, 1981.

85. Pawelczyk JA, Hanel B, Pawelczyk RA et al: Leg vasoconstriction during dynamic exercise with reduced cardiac output, *J Appl Physiol* 73(50):1838-1846, 1992.

86. Pellicia A, Maron BJ, Spataro A et al: The upper limit of physiologic cardiac hypertrophy in highly trained elite athletes, *N Eng J Med* 324(5):295-301, 1991.

87. Pendergast DR: Cardiovascular, respiratory, and metabolic responses to upper body exercise, *Med Sci Sports Exerc* 21(5):S121-S125, 1989.

88. Piper J, Pendergast DR, Marconi C et al: Blood flow distribution in dog gastrocnemius muscle at rest and during stimulation, *J Appl Physiol* 58(6):2068-2074, 1985.

89. Poole DC, Schaffartzik W, Knight DR et al: Contribution of exercising legs to the slow component of oxygen uptake kinetics in humans, *J Appl Physiol* 71(4):1245-1253, 1991.

90. Ray CA, Rea RF, Clary MP, Mark AL: Muscle sympathetic nerve responses to static leg exercise, *J Appl Physiol* 73(40):1523-1529, 1992.

91. Reitz BA: The history of heart and heart-lung transplantation. In Baumgartner WA, Reitz BA, Achuff SC: *Heart and heart-lung transplantation,* Philadelphia, 1990, WB Saunders.

92. Rerych SK, Scholz PM, Sabiston DC Jr, Jones RH: Effects of exercise training on left ventricular function in normal subjects: a longitudinal study by radionuclide angiography, *Am J Cardiol* 45(2):244-248, 1980.

93. Roberts RA, Appenzeller O, Qualls C et al: Increased endothelin and creatine kinase after electrical stimulation of paraplegic muscle, *J Appl Physiol* 75(6):2400-2405, 1993.

94. Roberts RA, Icenogle MV, Hudson TL, Greene ER: Brachial artery blood flow during wrist flexion exercise, *Med Sci Sports Exerc* 24(5)(abstract988) 1992.

95. Roca J, Agusti AGN, Alonso A et al: Effects of training on muscle O_2 transport at VO_2max. *J Appl Physiol* 73(3):1067-1076, 1992.

96. Roca J, Hogan MC, Story D et al: Evidence for tissue diffusion limitation of VO_2max in normal humans, *J Appl Physiol* 67(1):291-299, 1989.

97. Rowell LB: Human cardiovascular adjustments to exercise and thermal stress, *Physiol Rev* 54:75-159, 1974.

98. Rowell LB: What signals govern the cardiovascular response to exercise, *Med Sci Sports Exerc* 12(5):307-315, 1980.

99. Rowell LB: *Human circulation: regulation during physical stress,* New York, 1986, Oxford University.

100. Rowell LB: Muscle blood flow in humans: how high can it go? *Med Sci Sports Exerc* 29(5):S97-S103, 1988.

101. Rowell LB, O'Leary DS: Reflex control of the circulation during exercise: chemoreflexes and mechanoreflexes, *J Appl Physiol* 69(2):407-418, 1990.

102. Rowell LB, Saltin B, Kiens B, Christensen NJ: Is peak quadriceps blood flow in humans even higher during exercise with hypoxemia? *Am J Physiol* 251(20):H1038-H1034, 1986.

103. Rubal BJ, Al-Muhailani AR, Rosentsweig J: Effects of physical conditioning on the heart size and wall thickness of college women, *Med Sci Sports Exerc* 19(5):423-429, 1987.

104. Safar ME, Daou JE, Safiavian A, London GM: Comparison of forearm plethysmographic methods with brachial artery pulsed Doppler flowmetry in man, *Clin Physiol* 8:163-170, 1988.

105. Saltin B: Hemodynamic adaptations to exercise, *Am J Cardiol* 55:42D-47D, 1985.

106. Sawka MN: Physiology of upper body exercise, *Exerc Sports Sci Rev* 14:175-211, 1986.

107. Sawka MN, Young AJ, Pandolf KB et al: Erythrocyte, plasma, and blood volume of healthy young men, *Med Sci Sports Exerc* 24(4):447-453, 1992.

108. Schmidt JA, Intaglietta M, Borgstrom P: Periodic hemodynamics in skeletal muscle during local arterial pressure reduction, *J Appl Physiol* 73(3):1077-1083, 1992.

109. Schumacker PT, Samsel RW: Analysis of oxygen delivery and uptake relationships in the Krogh tissue model, *J Appl Physiol* 67(3):1234-1244, 1989.

110. Seeley RR, Stephens TD, Tate P: *Anatomy and physiology,* St. Louis, 1995, Mosby.

111. Sjogaard G, Sauard G, Juel C: Muscle blood flow during isometric activity and its relation to muscle fatigue, *Eur J Appl Physiol* 57:327-335, 1988.

REFERENCES—Cont'd

112. Smolander J, Saalo J, Kohonen O: Effect of workload on cutaneous vascular response to exercise, *J Appl Physiol* 71(4):1614-1619, 1991.

113. Snoeckx LHEH, Abeling HFM, Lambregts JAC et al: Echocardiographic dimensions in athletes in relation to their training program, *Med Sci Sports Exerc* 14(60):428-434, 1982.

114. Somers MF: Spinal cord injury: functional rehabilitation, Norwalk, Conn, 1992, Appleton & Lange.

115. Spiers JP, Silke R, McDermott V et al: Time and frequency domain assessment of heart rate variability; a theoretical and clinical appreciation, *Clin Autonomic Res* 3:145-158, 1993.

116. Spriet LL, Gledhill N, Froese AB, Wilkes DL: Effect of graded erythrocythemia on cardiovascular and metabolic responses to exercise, *J Appl Physiol* 61(5):1942-1948, 1986.

117. Stainsby WN, Brechue WF, O'Drobinak DM, Barclay JK: Effects of ischaemic and hypoxic hypoxia on VO_2 and lactic acid output during tetanic contractions, *J Appl Physiol* 68(2):574-579, 1991.

118. Staubli M, Roessler B: The mean red cell volume in long distance runners, *Eur J Appl Physiol* 55:49-53, 1986.

119. Tankerlsey CG, Zappe DH, Meister TG, Kenney WL: Hypohydration affects forearm vascular conductance independent of heart rate during exercise, *J Appl Physiol* 73(4):1232-1237, 1992.

120. Thorsson O, Hemdal B, Lilja B, Westlin N: The effect of external pressure on intra-muscular blood flow at rest and after running, *Med Sci Sports Exerc* 19(5):469-473, 1987.

121. Traill TA: Physiology and function of the transplant allograft. In Baumgartner WA, Reitz BA, Achuff SC: *Heart and heart-lung transplantation,* Philadelphia, 1990, WB Saunders.

122. Tyml K, Mikulash K: Evidence for increased perfusion heterogeneity in skeletal muscle during reduced flow, *Microvasc Res* 35:316-324, 1988.

123. Vane JR, Anggard EE, Botting RM: Regulatory functions of the vascular endothelium, *N Engl J Med* 323(1):27-36, 1990.

124. Wagner PD: Gas exchange and peripheral diffusion limitation, *Med Sci Sports Exerc* 24(1):54-58, 1992.

125. Walloe L, Wesche J: Time course and magnitude of blood flow changes in the human quadriceps muscles during and following rhythmic exercise, *J Physiol* 405:257-273, 1988.

126. Wesche J: The time and magnitude of blood flow changes in the human quadriceps muscles following isometric contraction, *J Physiol* 377:445-462, 1986.

127. Wood SC, Doyle MP, Appenzeller O: Effects of endurance training and long distance running on blood viscosity, *Med Sci Sports Exerc* 23(11):1265-1269, 1991.

128. Zappe DH, Tankersley CG, Meister TG, Kenney WL: Fluid restriction prior to cycle exercise: effects on plasma volume and plasma proteins, *Med Sci Sports Exerc* 25(11):1225-1230, 1993.

129. Zierler BK, Kirkman TR, Kraiss LW et al: Accuracy of duplex scanning for measurement of arterial volume flow, *J Vasc Surg* 16:520-526, 1992.

RECOMMENDED READINGS

■ Brechue WF, Barklay JK, O'Drobinak DM, Stainsby WN: Difference between VO$_2$ maxima of twitch and tetanic contractions are related to blood flow, *J Appl Physiol* 71(1):131-135, 1991.

■ Coyle EF, Hemmert MK, Coggan AR: Effects of detraining on cardiovascular responses to exercise: role of blood volume, *J Appl Physiol* 60(1):95-99, 1986.

■ Gaebelein CJ, Senay LC, Jr: Influence of exercise type, hydration, and heat on plasma volume shifts in men, *J Appl Physiol* 49(1):119-123, 1980.

■ Gledhill N, Cox D, Jamnik R: Endurance athletes' stroke volume does not plateau: major advantage is diastolic function, *Med Sci Sports Exerc* 26(9):1116-1121, 1994.

■ Joyner MJ, Lennon RL, Wedel DJ et al: Blood flow to contracting muscles: influence of increased sympathetic activity, *J Appl Physiol* 68(4):1453-1457, 1990.

■ Kenney WL, Johnson JM: Control of skin blood flow during exercise, *Med Sci Sports Exerc* 24(3):303-312, 1992.

■ Levensen JA, Peroneau PA, Simon A, Safar ME: Pulsed Doppler: determination of diameter, blood flow velocity, and volume flow of brachial artery in man, *Cardiovas Res* 15:164-170, 1981.

■ Miles DS, Sawka MN, Hanpeter DE et al: Central hemodynamics during progressive upper and lower-body exercise and recovery, *J Appl Physiol* 57(2):366-370, 1984.

■ Mitchell J: Neural control of the circulation during exercise, *Med Sci Sports Exerc* 22(2):141-154, 1990.

■ Pendergast DR: Cardiovascular, respiratory, and metabolic responses to upper body exercise, *Med Sci Sports Exerc* 21(5):S121-S125, 1989.

■ Rowell LB: What signals govern the cardiovascular response to exercise? *Med Sci Sports Exerc* 12(5):307-315, 1980.

■ Rowell LB, O'Leary DS: Reflex control of the circulation during exercise: chemoreflexes and mechanoreflexes, *J Appl Physiol* 69(2):407-418, 1990.

■ Rowell LB, Saltin B, Kiens B, Christensen NJ: Is peak quadriceps blood flow in humans even higher during exercise with hypoxemia? *Am J Physiol* 251(20):H1038-H1034, 1986.

■ Spriet LL, Gledhill N, Froese AB, Wilkes DL: Effect of graded erythrocythemia on cardiovascular and metabolic responses to exercise, *J Appl Physiol* 61(5):1942-1948, 1986.

■ Vane JR, Anggard EE, Botting RM: Regulatory functions of the vascular endothelium, *N Engl J Med* 323(1):27-36, 1990.

■ Wagner PD: Gas exchange and peripheral diffusion limitation, *Med Sci Sports Exerc* 24(1):54-58, 1992.

■ Walloe L, Wesche J: Time course and magnitude of blood flow changes in the human quadriceps muscles during and following rhythmic exercise, *J Physiol* 405:257-273, 1988.

CHAPTER 12

Pulmonary Adaptations to Exercise

During exercise the contracting muscles produce carbon dioxide and consume oxygen to fuel mitochondrial respiration. The lungs function to provide a way for oxygen to be transferred between atmospheric air and the blood and for the majority of metabolically produced carbon dioxide to be removed from the body. Since carbon dioxide content in blood influences blood acid-base balance, the lungs are also important for regulating blood pH. The progression from rest to intense exercise causes the volumes of air inhaled and exhaled by the lungs to increase from 6 to 160 L/min, with larger values possible for larger and more endurance-trained individuals. These large and rapid changes in lung function require intricate and sensitive control systems that optimize the lung's ability to exchange gases between the blood and alveolar air and maintain normal blood pH. For a diverse range of exercise intensities, exercise actually improves lung function. However, moderate to extreme altitude and intense exercise in highly endurance-trained individuals may tax the lung's abilities to maintain optimal function. This chapter details the regulation of ventilation during exercise, explains how the function of the lungs changes during exercise to optimize the exchange of gases, and summarizes research on changes in lung function during different exercise conditions and in response to exercise training.

Basic Anatomy of the Lung and Pulmonary Circulation

The two lungs are located within the thoracic cavity. Each lung is further enclosed by two pleural membranes, between which is the pleural fluid (Figure 12.1). The inner surface of each internal pleural membrane is connected to its respective lung and the outer surface of the external pleural membrane is connected to the inner walls of the rib cage and diaphragm. The pleural fluid and the absence of air within this pleura allow the lungs to slide across the pleura, yet retain a tight connection between the two anatomic structures. The functional importance of this anatomic arrangement is discussed in the section on the mechanics of breathing. Air is directed to and from the lungs by the *trachea*, a long tube supported by cartilage that extends from the larynx to the diverging bronchi and bronchioles of the lungs. The trachea and the left and right *bronchi* have circumferentially layered smooth muscle and are structurally supported by numerous C-shaped rings of cartilage. Collectively, the mouth and nasal passages, trachea, bronchi, and *bronchioles* make up the **conducting zone** of the lungs (Figure 12.2), whereas the *respiratory bronchioles, alveolar ducts,* and *alveoli*, which are the sites of gas exchange and responsible for

conducting zone
the regions of the lung, comprising the trachea, bronchi, and bronchioles, that allow for the bulk flow of air into the lung yet are not involved in gas exchange

FIGURE 12.1

The position of the lungs within the thoracic cavity. Surrounding each lung are two pleural membranes that are separated by a thin lining of pleural fluid. The pleural membrane and fluid function to form an air tight closure around the lungs, effectively cementing the lungs to the inner walls of the thoracic cavity.

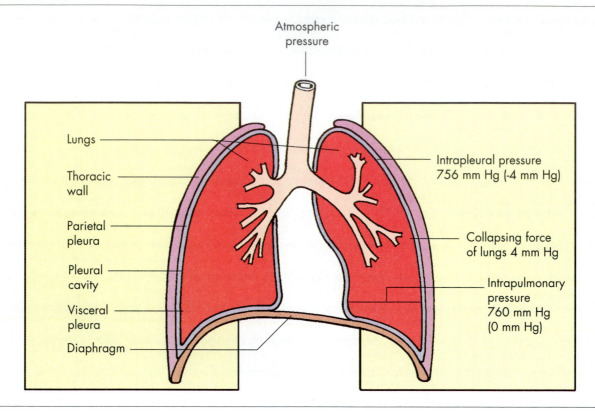

the largest lung gas volumes, are referred to as the **respiratory zone** of the lung (Figure 12.2). During the divergence from the conducting to respiratory zones of the lung the cross-sectional area of the airways greatly increases (Figure 12.3). This change results in largest air flow velocities in the upper regions of the conducting zone and a decrease in air flow velocity toward the respiratory zone. In addition, greatest air flow resistance occurs in the upper levels of the conducting zone, which is regulated by neural- and hormonal-induced vasodilation of the smooth muscle surrounding the trachea, bronchi, and bronchioles.

The respiratory zones of the lungs are the locations of lung inflation and, as their category name suggests, are the sites of *respiration* or gas exchange. The average diameter of an alveolus is approximately 0.25 mm, and the average membrane thickness of the respiratory structures is 0.5 μm. There are approximately 300 million respiratory bronchioles that diverge into numerous alveoli within the two lungs.[65] The alveoli and respiratory bronchioles are connected by openings or holes in their membranes, termed **pores of Kohn** (Figure 12.4). At one time it was believed that these holes allowed air to flow from one alveolus to another; however, recent research has shown that the pores are normally filled

with fluid and are responsible for the distribution of water and surfactant throughout the respiratory zone.[2] Collectively, the respiratory bronchioles and alveoli have a surface area of approximately 70 square meters, which is a phenomenally large area for gas exchange considering that it is contained within the thoracic cavity.

Blood from the heart is pumped through the pulmonary arteries to the lungs, and blood is directed back to the left side of the heart through the pulmonary veins. The circulation of blood to and through the lung is termed the **pulmonary circulation** and is a low-pressure circuit having a

respiratory zone
the regions of the lung, comprising the respiratory bronchioles and alveoli, that are involved in gas exchange

pores of Kohn
small holes between neighboring alveoli that allow for the even distribution of surfactant over the respiratory membranes

pulmonary circulation
the circulation between the right ventricle and left atrium

FIGURE 12.2

Lung structure can be divided into two zones. **A,** The conducting zone is composed of airways that direct air to and from the regions of the lung involved in gas exchange and the external environment. **B,** The respiratory zone consists of the regions of the lung involved in gas exchange, and are therefore comprised of highly vascularized inflatable structures, termed *alveoli*.

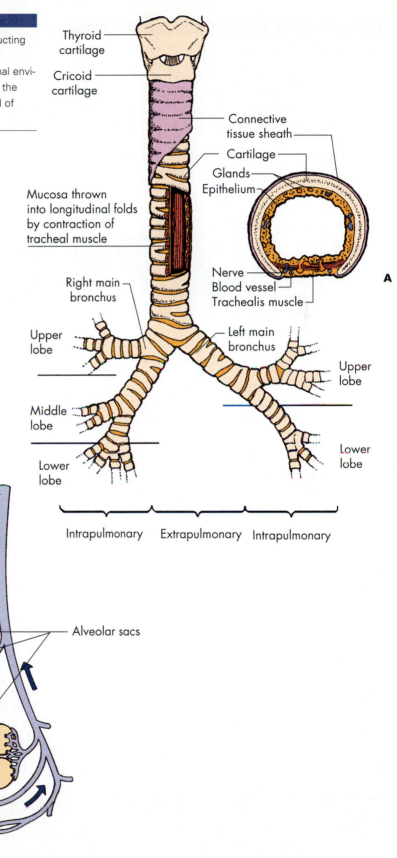

FIGURE 12.3

The progression along the lungs from the conducting to respiratory zones involves tremendous divergence, resulting in an exponential increase in the cross-sectional area of the lung. The greatest cross-sectional area corresponds to the alveoli, which are the main locations for gas exchange. (From West JB: *Respiratory physiology: the essentials,* 4 ed, Baltimore, 1990, Williams & Wilkins.)

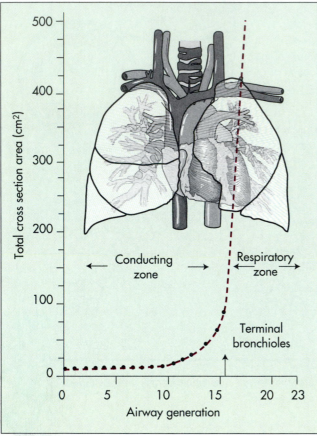

resting normal blood pressure of 25/8 mm Hg compared with the normal systemic blood pressure of 120/80 mm Hg. (See Chapter 11.) The respiratory zone of the lung is engorged with blood. A dense capillary bed surrounds the structures of the respiratory zone, providing a surface area of blood almost as large as that of the respiratory membranes. Obviously, optimal respiration would require a similarity between lung inflation and blood perfusion.

Fluid accumulation in the alveoli is prevented by fluid drainage within the lymphatic system. (See Chapter 15.) However, fluid drainage is a slow process,[64] and there is a risk for fluid accumulation in the interstitial spaces of the lung, or *edema.* Conditions that increase pulmonary blood pressure can increase the rate of fluid flow leaving the pulmonary vasculature, which increases the need for lymphatic drainage. If the pulmonary interstitial volume increases more than 100 ml, alveolar membranes may rupture, forcing fluid into the alveoli and resulting in the life-threatening condition *pulmonary edema.*[38] The retention of low pulmonary blood pressures during a wide range of systemic blood pressures and the function of the lymphatic system usually prevent this from happening. However, conditions that may cause minor and therefore structurally safe increases in pulmonary interstitial

FIGURE 12.4

Throughout the respiratory zone of the lung are small holes (pores of Kohn) that appear to connect alveoli and respiratory bronchioles to one another. When lung sections are prepared to reflect in vivo conditions, these pores are no longer visible and are presumably filled with fluid and surfactant.

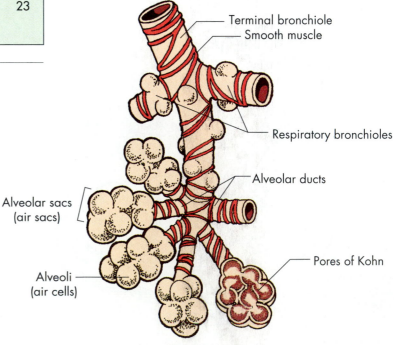

fluid volumes may hinder the ability to exchange gases between the alveoli and blood.

Lung Volumes and Capacities

The conducting zone of the lung is often referred to as the **anatomic dead space,** since it does not have a respiratory function. The anatomic dead space comprises an average volume of 150 ml, although this value varies depending on body size.

The remaining volumes of the lung (see Chapter 20) are subdivisions of the total lung capacity and essentially comprise the *residual volume* and *vital capacity.* The vital capacity is the maximal volume of air that can be exhaled from the lungs, and because it is measured during the forced expiration following a maximal inspiratory effort, it can be divided into inspiratory and expiratory components using *spirometry.* Normal resting breathing involves the inspiration and expiration of 500 ml of air, termed the **tidal volume.** It is the sum of the tidal volume and breathing frequency that determines *ventilation.* A detailed explanation of the measurement of lung volumes and function and the normal values for these volumes and functional capacities are given in Chapter 20.

Multiple Functions of the Lung

The functions of the two zones of the lung are listed in Table 12.1. As indicated, the functions of the lung are more diverse than the simple conduction and exchange of air between the blood and alveoli.

As air is conducted along the upper airways of the conducting zone of the lungs, it is warmed and humidified. These processes are so effective that by the time inhaled air reaches the trachea, it is warmed to 37° C and saturated with water vapor.[38] Inhaled air also contains particulate matter, which because of air turbulence is forced to the walls of the nose, mouth, trachea, bronchi, and bronchioles. The walls of the trachea, bronchi, and bronchioles are coated with cilia and a mucous layer that trap the particles and direct them back to the epiglottis where the mucus is swallowed. Foreign biologic particles, such as bacteria, are also destroyed by white blood cells that scavenge the mucous lining of the conducting airways. The cellular lining of the respiratory zone and the capillaries of the lung also have multiple functions. These cells can secrete substances that can dilate or constrict blood vessels or bronchioles, remove certain molecules from the circulation (e.g., serotonin), and enzymatically activate or deactivate substances. For example, the endothelial cells within the lung enzymatically convert angiotensin I to angiotensin II, which then stimulates the adrenal gland to produce and release aldosterone, a hormone involved in kidney function and fluid balance. These additional functions of the lungs are understandable considering that the lungs are exposed to the

TABLE 12.1	
Multiple functions of the two zones of the lung	
CONDUCTING ZONE	**RESPIRATORY ZONE**
Conduction of air	Respiration
Air humidification	Surfactant production (alveolar endothelium)
Air heating	Molecule activation (capillary endothelium)
Air particle filtration	Molecule inactivation (capillary endothelium)
Vocalization	Blood clotting regulation
Immunoglobulin secretion	Endocrine function

Modified from West JB: *Respiratory physiology: the essentials,* ed 4, Baltimore, 1990, Williams & Wilkins.

potentially infectious conditions of the external environment and are among the few organs that receive 100% of the body's cardiac output.

Ventilation

The term **ventilation** is synonymous with the process of breathing, but ventilation is very different from respiration, which is described in latter sections. Ventilation involves the movement of air into and out of the lungs by the process of bulk flow. During inspiration and expiration the lung compartments are opened to the external environment, and therefore to the pressure, temperature, and humidity of atmospheric air. The pressure differential that exists between the air within the lung is crucial to the process of ventilation, which can increase air flow through the lung from 6 L/min at rest to over 150 L/min during maximal exercise and to more than 200 L/min during maximal voluntary breathing.[25,43]

anatomical dead space
the conducting zone of the lung; typically 150 ml in the average-sized individual

tidal volume
the volume of air inhaled and exhaled with each breath; typically 500 ml at rest in the average-sized individual

ventilation (ven'til-a'shun)
the bulk flow of air into and out of the lung

FIGURE 12.5

At the end of expiration, intrapleural pressure approximates -5 cm H_2O. Inspiration is caused by the expansion of the thoracic cavity, which further decreases the intrapleural pressure, resulting in relatively negative pressures within the respiratory zone of the lung. During expiration, the compression of the thoracic cavity increases intrapleural pressure and the pressure within the respiratory zone, and air is forced to leave the lungs.

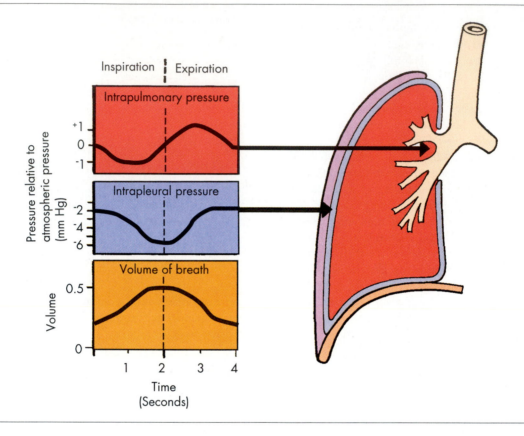

Alveolar Ventilation

As a result of the anatomic dead space, not all the air inspired actually reaches the respiratory zone and undergoes gas exchange. Of the normal 500 ml tidal volume, 350 ml of "fresh" air reaches the respiratory zone, but this value varies with the size of the individual and therefore the size of the tidal volume. The volume of fresh air that reaches the respiratory zone of the lung is termed **alveolar ventilation** (V_A). The greater the depth of breathing, the less impact the anatomic dead space has on alveolar ventilation.

Mechanics of Ventilation

The process of ventilation exemplifies how biologic function is often based on the application of physical principles. Ventilating air into the lungs, or *inspiration*, results from the expansion of the pleural cavity (Figure 12.5). This expansion lowers the pressure (relative to atmospheric) within the pleural cavity and connected alveoli and airways of the lung, and air moves by bulk flow down the airways along the pressure gradient that has developed to the respiratory zone. During resting ventilation, inspiratory effort can reduce the pleural pressure from –5 cm of H_2O to –7 cm H_2O (1 cm

$H_2O = 0.7352$ mm Hg; see Appendix A), which returns to resting values at the end of expiration. The relationships between changes in air pressure and volume are detailed in Appendix B.

During the expulsion of air from the lungs, or expiration, the reverse process occurs (Figure 12.5). The constriction of the pleural cavity increases pressure within and surrounding the lungs, generating a pressure gradient from the lung to the atmosphere and thus forcing air from the lungs. These mechanical processes are driven by muscle contractions, and as explained in later sections, involve work resulting from the conversion of metabolic energy expenditure to mechanical energy (changes in pressure). The work of breathing when applied to different exercise and environmental conditions is an interesting topic.

The muscles responsible for inspiration and expiration are illustrated in Figure 12.6. During resting ventilation, inspiration is driven by the contraction of the diaphragm, which enlarges the lower regions of the lungs. Expiration begins with the relaxation of the diaphragm, and elastic recoil returns the diaphragm and lung to their original end-expiration positions and volumes. During more forceful inspiration,

FIGURE 12.6

The muscles of **A,** inspiration and **B,** expiration, respectively. The inspiratory muscles cause the lowering of the diaphragm, and the flaring and raising of the rib cage, resulting in the expansion of the thoracic cavity. The muscles of expiration compress the thoracic cavity.

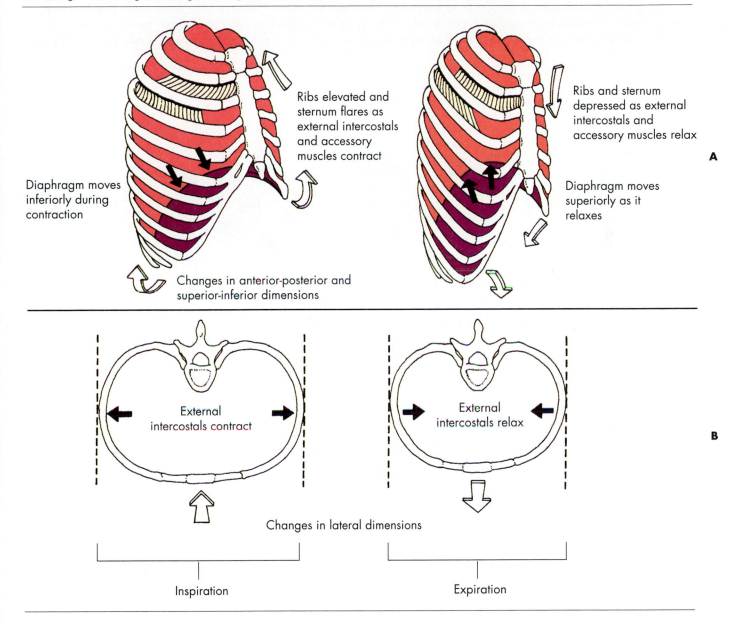

Ribs elevated and sternum flares as external intercostals and accessory muscles contract

Diaphragm moves inferiorly during contraction

Changes in anterior-posterior and superior-inferior dimensions

Ribs and sternum depressed as external intercostals and accessory muscles relax

Diaphragm moves superiorly as it relaxes

A

External intercostals contract

External intercostals relax

Changes in lateral dimensions

B

Inspiration

Expiration

such as that required during exercise, the diaphragm is assisted by the contraction of the external intercostal muscles, which function to raise and outwardly flare the rib cage, resulting in a further increase in lung volume and sustained decreases in pressure. Added lung inflation can result from the contraction of the muscles of the neck that have their origin on the sternum, clavicles, or upper ribs and further raise and expand the rib cage, such as the scalene, superior serratus posterior, and sternocleidomastoid muscles. These added pressure changes within the lung increase the volume of air that enters the airways and lungs and further increase the work of inspiration. The more rapid, large, and sustained the change in

pressure, the greater the functional and metabolic demands on the inspiratory muscles.

When the inspired volumes of air increase, enhanced expiration results from the elastic recoil of the rib cage. Added expiratory effort is obtained by the contraction of the internal intercostal, abdominal, transverse thoracic, and inferior serratus posterior muscles.

alveolar ventilation

that part of ventilation that reaches the respiratory zone of the lung

FIGURE 12.7

When modeling an alveolus as a small sphere, **A,** the law of Laplace states that as the radius of the sphere decreases, and surface tension remains unchanged, the pressure within the sphere increases dramatically. For an open alveolus, this would result in the expulsion of air and collapse the alveolus. For alveoli that are connected, this physical principle would result in the over inflation of the largest alveoli, causing marked inequality in the inflation of the lung. **B,** The presence of surfactant on the membranes decreases surface tension, prevents increases in intraalveolar pressure and decreases resistance to inflation, and allows for a more equal inflation of the millions of the alveoli in each lung.

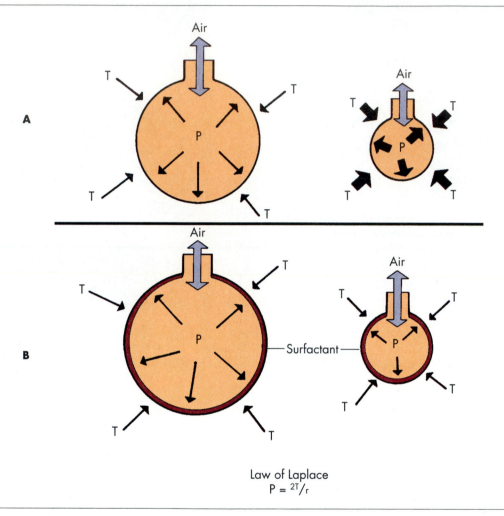

Law of Laplace
$$P = {}^{2T}/_r$$

Pressure-volume relationships. Different changes in pressure and volume of the lungs exist for inspiration and expiration. During inspiration the process of lung inflation is opposed by forces in the lung that resist inflation. These forces are illustrated in Figure 12.7. As previously mentioned, the main locations of lung inflation are the alveoli. When the alveolus is modeled as a sphere, the forces that resist inflation mainly comprise surface tension, as described by the law of Laplace.

12-1
$$P = 2\,T_S/r^4$$

The smaller the radius (r) of a sphere, the greater the surface tension (T_S) over the sphere and the greater the force required to overcome the pressure (P) within the sphere and cause inflation. Furthermore, as a sphere becomes smaller, surface tension increases and results in the expulsion of all air and the eventual collapse of the sphere. These physical characteristics would prevent lung inflation from occurring and result in collapsed alveoli and airways, or if the pores of Kohn increase in size, result in one overinflated alveolus. Obviously, for our lungs to operate as they do these conditions must be modified in vivo.

The processes of inflation and deflation of the respiratory structures are aided by the presence of **surfactant.** Surfactant is produced by a subset of alveolar epithelial cells and is a mixture of phospholipids, proteins, and calcium ions.[38] Surfactant mixes with the fluid that bathes the alveolar membranes and

FIGURE 12.8

The relationship between the change in lung volume for given changes in intrathoracic pressure during inspiration and expiration can be graphed as a pressure-volume curve. The pressure-volume relationship differs for inspiration and expiration. The ability a structure such as the lung has to change volume for a given pressure differential is referred to as compliance. At low lung volumes, the lung is more compliant during expiration than inspiration, and vice versa. (From West JB: *Respiratory physiology: the essentials,* 4 ed, Baltimore, 1990, Williams & Wilkins.)

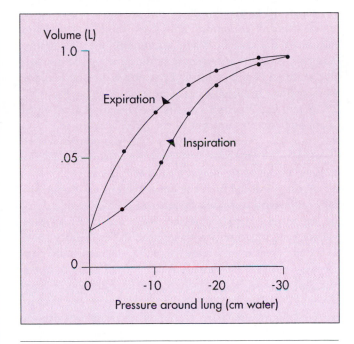

results in interruption of the water layer and reduction in surface tension. For example, the surface tension of water equals 70 dynes/cm², the tension of normal alveolar fluid (without surfactant) equals 50 dynes/cm², and the tension of alveolar fluid with surfactant is < 10 dynes/cm² (1 dyne/cm² = 0.1 N/m² = 0.750 × 10⁻³ mm Hg) (see Appendix A).

The presence of surfactant makes inflation of small alveoli easier. During inflation the alveolar surface area increases and the concentration of surfactant decreases, so that at higher lung volumes the resistance to inflation increases. This increased resistance is not disastrous, since it promotes a more even inflation of neighboring alveoli and respiratory bronchioles that are connected by the pores of Kohn and provides some elastic recoil force at the start of expiration.

As shown in Figure 12.5, during inspiration the lung is able to inflate with minimal generation of more negative intrapleural pressures and therefore has high *compliance.* Compliance is greatest during midinspiration and is less at the start and end of inspiration, even for resting ventilation (tidal) volumes (Figure 12.8). During expiration compliance is least at higher lung volumes, yet remains stable at moderate to low lung volumes.

The high compliance of the lung reduces the work of breathing. For example, a given volume of lung inflation requires one tenth of the work required to similarly inflate a balloon.[78] Data on the work of inspiration and expiration during rest and exercise conditions are presented in the section on acute respiratory adaptations to exercise.

What prevents lungs from collapsing during expiration?
As previously explained and as illustrated in Figure 12.5, the pleural pressure at end expiration is approximately –5 cm H₂O and therefore the lungs remain partially inflated. This requires added expiratory effort to cause further expiration and the generation of pressure gradients across the small airways of the lung. Eventually, these pressure gradients cause the small airways to collapse and retain air in the respiratory zone of the lungs. By preventing alveoli from deflating to dimensions that risk collapse, these processes give the lung its *residual volume* (see Chapter 20). Consequently, the functional role of surfactant in the normal lung is not to prevent alveolar collapse, but to increase lung compliance and thereby decrease the work of inspiration.

Regional Distribution of Ventilation

During the explanation of the mechanics of ventilation, it may have become obvious that the different muscles contributing to ventilation at different ventilation volumes alter the regional inflation of the lung. For example, normal resting ventilation is accomplished by the contraction of the diaphragm, which is connected to the bottom of the pleural membranes and lungs. This ventilation pattern results in greater volume changes in the lower regions of the lung and therefore increases alveolar ventilation in these regions more than in the upper regions (Figure 12.9). Conversely, increased depth of breathing increases inflation of the lateral and upper regions of the lung as a result of the flaring and elevation of the rib cage. A more even inflation of the lung results.

Regional Distribution of Blood Flow

Since the lungs are next to the heart and extend vertically above the heart, a force exerted by the vertical column of blood, or **hydrostatic force,** exists to oppose blood flow to and perfusion of the upper regions of the lung. For the superior regions of the lung this vertical distance can be as great as 30 cm, which amounts to a pressure differential of 23 mm Hg[38], which may equal or exceed pulmonary systolic blood pressure. Consequently, under resting conditions the

surfactant (sur-fak′tant)
 a lipoprotein secreted by tissue of the lung that reduces surface tension of the alveolar membranes

hydrostatic force
 force exerted by a column of water

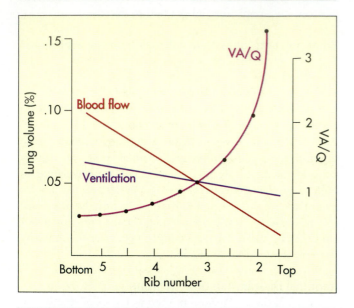

FIGURE 12.9

The distribution of ventilation and blood flow from the base to the upper regions of the lung. (From West JB: *Respiratory physiology: the essentials*, 4 ed, Baltimore, 1990, Williams & Wilkins.)

greatest perfusion of the lung occurs near the lower regions and practically zero flow occurs in the upper regions, as shown in Figure 12.9.

Respiration

The three main gases of air—nitrogen, oxygen, and carbon dioxide—diffuse between the alveolar air and blood, but because gaseous nitrogen is not metabolized within the body (see Chapter 6), only the latter two gases are of interest for normal physiologic conditions. The process of gas exchange, or **respiration,** involves the movement of oxygen and carbon dioxide down pressure gradients that exist between pulmonary capillary blood and the air of the alveoli, and between capillary blood of the systemic circulation and the cells perfused by this blood. Consequently, the locations of respiration can be either in the lung, which is referred to as **external respiration,** or at the level of the systemic tissues, which is referred to as **internal respiration.**

External Respiration

The processes of external respiration result in the movement of gases between alveolar air and the pulmonary capillary blood. This exchange occurs via diffusion through a fluid medium that contains several membranes. The success of this diffusion depends on the characteristics of the gases for diffusion in an aqueous environment and on the nature of the diffusion medium within the lung.

Gas partial pressures in atmospheric and alveolar air.

Dry atmospheric air contains 20.93% oxygen, 79.03% nitrogen, 0.03% carbon dioxide, and extremely small percentages of certain rare gases such as argon that make up the remaining 0.01%. When air contains moisture, or water vapor, the water vapor molecules force the gas molecules to disperse, resulting in an increased volume of air. For constant volumes of gas, the presence of water vapor occupies a pressure within the total gas pressure and the pressures of the gases decrease. As described in Appendix B, the water vapor pressure of air depends on relative humidity and the temperature of the gas.

Figure 12.10 presents the partial pressures of gases in air under standard conditions and how these gas pressures change in the alveoli. When accounting for the relative humidity (RH) and temperature of the atmospheric gas sample (at 55% RH and at 22° C, P_{H_2O} equals 18 mm Hg), the actual pressure occupied by the true gases decreases from 747 to 729 mm Hg. Within the alveoli the pressure remains equal to atmospheric pressure, but as the air is warmed to 37° C and completely humidified (100% RH), the partial pressure of water vapor increases to 47 mm Hg. Consequently, the pressure remaining for the true gases is 700 mm Hg.

As air is exhaled from the lungs, there is no change initially in the partial pressure of either oxygen or carbon dioxide, since a large portion of the air in the anatomic dead space has not been intermixed with air from the respiratory zone. As the air begins to mix, there is a gradual increase in the partial pressure of carbon dioxide and a gradual decrease in the partial pressure of oxygen until the air near the end of expiration *(end-tidal)* reflects alveolar air. Interestingly, end-tidal air gas fractions are often used as an indirect measure of alveolar gas fractions. When the alveolar partial pressure of carbon dioxide ($P_{A}CO_2$) and respiratory exchange ratio (RER) are known, the alveolar partial pressure of oxygen ($P_{A}O_2$) can be calculated from the alveolar gas equation:

12-2 $$P_{A}O_2 = P_{I}O_2 - (P_{A}CO_2 / RER) + [(P_{A}CO_2 \times F_{IO2} \times ([1 - RER] / RER)]$$

When no carbon dioxide is inspired, the right side of the equation can be removed[78]; this assumption is often used by researchers.

Diffusion of gases. Once air is in the alveoli, it is subject to gas diffusion between the alveoli and blood, or vice versa. The factors that govern the direction and magnitude of diffusion are the diffusion capacity of each of the gases, their partial pressure gradient between the alveoli and blood, and the characteristics of the medium through which diffusion occurs.

Physical Properties of Oxygen and Carbon Dioxide

The exchange of gases within the lung and body involves movement along a pressure gradient that exists in both liquid

FIGURE 12.10

A, The partial pressures of oxygen, carbon dioxide, and nitrogen in air under standard conditions. **B,** The change in these pressures is also shown when the respective air samples are inhaled and inflate the alveoli.

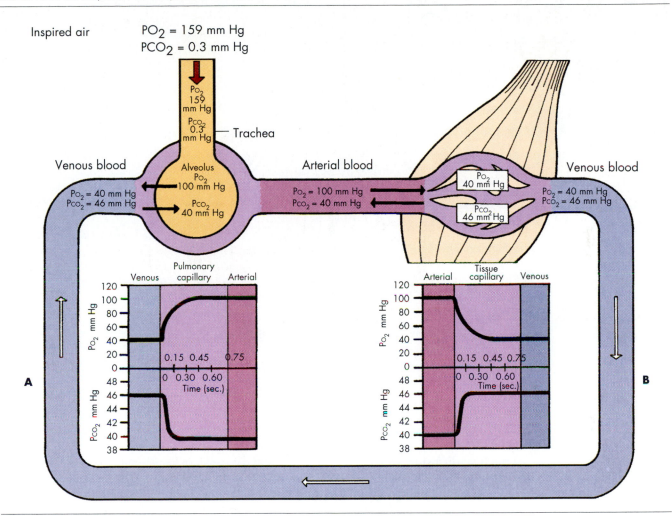

and gas mediums and encompasses several membranes (Figure 12.11). The solubility and diffusibility of gases through these membranes are therefore important for gas diffusion between the alveoli and blood (blood-gas interface).

Compared with carbon dioxide, oxygen is a relatively insoluble gas with a 20.3-fold lower solubility. The small thickness of the alveolar membranes and the large surface area of the respiratory zone (70 m²) make the lung suited to gas diffusion. However, the importance of gas solubility to the diffusion constant causes oxygen to have a relatively low capacity for diffusion.

Lung Diffusion Capacity

Researchers and clinical pulmonologists have measured the diffusion capacities of certain gases for the blood-gas

respiration (res′pi-ra′shun)

gas exchange at the tissue level; usually refers to the consumption of oxygen for use in oxidative phosphorylation

external respiration

gas exchange that occurs in the lung between the respiratory zone and blood

internal respiration

gas exchange that occurs by tissues for the purpose of energy metabolism

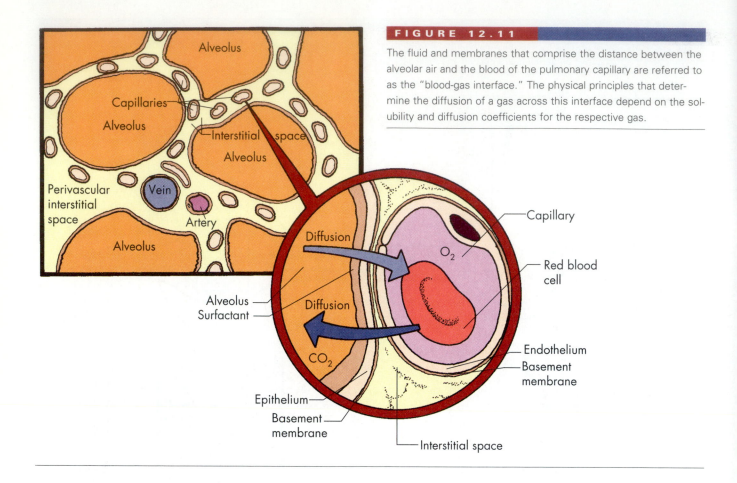

FIGURE 12.11

The fluid and membranes that comprise the distance between the alveolar air and the blood of the pulmonary capillary are referred to as the "blood-gas interface." The physical principles that determine the diffusion of a gas across this interface depend on the solubility and diffusion coefficients for the respective gas.

interface (Figure 12.12). Carbon dioxide and oxygen are not suited to the measurement of the lung **diffusion capacity** because the rate of diffusion is biased by their partial pressure gradients between the alveoli and blood. Conversely, carbon monoxide and nitrous oxide are suitable gases to use because they bind to hemoglobin within the lung with far greater affinity than oxygen, they are not soluble and therefore their respective blood partial pressures do not increase, and their exchange between the alveoli and blood is limited solely by diffusive properties.[37]

The diffusion capacity of the lung can be determined by having a subject inhale a given volume of CO or NO and measuring the rate of disappearance of the gas in expired air (see Chapter 17). As explained in later sections, the diffusion capacity of the lung increases from resting values during moderate exercise intensities but may decrease during more intense exercise.[59,61,70,72]

Gas Partial Pressure Gradients Between Alveoli and Blood

Figure 12.10 illustrates the difference in gas partial pressures between alveolar air and pulmonary capillary blood. A large gradient exists for the diffusion of oxygen from the alveoli to the blood, and a small gradient exists for the diffusion of carbon dioxide from the blood to the alveoli. When combined with the specific diffusive capacities for each gas, these partial pressure gradients result in similar diffusion profiles for oxygen and carbon dioxide (Figure 12.12). As blood flows through the pulmonary capillaries, the partial pressures of oxygen and carbon dioxide in the blood and alveoli reach an equilibrium after approximately 0.25 second under resting blood flow conditions (5 L/min). Clearly the larger partial pressure for oxygen overcomes the low diffusibility, yet such a gradient is necessary for adequate oxygen diffusion. The fact that alveolar and blood gas partial pressures reach equilibrium within the lung enables researchers to estimate arterial blood gas partial pressures from alveolar partial pressures.

Ventilation-perfusion relationships. For the lung to operate optimally in respiration, a balance between ventilation and perfusion is needed. Relative to blood flow, overinflation would cause the alveoli to be flushed with fresh air at a rate too high to maintain normal alveolar partial pressures. Conversely, underinflation would not provide adequate oxygen and remove adequate carbon dioxide. As explained previously, the regions of the lung are not ventilated or perfused equally. Furthermore, changes in ventilation and perfusion (Figure 12.9) in the progression from the bottom to top of the lung are not identical. Since an imbalance in alveolar ventilation and perfusion would impair gas exchange, a measure

FIGURE 12.12

A comparison between oxygen (O_2), nitrous oxide (NO), and carbon monoxide (CO) for the diffusion across the blood-gas interface of the lung. For the normal lung O_2 and NO are dependent on partial pressure gradients for diffusion; however, CO exchange is totally dependent on its poor diffusive properties. If the diffusion capacity of the lung changes, it would be more sensitively detected by a decreased capacity for the exchange of CO, rather than O_2 or CO_2, since diffusion is not modified by a partial pressure gradient. (From West JB: *Respiratory physiology: the essentials*, 4 ed, Baltimore, 1990, Williams & Wilkins.)

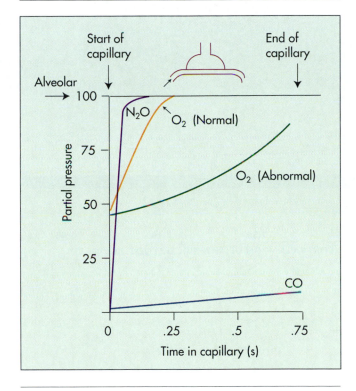

of the effectiveness of lung respiration is the **ventilation-perfusion ratio** $V_E/\dot{Q}$, which under optimal conditions equals 1.0.

The $V_E/\dot{Q}$ equals the ratio between regional alveolar ventilation and blood flow and because of measurement difficulty is calculated as follows:

12-3 $V_E/\dot{Q} = 0.863 \times RER \times [(CaO_2 - CvO_2) / P_ACO_2]$

This calculation needs to be made at several levels of the lung, and when the measurements required in this equation are completed in the vertical position, the results indicate that only a small region of the lung is at or close to $V_E/\dot{Q}$ unity (Figure 12.9). Apical gas exchange criteria reflect a relative overinflation and a resultant gas partial pressure profile that more *closely* resembles atmospheric air. Conversely, the basal regions of the lung reflect a relative underinflation and a

resultant gas partial pressure profile that more *closely* resembles central mixed venous blood.

In damaged regions of the lungs, either ventilation or perfusion may be reduced or completely absent. These regions are extreme examples of alterations in $V_E/\dot{Q}$ and when present constitute regions of *physiologic dead space.*

Transport of Oxygen and Carbon Dioxide in Blood

The equilibration of oxygen and carbon dioxide partial pressures between the alveoli and blood of the lung does not reflect gas volumes. To understand how gas partial pressures affect the volume of gases in blood, students must understand how blood transports oxygen and carbon dioxide.

Oxygen Transport

Oxygen is transported in blood bound to a specialized protein, **hemoglobin (Hb)** which is located on the surface of red blood cells. Hemoglobin consists of four polypeptide chain domains (globins) that each have a *heme* prosthetic group containing a central iron (Fe^{+2}) atom.[48] Each of these domains can bind one oxygen molecule, which amounts to the maximal binding of 1.34 ml of oxygen per gram of hemoglobin. Table 12.2 presents representative hemoglobin concentrations for certain athletic populations and clinical conditions, and the corresponding volume of oxygen transported at specific hemoglobin saturations. When the hemoglobin concentration equals 150 gm/L, the following calculations result in the maximal volume of oxygen that can be transported in arterial blood:

12-4   Blood oxygen   = [Hb] × O_2/gm Hb × HbO_2 saturation
carrying capacity = 150 gm/L × 1.34 ml/gm × 0.98
                  = 197 ml/L

The incomplete HbO_2 saturation is due to a combination of diffusion limitation, resulting from an average inequality between the lungs' $V_E/\dot{Q}$; a pulmonary arterial to venous shunt because of blood from the bronchioles that drains into the pulmonary veins without passing through the

diffusion capacity
the capacity for a gas to diffuse down a concentration gradient in the aqueous environment of the body

ventilation-perfusion ratio
the ratio between ventilation and blood flow for the lung, or for specific regions of the lung

hemoglobin (he-mo-globe′in)
the globular protein on red blood cells that contains four iron-containing heme groups that can bind oxygen and carbon dioxide

TABLE 12.2

Representative concentrations of hemoglobin and oxygen carrying capacity of the blood

POPULATION/CONDITION	HEMOGLOBIN	ml O$_2$/L BLOOD*
Males	14.0	183.8
Females	12.0	157.6
Blood doping	18.0	236.4
Anemia	<10.0	<131.3

*Assumes 98% Hb saturation and a blood pH equaling 7.4.

TABLE 12.3

Change in oxyhemoglobin saturation and blood oxygen carrying capacity for different values of Po$_2$ and blood pH

pH	7.35	7.40	7.45	7.35	7.40	7.45
Po$_2$	Hbo$_2$ SATURATION (%)			CONCENTRATION OF ARTERIAL OXYGEN* (ml/L)		
10	12.4	13.3	14.3	23.26	24.95	26.83
20	33.2	35.5	38.1	62.28	66.60	71.48
30	55.1	58.0	61.0	103.37	108.81	114.44
40	71.4	73.9	76.3	133.95	138.64	143.14
44	76.1	78.4	80.6	142.76	147.08	151.21
48	80.0	82.0	83.9	150.08	153.83	157.40
52	83.2	84.9	86.6	156.08	159.27	162.46
56	85.8	87.3	88.8	160.96	163.77	166.59
60	87.9	89.3	90.6	164.90	167.53	169.97
64	89.7	90.9	92.0	168.28	170.53	172.59
68	91.1	92.2	93.1	170.90	172.97	174.66
76	93.3	94.1	94.9	175.03	176.53	178.03
80	94.2	94.9	95.5	176.72	178.03	179.16
90	95.7	96.3	96.8	179.53	180.66	181.60
100	96.8	97.2	97.6	181.60	182.35	183.10

Modified from Jones NL: *Blood gases and acid-base physiology,* ed 2, New York, 1987, Thieme Medical.
*Assumes a concentration of hemoglobin of 140 gm/L.

The relationship between the saturation of hemoglobin with oxygen and the partial pressure of arterial oxygen (PaO_2). The resulting curve is called the oxy-hemoglobin dissociation curve. The curve is moved down and to the right during conditions that increase blood temperature, PCO_2, acidosis, and 2,3 bisphosphoglycerate.

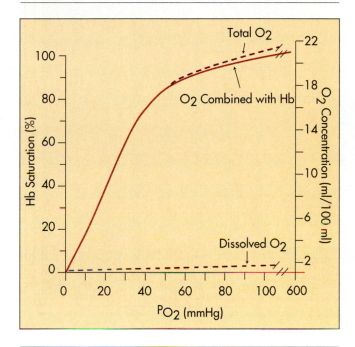

Figure: y-axis Hb Saturation (%), secondary y-axis O_2 Concentration (ml/100 ml), x-axis PO_2 (mmHg). Curves labeled Total O_2, O_2 Combined with Hb, and Dissolved O_2.

pulmonary capillaries of the respiratory zone; and a cardiac shunt involving the drainage of coronary venous blood into the left ventricle. The three deficiencies of pulmonary and cardiac circulation result in minor reductions in average arterial oxyhemoglobin saturation to 98%.

Another small source of oxygen transport in blood is the volume of dissolved oxygen. Of course, because of the low solubility of oxygen this store is minimal, amounting to 0.003 ml of oxygen for every mm Hg of gas partial pressure or approximately 0.3 ml of oxygen at sea level.

Oxyhemoglobin saturation. At sea level the normal P_AO_2 approximates 104 mm Hg. For conditions that lower P_AO_2, such as altitude or air pollution, the partial pressure gradient between the alveoli and blood decreases. Based on the low diffusion coefficient of oxygen and the data of Figure 12.10, this is disastrous for the exchange of oxygen between alveolar gas and blood, preventing the ability to equilibrate P_AO_2 and PaO_2.[41,70] It is important to understand how a decrease in the partial pressure gradient for oxygen affects the saturation of hemoglobin and therefore the oxygen carrying capacity of the blood.

Figure 12.13 illustrates the oxyhemoglobin dissociation curve, which essentially describes the change in hemoglobin saturation with a decrease in P_AO_2. For P_AO_2 values that range from 100 to 80 mm Hg there is almost no reduction in the saturation of hemoglobin. As P_AO_2 decreases from 80 to 60 mm Hg, hemoglobin saturation decreases from 94.9% to 89.3%. For P_AO_2 values below 60 mm Hg, dramatic decreases in hemoglobin saturation occur, which can result in large decreases in arterial oxygen transport (Table 12.3).

Additional Factors That Alter Oxyhemoglobin Saturation

Apart from a decreased saturation when the PO_2 is reduced, dissociation of oxygen and hemoglobin occurs at given PO_2 values by increases in blood temperature, PCO_2, and 2,3-bisphosphoglycerate (2,3-BPG, previously abbreviated as 2,3-DPG) and decreases in blood pH. These relationships are illustrated in Figure 12.13 and documented in Table 12.3.

The molecule 2,3-BPG is a by-product of glycolysis in the red blood cell, and its production increases during conditions of low PO_2 (hypoxia).[49,50] The 2,3-BPG produced by the red blood cell binds to the deoxygenated form of hemoglobin and therefore assists the unloading of oxygen from hemoglobin.[49,50] Temperature, PCO_2, 2,3-BPG, and pH are conditions that change at the level of the tissues, and the directions of these changes combine to decrease the affinity between oxygen and hemoglobin causing greater unloading of oxygen. The effects of temperature, pH, and PCO_2 on adjusting the oxyhemoglobin dissociation curve down and to the right is termed the **Bohr effect** in recognition of the scientist, Christian Bohr, who first observed the phenomenon.[3,65]

Carbon Dioxide Transport

The volume of carbon dioxide (CO_2) stored in the body (blood and tissues) is approximately tenfold greater than the oxygen stores[44] and is transported in the blood in several forms, some of which involve near-equilibrium chemical reactions (Figure 12.14).

Although carbon dioxide has a greater solubility than oxygen, the majority of CO_2 is not dissolved in plasma or the red blood cell, but reacts with water and is converted to carbonic acid through the **carbonic anhydrase** catalyzed reaction that occurs on the surface of red blood cells and inner walls of the vascular endothelium. Carbonic acid then dissociates to bicarbonate (HCO_3^-) and a free proton (H^+). The bicarbonate ions are transported in the plasma, and under

---

Bohr effect
the shift in the O_2-hemoglobin dissociation curve down and to the right by increases in temperature, PCO_2, and acidosis

carbonic anhydrase
the enzyme located on the surface of red blood cells that catalyzes the conversion of CO_2 and water (H_2O) to carbonic acid (H_2CO_3)

FIGURE 12.14

Carbon dioxide is transported in the blood dissolved in plasma and in the red blood cell, bound to hemoglobin and plasma proteins, and as bicarbonate ($HCO3^-$).

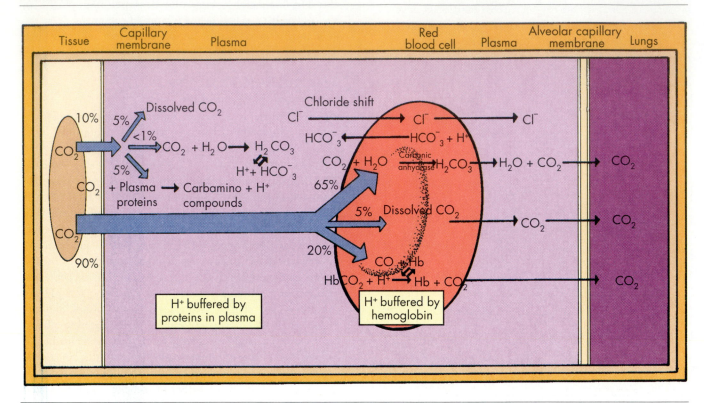

Internal Respiration

normal acid-base conditions the proton is bound to deoxygenated hemoglobin. The ability of hemoglobin to bind both carbon dioxide and protons is important for acid-base regulation of the blood (see Focus Box 12.1).

The exchange in hemoglobin binding for carbon dioxide and oxygen is based on the change in partial pressure of oxygen. When the partial pressure of oxygen increases, the affinity between hemoglobin and carbon dioxide decreases and carbon dioxide is forced from hemoglobin. This P_{O_2} effect on the blood's ability to store carbon dioxide is termed the **Haldane effect** in recognition of the scientist, John Scott Haldane, who first reported it.[45,65]

The changing content of blood CO_2 for a given P_{CO_2} can be graphed in a manner similar to the oxyhemoglobin dissociation curve. However, since CO_2 content in blood also depends on the oxygen saturation of hemoglobin, as explained by the Haldane effect, a family of CO_2 dissociation curves exists (Figure 12.15). For normal function of the lung and normal acid-base conditions the actual or "physiologic" curve for CO_2 dissociation from hemoglobin spans the normal range of blood P_{CO_2} and connects the two lines that span the normal range of oxyhemoglobin saturation. The resulting CO_2 dissociation curve is therefore a small curve compared with the curve of oxyhemoglobin dissociation, which is important for the role of blood P_{CO_2} in blood acid-base balance (Focus Box 12.1).

The exchange of gases at the cellular level is influenced by the Bohr and Haldane effects. In the tissues the partial pressure of oxygen is low (<5 mm Hg during intense exercise) resulting from the reduction of oxygen in the electron transport chain, and the partial pressure of carbon dioxide is high because of metabolic production of CO_2. The additional characteristics of an increased temperature and low pH favor the dissociation of oxygen from hemoglobin, and because of the Haldane effect, the affinity between hemoglobin and carbon dioxide increases.

The unloading of oxygen from hemoglobin is also aided by the molecule **myoglobin.** Myoglobin is found within skeletal muscle fibers and is a similar protein to hemoglobin in that it contains a *heme* prosthetic group, which has a central iron (Fe^{+2}) atom that binds oxygen.[48] At the cellular level

Text Continues on p. 326.

Haldane effect

the increasing affinity between hemoglobin and CO_2 during conditions of low P_{O_2}

myoglobin (my'o-globe'in)

the globular protein of muscle that contains one iron-containing heme group that can bind oxygen

FIGURE 12.15

The relationships between the partial pressure of alveolar carbon dioxide (P_ACO_2) and the saturation of hemoglobin with CO_2 in blood. Since the Haldane effect explains the role of PaO_2 on the affinity between hemoglobin and CO_2, there are a family of curves for the dissociation of CO_2 and hemoglobin based on the PaO_2. As the pressure gradient between P_ACO_2 and pulmonary PCO_2 is only 5 mm Hg, the physiologic range of CO_2 dissociation is small. (Adapted from Brooks GA et al: *Exercise physiology*, 2 ed, Mountain View, California, 1996, Mayfield; and Guyton AC: *Textbook of medical physiology*, Philadelphia, 1976, Saunders.)

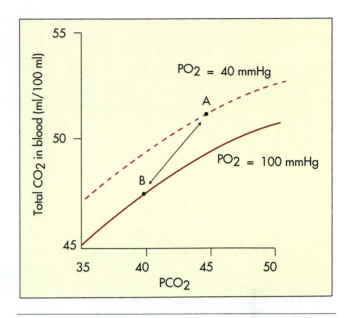

FOCUS BOX 12.1

Blood acid-base balance

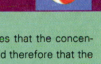

Acidosis is quantified by the pH scale, in which pH equals the negative logarithm of the hydrogen ion concentration (Figure 12.16).

$$pH = -\log [H^+] \text{ or } [H^+] = 10^{-pH}$$

Normal arterial blood pH equals 7.4, and normal muscle pH equals 7.0 The factors that combine to determine blood and muscle pH are the concentration of ions and other charged molecules between fluid compartments, the concentration of blood bicarbonate (HCO_3^-) and other weak acids and bases, the partial pressure of carbon dioxide, the ventilation of the lung, and the excretion or absorption of acid and base by the kidney. Since reactions of the body occur in an aqueous environment, the characteristics of water are also important in determining pH.

Dissociation of Water

Water has a tendency to dissociate (or release) a proton (H^+) and hydroxyl group (OH^-).

$$H_2O \Leftrightarrow H^+ + OH^-$$

At equilibrium the concentrations of these products are constant and a dissociation constant of water ($K'w$) can be calculated based on the relative concentrations of H_2O, H^+, and OH^-.

$$K [H_2O] = [H^+] \times [OH^-]$$
$$K'w = [H^+] \times [OH^-] = 1.008 \times 10^{-14} \text{ mol/L}$$

The $K'w$ is a very small number and indicates that the concentrations of H^+ and OH^- must be very small and therefore that the majority of water is in the form of H_2O. As the H^+ and OH^- are charged, these concentrations must be equal in pure water so that ionic neutrality is maintained.

$$[H^+] = [OH^-] = \sqrt{K'w} = 1.0 \times 10^{-7} \text{ (at 25° C)}$$

At 37° C, dissociation increases and $K'w$ increases to 4.4×10^{-14}, and the $[H^+]$ increases to 2.1×10^{-7}.

Since pH = -log [H$^+$], the pH of pure water at 25° C and 37° C is 7.0 and 6.6778, respectively. Clearly, temperature influences the pH of a water-based solution.

Ionic Distributions

Body fluids are not pure water because they contain many different ions and charged molecules. In solutions the law of electrical neutrality and the ion product of water must be maintained, so that the sum of all positively charged species equals the sum of all negatively charged species, and the sum of $[H^+]$ and $[OH^-]$ equals $K'w$. For example, in human plasma the above statement may be presented as follows:

12-5
$$[H^+] + [Na^+] + [Ca^{2+}] + [K^+] + [Mg^{2+}] =$$
$$[OH^-] + [Cl^-] + [PO_4^-] + [SO_4^-] +$$
$$[HCO_3^-] + [La^-] + [protein^-]$$

Continued.

Blood acid-base balance

If the concentration of any of these charged species changes, there is the potential for a change in [H+] or [OH-] and therefore for a change in pH. This is especially true if the charged species are not all free to change equally. For example, if the concentrations of several negatively charged species increased, this would increase the potential for an increase in [H+]. However, if certain positively charged species increased out of proportion while there were increases in the negatively charged species, a lesser increase in [H+] would result. In this way, movement of charged molecules between vascular compartments within the body can cause minor alterations in cellular and blood pH. Stewart[68] has proposed a mathematical model that takes into consideration all charged species (strong ions) in the calculation of pH (Figure 12.17), and this "physicochemical" approach has received widespread recognition and approval.[32]

Blood Bicarbonate

Traditionally, blood pH regulation has focused solely on the role of bicarbonate. The bicarbonate molecule can bind an H+ to form carbonic acid, as described in the text for carbon dioxide transport in the blood. When acid is produced from metabolism, as during the production of lactate, a proton is liberated, binds with bicarbonate, and eventually forms added carbon dioxide and water.

$$\text{lactate-H}^+ + \text{Na}^+\text{HCO}_3^- \Leftrightarrow \text{Na}^+\text{lactate-} + \text{H}_2\text{CO}_3$$

$$\text{H}_2\text{CO}_3 \overset{CA}{\Leftrightarrow} \text{CO}_2 + \text{H}_2\text{O}$$

This production of carbon dioxide from the bicarbonate buffering of acid accounts for the increase in RER above 1.0 during intense exercise. In addition, the production of carbon dioxide increases the partial pressure of carbon dioxide in the blood. Consequently, conditions of metabolic acidosis are accompanied by increases in $P_{V}CO_2$, and as discussed in the control of ventilation, severe acidosis may also cause slight increases in $P_{A}CO_2$.

Because a large volume of CO_2 is in the body fluids (see text), there is a large source of carbon for the formation of HCO_3^-. The equilibrium nature of the carbonic anhydrase (CA) reaction also enables excess CO_2 to be converted to bicarbonate. In addition, because of the removal of carbon dioxide from the lungs, large increases in carbon dioxide are prevented and the metabolic production of CO_2 allows for the reestablishment of normal bicarbonate levels and pH in the blood. The bicarbonate–carbon dioxide system relies on ventilation for proper function as a buffer system.

Characteristics of Acids and Bases

An acid is a molecule that can release a proton in solution. A base is a molecule that can bind a free proton from solution. The strength of an acid or base depends on the pH value at which it can release or bind a proton. A strong acid releases a proton at low pH values, whereas a strong base binds a proton at relatively low pH values. The measure of strength of an acid or base is the pH at which the molecule has removed or attained half of its protons, which is termed the *pK*.

TABLE 12.4

pK and chemical reactions of several physiologic and nonphysiologic acids and bases

NOMENCLATURE	REACTION	pK
ACIDS		
Acetic acid ⇔ acetate	$CH_3COOH \Leftrightarrow CH3COO^- + H^+$	4.76
Carbonic acid ⇔ bicarbonate	$H_2CO_3 \Leftrightarrow HCO_3^- + H^+$	3.77
Lactic acid ⇔ lactate	$CH_3CHOHCOOH \Leftrightarrow CH_3CHOHCOO^- + H^+$	3.86
Dihydrogen phosphate ⇔ hydrogen phosphate	$H_2PO_4^- \Leftrightarrow HPO_4^{2-} + H^+$	6.86
BASES*		
Ammonium	$NH_4+ \Leftrightarrow NH_3 + H^+$	9.25
Bicarbonate	$HCO_3^- \Leftrightarrow CO_3^{2-} + H^+$	10.2

*For the bases, a pK above 7.0 indicates that the product of the reaction readily binds protons and therefore acts as a base under physiologic conditions.

FOCUS BOX 12.1—Cont'd

Blood acid-base balance

FIGURE 12.16

The pH scale, with examples of solutions from everyday life. The rage of physiologic pH ranges from blood (pH=7.4) to skeletal muscle during intense exercise (pH=6.1). (From Thibodeau GA, Patton KT: *Anatomy and physiology*, 3 ed, St. Louis, 1996, Mosby.)

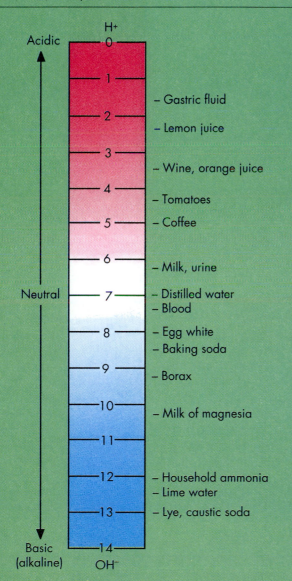

The reaction and pK of several acids and bases are listed in Table 12.4. Lactic acid has a low pK, and therefore almost all lactic acid molecules dissociate to lactate and a free proton.

Characteristics of Buffers

Dihydrogen phosphate has a pK close to intracellular pH and is termed a weak acid. A weak acid and its opposing base represent a buffering system and are termed a *conjugate acid-base pair*. A conjugate acid-base pair is a good physiologic buffer if it has a pK close to 7.0. However because of the small concentration of dihydrogen phosphate in vivo, it is not a very powerful buffer (see Chapter 10). The pK of carbonic acid is surprisingly low, but remember that carbonic acid is not a true buffer, since its buffering potential is based on the removal of carbon dioxide from the lung and the reestablishment of "normal" bicarbonate concentrations by the metabolic production of CO_2.

The effects of the concentrations of the acid and base of a conjugate acid-base on the pH of a solution can be calculated from the Henderson-Hasselbach equation.

$$pH = pK + \log ([base]/[acid])$$
$$= pK + \log ([A^-]/[HA])$$

FIGURE 12.17

The contribution of charged molecules and ions to the final determination of pH in the vascular compartments of the body. Based on the model proposed by Stewart[67].

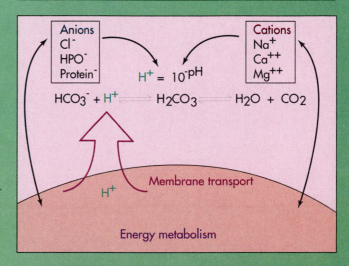

Continued.

FOCUS BOX 12.1—Cont'd

Blood acid-base balance

For example, when using the CO_2, H_2CO_3, HCO_3^- system, with the body's store of CO_2 as an acid, the following calculation can be made:

$$pH = 6.1 + \log [24 / (0.03 \times P_{CO_2})^*]$$
$$= 6.1 + \log (24 / 1.2)$$
$$= 6.1 + \log 20$$
$$= 6.1 + 1.3$$
$$= 7.4$$

*Represents the acid contribution from an increase in P_{CO_2}.

Thus, if the concentration and pK of a conjugate acid-base pair are known, the pH of the solution can be calculated. However, the result of the equation would be inaccurate if additional determinants of pH, such as positively and negatively charged ions and molecules, were present in a solution.

Responses to Metabolic and Respiratory Alkalosis and Acidosis

The effects of alkalosis and acidosis on ventilation can be detailed through the use of the Davenport diagram (Figure 12.18). This diagram presents the changes in blood bicarbonate and pH that occur during metabolic and ventilatory adjustments, and vice versa. Acidosis caused by a hypoventilation retains CO_2 in the blood, which increases both HCO_3^- and free H^+, and thereby reduces pH. The response by the kidney is to excrete acid and reabsorb base, thus further raising HCO_3^- and restoring normal blood pH. As previously explained, metabolic acidosis results in acid production, the release of free H^+, the binding of free H^+ to HCO_3^-, and its dissociation to CO_2 and H_2O. A respiratory compensation of metabolic acidosis involves hyperventilation and excess removal of carbon dioxide from the blood, which in turn causes further decreases in bicarbonate but also restores pH.

FIGURE 12.18

The Davenport diagram illustrating the ventilatory and renal responses to acidosis and alkalosis, and how these changes influence blood bicarbonate (HCO_3^-) and pH. (Adapted from Jones NL: *Blood gases and acid-base physiology,* 2 ed, New York, 1987, Theime Medical Publishers.)

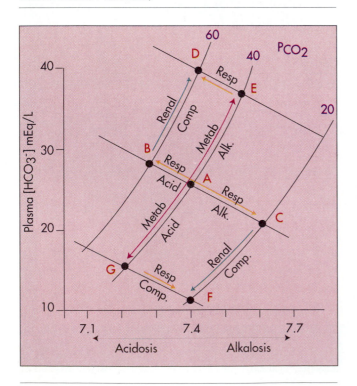

of the circulation in which oxygen is consumed and the partial pressure of oxygen in blood decreases, a sharp decrease in the affinity between oxygen and hemoglobin occurs. For oxygen partial pressures less than 60 mm Hg, myoglobin has a higher affinity for oxygen than does hemoglobin (Figure 12.19), which allows a unidirectional transfer of oxygen from hemoglobin to myoglobin within the muscle fibers.[3,75] Myoglobin can therefore be viewed as a "go-between," transferring oxygen molecules between hemoglobin and the mitochondria within the muscle fiber. The drastic decrease in oxygen and myoglobin affinity below an oxygen partial pressure of 10 mm Hg is interesting because some evidence exists to indicate that the intramuscular P_{O_2} may decrease to less than 5 mm Hg during intense exercise. At these low P_{O_2} values, there is a much higher capacity for oxygen to be released from myoglobin for use in mitochondrial respiration (see Chapter 4). Having more myoglobin would increase the reservoir of oxygen stored within muscle fibers and also increase the ability of muscle to continue mitochondrial respiration during intermittent periods of hypoxia (low Pa_{O_2}) or ischemia (reduced blood flow).

The cellular removal of carbon dioxide is driven by the Haldane effect and the concentration gradient between the cells and capillary blood. As previously explained, the relatively high solubility and diffusibility of carbon dioxide prevent diffusion limitation.

FIGURE 12.19

A comparison between oxyhemoglobin and oxymyglobin dissociation curves.

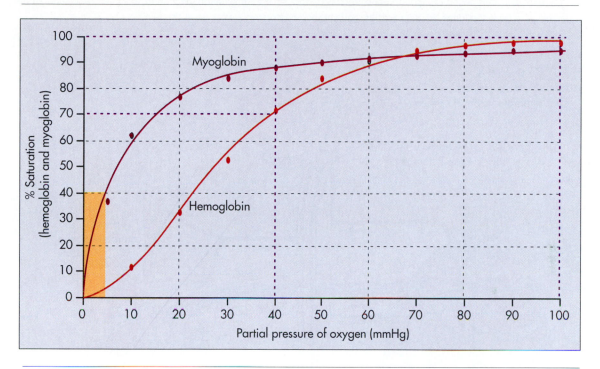

Acute Adaptations of Pulmonary Function During Exercise

As discussed earlier, the start of exercise is accompanied by immediate increases in ventilation. The factors that regulate this increase are numerous and need to be explained. In addition, the changes in ventilation can vary for different types of exercise and are affected by the acidosis generated during exercise at intensities above the lactate threshold. Low to moderate exercise intensities increase the effectiveness of external respiration, but for many individuals, intense exercise can impair external respiration. Research has focused on how exercise affects the lung diffusion capacity and $V_E/\dot{Q}$, and these results have provided valuable information about lung function during exercise.

Control of Ventilation during Rest and Exercise

The control of ventilation is an intricate and multifaceted regulatory characteristic of the human body. This is understandable given the importance of ventilation for maintaining optimal oxygen content of the blood and for regulating blood acid-base balance. Ventilation can be controlled by both voluntary and involuntary functions of the nervous system. Neural controls exist in the central and peripheral nervous system and exert their effects through input and alter-

ation to central controls of inspiration and expiration. Peripheral **chemoreceptors** that convert chemical stimuli into action potentials, which are then relayed to the control locations within the central nervous system, also exist. As a result of this anatomic diversity, an understanding of the anatomic distribution of the control sites involved in the regulation of ventilation is important. These multiple control systems combine to regulate ventilation, and their relative importance differs in the resting state compared with the exercise state.

Anatomic Organization of Ventilatory Control

Central nervous system. The main components of the neural circuitry within the central nervous system that are involved in the control of ventilation are presented in Figure 12.20. A collection of nerves within the medulla of the lower brain functions as the respiratory center. Within the respiratory center are localized regions that specifically influence inspira-

chemoreceptors (kem′o′re-sep′tor)
cells that can generate action potentials in response to changes in the chemical composition of their surroundings (usually blood)

FIGURE 12.20

The components of the nervous system and cranial and systemic circulations that are involved in the regulation of ventilation. The respiratory center of the medulla is composed of discrete neural regions responsible for inspiration, expiration, and their regulation. In the periphery, afferent nerves arise from the lungs, joints, muscles, and chemoreceptors, as explained in the text.

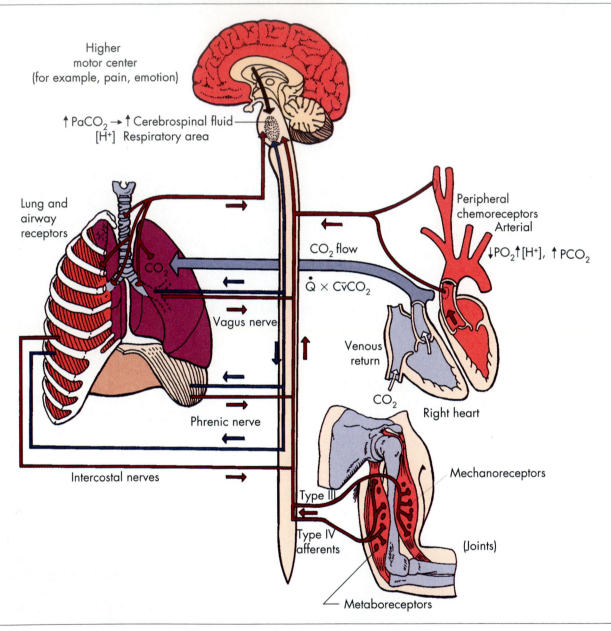

tion and expiration and are termed *inspiratory* and *expiratory centers,* respectively. As discussed, these two locations coordinate the sequence of inspiration and expiration during breathing.

Superior to the respiratory center are additional nerve regions, termed the *apneustic area* and *pneumotaxic area,* that influence the function of the respiratory center. Basically, input from the apneustic area prolongs the duration of inspiration, whereas input from the pneumotaxic area shortens the duration of inspiration and thereby increases the frequency of breathing. In addition, nerves that originate in the cortex

descend and innervate the respiratory center, as well as the apneustic and pneumotaxic areas, thus accounting for the voluntary control circuits of ventilation.

In close proximity to the respiratory center are a collection of nerve endings that are directly sensitive to hydrogen ions and indirectly sensitive to $PaCO_2$. The nerves from this location are termed *central chemoreceptors* and represent a method of ventilatory control based on a blood-borne, or humoral, factor. When $PaCO_2$ increases, as it does only slightly during conditions of metabolic acidosis, the CO_2 penetrates the blood-brain barrier, forms carbonic acid in the cerebrospinal fluid, and then dissociates to HCO_3^- and H^+. Since there is minimal bicarbonate in cerebrospinal fluid, even a small increase in $PaCO_2$ can decrease cerebrospinal fluid pH, which is detected by the central chemoreceptors.

Peripheral nervous system. Nerves from the periphery return from various locations to influence the pattern of ventilation. Free nerve endings exist in joints and within skeletal muscles that return action potentials to the respiratory center during muscle contraction and even passive limb movement. In addition, animal research has revealed the presence of chemoreceptors in the lung that are sensitive to CO_2.[35] Increasing PCO_2 in the pulmonary capillary blood stimulates these receptors, and action potentials are returned to the respiratory center to stimulate an increase in ventilation. It is unclear whether similar receptors exist in the human lung.

Additional chemoreceptors are located in the periphery. Located on the superior wall of the aortic arch are chemoreceptors termed **aortic bodies,** and on the carotid arteries in the region of the carotid bifurcation are additional chemoreceptors termed **carotid bodies.** Both sets of peripheral arterial chemoreceptors are stimulated by increases in $PaCO_2$ and decreasing pH (increasing $[H^+]$), with the carotid bodies capable of additional stimulation by potassium and decreased PaO_2.[9,55] However, decreases in PaO_2 cause only minor increases in ventilation until PaO_2 values are less than 65 mm Hg, after which stimulation to ventilation increases abruptly.[38] However, the hypoxic stimulation to ventilation is never as large as the increase caused by hypercapnia because of the excess CO_2 removed from the hypoxia-induced hyperventilation.

Controls of Ventilation at Rest

Normal resting breathing is characterized by infrequent shallow inspiratory and expiratory maneuvers. The transition between inspiration and expiration is controlled by a repetitive discharge of action potentials from the inspiratory center. Expiration involves the passive recoil of the diaphragm. During normal acid-base conditions, minimal additional regulation occurs from chemoreceptor stimulation.

Controls of Ventilation during Exercise

Exercise provides multiple stimuli for increases in ventilation. Depending on exercise intensity, all the components of Figure 12.20 become influential in determining the ventilatory rate. Considerable research has attempted to determine the most influential controls of ventilation during exercise, but the multiple regulation schemes have prevented the ability to rank each control system.

Neural factors. The relative importance of central neural versus peripheral neural controls of ventilation has been assessed by having humans exercise without intervention and exercise by artificial electrical stimulation.[10] Theoretically, if

voluntary control of muscle contraction is absent, conscious stimulation of the respiratory center will not occur and therefore the ventilatory pattern will be compromised. A similar model using individuals with complete spinal cord injury has been used for the same reasons.[11] Results have indicated that alveolar ventilation is optimal in either condition. Because spinal cord injury prevents afferent nerve return to the central nervous system, additional factors are also involved in regulating ventilation during exercise. Nevertheless, the role of neural factors in regulating ventilation has been extensively documented in animal research that is characterized by more invasive procedures and better control of other ventilatory stimulants.[28,29,31]

Humoral factors. A common model used with human subjects is to occlude blood flow from a limb and then to exercise the muscles from the limb. This model prevents the removal of a metabolite stimulant to ventilation, such as carbon dioxide.[42] Such research has shown that ventilation still increases in a similar manner to exercise in subjects with intact circulation.

Neurohumoral approach. A commonsense approach to the control of ventilation is to assume that multiple control systems function together. In 1954 the French physiologist DeJours[20] postulated that at the start of exercise neural mechanisms were of most importance, and then humoral factors fine-tuned the neural controls to provide a steady-state ventilatory profile (Figure 12.21). Consequently, because steady-state exercise implies being at an intensity below the lactate and ventilatory thresholds, the humoral factors were not determined by increasing $PaCO_2$, decreasing pH, or exercise-induced hypoxemia.[31] Recent evidence of lung CO_2 receptors that respond to increasing VCO_2 and alveolar CO_2 exchange may provide the functional explanation of a humoral effect of ventilatory control without hypercapnia and acidosis.[35]

When exercise intensity increases above the lactate or ventilatory thresholds, acidosis develops and is accompanied by small increases in $PaCO_2$. These stimuli exert action on the peripheral and central chemoreceptors, resulting in increased neural input to the respiratory center and increased ventilation. A general depiction of the changes in postulated humoral mediators of ventilation during incremental exercise is presented in Figure 12.22. The increase in ventilation occurs with increasing acidosis and is effective in reducing

aortic bodies
the mechanoreceptors and chemical receptors in the wall of the aorta, which respond to stretch of the artery wall and to PCO_2 and PO_2

carotid bodies
the chemical receptors in the walls of the carotid arteries

FIGURE 12.21

The classic DeJours model (DeJours) of ventilation expressed relative to the change in ventilation from rest to submaximal steady state exercise. When exercise is stopped the initial increase in ventilation and the rapid decrease in ventilation are rapid and are explained by the neural components of regulation. The fine-tuning of ventilation during exercise is believed to be due to humoral components of ventilation regulation.

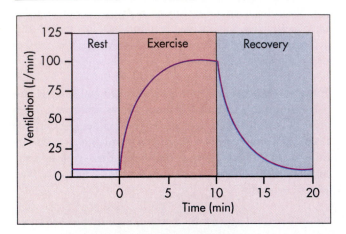

$PaCO_2$ at higher ventilatory rates. This response is paradoxic, given the belief that increasing $PaCO_2$ is a potent stimulator of ventilation. However, because of the multiple ventilatory stimulants that increase ventilation during exercise, the hyperventilation results in the removal of CO_2 from the blood and reduces $PaCO_2$ as a means to combat the increasing acidosis, as explained in Focus Box 12.1.

Ventilation during Transitions from Rest to Steady-State Exercise

As with oxygen consumption, the increase in ventilation during the transition to an increased steady-state exercise intensity is abrupt, exponential, and proportional to the change in intensity. Steady-state ventilation is attained earlier than steady-state VO_2 for a given bout of exercise (Figure 12.23), which is understandable given the effectiveness of both the neural and humoral controls of ventilation. The increase in ventilation is due to increases in tidal volume and breathing frequency.

The transition period following the increase in intensity is associated with slight increases in $PaCO_2$ and decreases in

FIGURE 12.22

The changes in the humoral stimulants of ventilation during incremental exercise to fatigue. As ventilation increases with an increase in intensity, there is a concomitant decrease in arterial blood pH. However, $PaCO_2$ actually decreases as a result of hyperventilation of exercise (hyperpnea). (Adapted from Brooks GA et al: *Exercise physiology*, 2 ed, Mountain View, California, 1996, Mayfield.)

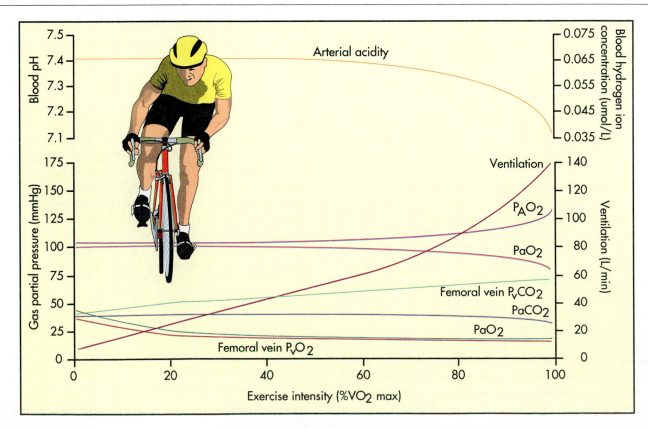

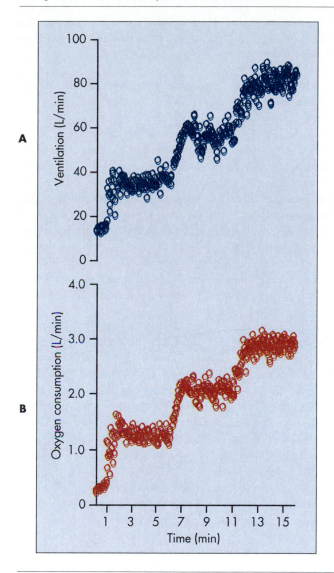

FIGURE 12.23

The increase in **A,** ventilation and **B,** oxygen consumption (VO$_2$) during different rest to steady state exercise intensities.

more evenly distributed throughout the lung.[14,17,25,26] Based on the previous discussion of $V_E/\dot{Q}$, these responses improve the $V_E/\dot{Q}$ of the lung and therefore improve the process of external respiration.

Ventilation during submaximal exercise at given loads is also known to differ for different types of exercise.[36,54] Arm or upper body exercise causes a relatively larger ventilation compared with cycling, and static exercise also causes ventilation to be larger than dynamic exercise. Data from Paek and McCool[54] also indicate that tidal volumes, inspiratory times, and end-expiratory lung volumes may differ among different types of exercise; however, their data were normalized to ventilation and not metabolic load (VO$_2$max). Finally, posture during exercise is known to affect ventilation, which has been of interest when different positions of the upper body during cycling were studied.

Ventilation during Incremental Exercise

The increase in ventilation during an incremental cycle ergometry exercise test for an endurance-trained individual is presented in Figure 12.24. The variables VE/VO$_2$ and VE/VCO$_2$ are the ventilatory equivalents for oxygen and carbon dioxide, respectively, and are obtained by dividing the VO$_2$ or VCO$_2$ into VE. During the initial intensities, ventilation increases linearly with intensity, and VO$_2$ and PaO$_2$ remain stable. After an individually specific intensity, the increase in VE is larger than the increase in VO$_2$ and by definition there is an abrupt increase in VE/VO$_2$. Depending on the protocol used, there is a short time delay (usually 2 minutes) before VE/VCO$_2$ also increases, and this time delay has been explained by the body's large storage capacity for CO$_2$ and the initial similarity between increased ventilation and VCO$_2$.[13]

Ventilatory Threshold

The exercise intensity at which there is a simultaneous deviation from linearity in ventilation and an increase in VE/VO$_2$ is termed the **ventilatory threshold (VT).**[*] Other measures can also be used to detect this point, such as an exponential increase in VCO$_2$ or RER and an abrupt increase in blood acidosis; however, Caizzeo[13] has demonstrated that the joint VE and VE/VO$_2$ criteria are most sensitive in detecting the VT.

The traditional explanation of the ventilatory threshold is that as exercise intensity increases, the abrupt increase in

PaO$_2$,[77] which indicate that although rapid, the increase in ventilation is still insufficient to overcome the instantaneous demands of the onset of exercise. Once again, as with oxygen consumption, ventilation continues to increase during intensities that are above the intensity at the lactate threshold.

Recent research has shown that increased ventilation rates are associated with the enlargement of the trachea during expiration,[43] which would decrease resistance to air flow. When this is combined with the dilation of the bronchi and bronchioles resulting from neural and circulatory catecholamine stimulation, the conducting zone of the lung is actually a very responsive component of the pulmonary system and therefore should not be viewed as a rigid structure.

Numerous studies have shown that both ventilation and perfusion of the lungs increase during exercise and become

---

* References 4, 13, 30, 34, 46, 52, 66, 74, 79, and 82.

ventilatory threshold
the increase in ventilation corresponding to the development of metabolic acidosis, usually detected during an incremental exercise test

FIGURE 12.24

The change in selective respiratory and ventilatory parameters during incremental exercise performed to volitional fatigue. The intensity corresponding to a nonlinear deviation in the increase in ventilation and the point where VE/VO$_2$ increases is termed the *ventilatory threshold* (VT).

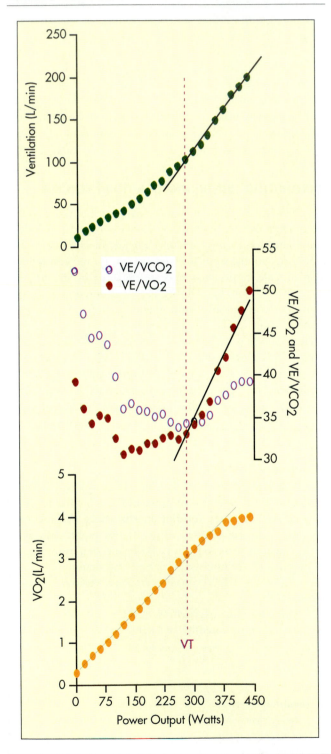

lactate acidosis that occurs after the lactate threshold causes an increase in blood acidosis and PaCO$_2$. Both the acidosis and the increased PaCO$_2$ stimulate the chemoreceptors to induce increased ventilation. This mechanism has been interpreted by many physiologists as evidence that the lactate and ventilatory thresholds occur at the same exercise intensity.

Is the ventilation threshold identical to the lactate threshold? Numerous studies have been conducted to compare the lactate and ventilatory thresholds. Researchers have concluded that the two measures are identical[13,19,73,74,79]; however, others have concluded that the two measures can differ under certain conditions and that the two criteria should not be used interchangeably.[1,34,39,42,52] Factors that can cause the two measures to deviate are altered carbohydrate nutrition, certain exercise test protocols, enzyme deficiency diseases, methodologic error, exercise training, and altered states of sympathetic stimulation.[1,33,34,52,82] Gladden et al.[34] have estimated that the variation in relative exercise intensity between two measures may be larger than 8% of VO$_2$max, which would be significant when using the measures to prescribe a training exercise intensity.

Mechanics and Metabolic Costs of Ventilation during Exercise

As alveolar ventilation increases, increased metabolic demands are placed on the muscles of inspiration and expiration. Both the frequency of ventilation and the tidal volume increase during increases in exercise intensity and ventilation and that further increases in ventilation rates are due to continued increases in the frequency of breathing and a plateau in tidal volume.

Various mechanical changes also occur as ventilation and exercise intensity increase. As intensity increases, so does the volume of air remaining in the lung after expiration, peak inspiratory pleural pressure, and the work of breathing. The exponential nature of the increased work of breathing during exercise is due predominantly to the cost of expiration at higher ventilation rates because the flow rate during expiration is limited by the constriction of the smaller airways (see Focus Box 12.2).[5,43]

Do the muscles of ventilation fatigue during exercise? The large increase in the work of breathing could cause respiratory muscle fatigue during maximal exercise. However, results indicate that for endurance-trained individuals the ability to generate inspiratory negative pleural pressures during maximal exercise is similar to the pleural pressures generated during maximal voluntary inspiratory maneuvers.[5,43] However, whether untrained individuals have near-optimal respiratory muscle and ventilatory function during fatiguing exercise remains to be researched.

Final comment needs to be given on the specific type of exercise performed. Some exercises, such as swimming and deep water exercise, have the upper body submerged in water, which provides an increased external pressure (compression) to the thoracic cavity. This would theoretically decrease the work of expiration but potentially increase the work of inspiration. Whether these changes would cause respiratory muscle fatigue and impair ventilation is unclear. Ventilation and external respiration during swimming are also compromised by forced entrainment of ventilation during specific intervals during a stroke. Although not thoroughly researched, such entrainment causes inspiration and expiration times to be longer but less frequent. It remains unclear how lung function, blood gases, and acid-base balance are affected by these constraints in trained or relatively untrained swimmers.

Exercise-Induced Hypoxemia

The partial pressure (PaO_2) and concentration of oxygen (CaO_2) in arterial blood remain stable in most individuals during all intensities of exercise. However, numerous reports have documented a lowering of the partial pressure of oxygen (hypoxia) resulting in a reduced CaO_2 **(hypoxemia)** during exhausting exercise at sea level in individuals with healthy lungs.

In 1984 it was observed that highly trained endurance athletes experience significant reductions in CaO_2, and this condition was termed **exercise-induced hypoxemia.**[22] Figure 12.25 reveals the change in arterial oxyhemoglobin saturation and CaO_2 in individuals of different cardiorespiratory endurance fitness levels during an incremental exercise test to volitional fatigue. The more endurance-trained the athlete, the larger the reduction in CaO_2, which indicates that for these individuals the lungs are not functioning optimally during intense exercise. Powers et al.[56,57,61] have shown that exercise-induced hypoxemia occurs in approximately 50% of well-trained endurance athletes during intensities above 80% VO_2max.

Since the healthy lung was always thought to function optimally during exercise, the initial explanation for this phenomenon was an imbalance between cardiac output and maximal pulmonary blood flow. It was assumed that endurance athletes were trained to the point at which their central blood volume and maximal cardiac output had exceeded the ability of their lungs to maintain pulmonary blood flow at a velocity required to equilibrate P_AO_2 and PaO_2. The velocity of blood flow in the pulmonary capillaries is important, since a high velocity would decrease the time of a given red blood cell within the blood-gas interface, termed the **pulmonary transit time,** and risk inequilibration. The time required for equilibration between P_AO_2 and PaO_2 in the healthy lung is believed to be 350 to 400 ms[72] (see Figure 12.12).

Warren et al.[72] indirectly measured pulmonary transit time in individuals known to exhibit exercise-induced hypoxemia. Although pulmonary transit time decreased during increases in exercise intensity, it did not reach critical levels in these subjects, indicating that the traditional explanation of

FIGURE 12.25

The decrease in oxy-hemoglobin saturation (hypoxemia) during incremental exercise in individuals with different VO_2max capacities. For individuals with increasing VO_2max there are larger reductions in oxy-hemoglobin saturation and indicate inadequacies in lung function. (Adapted from Powers SK, Williams J: *Exercise-induced hypoxemia in highly trained athletes, Sports Med* 4:46-53, 1987.)

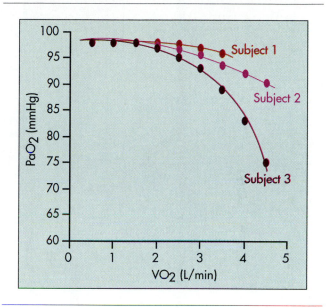

exercise-induced hypoxemia was inaccurate. The remaining explanations of inadequate hyperventilation, increasing venoarterial shunt, a decrease in lung diffusion capacity, or ventilation-perfusion inequality required investigation.

Inadequate ventilation would prevent the oxygenation of arterial blood and also limit the removal of CO_2 from the blood. Because there is no increase in $PaCO_2$ in individuals who experience hypoxemia, inadequate hyperventilation does not appear to be the cause.[36,49,51,52] In fact, Johnson et al.[43] have shown that highly trained endurance athletes (VO_2max > 70 ml/kg/min) reach the maximal mechanical limits of alveolar ventilation during maximal exercise yet

hypoxemia (hi-pok-se'mi-ah)
the decrease in the oxygen saturation of hemoglobin below normal

exercise-induced hypoxemia
the hypoxemia that occurs in highly endurance-trained individuals during intense exercise, even at sea level barometric pressures

pulmonary transit time
the time required for a red blood cell to pass through the pulmonary capillary; essentially the time available for gas exchange between the alveoli and blood circulating through the lung

FIGURE 12.26

The pathophysiology of asthma.

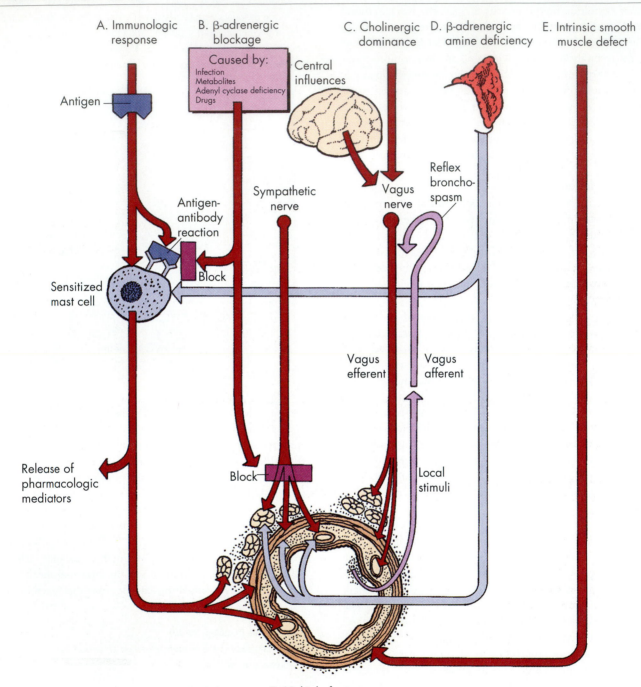

A. Immunologic response

B. β-adrenergic blockage

C. Cholinergic dominance

D. β-adrenergic amine deficiency

E. Intrinsic smooth muscle defect

Antigen

Caused by:
Infection
Metabolites
Adenyl cyclase deficiency
Drugs

Central influences

Reflex broncho-spasm

Antigen-antibody reaction

Sympathetic nerve

Vagus nerve

Block

Sensitized mast cell

Vagus efferent

Vagus afferent

Release of pharmacologic mediators

Block

Local stimuli

F. Multiple factors

Asthma is an obstructive disorder of the lung that has been difficult to define.[63,70] However, the U.S. Department of Health and Human Services[70] has developed a working definition that recognizes asthma as a lung disease with the following characteristics:

1. Airway obstruction that is reversible (although sometimes not completely) with treatment
2. Airway inflammation
3. Increased airway responsiveness to a variety of stimuli

The airway obstruction is caused by the combination of smooth muscle contraction and inflammation of the tissue surrounding the trachea and bronchioles. This response causes constriction of the large and small airways and a dramatic increase in the resistance to air flow in the conducting zone of the lungs. Some individuals who have mild asthma may be asymptomatic, with their condition detected only through pulmonary function testing (spirometry and peak expiratory flow rate), whereas others with more severe asthma experience concurrent episodes of cough and wheezing.[70] It has been estimated that 10 million individuals in the United States have asthma, that this incidence is increasing,[70] and that up to 25% of the population in the United States has experienced asthma at least once in their life.[63]

The pathophysiology of asthma varies (Figure 12.26). Asthma can be triggered by a hypersensitive reaction of the bronchial smooth muscle and endothelium to particles in the air. In young individuals, especially children, the asthma attack most often results from an allergic reaction, mainly to pollen from plants. In adults, asthma is more likely the result of a nonallergenic hypersensitivity to irritants in the air.

The initial trigger to asthma is thought to be the release of inflammatory mediators from mast cells, macrophages, and epithelial cells in the bronchiole lining. These mediators activate other inflammatory cells, which combine to produce changes in the epithelial lining of the bronchioles, interfere with the neural regulation of smooth muscle tone, and alter mucus secretion. The inevitable result from these changes is an inflammation of the bronchial lining.

Continued.

asthma (az'mah)
the condition of hypersenesitivity of the smooth muscle lining the bronchioles of the lung, causing constriction of these airways and increased difficulty in ventilating the lung

---

FIGURE 12.27

The evaluation of asthma symptoms and choices for treatment. (From Dept of Health and Human Services: *Guidelines for the diagnoses and management of asthma*, Pub No 91-3042, 1991, National Institutes of Health.)

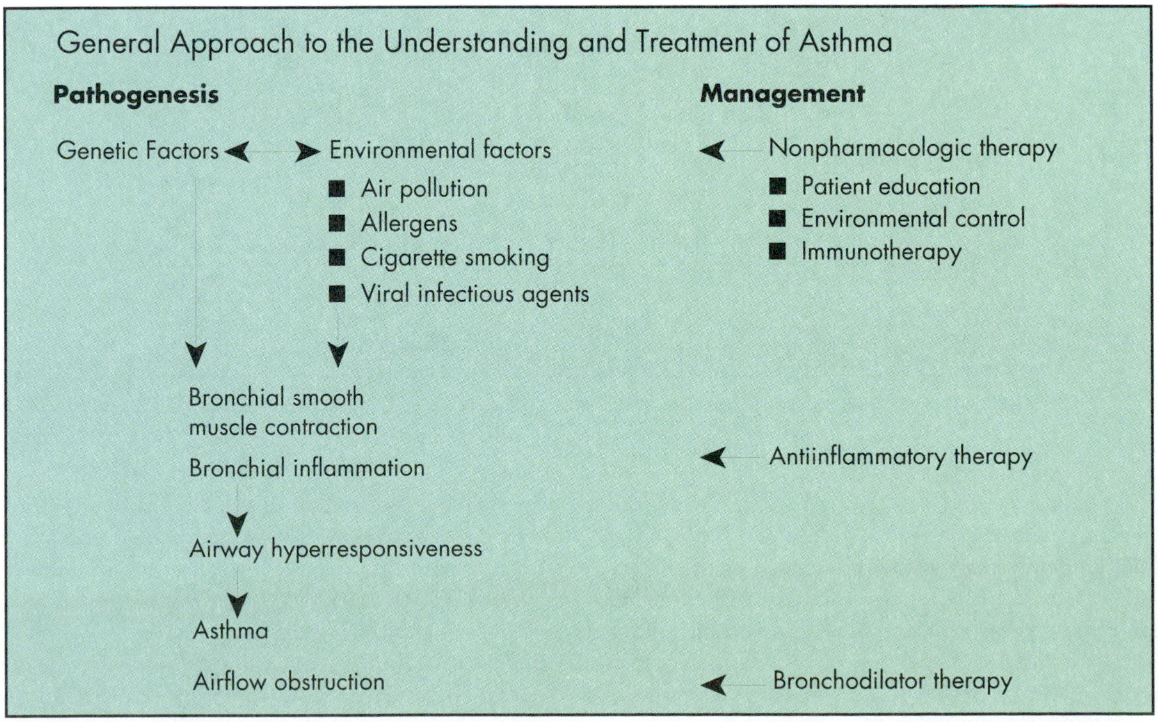

General Approach to the Understanding and Treatment of Asthma

Pathogenesis

Genetic Factors ◄———► Environmental factors
- Air pollution
- Allergens
- Cigarette smoking
- Viral infectious agents

Bronchial smooth muscle contraction

Bronchial inflammation

Airway hyperresponsiveness

Asthma

Airflow obstruction

Management

◄——— Nonpharmacologic therapy
- Patient education
- Environmental control
- Immunotherapy

◄——— Antiinflammatory therapy

◄——— Bronchodilator therapy

FOCUS BOX 12.2—Cont'd

Asthma, exercise-induced bronchoconstriction, and exercise

The aforementioned pathophysiology alludes to the treatment given for asthma (Figure 12.27). Since asthma results from the combination of airway hyperresponsiveness to stimuli, smooth muscle contraction, and inflammation, airway obstruction can be decreased if these events are prevented. Thus many individuals, especially children, are prescribed antiinflammatory preventative medications (usually intermittent use of inhaled corticosteroids). During an event of asthma, when obstruction is apparent, inhaled bronchodilators are used.[70]

Exercise is known to increase irritability of the bronchial network and increase the likelihood of asthma. However, unlike true asthma, asthma caused by exercise is not accompanied by inflammation and has therefore been termed *exercise-induced bronchoconstriction*. Exercise-induced bronchconstriction (EIB) results from irritation of the bronchial lining as a result of alterations in moisture and temperature caused by the increased air flow.[18] EIB usually does not occur until after exercise, reaching a

peak severity after 5 to 10 minutes of recovery and resolving completely after 30 minutes of recovery (Figure 12.28).[70] For individuals with EIB, graded exercise tests are often used to evaluate the onset of the condition or whether certain medications are effective in asthma prevention.[63,70]

Some research evidence exists for the decreased occurrence of EIB when exercise is performed in a warm, humid environment. Consequently, exercise such as swimming is highly recommended and exercise in cold or dry conditions is to be avoided for individuals susceptible to both EIB and asthma. When medications are used, the inhalation of a bronchodilator immediately before exercise and the use of corticosteroids as a preventative strategy can totally prevent asthma and EIB during and after exercise. Therefore individuals who are susceptible to asthma and EIB should not refrain from exercise participation. For example, during the 1984 Olympic games 67 athletes were asthmatics and many of these individuals received medals.[70]

FIGURE 12.28

The changes in FEV1 (forced expiration in 1 second) following a bout of exercise for an individual with exercise-induced bronchoconstriction. (From Dept of Health and Human Services: *Guidelines for the diagnoses and management of asthma,* Pub No 91-3042, 1991, National Institutes of Health.)

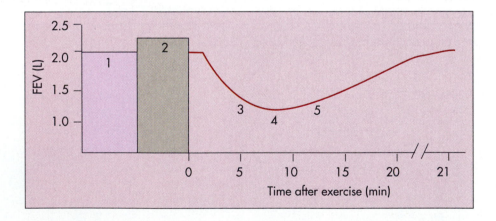

have an increasing $P_{A}O_2$ and a decreasing $PaCO_2$ during the development of arterial hypoxemia. At rest the venoarterial shunt of the lung and heart accounts for 50% of the difference between $P_{A}O_2$ and PaO_2, and researchers have estimated that the same could be true for exercise.[61] However, if a shunt explanation was valid, inspiring hyperoxic gas during exercise should not dramatically improve the hypoxemia. Dempsey[22] and Powers[56,58,60] have shown that breathing hyperoxic gas

does relieve the hypoxemia. The combined evidence presented earlier suggests that processes involved in the exchange of oxygen in the lung, such as diffusion limitations or ventilation–perfusion inequality, must be the causes.

The ventilation–perfusion ratio of the lung $V_E/\dot{Q}$ is difficult to measure during exercise however, researchers have documented evidence for the improvement and impairment of $V_E/\dot{Q}$ during increasing exercise intensities.[61] It is unclear whether an impaired $V_E/\dot{Q}$ contributes to hypoxemia, especially when this condition should also increase Pa_{CO_2}, which as previously described does not increase in this condition.

The final explanation, that of the lungs' decreasing diffusion capacity for oxygen, has received the most research support. Exercise challenges lung function by lowering the venous oxygen partial pressure and thus widening the pressure gradient for oxygen across the blood gas interface. In addition, exercise decreases the pulmonary transit time, thus decreasing the time for the equilibration of oxygen across an increased pressure gradient. If these conditions are accompanied by a decreased diffusibility of oxygen across the blood-gas interface, it is reasonable that an inequilibration between $P_{A_{O_2}}$ and Pa_{O_2} and hypoxemia might occur. However, these occurrences contradict the known increase in lung diffusion capacity during exercise.[16,40] A more likely explanation is that for a given diffusion capacity there is increased heterogeneity

FIGURE 12.29

The contribution of the possible causes of exercise-induced hypoxemia.

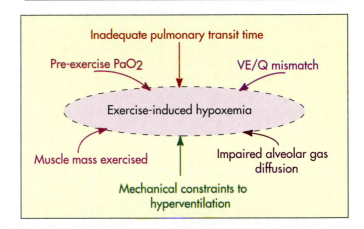

Efforts to Improve Exercise Tolerance and Training Adaptations in Individuals With Chronic Obstructive Pulmonary Disease

Chronic obstructive pulmonary disease (COPD) consists of numerous degenerative conditions of the lung characterized by the loss of compliance and increased resistance of the airways of either or both of the respiratory and conducting zones of the lung. In addition, alveoli can be damaged, thereby further impeding lung function by reducing the effective blood-gas interface. The most common forms of COPD are chronic bronchitis and emphysema.[18]

Individuals with COPD have labored breathing during both inspiration and expiration, and often have recurrent cough with expectorations. These conditions lower the maximal voluntary ventilatory volume. In addition, the obstruction to air flow and possible lung damage cause increased physiologic dead space, exaggerated ventilation-perfusion mismatch, and hypoxemia.[18] During exercise the damaged airways in individuals with COPD trap air and cause an increase in end-expiratory lung volume, which in turn decreases lung compliance during inspiration. Collectively, these responses cause an increase in the work of breathing.

The role of exercise in improving both central cardiovascular function and peripheral muscle endurance depends on the severity of COPD.[18] Mild COPD that causes minimal ventilatory restriction has been shown to improve systemic measures of improved endurance (e.g., decreased blood lactate, reduced

submaximal ventilation)[15,67]; however, individuals with severe COPD appear unable to train at a sufficient exercise intensity to induce central or peripheral chronic training adaptations.[6,7]

Strategies that have been used to overcome the limitations imposed by severe COPD are to generate positive pressure during inspiration (inspiratory positive airway pressure [IPAP]) or to produce continual (during both inspiration and expiration) positive airway pressure (CPAP). These conditions, if used during exercise or intermittently at rest, have been proposed to decrease the work of breathing, thereby providing increased blood flow and oxygen to the peripheral musculature. In addition, improved inspiratory function could partially improve the hypoxemia, as well as provide more time for expiration and normalize end-expiratory lung volume. Research has shown that use of IPAP in individuals with COPD prolonged exercise at 50% VO_2max and decreased ventilatory discomfort.[53] Other researchers have documented the reduced work of breathing with IPAP,[21,47] yet no data indicate that IPAP decreases end-expiratory lung volume. It is hoped that individuals with COPD will further benefit from advances made in equipment that aid in the overcoming of the central limitations to exercise tolerance, and thereby reap the improvements in quality of life that accompany increased exercise tolerance.

within the lung at very high exercise intensities,[40] and at best it remains unclear as to what actually causes the hypoxemia.

The best explanation of exercise-induced hypoxemia is that it is the result of several changes in lung function during intense exercise in well-trained endurance athletes (Figure 12.29). A decreasing pulmonary transit time, an increasing partial pressure gradient for oxygen, decreased or uneven diffusion capacities within the lung, venoarterial shunts, ventilation-perfusion inequality, and inadequate hyperventilation may combine to cause a significant arterial hypoxemia, although their separate influences are hard to detect experimentally.

Chronic Adaptations

The lungs and pulmonary circulation do not express the degree of long-term adaptation to exercise that was evident for the neuromuscular function and skeletal muscle energy metabolism. Efforts have been made to verify whether respiratory muscles can adapt to exercise training and improve lung function during exercise.[59] However, although respiratory muscles can adapt to exercise, it appears that their function remains near optimal, and there are no signs to support superior ventilatory function in the trained compared with the untrained state.

Numerous studies have shown that the ventilatory threshold improves with endurance training.[19,33,74] Because the causes for this improvement are determined more by muscular and cardiovascular function, as explained in Chapter 10 for the lactate threshold, no discussion is given in this chapter.

SUMMARY

- The lungs' main functions are to provide a means for oxygen to be transferred between atmospheric air and the blood, for the majority of metabolically produced carbon dioxide to be removed from the body, and for regulation of the blood pH.

- Air is directed to and from the lungs by the trachea. The mouth and nasal passages, trachea, bronchi, and bronchioles compose the **conducting zone** of the lungs, whereas the respiratory bronchioles, alveoli ducts, and alveoli, which are the sites of gas exchange and are responsible for the large lung gas volumes, are referred to as the **respiratory zone** of the lung. The conducting zone of the lung is often referred to as the **anatomic dead space,** since it does not have a respiratory function. The anatomic dead space comprises an average volume of 150 ml. The respiratory bronchioles and alveoli are the sites of lung inflation and deflation and collectively have a surface area of approximately 70 square meters.

- Blood from the heart is pumped through the pulmonary arteries to the lungs, and blood is directed back to the left side of the heart through the pulmonary veins. The circulation of blood to and through the lung is termed the **pulmonary circulation.**

- Normal resting breathing involves the inspiration and expiration of 500 ml of air, termed the **tidal volume.** It is the sum of the tidal volume and breathing frequency that determines **ventilation.** Because of the anatomic dead space, only 350 ml of "fresh" air reaches the respiratory zone during resting ventilation. The volume of fresh air that reaches the respiratory zone of the lung is termed **alveolar ventilation** (V_A).

- Ventilating air into the lungs, or *inspiration,* and expulsion of air from the lungs, or *expiration,* result from the expansion and compression of the pleural cavity, respectively. These maneuvers alter pressure gradients between the lung and atmospheric air, resulting in air movements along these gradients. These mechanical processes are driven by muscle contractions, and their role during ventilation increases during exercise.

■ Different changes in pressure and volume of the lungs exist for inspiration and expiration. During inspiration, the process of lung inflation is opposed by forces in the lung that resist inflation. the processes of inflation and deflation of the respiratory structures are aided by the presence of **surfactant,** which is evenly dispersed over the surfaces of the alveoli because of holes or **pores of Kohn,** that connect alveoli. Surfactant results in the interruption of the water layer and a reduction in surface tension, resulting in easier inflation of the lungs. The ability to inflate an object (such as the lung) with minimal force is termed *compliance.*

■ The resting pattern of ventilation results in greater volume changes in the lower regions of the lung, and therefore increases alveolar ventilation in these regions more than in the upper regions. Conversely, increased depth of breathing causes the added inflation of the lateral and upper regions of the lung because of the involvement of the flaring and elevation of the rib cage. A more even inflation of the lung results.

■ Because the two lungs are located beside the heart and extend vertically above the heart, a **hydrostatic force** exists to oppose blood flow to and perfusion of the upper regions of the lung. Consequently, under resting conditions greatest perfusion of the lung occurs near the lower regions and practically zero flow occurs in the upper regions.

■ The process of gas exchange, or **respiration,** involves the movement of oxygen and carbon dioxide down pressure gradients that exist between pulmonary capillary blood and the air of the alveoli, and between capillary blood of the systemic circulation and the cells perfused by this blood. Consequently, the locations of respiration can be either in the lung, which is referred to as **external respiration** (or pulmonary respiration), or at the level of the systemic tissues, which is referred to as **internal respiration** (or cellular respiration).

■ The factors that govern the direction and magnitude of gas diffusion in the lungs are the **diffusion capacity** of each of the gases, their partial pressure gradient between the alveoli and blood, and the characteristics of the medium through which diffusion occurs. The small thickness of the alveolar membranes and the large surface area of the respiratory zone (70 m^2) make the lung suited to gas diffusion. However, the low solubility and diffusion constant of oxygen may cause problems for oxygen diffusion.

■ The regions of the lung are not ventilated or perfused equally, and furthermore, the relationship between ventilation and perfusion varies in the progression from the bottom to the top of the lung. A measure of the effectiveness of lung respiration is the **ventilation-perfusion ratio** $V_E/\dot{Q}$, which under optimal conditions would equal 1.0.

■ Oxygen is transported in blood bound to a specialized protein, **hemoglobin,** which can carry 1.34 ml of oxygen per gram. Another small source of oxygen transport in blood is the volume of dissolved oxygen, which amounts to 0.003 ml of oxygen for every mm Hg of gas partial pressure, or 0.3 ml of oxygen at sea level.

■ The oxyhemoglobin dissociation curve describes the change in hemoglobin saturation with a decrease in $P_{A}O_2$. For $P_{A}O_2$ values that range from 100 to 80 mm Hg there is almost no reduction in the saturation of hemoglobin. As $P_{A}O_2$ decreases from 80 to 60 mm Hg, hemoglobin saturation decreases from 94.9% to 89.3%, and for $P_{A}O_2$ values below 60 mm Hg, dramatic decreases in hemoglobin saturation occur, which can result in large decreases in arterial oxygen transport.

■ Increased dissociation of oxygen and hemoglobin occurs at given P_{O_2} values in relation to increases in blood temperature, P_{CO_2}, and 2,3-bisphosphoglycerate and decreases in blood pH. These relationships are referred to as the **Bohr effect.** The volume of carbon dioxide stored in the body (blood and tissues) is approximately tenfold greater than oxygen stores. Carbon dioxide is transported in the blood in several forms, including bicarbonate, CO_2 bound to hemoglobin and blood proteins, and CO_2 dissolved in plasma and inside the red blood cells. The majority of CO_2 is transported as bicarbonate, and these reactions are driven by the enzyme **carbonic anhydrase,** located on the red blood cell membrane. The affinity between hemoglobin and CO_2 increases as the P_{O_2} decreases and vice versa, and this relationship is termed the **Haldane effect.**

SUMMARY—Cont'd

■ The unloading of oxygen from hemoglobin is also aided by the molecule **myoglobin.** Myoglobin is found within skeletal muscle fibers and is a protein similar to hemoglobin in that it can bind oxygen. In fact, the oxygen affinity of myoglobin is larger than that of hemoglobin, which allows a unidirectional transfer of oxygen from hemoglobin to myoglobin within the muscle fibers.

■ Ventilation can be controlled by both voluntary and involuntary functions of the nervous system. Neural controls exist in the central and peripheral nervous system and exert their effects through input and alteration to central controls of inspiration and expiration. The peripheral **chemoreceptors, aortic bodies** and **carotid bodies,** convert chemical stimuli into action potentials that are relayed to the control locations within the central nervous system. These multiple control systems combine to regulate ventilation, and their relative importance differs in the resting compared with exercise state.

■ Exercise provides multiple stimuli for increases in ventilation. At the start of exercise neural mechanisms are important, and then humoral factors fine-tune the neural controls to provide a steady-state ventilatory profile. When exercise intensity increases above the lactate or **ventilatory threshold,** acidosis develops and is accompanied by small increases in $PaCO_2$. These stimuli exert action on the peripheral and central chemoreceptors, resulting in increased neural input to the respiratory center and increased ventilation.

■ In 1984 it was observed that highly trained endurance athletes experience significant reductions in CaO_2 **(hypoxemia),** and this condition was termed **exercise-induced hypoxemia.** The more endurance trained the athlete, the larger the reduction in CaO_2, which indicates that for these individuals the lungs are not functioning optimally during intense exercise. The best explanation for exercise-induced hypoxemia is the combination of a decreasing **pulmonary transit time,** an increasing partial pressure gradient for oxygen, increasing pulmonary pressures and interstitial edema, venoarterial shunts, ventilation-perfusion inequality, and inadequate hyperventilation.

■ A common obstructive lung disorder is **asthma,** which is a temporary condition of increased sensitivity of the lining of the airways causing constriction of the small airways. There are many causes of asthma, and a common condition termed *exercise-induced bronchoconstriction* can occur during the initial recovery from exercise.

REVIEW QUESTIONS

1. What are the two zones of the lung, and how do their functions differ?

2. What is surfactant, where is it located within the lung, and what are its functions?

3. How does air move into and out of the lung?

4. Why is compliance of the lung important to ventilation at rest and during exercise?

5. Calculate the oxygen transported in the blood every minute for the following conditions:

    A) $[Hb]=120$ gm/L, $PaO_2=98$ mm Hg, $Q=25$ L/min

    B) $[Hb]=120$ gm/L, $PaO_2=75$ mm Hg, $Q=25$ L/min

    C) $[Hb]=145$ gm/L, $PaO_2=98$ mm Hg, $Q=25$ L/min

    D) $[Hb]=145$ gm/L, $PaO_2=75$ mm Hg, $Q=25$ L/min

When cardiac output is considered, do small changes in either hemoglobin concentration or hemoglobin saturation result in large changes in blood oxygen transport? How would small decreases in either $[Hb]$ or PaO_2 influence the ability to exercise at moderate to high intensities?

6. Are the Haldane and Bohr effects simply a reversal of each other? Explain.

7. Why are alveolar gas partial pressures different from those of atmospheric air?

8. Why is gas solubility important for diffusion between the alveoli and blood?

9. Why is carbon dioxide considered an acid in the balance of factors that can determine blood acid-base balance?

10. Why is PaO_2 less than P_AO_2?

11. Explain why ventilation and perfusion need to be balanced to optimize gas exchange in the lung. How does exercise improve ventilation–perfusion in the lung?

12. What are the central and peripheral regulators of ventilation?

13. How does ventilation change during incremental exercise, and what factors are believed to cause these changes?

14. Is the ventilation threshold identical to the lactate threshold? Explain.

15. Why does the metabolic cost of ventilation increase during exercise?

16. What is exercise-induced hypoxemia, why does it occur, and does it occur in all individuals?

APPLICATIONS

1. You are asked by an asthma sufferer why exercise seems to exacerbate the condition. What is your response, and what types of exercise would you recommend?

2. Given the limitations to gas exchange and blood gas transport induced by COPD, how would these conditions influence the status of skeletal muscle and its ability to tolerate exercise?

3. Why are clinical pulmonologists experimenting with positive inspiratory pressure to aid the rehabilitation and exercise tolerance of individuals with COPD?

4. Many well-trained endurance athletes experience decreases in PaO_2 during intense exercise. Does this response reflect an impairment of lung function or lung damage? Explain.

5. Many clinical exercise tests are conducted that use the ventilation threshold as an index of skeletal muscle metabolism and the lactate threshold. Is this a correct and accurate practice? Explain.

REFERENCES

1. Anderson GS, Rhodes EC: The relationship between blood lactate and excess CO_2 in elite cyclists, *J Sports Sci* 9:173-181, 1991.

2. Bastacky JB, Goerke J: Pores of Kohn are filled in normal lungs: low-temperature scanning electron microscopy, *J Appl Physiol* 73(1):88-95, 1992.

3. Baumann R, Bartels H, Bauer C: Blood oxygen transport. In Farhi LE, Tenney SM, editors: *Handbook of physiology,* Vol 1, Bethesda, Maryland, 1987, American Physiological Society.

4. Beaver W, Wasserman K, Whipp B: A new method for detecting anaerobic threshold by gas exchange, *J Appl Physiol* 60(6):2020-2027, 1986.

5. Beck KC, Babb TG, Staats BA, Hyatt RE: Dynamics of breathing during exercise. In Whipp BJ, Wasserman K, editors: *Exercise: pulmonary physiology and pathophysiology.* vol 52. *Lung biology in health and disease,* New York, 1991, Marcel Dekkes, pp 67-98.

6. Belman MJ, Kendregan BA: Exercise training fails to increase skeletal muscle enzymes inpatients with chronic obstructive pulmonary disease, *Am Rev Respir Dis* 123:256-261, 1981.

7. Belman MJ, Kendregan BA: Physical training fails to improve ventilatory muscle endurance in patients with chronic obstructive pulmonary disease, *Chest* 81:440-443, 1982.

8. Bennett F: A role for neural pathways in exercise hyperpnea, *J Appl Physiol* 56(6):1559-1564, 1984.

9. Boutellier U, Piwko P: The respiratory system as an exercise limiting factor in normal sedentary subjects, *Eur J Appl Physiol* 64:145-152, 1992.

10. Brice AG, Foster HV, Pan LG et al: Ventilatory and $PaCO_2$ responses to voluntary and electrically induced leg exercise, *J Appl Physiol* 64(1):218-225, 1988.

11. Brice AG, Foster HV, Pan LG et al: Is the hyperpnea of muscular contractions critically dependent upon spinal cord afferents? *J Appl Physiol* 64(1):226-233, 1988.

12. Busse M, Maassen N, Konrad H: Relation between plasma K^+ and ventilation during incremental exercise after glycogen depletion and repletion in man, *J Physiol* 443:469-476, 1991.

13. Caizzeo VJ, Davis JA, Ellis JF et al: A comparison of gas exchange indices used to detect the anaerobic threshold, *J Appl Physiol* 53(5):1184-1189, 1982.

14. Capen RL, Hanson WL, Latham LP et al: Distribution of pulmonary transmit times in recruited networks, *J Appl Physiol* 69(2):473-478, 1990.

15. Casaburi R, Patesio A, Franco I et al: Reduction in lactic acidosis and ventilation as a result of exercise training in patients with obstructive lung disease, *Am Rev Respir Dis* 143:9-18, 1991.

16. Cerretelli P, Di Prampero PE: Gas exchange in exercise. In Farhi LE, Tenney SM, editors: *Handbook of physiology,* vol 1, Bethesda, Maryland, 1987, American Physiological Society.

17. Cotton DJ, Taher F, Mink JT, Graham BL: Effect of volume history on changes in $DLco^{SB}$-3EQ with lung volume in normal subjects, *J Appl Physiol* 73(2):434-439, 1992.

18. Cox NJM, van Herwaarden CLA, Folgering H, Binkhorst RA: Exercise and training in patients with chronic obstructive lung disease, *Sports Med* 6(3):180-192, 1988.

19. Davis JA, Vodak P, Wilmore J et al: Anaerobic threshold and maximal aerobic power for three modes of exercise, *J Appl Physiol* 41(4):544-550, 1976.

20. Dejours P: Control of respiration in muscular exercise. In Fenn WO, Rahn H, editors: *Handbook of physiology,* vol 1, Washington, DC, 1964, American Physiological Society.

21. Dekhuijzin PNR, Foldering HTM, van Herwaarden CLA: Target-flow inspiratory muscle training during pulmonary rehabilitation in patients with COPD, *Chest* 99:128-133, 1991.

22. Dempsey JA, Hanson PG, Henderson KS: Exercise-induced arterial hypoxemia in healthy persons at sea level, *J Physiol* 355-161-175, 1984.

23. Dempsey JA, Mitchell G, Smith C: Exercise and chemoreception, *Am Rev Respir Dis* 129:31-34, 1984.

24. Dempsey JA, Virdruk E, Mitchell G: Pulmonary control systems in exercise: update, *Fed Proc* 44:2260-2270, 1985.

25. Dempsey JA: Is the lung built for exercise, *Med Sci Sports Exerc* 18(2):143-155, 1986.

26. Department of Health and Human Services: Guidelines for the diagnoses and management of asthma, Publication No. 91-3042, Washington, DC, 1991, National Institutes of Health.

27. Derion T, Guy HJB, Tsukimoto K et al: Ventilation-perfusion relationships in the lung during head-out water immersion, *J Appl Physiol* 72(1):64-72, 1992.

28. Eldridge F, Millhorn DE, Waldrop TG: Exercise hyperpnea and locomotion: parallel activation from the hypothalamus, *Science* 211:844-846, 1981.

29. Eldridge F, Millhorn DE, Kiley JP, Waldrop TG: Stimulation by central command of locomotion, respiration, and circulation during exercise, *Respir Physiol* 59:313-317, 1985.

30. Farrell SW, Ivy JL: Lactate acidosis and the increase in VE/VO_2 during incremental exercise, *J Appl Physiol* 62(4):1551-1555, 1987.

31. Favier R, Desplanches D, Frutoso J et al: Ventilatory and circulatory transients during exercise: new arguments for a neurohumoral theory, *J Appl Physiol* 54(3):647-653, 1983.

REFERENCES—Cont'd

32. Fencl V, Leith DE: Stewart's quantitative acid-base chemistry: applications in biology and medicine, *Respir Physiol* 91:1-16, 1993.

33. Gaesser GA, Poole DC: Lactate and ventilatory thresholds: disparity in time course of adaptations to training, *J Appl Physiol* 61(3):999-1004, 1986.

34. Gladden LB, Yates JW, Stremel RW, Stamford BA: Gas exchange and lactate anaerobic thresholds: inter- and intrae-valuator agreement, *J Appl Physiol* 58(6):2082-2089, 1985.

35. Green J, Schmidt N: Mechanism of hyperpnea induced by changes in pulmonary blood flow, *J Appl Physiol* 56:1418-1422, 1984.

36. Grucza R, Miyamoto Y, Nakazonto Y: Kinetics of cardiorespiratory response to rhythmic-static exercise in men, *Eur J Appl Physiol* 61:230-236, 1990.

37. Guenard H, Varene N, Vaida P: Determination of lung capillary blood volume and membrane diffusing capacity in man by the measurements of NO and CO transfer, *Respir Physiol* 70:113-120, 1987.

38. Guyton AC: *Textbook of medical physiology,* ed 8, Philadelphia, 1991, WB Saunders.

39. Hagberg JM, Coyle EF, Carrol JE et al: Exercise hyperventilation in patients with McArdle's disease, *J Appl Physiol* 52(4):991-994, 1982.

40. Hlastala MP: Diffusing capacity heterogeneity. In Farhi LE, Tenney SM, editors: *Handbook of physiology,* vol 1, pp 217-232 Bethesda, Maryland, 1987, American Physiological Society.

41. Hughes JMB: Diffusive gas exchange. In Whipp BJ, Wasserman K, editors: Exercise: pulmonary physiology and pathophysiology, Vol 52. *Lung biology in health and disease,* New York, 1991, Marcel Dekkes, pp 143-172.

42. Innes JA, Solarte I, Huszczuk A et al: Respiration during recovery from exercise: effects of trapping and release of femoral artery blood flow, *J Appl Physiol* 67(6):2608-2613, 1989.

43. Johnson BD, Saupe KW, Dempsey JA: Mechanical constraints on exercise hyperpnea in endurance athletes, *J Appl Physiol* 73(3):874-886, 1992.

44. Jones NL: *Blood gases and acid-base physiology,* ed 2, New York, 1987, Thieme Medical.

45. Klocke RA: Carbon dioxide transport. In Farhi LE, Tenney SM, editors: *Handbook of physiology,* vol 1, pp 173-198, Bethesda, Maryland, 1987, American Physiological Society.

46. Koike A, Weiler-Ravell D, McKenzie DK et al: Evidence that the metabolic acidosis threshold is the anaerobic threshold, *J Appl Physiol* 68(6):2521-2526, 1990.

47. Larson JL, Kim MJ, Sharp JT, Larson DA: Inspiratory muscle training with a pressure threshold breathing device in patients with chronic obstructive pulmonary disease, *Am Rev Respir Dis* 138:689-696, 1988.

48. Lehninger AL: *Principles of biochemistry,* New York, 1993, Worth Publishers.

49. Loat CER, Rhodes EC: Relationship between the lactate and ventilatory thresholds during prolonged exercise, *Sports Med* 15(2):104-115, 1993.

50. Mairbaurl H, Schobersberger W, Hasibeder W et al: Regulation of 2, 3-DPG and Hb-O$_2$-affinity during acute exercise, *Eur J Appl Physiol* 55:174-180, 1986.

51. McCool FD, Hershenson MB, Tzelepis GE et al: Effect of fatigue on maximal inspiratory pressure-flow capacity, *J Appl Physiol* 73(1):36-43, 1992.

52. Neary PJ, MacDougall JD, Bachus R, Wenger HA: The relationship between lactate and ventilatory thresholds: coincidental or cause and effect? *Eur J Appl Physiol* 54:104-108, 1985.

53. O'Donnell DE, Sanii R, Giesbrecht G, Younes M: Effect of continuous positive airway pressures on respiratory sensation in patients with chronic obstructive pulmonary disease during submaximal exercise, *Am Rev Respir Dis* 138:1185-1191, 1988.

REFERENCES—Cont'd

54. Paek D, McCool D: Breathing patterns during varied activities, *J Appl Physiol* 73(3):887-893, 1992.

55. Paterson D: Potassium and ventilation during exercise, *J Appl Physiol* 72(3):810-820, 1992.

56. Powers SK, Dodd S, Lawler J et al: Incidence of exercise induced hypoxemia in the elite endurance athlete at sea level, *Eur J Appl Physiol* 58:298-302, 1988.

57. Powers SK, Williams J: Exercise-induced hypoxemia in highly trained athletes, *Sports Med* 4:46-53, 1987.

58. Powers SK, Lawlor J, Dempsey JA et al: Effects of incomplete pulmonary gas exchange on VO_2max, *J Appl Physiol* 66(6):2491-2495, 1989.

59. Powers SK, Lawlor J, Criswell D et al: Endurance-training-induced cellular adaptations in respiratory muscles, *J Appl Physiol* 68(5):2114-2118, 1990.

60. Powers SK, Martin D, Cicale M et al: Exercise induced hypoxemia in athletes: role of inadequate hyperventilation, *Eur J Appl Physiol* 65:37-42, 1992.

61. Powers SK, Martin D, Dodd S: Exercise-induced hypoxemia in elite endurance athletes: incidence, causes and impact on VO_2max, *Sports Med* 16(1):14-22, 1993.

62. Reuschlein PS, Reddan WG, Burpee J et al: Effect of physical training on the pulmonary diffusing capacity during submaximal work, *J Appl Physiol* 24(2):152-158, 1968.

63. Roberts JA: Exercise-induced asthma in athletes, *Sports Med* 6(4):193-196, 1988.

64. Roselli RJ, Parker RE, Harris TR: A model of unsteady-state transvascular fluid and protein transport in the lung, *J Appl Physiol* 56(5):1389-1402, 1984.

65. Seeley RR, Stephens TD, Tate P: *Anatomy and physiology,* St. Louis, 1993, Mosby.

66. Skinner JS, McLellan TH: The transition from aerobic to anaerobic metabolism, *Res Quart Exerc Sport* 51(1):234-248, 1980.

67. Sonne LJ, Davis JA: Increased exercise performance in patients with severe COPD following inspiratory resistive training, *Chest* 81:436-439, 1982.

68. Stewart PA: Modern quantitative acid-base chemistry, *Can J Physiol Pharmacol* 61:1444-1461, 1983.

69. Terrados N, Jansson E, Sylven C, Kaijser L: Is hypoxia a stimulus for synthesis of oxidative enzymes and myoglobin? *J Appl Physiol* 68(6):2369-2372, 1990.

70. Torre-Bueono JR, Wagner PD, Saltzman HA, et al: Diffusion limitation in normal humans during exercise at sea level and simulated altitude, *J Appl Physiol* 58(3):989-995, 1985.

71. Wagner PD, Gale GE: Ventilation-perfusion relationships. In Whipp BJ, Wasserman K, editors: *Exercise: pulmonary physiology and pathophysiology.* Vol 52. *Lung biology in health and disease,* New York, 1991, Marcel Dekkes, pp 121-142.

72. Warren G, Cureton KJ, Middendorf WF, et al: Red blood cell pulmonary transit time during exercise in athletes, *Med Sci Sports Exerc* 23(12):1353-1361, 1991.

73. Wasserman K, McIlroy MB: Detecting the threshold of anaerobic metabolism in cardiac patients during exercise, *Am J Cardiol* 14:844-852, 1964.

74. Wasserman K, Whipp BJ, Koyal SN, Beaver WL: Anaerobic threshold and respiratory gas exchange during exercise, *J Appl Physiol* 35(2):236-243, 1973.

75. Wasserman K, Whipp BJ, Casaburi R: Respiratory control during exercise. In Cherniak NS, Widdicombe JG, editors: *Handbook of physiology,* vol II, Bethesda, Maryland, 1986, American Physiological Society.

76. Wasserman K, Casaburi R: Acid-base regulation during exercise in humans. In Whipp BJ, Wasserman K, editors: *Exercise: pulmonary physiology and pathophysiology.* Vol 52, *Lung biology in health and disease,* 1991, pp 405-448.

77. Weissman ML, Jones PW, Oren A et al: Cardiac output increase and gas exchange at the start of exercise, *J Appl Physiol* 52(1):236-244, 1982.

78. West JB: *Respiratory physiology: the essentials,* ed 4, Baltimore, 1990, Williams & Wilkins.

79. Whipp B, Ward S: Physiological determinants of pulmonary gas exchange kinetics during exercise, *Med Sci Sports Exerc* 22(1):62-71, 1990.

80. Whipp BJ, Ward SA: Coupling of ventilation to pulmonary gas exchange during exercise. In Whipp BJ, Wasserman K, editors: *Exercise: pulmonary physiology and pathophysiology,* Vol 52. *Lung biology in health and disease.* New York, 1991, Marcel Dekkes, pp 271-308.

81. Williams JH, Powers SK, Kelly Stewart M: Hemoglobin desaturation in highly trained athletes during heavy exercise, *Med Sci Sports Exerc* 18(2):168-173, 1986.

82. Yeh MP, Gardner RM, Adams TD et al: "Anaerobic threshold": problems of determination and validation, *J Appl Physiol* 55(4):1178-1186, 1983.

83. Younes M: Determinants of dynamic excursions during exercise. In Whipp BJ, Wasserman K, editors: *Exercise: pulmonary physiology and pathophysiology,* Vol 52. *Lung biology in health and disease,* New York, 1991, Marcel Dekkes, pp 1-66.

RECOMMENDED READINGS

▪ Baumann R, Bartels H, Bauer C: Blood oxygen transport. In Farhi LE, Tenney SM, editors: *Handbook of physiology,* vol 1, Bethesda, Maryland, 1987, American Physiological Society.

▪ Beaver W, Wasserman K, Whipp B: A new method for detecting anaerobic threshold by gas exchange, *J Appl Physiol* 60(6):2020-2027, 1986.

▪ Cerretelli P, Di Prampero PE: Gas exchange in exercise. In Farhi LE, Tenney SM, editors: *Handbook of physiology,* vol 1, Bethesda, Maryland, 1987, American Physiological Society.

▪ Dempsy JA: Is the lung built for exercise? *Med Sci Sports Exerc* 18(2):1423-155, 1986.

▪ Farrell SW, Ivy JL: Lactate acidosis and the increase in VE/VO$_2$ during incremental exercise, *J Appl Physiol* 62(4):1551-1555, 1987.

▪ Fencl V, Leith DE: Stewart's quantitative acid-base chemistry: applications in biology and medicine, *Respir Physiol* 91:1-16, 1993.

▪ Jones NL: *Blood gases and acid-base physiology,* ed 2, New York, 1987, Thieme Medical.

▪ Koike A, Weiler-Ravell D, McKenzie DK et al: Evidence that the metabolic acidosis threshold is the anaerobic threshold, *J Appl Physiol* 68(6):2521-2526, 1990.

▪ Powers SK, Martin D, Dodd S: Exercise-induced hypoxemia in elite endurance athletes: incidence, causes and impact on VO$_2$max, *Sports Med* 16(1):14-22, 1993.

▪ Stewart PA: Modern quantative acid-base chemistry, *Can J Physiol Pharmacol* 61:1444-1461, 1983.

▪ Warren G, Cureton KJ, Middendorf WF et al: Red blood cell pulmonary transit time during exercise in athletes, *Med Sci Sports Exerc* 23(12):1353-1361, 1991.

▪ West JB: *Respiratory physiology: the essentials,* ed 4, Baltimore, 1990, Williams & Wilkins.

CHAPTER 13 Neuroendocrine Adaptations to Exercise

OBJECTIVES

After studying this chapter, you should be able to :

- Explain the diversity of hormone secretion in the body and compare the different body tissues that secrete hormones.

- Classify hormones into the amine, peptide, or steroid category.

- Identify the different cellular response mechanisms of amine, peptide, and steroid hormones.

- Describe the hormonal responses to exercise that influence muscle energy metabolism, energy substrate mobilization, fluid balance, vascular hemodynamics, and protein synthesis.

- Explain the importance of circulating catecholamines to lung and muscle function during exercise.

- Explain why exercise intensity and duration influence the secretion of specific hormones.

- Explain the terms *insulin sensitivity* and *insulin responsiveness*, and how exercise and endurance training can alter either condition, as well as what these changes mean for individuals with either type I or type II diabetes.

- Identify the different reasons for hormone secretion during short-term compared with prolonged exercise.

- Describe the regulation of blood pressure and how certain drugs function to lower blood pressure in individuals with hypertension.

- Explain the changes in the secretion of specific hormones after endurance training.

- Describe the important roles played by the hypothalamic-pituitary axis in the body's acute and chronic responses to exercise.

KEY TERMS

neuroendocrinology	glucose-fatty acid cycle
gland	hyperglycemia
hormone	diabetes mellitus
down-regulation	osmoreceptor
up-regulation	antidiuretic
second messenger	diuresis
cyclic AMP (cAMP)	hypertension
GLUT-4	hypotension
hypoglycemia	vasomotor center
insulin sensitivity	endogenous opioids
insulin responsiveness	athletic amenorrhea

The body's acute adaptations to exercise have been explained extensively in the preceding chapters; these processes could not have taken place without the involvement of nerves or hormones, or both. Exercise induces a multitude of neural and hormonal adaptations, which are involved in changing the function of skeletal muscle, smooth muscle, the heart, lungs, liver, kidneys, brain, and other tissues. The large number of hormones involved in these responses requires a complete text to do justice to the topic. This chapter, then, is a summary of the field of exercise endocrinology. It is not intended to be a comprehensive review, but rather a concise organization of the most important theoretical issues and research findings. The study of exercise and endocrinology traditionally has been approached on a hormone-to-hormone or gland-to-gland basis. This is unfortunate, because often several hormones from different glands join forces to elicit a given biologic response to a particular exercise stress. Because of the multiplicity of endocrine regulation, the gland-by-gland approach is not the best means of presenting the overall picture of neurohumoral regulation of discrete biologic functions during exercise. This chapter provides a brief introduction to the science of neuroendocrinology. It also details the acute and chronic neuroendocrine adaptations to exercise, which are categorized by topics of regulation important to the body's response to exercise stress.

Neuroendocrine System

euroendocrinology is the study of the combined function of nerves and glands involved in the release of hormones that regulate the function of body tissues. Traditionally, the hormones of interest were secreted by glandular tissues grouped and classified as *endocrine glands*. The joint functioning of nerves and hormones is important because most of the body's glands are stimulated by nerves and metabolic conditions, resulting in the release (or inhibition of the release) of one or more hormones.

Glands

A **gland** is a tissue that secretes a substance within or from the body. The glands can be divided into *exocrine* or *endocrine*. Exocrine glands, which secrete substances from the body, are further divided into *apocrine* and *eccrine* glands. Apocrine and eccrine glands both have ducts. The apocrine gland secretes sebaceous fluid, such as the oil that is secreted to the surface of the skin, or the bile ducts of the liver. The eccrine gland secretes sweat.

neuroendocrinology (nu ro-en do-kri-**no'**l o-je)
   the study of the anatomy and function of the endocrine system and the components of the nervous system that regulate endocrine function

gland
   an organ that secretes one or more substances

TABLE 13.1

Traditional and nontraditional glands and hormones

TISSUE/GLAND	HORMONES		
	AMINE	**PEPTIDE**	**STEROID**
TRADITIONAL HORMONES			
Pituitary			
Anterior		Luteinizing hormone (LH), follicle-stimulating hormone (FSH), prolactin (PRL), growth hormone (GH), adrenocorticotropin (ACTH), β-lipoprotein, β-endorphin, thyroid-stimulating hormone (TSH)	
Intermediate		Melanocyte-stimulating hormone (MSH), β-endorphin	
Posterior		Antidiuretic hormone (ADH, or vasopressin), oxytocin	
Thyroid	Thyroxine (T_4), triiodothyronine (T_3)	Calcitonin	
Parathyroid		Parathyroid hormone (PTH)	
Adrenal			
Cortex			Cortisol, aldosterone, androstanedione
Medulla	Epinephrine, norepinephrine		
Gonads			
Testes			Testosterone, estradiol, androstanedione
Ovaries			Estradiol, progesterone, testosterone, androstanedione, FSH-releasing peptide
Placenta			Progesterone, estrogen
Pancreas		Insulin, glucagon, somatostatin, vasoactive intestinal peptide (VIP)	
NONTRADITIONAL HORMONES			
Hypothalamus		[ACTH]-releasing hormone (CRH), thyrotropin-releasing hormone (TRH), LH-releasing hormone (LHRH), GH-releasing hormone (GHRH), somatostatin	
Heart		Atrial natriuretic peptides (ANP)	
Kidney		Erythropoietin, renin, 1,25-dihydroxyvitamin D	
Liver		Insulin-like growth factor I (IGF-I)	
Gastrointestinal tract		Cholecystokinin (CCK), gastrin, secretin, VIP, enteroglucagon	
Lymphocytes		Interleukins	
Vascular endothelium,		Endothelin (ET), nitrous oxide (endothelial-derived relaxing factor [EDRF])	

FIGURE 13.1

An overview of the anatomic location of the major glands and gland-like tissues that are involved in the body's acute and chronic responses to exercise. (From Thibodeau GA, Patton KT: *Anatomy and physiology*, 3 ed, St. Louis, 1996, Mosby. Art by Joan Beck.)

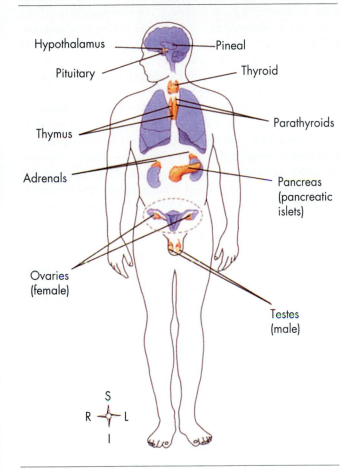

Endocrine glands, which are ductless, secrete a substance directly into the blood. Traditionally, a substance secreted from an endocrine gland was known as a **hormone.** Hormones were released in minor amounts that produced low concentrations in the blood (<1 μmol), and they exerted their function on tissues in other regions of the body. The science of endocrinology is the study of endocrine glands, their hormones, and the effects of specific hormones on various body tissues. A list of the traditional endocrine glands and their hormones is provided in Table 13.1, and the anatomic locations of these glands are illustrated in Figure 13.1.

Sources of Hormones

Research during the past decade has revealed that the traditional definition of a hormone may not be appropriate. It is now known that tissues other than true endocrine glands secrete substances that act as hormones. For example, the hypothalamus, heart, kidneys, liver, gastrointestinal (GI) tract,

lymphocytes, and endothelial cells all secrete substances that exert regulatory effects on other tissues; some of these substances influence neighboring tissues *(paracrine function)* and some influence the cells they are secreted from *(autocrine function).*[44]

A list of nontraditional hormones and the tissues from which they are secreted is provided in Table 13.1. Tissues such as the heart are involved in the regulation of blood pressure and fluid balance by means of the hormone atrial natriuretic peptide (ANP). The role of endothelial-derived substances that induce vasoconstriction and vasodilation is discussed in Chapter 11. Clearly, the traditional approach to and definitions of endocrinology are too simplistic and narrow to apply to the now-recognized complex hormonal regulation of many bodily functions.

Hormone Classification

Hormones differ in the way they stimulate cells. They are divided into three main categories: amine, peptide, and steroid.

Amine and Peptide Hormones

Amine hormones are derived from amino acids. Peptide hormones are proteins and therefore are structured by peptide bonds between multiple amino acids. The structures of the amine hormones epinephrine and norepinephrine and of the peptide hormones insulin and erythropoietin are illustrated in Figure 13.2. Epinephrine and norepinephrine are derived from the amino acid tyrosine. The peptide hormones are formed through protein synthesis (see Chapter 5). Insulin and erythropoietin are not synthesized as active hormones, but as larger hormone precursor molecules. The precursor molecule for insulin, called a *preprohormone,* requires the removal of an amino acid sequence (C peptide) within the molecule. Erythropoietin, a *prohormone,* requires enzymatic removal of an end sequence of amino acids.

Because amine and peptide hormones are soluble, they are transported in blood plasma in solution. However, being in solution, they are easily removed from the circulation by tissues such as the liver, kidneys, and lung; therefore they have only a few minutes to exert their function. The length of time it takes for the removal or destruction of half the hormone is called a *half-life.* For example, the half-life of epinephrine and norepinephrine is less than 3 minutes.[47] Although an amine, triiodothyronine has a half-life of about 7 days, because it binds to a special globulin protein in the plasma.[47] The half-life of cortisol, a steroid hormone that binds specific plasma proteins, is approximately 70 to 90 minutes.[44]

---

hormone (hor' mone)
a substance secreted from a tissue or cell that exerts a biologic effect on that tissue or cell, or on local or distant cells

FIGURE 13.2

The biochemical steps involved in the synthesis of the cate-cholamines. As indicated, both hormones are derivatives of the amino acid tyrosine, and the structure of epinephrine and norepinephrine are very similar. This slight structural difference explains the differing sensitivity of the two hormones to the various types of adrenergic receptors.

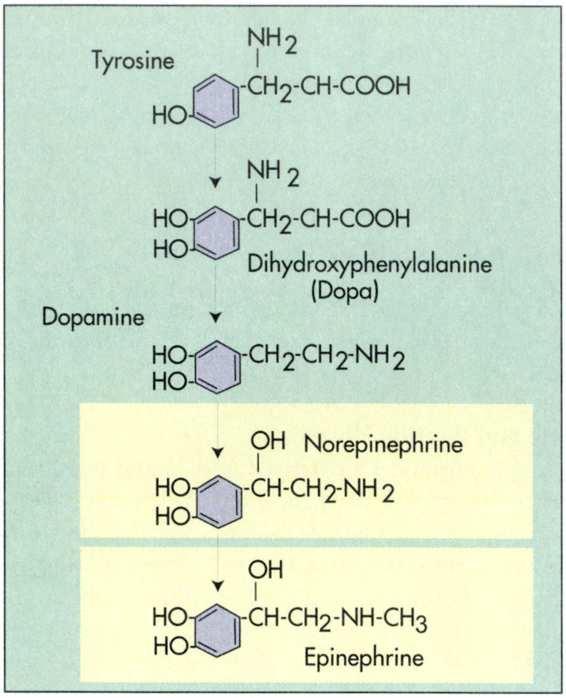

The biologic activity of hormones depends not only on their circulating concentration, but also on the number and density of receptors on cell membranes. Because hormone-receptor binding often destroys receptors, receptor production and positioning in the cell membrane is a continual process. Generally, an increase in circulating hormones causes a decrease in the number of receptors in the cell membrane, a process called **down-regulation.** Conversely, when a cell responds to a hormone by increasing receptor production and incorporation into the cell membrane, the process is called **up-regulation.** However, because thousands of excess receptors normally are present on a cell membrane relative to circulating hormone concentrations,[44] down- or up-regulation does little to influence the biologic response unless the number of receptors changes greatly. As with enzyme kinetics, *the greater the number of receptors, the lower the hormone concentration needed to elicit a given biologic response.* Table 13.2 identifies the hormones whose release from the glands of the body is influenced by exercise.

Cellular response mechanisms. Amine and peptide hormones exert their action on target cells by binding to specific

receptors on the cell membranes of the target tissue or tissues. Consequently, the correct receptors must be present on the cell membrane for the biologic response to the release of amine and peptide hormones to occur. Not only are receptors different and therefore specific for each hormone, but some hormones (e.g., epinephrine and norepinephrine) have several types of receptors, which further differentiate and specialize cellular biologic response. (This concept is explained in Chapter 8 for the α- and β-receptors of the neurotransmitter norepinephrine, as are the different affinities between norepinephrine and epinephrine for these receptors)

To elicit a cellular response, the binding of an amine or peptide hormone to a receptor must cause changes in cellular function. The molecules produced in a cell in response to hormone binding, which then stimulate a cellular response, are called **second messengers.** Figure 13.3 presents the main second messengers and a hormone-receptor example for each. As explained in Chapter 9, cyclic adenosine monophosphate (**cyclic AMP or cAMP**) is produced in response to the binding of epinephrine to a β_2-receptor on the sarcolemma of a skeletal muscle fiber; however, when epinephrine binds to an α_2-receptor, the production of cAMP is inhibited. When epinephrine binds to an α_1-receptor, an inositol phospholipid is broken down, and two additional second messengers are released (diacylglycerol and inositol triphosphate), which produce an increase in intracellular calcium and the activation and inhibition of various enzymes. A consistent theme in receptor binding and second-messenger production is activation of a membrane-bound enzyme that catalyzes the production of the second messenger. Second messengers then activate and inhibit certain enzymes, altering the metabolism of the cell. These processes of enzyme activation and inhibition are extremely fast, and the time between stimulation for the release of amine and peptide hormones and a cellular response is less than 1 minute.

down-regulation
a diminished biologic response to a given compound; usually involves a reduction in the number of receptors or an impaired cellular response to the binding of a hormone to its receptor.

up-regulation
an increased biologic response to a given compound

second messenger
an intracellular compound that increases in concentration during the amplification response to the binding of a hormone to its cell receptor

cyclic AMP (cAMP)
cyclic adenosine monophosphate; the second messenger produced by the activation of adenylate cyclase in response to the binding of certain hormones to their cell receptors

FIGURE 13.3

The two main second messenger systems of the body that are stimulated by hormones. **A,** The inositol triphosphate–diacylglycerol system that stimulates protein kinase c and the intracellular release of calcium, which in turn activate kinase enzymes within the cell and regulates muscle contraction.

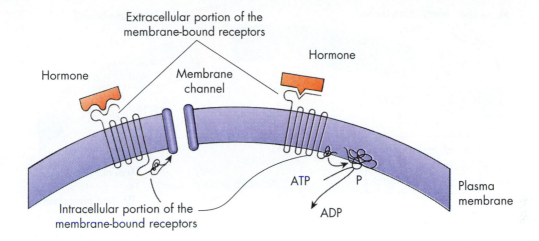

(1) When a hormone binds to the extracellular portion of its receptor, the intracellular portion of the receptor opens or closes a membrane channel (e.g. acetylcholine receptors open sodium ion channels).

(2) When a hormone binds to the extracellular portion of its receptor, the intracellular portion of the receptor phosphorylates proteins in the plasma membrane (e.g. insulin receptors phosphorylate proteins in the plasma membrane).

A

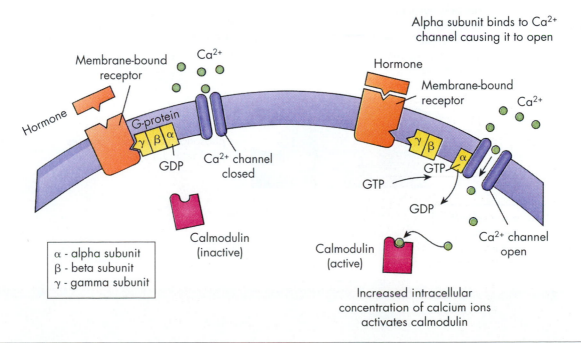

α - alpha subunit
β - beta subunit
γ - gamma subunit

Continued.

FIGURE 13.3—Cont'd

B, The adenylate cyclase–cyclic AMP (cAMP) system that activates kinase enzymes within the cell. (From Seeley RR, Stephens TD, Tate P: *Anatomy and physiology,* 3 ed, St. Louis, 1995, Mosby. Art by Rolin Graphics.)

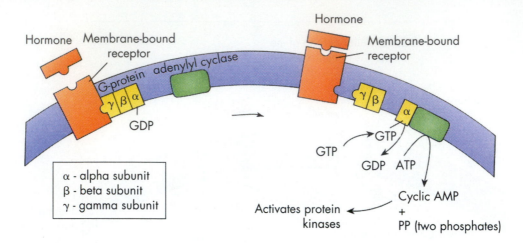

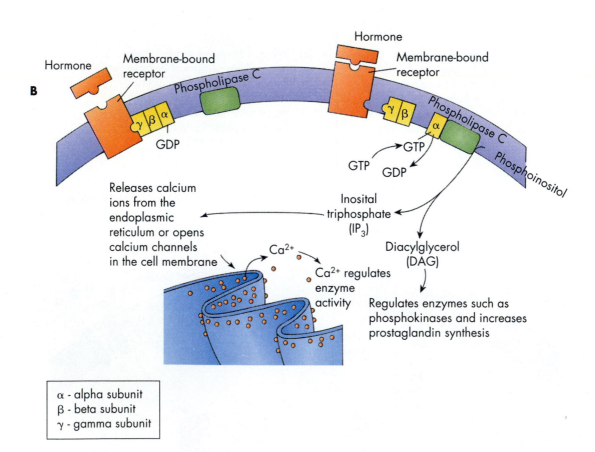

FIGURE 13.4

The cellular response to steroid hormones. Steroid hormones bind to a cytosolic receptor, and then migrate to the nucleus where they exert their function by stimulating the transcription of specific protein DNA sequences, and the resultant processes of protein synthesis. (From Seeley RR, Stephens TD, Tate P: *Anatomy and physiology,* 3 ed, St. Louis, 1995, Mosby. Art by Rolin Graphics.)

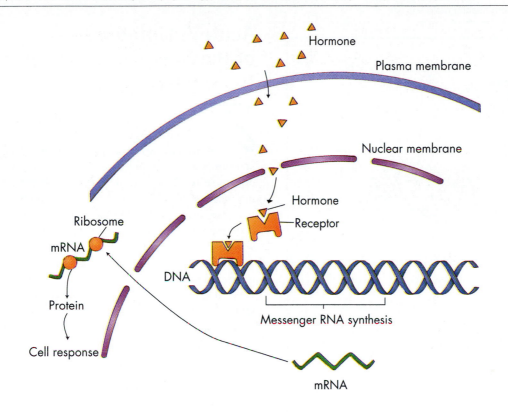

The receptor, when bound to its hormone, can bind to DNA near the site that codes for a specific messenger RNA.

Steroid Hormones

Steroid hormones are named after their chemical structure, which is based around four fused carbon rings, called a *steroid nucleus.*[13] Some examples of steroid hormones, aldosterone, and estrogen, were presented in Figure 13.2. As indicated, cholesterol is an important molecule in the synthesis of steroid hormones, and each of these hormones shares one or several intermediate molecules during synthesis.

Like other lipid molecules, steroid hormones are *hydrophobic* and therefore insoluble in water. They therefore must be bound to plasma proteins to be transported in the blood to their target tissues. Protein binding complicates the activity and half-life of these hormones. A protein-bound steroid hormone cannot enter a cell and stimulate a biologic response; the rate of hormone destruction or removal from the circulation is diminished and thus the half-life is prolonged.

Cellular response mechanisms. Steroid hormones do not bind to a cell membrane–bound receptor; rather, they pass through the cell membrane (Figure 13.4) and then bind to a specific cytoplasmic steroid receptor in the cell. The steroid-receptor complex migrates to the nucleus, where it enters and initiates the nuclear and cytosolic events required for the synthesis of specific proteins. The nuclear response to steroid hormones may require more than 45 minutes for a cellular response to be detected.[47]

Hormone Release Profiles

As with blood metabolites, hormone concentrations reflect a balance between release and removal from the circulation.[62] However, unlike with metabolites, the total concentration of a hormone in the blood may not necessarily reflect the amount of hormone needed to stimulate a cellular response. This fact applies to hormones that are circulated in the blood bound to plasma proteins (mainly steroid hormones). Unbound hormone, usually called the "free" hormone, is the biologically active form and represents a small fraction of the total.

FIGURE 13.5

A, Growth hormone, **B,** cortisol, and **C,** leutinizing hormone have characteristic pulsatile release profiles during the course of a normal day and are influenced by meals and exercise. The hormone profiles shown are from healthy male subjects.

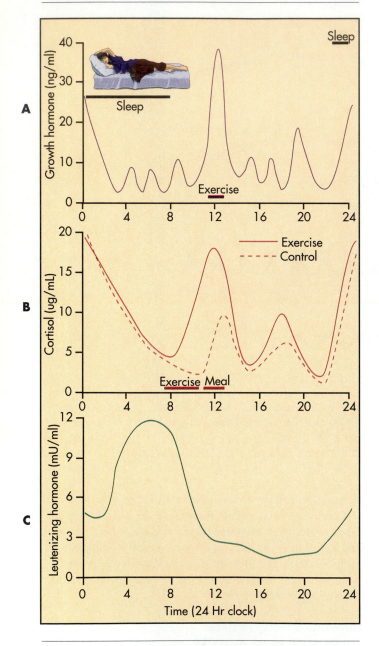

Certain hormones do not simply respond to a peripheral stimulus but are released at regular intervals during the 24-hour day (diurnal variation), as well as in cycles that may span several weeks (e.g., the menstrual cycle). These hormones are not confined to one category. For example, Figure 13.5 presents the changes in concentrations of growth hormone (GH), a peptide hormone; cortisol, a steroid hormone; and luteinizing hormone (LH), a peptide, during the 24-hour day. Definite surges of hormone release followed by periods of no

release are evident, resulting in a pulsatile profile.[12,49,92,104] Furthermore, the timing of exercise and meals relative to such surges changes the profile of these circulating hormones,[12] as is described in the following sections.

Acute Adaptations of the Neuroendocrine System to Exercise

The hormones and glandular tissues mainly involved in the body's response to different types of exercise and environmental stress are presented in Figure 13.1. A general summary of the body's responses to exercise that involve hormonal regulation would include energy metabolism, fuel mobilization, fluid balance, vascular hemodynamics, protein synthesis, immune function, and specific responses to select hormones, such as the gonadal hormones and endogenous opioids. These responses differ slightly for exercises of different intensities and between genders, and where appropriate these differences are highlighted in the following sections. A detailed discussion of immune function and exercise is presented in Chapter 15, and gender differences seen during and in response to exercise are detailed in Chapter 23.

Energy Metabolism

Incremental Exercise

Hormonal regulation of energy metabolism depends on the intensity and duration of exercise. For example, Figure 13.6 shows the increase in epinephrine and norepinephrine in the circulation during an incremental cycle ergometer exercise test to maximum oxygen uptake (VO$_2$max). Each hormone increases exponentially as exercise intensity increases. As explained in Chapter 6, increases in the catecholamine hormones stimulate lipolysis inside skeletal muscle and adipose tissue. They also increase the activity of phosphorylase, which catalyzes the breakdown of glycogen (glycogenolysis). As previously explained, low-intensity exercise is characterized by low catecholamine concentrations and the predominance of lipid catabolism. Higher intensity exercise is associated with cellular changes (increased inorganic phosphate) that combine with the increasing catecholamine stimulation of glycogenolysis to favor carbohydrate catabolism in skeletal muscle.

Intense Exercise

With more intense exercise (e.g., sprinting or weight lifting), the increase in catecholamine concentrations in the blood is more extreme. During these exercises the greater increase in catecholamines influences cellular metabolism in skeletal muscle, smooth muscle, the heart, adipose tissue, and the liver and overrides the opposing metabolic effects from increased cortisol and GH.[38,72]

FIGURE 13.6

The increase in epinephrine and norepinephrine during incremental exercise.

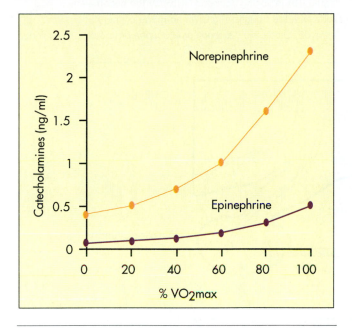

FIGURE 13.7

The changes in growth hormone, cortisol, insulin, and glucagon during incremental exercise.

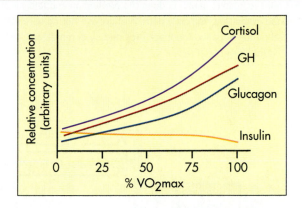

Fuel Mobilization

In addition to the catecholamine hormones' overriding influence on muscle metabolism during short-term moderate and intense exercise, these hormones also increase during prolonged submaximal exercise, as do other hormones. The main functions of the increase in these hormones are to regulate the concentrations of energy substrates (i.e., glucose, amino acids, and free fatty acids [FFAs]) in the blood and also to regulate indirectly the use of these substrates by the liver and skeletal muscle. The process of increasing circulating concentrations of energy substrates is called *mobilization*. As discussed in Chapter 4, each of these metabolites is a potential source of energy for skeletal muscle contraction.

Short-Term and Incremental Exercise

The concentrations of GH, cortisol, insulin, and glucagon in the blood change during incremental exercise, as illustrated in Figure 13.7. Insulin decreases and glucagon gradually increases with increasing exercise intensities.[6,41] In contrast, GH and cortisol increase, with the increase in GH being linear and the increase in cortisol exponential.[6]

The intensity-dependent increase in GH, glucagon, and cortisol reflects the primary control of these hormones by the central nervous system (CNS); however, the exact neural stimulation mechanism is unclear. Figure 13.8 illustrates the regulation of GH release, and Figure 13.9 illustrates the regulation of cortisol release. The benefit of increasing GH concentrations during intense exercise is difficult to explain. The

primary function of growth hormone is to increase circulating concentrations of free fatty acids and to inhibit glucose uptake by peripheral tissues, thus conserving blood glucose. During intense exercise, these effects are made redundant by the increase in catecholamines, the near-total reliance on carbohydrate catabolism in skeletal muscle, and the increase in glucose uptake into skeletal muscle.★ It would appear that increasing GH concentrations during exercise would aid in the recovery from exercise, because the half-life for growth hormone is several times longer than that of the catecholamines. Increasing GH also would result in glucose sparing, greater stimulation of muscle glycogen synthesis through the accompanying increases in insulin-like growth factor (IGF-I) (see Table 13.2), and rapid increases in skeletal muscle lipid catabolism.

The functions of GH are aided by increases in cortisol. Cortisol also increases the mobilization of free fatty acids from adipose tissue and reduces the uptake of amino acids by peripheral tissues, causing an increase in circulating amino acids. The increased free fatty acids and amino acids are predominately used by the liver in gluconeogenesis; however, during incremental or short-term intense exercise the body's carbohydrate stores are not depleted and there is little need for liver gluconeogenesis. Consequently, the metabolic benefit of cortisol release during intense exercise would also be confined to the immediate recovery period.

Intense exercise actually increases circulating blood glucose concentrations as a result of the epinephrine-induced increases in liver glycogenolysis (Figure 13-10). These increases are larger than can be explained by exercise-induced hemoconcentration. The increase in glucagon is

---

★References 22, 30, 46, 51, 63, 82, 109.

FIGURE 13.8

The factors that combine to regulate growth hormone (GH) release from the anterior pituitary. Release of GH is under the control of GH releasing hormone (GHRH), which is released during exercise and certain conditions, such as sleep, trauma, starvation, and hypoglycemia. GHRH release inhibits itself, as does the production and release of somatostatin (GH inhibiting hormone GHIH) by the hypothalamus. As mentioned in the text, the daily pattern of growth hormone release is pulsatile, with the troughs in growth hormone concentrations explained by the negative feedback provided by somatostatin. (Based on Griffin JE, Ojeda SR: *Textbook of endocrine physiology,* New York, 1988, Oxford University Press.)

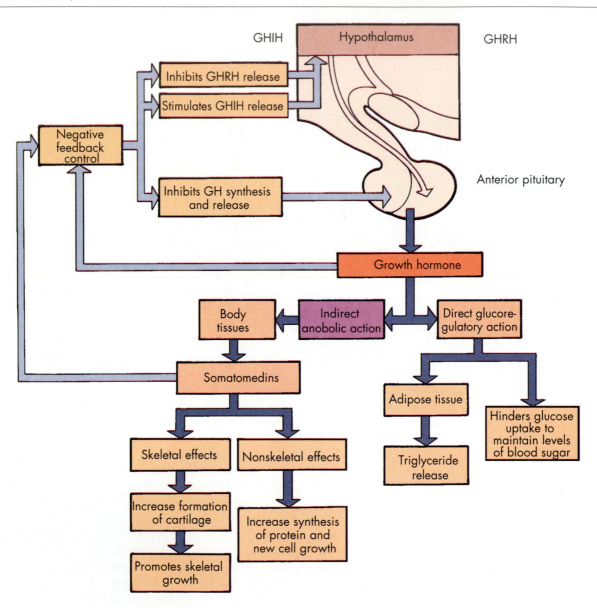

probably due to symathetic stimulation of the pancreas. The increasing blood glucose concentration would be interpreted to provide a stimulus for increasing insulin release from the β-cells of the pancreas (Figure 13-11). However, insulin does not increase for two main reasons: (1) exercise increases glucose uptake by skeletal muscle by increasing glucose transporter **(GLUT-4)** protein density on the sarcolemma independent of insulin, thereby increasing insulin sensitivity; and (2) intense exercise is accompanied by increasing blood lactate, acidosis, and IGF-I, all of which inhibit the release of insulin. Our understanding of glucose metabolism during exercise has been aided by research techniques involving the maintenance of blood glucose and insulin concentrations (Focus Box 13.1).

FIGURE 13.9

The factors that combine to regulate the release of cortisol. Adrenocorticotropic hormone (ACTH) is released from the anterior pituitary under control of a releasing hormone (corticotropin-releasing factor; CRF) from the hypothalamus during conditions of exercise, hypoglycemia, mental stress, pain, and feeding. ACTH then stimulates the synthesis and release of stored cortisol from the adrenal cortex. Increased circulating cortisol provides negative feedback to the hypothalamus. (From Seeley RR, Stephens TD, Tate P: *Anatomy and physiology,* 3 ed, St. Louis, 1995, Mosby. Art by Christine Oleksyk.)

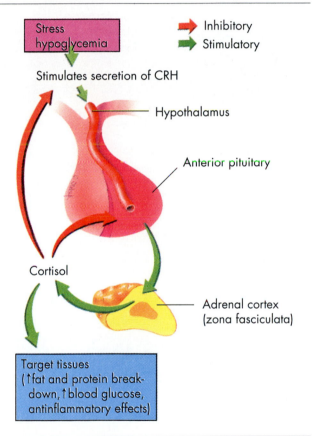

FIGURE 13.10

The change in blood glucose and epinephrine concentrations during the transition from steady state to intense exercise under adequate carbohydrate nutrition. Intense exercise and the increase in circulating epinephrine increases liver glycogenolysis, causing an increased release of glucose into the circulation. Part of the increase in blood glucose is due to an increased hemoconcentration accompanying intense exercise.

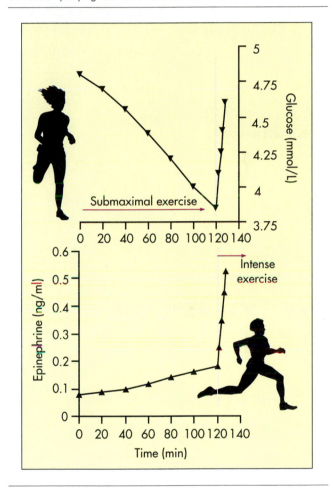

Prolonged Exercise

Prolonged exercise is accompanied by decreases in the body's skeletal muscle and liver glycogen stores. When skeletal muscle glycogen levels are low, skeletal muscle metabolism relies more on blood glucose concentrations; this can cause blood glucose levels to fall below normal (<4-5 mmol/L), a condition known as **hypoglycemia.** Because several body tissues rely solely on blood as their source of glucose for energy metabolism (e.g., red blood cells [RBCs] and neural tissue), the body must continually regulate blood glucose and, if possible, reduce the use of glucose by other tissues during low-carbohydrate conditions.

Figure 13.13, *A* shows the change in GH, cortisol, insulin, and glucagon during prolonged exercise accompanied by decreases in blood glucose. Similarly, Figure 13.13, *B*

and *C* show the changes in blood glycerol and β–hydroxybutarate during the same exercise condition. As explained in Chapter 6, glycerol is used as a marker of increased FFA mobilization, and β-hydroxybutarate is a ketone body produced during low-carbohydrate periods when the liver is overly reliant on lipid catabolism.

> **GLUT-4**
>
> *glucose transporter 4; the predominant glucose transport protein on the sarcolemma of skeletal muscle*
>
> **hypoglycemia (hi po-gli-se' me-ah)**
> *abnormally low blood glucose concentrations (<3.5 mmol/L)*

TABLE 13.2

Main functional responses to exercise and glandular tissues and hormones involved in acute adaptation

GLAND/HORMONES	STIMULANT FOR RELEASE	TARGET TISSUE	RESPONSE
CELLULAR ENERGY METABOLISM			
Adrenal Medulla			
Epinephrine	Stress, hypotension, moderate to intense exercise	Skeletal muscle	↑ Glycogenolysis
Norepinephrine	Hypoglycemia, moderate to intense exercise	Adipose tissue, liver	↑ Lipolysis, ↑ heart rate ↑ glycogenolysis, ↑ stroke volume, ↑ vascular resistance
FUEL MOBILIZATION			
Anterior pituitary			
ACTH	Injury, exercise	Adrenal cortex	↑ Cortisol release
GH	Exercise, hypoglycemia	Skeletal muscle, adipose tissue, liver	FFA mobilization, ↑ gluconeogenesis, ↓ glucose uptake
Adrenal cortex			
Cortisol	↑ ACTH; intense, prolonged exercise	Skeletal muscle, adipose tissue, liver	↑ gluconeogenesis, ↑ protein synthesis, ↓ glucose uptake
Pancreas			
Insulin	Hyperglycemia, ↑ circulating amino acids, autonomic nervous system (ANS)	Skeletal muscle, adipose tissue	↑ Glucose, amino acid, FFA uptake
Glucagon	Hypoglycemia, low amino acid concentrations, prolonged exercise	Liver	↑ Gluconeogenesis
Thyroid			
Triiodothyronine (T_3) Thyroxine (T_4)	Low T_3 and T_4 (?)	All	↑ Metabolic rate, GH; ↑ serum FFA, amino acids
Testes			
Testosterone	↑ FSH, LH; exercise (?)	Skeletal muscle, testes, bone	Protein synthesis, sperm production, ↑ sex drive
Ovaries			
Estrogen	↑ FSH, LH; light to moderate exercise	Skeletal muscle, adipose tissue	Inhibition of glucose uptake, fat deposition

TABLE 13.2—Cont'd

Main functional responses to exercise and glandular tissues and hormones involved in acute adaptation—Cont'd

GLAND/HORMONES	STIMULANT FOR RELEASE	TARGET TISSUE	RESPONSE
FLUID BALANCE			
Posterior pituitary			
Antidiuretic hormone (ADH; arginine vasopressin)	↑ Plasma osmolality	Kidneys	↑ Water reabsorption
Kidneys			
Renin	Urine flow	Blood	Converts angiotensinogen to angiotensin I
Adrenal cortex			
Aldosterone (ADH; arginine vasopressin)	Angiotensin II	Kidneys	↑ Sodium reabsorption ↑ Water reabsorption
Heart			
Atrial natriuretic peptide (ANP)	Hyperhydration ↑ venous return	Pituitary gland	Inhibition of ADH release
VASCULAR HEMODYNAMICS			
Adrenal medulla			
Norepinephrine	Stress, hypotension, moderate to intense exercise	Peripheral vascular smooth muscle	Vasoconstriction
Epinephrine	Hypoglycemia, moderate to intense exercise	Peripheral vascular smooth muscle	Vasoconstriction
Posterior pituitary			
ADH	↑ Plasma osmolality	Peripheral vascular smooth muscle	Vasoconstriction
Endothelium			
Endothelin	Tissue damage (?)	Local vasculature (??)	Vasoconstriction
Endothelial-derived relaxing factor (EDRF)	(??)	Local vaculature (??)	Vasodilation
MUSCLE REPAIR/HYPERTROPHY			
Anterior pituitary			
GH	↑ Stress	Mainly bone	Stimulation of growth
Various cells			
Insulin-like growth factor (IGF-I)	↑ GH	Almost all cells	Stimulation of growth
Testes and adrenal cortex			
Testosterone	↑ Stress	Skeletal muscle tissue	↑ Protein synthesis

FIGURE 13.11

The factors that combine to regulate the release of insulin from the pancreas. Each of an increase in blood glucose, increase in amino acids, increased gastrointestinal hormones, and increased stress hormones such as growth hormone and cortisol all increase insulin release. The ß-cells of the pancreas also have sympathetic and parasympathetic innervation; however it is unclear how neural innervation is involved in the overall regulation of insulin release. Insulin release is dampened by hypoglycemia, and by somatostatin, which is also produced by the pancreas.

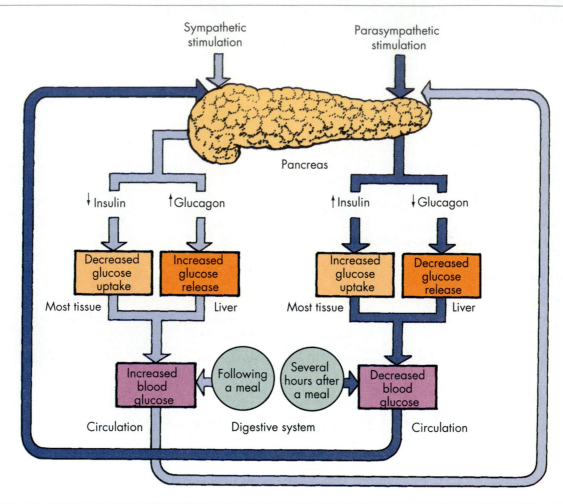

The increased release of GH from the anterior pituitary and of cortisol from the adrenal cortex occurs simultaneously with an increase in sympathetic activity, as explained previously. The increase in blood concentrations of FFAs and amino acids that accompanies increases in GH and cortisol provides substrates for gluconeogenesis and alternate fuels for skeletal muscle energy metabolism. However, unless the gluconeogenesis pathway is stimulated, these responses have little influence on the liver; stimulating this pathway is one of the main functions of glucagon. Glucagon increases liver glycogenolysis by a cAMP second-messenger system that eventually activates glycogen phosphorylase.[47] In addition, glucagon increases the rate of gluconeogenesis by causing the phosphorylation of PFK2/FBPase, which in turn reduces the rate of glycolysis and favors the dephosphorylation of fructose 1,6-bisphosphate to fructose 1-phosphate. Because the liver has relatively large concentrations of the enzymes pyruvate carboxylase and phosphoenolpyruvate carboxykinase (GTP), glycolysis can be reversed, allowing the formation of

insulin sensitivity

the ability of the body (usually skeletal muscle) to respond to insulin by increasing glucose uptake

insulin responsiveness

the ability of the pancreas to release insulin in response to hyperglycemia

FOCUS BOX 13.1

Use of glucose and insulin clamp methodology in understanding the effects of exercise and insulin on blood glucose kinetics in normal and diabetic subjects

A commonly used methodology to study the influence of exercise and insulin on glucose use by the body is to artificially control both the insulin and glucose concentrations in the blood. Typically, researchers maintain, or clamp, insulin at higher than normal concentrations, a condition called a *hyperinsulinemic clamp.* Once insulin is stable, the body's use of glucose can be measured by infusing glucose into the blood. When blood glucose is maintained at a near-constant concentration the condition is called a *euglycemic clamp.* Combined use of an insulin and a glucose clamp is called a *euglycemic-hyperinsulinemic clamp.*[27]

When the body can dispose of glucose better for a given insulin concentration, the capability is called **insulin sensitivity,** which is routinely measured by the euglycemic-hyperinsulinemic clamp. Another measurable capability relative to glucose and insulin responses is the body's insulin response to a constant hyperglycemia, called **insulin responsiveness.** Increased glucose uptake for a given insulin condition reflects increased insulin sensitivity (Figure 13.12, *A*). Increased insulin release for a given glucose condition reflects improved insulin responsiveness (Figure 13.12, *B*).

The glucose and insulin clamp procedures are research tools that have been used to quantify the difference in glucose utilization between individuals with and without diabetes, and between resting, exercise, and postexercise conditions. *A decrease in insulin sensitivity is evidence of a decreased ability of body cells to be stimulated by insulin for increased glucose uptake.* This is a common symptom of type II diabetes, which involves flaws in either the insulin receptor or the cellular response to insulin binding. *A decreased insulin responsiveness is evidence of impaired function of the β-cells of the pancreas.* This also is evident in a small percentage of type II diabetics and is totally the cause of type I diabetes.

Use of the euglycemic-hyperinsulinemic clamp in animals and humans has revealed that the increased glucose uptake that exists after exercise is due to simultaneous but independent exercise- and insulin-mediated processes that involve increased incorporation of GLUT-4 proteins in the sarcolemma.[5] The exercise response is retained for several hours into recovery,[51,73,77,100] and exercise training can induce further improvements in insulin sensitivity that have longer lasting effects.[30,56] These responses can occur in normal individuals as well as in individuals with either type I or type II diabetes.

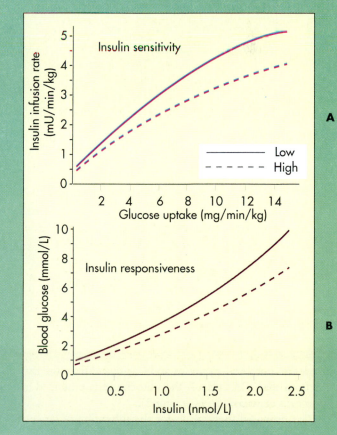

FIGURE 13.12

The difference between high and low **A,** insulin sensitivity and **B,** insulin responsiveness.

FIGURE 13.13

The change in **A,** growth hormone, cortisol, insulin, and glucagon during prolonged exercise, and the accompanied changes in the metabolites **B,** ß-hydroxybutarate and **C,** glycerol.

FIGURE 13.14

The interrelationships between increased blood glucose and free fatty acids on influencing metabolism in adipose tissue and skeletal muscle. These relationships were proposed in 1963 by Randle[79], and the scheme is referred to as the glucose-fatty acid cycle. (Adapted from Randle PJ et al: The glucose fatty-acid cycle, *Lancet* 785-789, 1963.)

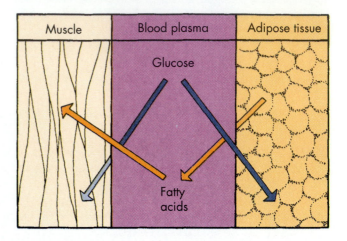

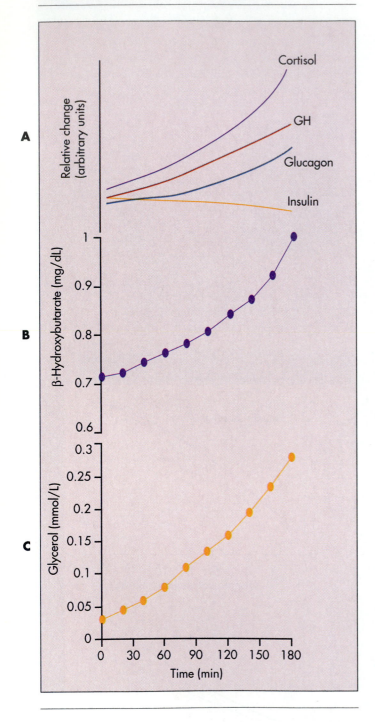

centrations is explained by the **glucose–fatty acid cycle,** as originally set forth by Randle et al.[79] (Figure 13.14). Increasing circulating FFAs inhibit the release of glucose from the liver, which in turn reduces glucose's availability to the periphery.[87,101] In addition, elevated circulating FFAs inhibit glucose uptake by peripheral tissues, such as skeletal muscle. During conditions of elevated blood glucose, called **hyperglycemia,** FFA release from adipose tissue is inhibited and a general condition of increased carbohydrate metabolism exists. These relationships in adipose tissue are aided by an increase in insulin during hyperglycemia and an increase in glucagon during hypoglycemia.[16,17,79] However, the relationships between blood glucose and FFAs are very different for a diabetic individual (Clinical Application, p. 363).

Estrogen is another hormone that influences substrate mobilization during exercise. "Estrogen" is a generic name for a number of hormones released from the ovaries that increase fertility. The most biologically active estrogen released by the ovary is estradiol–17β. It is produced from cholesterol, as are all the steroid hormones (see Figure 13.2). Most of the estradiol–17β in women is synthesized by the ovaries; however, small amounts are also synthesized in the adrenal cortex, and this source accounts for the estrogen produced in men. Because men have minimal estradiol–17β, this hormone's effect on substrate mobilization and energy metabolism is confined to women and is controlled by the menstrual cycle. (See Chapter 23.)

Estradiol–17β increases the mobilization of free fatty acids from adipose tissue and inhibits glucose uptake by the

glucose from glycerol, pyruvate, and lactate and from the carbons from the TCA cycle in the mitochondria produced by amino acid oxidation (see Chapter 5).

The proposed mechanism for the inhibition of glucose uptake during periods of increasing GH and cortisol con-

Role of Exercise in the Prevention of and Rehabilitation from Non–Insulin-Dependent (Type II) Diabetes Mellitus

Diabetes mellitus (or, simply, diabetes) is a disorder that develops when the glucose uptake capability of the body's tissues is reduced. Diabetes is expressed in two forms, type I and type II. *Type I* diabetes is characterized by the body's inability to produce and secrete insulin. This type of diabetes necessitates administration of insulin and usually manifests early in life; thus it often is called *juvenile-onset* or *insulin-dependent* diabetes.

Type II diabetes is the most common form, accounting for 90% of all cases of diabetes.[98] This type of diabetes usually occurs later in life and thus has been called *adult-onset* diabetes. Individuals with type II diabetes can be divided into two subgroups: (1) those with an impaired ability to secrete insulin resulting from a defect in the β-cells of the pancreas, which leads to diminished insulin responsiveness; and (2) those with a diminished cellular ability to respond to insulin, which results in reduced insulin sensitivity. Individuals in both subgroups eventually may require insulin administration. The peripheral tissue of the type II diabetic condition coincides with increases in body fat, and individuals with this condition therefore are typically overweight and have elevated blood concentrations of lipoprotein and triglycerides.[98]

Exercise combined with diet and insulin therapy has been a recognized treatment for diabetes since the early 1950s.[98] Since then, abundant research has isolated the effects of exercise on blood glucose regulation in people with either type I or type II diabetes. Because type II diabetes accounts for 90% of all cases, and because exercise is a more powerful treatment for the type II diabetic, the type II form is the focus of this section.

Exercise is characterized by an increase in glucose uptake by skeletal muscle; in normal individuals and type II diabetics. This increase in uptake is retained for up to 48 hours during the recovery from a single bout of exercise.[37,74,77] This response is a combination of increased insulin sensitivity and an endogenous effect in increased GLUT-4 transporters on the sarcolemmas of the exercised muscle fibers. The endogenous effect within skeletal muscle is related to the synthesis of muscle glycogen and can last up to 5 hours.[74] The exercise-induced increase in insulin sensitivity is greater when a larger muscle mass is exercised.[82] However, for individuals unaccustomed to exercise requiring an eccentric component to muscle contraction (e.g., running or weight lifting), the associated muscle damage causes a transient decline in insulin sensitivity.[60,61] The known prolonged effect of exercise in improving peripheral glucose disposal and insulin sensitivity is related to the insulin-stimulated mechanism.[98] Thus exercise can acutely alleviate inadequate insulin-mediated glucose disposal.

Long-term exercise training is also beneficial for type II diabetics, but not because of a continued improvement in exercise-induced insulin sensitivity. Insulin sensitivity is retained only in individuals who exercise and reduce body fat content.[98] In fact, loss of body fat in an overweight type II diabetic can reduce insulin release and increase sensitivity, regardless of exercise training. Nevertheless, in individuals who exercise daily, the continued increase in exercise-stimulated insulin sensitivity is retained from one bout of exercise to the next, producing a meaningful improvement in the control of blood glucose.

---

peripheral tissues.[44,86] Consequently, estradiol–17β and GH have similar metabolic effects during exercise. Exercise is known to increase circulating estrogen in both menstruating *(eumenorrheic)* and nonmenstruating *(amenorrheic)* women.[86] Furthermore, the higher circulating concentrations of estradiol–17β in endurance-trained women compared with equally endurance-trained men has been used to explain the greater dependence on lipid than on carbohydrate during exercise.[86,94] Chapter 23 presents evidence for differing metabolism in men and women during exercise.

glucose–fatty acid cycle
the theory that glucose uptake by skeletal muscle is inhibited by high circulating concentrations of fatty acid molecules

hyperglycemia (hi per-gli-se′ me ah)
abnormally high blood glucose concentrations (>5 mmol/L)

diabetes mellitus (di ah be′ tez mel li′ tus)
a condition characterized by a reduced ability to regulate blood glucose concentrations by means of insulin

The increase in renin activity, ADH, aldosterone, and atrial natri-uretic peptide during incremental exercise.

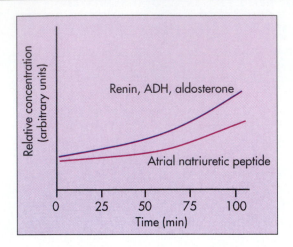

Fluid Balance

Short-Term and Incremental Exercise

Figure 13.15 illustrates the change in plasma renin activity, aldosterone, ANP, and antidiuretic hormone (ADH) during intermittent incremental exercise. Each component of the fluid balance and renal function regulatory scheme increases with an increase in exercise intensity. Although an increase in ANP and ADH appears contradictory, urine flow is reduced during moderate to high-intensity exercise.[39]

Prolonged Exercise and Dehydration

The increase in heat production during exercise initiates several neurally and locally controlled thermoregulatory reflexes that result in increased sweating and blood flow to the skin (see Chapter 11). Because sweating can occur at rates as high as 2 to 3 L/hour, large losses in body water are possible during prolonged exercise, especially in hot, humid environments. This reduces plasma volume, raises plasma osmolality, and evokes a complex hormonal response to conserve body water and ensure a long-term regulation of blood pressure (Figure 13.16).

Figure 13.17 illustrates the changing concentrations of ADH, renin, aldosterone, and ANP during prolonged exercise. The stimulus for ADH release is an increasing plasma osmolality, which is detected by **osmoreceptors** in the hypothalamus (see Figure 13.16). ADH functions by increasing the permeability of the kidney tubule from each of the juxtamedullary nephrons of the kidney. As this mechanism reduces urine flow and volume, it opposes urine formation and is called an **antidiuretic** function. A reduced urine flow through the kidney is detected by the specialized cells located around the distal tubule (macula densa) in the region of the glomerulus, called the *juxtaglomerular apparatus*. Low urine flow increases the absorption of sodium and chloride by the cells of the distal tubule, reducing the ionic concentrations exposed to the macula densa.[47] The neighboring juxtaglomerular cells secrete *renin* during these low ionic concentrations that surround the macula densa. Renin is actually an enzyme that removes angiotensin I from the prehormone angiotensinogen. Angiotensin I is then converted to angiotensin II in the circulation by the diffusely located, endothelium-bound *angiotensin-converting enzyme* (ACE).[44] Angiotensin II circulates to the adrenal cortex, where it stimulates the release of aldosterone.

Aldosterone is categorized as a *mineralocorticoid,* as are cortisol and the other hormones released by the adrenal cortex. Each of these hormones has a minor role in the regulation of blood potassium and sodium concentrations (hence their category name). Aldosterone exerts its function by increasing the synthesis of sodium transporter proteins by the epithelial cells of the distal tubule and collecting duct, eventually causing an increase in sodium reabsorption and a concomitant osmotic reabsorption of water. Because aldosterone is a steroid hormone, the cellular response to increased aldosterone is relatively slow, taking about 45 minutes.[47] Consequently, unless the exercise bout lasts at least 2 hours, the biologic effects of aldosterone would mainly occur in the recovery phase.

Under conditions of water excess, plasma volume expands, osmolality decreases, and the stimulus for ADH release declines. ADH release is further inhibited by the release of ANP from the atrial myocardium of the heart, which occurs in response to the increased filling pressures of the right atrium. Removing the ADH stimulus for water reabsorption increases urine flow, which in turn reduces renin output from the kidney and eventually the stimulation for aldosterone secretion. These conditions cause the formation of large urine volumes, which is called **diuresis.**

Vascular Hemodynamics

Exercise is accompanied by the regulation of blood vessels. As is explained in Chapter 11, this is required to regulate peripheral vascular resistance and blood pressures (Focus Box 13.2) and to redistribute blood flow to specific tissues. These

osmoreceptor (oz mo-re-**cep'** tor)
a cell that can generate an action potential in response to changes in the blood's osmolality

antidiuretic (an ti-di u-**ret'** ik)
a reduction in urine volume

diuresis (di u re' sis)
an increase in urine volume

FIGURE 13.16

The factors that combine to regulate fluid balance and systemic blood pressure.

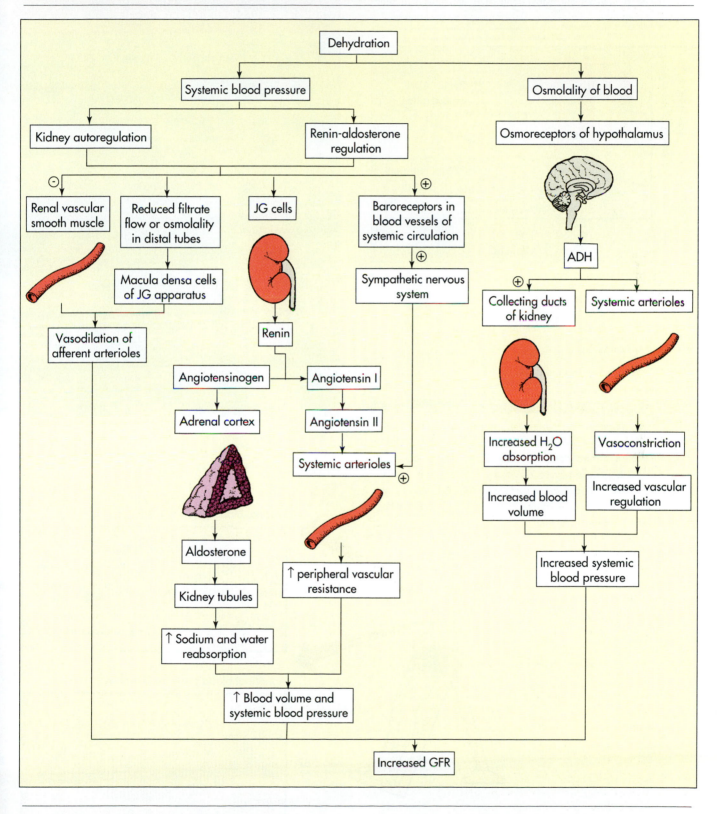

FIGURE 13.17

The change in renin activity, aldosterone, ADH, and atrial natriuretic peptide during prolonged exercise accompanied by dehydration.

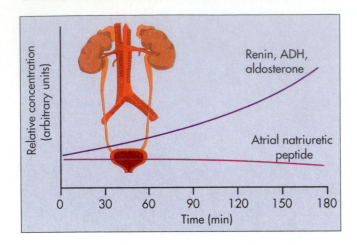

FOCUS BOX 13.2

Regulation of blood pressure

Exercise is a stress to the body that induces an increase in blood pressure, or a *hypertensive response*. During the recovery from exercise, the body can experience a dramatic decrease in blood pressure, or *hypotensive response*. Because the blood pressure increase during exercise is due to an increased systolic pressure without an increase in diastolic pressure, there is no increase in the afterload of the heart and therefore the exercise-induced hypertension is not detrimental to the functioning of a healthy heart. However, chronic exposure of the heart and vasculature to increases in blood pressure resulting from elevated systolic and diastolic pressures is called **hypertension,** which can damage the heart, vasculature, and organs these systems perfuse. Decreases in blood pressure below normal resting values, or **hypotension,** can occur during the immediate recovery from exercise or can be induced by postural adjustment *(orthostatic hypotension)*. This, too, can be potentially dangerous to the body. Hypotension often coincides with reduced venous return to the heart, which in turn decreases blood flow to the brain. An episode of syncope could and often does result. It is clear that regulation of blood pressure is important for optimal functioning of body organs and for the functioning of the body as a whole.

FIGURE 13.18

A, The near immediate sympathetic regulation of blood pressure prevents orthostatic hypotension in individuals during head-up tilt. **B,** Individuals who have a delayed or ineffective sympathetic response, such as hypertensive individuals resulting from chronic renal failure, exhibit decreases in systolic and diastolic blood pressure. This test is often instrumental in documenting abnormalities of sympathetic-adrenal function.

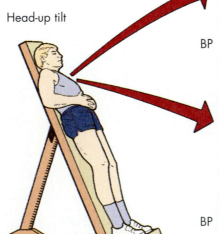

Head-up tilt

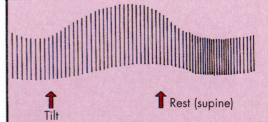

Normal blood pressure response

BP

Tilt   Rest (supine)

A

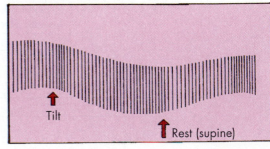

Abnormal blood pressure response

BP

Tilt

Rest (supine)

B

Blood pressure is regulated by a complex interaction between neural, endocrinologic, renal, cardiovascular, and behavioral functions (see Figure 3.16). The primary determinants of blood pressure are cardiovascular in origin and consist of cardiac output and peripheral vascular resistance. Such cardiovascular control of blood pressure by neural regulation is the most immediate, followed by endocrinologic regulation and then renal and behavioral factors. This time response is important, because neural regulation must obviously prevail during immediate perturbations that risk immediate changes in systemic blood pressure. For this reason, the function of the ANS in blood pressure regulation is an important area of research.

Neural Regulation

As cardiac output is influenced by the localized nuclei within the medulla, called the **vasomotor center,** increasing neural sympathetic stimulation and decreasing parasympathetic stimulation to the heart induces increases in heart rate and contractility, which in turn increases stroke volume. Increased sympathetic stimulation also increases peripheral vascular resistance by inducing catecholamine-stimulated vasoconstriction of blood vessels. Such sympathetic stimulation is very effective in stabilizing blood pressure and has a response time measured in seconds, as revealed during tilt table research (Figure 13.18).

Located in the walls of the ascending aorta and carotid arteries are baroreceptors sensitive to stretch. When the baroreceptors are exposed to stretch, such as occurs with an increase in stroke volume, the rate of afferent impulses that return to the cardiovascular center increases, causing an exaggerated inhibition of the vasomotor center. Conversely, when stretch to the wall of the aorta decreases, the rate of impulses directed to the vasomotor center decreases, resulting in less inhibition of the vasomotor center. The function of the baroreceptors is to protect the body against rapid changes in stroke volume.

Conditions that would evoke a baroreceptor reflex control of blood pressure are immediate extreme alterations in hydrostatic pressure accompanying postural changes, or rapid hemorrhage. Continuous stimulation to the baroreceptors is known to cause them to adapt and to reset to a higher level of stretch before increasing their rate of stimulation to the vasomotor center. It is this adaptation that overrides their effect during exercise and allows for a sustained increase in systemic blood pressure.

Behavioral Regulation

Because cardiovascular regulation of blood pressure is based on hemodynamic principles (see Focus Box 11.1 in Chapter 11), altering blood volume or blood viscosity would also influence the regulation of peripheral vascular resistance, which in turn would influence blood pressure. Behaviors that can influence blood volume and blood viscosity are exercise-induced dehydration, voluntary dehydration, and voluntary overhydration. These behavioral characteristics are obviously long-term adjustments to blood pressure regulation and therefore mostly external to baroreceptor involvement in ANS regulation of blood pressure. Such behaviors induce blood pressure regulation by endocrinologic and renal mechanisms.

Renal and Endocrinologic Regulation

Dehydration can result in the lowering of peripheral vascular resistance and a decrease in blood pressure. Dehydration produces an increase in plasma osmolality, which stimulates specific nerves of the posterior pituitary to secrete arginine-vasopressin, or antidiuretic hormone (ADH) (see text). ADH increases water reabsorption in the collecting ducts of the kidneys, causing a decreased urine volume (antidiuresis) and water conservation. Reduced urine flow in the tubules of the kidneys stimulates the release of renin from the juxtaglomerular apparatus. Renin release eventually leads to the release of aldosterone from the adrenal cortex, which circulates to the kidneys to stimulate increased synthesis of sodium receptors by the late distal tubule (see text). Increased sodium uptake induces an osmotic flux of water out of the tubule and also increases water conservation.

In addition to fluid conservation, angiotensin II and ADH cause vasoconstriction of arterioles, thus increasing peripheral vascular resistance. Dehydration is also accompanied by increased sympathetic stimulation, causing the increase in circulating epinephrine and norepinephrine. The catecholamines also increase peripheral vascular resistance and stabilize or slightly increase cardiac output. Thus the renal and endocrinologic responses influence peripheral vascular resistance and cardiac output, thereby providing a powerful delayed response to long-term decreases in blood pressure.

Overhydration increases blood volume, and this stimulus is overcome by decreased release of ADH, decreases in osmolality, increased release of ANP from the heart, and decreased release of aldosterone. These events result in an increase in urine volume, or diuresis.

---

hypertension (hi per-**ten'** shun)
abnormally high blood pressure

hypotension (hi po-**ten'** shun)
abnormally low blood pressure

vasomotor center
the neural region in the medulla that is responsible for regulating central and peripheral cardiovascular function

responses are elicited by neural, hormonal, and local regulators of arterioles and the microvasculature.

The increasing concentrations of the catecholamine hormones that accompany increasing exercise intensity are known to induce a general vasoconstriction of the vasculature as a result of the overwhelming α-receptor–induced vasoconstriction at high norepinephrine concentrations.[85]

Peripheral vascular resistance is also increased by increasing circulating concentrations of angiotensin I, ADH, and to a lesser extent aldosterone.[47] Angiotensin I is a potent vasoconstrictor of peripheral smooth muscle, as is ADH, whereas aldosterone exerts a minor influence on vascular smooth muscle contraction. The angiotensin, ADH, and aldosterone functions in vascular hemodynamics are more important during resting conditions characterized by dehydration or low blood volume resulting from hemorrhage. The influence of these hormones on vascular hemodynamics during exercise is less clear because of the overriding influence of the catecholamines and locally induced vasodilation in the vasculature of the contracting skeletal muscle.

Protein Synthesis and Reproductive Hormones

During Exercise

Contradictory research has been published concerning whether the gonadotropic stimulatory hormones, follicle-stimulating hormone (FSH), and luteinizing hormone (LH) increase during exercise.[18,24-26] Regardless, because the time required for FSH stimulation of the testes and resultant testosterone production may exceed 45 minutes, acute increases in FSH and LH during short-term exercise cannot account for increases in testosterone.[25] Recent findings indicate that testosterone does increase during short-term cycling and weight-lifting exercise,[25,88] which has been explained as the result of a direct catecholamine stimulation mechanism.[25] Prolonged exercise appears to cause a cortisol-induced inhibition of testosterone production.[24] In normally menstruating women, exercise-induced increases in estradiol-17β have also been detected.[103] How changes in estrogen and testosterone induced by short-term or prolonged exercises affect protein synthesis in men and women is unclear.

The other main androgenic stimulus for protein synthesis is the combined effects of GH and IGF-I (somatomedin C). Although GH does have some independent ability to induce growth in bone, most of the stimulus to protein synthesis and growth by GH results from its stimulation of the production of IGF-I in the tissues of interest. Increased concentrations of IGF-I then induce the cellular growth response. Most human research of GH responses during exercise have not included measurement of IGF-I in their design. However, research in both humans and animals has shown that IGF-I increases during exercise,[53] and this acute role is more for the insulin-like effects of the hormone rather than the anabolic effects. This interpretation is supported by the overwhelming evidence for protein catabolism and amino acid release from muscle during exercise. However, the state of protein metabolism during recovery is very different.

During Recovery

The protein synthesis response of IGF-I has been documented in resting individuals.[18] Data from Carraro et al.[18] also indicate that protein synthesis is impaired during exercise but stimulated during the recovery from exercise, resulting in a net protein gain. More research is needed to elucidate the hormonal regulation of postexercise muscle protein synthesis.

Endogenous Opioids

An opioid is a substance that produces an analgesic effect similar to that of morphine (which is also referred to as opium). The body produces opioid-like substances that can be categorized into three main types; β-endorphins, enkephalins, and α-endorphins (dynorphins).[45] The three molecules are produced in various regions of the brain, but secretion into the systemic circulation occurs mainly from the anterior pituitary. Research into the **endogenous opioids** has been based on blocking their receptor with the molecule *naloxone,* and this strategy mainly focuses on the effects of β-endorphin.

The secretion of β-endorphin from the anterior pituitary is linked to the secretion of ACTH. In fact, β-endorphin and ACTH share the same prehormone. β-Endorphin increases during times of hypoglycemia and therefore is involved in the body's multihormone regulation of blood glucose. β-endorphin and the enkephalins increase during exercise, and they have been associated with cardiovascular, ventilatory, metabolic, and thermoregulatory effects.[34,35,45,89] β-endorphin slightly inhibits ventilation, can suppress baroreceptor firing, and is associated with inhibition of the release of ACTH and GH.[45] However, the metabolic effects of β-endorphin have not been documented experimentally.

Despite the classification of β-endorphin, enkephalin, and dynorphin as opioid-like substances, there has been no research evidence connecting their increase in the circulation during exercise to pain suppression or psychologic states of euphoria or other similar mood alterations.[34,35]

Chronic Adaptations of the Neuroendocrine System to Exercise

*P*articipation in exercise training, no matter what type, has the potential to alter the secretion of hormones by changing (1) the stimuli that release hormones, (2) the cells' ability to respond to hormones, or (3) the maximal capacity of endocrine tissues to release hormones. The chronic adaptations of the neuroendocrine system to exercise are also categorized by their general biologic response.

FIGURE 13.19

The influence of endurance training on the circulating concentrations of catecholamines, growth hormone, and cortisol during prolonged exercise.

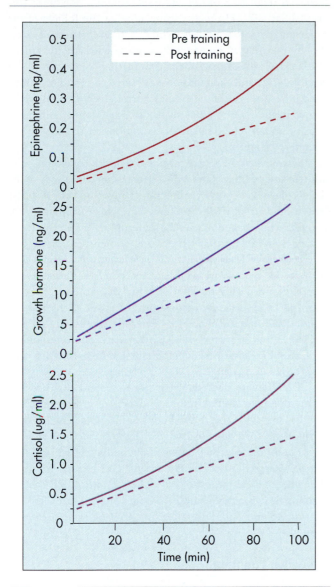

than adipose tissue, lower cortisol and GH concentrations do not detract from lipid catabolism.

When submaximal exercise is performed for longer periods, the reduced reliance on carbohydrate spares muscle and liver glycogen and therefore is not associated with the decreases in blood glucose that otherwise would occur. Consequently, serum glucagon concentrations are also lower after endurance training.[6,28] An additional factor that contributes to improved glucose kinetics during exercise is the chronic increase in glucose transporters (GLUT-4 proteins) on the sarcolemma of muscle fibers.[55,56]

During maximal exercise, several hormones circulate in larger concentrations in trained versus less-trained individuals. For example, after intense exercise, trained individuals have greater circulating concentrations of the catecholamines ACTH, β-endorphin, and cortisol.[15,69] Assuming that the sympathetic stimulation during maximal exercise is similar in trained and untrained individuals, these results have been interpreted to indicate a greater capacity for stress hormone synthesis and release after training.

Under resting conditions, the hormone balance between trained and untrained individuals is also different. Dela et al.[28] demonstrated that trained individuals have higher catecholamine concentrations during the active day than untrained individuals, although the functional implications of this difference are unclear. In addition, insulin responses to a meal are lower in the trained state, and one would expect consistently lower ACTH, cortisol, ADH, and aldosterone concentrations during the average day due to the plasma volume expansion that accompanies endurance training (see Chapter 11).

Reproductive Hormones

The secretion of LH and FSH from the anterior pituitary regulates gonadal hormone production and secretion. In women, the gonadal hormones of interest are estradiol-17β and progesterone; in men, the hormone of interest is testosterone. In both genders more that 90% of these hormones are secreted from the gonads, and the rest comes from the adrenal cortex.

Athletic Amenorrhea

Women biologically capable of menstruating who do not, have a condition known as *amenorrhea*. When the cause of the amenorrhea is related directly to exercise participation, the condition is called **athletic amenorrhea.** Historically,

Energy Metabolism and Fuel Mobilization

For a given submaximal exercise intensity, endurance training lowers the catecholamine, GH, and cortisol concentrations in the blood, as illustrated in Figure 13.19. As explained in Chapter 9, endurance training is also accompanied by an increased reliance on lipid catabolism for a given submaximal exercise intensity.[57] At first glance, these hormonal findings appear inconsistent with an increase in lipid catabolism. However, because the main source of FFAs during submaximal exercise is the active skeletal muscle rather

endogenous opioids

hormones released by the anterior pituitary gland that effect a biologic response similar to that of morphine

athletic amenorrhea

loss of menstrual cycle caused by excessive exercise training

FIGURE 13.20

The hormone 17ß-estradiol has potent effects on increasing lipid catabolism and decreasing carbohydrate catabolism during exercise. The effects of 17ß-estradiol administered by a patch on **A,** glucose turnover and **B,** glycerol turnover during treadmill running in ammenorrheic women.

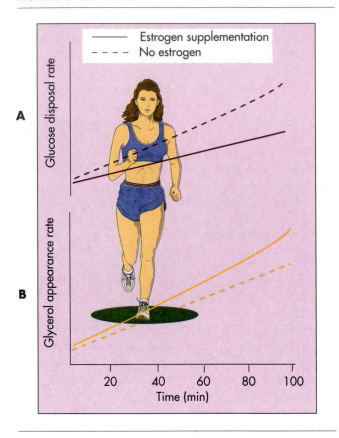

ever, the exact mechanism involved in athletic amenorrhea remains obscure.[68] Nevertheless, it is known that athletic amenorrhea is due to an altered release of LH and FSH, indicating that the irregularity resides in the hypothalamic-pituitary axis regulation of LH and FSH secretion. Reduced levels of FSH and LH prevent stimulation of the follicle of the ovary and therefore prevent synthesis and secretion of estradiol by the ovary. Consequently, women with athletic amenorrhea have lower than normal circulating concentrations of estradiol-17β and therefore do not have the estradiol-stimulated increases in lipid catabolism during exercise or the protective qualities of estradiol relative to bone density and high-density lipoprotein (HDL) concentrations in the blood (see Chapters 14 and 23).

Some researchers have proposed that the development of athletic amenorrhea starts with a decrease in the length of the luteal phase[90]; however, minimal changes in luteal phase length and menstrual function have been reported for women who engage in exercise training involving moderate distances and intensities.[83] Therefore women who participate in extremes of long-distance or high-intensity exercise may be more likely to develop athletic amenorrhea. This expectation is supported by research showing that athletic amenorrhea can be reversed by reducing the amount or intensity of training and that the incidence of athletic amenorrhea (1% to 44%) is higher in women who participate in more prolonged or metabolically stressful activities, such as long-distance running or ballet dancing.[31]

The dramatically reduced ability to secrete estradiol-17β in amenorrheic women results in decreases in the mobilization of fatty acids and in the body's ability to catabolize lipid during low to moderate exercise (Figure 13.20, *A* and *B*). This condition is further supported by reduced GH secretion during exercise and a disrupted daily GH release profile in the amenorrheic woman.[103,104] The condition of athletic amenorrhea essentially makes women more "male-like" in relation to the endocrinologic and metabolic responses to exercise.

Testicular Function

The male version of athletic amenorrhea is characterized by a chronic decrease in resting serum testosterone and chronically elevated resting cortisol concentrations.[24,33] In men, lowered testosterone may reduce sperm counts, and could also diminish bone mineral density, although no evidence has documented this as fact.[1,70]

the mechanism that causes athletic amenhorrhea was believed to be a reduction in the percentage of body fat, attributable to the added caloric demands of exercise.[3,31,59,68,75] However, it is now known that body fat content does not directly cause this condition.[31,55]

Women who train repeatedly expose themselves to increased concentrations of catecholamines, β-endorphin, and cortisol, which are known to exert some inhibition on anterior pituitary function and, more specifically, on the release of gonadotropin-releasing hormone (GnRH). How-

Conclusion

The diverse control exerted by the body's hormonal responses to exercise is illustrated in Figure 13.21. It is clear that during exercise, the pituitary gland is pivotal in the regulation of substrate mobilization, fluid balance and kidney function, protein synthesis, and gonadal function. The preceding sections of this chapter have discussed the research evidence that proves this to be true. Primary regulation of energy metabolism occurs through the catecholamines, and primary control over blood glucose regulation is exerted by the pancreas. However, prolonged exercise and the secretion of cortisol, GH, and estrogen in women also alter cellular metabolism and blood glucose regulation. The multiple functions of many of the body's hormones make the study of neuroendocrinology a difficult task. However, as this chapter has shown, knowledge of hormonal functioning during exercise is necessary to appreciate how the body can tolerate, and sometimes not tolerate, the various types, intensities, and durations of exercise.

FIGURE 13.21

An overview of the hormones released during exercise and their effects on the body's acute adaptations to exercise.

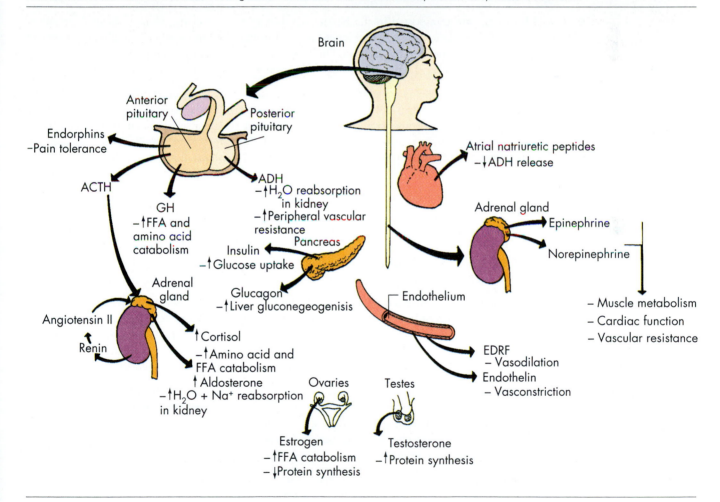

SUMMARY

- **Neuroendocrinology** is the study of the combined function of nerves and endocrine **glands** involved in the release of **hormones** that regulate the function of body tissues. Traditionally, the substances secreted by endocrine glands were each known as a hormone. These substances were released in minor amounts, resulting in very low concentrations in the blood (<1 μmol), and they exerted their function on tissues in other regions of the body. The traditional approach and definitions of endocrinology are too simplistic and narrow for application to the now-recognized complex hormonal regulation of many body functions.

- Hormones can be divided into three main categories: *amine, peptide,* and *steroid.* Amine and peptide hormones exert their action on target cells by binding to specific receptors on the cell membranes of the target tissue or tissues. Often, hormone release eventually leads to a decrease in the number of receptors, called **down-regulation.** An increase in receptor numbers is called **up-regulation.** The molecules produced in a cell in response to hormone binding, which then stimulate a cellular response, are called **second messengers.** Examples of second messengers are **cAMP,** inositol triphosphate, diacylglycerol, and calcium.

- Steroid hormones are transported in the blood bound to specific proteins, which reduces their rate of removal from the circulation. Steroid hormones can pass through the cell membrane and bind to a specific cytoplasmic steroid receptor within the cell. The steroid-receptor complex then migrates to the nucleus, where it enters and initiates the nuclear and cytosolic events required for synthesis of specific proteins.

- Hormonal regulation of energy metabolism and other functions depends on the intensity and duration of exercise and nutritional status. During an incremental cycle ergometer exercise test to VO_2 max, it was found that epinephrine, norepinephrine, cortisol, ACTH, and GH increase as intensity increases. These hormones either directly or indirectly alter metabolism within the skeletal muscle. With more intense exercise (e.g., sprinting or weight lifting), the increase in blood concentrations of catecholamines is more extreme.

- Increases in the catecholamines, GH, and cortisol increase the *mobilization* of free fatty acids (FFAs) and amino acids during exercise. Intense exercise increases circulating blood glucose concentrations because of the epinephrine-induced increases in liver glycogenolysis. Insulin is not released under these conditions because (1) exercise-induced increases in glucose uptake by contracting muscle ensure increased **GLUT-4** protein content on the sarcolemma, and (2) insulin release is inhibited by acidosis, lactate, and IGF-I.

- Prolonged exercise is accompanied by decreases in the body's skeletal muscle and liver glycogen stores, resulting in the condition of low blood glucose, or **hypoglycemia.** The increase in FFA and amino acid concentrations in the blood that accompanies increases in GH and cortisol provides substrates for gluconeogenesis and alternate fuels for skeletal muscle energy metabolism. Increases in glucagon increase liver glycogenolysis by a cAMP second-messenger system that eventually activates glycogen phosphorylase.

- Increasing circulating FFAs inhibit the release of glucose from the liver, which in turn reduces glucose availability to the periphery. These events have been called the **glucose–fatty acid cycle.** In addition, elevated circulating FFAs inhibit glucose uptake by peripheral tissues such as skeletal muscle. During conditions of elevated blood glucose, or **hyperglycemia,** free fatty acid release from adipose tissue is inhibited and a general condition of increased carbohydrate metabolism exists.

- Estrogen, or more specifically estradiol-17β, increases the mobilization of free fatty acids from adipose tissue and inhibits glucose uptake by the peripheral tissues. Consequently, estradiol-17β and GH exert similar metabolic effects during exercise. Exercise is known to increase circulating estrogen in both menstruating and amenorrheic women.

- **Diabetes mellitus** (or simply, diabetes) is a condition involving a decrease in the body tissues' glucose uptake capability. Diabetes is expressed in two forms: type I, which is characterized by an inability to produce and secrete insulin (poor **insulin responsiveness**), and type II, which involves either an impaired ability to secrete insulin because of a defect in the β-cells of the pancreas, or a decrease in the cells' ability to respond to insulin (poor **insulin sensitivity**).

■ Sweating can occur at rates as high as 2 to 3 L/hour during exercise. The resulting water loss from the body reduces plasma volume and increases plasma osmolality, thereby stimulating **osmoreceptors** in the hypothalamus, which stimulate the release of **antidiuretic** hormone (ADH) and aldosterone; these in turn act to conserve body water. During conditions of low blood volume and blood pressure, vasoconstriction of the vasculature is caused by the hormones ADH, angiotensin I, and aldosterone. With water excess, release of ADH is inhibited by atrial natriuretic peptides and by reduced osmolality, resulting in a net increase in urine volume, or **diuresis.**

■ The body's neural regulation of central and peripheral cardiovascular functioning is controlled by the **vasomotor center** of the medulla. The neural and endocrinologic regulation of fluid balance and cardiovascular function is vital for controlling blood pressure and preventing **hypotension** and **hypertension,** during both rest and exercise.

■ Circulating testosterone increases during short-term, intense cycling and weight-lifting exercise, but this response is not due to stimulation by LH. In normally menstruating women, exercise-induced increases in estradiol-17β have been detected. The main androgenic stimulus for protein synthesis is the combined effects of GH and *insulin-like growth factor I* (IGF-I or somatomedin C). During exercise protein synthesis is impaired, but during the recovery from exercise protein synthesis is increased, resulting in a net protein gain.

■ The body produces opioid-like substances **(endogenous opioids)**, which can be categorized into three main types: β-endorphins, enkephalins, and α-endorphins (dynorphins). β-Endorphin and the enkephalins increase during exercise, and they have been associated with cardiovascular, ventilatory, metabolic, and thermoregulatory effects. β-Endorphin slightly inhibits ventilation and can suppress baroreceptor firing.

■ Participation in exercise training, no matter what type, has the potential to alter the secretion of hormones by changing (1) the stimuli that release hormones, (2) the ability of cells to respond to hormones, or (3) the maximal capacity of endocrine tissues to release hormones. For a given submaximal exercise intensity, endurance training lowers the catecholamine, GH, glucagon, and cortisol concentrations in the blood. Endurance training also is accompanied by an increased reliance on lipid catabolism for a given submaximal exercise intensity.

■ Women who are biologically capable of menstruating but do not, have a condition known as *amenorrhea*. When the cause of the amenorrhea is directly related to exercise participation, the condition is called **athletic amenorrhea.** Athletic amenorrhea is caused by a negative feedback to the pituitary gland because of chronic exposure to the stress hormones epinephrine, norepinephrine, cortisol, and β-endorphin, resulting in decreased release of LH and FSH. Decreased levels of FSH and LH prevent stimulation of the follicle of the ovary, thereby preventing the synthesis and secretion of estradiol by the ovary. Consequently, women with athletic amenorrhea have lower than normal circulating concentrations of estradiol-17β and therefore do not have the estradiol-stimulated increases in lipid catabolism during exercise or the protective qualities of estradiol relative to bone density and HDL concentrations in the blood.

REVIEW QUESTIONS

1. Explain the differences between traditional and nontraditional endocrine function.

2. What are the structural and functional (cell response) differences between peptide and steroid hormones?

3. Which hormones predominantly control energy metabolism during exercise?

4. Which hormones influence substrate mobilization during exercise? Explain why exercise duration and carbohydrate nutritional status are important in these hormonal responses.

5. Explain the terms *insulin sensitivity* and *insulin responsiveness* with respect to the metabolic and endocrine differences between a type II diabetic and a nondiabetic individual.

6. Explain the multihormonal regulation of fluid balance during exercise.

7. How does exercise and exercise training influence the body's immune system?

8. What are endogenous opioids, and do they have a role in exercise-induced changes in mood or euphoria?

9. What is exercise amenorrhea, and what are the probable causes of the condition?

10. Explain how endurance training can influence the hormonal response to prolonged submaximal exercise.

APPLICATIONS

1. Why is exercise an important component in the prevention of and rehabilitation from type II diabetes?

2. You are an exercise physiologist at a university, and several women members of the swim team approach you for advice about the loss of their menstrual cycle. Apart from recommending that they see a gynecologist or the varsity athlete doctor, how would you explain this condition to them?

3. Why would estrogen supplementation be important for women athletes?

4. Very intense exercise and prolonged submaximal exercise are associated with increased protein breakdown. What endocrinologic characteristics of exercise and the recovery from exercise stimulate protein synthesis and an eventual increase in muscle mass?

REFERENCES

1. Bagatell CJ, Bremner WJ: Sperm counts and reproductive hormones in male marathoners and lean controls, *Fertil Steril* 53:688–692, 1990.

2. Bak JF, Moller N, Schmitz O: Effects of growth hormone on fuel utilization and muscle glycogen synthase activity in normal humans, *Am J Physiol* 260(23):E736–E742, 1991.

3. Bale P: Body composition and menstrual cycle irregularities of female athletes: are they precursors of anorexia? *Sports Med* 17(6):347–352, 1994.

4. Bertolli A, De Pirro R, Fusco AV et al: Differences in insulin receptors between men and menstruating women and influence of sex hormones on insulin binding during the menstrual cycle, *J Clin Endocrinol* 50(2):246–250, 1980.

5. Blok J, Gibbs M, Lienhard GE et al: Insulin-induced translocation of glucose transporters from post-Golgi compartments to the plasma membrane of 3T3-L1 adipocytes, *J Cell Biol* 106:69–76, 1988.

6. Bloom SR, Johnson RH, Park DM et al: Differences in the metabolic and hormonal response to exercise between racing cyclists and untrained individuals, *J Physiol* 258:1–18, 1976.

7. Bonen A: Exercise-induced menstrual cycle changes: a functional, temporary adaptation to metabolic stress, *Sports Med* 17(6):373–392, 1994.

8. Boyden TW, Pameter RW, Stanforth P et al: Sex steroids and endurance running in women, *Fertil Steril* 39(5):629–632, 1983.

9. Boulware SD, Tamborlane WV, Mathews LS, Sherwin RS: Diverse effects of insulin-like growth factor I on glucose, lipid, and amino acid metabolism, *Am J Physiol* 262(25):E130–E133, 1992.

10. Boyle PJ, Cryer PE: Growth hormone, cortisol, or both are involved in defense against, but not critical to recovery from, hypoglycemia, *Am J Physiol* 260(23):E395–E402, 1991.

11. Boyle PJ, Avogaro A, Smith L et al: Role of GH in regulating nocturnal rates of lipolysis and plasma mevalonate levels in normal and diabetic humans, *Am J Physiol* 263(26):E168–E172, 1992.

12. Brandenberger G, Follenius M, Hietter B: Feedback from meal-related peaks determines diurnal changes in cortisol response to exercise, *J Clin Endocrinol Metab* 54(3):592–596, 1982.

13. Brown WH: *Introduction to organic chemistry,* Boston, 1982, Willard Grant.

14. Bunt JC, Bioleau RA, Bahr JM, Nelson RA: Sex and training differences in human growth hormone levels during prolonged exercise, *J Appl Physiol* 61(5):1796–1801, 1986.

15. Butler P, Kryshak E, Rizza R: Mechanism of growth hormone–induced postprandial carbohydrate intolerance in humans, *Am J Physiol* 260(23):E513–E520, 1991.

16. Campbell PJ, Carlson MG, Hill JO, Nurjhan N: Regulation of free fatty acid metabolism by insulin in humans: role of lipolysis and reesterification, *Am J Physiol* 263(26):E1063–E1069, 1992.

17. Capaldo B, Nappoli R, Di Bonito P et al: Dual mechanism of insulin action on human skeletal muscle: identification of an indirect component not mediated by FFA, *Am J Physiol* 260(23):E389–E394, 1991.

18. Carraro F, Stuart CA, Hartl WH et al: Effect of exercise and recovery on muscle protein synthesis in human subjects, *Am J Physiol* 259(22):E470–E476, 1990.

19. Clark BA, Elahia D, Fish L et al: Atrial natriuretic peptide suppresses osmostimulated vasopressin release in young and elderly humans, *Am J Physiol* 261(24):E252–E256, 1991.

20. Convertino VA, Brock BJ, Keil LC et al: Exercise training–induced hypervolemia: role of plasma albumin, renin, and vasopressin, *J Appl Physiol* 48(4):665–669, 1980.

21. Convertino VA, Keil LC, Bernauer EM, Greenleaf JE: Plasma volume, osmolality, vasopressin, and renin activity during graded exercise in man, *J Appl Physiol* 50(1):123–128, 1981.

22. Cooper DM, Barstow TJ, Bergner A, Paul Lee WN: Blood glucose turnover during high- and low-intensity exercise, *Am J Physiol* 257():E405–E412, 1989.

23. Costill DL, Thomas R, Roberges RA et al: Adaptations to swimming training: influence of training volume, *Med Sci Sports Exerc* 23(3):371–377, 1991.

24. Cumming DC, Guigley ME, Yen SSC: Acute suppression of circulating testosterone levels by cortisol in men, *J Clin Endocrinol Metab* 57:671–677, 1983.

25. Cumming DC, Brunsting LA III, Strich G et al: Reproductive hormone increases in response to acute exercise in men, *Med Sci Sports Exerc* 18(4):369–373, 1986.

26. Cumming DC, Wheeler GD, McCall EM: The effects of exercise on reproductive function in men, *Sports Med* 7:1–17, 1989.

27. DeFronzo RA, Tobin JD, Andres R: Glucose clamp technique: a method for quantifying insulin secretion and resistance, *Am J Physiol* 237(3):E214–E233, 1979.

28. Dela F, Mikines KJ, Linstow MV, Galbo H: Effect of training on response to a glucose load adjusted for daily carbohydrate intake, *Am J Physiol* 260(23):E14–E20, 1991.

REFERENCES—Cont'd

29. Dela F, Mikines KJ, Linstow MV, Galbo H: Heart rate and plasma catecholamines during 24 hours of everyday life in trained and untrained men, *J Appl Physiol* 73(6):2389-2395, 1992.

30. Dela F, Mikines KJ, Von Linstow M et al: Effect of training on insulin-mediated glucose uptake in human muscle, *Am J Physiol* 263(26):E1134-E1143, 1992.

31. De Souza MJ, Metzger DA: Reproductive dysfunction in amenorrheic athletes and anorexic patients: a review, *Med Sci Sports Exerc* 23(9):995-1007, 1991.

32. Dohm GL, Elton CW, Friedman JE et al: Decreased expression of glucose transporter in muscle from insulin-resistant patients, *Am J Physiol* 260(23):E459-E463, 1991.

33. Eichner ER: Exercise and testicular function, *Sports Sci Exchange* 5(38):1-5, 1992.

34. Farrell PA, Gustafson AB, Morgan WP, Pert CB: Enkephalins, catecholamines, and psychological mood alternations: effects of prolonged exercise, *Med Sci Sports Exerc* 19(4):347-352, 1987.

35. Farrell PA, Kjaer M, Bach FW, Galbo H: β-endorphin and adrenocorticotropin response to supramaximal treadmill exercise in trained and untrained males, *Acta Physiol Scand* 130:619-625, 1987.

36. Felber J-P, Ferrannini E, Golay A et al: Role of lipid oxidation in pathogenesis of insulin resistance of obesity and type II diabetes, *Diabetes* 36:1341-1350, 1987.

37. Fell RD, Terblanche SE, Ivy JL, Holloszy JO: Effect of muscle glycogen on glucose uptake following exercise, *J Appl Physiol* 52:434-437, 1982.

38. Francesconi RP: Endocrinological responses to exercise in stressful environments, *Exerc Sport Sci Rev* 16:255-284, 1988.

39. Freund BJ, Shizuru EM, Hashiro GM, Claybaugh JR: Hormonal electrolyte and renal responses to exercise are intensity dependent, *J Appl Physiol* 70(2):900-906, 1991.

40. Froberg K, Pedersen PK: Sex differences in endurance capacity and metabolic response to prolonged, heavy exercise, *Eur J Appl Physiol* 52:446-450, 1984.

41. Galbo H, Holst JJ, Christensen NJ: Glucagon and plasma catecholamine responses to graded and prolonged exercise in man, *J Appl Physiol* 38(1):70-76, 1975.

42. Ganguly A: Atrial natriuretic peptide–induced inhibition of aldosterone secretion: a quest for mediators, *Am J Physiol* 263(26):E181-E194, 1992.

43. Goodyear LJ, Hirshman MF, Smith RJ, Horton ES: Glucose transported number, activity and isoform content in plasma membranes of red and white skeletal muscle, *Am J Physiol* 261(24):E556-E561, 1991.

44. Griffin JE, Ojeda SR: Organization of the endocrine system. In Griffin JE, Ojeda SR, editors: *Textbook of endocrine physiology,* New York, 1988, Oxford University Press.

45. Grossman A, Sutton JR: Endorphins: what are they? how are they measured? what is their role in exercise? *Med Sci Sports Exerc* 17(1):74-81, 1985.

46. Gulve EA, Cartee GD, Zierath JR et al: Reversal of enhanced muscle glucose transport after exercise: roles of insulin and glucose, *Am J Physiol* 259(22):E685-E691, 1990.

47. Guyton AC: *Textbook of medical physiology,* ed 8, Philadelphia, 1991, Saunders.

48. Hanson FM, Fahmy N, Nielsen JH: The influence of sexual hormones on lipogenesis and lipolysis in rat fat cells, *Acta Endocrinol* 95:566-570, 1980.

49. Hartman ML, Faria ACS, Vance ML et al: Temporal structure of in vivo growth hormone secretory events in humans, *Am J Physiol* 260(23):E101-E110, 1991.

50. Hatta H, Atomi Y, Shinohara S et al: The effects of ovarian hormones on glucose and fatty acid oxidation during exercise in female ovariectomized rats, *Horm Metab Res* 20:609-611, 1988.

51. Heath GW, Gavin JR III, Hinderliter JM et al: Effects of exercise and lack of exercise on glucose tolerance and insulin sensitivity, *J Appl Physiol* 55(2):512-517, 1983.

52. Heller SR, Cryer PE: Hypoinsulinemia is not critical to glucose recovery from hypoglycemia in humans, *Am J Physiol* 261(24):E41-E48, 1991.

53. Henriksen EJ, Louters LL, Stump CS, Tipton CM: Effects of prior exercise on the action of insulin-like growth factor I in skeletal muscle, *Am J Physiol* 263(26):E340-E344, 1992.

54. Highet R: Athletic amenorrhea: an update on aetiology, complications, and management, *Sports Med* 7:82-108, 1989.

55. Houmard JA, Egan PC, Neuffer PD et al: Elevated skeletal muscle glucose transporter levels in exercise-trained middle-aged men, *Am J Physiol* 261(24):E437-E443, 1991.

56. Houmard JA, Shinebarger MH, Dolan PL et al: Exercise training increases GLUT-4 protein concentration in previously sedentary middle-aged men, *Am J Physiol* 264(27):E896-E901, 1993.

57. Hurley BF, Nemeth PM, Martin WH III et al: Muscle triglyceride utilization during exercise: effect of training, *J Appl Physiol* 60(2):562-567, 1986.

58. Karagiorgos A, Garcia JF, Brooks GA: Growth hormone response to continuous intermittent exercise, *Med Sci Sports Exerc* 11(3):302-307, 1979.

59. Keizer HA, Rogol AD: Physical exercise and menstrual cycle alterations: what are the mechanisms? *Sports Med* 10(4):218-235, 1990.

REFERENCES—Cont'd

60. Kirwan JP, Bourey RE, Kohrt WM et al: Effects of treadmill exercise to exhaustion on the insulin response to hyperglycemia in untrained men, *J Appl Physiol* 70(1):246-250, 1991.

61. Kirwan JP, Hickner RC, Yarasheski KE et al: Eccentric exercise induces transient insulin resistance in healthy individuals, *J Appl Physiol* 72(6):2197-2202, 1992.

62. Kjaer M, Galbo H: The effect of physical training on the capacity to secrete epinephrine, *J Appl Physiol* 64:11-16, 1988.

63. Kjaer M, Kiens B, Hargreaves M, Richter EA: Influence of active muscle mass on glucose homeostasis during exercise in man, *J Appl Physiol* 71:552-557, 1991.

64. Kjaer M: Regulation of hormonal and metabolic responses during exercise in humans, *Exerc Sport Sci Rev* 20:161-184, 1992.

65. Kraemer WJ: Endocrine responses to resistance exercise, *Med Sci Sports Exerc* 20:S152-S157, 1988.

66. Kraemer WJ, Fleck SJ, Callister R et al: Training responses of plasma endorphin, adrenocorticotropin, and cortisol, *Med Sci Sports Exerc* 21(2):146-153, 1989.

67. Kujala UM, Alen M, Huhtaniemii IT: Gonadotropin-releasing hormone and human chorionic gonadotropin tests reveal both hypothalamic and testicular endocrine functions are suppressed during acute, prolonged physical exercise, *Clin Endocrinol* 33:219-225. 1990.

68. Loucks AB, Horvath SB: Athletic amenorrhea: a review, *Med Sci Sports Exerc* 17(1):56-72, 1985.

69. Luger A, Deuster PA, Kyle SB et al: Acute hypothalamic-pituitary-adrenal responses to the stress of treadmill exercise, *N Engl J Med* 316(21):1309-1315, 1987.

70. MacDougall JD, Webber CE, Martin J et al: Relationship among running mileage, bone density, and serum testosterone in male runners, *J Appl Physiol* 73(3):1165-1170, 1992.

71. Marieb EN: *Human anatomy and physiology,* ed 3, Redwood City, Calif, 1995, Benjamin/Cummings.

72. Methews DE, Pesola G, Campbell RG: Effect of epinephrine on amino acid and energy metabolism in humans, *Am J Physiol* 258:E948-E956, 1990.

73. Megeney LA, Neufer PD, Dohm GL et al: Effects of muscle activity and fiber composition on glucose transport and GLUT-4, *Am J Physiol* 264(27):E583-E593, 1993.

74. Mikines KJ, Sonne B, Farrell PA et al: Effect of physical exercise on sensitivity and responsiveness to insulin in humans, *Am J Physiol* 254(17):E248-E259, 1988.

75. Myerson M; Gutin B, Warren M et al: Resting metabolic rate and energy balance in amenorrheic and eumenorrheic runners, *Med Sci Sport Exerc* 23(1):15-22, 1991.

76. Naess PA, Christensen G, Kiil F: Atrial natriuretic factor reduces renin release by opposing α-adrenoreceptor activity, *Am J Physiol* 261(24):E240-E245, 1991.

77. Ploug T, Galbo H, Richter EA: Increased muscle glucose uptake during contraction: no need for insulin, *Am J Physiol* 247(10):E712-E731, 1984.

78. Plourde G, Rousseau-Migneron S, Nadeau A: Effect of endurance training on adrenergic system in three different skeletal muscles, *J Appl Physiol* 74(4):1641-1646, 1993.

79. Randle PJ, Hales CN, Garland PB, Newsholme EA: The glucose-fatty acid cycle: its role in insulin sensitivity and the metabolic disturbances of diabetes mellitus, *Lancet* (1):785-789, 1963.

80. Raz I, Katz A, Spencer MK: Epinephrine inhibits insulin-mediated glycogenesis but enhances glycolysis in human skeletal muscle, *Am J Physiol* 260(23):E430-E435, 1991.

81. Richter EA, Ruderman NB, Gravas H et al: Muscle glycogenolysis during exercise: dual control by epinephrine and contractions, *Am J Physiol* 242:E25-E32, 1982.

82. Richter EA, Kiens B, Saltin B et al: Skeletal muscle glucose uptake during dynamic exercise in humans: role of muscle mass, *Am J Physiol* 254(17):E555-E561, 1988.

83. Rogol AD: Growth hormone: physiology, therapeutic use, and potential for abuse, *Exerc Sport Sci Rev* 17:352-378, 1989.

84. Rogol AD, Weltman A, Weltman JY et al: Durability of the reproductive axis in eumenorrheic women during 1 year of endurance training, *J Appl Physiol* 72(4):1571-1580, 1992.

85. Rowell LB, O'Leary DS: Reflex control of the circulation during exercise: chemoreflexes and mechanoreflexes, *J Appl Physiol* 69(20):407-418, 1990.

86. Ruby BC, Robergs RA, Waters DL: Influence of estrogen supplementation on glucose and glycerol turnover during prolonged exercise in amenorrheic athletes, *Med Sci Sports Exerc* 1995 (in review).

87. Saloranta C, Koivisto V, Widen E et al: Contribution of muscle and liver to glucose–fatty acid cycle in humans, *Am J Physiol* 264(27):E599-E605, 1993.

88. Schwab R, Johnson GO, Housh TJ et al: Acute effects of different intensities of weight lifting on serum testosterone, *Med Sci Sports Exerc* 25(12):1381-1385, 1993.

89. Schwellnus MP, Gordon NF: The role of endogenous opioids in thermoregulation during submaximal exercise, *Med Sci Sports Exerc* 19(6):575-578, 1987.

REFERENCES—Cont'd

90. Shangold M, Freeman R, Thysen B, Gatz M: The relationship between long distance running, plasma progesterone, and luteal phase length, *Fertil Steril* 31(20):130-133, 1979.

91. Spencer MK, Katz A, Raz I: Epinephrine increases tricarboxylic acid cycle intermediates in human skeletal muscle, *Am J Physiol* 260(23):E436-E439, 1991.

92. Spratt DI, O'Dea LStL, Schoenfeld D et al: Neuroendocrine–gonadal axis in men: frequent sampling of LH, FSH, and testosterone, *Am J Physiol* 254(17):E658-E666, 1988.

93. Spriet LL, Ren JM, Hultman E: Epinephrine infusion enhances muscle glycogenolysis during prolonged electrical stimulation, *J Appl Physiol* 64:1439-1444, 1988.

94. Tarnopolsky LJ, MacDougall JD, Atkinson SA et al: Gender differences in substrate for endurance exercise, *J Appl Physiol* 68(1):302-308, 1990.

95. Vanhelder WR, Rodomski MW, Goode RC: Growth hormone responses during intermittent weight-lifting exercise in men, *Eur J Appl Physiol* 53:31-34, 1984.

96. Wade CE: Response, regulation, and actions of vasopressin during exercise: a review, *Med Sci Sports Exerc* 16(5):506-511, 1984.

97. Walker M, Fulcher GR, Sum CF et al: Effect of glycemia and nonesterified fatty acids on forearm glucose uptake in normal humans, *Am J Physiol* 261(24):E304-E311, 1991.

98. Wallberg-Henriksson H: Exercise and diabetes mellitus, *Exerc Sport Sci Rev* 20:339-368, 1992.

99. Warren MP, Brooks-Gunn J, Fox RP, Lancelon C: Lack of bone accretion and amenorrhea: evidence for a relative osteopenia in weight-bearing bones, *J Clin Endocrinol Metab* 72(4):847-853, 1991.

100. Wasserman DH, Geer RJ, Rice DE et al: Interaction of exercise and insulin action in humans, *Am J Physiol* 260(23):E37-E45, 1991.

101. Wasserman DH, Cherrington AD: Hepatic fuel metabolism during muscular work: role and regulation, *Am J Physiol* 260(23):E811-E824, 1991.

102. Watenpaugh DE, Yancy CW, Buckey JC et al: Role of atrial natriuretic peptide in systemic responses to acute isotonic volume expansion, *J Appl Physiol* 73(4):1218-1226, 1992.

103. Waters D, Robergs RA, Montner P: Growth hormone release during and after exercise in amenorrheic athletic women, *Med Sci Sports Exerc* 1995 (in press).

104. Weltman A, Weltman JY, Schurrer R et al: Endurance training amplifies the pulsatile release of growth hormone: effects of training intensity, *J Appl Physiol* 72(6):2188-2196, 1992.

105. Wilmore JH, Wambsgans KC, Brenner M et al: Is there energy conservation in amenorrheic compared with eumenorrheic distance runners? *J Appl Physiol* 72(1):15-22, 1992.

106. Winder WW, Hagberg JM, Hickson RC et al: Time course of sympathoadrenergic adaptation to endurance exercise training in man, *J Appl Physiol* 45:370-374, 1978.

107. Wolman RL, Clark P, McNally E et al: Menstrual state and exercise as determinants of spinal trabecular bone density in female athletes, *Br Med J* 301:516-518, 1990.

108. Yarasheski KE, Campbell JA, Smith K et al: Effect of growth hormone and resistance exercise on muscle growth in young men, *Am J Physiol* 262(25):E261-E267, 1992.

109. Young AA, Bogardus C, Stone K, Mott DM: Insulin response of components of whole-body and muscle carbohydrate metabolism in humans, *Am J Physiol* 254(17):E231-E236, 1988.

RECOMMENDED READINGS

▪ Brandenberger G, Follenius M, Hietter B: Feedback from meal-related peaks determines diurnal changes in cortisol response to exercise, *J Clin Endocrinol Metab* 54(3):592-596, 1982.

▪ Carraro F, Stuart CA, Hartl WH et al: Effect of exercise and recovery on muscle protein synthesis in human subjects, *Am J Physiol* 259(22):E470-E475, 1990.

▪ DeFronzo RA, Tobin JD, Andres R: Glucose clamp technique: a method for quantifying insulin secretion and resistance, *Am J Physiol* 237(3):E214-E223, 1979.

▪ Dela F, Mikines KJ, Linstow MV, Galbo H: Heart rate and plasma catecholamines during 24 hours of everyday life in trained and untrained men, *J Appl Physiol* 73(6):2389-2395, 1992.

▪ De Souza MJ, Metzger DA: Reproductive dysfunction in amenorrheic athletes and anorexic patients: a review, *Med Sci Sports Exerc* 23(9):995-1007, 1991.

▪ Dohm GL, Elton CW, Friedman JE et al: Decreased expression of glucose transporter in muscle from insulin-resistant patients, *Am J Physiol* 260(23):E459-E463, 1991.

▪ Grossman A, Sutton JR: Endorphins: what are they? how are they measured? what is their role in exercise? *Med Sci Sports Exerc* 17(1)74-81, 1985.

▪ Highet R: Athletic amenorrhea: an update on aetiology, complications, and management, *Sports Med* 7:82-108, 1989.

▪ Hartman ML, Faria ACS, Vance ML et al: Temporal structure of in vivo growth hormone secretory events in humans, *Am J Physiol* 260(23):E101-E110, 1991.

▪ Luger A, Deuster PA, Kyle SB et al: Acute hypothalamic-pituitary-adrenal responses to the stress of treadmill exercise, *N Engl J Med* 316(21):1309-1315, 1987.

▪ Rogol AD, Weltman A, Weltman JY et al: Durability of the reproductive axis in eumenorrheic women during 1 year of endurance training, *J Appl Physiol* 72(4):1571-1580, 1992.

▪ Spratt DI, O'Dea LStL, Schoenfeld D et al: Neuroendocrine-gonadal axis in men: frequent sampling of LH, FSH, and testosterone, *Am J Physiol* 254(17):E658-E666, 1988.

▪ Wallberg-Henriksson H: Exercise and diabetes mellitus, *Exerc Sport Sci Rev* 20:339-368, 1992.

▪ Weltman A, Weltman JY, Schurrer R et al: Endurance training amplifies the pulsatile release of growth hormone: effects of training intensity, *J Appl Physiol* 72(6):2188-2196, 1992.

CHAPTER 14

Bone Function and Adaptation to Exercise

OBJECTIVES

After studying this chapter you should be able to:

- Describe the functions of bone and the skeleton.

- Explain the processes of bone resorption and deposition.

- Describe the regulation of bone resorption and deposition.

- Explain the condition of osteoporosis and the risk of osteoporosis in certain groups.

- Explain how exercise influences bone remodeling and what types of exercises best maintain bone mineral density.

KEY TERMS

axial skeleton

appendicular skeleton

osseous tissue

compact bone

cancellous bone

osteocytes

haversian system

haversian canal

hydroxyapatite

hematopoiesis

ossification

epiphysis

epiphyseal plate

bone remodeling

dual x-ray absorptiometry (DEXA)

osteoporosis

Bone provides anchoring and support for the origin and insertion of skeletal muscle, which in turn allows movement of the limbs and provides the ability to resist movement. Stress applied to bone at junctions formed by muscle, tendon, and bone stimulates bone to alter itself, resulting in changed bone structure. As with exercise-induced improvements in cardiovascular, respiratory, and neuromuscular functions the exercise-induced improvements in bone have had ramifications in preventive and rehabilitative medicine. The ability of exercise to affect bone mineral content was first recognized in athletes. More recently, the importance of exercise to bone in women with abnormally low estrogen levels (postmenopausal or amenorrheic women) has been recognized. This chapter provides an overview of the morphology and function of bone and describes the regulation of bone growth, repair, and mineral content, as well as the effects of exercise on bone structure and function.

Skeletal System

*T*he *skeletal system* consists of the organized anatomic arrangement of the bones of the body. The human skeleton can be divided into the **axial skeleton** and the **appendicular skeleton** (Figure 14.1). The axial skeleton consists of the skull, vertebral column, and thorax (rib cage); the appendicular skeleton consists of the shoulder girdles and arms and the pelvic girdle and legs.

Different Types of Bone

Bone consists of two types of bone tissue, or **osseous tissue.** The osseous tissue can be **compact bone** or **cancellous bone** (also called spongy bone). The differences among the types of bone are illustrated in Figure 14.2.

---

axial skeleton
the skeletal structure comprising the bones of the head, thoracic cage, and vertebral column

appendicular skeleton
the skeletal structure comprising the bones of the legs, pelvis, and arms

osseous tissue
bone

compact bone
dense bone characterized by the arrangement of mineral and cells into haversian systems

cancellous bone
spongy (or trabecular) bone, which has no haversian system

FIGURE 14.1

The human skeleton, colored to indicate axial and appendicular components, and the different types of bones of the human skeleton.

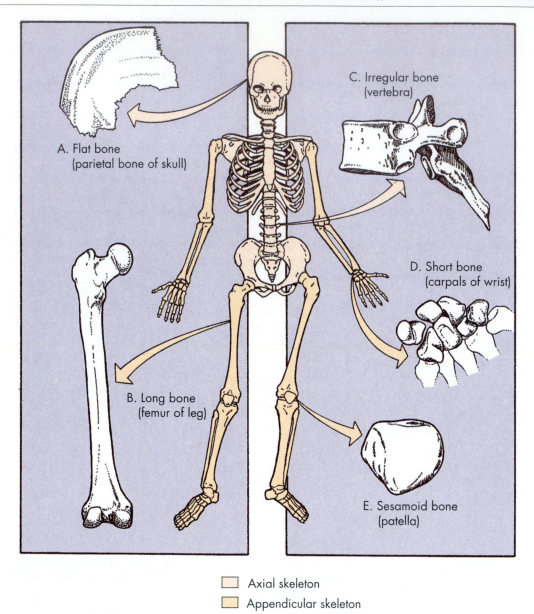

A. Flat bone
(parietal bone of skull)

C. Irregular bone
(vertebra)

D. Short bone
(carpals of wrist)

B. Long bone
(femur of leg)

E. Sesamoid bone
(patella)

☐ Axial skeleton

☐ Appendicular skeleton

Compact bone, which accounts for 80% of the skeletal mass[26] usually is localized to the outer layers of a given bone. The remaining 20% of the skeletal mass, made up of cancellous bone, forms in the inner regions, especially in areas exposed to stress. The smaller mass contribution by cancellous bone should not be viewed in terms of a minor role in bone function. Cancellous bone contributes 70% of the skeletal bone volume, and because of its *trabecular* arrangement, allows for marrow and fat storage and provides the microstructure that gives bone strength for a relatively low-mass tissue. As is discussed in later sections, loss of trabeculae and cancellous bone mass severely compromises bone strength and increases the risk of bone fractures.

Compact bone has a highly organized microscopic structure (Figure 14.3). Bone cells **(osteocytes),** nerves, and blood and lymph vessels collectively form structural units, each of which is called a **haversian system** (or osteon). Histologic stained cross-section specimens of bone reveal that the haversian systems are circular and have a central vascular supply **(haversian canal).** The osteocytes arrange themselves in small channels *(canaliculi),* which are positioned as successive circles around the haversian canal. Between each

FIGURE 14.2

A macroscopic comparison between compact cancellous bone. (From Thibodeau GA: *Anatomy and physiology*, 3 ed, St. Louis, 1996, Mosby. Art by Joan Beck.)

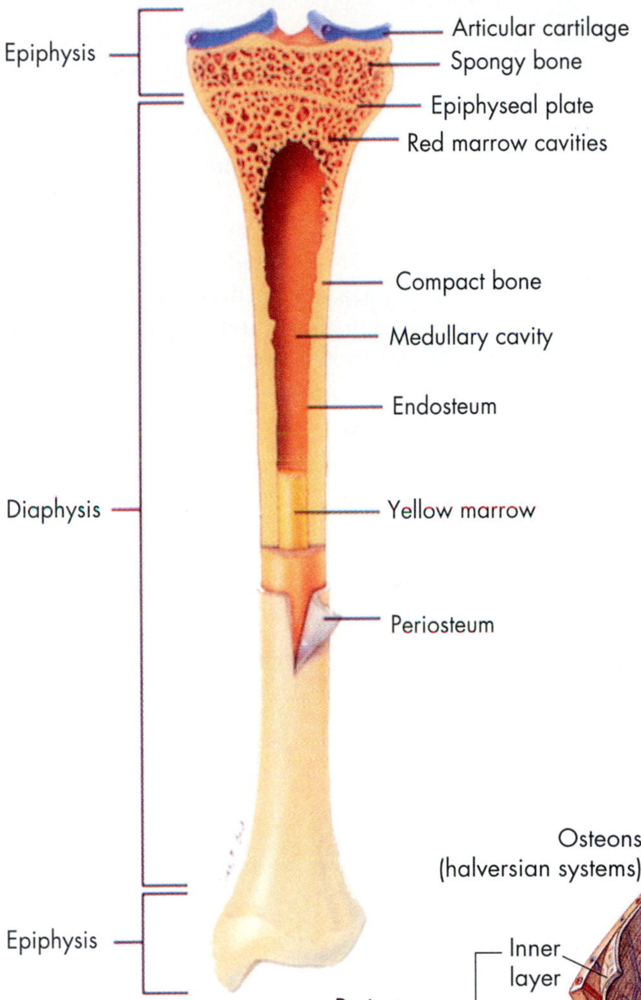

Epiphysis

Articular cartilage
Spongy bone
Epiphyseal plate
Red marrow cavities

Compact bone

Medullary cavity

Endosteum

Diaphysis

Yellow marrow

Periosteum

Epiphysis

two canaliculi is a matrix of bone mineral, and the circles formed by the bone mineral and canaliculi are called *lamellae*.

Cancellous bone is less structurally organized and less dense than compact bone. Cancellous bone is composed of separate threads of bone connected to each other in a three-dimensional array, much like the honeycomb of a bee hive but with open space rather than a filling in the pores.

osteocyte (os' te-o-**site**)

bone cell

haversian system

the organized circular, cellular, and vascular structure of compact bone

haversian canal

the central vascular component of the haversian system

FIGURE 14.3

The microscopic structure of compact bone. Osteocytes are identified as dark cells within the canaliculi that exist between the successive layers of lamellae. The lamellae combine to form the Haversian system, which encircles a central vascular canal (Haversian canal). (From Seeley RR, Stephens TD, Tate P: *Anatomy and physiology*, 3 ed, St. Louis, 1995, Mosby. Art by John V. Hagen.)

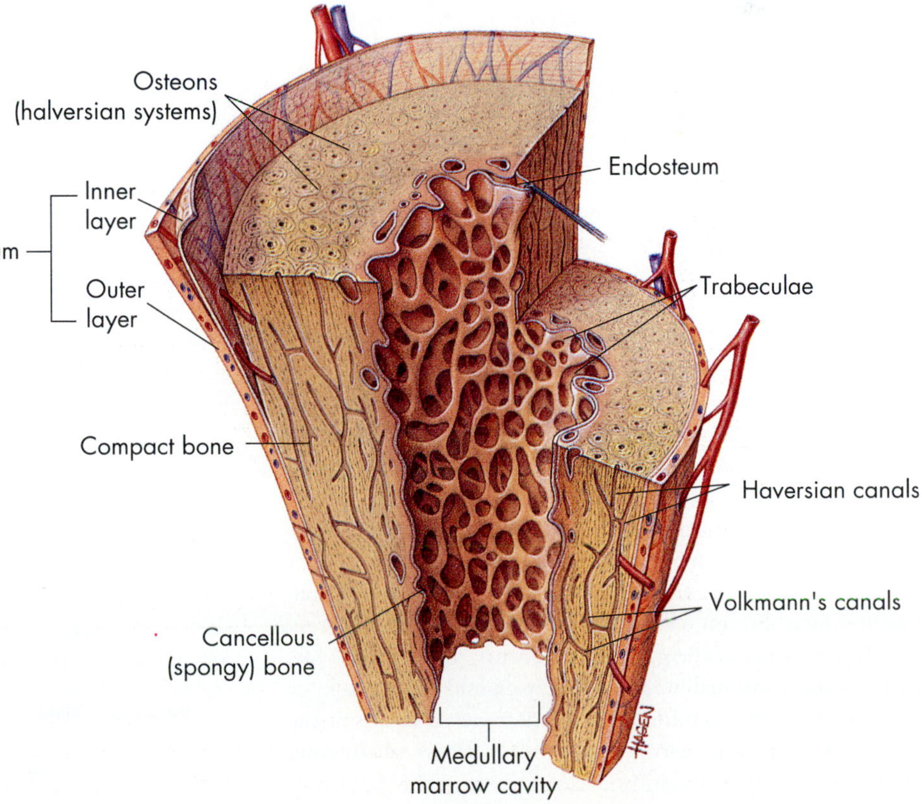

Osteons (halversian systems)

Periosteum
Inner layer
Outer layer

Compact bone

Cancellous (spongy) bone

Endosteum

Trabeculae

Haversian canals

Volkmann's canals

Medullary marrow cavity

The bone matrix itself consists of (1) three types of cells: osteoblasts, osteocytes, and osteoclasts, which contribute one third of the matrix; (2) organic elements (e.g., glycoproteins and collagen); and (3) inorganic mineral salts, which contribute 65% of the bone matrix. Although the organic elements represent a relatively minor component, they contribute to the strength and rigidity of bone. However, most of the strength and hardiness of bone is due to the inorganic mineral salts, which are collectively called **hydroxyapatites.** The main minerals are calcium salts and phosphates. The bone matrix is surprisingly strong, able to withstand more than 25,000 psi of compression.[14]

Function of Bone

The skeleton provides *support, protection,* and *leverage* for movement and the application of force; *storage* of fat and minerals; and the *production* of blood cells. Noted examples of these functions are the support given by the bones of the legs during locomotion; the protection provided by the skull for the brain; the leverage produced from muscle attachments near joints; the calcium and phosphate mineral stored in the bones; and the red blood cells (RBCs) produced in the *bone marrow.*

Bone marrow is found in the shafts of the long bones and in the inner cavity of certain flat and irregular bones, such as the sternum or ilium. Not all bone marrow produces blood cells **(hematopoiesis).** Yellow marrow is composed primarily of fat, whereas red marrow is involved in hematopoiesis. In adults, red marrow is located mainly in the head of the femur and humerus bones.

Bone Growth and Remodeling

Bone formation is called *osteogenesis,* or **ossification.** During the development of the human skeleton, ossification can be categorized into two types: formation of the skeleton and bone growth, and bone remodeling. During growth from infancy the skeleton is formed by the ossification of cartilage. Ossification begins in the middle of the shaft and extends to each end, or **epiphysis.** Once the long bone has formed, continued growth occurs from a retained line of cartilage at either epiphysis, called the **epiphyseal plate,** as well as laterally (outward to the sides). The long bones stop growing when the epiphyseal plates become completely ossified, which corresponds to late childhood or early adolescence. However, many of the flat or irregular bones continue to grow throughout life (e.g., skull, jaw, and facial bones).

Bone remodeling, which occurs throughout life, involves the continual breakdown, repair, and replacement of osteocytes and bone mineral. Bone deposition occurs at the sites of injury, or stress. Bone reabsorption occurs when bones are unstressed, or when an imbalance exists in the regulatory processes of bone mineral content. The regulation of bone remodeling, which is important for understanding the effects of exercise on bone structure and function, is discussed in a later section.

Cellular Events in Bone Remodeling

The balance of bone mineral results from the activity of the osteoblasts and osteoclasts. Recent evidence indicates that these cells do not function independently, but act as parts of a unit of cells *(basic multicellular unit; BMU)* that respond together to regulatory conditions (Figure 14.4). An increase in conditions favoring bone resorption increases osteoclast activity relative to osteoblast activity. Bone resorption occurs when catalytic enzymes are secreted by the osteoclasts. Osteoclasts also have a phagocytic action. The mineral salts released during reabsorption diffuse into the interstitial fluid, where they are removed by the circulation. During conditions of bone resorption, a negative bone mineral balance occurs. Conversely, stimuli that favor bone deposition increase osteoblast activity relative to osteoclast activity, and a net positive bone mineral balance is attained. Estimates indicate that most bone BMUs are in a state of quiescence,[6] with approximately 20% active in cancellous bone and less than 5% active in compact bone.

Regulation of Bone Remodeling

Bone remodeling occurs by means of a multiple-hormone regulation system and in response to physical stress (Table 14.1 and Figure 14.5).

---

hydroxyapatite (hi-drok se-**ap** a tite)
the mineral structure of the bone matrix

hematopoiesis (hem a-to-**poy**-e sis)
increased production of blood cells

ossification (os'-i-fi-**ka**-shun)
the replacement of cartilaginous bone with bone mineral

epiphysis (e-**pif**-i-sis)
either of the two end regions of long bones

epiphyseal plate
the cartilaginous region of the epiphysis, which is responsible for bone growth relative to a change in length

bone remodeling
the dynamic exchange between mineral deposition and resorption in bone

FIGURE 14.4

The basic multicellular unit (BMU) that is proposed to respond to hormonal and physical stress regulation during bone remodeling. (Adapted from Dalsky GP: Effect of exercise on bone: permissive influence of estrogen and calcium, *Med Sci Sports Exerc* 22(3):281-285, 1990.)

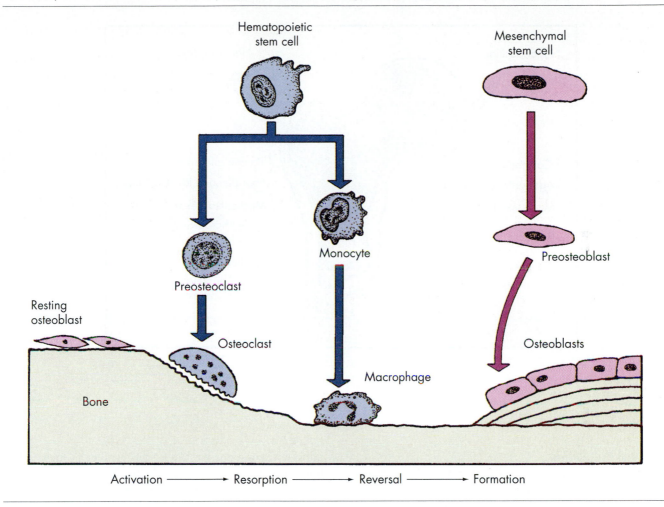

TABLE 14.1

Regulation of bone mineral content by hormones and physical stress

HORMONE	FUNCTION	MECHANISM
Calcitonin	↑ Bone deposition ↓ Bone resorption	↑ Osteoblast activity ↓ Osteoclast activity
Parathyroid hormone (PTH)	↑ Bone resorption	↑ Osteoclast activity
Estradiol-17β	↓ Bone resorption	↓ Sensitivity to PTH
Testosterone	↓ Bone resorption	↓ Sensitivity to PTH
Bone stress	↑ Bone deposition	↑ Osteoblast activity

FIGURE 14.5

An illustration of the overall regulation of bone remodeling. Factors that influence bone remodeling include hormonal, nutritional, and physical stress conditions.

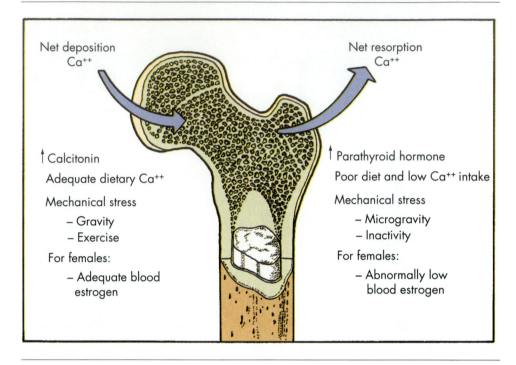

Hormonal Regulation

The hormonal regulation of bone remodeling is sensitive to blood calcium concentrations. Normal total blood calcium concentrations range between 85 and 105 mg/L. When blood calcium decreases, the parathyroid gland releases parathyroid hormone (PTH), which increases the activity of the osteoclasts, thereby increasing bone resorption. Conversely, when blood calcium concentrations are above normal, the thyroid gland releases calcitonin, which inhibits osteoclast activity, favoring osteoblast activity and bone deposition. In this hormonal system the primary element is blood calcium, because bone resorption will continue until a severely low bone mineral content develops if blood calcium concentrations remain low. This priority is understandable because blood calcium concentrations influence the membrane potential of excitable cells (e.g., nerves, myocardium, smooth muscle, and skeletal muscle), and optimal functioning of many of these tissues is essential for life. Also, excess blood calcium can be deposited in organs (e.g., kidneys and blood vessels), impairing their functioning.

Another hormone regulator of bone remodeling is estrogen. Estrogen reduces both the number of active BMUs and their sensitivity to PTH. This results in reduced osteoclast activity and bone resorption,[6] favoring the retention of bone

mineral. Testosterone has similar mechanisms in men. Other hormones also are known to influence bone mineral content through permissive and minor direct effects. These hormones are thyroxine (T_4), growth hormone (GH), somatomedin C (IGF-I), vitamin D, corticosteroids, prostaglandins, interleukin-1 (IL-1), and endothelial growth factors.[6,19]

Physical Stress

Physical stress on bone stimulates increased bone deposition. The physical stress can be a result of exercise, which can apply compressive and tensile (twisting) stress. In addition, simply overcoming the forces of gravity on the musculoskeletal system, or resisting impact, can stimulate bone deposition. Because of the large number of muscles (>600) that originate and insert on the numerous bones of the skeletal system (~206), muscle contraction, especially against resistance (gravity or external loads), can place large forces on the muscle tendon–bone joints, and these forces are relayed to the bone matrix. These facts are being revealed in astronauts in the U.S. space shuttle program, and efforts are being made to use exercise in zero gravity as a means to retard increased bone resorption during space flights (see Chapter 26).

There have been instances in sports when the impact, compression, or tensile forces have been too great for the

FIGURE 14.6

The change in bone mineral during growth, development, and aging throughout the lifecycle.

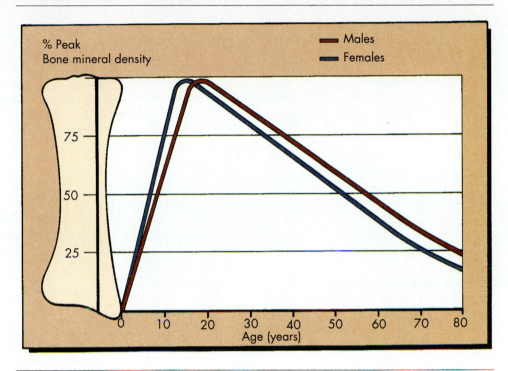

bones of certain athletes, resulting in fractures or complete breaks. Damage to bone occurs frequently in the contact sports of American football, Australian football, and rugby and in sports in which tensile forces are exaggerated because of restricted joint range of motion, such as water skiing and downhill snow skiing.

Changes in Bone Remodeling During the Life Cycle

Bone mineral content increases during adolescence and reaches a peak shortly after puberty.[26] It is unclear whether the earlier onset of pubescence in girls is associated with an earlier peak bone mineral content, which would also indicate an earlier onset of age-related bone mineral loss (Figure 14.6).

Research has clearly established an age-related loss in bone mineral content (Focus Box 14-1). This loss occurs first in cancellous bone, which begins to decline before the third decade of life. Compact bone is retained for another decade before resorption increases.[9,20,26] Given the differences in cellular arrangement and osteoclastic vulnerability between the different types of bone, this time difference is understandable.

The decline in trabecular bone mineral content is greater for women than men and greater again for post-

menopausal women[3,6,10,26,27] (Figure 14.9). After menopause the rate of trabecular bone mineral loss in women can increase to 7% per year, with the greatest loss in the first 5 years. This rate of loss is large compared with the average loss before menopause of less than 1% per year.[26]

Osteoporosis

The clinical condition known as **osteoporosis** does not have a precise definition; rather, it is a general state of the bones or skeleton in which bone mineral and the trabecular microarchitecture have deteriorated to such an extent that the risk of bone fractures is increased even during normal, everyday activities. Unfortunately, there is no known cure for osteoporosis. Once bone mineral has been lost, there is no evidence that any intervention can increase bone mineral content. This fact emphasizes that prevention not only is the best, it is the *only*, strategy for combating bone mineral loss

osteoporosis (os′ te-o-**po-ro**-sis)
a clinical condition characterized by a decrease in the mineral content of bone.

FOCUS BOX 14.1

Methods of measuring bone mineral density

Originally, bone mineral content and structure were studied by using bone samples from postmortem specimens. Bone samples from living individuals were obtained invasively by a biopsy of the iliac crest, and this remains the only way to determine bone structure (the arrangement of trabeculae in cancellous bone).

Since the 1980s, several noninvasive procedures have been used to estimate bone mineral content; single-photon and dual-photon absorptiometry, **dual x-ray absorptiometry (DEXA)**, quantitative computed tomography, and radiography. The equipment used in DEXA is illustrated in Figure 14.7. DEXA is a widely used method for evaluating regional and total bone mineral content. Subjects lie on a bench above a radionucleotide source that possesses dual energy (^{153}gadolinium). The filtered dual-energy radiation is scanned across the entire body for differences in absorption. The greater the bone mineral, the greater the interference in the passage of radiation from the source to the scanner. The image of the skeleton obtained from DEXA and the data from the analysis are illustrated in Figure 14.8.

As is explained in the text, knowing the bone mineral content does not completely reveal the risk of bone fracture. Risk evaluation would improve if an image of the trabecular arrangement of the cancellous bone could be obtained. Human and animal postmortem analysis reveals that a decrease in bone mineral content occurs mainly from the trabeculae of cancellous bone, because these bones have the largest area exposed to osteoclastic resorption.[26]

The regional information provided by DEXA is very useful, because there is considerable variability in the mass and volume of compact and cancellous bone (and therefore in bone mineral content) between the bones of the axial and appendicular skeletons.[9,20,26,27] For example, cancellous bone contributes approximately 35% of vertebral mass, compared with the average 20% for the skeleton.[26]

FIGURE 14.7

The equipment used in dual x-ray absorptiometry (DEXA); a common procedure used to indirectly measure total body and regional bone mineral density. (Courtesy, LUNAR Corporation, Madison, Wisconsin.)

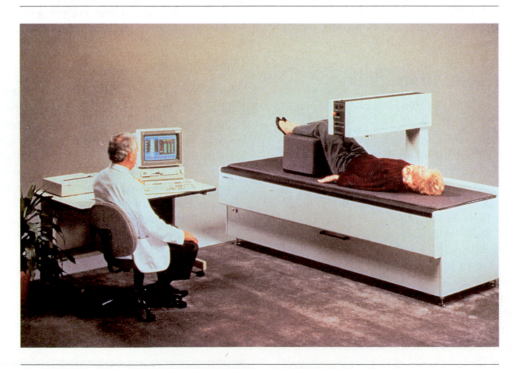

FIGURE 14.8

An image of the skeleton obtained from dual x-ray absorptiometry. The tabled data reveal values for bone mineral in different parts of the body. (Courtesy, LUNAR Corporation, Madison, Wisconsin.)

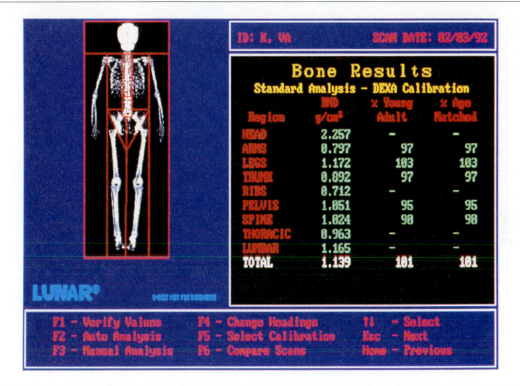

FIGURE 14.9

Representations of the relative amount of bone mineral in different populations. The zero percent reference line is based on the peak bone mineral content of an adolescent male. The specific site of the measurement is indicated.

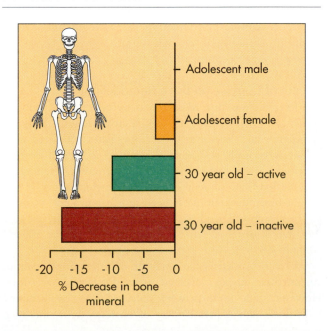

and the development of osteoporosis. Furthermore, the two main determinants in the development and severity of osteoporosis are peak bone mineral content and the rate of bone mineral loss.[23] Thus it is important to understand the factors that increase peak bone mineral content, as well as how to retard bone mineral loss.

Conditions That Influence the Age-Related Decrease in Bone Mineral Content

Besides aging, several conditions can exaggerate the loss of bone mineral content; these conditions consist of nutritional, endocrinologic, and exercise-related factors.

Effects of Nutrition on Bone Remodeling

Because bone is a storage site for calcium, and endocrine regulation of serum calcium involves modifying bone resorption and deposition, it is reasonable to hypothesize that an inadequate intake of calcium would favor increased bone resorption. However, available research data

dual x-ray absorptiometry (DEXA)
a method of measuring the mineral density of bone

do not indicate a clear role for dietary calcium in influencing bone mineral content.

First, it is important to focus on the age group most susceptible to nutrient sources of calcium. If nutritional intake of calcium is critical to bone mineral content, adolescence is the most important time during the life cycle for building bones; this is the period when the growth spurt in body mass and skeletal mineral mass occurs, when approximately 60% of the peak skeletal mineral mass is deposited.[26] Nutritional data indicate that the calcium intake of girls before pubescence is inadequate, which therefore may be limiting to skeletal mineral mass in adolescent girls.[26]

Despite media attention on calcium intake for individuals over 50 years of age, research indicates that nutritional influences on bone mineral status are minimal compared with endocrinologic influences.[22] However, since this study was done in Scandinavia, where calcium intake probably is very different from that of other countries, dietary supplementation of calcium during times of known bone mineral loss (over 30 years of age), regardless of gender, may be a safe recommendation. This is especially true given that calcium absorption by the small intestine is compromised by protein and caffeine ingestion. Thus getting enough calcium in the diet does not automatically ensure that this amount is available to the body. It is currently recommended that men and premenopausal women consume 1000 mg of calcium a day and that postmenopausal women increase this amount to 1500 mg/day.[6,26,27]

Effects of Endocrine Status on Bone Remodeling

The most important determinant of bone mineral content in women is the circulating concentration of estrogen. Consequently, any condition that reduces estrogen concentrations affects bone remodeling. The most prevalent conditions that influence estrogen concentrations in women are the normal menstrual cycle; menstrual cycle abnormalities, with complete lack of menses (*amenorrhea*) being the most influential; and *menopause*.

The changes in serum estrogen and progesterone concentrations during the menstrual cycle are large, especially during the estrogen surge portions of the follicular and luteal phases when menstrual function is normal (for a detailed description of the menstrual cycle, see Chapter 23). Drinkwater and colleagues[7] were the first to document the reduced bone mineral content (14%) in the vertebrae of amenorrheic women compared with eumenorrheic women. Subsequent research verified this finding, with relative reductions in bone mineral density reported to be as great as 25% compared with sedentary controls[6,27] (see Figure 14.9). These differences have been reported only for vertebral bone; the bone mineral content of bones from the appendicular skeleton (femoral neck, radius, trochanter) have shown no differences between eumenorrheic and amenorrheic women.

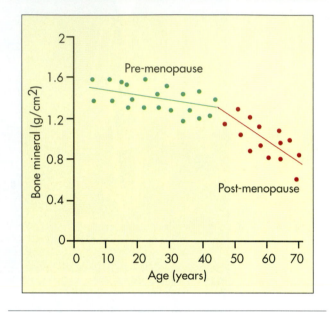

FIGURE 14.10

The relationship between lumbar spine bone mineral density and age for women who are either pre- or post-menopause (Adapted from Riggs BL et al: *J Clin Invest* 67:328-335, 1981; and Krolner B, Pors NS: *Clin Sci* 62:329-336. 1982.)

The influence of menopause on bone mineral content has revealed a negative correlation (Figure 14.10). The greatest bone mineral loss in postmenopausal women occurs during the first 5 years after menopause.[26,27] Interestingly, evidence from amenorrheic women who resume menstrual function and normal circulating estrogen indicates that the increased estrogen has the potential not only to retard bone resorption but also to slightly increase bone mineral content.[8] It remains to be proved whether estrogen supplementation in menopausal women significantly attenuates or reverses bone resorption.

Effects of Exercise on Bone Remodeling

Exercise was first reported to influence bone mineral content in a 1971 study that used a cross-sectional design.[16] Bone mineral density was higher in athletes compared with sedentary controls, and athletes involved in weight-bearing activities had the highest bone mineral content. The finding of increased bone mineral density in individuals involved in weight-bearing activities has been shown repeatedly in similar cross-sectional studies. Furthermore, it is believed that the amount of muscle mass is proportional to bone mineral content.[23]

Exercise can effect the retention of bone mineral even in amenorrheic athletes involved in weight-bearing activities. However, these findings were obtained using well-trained individuals, and a prescription of exercise (type, intensity, duration) adequate to retain bone mineral cannot be given at this time. Nevertheless, it is safe to say that exercise involving weight-bearing is more likely to retain more bone mineral than non-weight-bearing exercise.

For individuals between 40 and 60 years of age, long-term involvement in exercise (for decades) has been shown to be associated with greater bone mineral density (decreased resorption) compared to sedentary controls. It is unclear how exercise affects bone mineral content in more elderly individuals.

SUMMARY

- The human skeleton can be divided into the **axial skeleton** and the **appendicular skeleton.** The axial skeleton consists of the skull, vertebral column, and thorax (rib cage). The appendicular skeleton consists of the shoulder girdles and arms and the pelvic girdle and legs.

- Within bone there are two types of bone tissue **(osseous tissue): compact bone** or **cancellous bone** (also called spongy or trabecular bone). Compact bone accounts for 80% of the skeletal mass and usually is localized to the outer layers of a bone. Cancellous bone forms in the inner regions of bone. Cancellous bone contributes 70% of the skeletal bone volume, and because of its trabecular arrangement, provides the microstructure that gives bone strength for a relatively low-mass tissue.

- Histologic stained cross-section specimens of bone reveal circular **haversian systems,** with a central vascular system **(haversian canal).** The **osteocytes** arrange themselves in small channels *(canaliculi),* which are positioned as successive circles around the haversian canal. Between each two canaliculi is a matrix of bone mineral, and the circles formed by the bone mineral and canaliculi are called *lamellae.*

- Cancellous bone is less structurally organized and less dense than compact bone. Cancellous bone is made up of separate threads of bone connected to each other in a three-dimensional array, much like the honeycomb of a bee hive.

- The bone matrix consists of (1) three types of cells: *osteoblasts, osteocytes,* and *osteoclasts,* which contribute one third of the matrix; (2) organic elements, such as glycoproteins and collagen; and (3) inorganic mineral salts, which make up 65% of the bone matrix. Most of the strength and hardiness in bone is due to the inorganic mineral salts, which are collectively called **hydroxyapatites.** The main minerals are calcium salts and phosphates. The bone matrix is surprisingly strong, able to withstand more than 25,000 psi of compression.

- The skeleton provides support, protection, and leverage for movement and the application of force; storage of fat and minerals; and production of blood cells **(hematopoiesis).** Bone marrow is found in the shafts of the long bones and in the inner cavity of certain flat and irregular bones such as the sternum or ilium. Yellow marrow is composed primarily of fat, whereas red marrow is involved in hematopoiesis.

- Bone formation is called osteogenesis, or **ossification.** During the development of the human skeleton, ossification can be categorized into two types: formation of the skeleton and bone growth, and bone remodeling. During growth from infancy, the skeleton is formed by the ossification of cartilage. Ossification begins in the middle of the shaft of a long bone and extends to each end, or **epiphysis,** where growth plates **(epiphyseal plates)** are located.

- **Bone remodeling,** which occurs throughout life, involves the continual breakdown, repair, and replacement of osteocytes and bone mineral. Bone deposition occurs at the site of injury or stress. Bone reabsorption occurs when bones are unstressed or when there is an imbalance in the regulatory processes of bone mineral content.

- The balance of bone mineral depends on the activity of basic multicellular units (BMUs), which contain the osteoclasts and osteoblasts. Bone resorption occurs when catalytic enzymes are secreted by the osteoclasts. Osteoclasts also have a phagocytic action. The mineral salts released during resorption diffuse into the interstitial fluid, from which they are removed by the circulation, altering blood calcium concentrations.

SUMMARY—Cont'd

■ Bone remodeling occurs by means of a multiple-hormone regulation system and in response to physical stress. When blood calcium decreases, the parathyroid gland releases parathyroid hormone (PTH), which increases the activity of the osteoclasts, thereby increasing bone reabsorption. Conversely, when blood calcium concentrations are above normal, calcitonin is released from the thyroid gland, inhibiting osteoclast activity and thus favoring osteoblast activity and bone deposition.

■ An additional hormone regulator of bone remodeling is estrogen. Estrogen reduces the sensitivity of the BMUs to PTH, thereby reducing osteoclast activity and bone resorption. Testosterone serves the same function in men.

■ Physical stress on bone also stimulates increased bone deposition. The physical stress can be due to exercise, which can apply compressive and tensile (twisting) stress. In addition, simply overcoming the forces of gravity on the musculoskeletal system, or resisting impact, can stimulate bone deposition.

■ Bone mineral content increases during adolescence and reaches a peak shortly after puberty. It is unclear whether the earlier onset of pubescence in girls is associated with an earlier peak bone mineral content, which would also indicate an earlier onset of age-related bone mineral loss. Age-related loss in bone mineral content occurs first in cancellous bone, which begins to decline before the third decade of life. Compact bone is retained for another decade before increased resorption ensues.

■ The decline in the mineral content of trabecular bone is greater for women than men and greater again for postmenopausal women. After menopause the rate of trabecular bone mineral loss in women can increase to 7% a year, with greatest loss in the first 5 years. This rate of loss is large compared to the average loss before menopause of less than 1% a year.

■ The clinical condition of **osteoporosis,** which does not have a precise definition, is a general state of the bones or skeleton in which bone mineral and the trabecular microarchitecture have deteriorated to such an extent that the risk for bone fractures is increased even during normal, everyday activities. A common method of evaluating bone mineral density is **dual x-ray absorptiometry (DEXA).**

■ Besides aging, several conditions can exaggerate the loss of bone mineral content, and these conditions involve nutritional, endocrinologic, and exercise-related factors. Available research data do not indicate a clear role for dietary calcium in influencing bone mineral content in adults; however, inadequate calcium intake in girls before pubescence may be limiting to skeletal mineral mass in adolescent girls.

■ The most important determinant of bone mineral content in women is the circulating concentration of estrogen. Consequently, any condition that reduces estrogen concentrations influences bone remodeling. The most prevalent conditions that influence estrogen concentrations in women are the normal menstrual cycle; menstrual cycle abnormalities, with complete lack of menses (amenorrhea) being most influential; and menopause.

■ Bone mineral content in the vertebrae of amenorrheic compared to eumenorrheic women can be as low as 25% less. Bone mineral content of bones from the appendicular skeleton (femoral neck, radius, trochanter) have shown no differences between eumenorrheic and amenorrheic women.

■ The influence of menopause on bone mineral content has revealed a negative correlation. The greatest bone mineral loss in women occurs during the first 5 years after menopause. It remains to be proved whether estrogen supplementation in menopausal women significantly attenuates or reverses bone resorption.

■ Bone mineral density is higher in athletes compared to sedentary controls, and athletes involved in weight-bearing activities have the highest bone mineral content. Exercise can effect the retention of bone mineral even in amenorrheic athletes involved in weight-bearing activities. However, these findings were obtained using well-trained individuals, and a prescription of exercise (type, intensity, duration) adequate for retaining bone mineral cannot be given at this time. Nevertheless, it is safe to say that exercise involving weight-bearing is more likely to retain more bone mineral than non–weight-bearing exercise.

■ For individuals between 40 and 60 years of age, long-term involvement in exercise (for decades) has been shown to be associated with greater bone mineral density (decreased resorption) compared to sedentary controls. It is unclear how exercise affects bone mineral content in more elderly individuals.

REVIEW QUESTIONS

1. What are the two divisions of the skeleton, what are the four types of bone, and what are the differences between the two types of bone matrix?

2. Explain the differences between the microanatomy of compact bone and that of cancellous bone. How do these differences influence the multiple functions of bone?

3. Explain the growth process of bone.

4. Explain the term *bone remodeling*.

5. What factors can detrimentally influence bone mineral content? Explain these influences.

6. What factors can positively influence bone mineral content? Explain these influences.

7. According to research studies, what type of exercise would be most likely to best promote retention of bone mineral throughout the aging process?

APPLICATIONS

1. Is peak bone mineral content an important variable in the development of osteoporosis? Why or why not?

2. Given that it may take up to 1 year before changes in bone mineral density can be detected by current methods, how might this detract from good quality research and the application of the results?

3. It is generally accepted that weight training offers the greatest resistance to muscle contraction, thereby exposing bone-tendinous junctions and the bone matrix to the greatest stimulus for retaining or even increasing bone mineral. Do we really know enough to recommend weight-lifting exercise as the best exercise for stimulating bone mineral content? What research has to be done before we can correctly recommend specific types of exercise?

4. Why is it important to promote exercise and adequate nutrition during adolescence for the purpose of optimizing bone mineral content, when decreases in bone mineral may not be detected until after 30 to 40 years of age?

REFERENCES

1. Blocker JE, Genant HK, Black D: Greater vertebral bone mineral mass in exercising young men, *West J Med* 145:39-42, 1986.

2. Block JE, Friedlander AL, Brooks GA et al: Determinants of bone density among athletes engaged in weight-bearing and non-weight-bearing activity, *J Appl Physiol* 67(3):1100-1105, 1989.

3. Buchanan JR, Myers C, Lloyd T et al: Determinants of trabecular bone density in women: the role of androgens, estrogen, and exercise, *J Bone Miner Res* 3:673:680, 1988.

4. Conroy BP, Kraemer WJ, Merish CM et al: Bone mineral density in elite junior Olympic weightlifters, *Med Sci Sports Exerc* 25(10):1103-1109, 1993.

5. Dalsky GP, Stocke KS, Ehsani AA: Weight-bearing exercise training and lumbar bone mineral content in postmenopausal women, *Ann Intern Med* 108:824-828, 1988.

6. Dalsky GP: Effect of exercise on bone: permissive influence of estrogen and calcium, *Med Sci Sports Exerc* 22(3):281-285, 1990.

7. Drinkwater BL, Nilson K, Chesnut CH, III et al: Bone mineral content of amenorrheic and eumenorrheic athletes, *N Eng J Med* 311(5):277-281, 1984.

8. Drinkwater BL, Nilson K, Ott S, Chesnut CH III: Bone mineral density after resumption of menses in amenorrheic athletes, *JAMA* 256:380-382, 1986.

9. Geusens P, Dequeker J, Verstraeten A, Nijs J: Age-, sex-, and menopause-related changes of vertebral and peripheral bone: population study using dual- and single-photon absorptiometry and radiogrammetry, *J Nucl Med* 27:1540-1549, 1986.

10. Grove KA, Londeree BR: Bone density in postmenopausal women: high-impact versus low-impact exercise, *Med Sci Sports Exerc* 24(11):1190-1194, 1992.

11. Guyton AC: *Textbook of medical physiology,* ed 8, Philadelphia, 1991, WB Saunders.

12. Heinrich CH, Going SB, Pamenter RW et al: Bone mineral content of cyclically menstruating female resistance- and endurance-trained athletes, *Med Sci Sports Exerc* 22(5):558-563, 1990.

13. Marcus R: The relationship of dietary calcium to the maintenance of skeletal integrity in man: an interface of endocrinology and nutrition, *Metabolism* 31(1):93-101, 1982.

14. Marieb EN: *Human anatomy and physiology,* ed 3, Redwood City, Calif, 1995, Benjamin Cummings.

15. Mosekilde L: Age-related changes in vertebral trabecular bone architecture: assessed by a new method, *Bone* 9:247-250, 1988.

16. Nilsson BE, Westline NE: Bone density in athletes, *Clin Orthop* 77:179-182, 1971.

17. Orwoll ES, Ferar J, Oviatt SK et al: The relationship of swimming exercise to bone mass in men and women, *Arch Intern Med* 149:2197-2200, 1989.

18. Parfitt AM: Bone remodeling and bone loss: understanding the pathophysiology of osteoporosis, *Calcif Tissue Int* 36:S37-S45, 1984.

19. Raisz LG, Smith J: Pathogenesis, prevention, and treatment of osteoporosis, *Ann Rev Med* 40:251-267, 1989.

20. Riggs BL, Wahner HW, Dann WL et al: Differential changes in bone mineral density of the appendicular and axial skeleton with aging, *J Clin Invest* 67:328-335, 1981.

21. Riggs BL, Wahner HW, Melton LJ III et al: Rates of bone loss in the appendicular and axial skeletons of women, *J Clin Invest* 77:1487-1491, 1986.

22. Rus B, Thomsen K, Christiansen C: Does calcium supplementation prevent postmenopausal bone loss? a double-blind controlled clinical study, *N Eng J Med* 316:173-177, 1987.

23. Sanborn CF: Exercise, calcium, and bone density, *Gatorade Sports Science Exchange* 2(24):1-5, 1990.

24. Seldin DW, Esser PD, Alderson PO: Comparison of bone density measurements from different skeletal sites, *J Nuc Med* 29:168-173, 1988.

25. Snead DB, Weltman A, Weltman JY et al: Reproductive hormones and bone mineral density in women runners, *J Appl Physiol* 72(6):2149-2156, 1992.

26. Snow-Harter C, Marcus R: Exercise, bone mineral density, and osteoporosis, *Exerc Sport Sci Rev* 19:351-388, 1991.

27. Suominen H: Bone mineral density and long-term exercise, *Sports Med* 16(5):316-330, 1993.

28. Suominen H, Rahkila P: Bone mineral density of the calcaneus in 70- to 80-year old male athletes and a population sample, *Med Sci Sports Exerc* 23(11):1227-1233, 1991.

RECOMMENDED READINGS

■ Block JE, Friedlander AL, Brooks GA et al: Determinants of bone density among athletes in weight-bearing and non-weight-bearing activity, *J Appl Physiol* 67(3):1100-1105, 1989.

■ Buchanan JR, Myers C, Lloyd T et al: Determinants of trabecular bone density in women: the role of androgens, estrogen, and exercise, *J Bone Miner Res* 3:673-680, 1988.

■ Dalsky GP: Effect of exercise on bone: permissive influence of estrogen and calcium, *Med Sci Sports Exerc* 22(3):281-285, 1990.

■ Snead DB, Weltman A, Weltman JY et al: Reproductive hormones and bone mineral density in women runners, *J Appl Physiol* 72(6):2149-2156, 1992.

■ Snow-Harter C, Marcus R: Exercise, bone mineral density, and osteoporosis, *Exerc Sport Sci Rev* 19:351-388, 1991.

■ Suominen H: Bone mineral density and long-term exercise, *Sports Med* 16(5):316-330, 1993.

CHAPTER 15

Immune Function Adaptations to Exercise

OBJECTIVES

After studying this chapter you should be able to:

- Identify the main cellular components of the immune system.

- Compare the functions and interrelationships of phagocytes and lymphocytes.

- Explain the differences between nonspecific and specific immune protection.

- Explain the change in circulating leukocytes during and after exercise of different intensities and durations.

- Defend your opinion about whether exercise depresses or enhances immune protection and whether this is an acute or a chronic effect.

KEY TERMS

lymphatic system

lymph

lymph nodes

phagocytes

natural killer cells
  (NK cells)

lymphocytes

pathogen

complement proteins

interferon

antigen

humoral immune response

cell-mediated immune
  response

antibodies

immunoglobulins

leukocytosis

he influence of exercise on the body's immune system is not a new topic. Some of the earliest research into the effect of exercise on white blood cell (WBC) populations dates back to the early 1900s.[13] However, it was not until the 1970s and 1980s that advances in understanding and measurement of the components of the immune system improved our ability to measure changes in immune function. Today some textbooks are dedicated solely to the topic of exercise and immune function, and the continued research interest warrants a summary of exercise and immune function in an exercise physiology textbook. This chapter presents a concise explanation of immune function and documents the research findings on how exercise can acutely and chronically alter susceptibility to infection.

Immune System

The body's ability to resist infection is a culmination of the functions of the cardiovascular and lymphatic systems and of cellular immune mechanisms. In this chapter the roles of the lymph, lymph vessels, and lymph nodes are presented first. Then, based on this information, a concise review of cellular immune mechanisms follows. Finally, the chapter details how exercise intervenes in the operation of these components.

Lymphatic System

Chapter 11 described the functioning of the cardiovascular system. Although it is tempting to view fluid distribution in the body as a process involving the cells, interstitial spaces, and cardiovascular system, there is also a structurally and functionally organized vascular network within the interstitial spaces. This vascular network is called the **lymphatic system,** and it operates in concert with the cardiovascular system to distribute fluid throughout the body. The lymphatic system contains not only small vessels but also specialized tissues, called *lymphatic tissues,* that are profusely distributed throughout the body. It is the lymph tissue that gives the lymphatic system its important connection to the body's

lymphatic system
the combined fluid, cells, tissues, and organs that form the vascular system external to the systemic circulation; the lymphatic system is responsible for fluid distribution in the body, as well as the body's immune capabilities

FIGURE 15.1

The lymphatic system of the body. The diffuse location of lymph nodes are shown, as well as the location of larger lymph organs such as the tonsils, spleen, and thymus. (From Thibodeau GA, Patton KT: *Anatomy and physiology*, 3 ed, St. Louis, 1996, Mosby. Art by Barbara Cousins.)

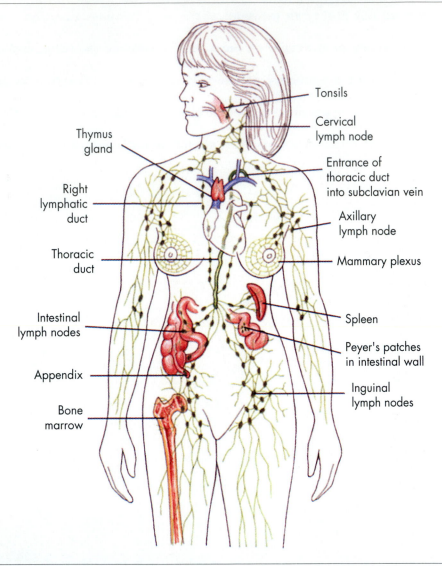

immune system. However, another important function of the lymph vessels is to provide the body with an extensive network of low-pressure vessels that can distribute molecules and specialized cells throughout the interstitial spaces, where there is greater proximity to cells. This feature, too, is important to the body's immune response to infection.

Figure 15.1 presents an illustration of the body's lymphatic system. Once interstitial fluid drains into the capillaries of the lymphatic system, it is called **lymph.** Lymph circulates toward the heart, where it is filtered through specialized structures called **lymph nodes.** Because a type of white blood cell, the *lymphocyte,* also is present in lymph nodes, these nodes have an immune function, as is detailed later. The spleen, thymus, and tonsils are all examples of enlarged lymph

nodes; typical lymph nodes are much smaller and located diffusely throughout the body.

The flow of lymph to the heart is problematic because, as was discussed in Chapter 11, pressures are very low in the capillary beds of the systemic circulation. Thus lymph vessels have one-way valves and rely on posture and the muscle

lymph (limf)
the fluid of the lymphatic system

lymph nodes
aggregations of lymph tissue that form and store lymphocytes

TABLE 15.1

Main blood cells and proteins involved in immune responses*

COMPONENT	SOURCE	FUNCTION
CELLS		
Phagocytes		
Granulocytes	Bone marrow	To ingest foreign particles *(phagocytosis)*
Monocytes	Bone marrow	Phagocytosis
Macrophages	Monocytes	Phagocytosis; also, to secrete interleukin-2 (IL-2)
Eosinophils	Bone marrow	Weak phagocytosis, detoxification
Neutrophils	Bone marrow	Phagocytosis
Basophils	Bone marrow	To secrete heparin and histamine and to stimulate additional allergic/infectious responses
Natural killer (NK) cells		
	Blood, lymph	To destroy infected cells
Lymphocytes		
T cells	Lymph tissue (cells then modified by the thymus gland)	Cell-mediated immunity
Helper T cells	Lymph tissue (cells then modified by the thymus gland)	To secrete interleukin-1 (IL-1) and γ-interferon
Cytotoxic T cells (killer cells)	Lymph tissue (cells then modified by the thymus gland)	To rupture and destroy foreign and virus-infected cells
Supressor T cells	Lymph tissue (cells then modified by the thymus gland)	To decrease function of other T cells
Memory T cells	T cells	Stored T cells for specific antibodies
B cells	Lymph tissue	Antigen-specific immunity
Plasma cells	B cells	To produce and secrete antibodies
Memory B cells	B cells	Stored B cells for specific antibodies
PROTEINS		
Antibodies (Immunoglobulins-Ig†)	Plasma cells	To inactivate antigens and stimulate complement proteins
Complement (Inactive enzymes)	Blood	To stimulate phagocytes and basophils, rupture bacteria, and increase inflammation
Lymphokines		
Interleukins	T-helper cells, macrophages	To stimulate growth and proliferation of cytotoxic and suppressor T cells, as well as B cells
γ-interferon	T-helper cells	To stimulate growth and proliferation of cytotoxic and suppressor T cells, as well as B cells, and to protect uninfected cells

*Data modified from 12, 13, and 20.
†The five classes of immunoglobulins are abbreviated IgM, IgG, IgA, IgD, and IgE.

pump to propel lymph against gravity to the heart. The lymph enters the systemic circulation in the left and right subclavian veins.

Cellular Components of the Immune System

The cells of the immune system can be classified as **phagocytes, natural killer cells (NK cells),** and **lymphocytes** (see Chapter 11 and Table 15.1). Of the numerous types of phagocytes, *macrophages* play the largest role in removing debris and foreign material. Phagocytes and NK cells are important in the body's immediate immune protection and therefore provide a nonspecific protection against infection. Lymphocytes can be subdivided into B lymphocytes *(B cells)* and T lymphocytes *(T cells)*. The B cells and T cells are involved in the body's response to specific infections.

Immune Function

"Immune function" refers to the body's defenses against a foreign material **(pathogen)** in the body.[21] The functioning of the body's immune system is very complex, as shown by the cellular components listed in Table 15.1. The body has essentially two main ways to fight infection: first through a nonspecific response, which involves the phagocytes and NK cells; and second, through a specific response, which involves the B cells and T cells.

Nonspecific Immune Protection

The nonspecific immune response is analogous to a first line of defense. When the body's external protective coat, the skin, is broken, internal body tissues are injured (see Focus Box 15.1) or, when bacterial or viral infection occurs, an inflammatory response develops, which initially is caused by local release of molecules from the damaged tissue. These events result in increased localized blood flow and migration of phagocytes to the damaged tissue. The phagocytes are assisted by several proteins. **Complement proteins** become activated during inflammation and assist in the rupturing of bacterial walls. **Interferon** is released by infected cells and acts to stimulate other cells to improve their resilience to viral infection.

Specific Immune Protection

The previously described response to infection differs from the B-cell and T-cell response in three important ways: (1) the phagocyte, complement, and interferon responses are not specific to a given pathogen; (2) no "memory" of the response to a specific pathogen results; and (3) the inflammation is localized to the region of initial infection of damage. Unlike the nonspecific response systems, B–cell and T–cell functions interact to induce a specific, memorized, and systemic response to infection.

The body's ability to mount a specialized immune response is based on specific proteins that exist on the membranes of host cells, as well as pathogens. One's own body cells are labeled with a special class of proteins recognized by the immune system as "safe"; these proteins are called *major histocompatibility (MHC) proteins*. Because MHC proteins are different in each individual except for identical twins, they induce an immune response triggered by tissue donation between individuals. This immune response occurs because the recipient's immune system does not recognize the MHC protein as safe, but rather interprets it to be a foreign protein **(antigen).** The B cells and T cells launch a specific response when they recognize the antigen of a given pathogen. Recognition of an antigen stimulates either a **humoral immune response** or a **cell-mediated immune response.**

Humoral Immune Response

If an antigen and a B cell can bind, an activation response occurs in the B cell that results in the rapid growth and multiplication of the B cell, causing the formation of identical B cells receptive to that antigen. These cells then circulate in the blood and lymph and develop the ability to synthesize and

---

phagocytes (fag'o-sites)
a type of leukocyte that engulfs foreign or damaged substances in the body

natural killer cells (NK cells)
leukocytes that assist in the destruction of foreign substances in the body

lymphocytes (lim'fo-sites)
a class of leukocytes formed in the lymphoid tissue; subdivided into B cells and T cells

pathogen (path'o-jen)
a foreign substance in the body

complement proteins
proteins in the blood and other body fluids that become activated during an immune response and assist in the destruction of a pathogen

interferon (in-ter-fer'on)
a glycoprotein released by infected cells that acts to increase the resistance to infection of "healthy" cells

antigen (an'ti-jen)
a substance that induces an immune response

humoral immune response
the defensive response triggered by the presence of free pathogens in the blood or interstitial spaces of the body

cell-mediated immune response
the defensive response triggered by activation of phagocytes and lymphocytes and specifically directed toward infected cells

FOCUS BOX 15.1

Exercise-induced muscle damage: an example of localized inflammation and immune response

When exercise is performed that involves eccentric muscle contractions, especially when a person is unaccustomed to the activity's duration or intensity, microscopic muscle damage occurs. This damage is associated with elevated serum creatine kinase activity, swelling, soreness, and restricted range of motion during the ensuing 48 hours.[2-4,11] Originally this condition was called delayed-onset muscle soreness (DOMS); however, research conducted since the early 1980s has indicated that the muscle damage that accompanies DOMS can be quite severe; that it induces an immune response; and that the biochemical events that coincide with this response probably induce the inflammation and soreness. In short, delayed-onset muscle soreness is a nondescript name for the condition, and the term *exercise-induced muscle damage* is becoming more accepted.

Figure 15.2 presents electron micrographs of damaged skeletal muscle. The disruption of the Z lines, called Z-line streaming,

probably results from damage to the nebulin and titin protein stabilization of the actin and myosin molecules of the Z line proteins. After approximately 12 hours, macrophages and lymphocytes infiltrate the damaged muscle region, resulting in the destruction of the damaged region of muscle. It has been theorized that chemicals released through the immune response induce the symptoms of swelling and pain. The influence of WBC presence on muscle glycogen synthesis and carbohydrate nutrition is discussed in Chapter 17.

Clarkson and Tremblay[3] have documented that recovery from even a single bout of exposure to eccentric muscle contractions protects the muscle from the same damage during a second bout of eccentric muscle contractions. This rapid adaptability to eccentric contractions is remarkable; however, the cellular events and changes that affect this tolerance are unknown.

FIGURE 15.2

Electron micrographs of damaged skeletal muscle resulting from excessive eccentric exercise. **A,** Z line streaming. **B,** The infiltration of macrophages and lymphocytes into the damaged region. (A, From Hikida RS et al: Muscle fiber necrosis associated with human marathon runners, *J Neuro Sci* 59:185-203, 1983.)

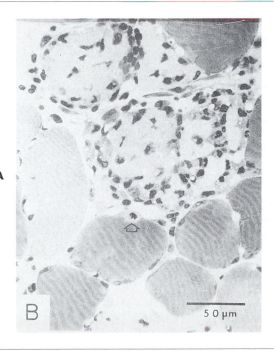

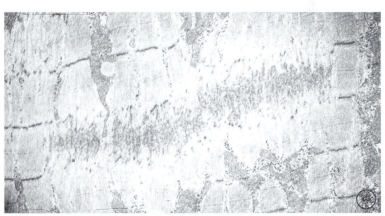

secrete proteins that can bind to the pathogen (**antibodies**). These developed B cells are called *plasma cells*. The interval from infection to peak circulating levels of antibodies may be as long as 10 days.[12] Many of the plasma cells remain stored in the lymph tissue and are released when exposed to their antibody, thereby providing a type of "memory" to the immune response.

Antibodies, which are also called **immunoglobulins** (Ig), can be grouped into five classes—IgD, IgM, IgG, IgA, and IgE—which differ according to structural size and complexity and functions. Of the immunoglobulins, IgG is the most abundant and functional in protecting the body against bacteria, viruses, and toxins. Interestingly, IgE is involved in histamine release in the lung airways during allergic reactions and asthma (see Chapter 12). The diversity of the antibodies within each class is due to the continual rearrangement of the genes of the B cells. Thus B-cell membrane proteins have a natural genetic diversity, which is extended into a diversity of plasma cell proteins and the antibodies they manufacture.

When the antibody binds to the pathogen, complement proteins attach to the antigen. This binding causes further stimulation of B cells and promotes the destruction of the antigen through phagocytosis.

Cell-Mediated Immune Response

The body's T cells are involved in *cell-mediated immunity* (Figure 15.3). However, unlike the B cells and phagocytes, which prey on the antibodies of exposed pathogens, the T cells target the exposed antigens of infectious organisms that penetrate cells to reproduce and interfere with cell functioning.

T cells are divided into three functional classes: helper T cells, cytotoxic T cells, and suppressor T cells. Helper T cells are activated by binding to antigen fragments associated with class I MHC proteins, as well as to B cells attached to antigens. After binding, the T-helper cells release proteins *(lymphokines)* (e.g., interleukin-2 [IL-2]), which mobilize phagocytes and stimulate their release of interleukin-1 (IL-1). IL-1 stimulates the activity of the bound T cells, thereby increasing the release of IL-2 and creating a positive feedback loop that amplifies the immune response.

Cytotoxic T cells, or killer T cells, are activated by binding to antigen fragments associated with class I MHC proteins. This association occurs when the pathogen (e.g., virus) enters a host cell. When bound to the infected cell, the cytotoxic T cell impregnates the target cell with a chemical that results in cell lysis. This process is enhanced by stimulation from lymphokines (e.g., IL-1).

Because the body's cell-mediated immune response is based on positive feedback, something must "turn off" the process. This is the function of the T-suppressor cells. As yet it is unclear what guides these cells to down-regulate the T-cell immune response, or how this down-regulation is made to coincide with complete destruction of the pathogens.

FIGURE 15.3

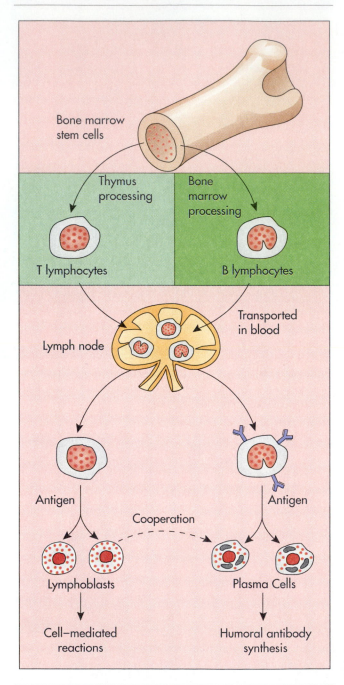

The cellular events of cell-mediated immunity. (From Atlas R: *Principles of microbiology*, St. Louis, 1995, Mosby.)

Exercise and Changes in the Immune System

The concentration and regulation of circulating macrophages and lymphocytes are known to change during exercise, during the immediate recovery period after an exercise bout, and chronically in response to exercise training. The research into altered immune conditions and functioning is presented based on acute and chronic exercise conditions.

Acute Effects of Exercise on the Immune System

The increase in circulating leukocytes (phagocytes and lymphocytes) that occurs in response to moderate to intense exercise has been well established.[13] This increase is greater for more prolonged exercise and returns to normal resting values within the first 2 hours of recovery.[8,13] Figure 15.4, *A*, illustrates the changes in circulating leukocytes in response to varied exercise intensities. Exercise that lasts less than 1 hour reveals a linear increase in leukocyte counts with increases in intensity. For exercise bouts that last longer than 2 hours, leukocyte counts increase gradually and reach peak values similar to those for more intense exercise.[1,5,13,20,21]

The fact that exercise-induced **leukocytosis** is related separately to both the intensity and the duration of exercise indicates a possible connection to the hormonal response to exercise. In fact, this connection has been documented,[1,13,22] with increased circulating catecholamines being responsible for the relationship between leukocyte counts and exercise intensity. The sites of action of the catecholamines are believed to be a combination of systemic effects plus direct sympathetic innervation of the spleen and pulmonary and systemic blood vessels.[13] The increase in cortisol release during prolonged exercise is believed to cause the rapid increase in leukocytes after 2 hours, attributable to an increased release of leukocytes from bone marrow[13] (Figure 15.5).

Obviously, simply measuring total leukocyte concentrations is a poor reflection of the specific functions of the phagocytes, NK cells, B cells, and T cells. Also, an increase in either the phagocyte or lymphocyte category may not necessarily reflect an alteration of immune function.

Research that has specifically measured phagocyte and lymphocyte classes has shown that prolonged exercise that increases serum cortisol primarily increases eosinophils.[7] Furthermore, individuals who are more cardiorespiratory endurance trained (higher VO$_2$max) have a larger increase in neutrophils during a given exercise intensity, whereas less-trained individuals have a greater increase in lymphocytes.[5]

Research into changes in lymphocyte classes during exercise have produced varied results, and no clear pattern has emerged relative to training status, exercise intensity, or exer-

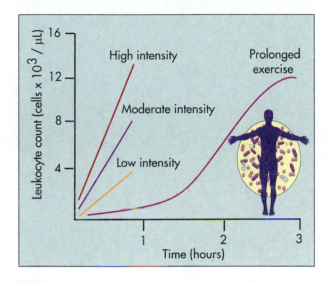

FIGURE 15.4

During exercise, the increase in leukocytes in blood is somewhat proportional to exercise intensity and duration. For duration less than 1 hour, greatest increases occur for higher exercise intensities. For prolonged exercise in excess of 2 hours, leukocyte concentrations increase dramatically, even though exercise intensity is relatively low. (Adapted from McCarthy DA, Dale MM: The leucocytosis of exercise, *Sports Med* 6:333-363, 1988.)

cise duration. Nevertheless, in vitro activity of NK cells increases with acute exercise,[6] and evidence of a decreased responsiveness of B cells and T cells to pathogens has been seen in vitro.[10]

Surprisingly, the in vitro activities of macrophages and lymphocytes have not revealed the enhanced immune function theorized from the large increases in circulating leukocyte concentrations. It is unclear whether the limited activities reflect methodologic limitations or in vivo function.

antibodies (an'ti-bod'is)
immune proteins that bind to an antigen to evoke an immune response

immunoglobulins (im'un-o-glob'u-lins)
antibodies, abbreviated Ig: the five classes are IgD, IgM, IgG, IgA, and IgE

leukocytosis (lu'ko-si-to-sis)
an increase in the blood's leukocyte concentration

FIGURE 15.5

A schematic illustrating the involvement of catecholamine hormones and cortisol in the exercise-induced luekocytosis. (Adapted from references 13, 20, and 21.)

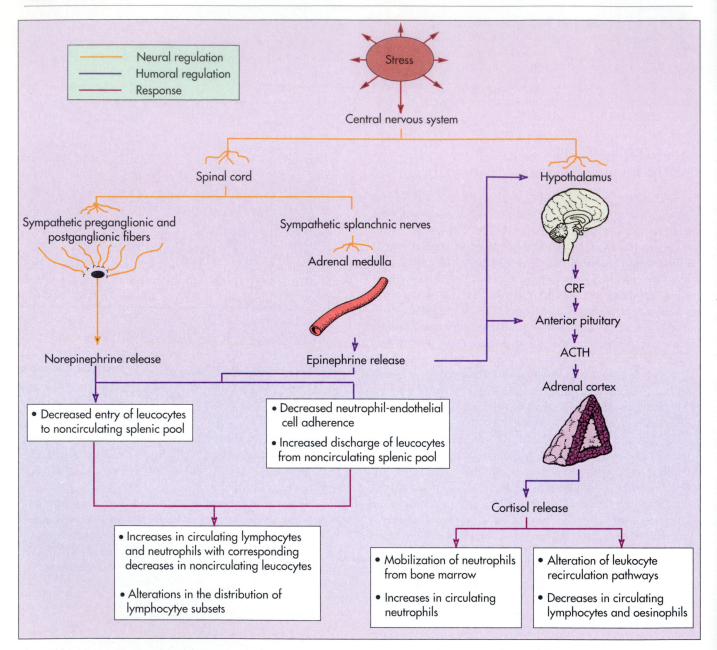

Chronic Effects of Exercise on the Immune System

Unlike what might be a positive response of the immune systems to acute exercise, long-term exposure to exercise actually causes a suppression of immune function. Studies generally have been consistent in finding lower total leukocyte counts, lymphocyte counts, and immunoglobulins in well-trained athletes at rest and during exercise.[20] Longitudinal training studies have provided inconsistent findings com-

pared to the previous cross-sectional data, probably because of the poorly controlled influence of the previous bout of training on immune function.

Well-trained athletes often report a higher incidence of upper respiratory infections than their more sedentary counterparts. This has been explained as being a result of a mechanism that suppresses immune response[17,20]; however, no experimental evidence of such a mechanism exists.

SUMMARY

■ A structurally and functionally organized vascular network exists within the interstitial spaces. This vascular network is called the **lymphatic system,** and it operates in concert with the cardiovascular system to distribute fluid throughout the body. The lymphatic system contains small vessels and specialized tissues and organs *(lymphatic tissues)* that are profusely distributed throughout the body.

■ Once interstitial fluid drains into the capillaries of the lymphatic system, it is called **lymph.** Lymph circulates toward the heart, where it is filtered through specialized structures called **lymph nodes.** The spleen, thymus, and tonsils are all examples of enlarged lymph nodes; typical lymph nodes are much smaller and are located diffusely throughout the body.

■ The cells of the immune system can be classified as **phagocytes, natural killer cells (NK cells),** and **lymphocytes.** Of the numerous types of phagocytes, *macrophages* play the largest role in removing debris and foreign material. Phagocytes and NK cells are important in the body's immediate immune protection and therefore provide a nonspecific protection against infection. Lymphocytes can be subdivided into B lymphocytes *(B cells)* and T lymphocytes *(T cells).* The B cells and T cells are involved in the body's response to specific infections.

■ "Immune function" refers to the body's defenses against a foreign material (pathogen) in the body. The body has essentially two main ways to fight infection: first, through a nonspecific response, which involves the phagocytes and NK cells; and second, through a specific response, which involves the B cells and T cells.

■ The nonspecific immune response is analogous to a first line of defense. When the body's external protective coat, the skin, is broken or an internal injury occurs, an inflammatory response develops, which initially is caused by local release of molecules from the damaged tissue. These events result in increased localized blood flow and migration of phagocytes to the damaged tissue. The phagocytes are assisted by several proteins. **Complement proteins** become activated during inflammation and assist in the rupturing of bacterial walls. **Interferon** is released by infected cells and acts to stimulate other cells to improve their resilience to viral infection.

■ One's own body cells are labeled with a special class of proteins recognized by the immune system as "safe"; these proteins are called *major histocompatibility (MHC) proteins.* MHC proteins are different in each individual except for identical twins. A foreign protein in the body is called an **antigen.** The B cells and T cells launch a specific response when they recognize the antigen of a given pathogen. Recognition of an antigen stimulates either a **humoral immune response** or a **cell-mediated immune response.**

■ When B cells are exposed to an antigen, they circulate in the blood and lymph and develop the ability to synthesize and secrete proteins **(antibodies)** that can bind to the pathogen. These developed B cells are called *plasma cells.* Antibodies, which are also called **immunoglobulins** (Ig), can be grouped into five classes—IgD, IgM, IgG, IgA, and IgE—which differ according to structural size and complexity and functions.

■ The body's T cells are involved in *cell-mediated immunity.* However, unlike the B cells and phagocytes, which prey on the antibodies of exposed pathogens, the T cells target the exposed antigens of infectious organisms that penetrate cells to reproduce and interfere with cell function.

■ The increase in circulating leukocytes (phagocytes and lymphocytes) that occurs in response to moderate to intense exercise has been well established. This increase is greater for more prolonged exercise and returns to normal resting values within the first 2 hours of recovery. Exercise that lasts less than 1 hour causes a linear increase in leukocyte counts with increases in intensity. For exercise bouts that last longer than 2 hours, leukocyte counts increase gradually and reach peak values similar to those for more intense exercise.

SUMMARY—Cont'd

- The **leukocytosis** of exercise is caused by an increase in circulating catecholamines. The sites of action of the catecholamines are believed to be a combination of systemic effects plus direct sympathetic innervation of the spleen and pulmonary and systemic blood vessels. The increase in cortisol release during prolonged exercise is believed to cause the rapid increase in leukocytes after 2 hours, attributable to an increased release of leukocytes from bone marrow.

- In vitro activity of NK cells increases with acute exercise, and evidence of a decreased responsiveness of B cells and T cells to pathogens in vitro has been noted. Surprisingly, in vitro activities of macrophages and lymphocytes have not revealed the enhanced immune functioning theorized from the large increases in circulating leukocyte concentrations.

- Long-term exposure to exercise may cause suppression of immune function. Studies have consistently found lower total leukocyte counts, lymphocyte counts, and immunoglobulins in well-trained athletes at rest and during exercise. Well-trained athletes frequently report a higher incidence of upper respiratory infections than their more sedentary counterparts. This has been explained as being a result of a mechanism that suppresses immune response, but no experimental evidence of such a mechanism exists.

REVIEW QUESTIONS

1. Why is the lymphatic system integral to the functioning of the immune system?

2. How are pathogens, antigens, antibodies, and lymphokines different?

3. List the differences between the humoral immune response and the cell-mediated immune response.

4. How does exercise acutely influence the immune system?

5. Is retained enhancement of the immune system a by-product of exercise?

6. Has an adequate amount of research been done to determine whether exercise training can suppress the immune system? Explain.

APPLICATIONS

1. The precision and sensitivity of the body's antibodies have been exploited in the development of techniques for measuring molecules that exist in very small concentrations. For example, many hormone concentrations are measured by radioactively labeling a hormone sample and adding this to a sample of human serum. This mixture is placed in a vial that has a specific antibody to the hormone (obtained from laboratory animals) bound to the side of the tube. The greater the hormone concentration in a blood sample, the greater the competition for the antibody between the natural and radioactively labeled hormone, and the lower the radioactivity measured in the vial. This technique is based on the procedure for developing *monoclonal antibodies*. Find two other experimental uses of the monoclonal antibody technique that can be applied to further our understanding of the body's adaptations to exercise.

APPLICATIONS—Cont'd

2. AIDS is caused by an immune system infection that eventually destroys the body's T cells. Using the cell-mediated immune response system as a basis, explain in detail why AIDS eventually causes death from complications of infection.

3. According to the research on how exercise influences the immune system and immune functioning, there is no clear answer as to whether exercise suppresses or improves immune protection from infection. What research needs to be done, for both acute and chronic exercise, to clarify the role of exercise in immune functioning?

REFERENCES

1. Ahlborg B, Ahlborg G: Exercise leukocytosis with and without β-adrenergic blockage, *Acta Med Scand* 187:241-246, 1970.

2. Byrnes WC, Clarkson PM, Spencer White J et al: Delayed-onset muscle soreness following repeated bouts of downhill running, *J Appl Physiol* 59:710-715, 1985.

3. Clarkson PM, Tremblay I: Exercise-induced muscle damage, repair, and adaptation in humans, *J Appl Physiol* 65(1):1-6, 1988.

4. Costill DL, Pascoe DD, Fink WJ et al: Muscle glycogen resynthesis after eccentric exercise, *J Appl Physiol* 69:46-50, 1990.

5. Dorner H, Heinold D, Hilmer W: Exercise-induced leucocytosis: its dependence on physical capability, *Sports Med* 8:152, 1987.

6. Edwards AJ, Bacon TH, Elms CA et al: Changes in the populations of lymphoid cells in human peripheral blood following physical exercise, *Clin Exp Immunol* 58:420-427, 1984.

7. Fauci AS, Dale DC: The effect of hydrocortisone on the kinetics of normal human leucocytes, *Blood* 46:235-243, 1975.

8. Fry RW, Morton AR, Keast D: Acute intensive interval training and T-lymphocyte function, *Med Sci Sports Exerc* 24(3):339-345, 1992.

9. Heath GW, Ford ES, Craven TE et al: Exercise and the incidence of upper respiratory tract infections, *Med Sci Sports Exerc* 23(2):152-157, 1991.

10. Hedfors E, Holm G, Ivansen M, Wahren J: Physiological variation of blood lymphocyte reactivity: T-cell subsets, immunoglobulin production, and mixed lymphocyte reactivity, *Clin Immunol Immunopharm* 27:9-14, 1983.

11. Hortobagyi T, Denaham T: Variability in creatine kinase: methodological, exercise, and clinically related factors, *Int J Sports Med* 10:69-80, 1989.

12. Marieb EN: *Human anatomy and physiology,* ed 3, Redwood City, Calif, 1995, Benjamin Cummings.

13. McCarthy DA, Dale MM: The leucocytosis of exercise, *Sports Med* 6:333-363, 1988.

14. Nehlsen-Cannarella SL, Nieman DC, Balk-Lamberton AJ et al: The effects of moderate exercise training on immune response, *Med Sci Sports Exerc* 23(1):64-70, 1991.

15. Nieman DC, Nehlsen-Cannarella SL, Donahue KM et al: The effects of acute and moderate exercise on leukocyte and lymphocyte subpopulations, *Med Sci Sports Exerc* 23(5):578-585, 1991.

16. Nieman DC, Miller AR, Hensen DA et al: Effects of high versus moderate-intensity exercise on natural killer cell activity, *Med Sci Sports Exerc* 25(10):1126-1134, 1993.

17. Peters EM, Goetzsche JM, Grobbelaar B, Noakes TD: Vitamin C supplementation reduces the incidence of upper respiratory tract infection in ultramarathon runners, *Am J Clin Nutr* 57:170-174, 1993.

18. Richter EA, Kiens B, Raben A et al: Immune parameters in male athletes after a lacto-ovovegetarian diet and a mixed Western diet, *Med Sci Sports Exerc* 23(5):517-521, 1991.

19. Shearer JD, Amarai JF, Caldwell MD: Glucose metabolism of injured skeletal muscle: contribution of inflammatory cells, *Circ Shock* 25:131-138, 1988.

20. Shepherd RJ, Verde TJ, Thomas SG, Shek P: Physical activity and the immune system, *Can J Appl Sport Sci* 16(3):163-185, 1991.

21. Shepherd RJ, Rhind S, Shek PN: Exercise and the immune system: natural killer cells, interleukins, and responses, *Sports Med* 18(5):340-368, 1994.

22. Soppi E, Varjo P, Eskola J, Laitinen LA: Effect of strenuous physical stress on circulating lymphocyte number and function before and after training, *J Clin Lab Immuno* 8:43-46, 1982.

23. Sternfeld B: Cancer and the protective effect of physical activity: the epidemiological evidence, *Med Sci Sports Exerc* 24(11):1195-1209, 1992.

RECOMMENDED READINGS

■ Clarkson PM, Tremblay I: Exercise-induced muscle damage, repair, and adaptation in humans, *J Appl Physiol* 65(1):1-6, 1988.

■ Fry RW, Morton AR, Keast D: Acute intensive interval training and T-lymphocyte function, *Med Sci Sports Exerc* 24(3):339-345, 1992.

■ Heath GW, Ford ES, Craven TE et al: Exercise and the incidence of upper respiratory tract infections, *Med Sci Sports Exerc* 23(2):152-157, 1991.

■ McCarthy DA, Dale MM: The leucocytosis of exercise, *Sports Med* 6:333-363, 1988.

■ Nehlsen-Cannarella SL, Nieman DC, Balk-Lamberton AJ et al: The effects of moderate exercise training on immune response, *Med Sci Sports Exerc* 23(1):64-70, 1991.

■ Nieman DC, Nehlsen-Cannarella SL, Donahue KM et al: The effects of acute and moderate exercise on leukocyte and lymphocyte subpopulations, *Med Sci Sports Exerc* 23(5):578-585, 1991.

■ Shearer JD, Amarai JF, Caldwell MD: Glucose metabolism of injured skeletal muscle: contribution of inflammatory cells, *Circ Shock* 25:131-138, 1988.

■ Shepherd RJ, Verde TJ, Thomas SG, Shek P: Physical activity and the immune system, *Can J Appl Sport Sci* 16(3):163-185, 1991.

■ Shepherd RJ, Rhind S, Shek PN: Exercise and the immune system: natural killer cells, interleukins and responses, *Sports Med* 18(5):340-368, 1994.

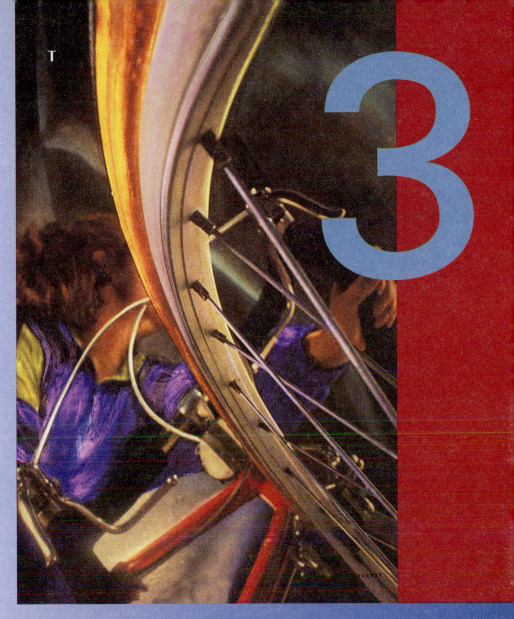

Aids to

Exercise

Performance

CHAPTER 16

Training for Sport and Performance

OBJECTIVES

After studying this chapter you should be able to:

- Explain the multiple theories and training concepts.

- Describe the principles behind the methods of training for specific sports and athletic activities.

- Explain the concept of overtraining, and provide indirect methods for detecting symptoms of overtraining.

- Explain the importance of the taper to a training program and optimal prerace preparation.

- Describe the process of detraining for each type of fitness component.

- Develop training programs based on applied muscle biochemistry and the findings from published scientific research.

- Explain how to modify training programs to emphasize long-term endurance, muscle power, muscle strength, or muscle hypertrophy.

KEY TERMS

training	overload
fitness	overtraining
adaptation	taper
specificity	reversibility
cross-training	detraining

*T*raining for improved performance can be applied to sports, athletics, or work environments such as fire fighting, the police, or the military. Athletes and individuals involved in strenuous vocations are more interested in the principles that apply to *performance-related fitness* rather than *health-related fitness* because their physical demands exceed those of individuals training for the development of accepted minimal standards of fitness for decreased risk for certain diseases (e.g., cardiovascular disease). To perform well in athletic competition, athletes must be pushed to extremes of training that far exceed those required for acceptable health standards (see Chapters 27 and 30). Consequently, the training programs that develop performance-related fitness are very different from those that develop health-related fitness. For athletes at all levels of competition, adequate training cannot be overemphasized. For elite athletes, proper training can mean the difference between remaining in obscurity or becoming internationally competitive and recognized in their events. In addition, for both elite and recreational athletes, proper training not only optimizes race performance, but also decreases the likelihood for injury, prevents *overtraining,* and provides greater satisfaction. The importance given to training by today's elite and recreational athletes striving for their personal best performances has demanded research on how best to train for a given event. Scientists of exercise physiology have responded to these needs, and numerous academic journals have published research on optimal training practices and on practices detrimental to improved performance. The purpose of this chapter is to present the scientifically proven principles and training practices that are known to influence exercise performance for the recreational and elite, competitive athlete.

Defining Fitness and Training

*T*he process of **training** is performed to improve **fitness.** Training involves the organized sequence of exercise that stimulates improvements, or **adaptations,** in anatomy and physiology. Depending on the quality of training and the duration of intervals between exercise sessions, these training-induced improvements are developed and retained, thereby providing improved tolerance of the exercise. In most circumstances, improved exercise tolerance results in improved exercise performance. Throughout the text, these retained training adaptations have been termed *chronic adaptations.*

The term *fitness* is harder to define. Fitness involves many components, including cardiorespiratory endurance, muscular endurance, muscular strength, muscular power, flexibility, body composition, and emotional and psychologic qualities. Typically the term fitness is used to express components of

---

training (tray'ning)
an organized program of exercise designed to stimualte chronic adaptations

fitness (fit'ness)
a state of well-being that provides optimal performance

adaptation (ad-ap-ta'shun)
a modification in structure or function that benefits life in a new or altered environment

cardiorespiratory and muscle function, whether the components be endurance, strength, or power. Thus the athlete may be concerned with training one of these components for the purpose of improving exercise performance. As explained, the term fitness means different things to different athletes, since it is very specific to the demands placed on the body. For example, an elite rower may train to improve fitness for rowing distances greater than 2000 m, but can a rower be classified as fit for the marathon running race?

An understanding of the important connections between training, chronic adaptation, and improved exercise performance is crucial if a high-quality training program is to be developed. In addition, this knowledge has to be applied to the specific demands of an exercise stress for the development of a successful training program. Therefore knowledge of the types, intensities, durations, and frequencies of exercise required to optimize training adaptations is essential. This knowledge is acquired from the study of skeletal muscle energy metabolism and from understanding the principles and terminology of training.

Important Principles of Training and Training Terminology

Optimizing training requires knowledge of such principles as specificity, overload, progression, recovery, diminishing returns, the taper, reversibility, detraining, and overtraining. In addition, knowledge of specific types of training programs is required.

Specificity

Specificity implies that the training should be devised to "train" the appropriate muscles and systems of the body, in a manner that is similar to how these systems are used during competition. Thus the specificity principle has implications to anatomy, neuromuscular recruitment, motor skill patterns, cardiorespiratory function, and muscle energy metabolism. The different movement components of the specificity principle are illustrated in Figure 16.1.

Traditionally, the most emphasized component of specificity has been skeletal muscle metabolism. In Chapter 10, Figure 10.1 illustrated the time dependence of the reliance on specific energy pathways for adenosine triphosphate (ATP) regeneration. Such an approach is useful for categorizing the metabolic demands of specific events. The shorter the time duration, the greater the dependence on glycolytic and creatine phosphate ATP regeneration. The longer the duration, the greater the reliance on ATP regeneration from mitochondrial respiration.

Figure 16.2 is a modification of Figure 10.1 and reveals the types of events that predominantly use either metabolic pathway in addition to the main limitations of exercise performance associated with these time frames. The metabolic objectives of training for an activity of a given duration would therefore be to optimize the capacity of ATP regeneration from the pathways most relied on for ATP regeneration or to stimulate adaptations that decrease the limitations (causes of fatigue) (see Chapters 27 and 30). Of course, the difficulty is that few events have a near-total reliance on just one metabolic pathway. Furthermore, one could also argue that for the activities that do rely on one metabolic pathway, such as throwing or jumping events, metabolic capacities are not the determining factor for success. In throwing events muscle power, strength, and technique could be argued to be most important. However, for the 100 meter sprint, which has a duration that can completely tax muscle creatine phosphate stores, metabolic factors may limit performance. In addition, for prolonged endurance events in which VO_2max and the lactate threshold combine to determine exercise performance, metabolic limitations are obvious.

Research of Training Specificity

When concerned with cardiorespiratory endurance and prolonged exercise performance, researchers have asked the question of whether the mode of exercise training is important. For example, is training by cycling as effective as training by running for running exercise performance? Obviously, the measures of VO_2max and the lactate threshold (LT) have been evaluated to answer this question. This question also is important for athletes involved in multi-mode events, such as biathlons, triathlons, and quadrathlons, since it is important to know how to distribute training among the multiple exercise modes for optimal performance.

VO_2max. In either run or cycle training, VO_2max improvements are largest in the exercise mode that is trained.[28,29] Consequently, if the training stimulus and muscles are used similarly, there is a transfer of fitness from one mode to another. Furthermore, despite the fact that VO_2max is larger for running than cycling in recreationally trained individuals, well-trained cyclists have a larger VO_2max during cycling than running, which further emphasizes the importance of training specificity.

For individuals who train in both cycling and running, VO_2max measurements in well-trained triathletes have shown that running VO_2max is larger than cycling VO_2max,[33] and for only moderately trained triathletes VO_2max between running and cycling is similar.[1] It is unclear whether the level of fitness and training of an individual influences the specificity of training adaptations in a given exercise mode.

Research comparing training from arm ergometry with either cycling or running has been used to indirectly evaluate the contribution of central cardiovascular adaptations (e.g., maximal cardiac output, increased blood volume) to increased exercise tolerance. If cycle or run training increases VO_2max during arm ergometry, it is evidence of the contribution of central adaptations to improved cardiorespiratory endurance. Research has reported 0% to 10% improvements

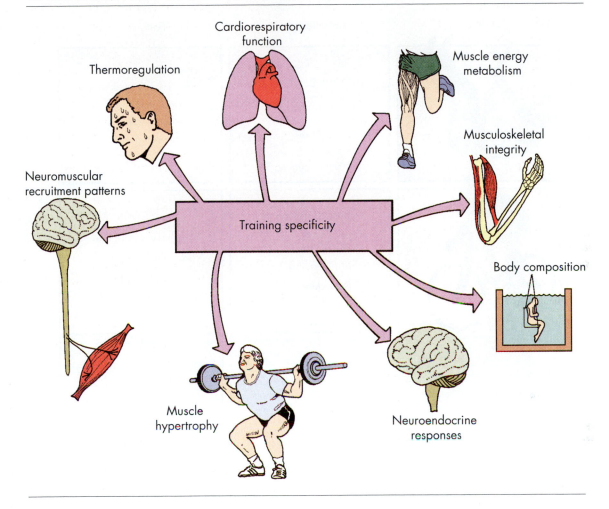

FIGURE 16.1

The different components of the specificity principle applied to exercise training.

Cardiorespiratory function

Thermoregulation

Muscle energy metabolism

Musculoskeletal integrity

Neuromuscular recruitment patterns

Training specificity

Body composition

Muscle hypertrophy

Neuroendocrine responses

in VO_2max during arm ergometry after cycle training.[26] The variability in these results probably reflects different training intensities and durations, thereby indicating that central cardiovascular adaptations may contribute to training improvements in VO_2max and offer a transfer of cardiorespiratory endurance between different exercise modes if the training stimulus is large enough.

Lactate threshold. In well-trained individuals, the LT and ventilation threshold (VT) are more sensitive indices of training improvement than VO_2max. Moreira et al.[27] and Withers et al.[38] revealed that trained runners have a significantly higher VT during treadmill running compared with cycle ergometry, whereas the VT in trained cyclists does not differ between running and cycling. Fewer differences would be expected between the LT during running and cycling for triathletes or biathletes, since these individuals are trained in both modes. Although minimal research has been done on this topic,[1] results indicate that no differences exist in the VT or LT between running and cycling in triathletes.

Intense exercise and weight lifting. Research on the specificity of exercise training mainly has been focused on cardiorespiratory endurance and prolonged exercise performance. Whether intense exercise training should be performed in a specific mode and how much carryover occurs between different modes are unknown. Furthermore, the influence of resistance exercise on muscular endurance and that of endurance exercise on muscle strength are topics that have not received considerable research attention.

Long-distance running training is known to decrease muscle power so much that endurance-trained individuals have lower muscle power than sedentary individuals. This information indicates that although training for muscular strength and power, as well as endurance, may at first seem in

specificity (spes'i-fis'i'ti)
having a fixed relation to a single cause or definite result

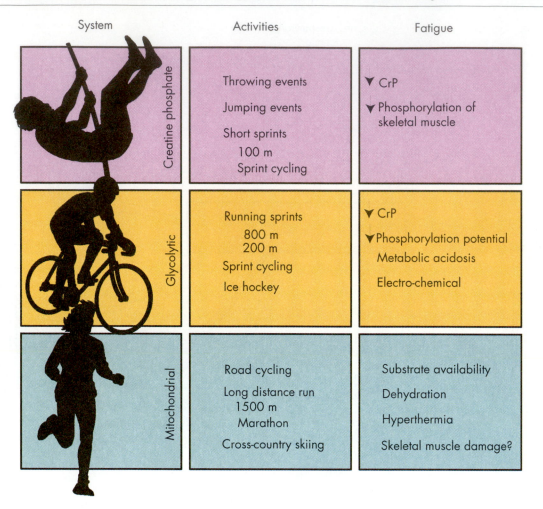

FIGURE 16.2

The activities that predominantly rely on given energy systems and their main causes of fatigue.

System	Activities	Fatigue
Creatine phosphate	Throwing events Jumping events Short sprints 100 m Sprint cycling	▼ CrP ▼ Phosphorylation of skeletal muscle
Glycolytic	Running sprints 800 m 200 m Sprint cycling Ice hockey	▼ CrP ▼ Phosphorylation potential Metabolic acidosis Electro-chemical
Mitochondrial	Road cycling Long distance run 1500 m Marathon Cross-country skiing	Substrate availability Dehydration Hyperthermia Skeletal muscle damage?

opposition and therefore have low specificity, both training strategies may combine to improve running performance by maintaining a more optimal muscle power. Thus the concept of specificity must always be used in reference to the demands of the exercise, rather than the main metabolic pathway used during exercise.

The principle of specificity is probably the most important training guideline. As previously explained, it not only encompasses energy metabolism but can also be applied to anatomic demands, neuromuscular function, and motor skill development. For sports that have a high skill component, such as swimming, tennis, golf, gymnastics, basketball, and soccer, training that improves all aspects of performance (metabolic to motor performance) must be devised. Often this is a difficult process, and coaches or trainers who can successfully orchestrate training programs that optimize improvement in all areas for specific individuals are those who experience success.

Cross-training.   An interesting topic that pertains to the principle of specificity is that of **cross-training.** This term can be defined in several ways because of different exercise mode and exercise intensity and duration options. Training in different modes of exercise can be performed either to stimulate similar metabolic adaptations in the same muscles (e.g., cardiorespiratory and muscular endurance for long-term running and cycling, or weight lifting and swimming for the development of muscle power) or to refer to the practice of completing resistance exercise by muscles that are being trained for long-term endurance.

The concept of cross-training developed from the previously described research on training improvements resulting from exercising by a different mode. Thus cross-training is really a way to improve the quality of training. Cross-training may do this by increasing the stimulus or overload for adaptation, by preventing overuse and maintaining muscle power (especially for runners), and by preventing overuse injuries.

The potential benefit has not been conclusively documented by research.

Overload and Overtraining

Training implies improved exercise tolerance and performance. Obviously, even if specificity principles are applied and therefore appropriate intensities used, unless sufficient durations and frequencies of training are performed, there may be no improvement in performance. A level of training above which there is a sufficient training stimulus must exist for chronic improvement. The principle of **overload** is based on the need to train above this stimulus threshold for the development of chronic training adaptations. In short, *the body does not improve unless it experiences more stress than it is accustomed to.* Coaches and athletes need the ability to determine the training program that provides an overload stimulus that optimizes training adaptation rather than overstressing the athlete, which leads to a condition known as **overtraining.**

The overload principle is based in part on the research of Dr. Hans Selye.[32,34] Dr. Selye identified a pattern of physical stress referred to as the *general adaptation syndrome* (GAS). The GAS reveals how the human body responds to and adapts to physical stress over time. Initially a physical stress causes the body to respond and to adapt to that stress. With exercise, signs of adaptation to training are muscles getting stronger and heart and lungs working more efficiently. When the stress is too great for too long, the body is not able to respond adequately and the stress leads to exhaustion.

Minimal Training Intensities and Frequencies

The nature of the overload stimulus depends on a variety of factors that include the following:

- Exercise intensity
- Exercise duration
- Frequency of exercise sessions and duration of recovery
- Type of exercise
- Initial level of fitness

Exercise intensity can be expressed relative to VO_2max or maximal heart rate for endurance exercise or relative to maximal muscle strength (maximal voluntary contraction), peak torque, or peak power for strength- and power-related activities. For endurance exercise a minimal training overload stimulus is attained at exercise intensities that elicit greater than 50% VO_2max, 70% of maximum heart rate, or 60% of the heart rate reserve and are maintained for greater than 15 minutes. Although evidence exists to indicate training improvements from less exercise or the accumulation of exercise throughout the day, this minimal training stimulus has limited application to recreational or elite athletes.

Exercise performed at or slightly above the LT is most beneficial in increasing both VO_2max and the LT. However, the way that increases in exercise intensity translate to gains in cardiorespiratory endurance is unclear.

FIGURE 16.3

Training programs provide a gradual increase in training volume, which includes periods of constant or decreasing training. As a person adapts to training, further improvements either require larger increases in training volume or more time at a given training volume.

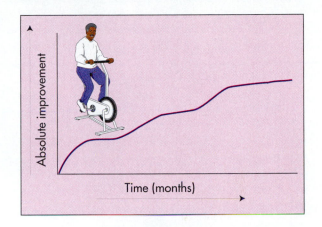

For muscular strength and power, the specific nature of overload that favors strength, power, or muscular endurance is manipulated by altering the number of repetitions, the resistance lifted, and the recovery duration (see Focus Box 16.1). A similar approach can be used to train for muscular power in cycling, running, swimming, rowing, and other activities. However, rather than resistance being modified, speed and exercise duration are altered.

Planning the Overload Stimulus

The principle of overload requires developing a training program in which the training stimulus increases in conjunction with improvements in training adaptation, yet in which recovery time is still adequate (Figure 16.3). Knowledge of the rate of training adaptation for long-term cardiorespiratory and muscular endurance, muscular strength, or muscular power is necessary. As discussed in Chapters 9 through 12, chronic adaptations to exercise involve alterations in neuro-

cross-training
the practice of exercise training with more than one exercise mode

overload (o'ver-lode)
exposure of the body to stress to which it is unaccustomed

overtraining (o'ver-tray'ning)
training that causes excess overload to which the body is unable to adapt, resulting in decreased exercise performance

FOCUS BOX 16.1

Application of the interval concept to resistance and endurance training programs

Interval training requires the completion of exercise bouts, separated by recovery periods. The relationship between the intensity and duration of exercise and the duration of recovery determines the specific training stimulus. For dynamic exercises, interval training can be used for developing varying degrees of endurance or power, whereas for resistance exercise, interval training can be used to develop strength, power, or general physical conditioning.

Training For Endurance and Power

Typically, interval training is suited to dynamic activities such as running, cycling, rowing, and wrestling. A training session would involve standard features of training, such as a warm-up, stretching, the training session, and a cool-down and further stretching. The training session involves a given number of work intervals, each followed by a rest interval.

An example of a weekly training schedule for a marathon runner, which includes interval training is provided in Table 16.1.

Training For Muscular Strength and Hypertrophy

The practice of weight lifting involves the organization of exercises into the resistance (weight) used, the number of times the weight is lifted (repetitions), the number of times a given repetition number is completed (sets), and the recovery between sets.

Manipulating any component alters the specific training stimulus. Typically, repetition numbers less than 10 are used with heavy weights for the development of muscular strength and hypertrophy. Increasing the number of repetitions decreases the amount of weight that can be lifted and the stimulus for hypertrophy but further increases metabolism and the development of improved muscular endurance and tone. The following terms are used frequently in weight training:

TABLE 16.1

An example of a training schedule for a marathon runner

DAY	TRAINING
1	0.5 hr easy run in morning Leg-weight workout in afternoon
2	1.0 hr easy run
3	1.5 hr road run, approximately 12-15 miles
4	6 mile run in morning (easy) Track interval workout in afternoon— 3 × 1000 m, 1 × 5000, 2 × 1000 m (110% race pace): 5 min rest intervals
5	1.0 hr run at desired pace
6	Rest
7	5 miles in morning 50 min of hard running in afternoon

- **Load**—the amount of resistance or weight used
- **Repetition**—the number of times an exercise is performed without recovery
- **Sets**—the number of times a series of repetitions is completed
- **Volume**—the total number of repetitions performed in a given time period
- **Recovery**—the duration between sets, which can be either active or passive
- **Frequency**—the number of training sessions per week

muscular, skeletal muscle, pulmonary, and cardiovascular structure and function. Figure 16.4 presents the changes that occur in specific aspects of body function during endurance and strength training. Cardiovascular adaptations to endurance training are immediate, with evidence of an increased plasma volume as early as after the first bout of exercise,[7,18] a polycythemia that may take approximately 2 weeks, and skeletal muscle metabolic adaptations that are detected as early as 6 weeks into a training program and that persist after a plateau in cardiorespiratory endurance.[9,12,25] As discussed in Chapter 11, research indicates that the initial improvements in VO_2max and endurance–exercise performance are more attributable to the initial cardiovascular adaptations than to

muscle metabolic adaptations.[7,13] These training improvements are of a larger magnitude for individuals who begin the training at a lower relative level of specific fitness.

The rapidity of exercise-induced training adaptations is astounding and stresses not just the need for a rapid progression in training quality, but also the recovery time needed to allow these adaptations to occur. It is important to remember that training provides the stimulus to adapt and that adaptation occurs during the recovery.

For strength training the initial increase in strength occurs from improved neuromuscular function (see Chapter 9), followed by muscular hypertrophy. The dose-response curve for strength training is considerably slower in time

FIGURE 16.4

The improved function and exercise performance resulting from endurance and strength training. Cardiovascular adaptations to endurance training occur rapidly, and explain the initial improved exercise performance. Later improvements are related to adaptations in skeletal muscle. For strength training, initial improvement has neuromuscular determinants, and subsequent increases in strength are slow and a result of muscle hypertrophy.

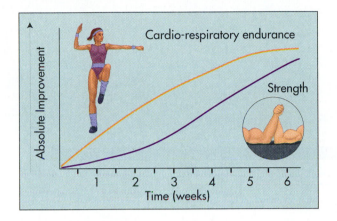

- An increased resting heart rate
- A loss of body weight
- A decrease in appetite
- Muscle soreness that lasts more than 24 hours
- Increased serum enzyme activity for creatine kinase and lactate dehydrogenase
- Worse running economy and increased submaximal heart rate
- An increase in illness, such as colds or flu
- Constipation or diarrhea
- A decrease in performance
- A lack of desire in training or competing

Most of these symptoms indicate overtraining, and therefore when present they indicate the need to decrease training volume immediately. Of these symptoms, the resting and submaximal exercise heart rate are most sensitive to the development of overtraining, whereas the remainder occur when overtraining is evident. Unfortunately, science has yet to provide a sensitive gauge of overtraining that is noninvasive, inexpensive, and applicable to all athletes.

The Taper

The **taper** involves a period of reduced training, usually scheduled for the weeks before athletic competition. For swimmers, cyclists, and runners the taper does not decrease conditioning but actually can increase muscle power, improve psychologic state, and heighten performance.[8]

Research has shown that periods of reduced training do not decrease VO_2max.[20] For example, after 10 weeks of endurance training, subjects who either decreased training from 6 to 2 days per week or reduced training duration from 40 to 13 minutes per day retained cardiovascular conditioning as measured by VO_2max for an additional 4 to 8 weeks. Clearly the maintenance of a given level of conditioning can be done on less training than what is needed to improve fitness. Given these facts, the taper, even during a training program for the purposes of improving recovery and decreasing the risk of overtraining, is a practice that has support from research. Athletes should not fear intermittent periods of reduced training to their long-term training program.

Reversibility and Detraining

When muscles are overloaded, they adapt by getting stronger and larger. When the exercise stimulus is removed, the training adaptations are reversed. If athletes do not remain active, changes in strength or aerobic endurance levels may be noticed.

development, especially after the initial neuromuscular improvement. The rate of strength improvement is variable depending on gender, hormonal status, genetics, and diet. In either case the overload used in training must be applied progressively by manipulating the intensity, duration, and frequency of exercise.

Research of Overload and Overtraining

Unfortunately, research that evaluates the volume of training performed by athletes is limited. Costill et al. studied swimmers to determine whether decreasing the volume of training detracted from conditioning and race performance. Interestingly, swimmers who trained once a day at 15,000 m/week rather than twice per day peaking at 30,000 m/week did not decrease in markers of conditioning (VO_2max, submaximal blood lactate levels, race performance).[11] Conversely, the swimmers who trained at the greater distances did not experience increased symptoms of overtraining. These findings raised questions concerning the efficacy of swim training using large distances. However, concerns exist regarding whether these results would have been found in more elite athletes and whether these results can be applied to other forms of exercise such as running, cycling, and weight lifting.

When there has been too great an overload training stimulus relative to the recovery, overtraining occurs. During overtraining, exercise performance decreases and there is actually a loss in training adaptations, causing a partial detraining effect. Overtraining can be detected by the presence of symptoms that include the following:

taper (tape′er)
a period of reduced training before athletic competition

An extreme example of **reversibility** and **detraining** occurs during bed rest.[31] Under this condition of forced inactivity, VO$_2$max has been shown to decrease by 27%[31] in as little as 20 days. Decreases in VO$_2$max have also been shown for prolonged periods in which no training has occurred. Based on research of swimmers, runners, and cyclists, decrements in VO$_2$max resulting from training cessation initially result from reductions in plasma volume[13] and then from marked reductions in muscle mitochondrial enzyme activity[9,12] (Figure 16.5).

Since reductions in glycolytic enzyme activities have not been shown during detraining, the metabolic causes of decreased performance during strength- or power-related exercises are minimal. Furthermore, because of this fact, it is no surprise that strength and muscle power exhibit slower detraining curves compared with endurance fitness. For example, in one study no loss of strength occurred after 6 weeks of detraining from a strength-training program.[35,36]

FIGURE 16.5

The physiologic events associated with detraining from cardiorespiratory and muscular endurance.

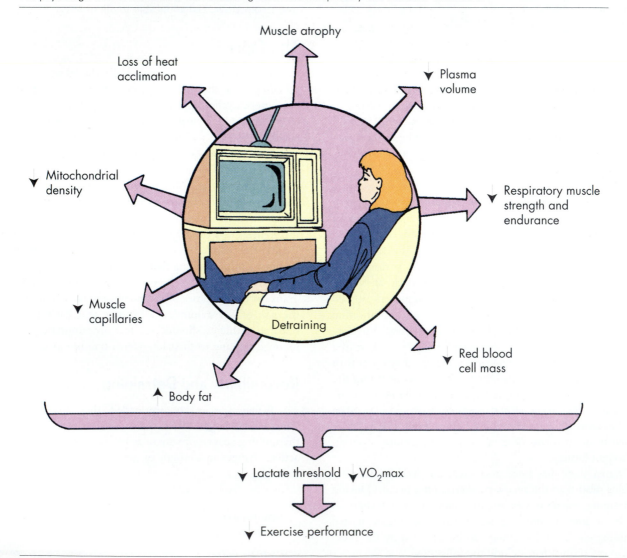

Training For Specific Performance Improvement

Given the previously explained requirements of a training program, how should an athlete train to optimally develop specific performance capacities, such as long-term endurance, muscular strength, or muscular power?

Cardiorespiratory and Muscular Endurance

Athletes can increase cardiorespiratory and muscular endurance, or muscle power, by performing one or a combination of interval, continuous, or fartlek training protocols. Focus Box 16.2 provides an example of a fartlek training program.

Interval training, as explained in Focus Box 16.1, pertains to the completion of exercise at an intensity that is above steady state, or race pace, and therefore requires a recovery period between exercise bouts. The faster or more intense the exercise, the longer the recovery interval. Consequently, athletes involved in long-duration exercise typically have a short recovery interval, whereas events of a shorter duration (e.g., the mile) have longer recovery intervals as a result of the greater need to recover muscle metabolites and restore more normal muscle and blood acid-base balance.

Controversy exists regarding the best way to increase aerobic power. Training programs that stress intensity over duration have been shown to be effective in increasing aerobic power.[5,15] Lower intensity, long-duration training was made popular in the 1960s and 1970s. This type of training was referred to as LSD training, or long slow distance training. Today most endurance athletes use a combination of periods of high-intensity training, LSD training, and interval workouts on a track.

FOCUS BOX 16.2

Example of a fartlek training schedule

1. Warm-up (dynamic exercise and stretching)

2. Running, with sprint bouts of 50 to 100 meters repeated continuously until fatigue is evident

3. Running at full speed for 100 to 200 meters

4. Recovery with slow jogging

5. Running, with bouts of increased speed and a duration specific to the race pace and duration, repeated continuously until fatigue is evident

---

reversibility (re-ver′si-bil′i-ti)
the loss of training adaptations when exercise training ceases

detraining (de-tray′ning)
the absence of training, usually occuring after the attainment of training adaptations

Different strength training terminology and protocols

Terminology
Power lifting

Power lifting, or lifting in a competitive setting to determine the maximum amount of weight an individual can lift, is not recommended for young or elderly people or individuals just starting a strength-training program. Power lifting generally involves core weight-lifting exercises, such as the bench press, squat, clean and jerk, and snatch. These types of exercises are commonly used by athletes to develop overall strength and explosive power. Power lifting is effective but can also be dangerous if not performed correctly. Athletes should be gradually introduced to power lifting.

One repetition maximum (1RM)

The 1RM is used to establish starting weights for different exercises. It involves an individual lifting the maximum amount of weight he or she can lift for a particular exercise. Once an individual's 1RM is established, different percentages of the 1RM weight are used when performing selected exercises.

Circuit training

Circuit training is a form of strength training and consists of a series of strength-training exercises. Circuit training is an effective way of developing strength and flexibility and can cause minor increases in cardiorespiratory endurance (VO_2max).

Periodization

Periodization is a technique used by virtually all athletes. Periodization is a way to plan training sessions systematically to avoid overtraining and to maximize workout sessions. With periodization, athletes vary the type, amount, and intensity of training for several weeks, a month, or a whole year.

Pyramid system

The pyramid system has become a popular technique among athletes and body builders. In this system the athlete performs continuous sets of exercises, progressing from light to heavy resistance, while decreasing the number of repetitions during the session.

Split-routine system

A split-routine system trains different body parts on alternate days in an effort to stimulate hypertrophy of all muscles in a particular area of the body. A typical training routine might be—chest, shoulders, and back on Monday, Wednesday, and Friday; arms, legs, and abdominal muscles on Tuesday, Thursday, and Saturday.

Eccentric loading

Eccentric loading or performing "negatives" allows athletes to develop strength while maintaining control of the weight. Negatives are a popular and effective technique to develop strength and overcome "sticking points," but they also seem to cause more fatigue and soreness than other methods.

Plyometric training

Plyometric training is a technique used to develop explosive strength and power. A plyometric exercise consists of a quick eccentric stretch followed by a powerful concentric contraction.

Super set system

With the super set system, opposing muscle groups are worked through exercises performed immediately after one another. An example of a super set workout would be to perform biceps curls immediately followed by triceps extensions, or leg extensions immediately followed by leg curls. Super setting is a popular way to increase muscle hypertrophy.

Muscular Strength and Hypertrophy

Apart from increasing the resistance and lowering the number of repetitions, using dynamic rather than isometric contractions[16] and incorporating eccentric contractions into the training program[24] can increase strength gains. Similar increases in strength occur from variable resistance and constant resistance exercise.[16]

There are numerous ways to design a strength-training program, and these are summarized in Focus Box 16.3. Essentially, training programs differ depending on the purpose of the weight lifting (strength versus general conditioning) and the number of body parts used. Different types of weight-lifting exercises are presented in Focus Box 16.4.

FOCUS BOX 16.4

Weight-training exercises

Exercises to Develop the Chest Muscles

1. Bench press (barbell)
2. Incline bench press (barbell)
3. Incline bench press (dumbbell)
4. Decline bench press
5. Dumbbell flys

Exercises to Develop the Shoulder Muscles

1. Dumbbell shoulder press
2. Dumbbell lateral raise
3. Dumbbell front raise
4. Medial rotation
5. Lateral rotation

Exercises to Develop the Arm Muscles

1. Tricep extension
2. One arm french curls
3. Dumbbell kickback
4. Seated dumbbell curl
5. Preacher curl with dumbbells
6. Standing dumbbell curl
7. Concentration curl
8. Wrist curls

Exercises to Develop the Upper and Lower Back Muscles

1. Upright rowing (barbell)
2. Upright rowing (dumbbells)
3. Shoulder shrugs
4. Lat pulls (machine)
5. Low back extensions

Exercises to Develop the Lower Body Muscles

1. Squats
2. Lunges
3. Calf raises
4. Knee Extensions (machine)
5. Hamstring curls (machine)

SUMMARY

- The process of **training** is performed to improve **fitness.** Training involves the organized sequence of exercise that stimulates improvements, or **adaptations,** in anatomy and physiology. Fitness involves many components, including cardiorespiratory endurance, muscular endurance, muscular strength, muscular power, flexibility, body composition, and emotional and psychologic qualities. The term *fitness* means different things to different people and athletes because it is specific to the demands placed on the body.

- **Specificity** implies that the training should be devised to "train" the appropriate muscles and systems of the body in a manner that is similar to how these systems are used during competition. The specificity principle has implications to anatomy, neuromuscular recruitment, motor skill patterns, cardiorespiratory function, and muscle energy metabolism.

- When concerned with either run or cycle training, VO_2max improvements are largest in the exercise mode that is trained. Consequently, there is a transfer of fitness from one mode to another if the training stimulus and muscles used are similar.

- **Cross-training** can be defined in several ways because of different exercise mode and exercise intensity and duration options. Training in different modes of exercise can either be performed to stimulate similar metabolic adaptations in the same muscles (e.g., cardiorespiratory and muscular endurance for long-term running and cycling, or weight lifting and swimming for the development of muscle power) or refer to the practice of completing resistance exercise by muscles that are being trained for long-term endurance.

- The principle of **overload** is based on the need to train above this stimulus threshold for the development of chronic training adaptations. In short, *the body does not improve unless it experiences more stress than it is accustomed to.* Coaches and athletes require the ability to determine a training program in which the overload stimulus optimizes training adaptation rather than overstressing the athlete, which leads to a condition known as **overtraining.**

- The nature of the overload stimulus depends on a variety of factors that include exercise intensity, exercise duration, frequency of exercise sessions and duration of recovery, the type of exercise, and the initial level of fitness. Overtraining can be detected by the presence of symptoms that include increased resting heart rate; a loss of body weight; a decrease in appetite; muscle soreness that is retained for more than 24 hours; increased serum enzyme activity for creatine kinase and lactate dehydrogenase; worse running economy and increased submaximal heart rate; an increase in illness, such as colds, flu, etc.; constipation or diarrhea; a decrease in performance; and a lack of desire in training or competing.

- Research has shown that exercise performed at or slightly above the LT is most beneficial in increasing both VO_2max and the LT. However, the transition in the gains in cardiorespiratory endurance and further increases in exercise intensity are unclear.

- The **taper** involves a period of reduced training, usually timed in the weeks before athletic competition. An extreme example of **reversibility** and **detraining** occurs during bed rest. Under this condition of forced inactivity, VO_2max has been shown to decrease by 27% in as little as 20 days. Decrements in VO_2max resulting from training cessation initially result from reductions in plasma volume and then from marked reductions in muscle mitochondrial enzyme activity.

- Athletes can increase cardiorespiratory and muscular endurance, or muscle power, by performing one or a combination of interval, continuous, or fartlek training protocols. Strength gains can be increased when dynamic rather than isometric contractions are used and when eccentric contractions are incorporated into the training program. Similar increases in strength occur from variable resistance and constant resistance exercise.

REVIEW QUESTIONS

1. Why is overload required to induce chronic training adaptations?

2. Why are the risks and repercussions of overtraining so severe in elite athletes?

3. What differentiates the taper from detraining?

4. Why is the taper an important component of a training program for competitive athletes?

5. What is cross-training?

6. How would you plan a training schedule for a runner preparing to compete in a 15 km road race (hilly course) in 4 months? How would this training program change if the event were for a weight lifter preparing for a power lifting competition?

7. Explain how changing repetition number, resistance, and the number of sets can alter the specificity of resistance training.

8. Why is interval training so widely used by athletes involved in training that ranges from resistance training to sprint cycling to marathon running?

APPLICATIONS

1. Do you think the extra training completed by competitive athletes compared with recreationally active individuals adds to increased health and disease prevention?

2. How would you change a cardiorespiratory endurance-training program to suit a more elderly individual with risk factors for coronary artery disease? Why?

REFERENCES

1. Albrecht TJ, Foster VL, Dickinson AL, DeBever JM: Triathletes: exercise parameters measured during bicycle, swim bench, and treadmill testing, *Med Sci Sports Exerc* 18(2):S86, 1986.

2. American College of Sports Medicine: *ACSM's guidelines for exercise testing and prescription,* Baltimore, 1995, Williams & Wilkins.

3. Barnett A: Periodization training with exercise machines, *NSCA* 15(5), 14-16, 1993.

4. Boutcher SS, Seip RL, Hetzler RK et al: The effects of specificity of training on rating of perceived exertion at the lactate threshold, *J Appl Physiol* 59:365-369, 1989.

5. Burke E, Franks BD: Changes in VO$_2$max resulting from bicycle training at different intensities holding total mechanical work constant, *Res Quart* 46:31-37, 1975.

6. Chi MY, Hintz CS, Coyle EF et al: Effects of detraining on enzymes of energy metabolism in individual human muscle fibers, *Am J Physiol* 244(13):C276-C287, 1983.

7. Convertino VA, Brock PJ, Keil LC, Bernauer EM: Exercise training-induced hypervolemia: role of plasma albumin, renin, and vasopressin, *J Appl Physiol* 48(4):665-669, 1980.

8. Costill DL, King DS, Thomas R, Hargreaves M: Effects of reduced training on muscular power of swimmers, *Phys Sports Med* 13:94-101, 1985.

9. Costill DL, Fink WJ, Hargreaves M et al: Metabolic characteristics of skeletal muscle during detraining from competitive swimming, *Med Sci Sports Exerc* 17:339-343, 1985.

10. Costill DL, Flynn MG, Kirwan JP: Effects of repeated days of intensified training on muscle glycogen and swimming performance, *Med Sci Sports Exerc* 20:249-254, 1988.

11. Costill DL, Thomas R, Robergs RA et al: Adaptations to swimming training: influence of training volume, *Med Sci Sports Exerc* 23(3):371-377, 1991.

REFERENCES—Cont'd

12. Coyle EF, Martin III WH, Sinacore DR et al: Time course of loss of adaptations after stopping prolonged intense endurance training, *J Appl Physiol* 57:1857-1864, 1984.

13. Coyle EF, Hemmert MK, Coggan AR: Effects of detraining on cardiovascular responses to exercise: role of blood volume, *J Appl Physiol* 60:95-99, 1986.

14. Davies C, Knibbs A: The training stimulus: the effects of intensity, duration, and frequency of effort on maximum aerobic power output, *Int Z Angew Physiol* 29:299-305, 1971.

15. Dudley G, Abraham W, Terjung R: Influence of exercise intensity and duration on biomechanical adaptations in skeletal muscle, *J Appl Physiol* 59:844-850, 1982.

16. Fleck SJ, Kraemer WJ: *Designing resistance training programs,* Champaign, Illinois, 1987, Human Kinetics Books.

17. Fox EL, Bartels RL, Billings C et al: Intensity and distance of interval training programs and changes in aerobic power, *J Appl Physiol* 38:481-484, 1975.

18. Gillen CM, Lee R, Mack GW et al: Plasma volume expansion in humans after a single intense exercise protocol, *J Appl Physiol* 71(5):1914-1920, 1991.

19. Gonyea WJ, Sale D: Physiology of weightlifting, *Arch Phys Med Rehab* 63:235-237, 1982.

20. Hickson RC, Rosenkoetter MA: Reduced training frequencies and maintenance of aerobic power, *Med Sci Sports Exerc* 13:13-19, 1981.

21. Jensen CR, Fisher AG: *Scientific basis of athletic conditioning,* Philadelphia, 1979, Lea & Febiger.

22. Kirwan JP, Costill DL, Flynn MG: Physiological responses to successive days of intense training in competitive swimmers, *Med Sci Sports Exerc* 20:255-259, 1988.

23. Kojima T: Force-velocity relationship of human elbow flexors in voluntary isotonic contraction under heavy loads, *Int J Sports Med* 12:208-213, 1991.

24. Komi PV, Buskirk ER: Effect of eccentric and concentric muscle conditioning on tension and electrical activity of human muscle, *Ergonomics* 15:417-434, 1972.

25. MacDougall JD, Ward GR, Sale DG, Sutton JR: Biochemical adaptation of human skeletal muscle to heavy resistance training and immobilization, *J Appl Physiol* 43:700-703, 1985.

26. McKenzie DC, Fox EL, Cohen D: Specificity of metabolic and circulatory responses to arm and leg training, *Eur J Appl Physiol* 39:241-248, 1978.

27. Moreira CM, Russo AK, Picarro IC et al: Oxygen consumption and ventilation during constant-load exercise in runners and cyclists, *J Sports Med Phys Fit* 29(1):36-44, 1980.

28. Pechar GS, McArdle WD, Katch FI et al: Specificity of cardiorespiratory adaptation to bicycle and treadmill running, *J Appl Physiol* 36(6):753-756, 1974.

29. Pierce EF, Seip RL, Shead D, Weltman A: Specificity of training on the lactate threshold (LT) and VO_2max, *Med Sci Sports Exerc* 20(2):S38, 1988.

30. Roberts JA, Alspaugh JW: Specificity of training effects resulting from programs of treadmill running and bicycle ergometer riding, *Med Sci Sports Exerc* 4(1):6-10, 1972.

31. Saltin B, Blomqvist G, Mitchell JH et al: Response to submaximal and maximal exercise after bed rest and training, *Circulation* 38(Suppl 7), 1968.

32. Schafer W: *Wellness through stress management,* Davis, California, 1983, International Dialogue Press.

33. Schnieder DA, Lacroix KA, Atkinson GR et al: Ventilatory threshold and maximal oxygen uptake during cycling and running in triathletes, *Med Sci Sports Exerc* 22(2):257-264, 1990.

34. Selye H: *The stress of life,* New York, 1956, McGraw-Hill.

35. Thorstensson A, Larsson L, Tesch P, Karlsson J: Muscle strength and fiber composition in athletes and sedentary men, *Med Sci Sports Exerc* 9:26-30, 1977.

36. Thorstensson AL: Observations on strength training and detraining, *Acta Physiol Scand* 100:491-493, 1977.

37. Tesch PA, Karlsson L: Muscle fiber type and size in trained and untrained muscles of elite athletes, *J Appl Physiol* 59:1716-1723, 1985.

38. Withers RT, Sherman WM, Miller JM, Costill DL: Specificity of the anaerobic threshold in endurance trained athletes, *Eur J Appl Physiol* 47:93-104, 1981.

RECOMMENDED READINGS

■ American College of Sports Medicine: *ACSM's guidelines for exercise testing and prescription,* Baltimore, 1995, Williams & Wilkins.

■ Convertino VA, Brock PJ, Keil LC, Bernauer EM: Exercise training-induced hypervolemia: role of plasma albumin, renin, and vasopressin, *J Appl Physiol* 48(4):665-669, 1980.

■ Costill DL, Fink WJ, Hargreaves M et al: Metabolic characteristics of skeletal muscle during detraining from competitive swimming, *Med Sci Sports Exerc* 17:339-343, 1985.

■ Costill DL, Thomas R, Robergs RA et al: Adaptations to swimming training: influence of training volume, *Med Sci Sports Exerc* 23(3):371-377, 1991.

■ Coyle EF, Martin III WH, Sinacore DR et al: Time course of loss of adaptations after stopping prolonged intense endurance training, *J Appl Physiol* 57:1857-1864, 1984.

■ Coyle EF, Hemmert MK, Coggan AR: Effects of detraining on cardiovascular responses to exercise: role of blood volume, *J Appl Physiol* 60:95-99, 1986.

■ Hickson RC, Rosenkoetter MA: Reduced training frequencies and maintenance of aerobic power, *Med Sci Sports Exerc* 13:13-19, 1981.

■ Kirwan JP, Costill DL, Flynn MG: Physiological responses to successive days of intense training in competitive swimmers, *Med Sci Sports Exerc* 20:255-259, 1988.

■ Pierce EF, Seip RL, Shead D, Weltman A: Specificity of training on the lactate threshold (LT) and VO$_2$max, *Med Sci Sports Exerc* 20(2):S38, 1988.

■ Withers RT, Sherman WM, Miller JM, Costill DL: Specificity of the anaerobic threshold in endurance trained athletes, *Eur J Appl Physiol* 47:93-104, 1981.

CHAPTER **17** # Nutrition and Exercise

OBJECTIVES

After studying this chapter you should be able to:

- List the main macronutrients and micronutrients, and explain why they are important to the body during exercise.

- Detail the importance of the carbohydrate content of the diet for promoting adequate stores of muscle and liver glycogen, and describe how this is obtained.

- List the quantities and types of carbohydrate that best replenish muscle glycogen after exercise.

- State the required types and quantities of carbohydrate to be ingested during exercise, and list the types and durations of exercise in which carbohydrate supplementation may be needed.

- Explain how researchers measure gastric emptying and intestinal absorption, and how these techniques have contributed to research into carbohydrate and fluid nutrition during exercise.

- Describe the types and quantities of carbohydrate that should be ingested to maximize muscle glycogen synthesis during the recovery from prolonged exercise, and explain the nonnutritional factors that influence the rate of muscle glycogen synthesis during recovery.

- Explain why protein amounts above the Recommended Daily Allowance (RDA) might be needed for individuals involved in prolonged endurance exercise or intense exercise.

- Describe the nutritional requirements for prolonged exercise and those for intense exercise, and explain the differences between the two sets of requirements.

KEY TERMS

nutrients	glucose polymers
nutrition	gastric emptying
micronutrients	intestinal absorption
macronutrients	dehydration
vitamins	water intoxication
minerals	hyponatremia
complete proteins	rehydration
glycogen supercompensation	free radicals
rebound hypoglycemia	antioxidants
glycemic index	3-methylhistidine
hyperhydration	nitrogen balance

he movement involved in exercise results from muscle contraction, which requires the breakdown of adenosine triphosphate (ATP) and therefore expends calories. These calories used to regenerate ATP come from a few select molecules, which have been called energy substrates. The body therefore must have a continual supply of energy substrates for optimal exercise performance. There are other molecules, in addition to energy substrates, that the body must have to optimize cellular function during exercise. Essential molecules required for normal bodily function are called *nutrients,* and the study of nutrients and their roles in the body is the science of *nutrition.* Exercise places added nutritional demands on the body, and the exercise physiologist must understand what these demands are, how best they can be met, and how they differ for different exercises and intensities. This chapter presents a review of the nutrients the body requires during exercise and the results of research that has revealed the importance of these nutrients to bodily function before, during, and after exercise.

Nutrients of the Body

utrients can be divided into **micronutrients,** the small compounds that are not catabolized to release free energy during energy metabolism, and **macronutrients,** the nutrients that can be used during energy metabolism. Many of the micronutrients are necessary for optimal catabolism of macronutrients. The important micronutrients and macronutrients of the body and their major functions are presented in Table 17.1.

Micronutrients

The micronutrients can be divided into *vitamins* and *minerals.* **Vitamins** are organic compounds that the body requires in small amounts for health. Vitamins themselves are not used as substrates for energy metabolism; rather, as indicated in Table 17.1, they are required for the catabolism of

nutrients (nu′tri-ents)
food components that can be used by the body

nutrition (nu-trish′un)
the study of the foods and liquids the body needs for optimal functioning

micronutrients (my-kro-nu′tri-ents)
essential food components that are required only in small quantities

macronutrients (ma-kro-nu′tri-ents)
essential food components that are required in large quantities

vitamins (vi′ta-mins)
organic micronutrients of food that are essential to normal bodily functions

TABLE 17.1

Major micronutrients and macronutrients and their functions that support exercise

NUTRIENT	FUNCTIONS SUPPORTING EXERCISE	MAIN NUTRIENT SOURCES
MICRONUTRIENTS		
VITAMINS		
Water soluble		
Thiamine (B_1)	Coenzyme in cellular metabolism	Pork, organ meats, whole grains, legumes
Riboflavin (B_2)	Component of FAD^+ and FMN of the electron transport chain	Most foods
Niacin	Component of NAD^+ and $NADP^+$	Liver, lean meats, grains, legumes
Pyridoxine (B_6)	Coenzyme in metabolism	Meat, vegetables, whole grains
Pantothenic acid	Component of coenzyme A (e.g., acetyl-CoA, fatty acyl-CoA	Most foods
Folacin	Coenzyme of cellular metabolism	Legumes, green vegetables, whole wheat
(B_{12})	Coenzyme of metabolism in nucleus	Muscle meat, eggs, dairy products
Biotin	Coenzyme of cellular metabolism	Meats, vegetables, legumes
Ascorbic acid (C)	Maintains connective tissue; immune protection (?)	Citrus fruits, tomatoes, green peppers
Fat soluble		
ß-carotene (provitamin A)		Green vegetables
Retinol (A)	Sight; component of rhodopsin (visual pigment); maintains tissues	Milk, butter, cheese
Cholecalciferol (D)	Bone growth and maintenance; calcium absorption	Cod liver oil, eggs, dairy products
Tocopherol (E)	Antioxidant; protects cellular integrity	Seeds; green, leafy vegetables; margarine
Phylloquinone (K)	Role in blood clotting	Green, leafy vegetables; cereals; fruits; meat
MAJOR MINERALS		
Calcium (Ca^{2+})	Bone and tooth formation; muscle contraction; action potentials	Milk, cheese, dark green vegetables
Phosphorus (PO^{3-})	Bone and tooth formation; acid-base; chemical energy	Milk, cheese, yogurt, meat, poultry, grains, fish
Potassium (K^+)	Action potential; acid-base; body water balance	Leafy vegetables, cantaloupe, lima beans, potatoes, milk, meat
Sulfur (S)	Acid-base; liver function	Proteins, dried food
Sodium (Na^+)	Action potential; acid-base; osmolality; body water balance	Fruits, vegetables, table salt
Chlorine (cl^-)	Membrane potential; fluid balance	Fruits, vegetables, table salt
Magnesium (Mg^{2+})	Cofactor for enzyme function	Whole grains; green, leafy vegetables
MINOR MINERALS		
Iron (Fe)	Component of hemoglobin, myoglobin, and cytochromes	Eggs; lean meats; legumes; whole grains; green, leafy vegetables
Fluorine (F)	Bone structure (?)	Water, sea food
Zinc (Zn)	Component of enzymes of digestion	Most foods
Copper (Cu)	Component of enzymes of iron metabolism	Meat, water

TABLE 17.1—Cont'd

Major micronutrients and macronutrients and their functions that support exercise

NUTRIENT	FUNCTIONS SUPPORTING EXERCISE	MAIN NUTRIENT SOURCES
Selenium (Se)	Functions with vitamin E	Seafood, meat, grains
Iodine (I)	Component of thyroid hormones	Marine fish and shellfish, dairy products, vegetables, iodized salt
Chromium (Cr)	Required for glycolysis	Legumes, cereals, organ meats
Molybdenum (Mo)	Cofactor for several enzymes	Fats, vegetable oils, meats, whole grains
MACRONUTRIENTS		
CARBOHYDRATES		
Monosaccharides		
Glucose	Essential for neural tissue and blood cell metabolism; required for optimal cellular metabolism	Candies, fruit, processed food, soda
Fructose	Metabolic substrate for the liver	Honey, corn
Galactose	Metabolic substrate for the liver	Breast milk
Disaccharides		
Sucrose	Provides glucose and fructose for energy metabolism	Table sugar, maple syrup, sugar cane
Lactose	No essential role in nutrition	Dairy products
Maltose	No essential role in nutrition	Formed during digestion
Polysaccharides		
Starch	Source of glucose, for storage as glycogen or conversion to fat	Corn, cereal, pasta, bread, beans, peas, potatoes
Fiber	Increases intestinal motility	Fruits, vegetables
LIPIDS		
Cholesterol	Component of cell membrane; precursor for steroid hormone synthesis	Beef liver, eggs, butter, shrimp
Triglycerides and fatty acids	Energy source; insulation; organ protection	Meats, oils, nuts, cheese, whole milk and other dairy products
Omega-3 fatty acids	May improve blood cholesterol and decrease atherosclerosis	Cold-water fish oils
Saturated fat	?	Coconut oil, butter, cream, animal fat
Monounsaturated fat	?	Olives, almonds, avocados, peanuts
Polyunsaturated fat	?	Safflower and sunflower oil, sesame seeds
PROTEIN		
Complete proteins	Cell maintenance, structure, and repair; immune function	Meats, poultry, eggs, cheese, fish, milk
Incomplete proteins	Cell maintenance, structure, and repair; immune function	Legumes, cereal, seeds, leafy vegetables
WATER	Medium for cell reactions, blood, circulation, thermoregulation	Drinking water, juices, sodas, fruits, vegetables

carbohydrates, fats, and protein. In fact, most vitamins are the principal component of coenzymes.

The vitamins are grouped according to their solubility characteristics. The *water-soluble* vitamins consist of the B vitamins and vitamin C. The *fat-soluble* vitamins consist of vitamins A, D, E, and K. Water-soluble vitamins can be stored in the body in small amounts bound to protein structures; however, because this capacity is small, most excess intake is excreted in the urine. Except for vitamin K, fat-soluble vitamins are stored in adipose tissue (fat), and excess intake can lead to symptoms of toxicity. Of the fat-soluble vitamins, vitamins D and K are produced in the body.

Minerals are elements the body needs for a variety of functions. The body requires some minerals in relatively large amounts (calcium, phosphorus, potassium, sulfur, sodium, chloride, and magnesium). Other minerals are needed only in small, or trace, amounts (iron, iodine, manganese, copper, zinc, cobalt, fluorine, selenium, and chromium); these minerals are also known as *trace elements*.

The Recommended Daily Allowance (RDA) of vitamins and minerals is determined by the Food and Nutrition Board of the National Academy of Sciences (see inside front cover). The RDAs are small, vary for individuals of different gender and age, and can range from 0.002 mg for vitamin B_{12} to more than 1 g for sodium, calcium, and phosphorus.

Macronutrients

The macronutrients are carbohydrates, lipids, and proteins. The chemical structure of the common types of each was discussed in Chapters 4 and 5; the functions of the macronutrients are presented in Table 17.1.

It is recommended that a normal, balanced diet get 60% of its total kilocalories (Kcals) from carbohydrates, 30% from fat, and 10% from protein.[144] Of the carbohydrate component, 48% should be from complex carbohydrates and 12% from simple carbohydrates (sucrose, fructose, glucose). Of the fat component, 10% should be from saturated fat, 10% from monounsaturated fat, and the remaining 10% from polyunsaturated fat. As discussed in Chapter 29, saturated fats present a greater risk of the development of increased blood cholesterol and atherosclerotic cardiovascular disease. In reality, the diet of the average citizen in the United States consists of 46% carbohydrates (24% from simple carbohydrates), 42% fat, and 12% protein.[145] The absolute number of calories derived from each food source depends on the total caloric intake, which may vary between 1200 Kcal/day for a small individual who is dieting to more than 5000 Kcal/day for a competitive athlete involved in 3 to 4 hours of training a day.

Of the three macronutrients (carbohydrates, fat, and protein) there is an RDA only for protein: 0.8 g/kg body weight/day.[145] Because the protein RDA is expressed relative to body weight, larger individuals would have increased protein needs. Ironically, the average American eats about twice the RDA for protein.

The *essential amino acids* are those that the body cannot synthesize; for adults this involves eight amino acids: leucine, isoleucine, threonine, lysine, methionine, phenylalanine, tryptophan, and valine. Individuals who do not consume animal or dairy products, which are the main sources of **complete proteins** (those that contain all the essential amino acids), must eat a careful selection of grains, nuts, and legumes to receive all essential amino acids (see Table 17.1).

Fat is categorized into saturated, monounsaturated, and polyunsaturated forms. These divisions relate to the presence of carbon-carbon double bonds. When double bonds are absent from the fatty acid chain, more hydrogen atoms can bind to the carbon chain, creating a *saturated* fat. When one double bond is present, the fat is *monounsaturated*; when more than two double bonds are present, the fat is *polyunsaturated*. The more double bonds and the more polyunsaturated the fat, the more likely it is to be a liquid (oil) at room temperature. Categorizing fats according to saturation has practical application, because saturated fat intake is associated with the development of high blood concentrations of cholesterol and an increased risk of atherosclerotic cardiovascular disease (see Chapter 27).

Humans need some fat in their diet to get the one essential fatty acid, linoleic acid. However, very little fat is required to meet this need. Most people are interested in how to lower the fat contribution to their diet.

Water

Water is an important nutrient because it accounts for approximately 70% of the lean body mass.[84] Water provides the aqueous medium within which the body's reactions occur, and the interactions between charged and uncharged regions of proteins in an aqueous environment produce the structure of many of the body's proteins, as well as many lipid-containing structures, such as the cell membrane.

The body continually replenishes its water content (Figure 17.1). Water is lost through the excretion of urine, the evaporation of sweat, and the humidification of inhaled air. Water is used as a substrate in many chemical reactions and is a product of other chemical reactions. It is recommended that normally active people in a temperate climate get approximately 2.5 L of water a day.[145] This value increases for individuals who live in a hot, humid, or high-altitude environment or who exercise daily. The specific details on the type of fluid and the amounts required during and after exercise are presented in the following sections.

minerals (min'er-als)
inorganic micronutrients that are essential to normal bodily functions

complete proteins
proteins that contain all of the essential amino acids

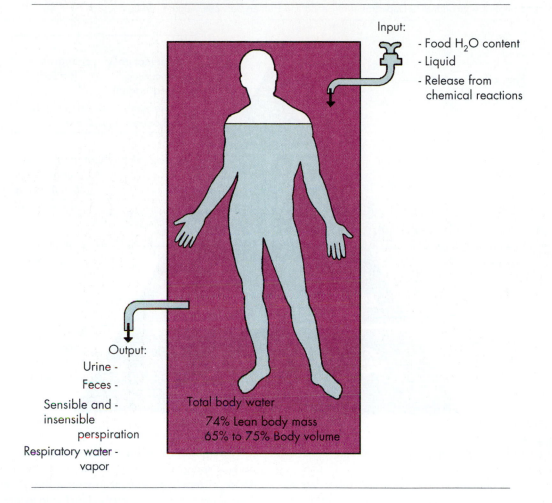

FIGURE 17.1

The various uses of body water, and the sources from which it is replaced within the body.

Input:
- Food H_2O content
- Liquid
- Release from chemical reactions

Output:
Urine -
Feces -
Sensible and - insensible perspiration
Respiratory water - vapor

Total body water
74% Lean body mass
65% to 75% Body volume

Meeting the Body's Nutrient Needs

The need to ingest calories, vitamins, minerals, and water, yet restrict the intake of fat and protein, requires that individuals be selective in their choices of food and liquid. This is true even for athletes because a sound diet provides the foundation for both tolerance of exercise training and optimal performance.

Dividing foods into groups has proved to be a time-tested, successful approach to establishing a balanced diet. Foods have been divided into six main classes: whole-grain cereals, vegetables, fruits, dairy products, meat and poultry, and fats and simple carbohydrates (mainly glucose, sucrose, and fructose). The macronutrients and micronutrients provided by each food group are used to determine the amount of food needed from each group to attain the RDA for micronutrients. For a healthy, low-fat diet that derives at least 60% of kilocalories from carbohydrates, the whole-grain cereals should provide most of the calories, followed by fruits and vegetables, dairy products, and meat and poultry; fats and simple carbohydrates should provide minimal calories (Figure 17.2).

Individuals who exercise regularly especially need a sound diet based on the previously mentioned food groups. However, as is discussed later, participation in regular exercise for extended periods places additional nutritional demands on the body, and depending on the type of exercise performed, minor nutritional modifications can enhance exercise performance.

Optimizing Nutrition For Exercise

The nutritional requirements of exercise place immediate and long-term nutrient intake demands on the body. For example, a single bout of exercise would be tolerated better if an individual had optimal carbohydrate stores and hydration before commencing exercise. Similarly, if this person has been training for several weeks or months, he or she may have long-term nutritional needs that extend beyond the time of an exercise session. For these reasons the information to follow is broadly categorized into

FIGURE 17.2

The USDA's Food Guide Pyramid, which lists and illustrates the recommended number of servings of each major food group for adults. (From: US Department of Agriculture/US Department of Health and Human Services, August, 1992.)

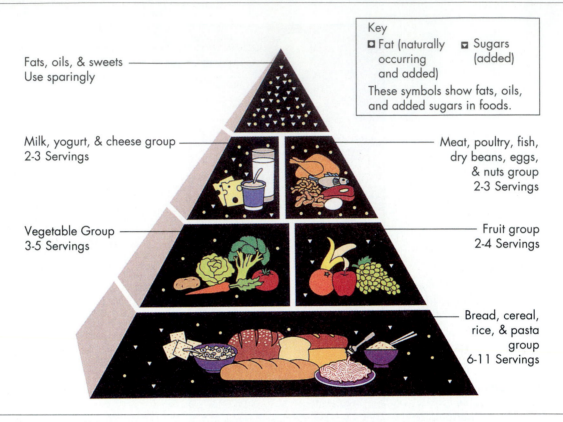

nutritional needs before, during, and after exercise, as well as long-term needs.

These sections contain further categories that relate to micronutrients and macronutrients, the duration and intensity of exercise, and special topics such as the optimal composition of liquid carbohydrate beverages; optimal amounts of carbohydrates before, during, and after exercise; and the factors that determine the rate of postexercise muscle glycogen synthesis.

Macronutrient Concerns Before, During, and After Exercise

From an exercise perspective, the intake of macronutrients serves to replenish muscle and liver glycogen, maintain normal blood glucose concentrations, replenish muscle and adipose tissue triglycerides, maintain cell membrane integrity, and maintain or increase muscle protein. The importance of each of these components changes for exercise of different intensities and the time of ingestion relative to when the exercise is performed.

Prolonged Submaximal Exercise

During prolonged exercise, muscle and liver glycogen, blood glucose, blood free fatty acids (FFAs), muscle FFAs, and blood and muscle amino acids are the substrates used to fuel muscle energy metabolism. The relative priority of these substrates changes for different intensities and durations of exercise, as explained in Chapter 4. During low-intensity exercise, lipid predominates as the primary substrate; the reliance on carbohydrate increases as exercise intensity increases. When the body's stores of carbohydrate become low, the use of lipid and amino acids as substrates for energy metabolism increases[143] (Figure 17.3). The metabolic and hormonal explanations of the regulation of substrate selection and use during different exercise conditions are offered in Chapters 4 and 13.

Because of the body's general need to conserve its stores of amino acids, low-carbohydrate conditions are not recommended during exercise. Low-carbohydrate conditions also diminish exercise performance and increase the perception of fatigue.[1,2,40,99] Understandably, emphasis is placed on having an adequate intake of carbohydrate before exercise to ensure optimal reserves of muscle and liver glycogen.

Preexercise nutrition. The importance of muscle glycogen to exercise performance was first documented by Scandinavian researchers in 1967.[7,8,10,69,76] Since then, hundreds of research studies have been done to further evaluate the importance of carbohydrate intake to muscle glycogen and to

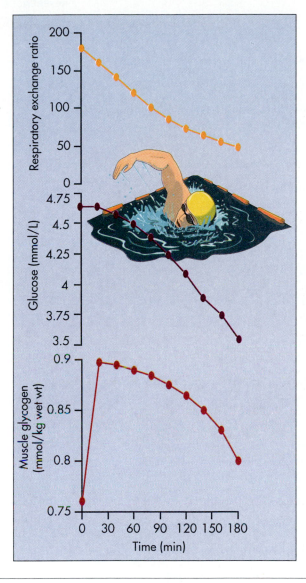

FIGURE 17.3

As muscle glycogen decreases, the body is forced to rely on lipid and amino acid catabolism. As explained in the text, low carbohydrate conditions are detrimental to exercise performance.

prolonged exercise performance (Figure 17.4). The general findings of this research, and the developments in research into nutrition and exercise, are presented in Table 17.2.

In 1967 researchers from Scandinavia also provided evidence that a modified diet strategy in the days preceding an athletic event could increase skeletal muscle glycogen stores.[10] Because this strategy could increase muscle glycogen concentrations above those usually attained with normal dietary practices, this regimen was called **glycogen supercompensation.** As indicated in Figure 17.5, this regimen involved depleting the body's carbohydrate stores through a combination of exhaustive exercise and a low-carbohydrate diet. After this, the athlete was required to reduce training, eat a high-carbohydrate diet, and have a rest day before competition. This regimen took approximately 1 week. The prob-

glycogen supercompensation

a regimen of increased carbohydrate ingestion and modified exercise training that results in maximal storage of glycogen in skeletal muscle

FIGURE 17.4

As an individual increases carbohydrate intake in the days preceeding prolonged exercise, muscle glycogen concentrations increase and the duration at which exercise at approximately 70% VO_2max can be sustained is increased.

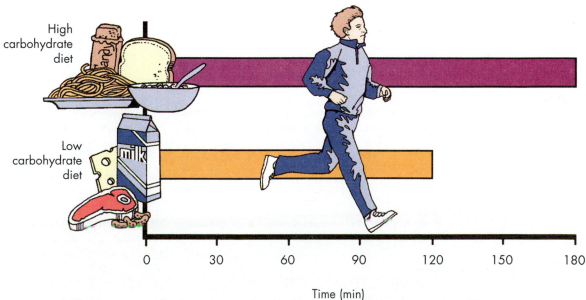

TABLE 17.2

Summary of research findings important to carbohydrate ingestion* before, during, and after exercise

CATEGORY	FINDINGS	REFERENCES
BEFORE EXERCISE		
1960s		
	An increase in the carbohydrate content of the diet before exercise prolongs endurance	10
	An increase in the carbohydrate content of the diet increases muscle glycogen	8-10
	Muscle glycogen stores can be further increased after depletion of muscle glycogen by a low-carbohydrate diet and exhaustive exercise	10
1970s and 1980s		
	Replication of above findings on diet, muscle glycogen, and exercise performance	32,137
	Adequate maximal muscle glycogen concentrations are obtained by decreasing training volume and intensity and increasing the carbohydrate content of the diet	137
	Ingesting fructose before exercise does not increase muscle glycogen or improve exercise performance	48,63,64
DURING EXERCISE		
1980s		
	Carbohydrate ingestion during exercise prevents hypoglycemia and prolongs endurance	25-27,36,37, 47,58,65,100
	Carbohydrate ingestion during continuous submaximal exercise at intensities >65% VO_2max does not spare muscle glycogen	36,47
	Despite carbohydrate ingestion during exercise and normoglycemia, fatigue still develops	25,27
	Giving carbohydrate late in exercise before fatigue develops is just as beneficial as ingestion throughout continuous submaximal exercise	27
	For purposes of hydration and blood glucose supplementation, the optimal concentration and ingestion rate of a carbohydrate beverage is approximately 60 g/L at 1 L/hr	36,53,99, 103,128
1990s		
	The primary determinant of gastric emptying is the volume of the drink	98,111
	Carbohydrate in a drink increases the absorption of water by the small intestine	51-54
	A drink's electrolyte content does not increase carbohydrate delivery to the body	64
	Carbohydrate ingestion during intermittent exercise "spares" muscle glycogen	148
	Solid carbohydrate is just as beneficial as liquid carbohydrate in increasing blood glucose during exercise	91
	The benefits of ingesting carbohydrate and fluid during exercise are independent and additive	59
AFTER EXERCISE		
1980s		
	During the initial hours of recovery, muscle glycogen synthesis is optimized when approximately 0.7 g/kg/hr of carbohydrate is ingested	11-15,71,72,124
	For optimal muscle glycogen synthesis, carbohydrate must be ingested immediately after exercise	72
	Solid and liquid carbohydrate are equally beneficial for postexercise muscle glycogen synthesis	122
	If muscle damage occurs during the exercise, glycogen synthesis is impaired	34,44
	High rates of muscle glycogen synthesis occur immediately after intense exercise to fatigue without carbohydrate ingestion	69,131
1990s		
	Having protein in the carbohydrate beverage increases the rate of muscle glycogen synthesis	150

*Carbohydrate refers to ingestion predominantly of glucose (see Chapter 22).

FIGURE 17.5

The original Scandinavian regimen to increase skeletal muscle glycogen concentrations before exercise and the modified regimen of glycogen supercompensation. (Adapted from Sherman WM et al: *Int J Sports Med* 2(2):114-118, 1981.)

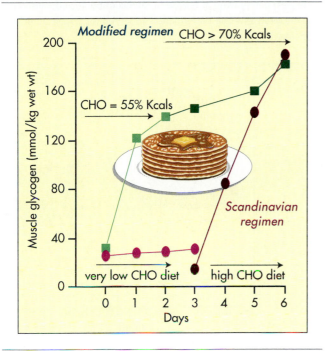

ing muscle glycogen storage as the original Scandinavian approach. Recommendations for optimizing muscle glycogen stores before exercise are presented in Focus Box 17.1.

The preceding guidelines raise questions about the amount of carbohydrate that should be included in a diet for endurance athletes, the extent to which this proportion should be increased during the days before competition, and what types of carbohydrate should be ingested.

Recommended Quantities and Types of Carbohydrate

For an athlete the macronutrient recommendations based on a percentage of total kilocalories are inappropriate because a 5000 Kcal diet would require that these athletes consume 167 g of fat and 125 g of protein and restrict carbohydrate intake to 750 g. For a 75 kg person, this protein intake would be more than twice the RDA of 0.8 g/kg, would waste caloric intake in excess fat, and would equal a daily carbohydrate intake of 10 g/kg. Because carbohydrate is the primary nutrient used during prolonged exercise at moderate to high intensities and because most people have adequate triglyceride stored in adipose tissue, athletes should try to increase caloric intake by increasing carbohydrate. A more realistic comparison of caloric intake is presented in Figure 17.6, in which the percentage of calories from carbohydrate is increased to 70%, with fat intake approximating 20%, and protein intake remaining at 10%. The increase in carbohydrate calories may be achieved in the form of complex or simple carbohydrates, in either liquid or solid form.[61,65,77,91]

One could argue that for individuals expending more than 5000 Kcal/day, less fat intake could be recommended; however, a diet lower than 20% fat in today's society would require considerable effort in planning and preparation and therefore would be time consuming. One has to admire the individuals who succeed in following a diet in which fat contributes less than 20% of total kilocalories. The dietary concerns of exercise, food intake, and body fat reduction are discussed in Chapter 29.

lem was that the process of carbohydrate depletion is physically and mentally uncomfortable, especially in the week before competition. For this reason, other researchers studied athletes' ability to increase muscle glycogen stores simply by altering the number of training sessions and intensities and by increasing the carbohydrate content of the diet during the week before competition[137] (Figure 17.5). For trained athletes this modified regimen was just as beneficial in increas-

FOCUS BOX 17.1

Recommendations for increasing muscle glycogen stores in the days before prolonged exercise

1. Plan to taper at least 1 week before the event.

2. In the final week, train as planned and eat your typical diet during the first 3 days.

3. For the 3 days before the day of the event, increase the carbohydrate content of the diet to more than 10 g/kg body weight/day.

4. Refrain from training the day before the event.

5. Eat your final meal at least 3 hours before the event.

Adapted from Bergstrom J, Hermansen L, Saltin B: *Acta Physiol Scand* 71:140-150, 1967; Sherman Wm, Costill DL, Fink WJ, Miller JM: *Int J Sports Med* 2(2):114-118, 1981.

FIGURE 17.6

For athletes, the recommended percentage contributions of carbohydrate, fat, and protein should be altered to reflect greater carbohydrate content, less fat content, and similar protein content.

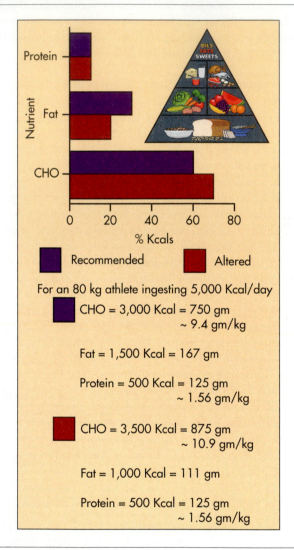

For an 80 kg athlete ingesting 5,000 Kcal/day

CHO = 3,000 Kcal = 750 gm
~ 9.4 gm/kg

Fat = 1,500 Kcal = 167 gm

Protein = 500 Kcal = 125 gm
~ 1.56 gm/kg

CHO = 3,500 Kcal = 875 gm
~ 10.9 gm/kg

Fat = 1,000 Kcal = 111 gm

Protein = 500 Kcal = 125 gm
~ 1.56 gm/kg

FIGURE 17.7

When exercise is performed within 30 to 45 minutes after the
ingestion of simple carbohydrate, the muscle contraction combined with increased circulating insulin can lower blood glucose
concentrations. This hypoglycemia can be accompanied by
increased perceptions of fatigue or ratings of perceived exertion
and impaired exercise performance. (Adapted for Costill DL et al: *J
Appl Physiol* 43:965-999, 1977.)

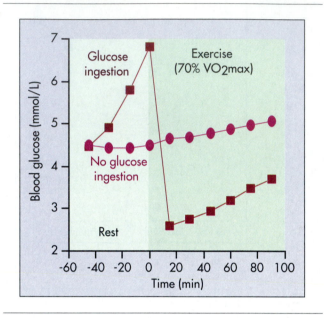

Ingestion of fat or protein before exercise is not beneficial for optimizing muscle and liver glycogen stores. Also,
when a meal is high in fat and protein, gastric emptying is
delayed and the blood acid–base balance in the resting state
can be detrimentally affected, impairing subsequent exercise
performance.[57-59,94] Nevertheless, research done on increasing
FFA concentrations in the blood during exercise, by ingesting lipid, infusing heparin to increase blood FFA mobilization from circulating triglycerides, or both, has shown that
high FFA concentrations in the blood increase lipid catabolism for a given exercise intensity and even spares muscle
glycogen.[33,62,142] These findings are tempting to recommend
as not even glucose ingestion during continuous exercise
spares muscle glycogen. However, there is no evidence that

such a dietary strategy can support exercise performance similar to the way carbohydrate does, and based on muscle biochemistry, a reduction in exercise performance would be
expected from a decreased capacity of contracting skeletal
muscle to catabolize carbohydrate (see Chapter 4).

Timing of Carbohydrate Ingestion Before Exercise

Evidence exists to question the use of carbohydrate at
certain times before the start of exercise. In 1977 Costill et
al.[33] reported that ingesting carbohydrate and increasing
blood glucose 30 to 60 minutes before exercise can increase
blood insulin concentrations. When exercise commences, the
increased uptake of glucose by skeletal muscle from contraction and the increased insulin can rapidly lower blood glucose concentrations, causing what was called **rebound
hypoglycemia** (Figure 17.7). Evidence has also been presented that muscle glycogenolysis increases under these conditions, resulting in the risk of prematurely lowered muscle

rebound hypoglycemia

*the decrease in blood glucose that occurs when a person
exercises at least 30 minutes after ingesting carbohydrate*

Glycemic Index: Clinical and Applied Use

Nutritionists have developed a rating that compares different foods' ability to raise blood glucose concentrations. This value is called the **glycemic index,** and the blood glucose response to the ingestion of different foods is illustrated in Figure 17.8. The reference standard for the glycemic index is the blood glucose response to the ingestion of white bread.[145] This reference point is the area under the blood glucose concentration curve and is a value of 100. Other foods that have the same quantity of carbohydrate are compared as a percentage of this reference. Table 17.3 lists the glycemic index values for several carbohydrate-containing foods.

In general, more complex carbohydrates yield a lower glycemic index value than simple forms. However, the glycemic index does not just reflect the type of carbohydrate in the food; foods with a greater fat or fiber content than white bread produce a slower digestion of carbohydrate and less of an increase in blood glucose.

Use of the glycemic index has proved important for both type I and type II diabetics. An individual with diabetes has an enlarged blood glucose response to a given carbohydrate food owing to an inadequate insulin response, or an impaired ability at the cellular level to respond to insulin (see Chapter 13). This impairment can easily be documented following a standard ingestion of glucose (Figure 17.9). For example, in the glucose tolerance test the person ingests 75 g of glucose, and blood samples are drawn at repeated intervals for analysis of blood glucose concentrations.[145] Compared to normal controls, type II diabetics have a much greater and more prolonged increase in blood glucose. Thus, to avoid large increases in blood glucose, individuals with diabetes should avoid foods with a high glycemic index value.

The glycemic index also has been used to determine the best type of carbohydrate for promoting increases in muscle glycogen during the hours immediately after exercise.[20,73,78] As explained in the text, foods with a high glycemic index value are better for optimizing muscle glycogen synthesis in the first 2 hours after exercise.[20,72]

glycemic index

a rating of the increase in blood glucose after ingestion of a standard amount of carbohydrate; the rating is based on a comparison to the blood glucose response after ingestion of an equivalent amount of carbohydrate in the form of white bread

FIGURE 17.8

The different blood glucose responses to the ingestion of equal carbohydrate amounts from different food sources. The expression of the blood glucose response as a percentage of the glucose response to white bread ingestion is referred to as the glycemic index.

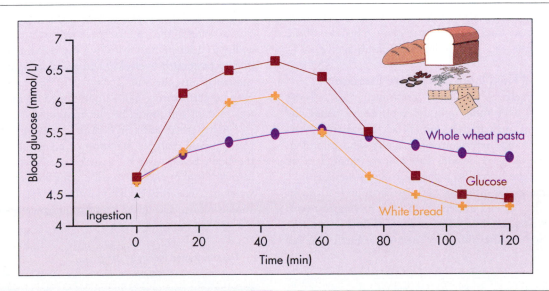

TABLE 17.3

Glycemic index of some sources of carbohydrate

FOOD	GLYCEMIC INDEX VALUE
Cornflakes	121
Instant mashed potatoes	120
Whole wheat bread	100
Baked beans	70
Skim milk	46
White pasta (boiled)	45
Lentils (boiled)	36

Adapted from Burke L, Collier GR, Hargreaves M: *J Appl Physiol* 75(2):1019-1023, 1993.

FIGURE 17.9

The difference in blood glucose response to an identical amount of ingested glucose between an individual with type II diabetes and a normal control. (Source: Wardlaw GM, Insel PM: *Perspectives in nutrition*, 3 ed, St. Louis, 1996, Mosby.)

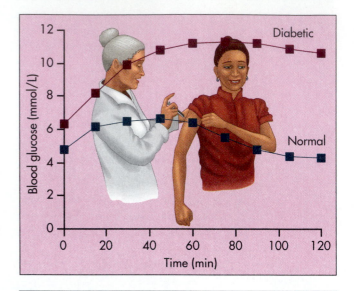

glycogen concentrations and diminished prolonged exercise performance.[33]

Despite the risk of rebound hypoglycemia, ingesting carbohydrate before exercise should not be totally avoided. A large meal can be eaten up to 6 hours before competition, and smaller meals that provide less than 100 g of carbohydrate can be ingested up to 45 minutes before exercise without impairing performance.[*] Such added carbohydrate ingestion can further ensure maximal muscle and liver glycogen stores. Added carbohydrate also can be ingested in a liquid or carbohydrate form within 15 minutes before exercise. This short interval, especially if it includes a warm-up, does not provide enough time for insulin to increase in the blood. In addition, exercise performed during or shortly after carbohydrate ingestion depresses the body's insulin response to a given increase in blood glucose, and the rebound hypoglycemic response is avoided. Ingestion of fructose before exercise does not have the same time constraints as glucose because of the low glycemic response[117] (see Clinical Application on p. 437).

Hydration and Fluid Ingestion Before Exercise

During exercise, the body continually loses water through sweat. This fluid must be replaced to retard the development of dehydration and its accompanying detriments to endurance performance. Athletes who intend to exercise for prolonged periods can prepare themselves by ensuring adequate hydration before starting to exercise.

One strategy for ensuring optimal nutrition is to ingest excess fluid the day and evening before the prolonged event. This ensures adequate hydration, and excess fluid is removed from the body by the kidneys. However, research also has identified procedures to increase the body's fluid stores, a process called **hyperhydration**.

For hyperhydration to occur, the intravascular and extravascular compartments must be able to attract and retain added water, and in doing so prevent it from being filtered by the kidneys. Experimental procedures have succeeded in achieving this by infusing an osmotic agent into the blood to retain water in the vascular space; this method has been shown to increase blood volume by 400 ml.[101] Expanding the blood volume by this method results in increased venous return and associated improvements in cardiovascular function (increased stroke volume, lowered heart rate) and enhances endurance performance. However, osmotic retention of water in the vascular space neither increases the body's ability to dissipate heat nor slows the rise in core temperature during prolonged exercise.[101] In addition, infusing a foreign substance into the vascular space of the body to enhance exercise performance can be questioned on medical and ethical grounds and should not be condoned.

A hyperhydration procedure based on nutritional supplementation involves ingestion of glycerol, a metabolite of the body, before exercise. Ingestion of glycerol in a liquid form (<50 g/L) also has been proven to increase total body water and, like artificial plasma volume expansion, it increases venous return during exercise and enhances exercise perfor-

[*]References 39, 48, 55, 56, 64, 82, 102, 135, and 136.

hyperhydration (hi'per-hy'dra-shun)
an increase in body water content to above normal

FIGURE 17.10

Before exercise, increased total body water stores can be attained from the ingestion of fluid containing less than 50 gm/L of glycerol. This process of hyperhydration can decrease urine output and increase total body weight (body fluid content), and result in improved exercise performance as measured by decreased heart rates, lower rectal temperatures, and prolonged exercise durations until volitional fatigue.

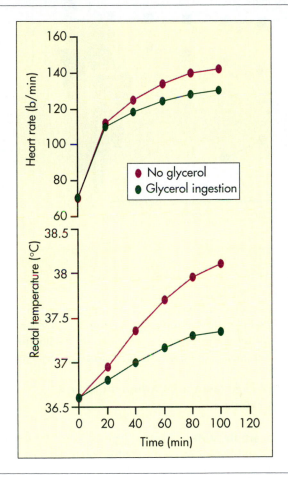

tal muscle. The duration that optimal muscle glycogen stores can supply substrate for energy metabolism can be estimated. For running, we can assume a prime moving muscle mass of 20 kg; if an individual is running at an exercise intensity requiring 2 LO$_2$/min at a respiratory exchange ratio (RER) of 1.0, the energy expenditure would be 10.1 Kcal/min.[116] For an efficiency of 40% for the complete oxidation of glucose from glycogen (–277.4/–686 Kcal/mol), these values would enable muscle glycogen stores to support running for a duration of 110 minutes (see calculation). The contribution of blood glucose derived from the liver to skeletal muscle metabolism would prolong this time.

Kilocalories from glycogen:

$$\underset{\text{(Kcal/mol)}}{277.4} \times \underset{\text{(mol glycogen/kg muscle)}}{0.2} \times \underset{\text{(kg)}}{20} = \underset{\text{(Kcal)}}{1{,}109.6}$$

Kilocalories expended during exercise when:
VO$_2$ = 2 L/min and RER = 1:

$$\underset{\text{(LO}_2\text{/min)}}{2} \times \underset{\text{(Kcal/min)}}{5.05} = \underset{\text{(Kcal/min)}}{10.1}$$

Exercise duration:

$$\underset{\text{(Kcal)}}{1{,}109.6} \div \underset{\text{(Kcal/min)}}{10.1} = \underset{\text{(min)}}{109.86,\text{ or }110}$$

The main interpretation of the previous calculation is this: when carbohydrate is used as the predominant substrate, exercise cannot be maintained for much longer than 2 hours. After this time muscle and liver glycogen stores are at risk of being depleted and continued exercise will require ingestion of carbohydrate to prevent hypoglycemia, as well as to delay fatigue and its accompanying detriments to exercise performance.

Figure 17.11 illustrates the ergogenic benefit provided by ingestion of carbohydrate during prolonged exercise. Research has shown that this benefit can be obtained when carbohydrate is ingested at repeated intervals during exercise,* or simply 30 minutes before the expected time of fatigue[27] (Figure 17.11). The interpretation of this finding is that carbohydrate ingestion during prolonged, continuous exercise at 65% to 75% VO$_2$max does not spare muscle glycogen, but simply provides an added supplement to blood glucose, which becomes important only when muscle glycogen stores are near depletion and blood glucose then becomes the main source of glucose for the contracting muscle.[27,28,38] Conversely, research into continuous exercise performed at low intensities (<60% VO$_2$max) indicates that muscle glycogen is spared because of a larger insulin response from ingesting carbohydrate, compared with exercise performed at or above 70% VO$_2$max.[64,148] Because continuous exercise during competition is performed at or above 70% VO$_2$max, the findings of glycogen sparing during carbohydrate ingestion have

mance[87,103,129] (Figure 17.10). Unlike artificial plasma volume expansion, glycerol hydration does dampen the increase in core temperature during prolonged exercise and therefore has thermoregulatory as well as cardiovascular benefits.[87] When combined with carbohydrate ingestion during exercise (see sections to follow), hyperhydration may provide an athlete with a distinct advantage during prolonged exercise or exercise in a hot or humid environment, compared with athletes who rely on fluid ingestion during exercise to offset dehydration.[101,129]

Nutrition during exercise. The store of glycogen is limited in skeletal muscle and the liver; it is approximately 150 to 250 mmol/kg and 300 to 350 mmol/kg wet weight, respectively. Because of the much larger mass of muscle tissue relative to the liver, far greater total glycogen stores are found in skele-

---

*References 25, 28, 40, 42, 45, 47, 49, 87, 95, 100, 104, 108, 118, and 147.

FIGURE 17.11

The ingestion of carbohydrate high in glucose content during exercise can increase blood glucose concentrations, and prolong the exercise duration to volitional fatigue. Carbohydrate ingestion late in exercise can produce similar results. (Adapted from references 25, 27, 37, and 106.)

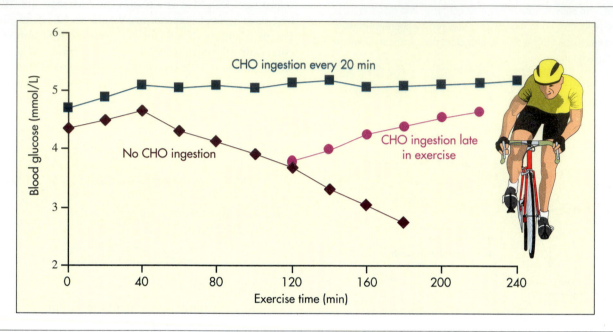

FIGURE 17.12

The different rates of gastric emptying for different volumes of liquid for different types and concentrations of carbohydrate. For a given carbohydrate content and type, greater emptying occurs when the drink volume is increased.

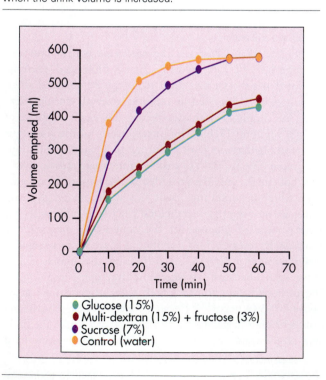

limited practical significance. Carbohydrate ingestion during intermittent exercise also may increase muscle glycogen synthesis during the recovery intervals, thereby prolonging the time until muscle and liver glycogen stores are depleted.[148]

Optimal Fluid and Carbohydrate Ingestion During Exercise

Liquid carbohydrate. Various types of carbohydrate are available, and these can be ingested in either liquid or solid forms. Research of liquid carbohydrate ingestion during exercise reveals the preference of glucose as the main form of carbohydrate. Drinks too high in fructose may irritate the stomach, thereby slowing gastric emptying[19,31,93] (see Table 17.4 and Figure 17.12). In addition, fructose is poorly taken up by skeletal muscle and poorly incorporated into glycolysis, and it is not effective in raising blood glucose concentrations. Conversely, fructose is a good gluconeogenic substrate for the liver. Drinks can also contain connected chains of glucose molecules, called **glucose polymers**, such as *multidextran*. Originally these forms of carbohydrate were thought to aid gastric emptying by providing carbohydrate calories with fewer particles in solution, or a lower *osmolality* (see Focus Box 17.2.) However, research has shown that drinks with this form of carbohydrate do not empty faster than pure glucose or glucose-fructose solutions of a similar carbohydrate content.[93,99]

The amount of carbohydrate that must be ingested to provide an ergogenic effect is approximately 45 to 60 g/hr.[28,36]

TABLE 17.4

Carbohydrate and electrolyte contents of selected liquid carbohydrate beverages and solid foods that contain high amounts of carbohydrate

	CARBOHYDRATE		FAT	PROTEIN	ELECTROLYTE CONTENT (mEq/L)			OSMOLALITY*
	g/L	(MAIN SOURCE)	(g)	(g)	NA⁺	K⁺	OTHER	(mOsm/L)
BEVERAGE								
Gatorade	6	Sucrose, glucose powder	—	—	110	25	Cl, P	280-360
Exceed	7.2	Glucose polymers, fructose	—	—	50	45	Cl, Ca, Mg, P	250
10K	6.3	Sucrose, fructose, glucose	—	—	52	26	Vitamin C; Cl, P	350
Coca-Cola	10.7-111.3	High-fructose corn syrup	—	—	9.2	Trace	P	600-715
Sprite	10.2	High-fructose corn syrup, sucrose	—	—	28	Trace		695
Cranberry juice	15	High-fructose corn syrup, sucrose	—	—	10	61	Vitamin C	890
Orange juice	11.8	Fructose, sucrose, glucose	—	—	2.7	510	P, Ca; vitamins C, A, niacin, riboflavin, thiamine; Fe	690
Water	—	—			Low†	Low†	Low†	10-20
SOLID CARBOHYDRATE‡								
Power Bar (65 g)	42	High-fructose corn syrup, oat bran, maltodextrin	10	2	60	120	Niacin; Ca, P, Mg, Zn, Fe, Cu, Cr; vitamins D, E, B₅, B₆, B₁₂	—
Banana (medium)	26.7	Starch	0.6	1.2	1	11.5	Ca, Fe; vitamins B₁, B₂, B₆, A, C; Zn	—
Orange (medium)	17.4	Fructose	0.3	1.1	1	254	Ca, Fe; vitamins B₁, B₂, B₆, A, C; Zn	—

* The osmolality of body fluids is 280 mOsm/L.
† Depending on water source.
‡ Ingredient concentrations are in g/serving or mEq/serving.
Ca, calcium; *Cl*, chloride; *Cr*, chromium; *Cu*, cooper; *Fe*, iron; *K⁺*, potassium; *Mg*, magnesium; *Na⁺*, sodium; *P*, phosphorus; *Zn*, zinc.

Presumably, enough carbohydrate is needed to raise blood glucose concentrations and in turn increase glucose uptake by skeletal muscle.

The optimal carbohydrate concentration for a drink to be ingested during exercise is specific to the individual and the environmental conditions that predominate during the exercise session. Research has presented contradictory findings on the carbohydrate concentrations that result in slower rates of gastric emptying compared with a water–electrolye solution. When different sampling methods are considered, it generally is accepted that drink concentrations over 80 g/L empty more slowly from the stomach than water, may cause gastric distress, and obviously may be detrimental to exercise performance.[38,93,111,112] Research on intestinal absorption also supports these findings.[42,51-54,93] However, there is marked individual variability in the gastric emptying of carbohydrate solutions and the incidence of GI distress.[4,93] A carbohydrate concentration approximating 60 g/L or less is more appropriate for fluid delivery than more concentrated solutions.

Table 17.5 presents a range of carbohydrate concentrations and volumes in drinks that can be ingested to hydrate the body and support energy metabolism during exercise. The higher the carbohydrate concentration, the greater the carbohydrate delivery to the body—but the lower the fluid delivery is, due to impaired gastric emptying, especially for drinks that provide more than 120 g/L of carbohydrate (Figure 17.13). Nevertheless, because of the overriding influence of the volume of a drink on gastric emptying, it is unclear whether frequent ingestion that maintains a larger gastric

glucose polymers

glucose residues that connect to form a chain structure

TABLE 17.5

Volume of drink at given carbohydrate concentrations that must be ingested every 20 minutes to provide certain amounts of carbohydrate per hour

DRINK CARBOHYDRATE CONCENTRATION (g/L)	DRINK VOLUME (ml) HOURLY AMOUNT OF CARBOHYDRATE INGESTION (g)						
	30	35	40	45	50	55	60
20	500	583	667	750	833	917	1000
30	333	389	444	500	555	611	667
40	250	291	333	375	416	458	500
50	200	233	267	300	333	367	400
60	167	194	222	250	278	306	333
70	142	167	190	214	238	262	286
80	125	145	166	187	208	227	250
90	111	130	148	167	185	204	222
100	100	116	133	150	166	183	200
110	91	106	121	135	151	167	182
120	83	97	111	125	139	153	166
150	67	78	89	100	111	122	133
200	50	65	74	75	83	91	100

Adapted from Coyle EF, Montain SJ: *Med Sci Sports Exerc* 24(6):671-678, 1992.

volume or infrequent, larger fluid intakes are more desirable for fluid delivery. Figure 17.14 illustrates the results from research that demonstrates the exponential decline in gastric volume after ingestion and that repeated ingestion increases gastric volume. It is reasonable to assume that if an individual can tolerate maintained moderate volumes of gastric contents during exercise, fluid and carbohydrate delivery to the body would be increased.

Since research has shown that provision of carbohydrate may not be important until late in exercise for prolonged, continuous events,[27,28] a low-concentration drink may be recommended for the first 60 to 90 minutes for fluid replenishment purposes. During the last 30 to 60 minutes of a long-term activity, a drink with an increased carbohydrate concentration would be needed. Similarly, if environmental conditions are hot and humid, a drink low in carbohydrate would favor fluid delivery to the body and therefore help prevent dehydration and hyperthermia. Because the maximal rate of gastric emptying approximates 1200 ml/hour,[36] a carbohydrate concentration and drink volume association that provides close to 1 L/hour would be recommended for hydration purposes. As indicated in Table 17.5, drinks with a carbohydrate concentration between 40 to 80 g/L would satisfy these requirements.

It must be understood that research has shown only that carbohydrate ingestion during exercise is beneficial during prolonged exercise when muscle glycogen concentrations are near depletion and blood glucose concentrations decline to less than 3 mmol/L.[28,40] With adequate preexercise nutrition, there is no metabolic or ergogenic need to ingest carbohydrate during continuous exercise that lasts less than 90 minutes. This is important because carbohydrate ingestion during short-term exercise becomes a situation of excess caloric intake, and this is counterproductive for individuals who exercise as a means to generate a caloric deficit. However, since carbohydrates and fluids during exercise have independent benefits for exercise performance,[6] fluid intake should always be of concern during exercise.

Solid carbohydrate. Although the research into carbohydrate ingestion before, during, and after exercise has predominantly focused on beverages, blood glucose is also maintained during exercise when solid carbohydrate supplementation is provided.[65,73,91] Of course, water is also recommended to aid

FIGURE 17.13

The relationship between the carbohydrate content of a drink and each of carbohydrate and fluid delivery to the body. (Adapted from Mitchell JB: et al: *Med Sci Sports Exerc* 21:269-274, 1989.)

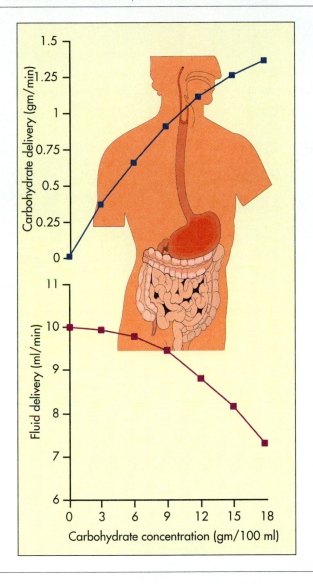

FIGURE 17.14

The exponential decrease in gastric emptying after the ingestion of liquid carbohydrate. These decreases are presented when **A,** drinks are repeatedly ingested during exercise, and **B,** when one large bolus of liquid is ingested. (Adapted from Rehrer NJ et al: *Med Sci Sports Exerc* 21:540-549, 1989.)

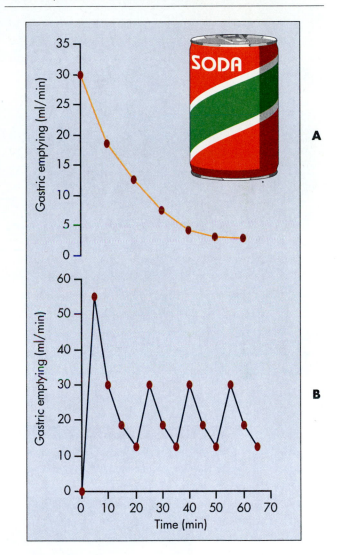

digestion of food and emptying from the stomach and to prevent exercise-induced dehydration.

Hydration and fluid ingestion during exercise. The importance of fluid ingestion before exercise was discussed previously. When a person exercises in a hot or humid environment, the body can lose water at a maximal rate of 2 to 3 L/hour through sweat (Figure 17.18); most of this fluid comes from the cells and interstitial spaces of the body,[29,110] resulting in **dehydration.** However, the largest relative decrease in fluid volume occurs from the vascular compartment (decreased plasma volume). Obviously, without fluid

replacement these rates of water loss cannot be maintained for long. Figure 17.18 illustrates the decrease in performance and the greater physiologic strain on the body during exercise when fluid ingestion is prevented. If fluid is not provided, the rate of sweating declines, which adds to the risks of heat illness, as is explained in Chapter 26.

Text Continues on p. 447.

dehydration (de-hi-dra'shun)
a decrease in body water content to below normal

FOCUS BOX 17.2

Measurement and regulation of gastric emptying and intestinal absorption

The knowledge we have of the suitability of certain drinks to provide carbohydrate and electrolytes to the body is based on research using techniques that measure the emptying of solutions from the stomach **(gastric emptying),** and the absorption of carbohydrate and electrolytes by the small intestine **(intestinal absorption).**

Gastric Emptying

Gastric emptying can be measured in a variety of ways, including expiration of gastric contents via a nasogastric tube[31] (Figure 17.15) or repeated sampling of gastric contents via a nasogastric tube[125-128], or by methods involving adding radioactive substances to a drink and monitoring gastric emptying from the movement of the radioactivity into the small intestine.[4]

The nasogastric tube method is the most common technique. A tube is placed up the nose and down the esophagus into the stomach. The tube has many openings near the distal end, and a suction syringe is attached to the start of the tube. The subject drinks the required solution and then performs exercise or the activity of interest for the study. The drink is usually modified by the addition of a dye. The dye is needed to allow detection of fluid that is secreted by the stomach and therefore allow calculation of the fluid and carbohydrate that are emptied. The remain-ing gastric contents usually are completely removed at the end of the study, after all the fluid has been ingested. Basically, the solution remaining in the stomach, when corrected for gastric secretion, is subtracted from the total volume ingested and is the volume that was emptied.

Scientists from Holland modified a similar strategy,[126] allowing sampling during exercise, called the *double-sampling* technique. This technique allows repeated measurement of gastric emptying to be obtained during the exercise conditions (Figure 17.16). This method allows calculation of gastric emptying at repeated intervals, providing knowledge of how emptying occurs after each ingestion of liquid or of the consistency of gastric emptying under different conditions of hydration or fatigue within the same exercise bout.

gastric emptying
the emptying of the stomach contents into the small intestine

intestinal absorption
the absorption of water and organic and inorganic nutrients from the small intestine

FIGURE 17.15

The sampling of gastric contents through a naso-gastric tube, and the accompanying results that can be obtained (volume emptied, gastric secretion, and carbohydrate delivery).

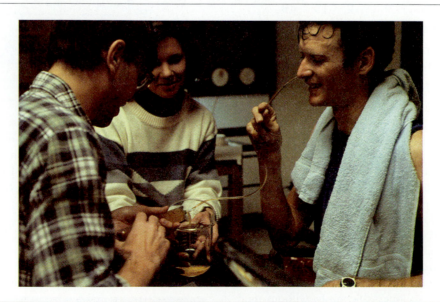

FOCUS BOX 17.2—Cont'd

Measurement and regulation of gastric emptying and intestinal absorption

Finally, researchers have determined the rate of gastric emptying by detecting the movement of a radioactive tracer in the drink as it passes from the stomach to the duodenum.[4] Although arguably the most accurate method, it exposes the subject to greater risk, presents postural restrictions on the subject during exercise, and must be done in a hospital. Also, research has shown that the double-sampling gastric intubation method provides similar results.[4]

Regulation

Many factors combine to influence the rate at which fluid empties from the stomach (Figure 17.17). Of these, the main factors are the volume of the drink and the carbohydrate content.* The stomach's maximal ability to empty fluid has not been adequately researched and is a difficult capacity to measure and interpret because of the differences in drink volumes and carbohydrate contents used in previous research. Nevertheless, researchers have approximated this capacity to be 1 to 1.2 L/hour, and repeated ingestion of fluid is required so that gastric volume remains greater than 100 to 200ml.[93,125-128] For many individuals, such a sustained high gastric volume may cause symptoms of gastric distress,[19] which would not be conducive to optimal exercise performance. It is important

*References 18, 70, 93, 94, 96, 107, and 111.

Continued.

Data obtained from the repeated sampling of gastric contents using a naso-gastric tube.

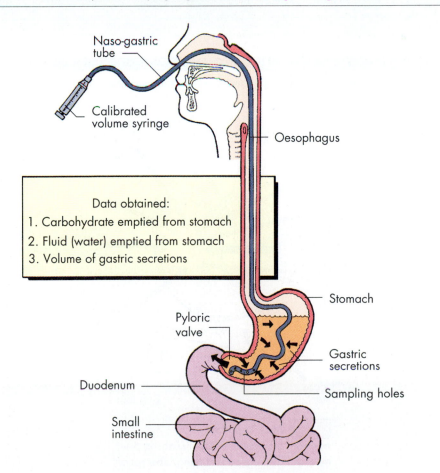

FOCUS BOX 17.2—Cont'd

Measurement and regulation of gastric emptying and intestinal absorption

that individuals experiment within themselves to find the carbohydrate concentration and gastric volume they can tolerate during exercise.[120]

Intestinal absorption

The emptying of fluid from the stomach may not mean that the fluid and carbohydrate will enter the blood at a similar rate. Research done on the measurement of carbohydrate and fluid absorption by the small intestine has confirmed this concern.

To measure the intestinal absorption of carbohydrate and electrolyte solutions, researchers place a special nasogastric tube down the esophagus, into the stomach, and through the pylorus into the duodenum.[51,53,54] This tube is actually several tubes in one, with each tube being of different length and having a separate end opening. The placement of the tube is confirmed by x-ray or other imaging techniques. Because the multiple openings at the end of the tube are located at different distances, sampling of the intestinal contents can occur at different positions within the duodenum. The farther the sampling from the pylorus, the greater the time for absorption of water, carbohydrate, and electrolytes by the intestinal mucosa that lines the lumen of the duodenum or jejunum of the small intestine. The absorption of water and carbohydrate are calculated according to the different concentrations of the sample contents and nonabsorbable marker in the solutions from each tube.

Regulation

Absorption of water, electrolytes, and glucose by the intestinal mucosa occurs in concert (Figure 17.17). Glucose is absorbed by a sodium-glucose active cotransport process, which is why several researchers propose that glucose absorption should be aided by drinks containing sodium.[93] However, as explained in the text, there is no research evidence to support this. Water moves across the intestinal border in either direction by the processes of diffusion and osmosis. Thus, when nutrients are absorbed, water is also absorbed. However, if the stomach releases hyperosmotic solutions into the small intestine, water moves from the intestinal mucosal cells into the chyme, reducing the osmolality of the chyme.[110] Conversely, when hypotonic solutions are released into the small intestine, electrolytes are released into the chyme.

FIGURE 17.17

The multiple factors that combine to regulate gastric emptying and intestinal absorption of liquid carbohydrate beverages.

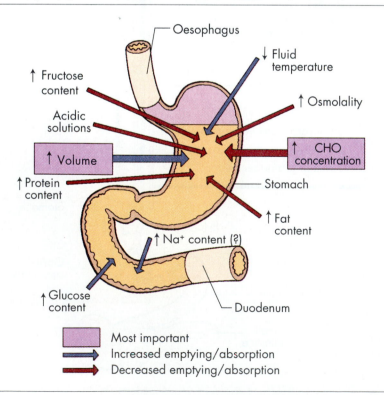

fluid delivery to the body.[53,54] Gisolfi et al.[53] demonstrated that water absorption by the small intestine was increased sixfold by the presence of 60 g CHO/L and of electrolytes (20 mEq Na^+ and 2.6 mEq K^+) in the drink, and this was the basis for the previous recommendation of ingesting low-carbohydrate-concentrated drinks during the early stages of a prolonged endurance event (Table 17.6).

Despite the difficulty in ingesting large amounts of fluid during prolonged exercise, some individuals have accomplished this. If the fluid ingested at such large volumes has a low osmolality, individuals are at risk of developing **water intoxication.**[106] This condition can be dangerous because large volumes of fluid with a low osmolality attract electrolytes from the blood bathing the stomach and small intestine, resulting in a lowering of the serum sodium concentration to below 130 mEq/L; this condition is called **hyponatremia.**[109,112] During ultraendurance events the incidence of hyponatremia has been reported to be 0.03% of all competitors, with at least a 10% incidence among runners who collapse and require medical assistance.[109]

Based on previous information, most individuals are in a constant state of fluid deficit during exercise that is intense enough to induce profuse sweating. Clearly, adequate hydration must be ensured during exercise, in combination with adequate hydration before exercise, to reduce the magnitude of dehydration during exercise more effectively. Despite the media and research interest in carbohydrate ingestion during exercise, failing to ingest fluid during exercise is more detrimental to exercise performance than is failing to ingest carbohydrate. Consequently, for all endurance events, fluid ingestion should be the primary concern.

Postexercise nutrition. Many athletes need to train several times in one day, or they compete within events that require them to perform prolonged exercise bouts on consecutive days (e.g., Tour de France cycle race). These demands require that the individual attempt to optimize the recovery process with regard to hydration and muscle glycogen synthesis.

Rehydration after Exercise

Of course, the best strategy for treating dehydration is prevention. However, as previously explained, most individuals have difficulty replacing fluid equal to its loss during prolonged exercise, especially in a competitive environment. Therefore exercise-induced dehydration is always a concern, and for this reason research has been conducted to determine

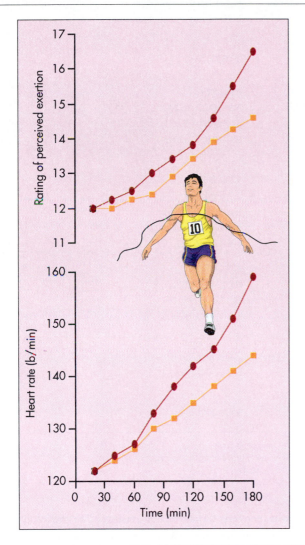

FIGURE 17.18

During prolonged exercise inducing profuse sweating, the body can become dehydrated, resulting in increases in heart rate and perceptions of fatigue. When liquid is ingested during exercise, the increase in heart rate and perceptions of fatigue are each depressed and exercise can be performed for longer durations until volitional fatigue.

Another confounding variable in the issue of hydration during exercise is that there are limits to the ingestion and emptying of fluid from the stomach. Research has shown that maximal rates of gastric emptying approximate 1200 ml/hour.[36] This rate is considerably less than the maximal sweat rate (~3 L/hour), and for certain types of exercise (e.g., running, cross-country skiing, cycling) in which transportation of adequate volumes of water is difficult, it is unrealistic to expect fluid ingestion of more than 1 L/hour. Research into delivery of carbohydrate (CHO) and water to the small intestine and the uptake of water and carbohydrate by the small intestine indicates that carbohydrate solutions can aid in

> **water intoxication**
> *water ingestion that causes diminished blood concentrations of electrolytes, especially sodium*
>
> **hyponatremia (hi′po-na-tre′mi-ah)**
> *a decrease in the serum concentration of sodium below 135 mEq/L*

TABLE 17.6

Recommendations for ingestion of fluid, carbohydrate, and electrolytes before, during, and after prolonged submaximal exercise

ISSUES	EXERCISE <60 MIN	EXERCISE 60-180 MIN	EXERCISE >180 MIN	POSTEXERCISE
Exercise intensity	80%-130% VO_2max	60%-90% VO_2max	30%-70% VO_2max	Passive rest
Primary concerns	Dehydration, hyperthermia	Dehydration, CHO nutrition	Hyperthermia, dehydration, CHO nutrition, hyponatremia	
Proposed Formulation:				
Preevent*	30-50 g CHO	30-50 g CHO	30-50 g CHO	
During exercise				
Initial 60 min	6% CHO	6% CHO Na^+:10-20 mEq/L Cl^-:10-20 mEq/L	6% CHO Na^+:10-20 mEq/L Cl^-:10-20 mEq/L	
After 60 min	—	8%-12% CHO	8%-12% CHO	
Recovery				
Initial 120 min	6% CHO Na^+: 10-20 mEq/L Cl^-: 10-20 mEq/L 8%-12% CHO	12% CHO at 0.7 gm/kg/hr Na^+: 10-20 mEq/L Cl^-: 10-20 mEq/L 8%-12% CHO	12% CHO at 0.7 gm/kg/hr Na^+: 10-20 mEq/L Cl^-: 10-20 mEq/L 8%-12% CHO	
After 120 min	6% CHO Na^+: 10-20 mEq/L Cl^-: 10-20 mEq/L 8%-12% CHO	6% CHO Na^+: 10-20 mEq/L Cl^-: 10-20 mEq/L 8%-12% CHO	6% CHO Na^+: 10-20 mEq/L Cl^-: 10-20 mEq/L 8%-12% CHO	
Volume†				
Preevent‡	300-500 ml	300-500 ml	300-500 ml	
During exercise	500-1000 ml	500-1000 ml/hr	500-1000 ml/hr	
Volume				
Recovery	500-1000 ml/hr	500-1000 ml/hr	500-1000 ml/hr	

* Carbohydrate can be in solid or liquid form. If solid, carbohydrate should be ingested with stated volumes of water.
† The frequency of ingestion is not stated. More frequent ingestion of smaller volumes is recommended to prevent gastric distress.
‡ Hyperhydration with glycerol solutions at low concentrations (1%-4%) has also been shown to be beneficial.
Adapted from Gisolfi CV, Duchman SM: *Med Sci Sports Exerc* 24(6):679-687, 1992.

procedures for optimal fluid replacement, or **rehydration,** during the recovery.

When an individual is dehydrated, ingestion of pure water causes less fluid retention in the body than does a carbohydrate–electrolyte drink because carbohydrate–electrolyte drinks maintain a higher osmolality of the blood. Higher osmolality means more of the antidiuretic hormone stimulus for water conservation by the kidneys is retained and therefore less fluid is lost in the urine. Data also show that carbonated beverages are just as beneficial for rehydration as noncarbonated beverages.[84]

Factors that Determine Postexercise Muscle Glycogen Synthesis

Figure 17.19 presents the theorized pattern of the rate of postexercise muscle glycogen synthesis during the first 24 hours of recovery. Unfortunately, research has provided only estimations of the maximal rate of synthesis after 2 hours of recovery.[130] Nevertheless, based on in vitro research of the regulation of glycogen synthetase (see Chapter 5) and the fact that glucose uptake and synthetase activity are inversely affected by the amount of glycogen present,[46,81,149] it is likely that this inverse exponential relationship is appropriate.

Based on Figure 17.19, it is obvious that optimal conditions need to be fostered as early after exercise as possible. These optimal conditions were listed in Table 17.6 and consist of exercise-related and nutritional factors.

rehydration (re-hi-dra'shun)
the return of water to the body during recovery from dehydration

FIGURE 17.19

The hypothesized exponential decrease in skeletal muscle glycogen synthesis during the recovery from exercise. The initial rapid decline in glycogen synthesis is due to blood flow reductions and the powerful biochemical inverse relationship among muscle glycogen concentrations, glucose uptake, and glycogen synthetase activity. Depending on the carbohydrate nutrition and extent of muscle glycogen depletion after exercise, the shape of the curve will differ, since muscle glycogen concentrations after 24 hours of recovery are similar regardless of whether simple carbohydrate is ingested immediately after exercise.

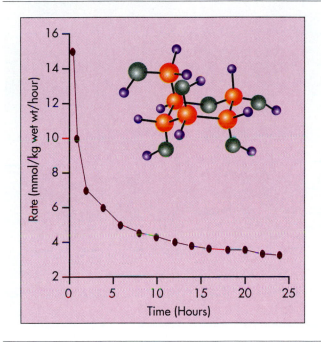

Exercise determinants. The rate of postexercise muscle glycogen synthesis depends on whether the previous bout of exercise has damaged skeletal muscle. Exercise that has an eccentric component (e.g., running) or involves body contact (e.g., football or ice hockey) can result in microscopic damage to skeletal muscle fibers. This damage is known to stimulate the infiltration of white blood cells (WBCs), which rely on blood glucose as their sole energy substrate (see Chapter 15). Consequently, the local increase in WBCs within skeletal muscle means increased competition for blood glucose, resulting in a decreased rate of muscle glycogen synthesis. However, because infiltration of WBCs requires at least 12 hours,[34,43,109] it is known that carbohydrate intake during the hours immediately after the exercise bout can sustain comparable rates of glycogen synthesis to conditions of no muscle damage. In addition, increasing the carbohydrate ingested during recovery can further increase blood glucose, which in turn makes additional glucose available for the muscle, despite increasing WBC proliferation.[34,43]

Muscle glycogen synthesis is reduced during an active recovery[14,17]; however, if the active recovery is done at a low intensity ($<35\%$ VO_2max), some glycogen can be stored in fast-twitch muscle, which is not recruited at these low intensities.[114,121,144] (see Chapter 9).

Nutritional determinants

The optimal rate of carbohydrate ingestion after exercise approximates 0.7 g/kg body weight/hour.* Increasing carbohydrate does not increase glycogen synthesis[13,71,124,130]; however, adding protein to the liquid carbohydrate solution may further increase the rate of glycogen synthesis as a result of an increased release of insulin.[150] The carbohydrate should be in the form of glucose, sucrose, or glucose polymers in liquid form or, if in solid form, should have a high glycemic index value.[19,91]

The maximal rate of postexercise glycogen synthesis after prolonged submaximal exercise is 7 to 9 mmol/kg/hour.† The carbohydrate can be ingested in a bolus feeding or dispersed in intervals. However, if ingestion of the carbohydrate is delayed, the rate of glycogen synthesis is reduced considerably. For example, delaying carbohydrate ingestion for 2 hours after exercise can reduce the rate of synthesis from 7 mmol/kg/hour to less than 3 mmol/kg/hour.[72]

Demands of exercise performed on consecutive days. When exercise is performed on consecutive days, muscle glycogen must be replenished within a 24-hour period.[79] Research has clearly shown that muscle glycogen can be returned to normal resting values within 24 hours[10,69,89,130]; however, when muscle damage is a factor, muscle glycogen replenishment may take several days.[35,44,138]

Short-term intense exercise

Intense exercise requires rapid degradation of muscle glycogen, as explained in Chapter 10. This fact is true even for exercise performed to volitional fatigue for durations as short as several minutes.[130,131] These facts emphasize that carbohydrate nutrition may also be important for intense exercise.[16] Also, the muscle damage incurred during intense exercise and the subsequent hypertrophy may increase the need for protein in the diet.

Nutrition before, during, and after exercise. Compared with preexercise nutrition for prolonged exercise, minimal research has addressed the nutritional needs for intense exercise[16,57-59] or for individuals who need to lose weight or gain lean body mass (see Focus Box 17.3). In a series of studies conducted by scientists in Scotland, the influence of preexercise diet composition on muscle, blood, and performance variables during intense exercise was investigated. The ingestion of either a high-fat and protein diet (3% CHO by kilocalorie) or a high-carbohydrate diet (87% of kilocalories) for 4 days before intense cycle ergometer exercise (3 minutes at

---

*References 13, 14, 71, 72, 119, 124, 132, 138, and 149.
†References 13, 15, 71, 72, 119, 126, 130, 138, and 149.

FOCUS BOX 17.3

Nutritional concerns for athletes involved in weight maintenance, reducing body weight, or increasing body weight

For athletes who participate in wrestling, boxing, ballet dancing, horse racing, rowing, or other sports requiring performance categories based on body weight or aesthetics, practices for losing weight rapidly are promoted and condoned. In certain circumstances, routine use of these practices may be detrimental to long-term nutrition and health. Conversely, some individuals are required to increase body mass, preferably by a selective increase in lean body weight. Unfortunately, for some sports the health and body composition implications of weight gain are not always the most performance-enhancing end objective (e.g., sumo wrestling). The specific nutritional demands of either dietary or exercise intervention require clarification.

Body weight maintenance and reduction

The mass of water (1 g/ml), its contribution to total body mass (65% to 75% by weight), and the relative ease of removing it from the body (exercise-induced sweating can expend 1 to 3 L/hour), result in dehydration being the preferred means of weight loss. Dehydration is problematic to individuals who must exercise. Dehydration to levels at which more than 3% of the body weight has been lost is known to be detrimental to both prolonged and short-term intense exercise.[139]

The more serious nutritional concern for individuals who must constantly lose or retain a low weight is the development of mal-nutrition.[139] Numerous studies have reported that athletes who routinely lose weight rapidly have poor diets (resulting in ingestion of micronutrients at amounts less than the RDA) and clinically diagnosed eating disorders.[22,139] The main micronutrients of concern are iron and calcium, which for women is bothersome as a result of the already relatively low iron stores and the connection between low dietary calcium and an increased risk of osteoporosis. For these individuals, it is not the exercise that demands increased macronutrient and micronutrient intake, but the unbalanced diet that mainly is caused by an insufficient caloric intake.[139]

Gaining weight

Unfortunately, the specific dietary and exercise strategies best used for weight gain while still promoting cardiovascular health have not been researched with the fervor of weight loss. For both the athlete and the nonathletic individual, weight gain by increasing lean body mass is the most desirable method for health reasons. Commonsense recommendations include selecting foods with a high caloric density that do not induce a high glycemic response. Increases in lean body mass would be maximized by adding a resistance exercise training program to the weight gain program. Research is needed on the effect on weight gain on the interaction between different types and intensities of exercise and diets.

100% VO_2max) resulted in greater preexercise muscle glycogen concentrations in the high-carbohydrate diet trial and greater use of glycogen during the exercise.[57-59] With the high-fat and protein diet, muscle acidosis was more severe after exercise than with the high-carbohydrate diet, indicating that muscle buffer capacity is reduced by a high-fat and protein diet. When a normal carbohydrate diet and a high-carbohydrate diet were compared, greater acidosis occurred with the high-carbohydrate diet.[57] These results indicate that intense exercise may be detrimentally affected by a diet that is either low or very high in carbohydrates. Therefore individuals involved in intense exercise should eat moderate amounts of carbohydrate and should not complete a regimen of carbohydrate supercompensation in preparation for intense exercise.

Finally, as explained in Chapter 10, muscle glycogen stores as low as 50 mmol/kg wet weight have not been shown to detrimentally affect intense exercise performance. This provides further evidence supporting the lessened importance of preexercise carbohydrate nutrition for intense compared with prolonged steady-state exercise.

Factors that Determine Postexercise Muscle Glycogen Synthesis

The large degradation of muscle glycogen during intense exercise demands that glycogen stores be replenished as quickly as possible during the recovery from exercise. However, research has shown that carbohydrate ingestion during the recovery from high-intensity exercise is not necessary because glycogen synthesis rates as high as 15 mmol/kg wet weight/hour have been reported without carbohydrate ingestion.[69,131] These relatively high rates of synthesis have been explained by a reversal of the reactions of the hexose-phosphate intermediates of glycolysis, which enables these intermediates to be used as endogenous substrates for glycogen synthesis.*

---

*References 41, 50, 88, 96, 130, 131.

TABLE 17.7

Concentrations of electrolytes in plasma and sweat, and loss of electrolytes during exercise*

ELECTROLYTE	PLASMA (mEq/L)	SWEAT (mEq/L)	LOSSES* (mEq)
Sodium (Na+)	140	40-60	155
Potassium (K+)	4	4-5	16
Chloride (Cl-)	101	30-50	137
Magnesium (Mg++)	1.5	1.5-5	13
Osmolality	302	80-185	—

Data from Costill DL: *Ann NY Acad Sci* 301:160-174, 1977.
*From exercise-induced dehydration of 5.8%.

Micronutrient Concerns Before, During, and After Exercise

From the previous discussion, it should be clear that a well-balanced diet that provides sufficient calories also provides all the micronutrients, in adequate amounts, required to sustain exercise of different types, intensities, and durations. Nevertheless, questions remain as to whether vitamin and mineral supplementation can improve exercise performance.

Based on research concerning fluid ingestion during or after exercise and body hydration, an argument can be made for the need for sodium. However, this need applies only to prolonged exercise performed in an environment that causes high sweat rates, resulting in losses of 1 to 3 L/hour of body water. Under these circumstances, sodium ingestion in liquid beverages improves drink palatability,[74] assists in the absorption of fluid from the small intestine,[51-53,55,93] and prevents excess fluid loss in the urine.[114,115,133] Although it has been theorized that sodium should increase glucose absorption by the small intestine, no experimental evidence supports this effect.[64]

Another issue raised about electrolytes is whether sufficient electrolytes are lost in sweat to require supplementation for replacement during or after exercise. Table 17.7 presents the concentration of the electrolytes in sweat and plasma and the amount of these electrolytes lost during exercise-induced dehydration. Because the duct of the sweat gland absorbs most of the electrolytes before excretion to the skin's surface, electrolyte loss through sweat is minimal. The main electrolyte of concern is sodium, and as has been previously discussed, sodium reductions in blood are caused by a combination of loss through sweat and redistribution within the body. Sodium redistribution into the small intestine increases when a hypotonic drink (a drink with an osmolality less than blood osmolality) is ingested.[109]

This evidence does not indicate a need to ingest salt tablets during exercise, which would cause a large loss of water into the small intestine, decreasing the osmolality of the chyme, which in turn would exacerbate the effects of dehydration on exercise performance. Similarly, the evidence does not indicate a need for increasing the intake of sodium after exercise. Ingesting a rehydration beverage that contains sodium provides adequate sodium replenishment in the initial hours of recovery, and since the typical diet provides sodium in excess of the RDA, body sodium stores rapidly return to normal.

Although some claim that added vitamins can increase exercise performance, probably based on their major roles in energy metabolism (see Table 17.1), no research evidence exists to support this claim.[5] However, current research interest has focused on the potential need to destroy tissue-damaging by-products of metabolism, called **free radicals.**[75] Free radicals have only a short half-life (<1 second) but are believed to be responsible for some of the microscopic tissue damage that can accompany exercise.[3] Vitamins E and C, ß-carotene, and selenium, which are known to protect the body against tissue damage from free radicals are called **antioxidants.** However, it is unknown how this antioxidant protection functions and what levels of these micronutrients offer greatest protection.[75]

free radicals
small molecules in the body with an extremely high affinity for electrons

antioxidants (an'ti-ok'si-dants)
substances that provide electrons to reduce free radicals, thus preserving other, more important molecules

Long-Term Macronutrient Concerns for Exercisers

We have already commented on the need to raise the carbohydrate content and lower the fat content of the diet for individuals who participate in prolonged exercise. Of more interest to the long-term dietary macronutrient needs of athletes is the amount of protein to ingest.

Traditionally the RDA for protein has been reputed to be adequate, even for individuals involved in intense exercise that induces increases in muscle mass. However, recent research has shown that the RDA may not be appropriate for highly trained endurance athletes, as well as athletes involved in intense exercise training.[85,86] Highly trained individuals have an increase in protein catabolism that must be compensated for by an increased protein intake. For example, during training involving weight resistance exercise, urinary excretion of **3-methylhistidine** (a marker of skeletal muscle actin and myosin catabolism) increased after only 3 days of training[123] (Figure 17.20). Research using **nitrogen balance** techniques,[86] which are necessary to determine if subjects are gaining or losing protein, has shown that weight-training exercise may require a protein intake of approximately 1.6 to 1.7 g/kg/day to maintain nitrogen balance, which is more than double the RDA. Current evidence indicates that additional strength or hypertrophy does not occur when the RDA is exceeded for periods of less than 6 weeks. However, it remains to be proved that added hypertrophy does not occur when athletes are in positive nitrogen balance for extended periods, as is the claim by individuals who train for body building.

Since a well-balanced diet that is sufficient in calories generally provides almost double the RDA for protein, these results indicate that although an increased RDA is necessary, the typical diet does not need supplementation to attain this.[21] Consequently, although some research has indicated that increases in protein intake to 2 g/kg body weight/day may be inadequate for some individuals,[21] the combined effects of caloric intake, energy expenditure, and training adaptation on influencing nitrogen balance make it impossible at this time to provide a definitive recommendation for the protein needs of athletes.[140]

Long-Term Micronutrient Concerns for Exercisers

Long-term micronutrient concerns apply mainly to individuals who exercise and have poor dietary habits. For example, the need for vitamins C and B_6 may increase during exercise, but usually the body has adequate stores. For individuals with a low vitamin C or B_6 intake, supplemental ingestion of these vitamins is known to be beneficial.[83] Also, as discussed in Chapter 14, added vitamin C intake for individuals who train and compete in marathon and ultraendurance events has been shown to reduce the incidence of upper respiratory tract infection.

FIGURE 17.20

Intense exercise, such as weight lifting, can increase markers of the catabolism of muscle contractile proteins (3-methylhistidine). Similar evidence of increased protein catabolism exists during endurance training.

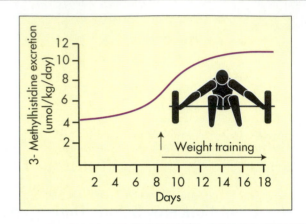

Of greatest concern to individuals is the intake of iron. Iron is an important component of hemoglobin and myoglobin. It is therefore essential for the transport of oxygen in the blood and the delivery of oxygen from the blood to the muscle tissues and then to the mitochondria of the muscle fibers. Depleted iron stores have been reported in both men and women runners,[23,90,91] although the incidence is greater in women; ironically, the incidence in athletes is generally no greater than that in sedentary controls.[23] Early stages of iron deficiency are measured as a decrease in serum ferritin levels (the main storage form of iron). Serum ferritin levels are known to decline during periods of intense training,[90] but these decreases are not associated with decrements to exercise performance.[92] Supplementation of iron improves body iron stores but increases exercise performance only in individuals who are iron deficient (anemic), that is, having low serum ferritin and blood hemoglobin concentrations.[23,80]

Despite reports that 72% of athletes take vitamin and mineral supplements,[58] studies on the effects of vitamin and mineral supplementation on exercise performance have shown no benefit.[146] Athletes who consume a balanced diet do not need micronutrient supplementation.[3,5,83]

3-methylhistidine (3-meth'il-his'ti-deen)
a methylated amino acid used as a urine marker for muscle protein catabolism

nitrogen balance
the state in which nitrogen intake equals nitrogen excretion from the body

SUMMARY

- **Nutrients** can be divided into **micronutrients,** the small compounds that are not catabolized to release free energy during energy metabolism (i.e., **vitamins** and **minerals**) and **macronutrients** (carbohydrate, fat, protein, water), which can be used during energy metabolism. The study of the nutrients needed by the body is called **nutrition.**

- The Recommended Daily Allowance (RDA) of vitamins and minerals is determined by the Food and Nutrition Board of the National Academy of Sciences. The American Dietetics Association recommends that a normal balanced diet have 60% of total kilocalories from carbohydrate, 30% from fat, and 10% from protein. Of the macronutrients carbohydrate, fat, and protein, there is an RDA only for protein, about 0.8 g/kg body weight/day. Proteins that contain all the essential amino acids are called **complete proteins.**

- Water makes up approximately 70% of the lean body mass. It is used as a substrate in many chemical reactions and is a product of other chemical reactions. It is recommended that normally active people in a temperate climate consume approximately 2.5 L of water a day.

- Low-carbohydrate conditions for the body diminish exercise performance and increase perceptions of fatigue. A modified diet strategy in the days preceding an athletic event can increase skeletal muscle glycogen stores. For trained athletes, simply reducing training and increasing the carbohydrate content of the diet to more than 10 g/kg/day during 3 days before competition increases muscle glycogen stores to their maximal values. This process has been called **glycogen supercompensation.**

- Ingesting carbohydrate 20 to 60 minutes before the start of exercise can increase both blood glucose and insulin concentrations and result in a rapid fall in blood glucose after the start of exercise, or **rebound hypoglycemia.** Carbohydrate should be ingested in a meal 3 to 6 hours before competition. If carbohydrate is to be ingested within the hour of competition, these feedings should be less than 100 g of carbohydrate, should occur within 30 minutes of exercise, and should be immediately followed by an active warm-up.

- Procedures designed to optimize fluid status have been called **hyperhydration,** and the ingestion of fluid-retaining substances, such as solutions of glycerol (<50 g/L), have been shown to increase body water, improve thermoregulation during exercise, and prolong the time until fatigue during cycling at less than 70% VO_2max.

- When a person is exercising for longer than $1^1/2$ hours, ingesting carbohydrate prevents hypoglycemia and delays fatigue and therefore can improve exercise performance. This benefit can be obtained when carbohydrate is ingested at repeated intervals during exercise or 30 minutes before the expected time of fatigue. The amount of carbohydrate required is estimated at 30 to 60 g/hour, and it can be in liquid or solid form; if in solid form, it should have a high **glycemic index** value.

- Ingestion of drinks that are too high in fructose may irritate the stomach, thereby decreasing **gastric emptying.** Drinks can also contain connected chains of glucose molecules, called **glucose polymers.** However, research has shown that drinks with this form of carbohydrate do not empty from the stomach faster than pure glucose or glucose-fructose solutions of a similar carbohydrate content and drink volume.

- Drink concentrations in excess of 80 g/L empty more slowly from the stomach than water; these may cause gastric distress and obviously would be detrimental to exercise performance. Research into **intestinal absorption** supports these findings. Because the maximal rate of gastric emptying is about 1200 ml/hour, a carbohydrate concentration and drink volume association that provides close to 1 L/hour would be recommended for hydration purposes. Drinks with a carbohydrate concentration between 40 and 80 g/L would satisfy these requirements.

SUMMARY—Cont'd

■ Although the research into carbohydrate ingestion before, during, and after exercise has predominantly used liquid beverages, blood glucose is also maintained during exercise when solid carbohydrate supplementation is provided. Of course, water is also recommended to aid the digestion of the food and emptying from the stomach and to prevent exercise-induced **dehydration.**

■ Water absorption by the small intestine can increase sixfold if a drink has 60 g CHO/L and electrolytes (20 mEq Na^+ and 2.6 mEq K^+). Despite the difficulty of ingesting large fluid volumes during prolonged exercise, some individuals have accomplished this. If the fluid ingested in such large volumes has a low osmolality, the person could be at risk of developing **water intoxication,** which can lead to a life-threatening reduction in serum sodium concentrations, or **hyponatremia.**

■ For purposes of **rehydration** the ingestion of pure water by a dehydrated individual causes less fluid retention in the body than a carbohydrate-electrolyte drink because a carbohydrate-electrolyte drink maintains a higher osmolality of the blood than does water. A higher osmolality retains more of the antidiuretic hormone stimulus for water conservation by the kidneys, and therefore less fluid is lost in the urine.

■ The optimal rate of carbohydrate ingestion after exercise is approximately 0.7 g/kg/hour. Increasing the carbohydrate does not increase glycogen synthesis. The carbohydrate should be taken in the form of glucose, sucrose, or glucose polymers in liquid form or, if in solid form, it should have a high glycemic index value. The carbohydrate can be ingested in a bolus feeding or be dispersed in intervals. However, if ingestion of the carbohydrate is delayed, the rate of glycogen synthesis is reduced considerably.

■ Intense exercise can be detrimentally affected by a diet that is either low or very high in carbohydrates. Therefore individuals involved in intense exercise should eat moderate amounts of carbohydrate and should not undergo a regimen of carbohydrate supercompensation in preparation for intense exercise.

■ A well-balanced diet that provides sufficient calories also provides all the micronutrients, in adequate amounts, required to sustain exercise of different types, intensities, and durations. Although vitamin E is a known **antioxidant** and can protect the body against tissue damage from **free radicals,** it is unknown how this protection functions and what levels of vitamin E offer greatest protection.

■ Highly trained individuals have an increased protein catabolism, as measured by increased urinary **3-methylhistidine** and amino acid release from skeletal muscle; this must be compensated for by an increased protein intake that exceeds the RDA for protein. For example, weight-training exercise may require a protein intake of 2 g/kg/day to maintain **nitrogen balance,** an amount more than double the RDA. Although an increased protein RDA is necessary for many athletes, the typical diet already provides protein in excess of the RDA and thus protein supplementation is not necessary.

■ Athletes who consume a well-balanced diet do not need vitamin and mineral supplementation. However, iron supplementation is recommended for athletes known to be low in iron stores, or anemic.

REVIEW QUESTIONS

1. What roles do vitamins play in nutrition and in supporting energy metabolism?

2. What are the functions of the many minerals of the body that are important during exercise?

3. For healthy individuals concerned with exercise performance, why is carbohydrate the main macronutrient of interest?

4. Explain the procedure of glycogen supercompensation.

5. What is rebound hypoglycemia?

6. What is the glycemic index? Explain how it has been used clinically and applied to exercise.

7. What methods have been used to hyperhydrate the body? Have these methods been equally effective in improving exercise performance? Explain.

8. What factors determine how fast a liquid sports beverage empties from the stomach?

9. How do researchers measure gastric emptying and intestinal absorption?

10. Try to explain why adding carbohydrate to a drink increases the rate of fluid absorption by the small intestine.

11. What is the optimal carbohydrate concentration of a sports drink for increasing fluid intake by the body, thereby delaying dehydration? Why?

12. Is there a limit to the amount of fluid that should be ingested during exercise? Why or why not? What problems might arise if individuals drink too much fluid, especially water?

13. What would be your dietary recommendations to an individual who needs to replenish muscle glycogen as fast as possible after exercise because of the need to compete again the same day?

14. Is the RDA for protein adequate for all individuals? Explain.

15. Why are free radicals and antioxidants of interest to exercise physiologists?

16. Is there any research evidence that certain populations need to supplement micronutrient intake for improved exercise performance? Explain.

APPLICATIONS

1. Would the greater blood glucose concentration of a type II diabetic be associated with impaired or increased muscle glycogen synthesis compared with a nondiabetic individual?

2. Although high glycemic-index foods may be better for postexercise muscle glycogen synthesis, what is the fate of glucose not taken up by muscle? What might be the health consequences of this scenario for the untrained person?

3. Many clinical disorders can reduce lean body mass (AIDS, diabetes, renal failure, cardiac failure), resulting in the need for a special diet. How might exercise training interact with improved diet to retard the loss of lean body mass in these individuals?

REFERENCES

1. Ahlborg G, Felig P: Substrate utilization during prolonged exercise preceded by ingestion of glucose, *Am J Physiol* E188-E194, 1977.

2. Ahlborg B, Bergstrom J, Ekelund LG, Hultman E: Muscle glycogen and muscle electrolytes during prolonged physical exercise, *Acta Physiol Scand* 70:129-142, 1967.

3. Anderson RA: New insights on the trace elements, chromium, copper, and zinc, and exercise. In Brouns F, editor: Advances in nutrition and top sport, *Med Sport Sci* 32:38-58, Basel, 1991, Karger.

4. Beckers ET, Leiper JB, Davidson J: Comparison of aspiration and scintigraphic techniques for the measurement of gastric emptying. *Gut* 33:115-117, 1992.

5. Belko AZ: Vitamins and exercise: an update, *Med Sci Sports Exerc* 19(5):S191-S196, 1987.

6. Below PR, Mora-Rodriguez R, Gonzalez-Alonso J, Coyle EF: Fluid and carbohydrate ingestion independently improve performance during 1 h of intense exercise, *Med Sci Sports Exerc* 27(20):200-210, 1995.

7. Bendich A: Exercise and free radicals: effects of antioxidant vitamins. In Brouns F, editor: Advances in nutrition and top sport, *Med Sport Sci* 32:59-78, Basel, 1991, Karger.

8. Bergstrom J, Hultman: Muscle glycogen synthesis after exercise: an enhancing factor localized to the muscle cells in man, *Nature* 210:309-310, 1967.

9. Bergstrom J, Hultman E: Synthesis of muscle glycogen in man after glucose and fructose infusion, *Acta Medica Scand* 182(1):93-107, 1967.

10. Bergstrom J, Hermansen L, Saltin B: Diet, muscle glycogen, and physical performance, *Acta Physiol Scand* 71:140-150, 1967.

11. Blom PCS: Post exercise glucose uptake and glycogen synthesis in human skeletal muscle during oral or IV glucose intake, *Eur J Appl Physiol* 59:327-333, 1989.

12. Blom PCS, Costill DL, Vollestad NK: Exhaustive running: inappropriate as a stimulus of muscle glycogen supercompensation, *Med Sci Sports Exerc* 19(4):398-403, 1987.

13. Blom PCS, Vaage O, Kardel K, Hermansen L: Effect of increasing glucose loads on the rate of muscle glycogen resynthesis after prolonged exercise, *Acta Physiol Scand* 108(2):C12, 1980.

14. Blom PCS, Vollestad NK, Costill DL: Factors affecting changes in muscle glycogen concentration during and after prolonged exercise, *Acta Physiol Scand* 128(suppl 556):67-74, 1986.

15. Blom PCS, Hostmark AT, Vaage O et al: Effect of different postexercise sugar diets on the rate of muscle glycogen resynthesis, *Med Sci Sports Exerc* 19(5):491-496, 1987.

16. Bonen A, Malcom SA, Kilgour RD et al: Glucose ingestion before and during intense exercise, *J Appl Physiol* 50(4):766-771, 1981.

17. Bonen A, Ness GW, Belcastro AN, Kirby RL: Mild exercise impedes glycogen repletion in muscle, *J Appl Physiol* 58(5):1622-1629, 1985.

18. Brenner W, Hendrix TR, McHugh PR: Regulation of the gastric emptying of carbohydrates, *Gastroenterology* 85(1):76-82, 1983.

19. Brouns F: Gastrointestinal symptoms in athletes: physiological and nutritional aspects. In Brouns F, editor: Advances in nutrition and top sport, *Med Sports Sci* 32:166-199, Basel, 1991, Karger.

20. Burke L, Collier GR, Hargreaves M: Muscle glycogen storage after prolonged exercise: effect of the glycemic index of carbohydrate feedings, *J Appl Physiol* 75(2):1019-1023, 1993.

21. Butterfield GE: Whole-body protein utilization in humans, *Med Sci Sports Exerc* 19(5):S157-S165, 1987.

22. Calabrese LH, Kirkendall DT, Floyd M et al: Menstrual abnormalities, nutritional patterns, and body composition in female classical ballet dancers, *Physician Sports Med* 11(2):86-98, 1983.

23. Clarkson PM: Tired blood: iron deficiency in athletes and effects of iron supplementation, *Sports Sci Exchange* 1(28):1-5, 1990.

24. Clarkson PM: Trace mineral requirements for athletes: to supplement or not to supplement? *Sports Sci Exchange* 4(33):1-6, 1991.

25. Coggan AR, Coyle EF: Reversal of fatigue during prolonged exercise by carbohydrate infusion or ingestion, *J Appl Physiol* 63(6):2388-2395, 1987.

26. Coggan AR, Coyle EF: Effects of carbohydrate during high-intensity exercise, *J Appl Physiol* 65(4):1703-1709, 1988.

27. Coggan AR, Coyle EF: Metabolism and performance following carbohydrate late in exercise, *Med Sci Sports Exerc* 21(1):59-65, 1989.

28. Coggan AR, Coyle EF: Carbohydrate ingestion during prolonged exercise: effects on metabolism and performance, *Exerc Sport Sci Rev* 19:1-40, 1991.

29. Coleman E: Sports drink update, *Sports Sci Exchange* 1(5):1-5, 1988.

30. Costill DL: Sweating: its composition and effect on body fluids, *Ann NY Acad Sci* 301:160-174, 1977.

31. Costill DL, Saltin B: Factors limiting gastric emptying during rest and exercise, *J Appl Physiol* 37:679-683, 1974.

REFERENCES—Cont'd

32. Costill DL, Bowers R, Branam G, Sparks K: Muscle glycogen utilization during prolonged exercise on successive days, *J Appl Physiol* 31:834-838, 1971.

33. Costill DL, Coyle EF, Dalsky G et al: Effects of elevated plasma FFA and insulin on muscle glycogen usage during exercise, *J Appl Physiol* 43:695-699, 1977.

34. Costill DL, Pascoe DD, Fink WJ et al: Impaired muscle glycogen resynthesis after eccentric exercise, *J Appl Physiol* 69(1):46-50, 1990.

35. Costill DL, Sherman WM, Fink WJ et al: The role of dietary carbohydrates in muscle glycogen resynthesis after strenuous running, *Am J Clin Nutr* 34:1831-1836, 1981.

36. Coyle EF, Montain SJ: Carbohydrate and fluid ingestion during exercise: are there trade-offs? *Med Sci Sports Exerc* 24(6):671-678, 1992.

37. Coyle EF, Coggan AR, Hemmert MK, Ivy JL: Muscle glycogen utilization during prolonged strenuous exercise when fed carbohydrate, *J Appl Physiol* 61(1):165-172, 1986.

38. Coyle EF, Costill DL, Fink WJ, Hoopes DG: Gastric emptying rates of selected athletic drinks, *Res Q Exerc Sport* 49:119-124, 1978.

39. Coyle EF, Coggan AR, Hemmert MK et al: Substrate usage during prolonged exercise following a preexercise meal, *J Appl Physiol* 59(2):429-433, 1985.

40. Coyle EF, Hagberg JM, Hurley BF et al: Carbohydrate feedings during prolonged exercise can delay fatigue, *J Appl Physiol* 55(1):230-235, 1983.

41. Crabtree B, Higgins SJ, Newsholme EA: The activities of pyruvate carboxylase, phosphoenolpyruvate carboxylase, and fructose diphosphatase in muscle from vertebrates and invertebrates, *Biochem J* 130:391-396, 1972.

42. Davis JM, Burgess WA, Slentz CA et al: Effects of ingesting 6% and 12% glucose-electrolyte beverages during prolonged intermittent cycling exercise in the heat, *Eur J Appl Physiol* 57:563-569, 1988.

43. Doyle JA, Sherman WM: Eccentric exercise and glycogen synthesis, *Med Sci Sports Exerc* 23(4):S98, 1991 (abstract 587).

44. Doyle JA, Sherman WM, Strauss RL: Effects of eccentric and concentric exercise on muscle glycogen replenishment, *J Appl Physiol* 74(4):1848-1855, 1993.

45. Erikson MA, Schwarzkopf RJ, McKenzie RD: Effects of caffeine, fructose, and glucose ingestion on muscle glycogen utilization during exercise, *Med Sci Sports Exerc* 19:579-583, 1987.

46. Fell RD, Terblanche SE, Ivy JL et al: Effect of muscle glycogen content on glucose uptake following exercise, *J Appl Physiol* 52:434-437, 1982.

47. Fielding RA, Costill DL, Fink WJ et al: Effect of carbohydrate feeding frequency and dosage on muscle glycogen use during exercise, *Med Sci Sports Exerc* 17:472-476, 1985.

48. Fielding RA, Costill DL, Fink WJ et al: Effects of preexercise carbohydrate feedings on muscle glycogen use during exercise in well-trained runners, *Eur J Appl Physiol* 56:225-229, 1987.

49. Flynn MG, Costill DL, Hawley JA et al: Influence of selected carbohydrate drinks on cycling performance and glycogen use, *Med Sci Sports Exerc* 19(1):37-40, 1987.

50. Gaesser GA, Brooks GA: Glycogen repletion following continuous and intermittent exercise to exhaustion, *J Appl Physiol* 49:722-728, 1980.

51. Gisolfi CV: Exercise, intestinal absorption, and rehydration, *Sports Sci Exchange* 4(32):1-5, 1991.

52. Gisolfi CV, Duchman SM: Guidelines for optimal replacement beverages for different athletic events, *Med Sci Sports Exerc* 24(6):679-687, 1992.

53. Gisolfi CV, Summers RW, Schedl HP, Bleiler TL: Intestinal water absorption from select carbohydrate solutions in humans, *J Appl Physiol* 73(5):2142-2150, 1992.

54. Gisolfi CV, Spranger KJ, Summers RW et al: Effects of cycle exercise on intestinal absorption in humans, *J Appl Physiol* 71(6):2518-2527, 1991.

55. Gleeson M, Maughan RJ, Greenhaff PL: Comparison of the effects of preexercise feedings of glucose, glycerol, and placebo on endurance and fuel homeostasis in man, *Eur J Appl Physiol* 55:645-653, 1986.

56. Gollnick PD, Piehl K, Saubert CW IV et al: Diet, exercise, and glycogen changes in human muscle fibers, *J Appl Physiol* 33(4):421-425, 1972.

57. Greenhaff PL, Gleeson M, Maughan RJ: The effects of a glycogen-loading regimen on acid-base status and blood lactate concentration before and after a fixed period of high-intensity exercise in man, *Eur J Appl Physiol* 57:254-259, 1988.

58. Greenhaff PL, Gleeson M, Maughan RJ: The effects of diet on muscle pH and metabolism during high-intensity exercise, *Eur J Appl Physiol* 57:531-539, 1988.

59. Greenhaff PL, Gleeson M, Maughan RJ: Diet-induced metabolic acidosis and the performance of high-intensity exercise in man, *Eur J Appl Physiol* 57:583-590, 1988.

60. Guyton AC: *Textbook of medical physiology*, ed 8, Philadelphia, 1991, Saunders.

61. Hargreaves M, Briggs CA: Effects of carbohydrate ingestion on exercise metabolism, *J Appl Physiol* 65:1553-1555, 1988.

REFERENCES—Cont'd

62. Hargreaves M, Kiens B, Richter EA: Effect of increased plasma free fatty acid concentrations on muscle metabolism in exercising man, *J Appl Physiol* 70(1):194-201, 1991.

63. Hargreaves M, Costill DL, Katz A, Fink WJ: Effect of fructose ingestion on muscle glycogen usage during exercise, *Med Sci Sports Exerc* 17(3):360-363, 1985.

64. Hargreaves M, Costill DL, Burke G et al: Influence of sodium on glucose bioavailability during exercise, *Med Sci Sports Exerc* 26(3):365-368, 1994.

65. Hargreaves M, Costill DL, Coggan AR et al: Effects of carbohydrate feedings on muscle glycogen utilization and exercise performance, *Med Sci Sports Exerc* 16:219-222, 1984.

66. Hargreaves M, Costill DL, Fink WJ et al: Effect of preexercise carbohydrate feedings on endurance cycling performance, *Med Sci Sports Exerc* 19:33-36, 1987.

67. Houmard JA, Egan PC, Anderson Johns R et al: Gastric emptying during 1 hour of cycling and running at 75% VO_2max, *Med Sci Sports Exerc* 23(3):320-325, 1991.

68. Hudlicka O, Zweilach BW, Tyler RR: Capillary recruitment and flow velocity in skeletal muscle after contraction, *Microvasc Res* 23:209-217, 1982.

69. Hultman EH: Carbohydrate metabolism during hard exercise and in the recovery period after exercise, *Acta Physiol Scand* 128(suppl 556):75-82, 1986.

70. Hunt JN, Smith JL, Jiang CL: Effect of meal volume and energy density on the gastric emptying of carbohydrate, *Gastroenterology* 89:1326-1330, 1985.

71. Ivy JL, Lee MC, Bronzinick JT Jr, Reed MC: Muscle glycogen storage following different amounts of carbohydrate ingestion, *J Appl Physiol* 65(5):2018-2023, 1988.

72. Ivy JL, Katz AL, Cutler CL et al: Muscle glycogen synthesis after exercise: effect of time of carbohydrate ingestion, *J Appl Physiol* 64(4):1480-1485, 1988.

73. Jarvis JK, Pearsall D, Oliner CM, Schoeller DA: The effect of food matrix on carbohydrate utilization during moderate exercise, *Med Sci Sports Exerc* 24(3):320-326, 1992.

74. Johnson HL, Nelson RA, Consolazio CF: Effects of electrolyte and nutrient solutions on performance and metabolic balance, *Med Sci Sports Exerc* 20(1):26-33, 1988.

75. Kanter M: Free radicals and exercise: effects of nutritional antioxidant supplementation, *Exerc Sport Sci Rev* 23:375-397, 1995.

76. Karlsson J, Saltin B: Diet, muscle glycogen, and endurance performance, *J Appl Physiol* 31:203-206, 1971.

77. Keizer HA, Kuipers H, Van Kranenburg G, Guerten P: Influence of liquid and solid meals on muscle glycogen resynthesis, plasma fuel hormone response, and maximal physical work capacity, *Int J Sports Med* 8:99-104, 1986.

78. Kiens B, Raben AB, Valeur AK, Richter EA: Benefit of dietary simple carbohydrates on the early postexercise muscle glycogen repletion in male athletes, *Med Sci Sports Exerc* 22(2):S88, 1990 (abstract 524).

79. Kirwan JP, Costill DL, Mitchell JB et al: Carbohydrate balance in competitive runners during successive days of intense training, *J Appl Physiol* 65(6):2601-2606, 1988.

80. Klingshirn LA, Pate RR, Bourque SP et al: Effect of iron supplementation on endurance capacity in iron-depleted female runners, *Med Sci Sports Exerc* 24(7):819-824, 1992.

81. Kochan RG, Lamb DR, Lutz SA et al: Glycogen synthetase activation in human skeletal muscle: effects of diet and exercise, *Am J Physiol* 236(6):E660-E666, 1979.

82. Koivisto V, Karonen SL, Nikkila EO: Carbohydrate ingestion before exercise: comparison of glucose, fructose, and sweet placebo, *J Appl Physiol* 51:783-787, 1981.

83. Kris Etherton PM: The facts and fallacies of nutritional supplements for athletes, *Sports Sci Exchange* 2(18):1-5, 1989.

84. Lambert CP, Costill DL, McConnell GK et al: Fluid replacement after dehydration: influence of beverage carbonation and carbohydrate content, *Int J Sports Med* 13(4):285-292, 1992.

85. Lemon PWR: Does exercise alter dietary protein requirements? In Brouns F, editor: Advances in nutrition and top sport, *Med Sport Sci* 32:15-37, Basel, 1991, Karger.

86. Lemon PWR, Tarnopolsky MA, MacDougall JD, Atkinson SA: Protein requirements and muscle mass/strength changes during intensive training in novice body builders, *J Appl Physiol* 73(2):767-775, 1992.

87. Lyons TP, Riedesel ML, Meuli LE, Chick TW: Effects of glycerol-induced hyperhydration prior to exercise in the heat on sweating and core temperature, *Med Sci Sports Exerc* 22(4):477-483, 1990.

88. MacDougall JD, Ward GR, Sale DG, Sutton JR: Muscle glycogen repletion after high-intensity intermittent exercise, *J Appl Physiol* 42(2):129-132, 1977.

89. Maehlum S, Hermansen L: Muscle glycogen concentration during recovery after prolonged severe exercise in fasting subjects, *Scand J Clin Lab Invest* 38:557-560, 1978.

90. Magazanik A, Weinstein Y, Dlin RA et al: Iron deficiency caused by 7 weeks of intensive physical exercise, *Eur J Appl Physiol* 57:198-202, 1988.

91. Mason WL, McConell G, Hargreaves M: Carbohydrate ingestion during exercise: liquid versus solid feedings, *Med Sci Sports Exerc* 25(8):966-969, 1993.

92. Matter M, Stittfall T, Graves J et al: The effect of iron and folate therapy on maximal exercise performance in female marathon runners with iron and folate deficiency, *Clin Sci* 72:415-422, 1987.

REFERENCES—Cont'd

93. Maughan RJ: Gastric emptying during exercise, *Sports Sci Exchange* 6(5):1-6, 1993.

94. Maughan RJ, Greenhaff PL: High-intensity exercise performance and acid-base balance: the influence of diet and induced metabolic acidosis. In Brouns F, editor: Advances in nutrition and top sport, *Med Sports Sci* 32:147-165, Basel, 1991, Karger.

95. Maughan RJ, Fenn CE, Leiper LB: Effects of fluid, electrolyte, and substrate ingestion on endurance capacity, *Eur J Appl Physiol* 58:481-486, 1989.

96. McLane JA, Holloszy JO: Glycogen synthesis from lactate in the three types of skeletal muscles, *J Biol Chem* 254:6548-6553, 1979.

97. Millard-Stafford M, Sparling PB, Rosskopf LB, Dicarlo LJ: Carbohydrate-electrolyte replacement improves distance running performance in the heat, *Med Sci Sports Exerc* 24(8):934-940, 1992.

98. Mitchell JB, Voss KW: The influence of volume on gastric emptying and fluid balance during prolonged exercise, *Med Sci Sports Exerc* 23(3):314-319, 1991.

99. Mitchell JB, Costill DL, Houmard JA et al: Gastric emptying: influence of prolonged exercise and carbohydrate concentration, *Med Sci Sports Exerc* 21:269-274, 1989.

100. Mitchell JB, Costill DL, Houmard JA et al: Influence of carbohydrate dosage on exercise performance and glycogen metabolism, *J Appl Physiol* 67:1843-1849, 1989.

101. Montain SJ, Coyle EF: Fluid ingestion during exercise increases skin blood flow independent of increases in blood volume, *J Appl Physiol* 73(3):903-910, 1992.

102. Montain SJ, Hooper MK, Coggan AR, Coyle EF: Exercise metabolism at different time intervals following a meal, *J Appl Physiol* 70(2):882-888, 1991.

103. Montner P, Chick T, Riedesel M et al: Glycerol hyperhydration and endurance exercise, *Med Sci Sports Exerc* 24(4):S157, 1992.

104. Murray R, Paul GL, Seifert JG et al: The effects of glucose, fructose, and sucrose ingestion during exercise, *Med Sci Sports Exerc* 21:275-282, 1989.

105. Murray R, Seifert JG, Eddy DE et al: Carbohydrate feeding and exercise: effect of beverage carbohydrate content, *Eur J Appl Physiol* 59:152-158, 1989.

106. Natali A, Santoro D, Brandi LS et al: Effects of acute hypercarnitinemia during increased fatty substrated oxidation in man, *Metabolism* 42(5):594-600, 1993.

107. Neufer PD, Costill DL, Fink WJ et al: Effects of exercise and carbohydrate composition on gastric emptying, *Med Sci Sports Exerc* 18:658-662, 1986.

108. Neufer PD, Costill DI, Flynn MG et al: Improvements in exercise performance: effects of carbohydrate feedings and diet, *J Appl Physiol* 62:983-988, 1987.

109. Noakes TD: Hyponatremia during endurance running: a physiological and clinical interpretation, *Med Sci Sports Exerc* 24(4):403-405, 1992.

110. Noakes TD: Fluid replacement during exercise, *Exerc Sport Sci Rev* 21:297-330, 1993.

111. Noakes TD, Rehrer NJ, Maughan RJ: The importance of volume in regulating gastric emptying, *Med Sci Sports Exerc* 23(3):307-313, 1991.

112. Noakes TD, Norman RJ, Buck RH et al: The incidence of hyponatremia during prolonged ultraendurance exercise, *Med Sci Sports Exerc* 22(2):165-170, 1990.

113. Nordheim K, Vollestad NK: Glycogen and lactate metabolism during low-intensity exercise in man, *Acta Physiol Scand* 139:475-484, 1990.

114. Nose H, Mack GW, Shi X, Nade ER: Role of osmolality and plasma volume during rehydration in humans, *J Appl Physiol* 65:325-331, 1988.

115. Nose H, Mack GW, Shi X, Nadel ER: Involvement of sodium retention hormones during rehydration in humans, *J Appl Physiol* 65:332-336, 1988.

116. O'Brien MJ, Vivuie CA, Mazzeo RS, Brooks GA: Carbohydrate dependence during marathon running, *Med Sci Sports Exerc* 25(9):1009-1017, 1993.

117. Okano G, Takeda H, Morita I et al: Effect of preexercise fructose ingestion on endurance performance in fed men, *Med Sci Sports Exerc* 20(2):105-109, 1988.

118. Owen MD, Kregal KC, Wall PT, Gisolfi CV: Effects of ingesting carbohydrate beverages during exercise in the heat, *Med Sci Sports Exerc* 18(5):568-575, 1986.

119. Pascoe DD, Costill DL, Fink WJ et al: Effects of exercise mode on muscle glycogen restorage during repeated bouts of exercise, *Med Sci Sports Exerc* 22(5):593-598, 1990.

120. Peters HP, Van Schelven FW, Verstappen PA et al: Gastrointestinal problems as a function of carbohydrate supplements and mode of exercise, *Med Sci Sports Exerc* 25(11):1211-1224, 1993.

121. Peters Futre EM, Noakes TD, Raine RI, Terblanche SE: Muscle glycogen repletion during active postexercise recovery, *Am J Physiol* 253(16):E305-E311, 1987.

122. Piehl K, Adolfsson S, Nazar K: Glycogen storage and glycogen synthase activity in trained and untrained muscle of man, *Acta Physiol Scand* 90:779-788, 1974.

123. Pivarnik JM, Hickson JF, Wolinsky I: Urinary 3-methylhistidine excretion increases with repeated weight-training exercise, *Med Sci Sports Exerc* 21(3):283-287, 1989.

REFERENCES—Cont'd

124. Reed MJ, Bronzinick JT Jr, Lee MC, Ivy JL: Muscle glycogen storage postexercise: effect of mode of carbohydrate administration, *J Appl Physiol* 66(2):720-726, 1989.

125. Rehrer NJ: Aspects of dehydration and rehydration during exercise. In Brouns F, editor: Advances in nutrition and top sport, *Med Sport Sci* 32:128-146, Basel, 1991, Karger.

126. Rehrer NJ, Beckers E, Brouns F et al: Exercise and training effects on gastric emptying of carbohydrate beverages, *Med Sci Sports Exerc* 21:540-549, 1989.

127. Rehrer NJ, Brouns F, Beckers EJ: Gastric emptying with repeated drinking during running and bicycling, *Int J Sports Med* 11:238-243, 1990.

128. Rehrer NJ, Wagenmakers AJM, Beckers EJ et al: Gastric emptying, absorption, and carbohydrate oxidation during prolonged exercise, *J Appl Physiol* 72:468-475, 1992.

129. Riedesel ML, Allen DY, Peake GT, Al-Qattan K: Hyperhydration with glycerol solutions, *J Appl Physiol* 63(6):2262-2268, 1987.

130. Robergs RA: Nutrition and exercise determinants of postexercise glycogen synthesis, *Int J Sport Nutr* 1(4):307-337, 1991.

131. Robergs RA, Pearson DR, Costill DL et al: Muscle glycogenolysis during differing intensities of weight-resistance exercise, *J Appl Physiol* 70(4):1700-1706, 1991.

132. Ryan AJ, Bleiler TL, Carter JE, Gisolfi CV: Gastric emptying during prolonged cycling exercise in the heat, *Med Sci Sports Exerc* 21(1):51-58, 1989.

133. Sawka MN, Greenleaf JE: Current concepts concerning thirst, dehydration, and fluid replacement: overview, *Med Sci Sports Exerc* 24(6):643-644, 1992.

134. Shearer JD, Amarai JF, Caldwell MD: Glucose metabolism of injured skeletal muscle: contribution of inflammatory cells, *Circ Shock* 25:131-138, 1988.

135. Sherman WM: Pre-event nutrition, *Sports Sci Exchange* 1(12):1-5, 1989.

136. Sherman WM: Muscle glycogen supercompensation during the week before athletic competition, *Sports Sci Exchange* 2(16):1-6, 1989.

137. Sherman WM, Costill DL, Fink WJ, Miller JM: Effect of exercise-diet manipulation on muscle glycogen and its subsequent utilization during performance, *Int J Sports Med* 2(2):114-118, 1981.

138. Sherman WM, Costill DL, Fink WJ et al: Effect of a 42.2 km foot race and subsequent rest or exercise on muscle glycogen and enzymes, *J Appl Physiol* 55:1219-1224, 1983.

139. Steen SN: Nutritional concerns for athletes who must reduce body weight, *Sports Sci Exchange* 2(20):1-6, 1989.

140. Tarnopolsky MA, Atkinson SA, MacDougall JD et al: Evaluation of protein requirements for trained strength athletes, *J Appl Physiol* 73(5):1986-1995, 1992.

141. Vollestad NK, Blom PCS, Gronnerod O: Resynthesis of glycogen in different muscle fiber types after prolonged exhaustive exercise in man, *Acta Physiol Scand* 137:15-21, 1989.

142. Vukovich MD, Costill DL, Hickey MS et al: Effect of fat emulsion infusion and fat feeding on muscle glycogen utilization during cycle exercise, *J Appl Physiol* 75(4):1513-1518, 1993.

143. Wagenmakers AJM, Beckers EJ, Brouns R et al: Carbohydrate supplementation, glycogen depletion, and amino acid metabolism during exercise, *Am J Physiol* 260(23):E883-E890, 1991.

144. Walberg JL, Ruiz VK, Tarlton SL et al: Exercise capacity and nitrogen loss during a high- or low-carbohydrate diet, *Med Sci Sports Exerc* 20(1):34-43, 1988.

145. Wardlaw GM, Insel PM: *Perspectives in nutrition,* St. Louis, 1993, Mosby.

146. Weight LM, Noakes TD, Labadorios D et al: Vitamin and mineral status of trained athletes, including the effects of supplementation, *Am J Clin Nutr* 47:186-191, 1988.

147. Williams C, Nute MG, Broadbank L, Vinall S: Influence of fluid intake on endurance running performance: a comparison between water, glucose, and fructose solutions, *Eur J Appl Physiol* 60:112-119, 1990.

148. Yaspelkis BB III, Paterson JG, Anderla PA et al: Carbohydrate supplementation spares muscle glycogen during variable-intensity exercise, *J Appl Physiol* 75(4):1477-1485, 1993.

149. Zachweija J, Costill DL, Pascoe DD et al: Influence of muscle glycogen depletion on the rate of resynthesis, *Med Sci Sports Exerc* 23(1):44-48, 1990.

150. Zawadzki KM, Yaspelkis BB, Ivy JL: Carbohydrate-protein complex increases the rate of muscle glycogen storage after exercise, *J Appl Physiol* 72(5):1854-1859, 1992.

RECOMMENDED READINGS

■ Coggan AR, Coyle EF: Carbohydrate ingestion during prolonged exercise: effects on metabolism and performance, *Exerc Sport Sci Rev* 19:1-40, 1991.

■ Coyle EF, Montain SJ: Carbohydrate and fluid ingestion during exercise: are there trade-offs? *Med Sci Sports Exerc* 24(6):671-678, 1992.

■ Doyle JA, Sherman WM, Strauss RL: Effects of eccentric and concentric exercise on muscle glycogen replenishment, *J Appl Physiol* 74(4):1848-1855, 1993.

■ Gisolfi CV, Duchman SM: Guidelines for optimal replacement beverages for different athletic events, *Med Sci Sports Exerc* 24(6):679-687, 1992.

■ Gisolfi CV, Summers RW, Schedl HP, Bleiler TL: Intestinal water absorption from select carbohydrate solutions in humans, *J Appl Physiol* 73(5):2142-2150, 1992.

■ Ivy JL, Katz AL, Cutler CL et al: Muscle glycogen synthesis after exercise: effect of time of carbohydrate ingestion, *J Appl Physiol* 64(4):1480-1485, 1988.

■ Ivy JL, Lee MC, Bronzinick JT Jr, Reed MC: Muscle glycogen storage following different amounts of carbohydrate ingestion, *J Appl Physiol* 65(5):2018-2023, 1988.

■ Kochan RG, Lamd DR, Lutz SA et al: Glycogen synthetase activation in human skeletal muscle: effects of diet and exercise, *J Appl Physiol* 236(6):E660-E666, 1979.

■ Lyons TP, Riedesel ML, Meuli LE, Chick TW: Effects of glycerol-induced hyperhydration prior to exercise in the heat on sweating and core temperature, *Med Sci Sports Exerc* 22(4):477-483, 1990.

■ Noakes TD: Fluid replacement during exercise, *Exerc Sport Sci Rev* 21:297-330, 1993.

■ Noakes TD, Rehrer NJ, Maughan RJ: The importance of volume in regulating gastric emptying, *Med Sci Sports Exerc* 23(3):307-313, 1991.

■ Robergs RA: Nutrition and exercise determinants of postexercise glycogen synthesis, *Int J Sport Nutr* 1(4):307-337, 1991.

■ Sawka MN, Greenleaf JE: Current concepts concerning thirst, dehydration, and fluid replacement: overview, *Med Sci Sports Exerc* 24(6):643-644, 1992.

■ Sherman WM, Costill DL, Fink WJ, Miller JM: Effect of exercise-diet manipulation on muscle glycogen and its subsequent utilization during performance, *Int J Sports Med* 2(2):114-118, 1981.

CHAPTER **18**

Ergogenic Aids To Exercise Performance

OBJECTIVES

After studying this chapter you should be able to:

- Define the terms *ergogenic aid* and *ergolytic aid*.

- List the different drugs, nutrients, and practices that can enhance exercise performance.

- Explain the mechanisms by which the different ergogenic aids function.

- Identify the dangers of using specific types of ergogenic aids.

- Describe how certain ergogenic aids specifically help with prolonged or intense exercise.

- Apply your knowledge of muscle biochemistry and systems physiology to the function of ergogenic aids.

KEY TERMS

ergogenic aid

ergolytic

warm-up

caffeine

glycerol

carnitine

phosphate loading

sodium bicarbonate

dichloroacetate

erythropoietin

blood doping

autologous transfusion

homologous transfusion

polycythemia

erythrocythemia

growth hormone

anabolic-androgenic steroids

amphetamines

The quest to improve exercise performance has characterized athletic competition throughout history. Improvements in training techniques, clothing, and nutritional practices, as well as new tactics, medical interventions, and use of illegal drugs, all have abetted the drive to win, at what seems to be an ever-increasing cost to tradition, health, moral beliefs, and a clear conscience. Not all of these changes are unethical; for example, the innovations in equipment, such as those seen in cycling, rowing, and skiing, are the results of scientific invention applied to athletic endeavor to push the limits of human performance. On the other hand, certain nutritional practices (ingestion of caffeine, sodium bicarbonate, or dichloroacetate), medical interventions (blood doping), prescription drugs (ß-blockers, antihistamines), and nonprescribed medications (anabolic steroids, growth hormone, erythropoietin) are less accepted or even illegal, and they foster a "win at all costs" attitude toward sports and athletics. Agents and practices that can improve exercise performance, such as those listed previously, have been called *ergogenic aids*. This chapter presents the ergogenic aids that have been used by athletes, as well as the research evidence documenting their effects on exercise performance and, where appropriate, their long-term effects on the human body.

Ergogenic Aids in Sports and Athletics

The term *ergogenic* means "tending to increase work." This definition has been modified to apply to exercise performance, resulting in the term **ergogenic aid,** which is a physical, mechanical, nutritional, psychologic, or pharmacologic substance or treatment that either directly improves physiologic variables associated with exercise performance or removes subjective restraints that may limit physiologic capacity.[3,4,68] Thus any substance, practice, or piece of equipment that can increase the work performed during exercise, or enhance exercise performance, is an ergogenic aid. Table 18.1 lists substances athletes can ingest and practices they can perform that fit the definition of an ergogenic aid. Focus Box 18.1 presents the recommendations

of the American College of Sports Medicine concerning the use of ergogenic aids for improved exercise performance.

As indicated in Table 18.1, all the main ergogenic aids, except for ingestion of carnitine, are known to improve attributes of function that can influence exercise performance. However, the exercise conditions associated with improved function are often limited, and several ergogenic aids are known to pose health risks when used excessively or

ergogenic aid
a physical, mechanical, nutritional, psychologic, or pharmacologic substance or treatment that either directly improves physiologic variables associated with exercise performance or removes subjective restraints that may limit physiologic capacity

TABLE 18.1

Potential and known ergogenic aids to exercise performance

ERGOGENIC AID	PROPOSED BENEFIT	PROVEN BENEFIT	BEST USE
Warm-up	Stimulates muscle metabolism and cardiorespiratory function	Yes	Both low- and moderate-intensity exercise performed 5-30 min before main exercise bout
Caffeine ingestion	Lipid mobilization	Yes	Before prolonged exercise
	Glycogen sparing	Yes	
Carbohydrate ingestion	Prevents hypoglycemia	Yes	Increased intake 3 days before event; also immediately before and during event
	Increases carbohydrate metabolism	Yes	
Liquid ingestion	Improves thermoregulation and cardiovascular function	Yes	Before and during prolonged exercise
Saline infusion	Improves thermoregulation and cardiovascular function	Yes	Before and during prolonged exercise
Glycerol hyperhydration	Increases interstitial and vascular water	Yes	Before and during prolonged exercise
	Improves thermoregulation and cardiovascular function	Yes	
Carnitine ingestion	Increases lipid catabolism	No	—
	Spares muscle glycogen	No	
Phosphate ingestion	Delays muscle fatigue	?	Supplementation 3-6 days before event
	Increases VO$_2$max and ventilatory threshold	Yes	
Pure oxygen inhalation	Improves intense exercise	Yes	Only if done during non-steady-state exercise
	Speeds recovery from intense exercise	No	
Sodium bicarbonate ingestion*	Increases blood buffering capacity	Yes	Immediately before intermittent intense exercise
Dichloroacetate ingestion†	Increases oxidation of pyruvate	Yes	Up to 2 hours before exercise
	Reduces peripheral vascular resistance	Yes	
	Decreases lactate production	Yes	
Blood doping*	Increased oxygen transport	Yes	1 week before prolonged exercise
Erythropoietin*	Increases red blood cells and oxygen transport	Yes	1-2 weeks before prolonged exercise
Growth hormone*	Increases muscle hypertrophy	Yes	
Testosterone*	Increases muscle hypertrophy	Yes	
Amphetamines*	Increases pain tolerance	Yes	

* Medical evidence of detrimental side effects when used in excess or administered incorrectly.
† Not yet approved by the FDA.

FOCUS BOX 18.1

Position stands of the American College of Sports Medicine on the use of ergogenic aids and alcohol to improve exercise performance

The American College of Sports Medicine (ACSM) has published several statements on the use of blood doping, anabolic-androgenic steroids, and alcohol to improve exercise performance. Each statement is supported by research and was written to justify the current opinion of the world's leading experts on the use of the specific substance. The recommendations of the statements follow.

Use of Alcohol in Sports[2]

Alcohol has been used by athletic and nonathletic individuals for centuries. Alcohol's reported ability to increase relaxation and reduce the perception of stress has given rise to the belief that alcohol may improve exercise performance. However, alcohol is not an ergogenic aid, but rather an ergolytic substance. In 1982 ACSM published the following findings on the use of alcohol as a possible ergogenic aid.

1. Acute ingestion of alcohol can exert a deleterious effect on a wide variety of psychomotor skills, such as reaction time, hand-eye coordination, accuracy, balance, and complex coordination.

2. Acute ingestion of alcohol will not substantially influence metabolic or physiologic functions essential to physical performance, such as energy metabolism, maximal oxygen consumption (VO_2max), heart rate, stroke volume, cardiac output, muscle blood flow, arteriovenous oxygen difference, or respiratory dynamics.

3. Alcohol consumption may impair body temperature regulation during prolonged exercise in a cold environment. Acute alcohol ingestion will not improve and may decrease strength, power, local muscular endurance, speed, and cardiovascular endurance.

4. Alcohol is the most abused drug in the United States and is a major factor in accidents and their consequences. Also, it has been widely documented that prolonged, excessive alcohol consumption can elicit pathologic changes in the liver, heart, brain, and muscle, which lead to disability and death.

5. Serious and continuing efforts should be made to educate athletes, coaches, health and physical educators, physicians, trainers, the sports media, and the general public about the effects of acute alcohol ingestion on human physical performance and on the potential acute and chronic problems of excessive alcohol consumption.

Use of Anabolic-Androgenic Steroids in Sports[3]

Evidence that athletes were using steroids to enhance performance was first detected in the early 1950s.[3] Despite research

evidence and medical warnings regarding the dangers of using exogenous steroid compounds, use of these drugs has increased, fueled in recent years by the development of steroids that maximize the anabolic effects while minimizing (although not eliminating) the androgenic effects. The following ACSM findings are based on research completed up to 1986.

1. Anabolic-androgenic steroids in the presence of an adequate diet can contribute to increases in body weight, often in the lean mass compartment.

2. The gains in upper body strength achieved through high-intensity exercise and proper diet can be increased by the use of anabolic-androgenic steroids in some individuals.

3. Anabolic-androgenic steroids do not increase aerobic power or capacity for muscular exercise.

4. Anabolic-androgenic steroids have been associated with adverse effects on the liver, cardiovascular system, reproductive system, and psychologic status in therapeutic trials and in limited research on athletes. Until further research is completed, the potential hazards of the use of the anabolic-androgenic steroids in athletes must include those found in therapeutic trials.

5. Use of anabolic-androgenic steroids by athletes is contrary to the rules and ethical principles of athletic competition, as set forth by many of the sports' governing bodies. The American College of Sports Medicine supports these ethical principles and deplores the use of anabolic-androgenic steroids by athletes.

Blood Doping as an Ergogenic Aid[4]

Scientific inquiry into homologous and autologous blood reinfusion has provided extensive evidence of normal physiologic function, the body's response to high and low erythrocyte content of blood, and the importance of blood oxygen transport in determining both maximal and submaximal exercise performance. However, because research has proved the benefits of blood reinfusion to performance of endurance exercise, athletes have adopted this procedure as a means of enhancing training and competitive performance. In 1984 ACSM published a statement on this practice:

It is the position of the American College of Sports Medicine that the use of blood doping as an ergogenic aid for athletic competition is unethical and unjustifiable, but that autologous RBC infusion is an acceptable procedure to induce erythrocythemia in clinically controlled conditions for the purpose of legitimate scientific inquiry.

improperly. Each ergogenic aid is discussed specifically in the sections that follow.

Substances that impair exercise performance are called **ergolytic** substances.[23] These include alcohol, marijuana, smokeless and cigarette tobacco, cocaine, ß-blockers, calcium channel blockers, and diuretics. This chapter does not cover the use and functions of these substances.

Warm-Up

The ergogenic benefits of a **warm-up** are supported by a vast array of research dating back to the 1950s.[49] In the 1970s, research focused on determining the best type of warm-up for improving exercise,[37] the effect of muscle temperature on subsequent energy metabolism,[22] and the specificity of warm-up benefits to muscle groups of the body.[41] More recently research has centered on whether warming up is beneficial for certain types of more intense exercise.[54,56] Based on this research, warm-ups can be divided into several categories: active versus passive, general versus specific, and submaximal versus intense.

Active Versus Passive Warm-Up

There are several ways to warm up the body before competition. One important question answered by research was whether exercise was a better warm-up than more passive forms of increasing body temperature (hot shower or bath). Passive body heating proved better than not warming up at all, but it was not as effective as an active warm-up at increasing the quickness of the body's responses to exercise.[39]

Table 18.2 lists the benefits (both proven and unsubstantiated) derived from a warm-up before prolonged submaximal or short-term intense exercise. These benefits are related to improved exercise performance, because raising muscle temperature (1) increases muscle energy metabolism (as a result of the Q_{10} effect [see Chapter 4]); (2) increases tissue elasticity; (3) aids in oxygen delivery (because of the Bohr effect); (4) increases local blood flow and oxygen delivery, to support increases in exercise intensity; and (5) may improve the recruitment profile of motor units. Of course, many athletes maintain that they also gain psychologic benefits from a warm-up, but research has not adequately addressed this issue.

Karlsson et al.[39] conducted a classic study of the effects of an intense warm-up before submaximal exercise. They used either arms or legs to perform exhaustive exercise, and then exercised the legs. The prior intense exercise actually reduced performance in both muscle that was previously exercised, and muscle that was not. Consequently, an active warm-up that is too intense and that is separated from the main exercise bout by only 6 minutes of recovery can do more harm than good. That detriment may be a result of the acidosis generated by the intense warm-up.

TABLE 18.2	
Benefits of an active warm-up before submaximal and intense exercise	
BENEFIT	**VERIFIED BY RESEARCH**
SUBMAXIMAL EXERCISE	
Increased muscle temperatures	Yes
Increased muscle blood flow	Yes
Reduced oxygen deficit	Yes
Improved neuromuscular function	Not yet substantiated
Increased lipid catabolism	Yes
Decreased carbohydrate catabolism	Yes
Muscle glycogen sparing	Not yet substantiated
Reduced risk of musculoskeletal injury	Not yet substantiated
INTENSE EXERCISE	
Improved neuromuscular function	Yes
Increased lipid catabolism	Not yet substantiated
Decreased carbohydrate catabolism	Not yet substantiated
Improved acid-base balance	Yes
Reduced oxygen deficit	Yes
Muscle glycogen sparing	Not yet substantiated
Reduced risk of musculoskeletal injury	Not yet substantiated

General Versus Specific Warm-Up

A warm-up should be active, not too intense,[41] and should engage the muscles that will be the prime movers in the exercise bout. A general warm-up, such as muscle stretching and total body exercise, can provide some of the benefits shown in Table 18.2, but it is not as effective in stimulating increased blood flow and muscle mitochondrial respiration as a specific warm-up.

Warm-up strategies have been devised for activities that demand more neuromuscular precision than physiologic function (e.g., gymnastics, dancing, diving, ice skating, and other high-skill activities). Athletes in these sports often use psychologic imagery, which is believed to prompt the correct sequence of motor pattern stimulation in the central nervous system. Based on the extent of its use by these athletes, this form of general warm-up seems to be important, but there is no scientific evidence supporting its effectiveness.

Submaximal Versus Intense Warm-Up

Because a specific, active warm-up can increase local blood flow and muscle temperature and reduce the oxygen deficit, it has been proposed that a warm-up may also be beneficial for intense exercise performance.[54,56] An active warm-up before intense swimming or cycling has been shown to increase oxygen consumption, improve muscle metabolism,[56] and reduce the acid–base disturbance caused by intense exercise.[54] Despite these improvements, however, no evidence was found of improved exercise performance.

Clinical Considerations

Not all exercisers are young, healthy, or highly trained. Research has shown that an active warm-up has certain benefits for cardiovascular function that may prevent abnormal heart responses and, in fact, save lives.[6] In one study, men who had no symptoms of heart disease performed intense treadmill running, some with and some without a warm-up; significantly more arrhythmias occurred among those who did not warm up, which was interpreted to indicate impaired coronary blood flow. These findings suggest that a warm-up may be especially important for individuals who have cardiovascular disease or risk factors for cardiovascular disease.

Nutritional Ergogenic Aids

Caffeine

Caffeine is a chemical constituent of many foods, especially coffee, tea, and cocoa. Because these substances and foods are very popular in Western societies, caffeine ingestion is high; caffeine is arguably the most widely consumed drug in North America and Europe.[63] It is a central nervous system (CNS) stimulant, a stimulator of adipocyte lipolysis, a mild diuretic, and a potentiator of muscle contractile force at low frequencies (contraction rate <10 Hz)[63] (Figure 18.1).

Caffeine functions in the CNS and in adipocytes by binding to adenosine receptors and increasing intracellular concentrations of cyclic adenosine monophosphate (cAMP). In the CNS this function improves alertness, concentration, and vigor and may increase maximal motor unit recruitment. The increase in cAMP concentrations in adipose tissue increases lipolysis, increasing the mobilization of free fatty acids (FFAs) and the availability of FFA for muscle catabolism. In skeletal muscle, caffeine facilitates the release of calcium from the sarcoplasmic reticulum, thereby increasing the muscles' ability to generate force during contraction.[63] Caffeine's inhibition of phosphodiesterase in skeletal muscle and adipose tissue has been identified as its mechanism for

FIGURE 18.1

The actions of caffeine on the liver, skeletal muscle, adipose tissue, and central nervous system.

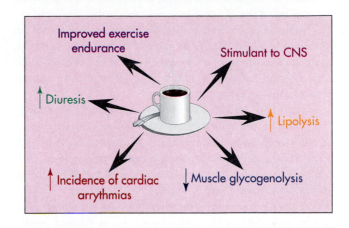

increasing intracellular cAMP, but convincing evidence indicates that this mechanism is incorrect,[68] and Tarnopolsky[59] recommends that the phosphodiesterase connection no longer be promoted.

Research into the ergogenic effects of caffeine during exercise was based on the metabolic implications of an increased reliance on lipid for energy catabolism during exercise.[14] According to this hypothesis, if caffeine increased FFA mobilization and reliance on lipid catabolism, muscle glycogen would be spared and exercise could be performed at higher intensities or for longer periods. However, research has yielded contradictory evidence on the ergogenic benefits of caffeine.* The main reasons suggested for the discrepancies are different caffeine tolerances among study subjects, different doses of caffeine, and the often uncontrolled dietary state of the subjects before exercise. Nevertheless, in studies that measured the effects of preexercise caffeine ingestion on muscle glycogen use during exercise,[26,27,59] caffeine consis-

---

*References 8, 14, 18, 19, 26, 31, 49, and 67.

---

ergolytic (er-go-lit′ik)
having the ability to impair exercise performance

warm-up
a general term for practices performed before exercise to prepare the body for the exercise activity

caffeine (kaf′een)
a naturally occuring substance that acts as a central nervous system (CNS) stimulant and a competitive antagonist for adenosine receptors in the CNS and periphery

tently effected sparing of muscle glycogen. Given the recent findings that carbohydrate intake immediately before or during exercise negates the metabolic effects of caffeine,[60] the influence of caffeine on exercise performance secondary to the sparing of muscle glycogen requires further research.

Some research indicated that a person could exercise longer after ingesting caffeine, compared with a control trial, and that perceptions of effort were lower with caffeine.[14] This latter effect is believed to be due to sympathetic stimulation of the central nervous system.[14,26]

The main drawback of caffeine ingestion is its diuretic function. This response is problematic when exercise is done in a hot or humid environment or for a prolonged period, since it will exacerbate the development of dehydration. Caffeine can also be addictive, resulting in withdrawal symptoms of headache, nausea, and irritability.[63]

Based on research findings and subjective feelings about caffeine as an ergogenic aid for long-term endurance events, the International Olympic Committee (IOC) classified caffeine as a banned substance in 1962; it was removed from this list in 1972. Currently, caffeine ingestion that results in urinary caffeine concentrations of 12 mg/L or higher would be considered unethical by the IOC and grounds for confiscating Olympic medals.

Ironically, such a urinary concentration would require extreme dosages, since a caffeine intake greater than 13.5 mg/kg generally is required to exceed the urinary concentration set by the IOC.[63] To give an example, if the caffeine source is a 250 ml (7 $\frac{1}{2}$ oz) cup of instant coffee (80 mg of caffeine), a man weighing 67.5 kg (150 lb) would have to drink more than 11 cups to violate the IOC standard; a woman weighing 54 kg (120 lb) would have to drink more than 9 cups. Furthermore, in research studies a caffeine dose as low as 4.4 mg/kg was shown to have an ergogenic effect.[10]

Research also has shown that caffeine is not an ergogenic aid for intense exercise.[63]

Carbohydrate, Fluid, and Glycerol

The importance of muscle glycogen and of maintaining blood glucose and preventing dehydration during prolonged exercise is discussed in depth in previous chapters. Furthermore, the practice of consuming carbohydrates and liquid during exercise is accepted in most athletic competitions and therefore is not an ethical issue. Chapter 17 presents the research on exercise performance after ingestion of carbohydrate and fluid.

Recently, in comparing the effects of carbohydrate ingestion with glycerol ingestion, researchers discovered that prolonged exercise was better enhanced by ingestion of the **glycerol** solution.[48,52] Glycerol has an ergogenic benefit because it retains water in interstitial and vascular spaces, improving cardiovascular function and thermoregulation. Only minimal research has been completed on the ergogenic benefits of glycerol, but the current recommendation is ingestion of a 5% solution providing 1.2 g/kg glycerol

during the 2 hours before competition, followed by ingestion of a 1% glycerol and carbohydrate solution during the event in volumes that apply for carbohydrate solutions (see Chapter 17).

Carnitine

The molecule **carnitine** is essential for transportation of acylated FFAs into mitochondria (Figure 18.2; also see Chapter 4). During exercise of increasing intensity, a metabolic transition occurs resulting in a shift from reliance on fat catabolism to reliance on carbohydrate catabolism. It has been proposed that the limiting step for continued fatty acid entry into mitochondria and its subsequent degradation in ß-oxidation is the availability of carnitine. However, research evaluating this hypothesis has shown no ergogenic benefit to ingestion of carnitine.[64]

Phosphate

During intense exercise, muscle fatigue develops because of the muscles' inability to regenerate adenosine triphosphate (ATP) from oxidative phosphorylation at a rate that matches demand. Thus ATP regeneration relies more on glycolysis and creatine phosphate. It has been hypothesized that if phosphate can be provided to the muscles during intense exercise, it would take longer to exhaust creatine phosphate stores, and intense exercise could be performed longer before fatigue. In addition, added phosphate levels in the blood have been hypothesized to increase production of 2,3-bisphosphoglycerate and to facilitate oxygen dissociation from hemoglobin, thereby improving oxygen delivery to skeletal muscle.

Despite evidence of no benefit from **phosphate loading** during intense isokinetic resistance exercise and treadmill running to exhaustion (214.4 m/min at 6%),[20] Kreider et al.[42] reported that phosphate ingestion significantly improved maximum oxygen consumption (VO_2max) andthe ventilation threshold, and may improve 5-mile run performance. Further research is needed, especially at the muscle level, to clarify the influence of phosphate loading on exercise performance.

Sodium Bicarbonate and Sodium Citrate

Because the body's main buffering agent is bicarbonate (HCO_3^-), and because metabolic acidosis contributes to the development of muscle fatigue and cognitive perception of fatigue (see Chapter 22), it would seem possible that increasing the body's bicarbonate stores would improve intense exercise performance.

A common method of increasing circulating HCO_3^- is to ingest **sodium bicarbonate** (baking soda). Although this is effective, it also carries a greater likelihood of gastrointestinal (GI) distress. Initial research on the use of bicarbonate for intense exercise did not support previous claims[31,38]; however, when intense exercise is performed for 1 to 7 minutes and when the exercise is intermittent, definite improvements in performance have been documented (Figure 18.3).[15,45,58,66]

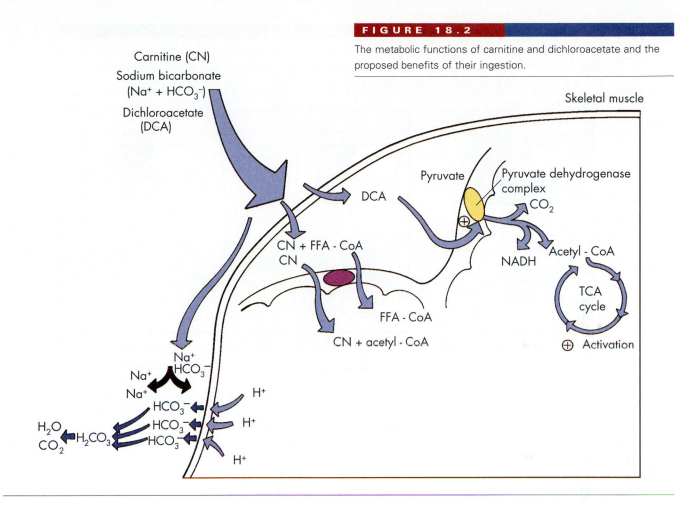

FIGURE 18.2

The metabolic functions of carnitine and dichloroacetate and the proposed benefits of their ingestion.

Intermittent exercise is important because without the recovery in blood flow during the rest periods, limited blood (and therefore HCO_3^-) becomes available to buffer the acid that accumulates in muscle and the extracellular space.

Research on sodium citrate has also shown a beneficial role in increasing the blood's buffering capacity and improving exercise performance.[43,51] In addition, no GI distress has been reported with sodium citrate ingestion.[43]

Dichloroacetate

Dichloroacetate (DCA) is an artificial derivative of a substrate that occurs in the body (acetate) during lipid catabolism in the liver. DCA has not been approved by the Food and Drug Administration (FDA) for general use; however, many researchers have been given approval to use it to combat metabolic acidosis arising from several clinical disorders, such as heart failure and certain kidney and liver conditions that contribute to metabolic acidosis. DCA has also been used in research involving exercise that stressed muscle metabolic and cardiovascular function. Evidence indicates that DCA reduces peripheral vascular resistance, thereby increasing muscle blood flow, and stimulates pyruvate dehydrogenase, which increases pyruvate oxidation, reduces the pro-

glycerol (glis′er-ol)

a by-product of glycolysis that is used in triacylglycerol synthesis; Glycerol is released during the mobilization of fatty acids in lipolysis and often is considered an indirect reflection of the mobilization of fatty acids in blood and adipose tissue

carnitine (kar′ni-teen)

a molecule required for the transport of medium- to long-chain fatty acids in the mitochondria

phosphate loading

the practice of ingesting phosphate to improve exercise performance

sodium bicarbonate

the molecule in blood with the greatest buffering power against acid

dichloroacetate (di-klor′o-ass′e-tate)

an artificial, chlorinated derivative of acetyl-CoA that stimulates the activity of pyruvate dehydrogenase, reduces lactate accumulation in the blood, and decreases peripheral vascular resistance

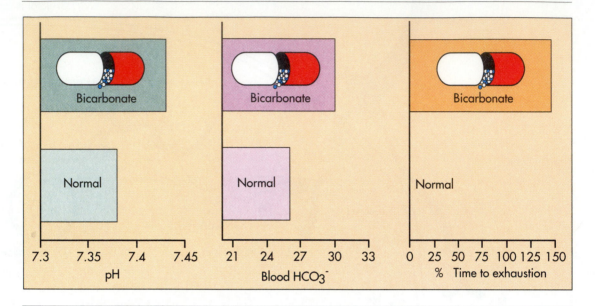

FIGURE 18.3

The increased blood bicarbonate, decreased acidosis, and improved exercise tolerance of intense exercise when sodium bicarbonate was ingested before exercise. (Adapted from Costill DL et al: *Int J Sports Med* 5:228-231, 1984; and Horswill CA et al: *Med Sci Sports Exerc* 20(6):566-569, 1988.)

duction of lactate, (see Figure 18.2) and theoretically should increase the rate of ATP regeneration from oxidative phosphorylation.[11,17,47,61] Unfortunately, because minimal research in human subjects has been completed using DCA during exercise, it is unclear whether dichloroacetate improves exercise performance.[11]

Inhalation of Pure Oxygen

Athletes have inhaled pure oxygen immediately before an athletic event to better prepare themselves, to improve performance during exercise, and to improve recovery from intense exercise. Pure oxygen is used because of its increased partial pressure relative to oxygen in normal atmospheric air. Inhaling pure oxygen raises the partial pressure of arterial oxygen (PaO_2) from approximately 98 mm Hg to over 600 mm Hg, depending on the barometric pressure and extent of mixing with atmospheric air during inhalation. However, because hemoglobin (Hgb) is approximately 98% saturated in pulmonary capillary blood, at sea level pure oxygen can increase oxygen transported on erythrocytes only to approximately 3.5 ml O_2/L. Because some oxygen (about 0.003 ml/L/mm Hg) is also transported dissolved in plasma (see Chapter 12), the total added oxygen for an inspired PO_2 of 600 mm Hg is 21.5 ml/L for a person whose Hgb is 14 g/dl.

The increase in oxygen transport of 21.5 ml/L may not sound like much, but when multiplied by the cardiac output, which increases from 5 L/min to over 25 L/min at maximal exercise in trained individuals, this additional oxy-gen store can amount to an increase in oxygen transport of 0.65 L/min at maximal exertion, or an increase of 0.4 L/min at intensities corresponding to the lactate threshold. Given these numbers, it is no surprise that research on the use of pure oxygen during exercise has shown significant increases in VO$_2$max; oxygen consumption (VO$_2$) during the initial minutes of intense exercise; and time to exhaustion[28,37,62] (Figure 18.4).

Erythropoietin

Erythropoietin (EPO) is a hormone produced mainly by the kidneys (see Chapters 11 and 13) in response to hypoxia, and anemia that may result from increased blood losses (e.g., hemorrhage). Erythropoietin stimulates the bone marrow to specifically increase the differentiation of stem cells into erythrocytes. Clinically, EPO is used for patients with anemic conditions that often result from kidney damage. For example, there is a growing body of research on the effects of EPO on the exercise tolerance and hematology of renal dialysis patients.

As with most of the pharmacologic ergogenic aids, because EPO works, it has been exploited in athletics and sports. In late 1980s several Dutch cyclists attempted to use EPO to increase their blood oxygen transport capacities. Unfortunately, the EPO worked too well; it greatly increased red blood cell production, blood viscosity, and blood pressure, resulting in pulmonary embolism and eventually death. It is hoped that the deaths of these athletes have diverted attention from use of EPO.

FIGURE 18.4

When pure oxygen is inhaled during intense exercise, oxygen consumption increases more rapidly, causing a lower oxygen deficit, and intense exercise can be tolerated for longer before fatigue.

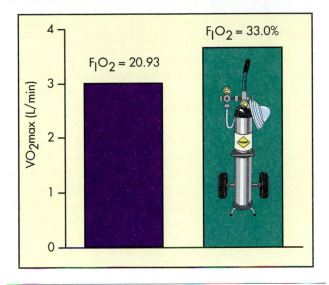

added 1.7 L O_2/min at a cardiac output of 20 L/min (as would occur at the lactate threshold for a moderately trained individual). This provides the potential for athletes to exercise at steady state at higher than normal intensities, to increase their maximal exercise intensity, and to improve endurance performance.

Research into the effects of blood transfusions on exercise performance has been going on since the 1970s.[25] Most of this work has stemmed from the known improvements in erythrocyte mass in blood after prolonged altitude exposure, a process called **polycythemia.** These early studies revealed that artificially raising the blood's erythrocyte content had the potential to improve endurance-exercise tolerance. The artificial increase in blood erythrocyte content has been called **erythrocythemia** to emphasize its difference from the natural increases that occur with polycythemia.

Figure 18.5 illustrates the change in hematologic parameters after transfusion of differing volumes of blood.[60] Autologous infusion of 1 U of blood did not increase oxygen transport or exercise capacities. However, infusion of 2 and 3 U improved these parameters, with 3 U providing the greatest improvement. It should also be noted that the improved hemoglobin and hematocrit values after autologous infusion are not the result of a simple additive effect, as previously explained for the theoretical increase in oxygen transport. Infusion of 2 or 3 U represents 20% or 27% additions (respectively) of red blood cells (assuming a blood volume of 4.5 L) but results in similar increases in hemoglobin and hematocrit (8% and 11%, respectively).[60]

Blood Doping

Blood doping is the procedure of removing blood from the body, allowing the body to reproduce new red blood cells (RBCs), and then reinfusing the blood. Usually 1 to 4 U of blood (450 to 1800 ml, or $^4/_5$ to 3 $^1/_3$ pt) is removed from the body.[4,60] One unit is removed every 4 to 8 weeks to prevent excessive lowering of blood's oxygen transport capacity and detriments to training quality. The plasma from the blood is reinfused into the athlete, and the remaining blood cells are processed to isolate the erythrocytes, which are stored in a special preservative solution. Approximately 1 week before an event the stored erythrocytes are reinfused into the athlete. This process is called an **autologous transfusion,** since the blood cells came from the same person. When blood cells from another person are infused, the process is called a **homologous transfusion.**

Blood doping can double the hemoglobin concentration. However, because of the increased viscosity of the blood, the potential increase in oxygen transport capacity is compromised by the increased demand on the cardiovascular system. Thus athletes usually wait at least 1 week after reinfusion to allow natural removal of some of the excess blood cells before competition. If the hemoglobin concentration has been increased from 14 g/dl to 20 g/dl, then when hemoglobin is 98% saturated, this extra oxygen transport capacity transports an added 84 ml O_2/L and circulates an

erythropoietin (e′rith-ro-**poy**′e-tin)
a hormone secreted by the kidneys that is responsible for stimulating the production of red blood cells (erythropoiesis)

blood doping
the process of removing blood from the body and reinfusing it at a later date for the purpose of increasing hematocrit and oxygen-carrying capacity

autologous transfusion
reinfusion of red blood cells into the individual from whom they were removed

homologous transfusion
infusion of red blood cells that were removed from another individual

polycythemia (pol′i-si-the′mi-ah)
increased concentration of red blood cells in the blood

erythrocythemia (e-rith′ro-si-the′mi-ah)
an artificially increased concentration of red blood cells in the blood

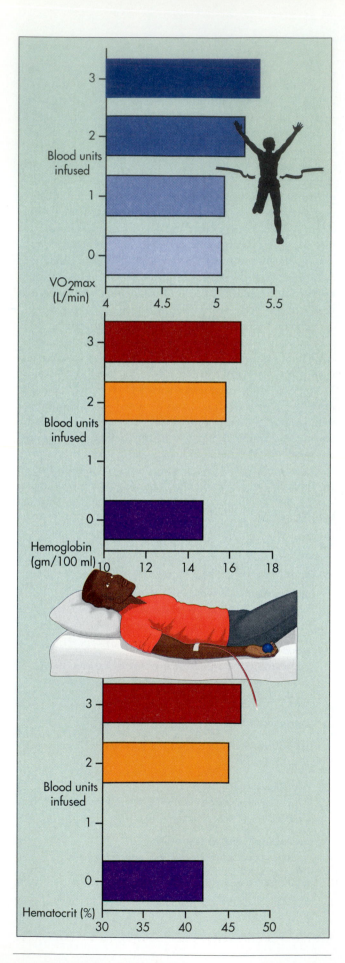

FIGURE 18.5

The different changes in hemoglobin concentration, hematocrit, and VO$_2$max following either 1, 2, or 3 units of autologous blood transfusion.

Growth Hormone

Growth hormone (GH) is a natural glucoregulatory, anabolic hormone. It has been and continues to be used to treat disorders that result in limited growth (e.g., dwarfism) or increased wasting of the body (e.g., AIDS). Use of GH to increase muscle hypertrophy made it attractive to athletes who could perform better with increased muscle mass. Other perceived benefits were increased use of FFAs, reducing body fat; increased bone growth in immature long bones and flat bones; and improved healing of musculoskeletal injury.

Research has shown that administering GH to elderly individuals (61 to 81 years of age) resulted in increased lean body mass, reduced fat mass, and minor increases in bone mineral density.[55] In another study, younger men were divided into two groups to perform resistance training; one group was given GH, the other was not. Those who received growth hormone showed the largest increases in lean body mass.

Anabolic-Androgenic Steroids

Anabolic steroids are a family of synthetic steroid hormones similar to natural steroid hormones (e.g., testosterone) that increase protein synthesis and resultant muscle hypertrophy *(anabolic)* and produce the male secondary sex characteristics *(androgenic)*, such as hirsutism (increased body hair), deepening of the voice, and aggressive behavior. Because of these characteristics, these drugs are called **anabolic-androgenic steroids.**

The natural increase in anabolic steroids in men increases lean body mass and promotes the development of the secondary sex characteristics. Additional use of anabolic-androgenic steroids is known to further increase lean body mass, reduce fat mass, and produce greater increases in training-related improvements in muscle strength.[3]

A research strategy adopted to investigate the influence of anabolic steroid use on physiology and exercise performance involves studying people who of their own free will are taking steroids in amounts that would not be allowed in randomized controlled designs.[34] The dosage of steroids used is important because research has shown that large gains in hypertrophy and strength occur only with very high doses.[29] It is unclear what the optimal protein intake would be to foster maximal gains in hypertrophy when anabolic steroids are used in conjunction with resistance training; however, an intake at least three times the current daily recommendations (i.e., 0.8 gm/kg) may be required. The same concerns are true with GH use.

FOCUS BOX 18.2

Medical problems associated with abuse of anabolic-androgenic steroids

- Early calcification of the epiphyseal plates of the long bones, resulting in stunted growth

- Prolonged suppression of gonadal hormone secretion

- Testicular atrophy in men

- Menstrual irregularities in women

- Reduced sperm count

- Prostate enlargement

- Liver damage (resulting from exaggerated need for metabolic removal of the steroids)

- Cardiomyopathy

- Decrease in HDL cholesterol

- Increased risk of atherosclerotic cardiovascular disease

- Increased risk of cancer

Other possible benefits of steroid use are their proposed ability to increase maximal oxygen uptake and improve tolerance to and recovery from intense training. However, the accuracy of the claims has not yet been clarified by research because results have been contradictory as to whether VO_2max is improved, and the influence of anabolic steroids in aiding muscle repair and recovery has not been adequately researched.

Use of large doses of anabolic-androgenic steroids is dangerous because it poses health risks. Regardless of this dilemma, athletes are often forced to decide to use anabolic steroids to remain competitive in an event associated with steroid abuse. For example, estimates of steroid use by athletes involved in power events (e.g., the throwing events of discus, shot put, and javelin) and pure strength sports (e.g., weight lifting and body building) exceed 50% of participants.[67] This incidence of use is problematic because well-documented medical risks are associated with abuse of steroids. Focus Box 18.2 lists possible medical problems associated with steroid abuse.

The health-related side effects of anabolic steroid use by women are unclear. Anabolic steroids produce similar developmental effects in women as in men, with the added effects of increased sebaceous gland activity and incidence of acne and enlargement of the clitoris. The long-term consequences of a disrupted menstrual cycle in women resulting from the steroid abuse are unknown, and it is also unclear whether the increased weight-bearing activity performed by women who also use anabolic steroids offsets the known potential for bone mineral loss caused by chronically low estradiol concentrations (see Chapters 13 and 23).

Amphetamines

Amphetamines are a group of CNS stimulants that are far more potent than caffeine. They reportedly have the effects of heightened arousal, euphoria, and increased alertness.[13,40] As with other potentially harmful ergogenic agents, minimal controlled scientific research has been completed on the use of amphetamines. However, studies that have been completed indicate that athletes may be able to increase their tolerance to fatigue, as indicated by increased muscular strength and time to fatigue.[12] In addition, amphetamines overcome CNS inhibition of movement, as indicated by increased acceleration and shortened response times. It is unknown whether these proven benefits improve actual athletic performance or whether larger doses of amphetamines induce greater changes in these or other parameters.

The danger of amphetamines is their excessive stimulation of the cardiovascular system. Possible effects include cardiac arrhythmias and excessive blood pressure response to exercise. Exercising beyond the normal limits imposed by symptoms of fatigue is also inherently dangerous for the musculoskeletal system, increasing the risk of orthopedic injury. Also, symptoms of amphetamine abuse range from dizziness, irritability, and headache for mild dosages to addiction, paranoid delusions, and neuropathy for habitual abuse.[65]

---

growth hormone

a hormone that primarily functions to regulate blood glucose, and secondarily functions in concert with somatomedins to stimulate bone and muscle growth

anabolic-androgenic steroids

hormones that stimulate growth and the development of secondary sex characterisitcs

amphetamines (am'**fet**-a'meens)

drugs that overcome the discomfort and some of the neuromuscular recruitment limitations experienced during intense exercise

SUMMARY

- An **ergogenic aid** has been defined as a physical, mechanical, nutritional, psychologic, or pharmacologic substance or treatment that either directly improves physiologic variables associated with exercise performance or removes subjective restraints that may limit physiologic capacity.

- Substances that impair exercise performance are known as **ergolytic** substances. These include alcohol, marijuana, smokeless and cigarette tobacco, cocaine, ß-blockers and calcium channel blockers, and diuretics.

- Accepted ergogenic aids are a **warm-up,** carbohydrate ingestion, fluid intake, **glycerol** ingestion, natural practices to induce **polycythemia** (e.g., altitude exposure), and sodium citrate ingestion. Illegal and therefore ethically questionable ergogenic aids are use of anabolic-androgenic steroids, amphetamines, or erythropoietin; excessive **caffeine** intake; and ingestion of sodium bicarbonate or dichloroacetate.

- Warm-up practices can be divided into several categories: active versus passive, general versus specific, and submaximal versus intense. Active warm-up of specific muscles used during exercise is most effective for prolonged exercise; for more skilled activities, completing specific movement patterns and rehearsing them mentally are believed to improve exercise performance (however, there are no research data documenting this effect). There also is no evidence that warming up improves the performance of intense exercise.

- The nutrient ergogenic aids are caffeine, carbohydrate, liquid, glycerol, **carnitine**, dichloroacetate, sodium phosphate (**phosphate loading**), sodium citrate, and **sodium bicarbonate.** Caffeine stimulates adipose and skeletal muscle tissue to increase lipolysis, thereby increasing serum free fatty acids (FFAs) and intramuscular catabolism of FFAs. Caffeine also has a mild diuretic effect, which is its main drawback. This effect becomes problematic when exercise is done in a hot or humid environment or for a prolonged period, because it exacerbates the development of dehydration. Caffeine also can be addictive, producing withdrawal symptoms of headache, nausea, and irritability.

- Research has shown that ingesting a glycerol solution better enhances the performance of prolonged exercise than does ingesting carbohydrate. The mechanism of glycerol's ergogenic benefit is that it retains water in interstitial and vascular spaces, improving cardiovascular function and thermoregulation. Ingesting sodium bicarbonate improves the performance of intense exercise by increasing blood buffering capacity.

- Carnitine is a molecule that is essential for the transportation of acylated free fatty acids into mitochondria; however, studies consistently have shown no ergogenic benefit to ingestion of carnitine. **Dichloroacetate** (DCA) is an artificial derivative of a substrate that occurs in the body (acetate) during lipid catabolism in the liver. The U.S. Food and Drug Administration (FDA) has not approved DCA for general use but has granted researchers permission to investigate it. So far, studies indicate that DCA reduces peripheral vascular resistance, thereby increasing muscle blood flow, and stimulates pyruvate dehydrogenase, which increases pyruvate oxidation, reduces the production of lactate, and theoretically should increase the rate of adenosine triphosphate (ATP) regeneration from oxidative phosphorylation. However, minimal research has been done using DCA during exercise, and it is unclear whether it improves exercise performance.

- Research into the use of pure oxygen *during* intense exercise has shown significant increases in VO_2, VO_2max, and time to exhaustion. However, there is no research evidence that inhaling pure oxygen *before* exercise improves performance or that it speeds recovery from intense exercise.

- **Erythropoietin** (EPO) is a hormone that stimulates the bone marrow to increase the differentiation of stem cells to form erythrocytes, a process called erythropoiesis. As with most of the pharmacologic ergogenic aids, because EPO works, it has been exploited in athletics and sports. Unfortunately, however, EPO works too well; it can cause large increases in the production and concentration of red blood cells, resulting in increased blood viscosity, greatly increased blood pressure, pulmonary embolism, and eventually death if used in an uncontrolled manner.

- A safer alternative to EPO is **blood doping,** which involves removing blood and infusing it at a later date. If an individual's own blood is reinfused, the process is known as an **autologous transfusion;** infusion of blood from another individual is a **homologous transfusion.** However, because of an artificial increase in red blood cell concentration (**erythrocythemia**), blood viscosity is increased and the potential increase in oxygen transport capacity is compromised by the increased demand on the cardiovascular system. Thus athletes usually wait at least 1 week after transfusion before competing, to allow natural removal of some of the excess blood cells. The added blood cells give athletes the potential to exercise at steady state at a higher than normal intensity, increase their maximal exercise intensity, and improve endurance.

- **Growth hormone** (GH) is a natural glucoregulatory and anabolic hormone. In research studies, elderly individuals (61 to 81 years of age) given GH showed increased lean body mass, reduced fat mass, and slightly increased bone mineral density. Another study was done with younger men who performed resistance training; one group was given GH, the other was not. Those who received growth hormone demonstrated the largest increases in fat-free body mass.

- **Anabolic-androgenic steroids** make up a family of steroid hormones similar to natural steroid hormones (e.g., testosterone) that increase protein synthesis and resultant muscle hypertrophy (*anabolic*) and produce the male secondary sex characteristics (*androgenic*), such as hirsutism (increased body hair), deepening of the voice, and aggressive behavior. Supplemental use of anabolic-androgenic steroids is known to further increase lean body mass, reduce fat mass, and produce greater increases in training-related improvements in muscle strength.

  However, the dangers of exogenous use of steroids are many and serious. In men it causes testicular atrophy, reduced sperm count, and prostate enlargement. In women it causes menstrual irregularities. In both sexes the consequences include calcification of the epiphyseal plates of the long bones, resulting in stunted growth; prolonged suppression of gonadal hormone secretion; liver damage (resulting from an exaggerated need for metabolic removal of the steroids); cardiomyopathy; a decrease in HDL cholesterol; increased risk of atherosclerotic cardiovascular disease; and increased risk of cancer.

- **Amphetamines** are a group of CNS stimulants far more potent than caffeine. Their reported effects include heightened arousal, euphoria, and increased alertness. The few studies that have been done indicate that amphetamines may allow athletes to increase their tolerance to fatigue (as indicated by increased muscular strength and time to fatigue) and overcome CNS inhibition to movement (as indicated by increased acceleration and shortened response times). It is not known whether these proven benefits improve actual athletic performance or whether larger doses of amphetamines induce greater changes in these or other parameters.

  The danger of amphetamines is their excessive stimulation of the cardiovascular system. Possible effects are cardiac arrhythmia, excessive blood pressure response to exercise, and increased risk of orthopedic injury. Also, symptoms of amphetamine abuse range from dizziness, irritability, and headache with mild dosages to addiction, paranoid delusions, and neuropathy with habitual abuse.

REVIEW QUESTIONS

1. What benefits does a warm-up have for both intense and prolonged submaximal exercise?

2. For what types of exercise does ingestion of sodium bicarbonate provide an ergogenic effect?

3. Does increasing the oxygen transported in the blood improve $\dot{V}O_2$max and endurance exercise performance? What ergogenic aids increase blood oxygen content?

4. What are the benefits to exercise performance—and the health risks of abuse—of growth hormone, anabolic steroids, and amphetamines?

5. Summarize the ergogenic aids that would apply either to short-term, intense exercise or to prolonged submaximal exercise.

APPLICATIONS

1. Although they were not covered in this chapter, several prescription drugs are known to have a positive effect on exercise performance; others are known to diminish it. Try to name some drugs in either category (or both), and explain the mechanism or mechanisms by which they would affect exercise performance.

2. Using what you learned in section 2 of this chapter, detail the cardiorespiratory complications inherent in blood doping.

REFERENCES

1. Alen M, Reinila M, Vihko R: Response of serum hormones to androgen administration in power athletes, *Med Sci Sports Exerc* 17(3):354-359, 1985.

2. American College of Sports Medicine: Position statement on the use of alcohol in sports, *Med Sci Sports Exerc* 14:(6):ix-xi, 1982.

3. American College of Sports Medicine: Position stand on the use of anabolic-androgenic steroids in sports, *Med Sci Sports Exerc* 19(5):534-539, 1987.

4. American College of Sports Medicine: Position stand on blood doping as an ergogenic aid, *Med Sci Sports Exerc* 19(5):540-543, 1987.

5. Bangsbo J, Jacobsen K, Nordberg N et al: Acute and habitual caffeine ingestion and metabolic responses to steady-state exercise, *J Appl Physiol* 72(4):1297-1303, 1992.

6. Barnard RJ: Ischemic response to sudden strenuous exercise in healthy men, *Circulation* 48:936-942, 1973.

7. Basuttil CP, Ruhling RO: Warm-up and circulo-respiratory adaptations, *J Sports Med* 17:69-74, 1977.

8. Berry MJ, Stoneman JV, Weyrich AS, Burney B: Dissociation of the ventilatory and lactate thresholds following caffeine ingestion, *Med Sci Sports Exerc* 23(94):463-469, 1991.

9. Bredle DL, Stager JM, Brechue WF, Farber MO: Phosphate supplementation, cardiovascular function, and exercise performance in humans, *J Appl Physiol* 65:1821-1826, 1988.

10. Cadarette BS, Levine L, Berube CL: Effects of varied dosages of caffeine on endurance exercise to fatigue, *Biochem Exerc* 13:871-877, 1983.

11. Carraro F, Klein S, Rosenblatt JI, Wolfe RR: Effect of dichloroacetate on lactate concentration in exercising humans, *J Appl Physiol* 66(2):591-597, 1989.

12. Chandler JV, Blair SN: The effect of amphetamines on selected physiological components related to athletic success, *Med Sci Sports Exerc* 12:65-69, 1980.

13. Conlee RK: Amphetamine, caffeine, and cocaine. In Lamb DR, Williams MH, editors: *Ergogenics enhancement of performance in exercise and sport,* Dubuque, Iowa, 1991, Brown & Benchmark.

14. Costill DL, Dalsky GP, Fink WJ: Effects of caffeine ingestion on metabolism and exercise performance, *Med Sci Sports Exerc* 10:155-158, 1978.

15. Costill DL, Verstappen F, Kuipers H et al: Acid-base balance during repeated bouts of exercise: influence of HCO_3, *Int J Sports Med* 5:228-231, 1984.

16. De Bruyn-Prevost P: The effects of varying warming up intensities and durations upon some physiological variables during an exercise corresponding to the WC170, *Eur J Appl Physiol* 43:93-100, 1980.

17. Delehanty JM, Naoaki M, Chang-Seng L: Effects of dichloroacetate on hemodynamic responses to dynamic exercise in dogs, *J Appl Physiol* 72(2):515-520, 1992.

18. Dodd SL, Herb RA, Powers SK: Caffeine and exercise performance: an update, *Sports Med* 15:14-23, 1993.

19. Doubt TJ, Hsieh SS: Additive effects of caffeine and cold water during submaximal leg exercise, *Med Sci Sports Exerc* 23(40):435-442, 1991.

20. Duffy DJ, Conlee RK: Effects of phosphate loading on leg power and high intensity treadmill exercise, *Med Sci Sports Exerc* 18(6):674-677, 1986.

21. Duthel JM, Vallon JJ, Martin G et al: Caffeine and sport: role of physical exercise upon elimination, *Med Sci Sports Exerc* 23(8):980-985, 1991.

22. Edwards HT, Harris RC, Hultman E et al: Effect of temperature on muscle energy metabolism and endurance during successive isometric contractions, sustained to fatigue, of the quadriceps muscle in man, *J Physiol* 220:335-352, 1972.

23. Eichner ER: Ergolytic drugs, *Sports Sci Exchange* 2(15):1-3, 1989.

24. Ekblom B, Berglund B: Effect of erythropoietin administration on maximal aerobic power, *Scand J Med Sci Sports* 1:88-93, 1991.

25. Ekblom B, Goldbarg AN, Gullbring B: Response to exercise after blood loss and reinfusion, *J Appl Physiol* 33:175-180, 1972.

26. Erikson MA, Schwartzkopf RJ, McKenzie RD: Effects of caffeine, fructose, and glucose ingestion on muscle glycogen

REFERENCES—Cont'd

utilization during exercise, *Med Sci Sports Exerc* 19:579-583, 1987.

27. Essig D, Costill DL, Van Handel PJ: Effects of caffeine ingestion on utilization of muscle glycogen and lipid during ergometer cycling, *Int J Sports Med* 1:86-90, 1980.

28. Forbes GB: The effect of anabolic steroids on lean body mass: the dose response curve, *Metabolism* 34:571-573, 1985.

29. Gledhill N: The influence of altered blood volume and oxygen transport capacity on aerobic performance, *Exerc Sport Sci Rev* 13:75-93, 1985.

30. Graham TE, Spriet LL: Performance and metabolic responses to a high caffeine dose during prolonged exercise, *J Appl Physiol* 71:2292-2298, 1991.

31. Gutin B, Stewart K, Lewis S, Kruper J: Oxygen consumption in the first stages of strenuous work as a function of prior exercise, *J Sports Med* 16:60-65, 1976.

32. Heath EM, Wilcox AR, Quinn CM: Effects of nicotinic acid on respiratory exchange ratio and substrate levels during exercise, *Med Sci Sports Exerc* 25(9):1018-1023, 1993.

33. Hervey GR, Knibbs AV, Burkinshaw L et al: Effects of methandienone on the performance and body composition of men undergoing athletic training, *Clin Sci* 60:457-461, 1981.

34. Hetzler RK, Knowlton RG, Kaminsky LA, Kamimori GH: Effect of warm-up on plasma free fatty acid responses and substrate utilization during submaximal exercise, *Res Q* 57:223-228, 1986.

35. Horswill CA, Costill DL, Fink WJ et al: Influence of sodium bicarbonate on sprint performance: relationship to dosage, *Med Sci Sports Exerc* 20(6):566-569, 1988.

36. Hultman E, Sahlin K: Acid-base balance during exercise, *Exerc Sport Sci Rev* 7:41-128, 1980.

37. Ingjer F, Stromme SB: Effects of active, passive, or no warm-up on the physiological responses to heavy exercise, *Eur J Appl Physiol* 40:273-282, 1979.

38. Ivy JL: Amphetamines. In Williams MH, editor: *Ergogenic aids in sport,* Champaign, Illinois, 1983, Human Kinetics.

39. Karlsson J, Bonde-Petersen F, Henriksson J, Knuttgen HG: Effects of previous exercise with arms or legs on metabolism and performance in exhaustive exercise, *J Appl Physiol* 38:763-767, 1975.

40. Katz RM: Prevention with and without the use of medications for exercise-induced asthma, *Med Sci Sports Exerc* 18(3):331-333, 1986.

41. Kowalchuk JM, Maltais SA, Yamaji K, Hughson RL: The effect of citrate loading on oxygen uptake, ventilatory anaerobic threshold, and run performance, *Eur J Appl Physiol* 58:858-864, 1989.

42. Kreider RB, Miller GW, Williams MH et al: Effects of phosphate loading on oxygen uptake, ventilatory anaerobic threshold, and run performance, *Med Sci Sports Exerc* 22(2):250-256, 1990.

43. Linderman J, Fahey TD: Sodium bicarbonate ingestion and exercise performance: an update, *Sports Med* 11:71-77, 1991.

44. Linderman JK, Gosselink KL: The effects of sodium bicarbonate ingestion on exercise performance, *Sports Med* 18(2):75-80, 1994.

45. Ludvik B, Peer G, Berzlanovich A: Effects of dichloroacetate and bicarbonate on hemodynamic parameters in healthy volunteers, *Clin Sci* 80(1):47-51, 1991.

46. Lyons TP, Riedesel ML, Meuli LE, Chick TW: Effects of glycerol-induced hyperhydration prior to exercise in the heat on sweating and core temperature, *Med Sci Sports Exerc* 22(4):477-483, 1990.

47. Malareck I: Investigation on physiological justification of so called "warming-up," *Acta Physiol Pol* 4:543-546, 1954.

48. McCartney N, Spriet LL, Heigenhauser GJF et al: Muscle power and metabolism in maximal intermittent exercise, *J Appl Physiol* 60:1164-1169, 1986.

49. McNaughton LR: Sodium citrate and anaerobic performance: implications of dosage, *Eur J Appl Physiol* 61:392-397, 1990.

50. Montner P, Chick T, Riedesel M et al: Glycerol hyperhydration and endurance exercise, *Med Sci Sports Exerc* 24(4):S157, 1992.

51. Riedesel ML, Allen DY, Peake GT, Al-Qattan K: Hyperhydration with glycerol solutions, *J Appl Physiol* 63(6):2262-2268, 1987.

52. Robergs RA, Costill DL, Fink WJ et al: Effects of warm-up on blood gases, lactate, and acid-base status during sprint swimming, *Int J Sports Med* 11(4):273-278, 1990.

53. Robergs RA, Pascoe DD, Costill DL et al: Effects of warm-up on muscle glycogenolysis during intense exercise, *Med Sci Sports Exerc* 23(1):37-43, 1991.

54. Signorile JF, Kaplan TA, Applegate B, Perry AC: Effects of acute inhalation of the bronchodilator, albuterol, on power output, *Med Sci Sports Exerc* 24(6):638-642, 1992.

55. Spriet LL, Gledhill N, Froese AB, Wilkes DL: Effect of graded erythrocythemia on cardiovascular and metabolic responses to exercise, *J Appl Physiol* 61(5):1942-1948, 1986.

56. Spriet LL, Lindinger ML, Heigenhauser GJF, Jones NL: Effects of alkalosis on skeletal muscle metabolism and performance during exercise, *Am J Physiol* 251(20):R833-R839, 1986.

57. Spriet LL, MacLean DA, Dyck DJ et al: Caffeine ingestion and muscle metabolism during prolonged exercise in humans, *Am J Physiol* 262(25):E891-E898, 1992.

58. Stacpoole PW: The pharmacology of dichloroacetate, *Metabolism* 38(11):1124-1144, 1989.

59. Tarnopolsky MA: Caffeine and endurance performance, *Sports Med* 18(2):109-125, 1994.

REFERENCES—Cont'd

60. Tarnopolsky MA, Atkinson SA, MacDougall JD et al: Physiologic response to caffine during endurance running in habitual caffine users, *Med Sci Sports Exerc* 21(4):418-424, 1989.

61. Vukovich MD, Costill DL, Fink WJ: L-Carnitine supplementation: effect on muscle carnitine content and glycogen utilization during exercise, *Med Sci Sports Exerc* 26(5):S8, 1994 (abstract 44).

62. Wadler GI, Hainline B: *Drugs and the athlete,* Philadelphia, 1989, FA Davis.

63. Webster MJ, Webster MN, Crawford RE, Gladden LB: Effects of sodium bicarbonate ingestion on exhaustive resistance exercise performance, *Med Sci Sports Exerc* 25(8):960-965, 1993.

64. Weir J, Noakes TD, Myburgh K, Adams B: A high-carbohydrate diet negates the metabolic effects of caffeine during exercise, *Med Sci Sports Exerc* 12:100-105, 1987.

65. Williams JH: Caffeine, neuromuscular function, and high-intensity exercise performance, *J Sports Med Phys Fitness* 31:481-489, 1991.

66. Williams MH: Bicarbonate loading, *Sports Sci Exchange* 4(36):1-4, 1992.

67. Winter FD, Snell PG, Stray-Gundersen J: Effects of 100% oxygen on performance of professional soccer players, *JAMA* 262:227-229, 1989.

68. Yesalis CE, Wright JE, Bahrke MS: Epidemiological and policy issues in the measurement of the long-term health effects of anabolic-androgenic steroids, *Sports Med* 8:129-138, 1989.

RECOMMENDED READINGS

■ American College of Sports Medicine: Position statement on the use of alcohol in sports, *Med Sci Sports Exerc* 14(6):ix-xi, 1982.

■ American College of Sports Medicine: Position stand on the use of anabolic-androgenic steroids in sports, *Med Sci Sports Exerc* 19(5):534-539, 1987.

■ American College of Sports Medicine: Position stand on blood doping as an ergogenic aid, *Med Sci Sports Exerc* 19(5):540-543, 1987.

■ Costill DL, Verstappen F, Kuipers H et al: Acid-base balance during repeated bouts of exercise: influence of HCO_3, *Int J Sports Med* 5:228-231, 1984.

■ De Bruyn-Prevost P: The effects of varying warming-up intensities and durations upon some physiological variables during an exercise corresponding to the WC170, *Eur J Appl Physiol* 43:93-100, 1980.

■ Duthel JM, Vallon JJ, Martin G et al: Caffeine and sport: role of physical exercise upon elimination, *Med Sci Sports Exerc* 23(8):980-985, 1991.

■ Ekblom B, Berglund B: Effect of erythropoietin administration on maximal aerobic power, *Scand J Med Sci Sports* 1:88-93, 1991.

■ Ekblom B, Goldbarg AN, Gullbring B: Response to exercise after blood loss and reinfusion, *J Appl Physiol* 33:175-180, 1972.

■ Gledhill N: The influence of altered blood volume and oxygen-transport capacity on aerobic performance, *Exerc Sport Sci Rev* 13:75-93, 1985.

■ Gutin B, Stewart K, Lewis S, Kruper J: Oxygen consumption in the first stages of strenuous work as a function of prior exercise, *J Sports Med* 16:60-65, 1976.

■ Linderman J, Fahey TD: Sodium bicarbonate ingestion and exercise performance: an update, *Sports Med* 11:71-77, 1991.

■ Lyons TP, Riedesel ML, Meuli LE, Chick TW: Effects of glycerol-induced hyperhydration prior to exercise in the heat on sweating and core temperature, *Med Sci Sports Exerc* 22(4):477-483, 1990.

■ McNaughton LR: Sodium citrate and anaerobic performance: implications of dosage, *Eur J Appl Physiol* 61:392-397, 1990.

■ Robergs RA, Costill DL, Fink WJ et al: Effects of warm-up on blood gases, lactate, and acid-base status during sprint swimming, *Int J Sports Med* 11(4):273-278, 1990.

■ Robergs RA, Pascoe DD, Costill DL et al: Effects of warm-up on muscle glycogenolysis during intense exercise, *Med Sci Sports Exerc* 23(1):37-43, 1991.

■ Rogol AD: Growth hormone: physiology, therapeutic use, and potential for abuse, *Exerc Sport Sci Rev* 17:352-378, 1989.

■ Spriet LL, Gledhill N, Froese AB, Wilkes DL: Effect of graded erythrocythemia on cardiovascular and metabolic responses to exercise, *J Appl Physiol* 61(5):1942-1948, 1986.

■ Spriet LL, Lindinger ML, Heigenhauser GJF, Jones NL: Effects of alkalosis on skeletal muscle metabolism and performance during exercise, *Am J Physiol* 251(20):R833-R839, 1986.

■ Spriet LL, MacLean DA, Dyck DJ et al: Caffeine ingestion and muscle metabolism during prolonged exercise in humans, *Am J Physiol* 262(25):E891-E898, 1992.

■ Tarnopolsky MA: Caffeine and endurance performance, *Sports Med* 18(20):109-125, 1994.

■ Winter FD, Snell PG, Stray-Gundersen J: Effects of 100% oxygen on performance of professional soccer players, *JAMA* 262:227-229, 1989.

■ Yesalis CE, Wright JE, Bahrke MS: Epidemiological and policy issues in the measurement of the long-term health effects of anabolic-androgenic steroids, *Sports Med* 8:129-138, 1989.

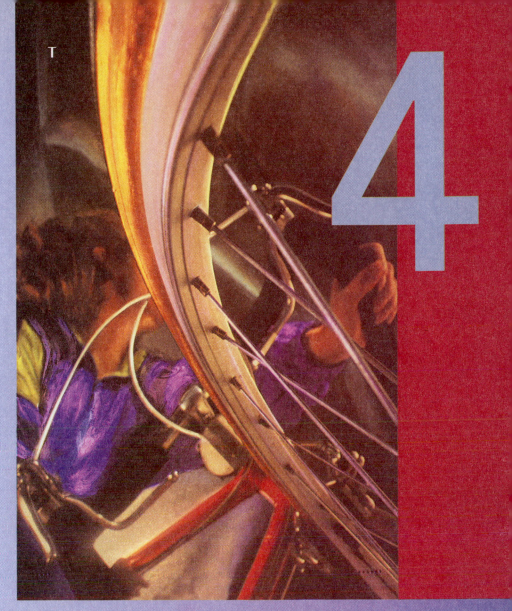

4

Measurements of Physiologic Composition and Capacities

CHAPTER 19

Measuring Endurance, Anaerobic Capacity, and Strength

OBJECTIVES

After studying this chapter you should be able to:

■ List the different tests that can be performed to measure cardiorespiratory and muscular endurance, peak muscle power, and anaerobic capacity.

■ List several examples of maximal and submaximal tests that estimate VO_2max from treadmill, cycle ergometer, and field methods.

■ Explain why tests that estimate VO_2max are never perfect.

■ Describe the suitability of VO_2max and the lactate threshold for prediction of endurance exercise performance.

■ Explain the different methods available for strength testing.

KEY TERMS

VO_2peak

prediction

criterion variable

multiple regression

muscle power

anaerobic capacity

accumulated oxygen deficit

muscular strength

dynamometer

1 repetition maximum (1 RM)

ests of endurance, power, and strength can be used to evaluate physical fitness, the potential for sport and athletic performance, and suitability for the demands of specific vocations (e.g., fire fighting, the military, police). Periodic physiologic testing can also help guide an exercise training program or provide motivation for behavioral change. For example, the results of a person's maximal endurance, power, or strength capacities reflect an individual's ability to perform daily physical tasks (e.g., climbing stairs) and potential success in most athletic events. In the medical community, these tests can be used to monitor rehabilitation from injury (e.g., physical therapy) or disease (e.g., cardiac rehabilitation). The purpose of this chapter is to present the different tests available to measure or estimate cardiorespiratory endurance, muscle power and related metabolic capacities, and strength. In addition, where appropriate, normal scores on these tests for specific populations are provided.

Metabolic Determinants of Physiologic Capacities

ests that measure or estimate cardiorespiratory endurance are used to evaluate an individual's capacity to acquire and transport oxygen in the blood to fuel muscle mitochondrial respiration. Conversely, tests that measure or estimate muscle power development evaluate the capacity for skeletal muscle adenosine-triphosphate (ATP) regeneration from creatine phosphate hydrolysis and glycolysis. Finally, tests that measure strength evaluate muscle mass and neuromuscular function. The metabolic and neuromuscular determinants of these functional capacities are explained and illustrated in Chapters 4, 9, and 10.

An individual's capacity for mitochondrial respiration depends on the proportion of slow-twitch motor units in the muscles of interest, muscle mitochondrial and capillary densities, cardiovascular function, and pulmonary function (see Chapters 11 and 12). The most common tests used for reflecting these capacities are the test of maximal oxygen consumption (VO_2max) and the test of the lactate or ventilatory threshold. These tests reflect a combination of cardiorespiratory and muscular endurance capacities.

An individual's capacity for generating and maintaining high muscle power is determined by muscular strength, fast-twitch motor unit proportions, and the ability to regenerate ATP at high rates through creatine phosphate hydrolysis and glycolysis. If performed in excess of 30 seconds, these tests also indirectly assess a person's acid-buffering capacity (muscle and blood) resulting from the metabolic acidosis that accompanies sustained high rates of glycolysis. Tests of muscle power can be performed at varying time lengths. For example, as few as five repetitions can be used to determine peak power at different contraction speeds during isokinetic testing. Intense exercise (e.g., running, cycling) can be performed for as short as 10 seconds, 30 seconds, or 1 to 2 minutes. The longer the duration is, the more the test reflects both glycolytic and mitochondrial respiration metabolic capacities.

The strength capacities of an individual are not dependent on the proportions of the different muscle motor units. As explained in Chapters 8 and 9, the ability to generate strength requires time for motor unit recruitment, and greatest muscular strength occurs during isometric contractions. Muscular strength reflects a combination of optimizing (increased amount) motor unit recruitment and the cross-sectional area of the skeletal muscles tested. Thus, compared with endurance and power, maximal strength is influenced minimally by metabolic capacities.

As previously explained, success in specific athletic events is directly linked to an individual's ability or potential to regenerate ATP using a particular metabolic pathway. Because of the influence of genetics on muscle motor unit proportions, and therefore metabolic capacities, an individual's genetic makeup is an important determinant of maximal cardiorespiratory and muscle endurance, muscle power, and strength.[9] For this reason, comparisons among individuals for a given measurement is a reflection of both training status and genetic potential. Comparisons of physiologic capacities among individuals of similar training would be more reflective of genetic limitation than training limitation. However, the progress of an individual during a training program can be monitored by comparing scores over time.

Measurement Versus Prediction

The direct measurement of physiologic capacities requires expensive equipment and highly trained personnel. Therefore the ability to indirectly estimate or predict the capacities has many advantages. Unfortunately, tests that predict rather than measure a capacity have the potential for relatively poor reliability and validity and therefore may not have acceptable accuracy. Table 19.1 lists some of the factors affecting the relationship between measured and predicted oxygen consumption (VO_2).

The choice of prediction versus measurement is highly dependent on the purpose of the testing. Research and clinical evaluation requires measurement of physiologic capacities; however, the determination of general fitness profiles for a large number of subjects may make prediction protocols the method of choice. If prediction methods are used, it is imperative that the accuracy and associated error of the testing be known and provided to the individuals who are tested. If an estimate of error of a prediction or estimation method cannot be provided, that test should not be performed. For example, does a person with an estimated VO_2max of 50 ml/kg/min have higher cardiorespiratory endurance than a person with an estimated value of 45 ml/kg/min? Although it is tempting to say yes, if the method for estimating VO_2max had an error of ±10%, a value of 50 ml/kg/min could actually be anything in a range of 45 to 55 ml/kg/min, and a value of 45 ml/kg/min could actually be anywhere in the range of 40 to 50 ml/kg/min. Clearly, it is invalid to claim with any confidence that these individuals had different levels of cardiorespiratory endurance resulting from the error associated with the method of prediction. Nevertheless, if a given individual demonstrates a change in VO_2max by the same method, there is more validity in interpreting the change as real. Thus prediction methods have more validity when used for intraindividual comparisons.

Measuring Cardiorespiratory and Muscular Endurance

Traditionally, the test used to measure cardiorespiratory and muscular endurance has been that of VO_2max.* However, research evidence indicates that VO_2max alone may not be an accurate assessment of the cardiorespiratory demands of submaximal exercise.[19,47,62,66] For example, research since the 1970s has shown that although VO_2max predicts endurance exercise performance in a large group of individuals with a large range of VO_2max values (r>0.85), it has less importance in determining exercise performance in a group of individuals with a similar VO_2max.[47] Obviously, other factors are involved in determining how well a person can perform in endurance exercise.

The best measure of success in running events longer than the 1500 meters and also in long-distance road cycling is the pace at the lactate threshold (LT).† As previously explained, the intensity at the LT reflects an individual's maximal steady-state intensity (see Chapter 10). Research has continually revealed very high correlations (>0.9) between the pace at the LT and some expression of race performance (e.g., time, average pace).† Similar findings have resulted from use of the ventilatory threshold (VT).[47,62] Furthermore, for individuals with a similar VO_2max, differences in the LT between the individuals provided a better measure of race performance than VO_2max alone. Because people function in daily activities and compete in endurance events at intensities that are well below VO_2max, the LT may be a more valid measure of cardiorespiratory endurance than is VO_2max. However, it should be noted that to have a high LT, an individual needs also to have a moderate to high VO_2max. Thus the measures of VO_2max and the LT combine to provide an accurate indication of cardiorespiratory and muscular endurance, as well as the potential for success in prolonged endurance events.

Each of VO_2max and the LT can be measured directly or be estimated by other methods. For example, VO_2max can be estimated or predicted from studies that have developed equations specific to certain protocols or exercise modes, and the LT can be estimated noninvasively from ratings of perceived exertion or heart rate.

---

*References 3, 5, 11, 15, 30, and 55.
†References 19, 24, 38, 43, 47, 60, 65, and 68.

TABLE 19.1	
Factors confounding the relationship between measured and predicted oxygen uptake	
CONFOUND	**CONSEQUENCE**
Habituation	Oxygen uptake and variablility decrease; reproducibility improves with treadmill familiarization
Fitness	Oxygen uptake and variability in oxygen uptake for a given workload decrease with increased fitness
Heart disease	Oxygen uptake is overpredicted in patients with heart disease
Handrail holding	Oxygen uptake is reduced by holding handrails and therefore is overpredicted
Exercise protocol	Oxygen uptake is overpredicted and variability is increased with rapidly incremental, more demanding protocols
Mechanical efficiency	Oxygen cost of work is increased by obesity (on treadmill) but reduced by stride length, training specificity, habituation, and coordination
Heart rate response	Heart rate response is usually lower for a given relative exercise intensity for endurance-trained compared with untrained individuals. Consequently, VO_2max is usually overpredicted for trained individuals and underpredicted for untrained individuals

Modified from Froelicher VF, Follansbee WP, Labovitz AJ: *Exercise and the heart,* ed 3, St Louis, 1993, Mosby.

Maximal Oxygen Consumption (VO_2max)

Direct measurement of VO_2 requires the measurement of expired gas fractions and ventilation during exercise. A variety of gas analyzing systems have been developed over the years, ranging from expired gas collection in Douglas bags with the chemical analysis of expired air for oxygen and carbon dioxide content to today's sophisticated computer-driven equipment with electronic analyzers that compute data for each breath (see Chapter 6).

The decision over whether a time-averaged or breath-by-breath system is to be used depends on the purpose of the test. If the purpose is simply to measure VO_2max, either method is suitable. However, if additional data of the rate of change (kinetics) of VO_2 are also required, a breath-by-breath system should be used.[71]

The test of VO_2max must meet several requirements for the peak VO_2 attained to be a maximal VO_2. First, the duration and increment magnitude of the test can influence the peak VO_2 obtained.[12,58] A total test duration in excess of 16 minutes can lower VO_2peak. Conversely, test durations less than 8 minutes involve large increments in intensity and lead to premature fatigue and a low VO_2peak. Buchfuhrer et al. recommended that test durations should be between 8 and 12 minutes to obtain a true VO_2max.[12]

In addition to test duration, criteria of a plateau in VO_2 with increasing exercise intensity, a respiratory exchange ratio (RER) greater than 1.1, and the attainment of age-predicted maximal heart rate (220-age) have also been used as criteria to validate VO_2peak as VO_2max. However, of these additional criteria, a plateau in VO_2max has not been conclusively demonstrated as valid because of the difficulty more than 40% of healthy individuals have in demonstrating a plateau in VO_2 during a maximal test.[3,4,55] Furthermore, individuals with cardiovascular diseases or chronic obstructive pulmonary disease will prematurely terminate a maximal test because of clinical symptoms of exercise intolerance, such as angina, abnormal ECG, dyspnea (breathlessness), or leg fatigue resulting from claudication. For the more clinically determined maximal VO_2 values, the expressions *symptom-limited VO_2max* or **VO_2peak** are more appropriate.

Finally, a decision on the exercise mode used to conduct the test is needed. As explained in Chapter 10, sedentary and moderately trained individuals attain a higher VO_2max during treadmill protocols. However, highly trained individuals on exercise modes that differ from running may have the same or a higher VO_2max than during treadmill running. In addition, if a treadmill protocol is chosen, there is evidence that individuals who train on hilly terrain do better on a protocol involving an incline than do runners who train on level ground.[1,29]

Testing Protocols

The need to maintain a test duration of 12 minutes would mean that increments in intensity would be different for individuals of differing cardiorespiratory fitness. This fact

VO_2peak

the largest VO_2 during an incremental exercise test

stresses the need to tailor a protocol to suit a given individual. Therefore estimations of a person's cardiorespiratory fitness and training history are important first steps in determining a protocol for a test of VO_2max. This estimation can then be applied to cycling or running using the equations of the American College of Sports Medicine, Wasserman and Whipp, or the others listed in Table 19.2.[2,70] For example, when estimating a VO_2max of 4 L/min during cycle ergometry, the maximal power output would approximate 390 W. When using 400 W as an estimated maximal intensity, a warm-up ending at 100 W would leave 300 W of increment to VO_2max. When dividing 300 by 12, the result is an increment of 25 W/min.

For the same person when running on a treadmill, VO_2 needs to be estimated in ml/kg/min (4000/75=53.3 ml/kg/min), and a running pace that is comfortable needs to be estimated. This is difficult, since it could be less than 7 kmh (4.4 mph) for an untrained individual or greater than 16 kmh (10 mph) for a highly trained endurance athlete. This pace is important, since it is recommended that the subject be warmed up to sustain this running pace during level running and thereafter have exercise intensity increased by increasing the grade of the treadmill. Thus if the individual of this example were able to run comfortably at 12 kmh (7.5 mph), which requires an approximate VO_2 of 43.8 ml/kg/min (Table 19.3), there is a remaining 9.5 ml/kg/min that must be met by an increasing grade. Although the energy demand of an increase in grade increases with increasing running speed, an approximation of 1.5 ml/kg/min/% grade indicates that the maximal exercise speed and grade required by this individual will approximate 12 kmh at 7% grade. A suitable protocol for this individual would therefore involve 1–minute stage durations requiring 1–kmh increments from 8 to 12 kmh, followed by 1%–grade increments to exhaustion. This test would take 11 minutes.

For individuals confined to walking on a treadmill, Table 19.4 can be used to develop a suitable protocol.

Estimations of energy expenditure and VO_2 can be made for other exercise modes as long as mechanical power output is known. Thus for arm ergometry, rowing, and stair climbing, mechanical power can be converted to kg/min, and then to Kcal/min. Assuming a given efficiency (30%), mechanical energy can be converted to chemical energy expenditure. When assuming a given RER, this energy expenditure can be converted to VO_2 (see Chapter 7).

The need to tailor a protocol to the fitness and health status of an individual indicates that using predetermined protocols is inappropriate. When testing healthy or highly trained athletes, this is true. However, the exercise testing of diseased individuals has been performed using standard protocols that allow comparison of data within and between populations. For example, during treadmill testing of individuals with cardiovascular diseases, the Bruce protocol is used routinely (see Focus Box 19.1), even despite the bias of this

TABLE 19.2

Summary of VO_2 prediction equations

EXERCISE MODE	STUDY	N	POPULATION AGES	POPULATION GENDER/HEALTH	EQUATION	R	SEE
SUBMAXIMAL VO_2*							
Treadmill walking (ml/kg/min)	ACSM[2]	—	—	M,F healthy	[0.1(m/min)] + [(grade;fraction)(m/min)(1.8) = 3.5	—	—
Treadmill running (ml/kg/min)	ACSM[2]	—	—	M,F healthy	[0.2(m/min)] + [(grade;fraction)(m/min)(1.8)(0.5) + 3.5	—	—
Cycle ergometry							
(ml/min)	ACSM[2]	—	—	M,F healthy	[2.0(kg/min)] + [3.5(wt;kg)]	—	—
(L/min)	ACSM[2]	—	—	M,F healthy	[0.012(Watts)] + 0.3	—	—
(ml/min)	Latin[45]	110	18-38	M healthy	[kg/min(1.9)] + [3.5(wt;kg)] + 260	0.96	154.0
	Legge[46]	15	20-29	M trained	[0.034(ΔHR)] + 1.03	—	0.39
		10		M untrained	[0.023(ΔHR)] + 1.09	—	0.32
(ml/min)	Wasserman[70]	—	—	—	[10(Watts)] + 500		
Arm ergometry							
(ml/min)	ACSM[2]	—	—	M,F healthy	[3(kg/min)] + [(3.5(body weight-kg)]	—	—
Bench stepping							
(ml/kg/min)	ACSM[2]	—	—	M,F healthy	[0.35(steps/min)] + [(height-m)(steps/min)(1.33)(1.8)	—	—

*Assumes steady state conditions.

TABLE 19.2—Cont'd

Summary of VO$_2$ prediction equations

EXERCISE MODE	STUDY	N	POPULATION AGES	POPULATION GENDER/HEALTH	EQUATION	R	SEE

MAXIMAL VO$_2$ (VO$_2$MAX)

A MAXIMAL TESTS
TREADMILL (ml/kg/min)

EXERCISE MODE	STUDY	N	AGES	GENDER/HEALTH	EQUATION	R	SEE
Bruce Protocol	Bruce[11]	44		M active	3.778(time) + 0.19	0.906	—
		94		M sedentary	3.298(time) + 4.07	0.906	—
		97		M cardiac	2.327(time) + 9.48	0.865	—
		295		M,F healthy	6.70 − [2.82(gender)] + [0.056(time)]	0.920	—
	Foster[27]	230		M varied	14.76 − [1.38(time) + [0.451(time^2)] − [0.12(time^3)]	0.977	3.35
Balke Protocol	Froelicher[30]	1,025	20-53	M healthy	11.12 + [1.51(time)]	0.72	4.26
Cycle ergometry (ml/min)	Patton[56]	15		M healthy	[(0.012)Watts] − 0.099	0.89	—
		12		F healthy	[(0.008)Watts] + 0.732	0.88	—
(ml/min)	Storer[67]	115	20-70	M healthy	[10.51(Watts;max)] + [6.35(wt;kg)] − [10.49(age;yr)] + 519.3	0.94	212.0
		116		F healthy	[9.39(Watts;max)] + [7.7(wt;kg)] − [5.88(age;yr)] + 136.7	0.93	147.0
Bench stepping none							

SUBMAXIMAL TESTS

EXERCISE MODE	STUDY	N	AGES	GENDER/HEALTH	EQUATION	R	SEE
Treadmill (ml/kg/min)	Ebbeling[22]	67	20-59	M	15.1 + p21.8(walk speed;mph)] − [0.327(HR)] − 0.263(speed)(age)] + [0.00504(HR)(age)] + [5.989(gender-F=0,M=1)]	0.96	5.0
		72		F			
	Widrick[72]	145	20-59	M healthy F healthy	see Kline[40]	0.91	5.26
	Wilmore[74]	42	18-30	M healthy		0.76	5.0
Cycle ergometry (ml/min)	Fox[28]	87	17-27	M	6,300 − [19.26(HR-at 5th min at 150 Watts)]	0.76	246.0
(L/min)	Åstrand[3]	27	18-30	M healthy	nomogram	—	0.28
		31		F healthy	nomogram	—	0.27
(L/min)	Siconolfi[64]	25	20-70	M healthy	[0.348(VO$_2$;Åstrand)] − [0.035(age) + 3.011	0.86	0.36
		28		F healthy	[0.302(VO$_2$;Åstrand)] − [0.019(age) + 1.593	0.97	0.20
	Legge[46]	25	2-29	M healthy	nomogram using ΔHR(maxHR-zero loadHR)	0.98	0.17
Bench stepping (ml/kg/min)	McArdle[50]	41	18-22	F healthy	65.81 − [0.1847(recovery HR)]	0.92	2.9
		—	18-22	M healthy	111.33 + [0.42(recovery HR)]	—	—
Field tests	Cooper[15]	115	17-52	M	35.97(miles after 12 min) − 11.29	0.90	—
	Kline[40]	343	18-23	M,F healthy	6.9652 + [0.0091(weight-kg)] − [0.02579(age) + (0.5955(gender-F=0,M=1)] − [0.224(time-1-mile walk)] − [0.0115(HR)]	0.93	0.325
	Coleman[16]	90	20-29	M,F healthy	see Kline[40]	0.79	5.68

TABLE 19.3

Estimated oxygen consumption for jogging and running on a level surface and uphill*

Equivalent rates		5.0	6.0	7.0	7.5	8	9	10
	mph	5.0	6.0	7.0	7.5	8	9	10
	kph	8.0	9.7	11.3	12.1	12.9	14.5	16.1
	m\min	134	161	188	201	215	241	268
PERCENT GRADE								
Outdoor terrain								
0		30.1	35.7	41.0	43.8	48.6	51.8	57.1
2.5		36.1	43.1	49.4	52.9	56.4	62.7	69.0
5.0		42.0	50.1	57.8	62.0	65.8		
7.5		48.3	57.4	66.2				
10.0		54.3	64.8					
Treadmill								
0		30.1	35.7	41.0	43.8	46.6	51.8	57.1
2.5		33.3	39.2	45.2	48.3	51.5	57.1	63.0
5.0		36.1	43.1	49.4	52.9	56.4	62.7	69.0
7.5		39.2	46.6	53.6	57.4	60.9	67.9	
10.0		42.0	50.1	57.8	62.0	66.5		
12.5		45.2	53.9	62.0	66.5			
15.0		48.3	57.4	66.2				

mph, Miles per hour; *kph*, kilometers per hour; *m/min*, meters per minute.
* Assumes steady-state conditions.
Modified from American College of Sports Medicine: *Guidelines for exercise testing and prescription*, ed 4, Philadelphia, 1991, Lea & Febiger.

protocol to an increasing grade and the increased likelihood for leg fatigue, limiting exercise duration. However, a walking protocol has advantages in decreasing electrical artifact during electrocardiogram evaluation of heart function and allowing more accurate monitoring of blood pressure. Other commonly used treadmill protocols for the exercise evaluation of high-risk individuals are those of Naughton et al. and Balke et al.[5,54]

Lactate and Ventilatory Thresholds

Since VO₂max represents an individual's maximal cardiorespiratory capacity, this is the available oxygen consumption that is possible during exercise. However, the development of metabolic acidosis, muscle fatigue, and possibly central fatigue (see Chapters 4, 10, and 22) prevent the ability to exercise at VO₂max for much more than 1 minute. Clearly, sustained steady-state exercise must be performed at exercise intensities below VO₂max. Because of this fact a measurement that reflects the ability of an individual to exercise while remaining at steady state would be an accurate measure of an individual's functional cardiorespiratory capac-

ity. As previously explained, such a measurement exists and is termed the *lactate threshold (LT)*.

The LT is typically measured during a test of VO₂max by sampling blood from one of several possible sites. As such, the LT is used to represent whole-body lactate kinetics and either central venous or central arterial blood is sampled for this purpose. However, because of the invasiveness, potential risk for complications to the procedure, and need for medical supervision, arterial and central venous blood samples are difficult to justify for the purpose of determining the LT. Alternative, more accessible sites for blood sampling are an antecubital vein, dorsal hand vein, finger capillary, or earlobe. The choice of a sampling site depends on the exercise mode. For example, during arm exercise, the blood from the antecubital vein, dorsal hand vein, or finger tip would have an increased lactate concentration resulting from the altered blood flow and increased lactate release from the working musculature. Furthermore, depending on the method used to detect the LT, venous, arterial, and capillary blood samples will have different lactate concentrations for a given exercise condition and may in turn cause different estimations of the LT.[61] Of course, the best way to avoid the complications of these issues

TABLE 19.4

Estimated oxygen consumption for walking on a level surface and uphill*

Equivalent rates {	mph	1.7	2.0	2.5	3.0	3.4	3.75
	kph	2.7	3.2	4.0	4.8	5.5	6.00
	m\min	45.6	53.7	67.0	80.5	91.2	100.5

PERCENT GRADE							
0		8.0	8.8	10.2	11.6	12.6	13.7
2.5		10.2	11.2	13.3	15.1	16.8	18.2
5.0		12.3	13.7	16.1	18.9	20.7	22.8
7.5		14.4	16.1	19.3	22.4	24.9	27.3
10.0		16.1	18.6	22.1	25.9	29.1	31.9
12.5		18.2	21.0	25.2	29.8	33.3	36.4
15.0		20.3	23.1	28.4	33.3	37.1	41.0
17.5		22.4	25.6	31.2	36.8	41.3	45.2
20.0		24.5	28.0	34.3	40.6	45.5	49.7
22.5		26.6	30.5	37.1	44.1	49.7	54.3
25.0		28.7	32.9	40.3	47.6	53.6	58.8

mph, Miles per hour; *kph*, kilometers per hour; *m/min*, meters per minute.
* Assumes steady-state conditions.
Modified from American College of Sports Medicine: *Guidelines for exercise testing and prescription*, ed 4, Philadelphia, 1991, Lea & Febiger.

is always to sample blood for a given exercise mode from the same site.

The detection of the LT is based on graphing blood lactate concentration (y-axis) versus some measure of exercise intensity (e.g., VO$_2$, Watts, running velocity) (x-axis). Thus there is increased precision in detecting the LT with more data points. Therefore it is recommended that at least eight blood samples be obtained during an incremental exercise test. As previously described, if the test of VO$_2$max is to be based on 1-minute stage durations, lasting a total of 12 minutes, this requires a blood sample every minute. Unless a catheter is being used, this is a demanding task for both the subject and researcher. A compromise is to make stage durations 2 minutes and include a warm-up in the protocol. Thus, if the first three stages of the protocol are the warm-up totaling 6 minutes, a 12-minute test would provide six additional 2-minute stages, and provide a total of nine blood samples.

Methods for Detecting the Lactate Threshold

The concept of an LT has received criticism because of the subjective methods for detecting the intensity at the LT and because blood lactate may not increase in a threshold manner but rather as an exponential function of exercise intensity.[7] Consequently, visual detection is no longer an acceptable method for detecting the LT.

Refer to Chapter 10 for an increasingly used method for decreasing the error of subjective detection of the LT. Both axes, or just the lactate axis units, can be converted into logarithm values. A purely exponential increase in lactate would then result in a straight line. Conversely, an increase in lactate that has two or more exponential components would reveal the same number of linear segments. Simple linear regression of two segments of the data set that results in least error reveals that the LT is the intensity at which the two lines intersect.[7]

Scientists from Europe have devised a method of LT detection that accounts for individual differences in lactate removal during the recovery from the exercise test (Figure 19.1).[66] Although more complicated than the log-conversion method, it has some merit in its use resulting from the important role of lactate removal in the total body kinetics of blood lactate accumulation. Research has indicated that the various methods of LT determination can produce slightly differing results, and although the implications these differences have on endurance exercise performance and training remain unclear, once again it is imperative that a given method be used consistently to avoid the potential error involved in comparisons between methods.[61]

There are numerous other methods for detecting the LT. Fixed blood lactate concentrations have been used, with 2 mmol/L referred to as the aerobic threshold and 4 mmol/L

Research has produced many equations that estimate VO₂ during exercise from other variables that are more easily measured (Table 19.2). The design of this type of research must first be explained briefly to emphasize the limitations and error associated with results.

To develop **prediction** equations, researchers need to complete measurements on large numbers of individuals (ideally >100). In this case the measurements would be VO₂max, other related variables, such as heart rate during the exercise, heart rate after the exercise, or exercise time on a given protocol, as well as demographic variables, such as gender, age, weight, height, and ethnicity. The purpose of developing prediction equations is to provide a simpler means of determining a complex measurement. The needed features of this research are large numbers of subjects, good research techniques and equipment, and the selection of important variables that are likely to influence the **criterion variable** (e.g., VO₂max). Large numbers of subjects are required to minimize the between-subjects error in the relationships between VO₂max and the prediction (independent) variables and to improve the generalizability of the results. Conversely, if subjects differ too much in the independent variables the accuracy of the study may decrease and therefore compromise application of the findings. Thus prediction equations are never perfect.

The purpose of using multiple independent variables is to decrease the error of the prediction. In doing this, statistical analyses can be performed that combine different combinations of variables that when treated together improve the prediction of the criterion. The main technique used is **multiple regression,** which results in a formula that may contain several variables that are used in the calculation of the criterion. The resulting correlation between the predicted and measured values of the criterion is denoted "R" (or multiple r), as distinct from "r," which concerns the correlation between two single variables.

Even if correlations close to 1 are obtained between predicted and measured values and the spread of data points about the regression line is small, there may still be poor accuracy. This is because correlation research does not assess accuracy but a relationship. This fact was well demonstrated by Latin et al., who reported a similar correlation and standard error of the estimate from a new equation to estimate VO₂max during cycle ergometry, compared with that recommended by ACSM (Table 19.2).[45] However, the new equation was significantly more accurate than the ACSM equation, with mean values differing by only 13 ml/min compared with a difference of 198 ml/min for the ACSM equation. This fact should be considered when evaluating research for prediction of variables.

termed the *anaerobic threshold,* or onset of blood lactate accumulation (OBLA).* These additional versions of the LT are also accurate predictors of endurance performance; however, the running pace at the LT best resembles the average race pace during endurance events.

Ventilatory Threshold

The LT can be noninvasively determined by plotting ventilation and respiratory data obtained from an incremental exercise test to VO₂max. Caiozzeo et al. have determined that the most accurate variables to use are minute ventilation (VE), the ventilatory equivalent for oxygen (VE/VO₂), and the ventilatory equivalent for carbon dioxide (VE/VCO₂) (see Chapter 12).[13]

---

*References 19, 47, 61, 65, and 66.

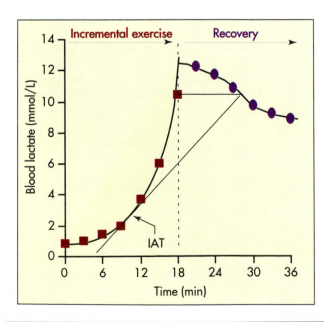

FIGURE 19.1

A method of detecting the lactate threshold that includes individual differences in blood lactate removal kinetics after a maximal incremental exercise test. This procedure is termed the *individual anaerobic threshold* (IAT).

The detection of the LT is very similar to the intensity in which there is a rate of increase in VE that exceeds the rate of increase in VO_2. For this reason the VE/VO_2 data set is usually most sensitive to detecting the change in ventilation and metabolism. Thus the ventilatory threshold (VT) is detected as the first increase in VE/VO_2 that corresponds to an increased rate of ventilation without a change in VE/VCO_2. Depending on the protocol used, VE/VCO_2 increases between 1 and 2 minutes after the increase in VE/VO_2. The delayed increase in VE/VCO_2 is a secondary criterion for detecting the VT.

The physiologic explanation for an increase in ventilation to correspond to an increase in blood lactate accumulation has been based on the acidosis and increased venous blood PCO_2 that accompany lactate production (see Chapters 10 and 12). However, the exact mechanisms that cause the increase in ventilation are unclear because $PaCO_2$ actually decreases during incremental exercise (see Chapter 12), and threshold increases in ventilation have been demonstrated in individuals who were not acidotic. Nevertheless, as previously explained, both LT and VT are known to be very accurate predictors of success in prolonged endurance exercise.

Running Economy

Several studies that have evaluated the contribution of multiple variables to prolonged endurance running performance have shown that running economy is an additional independent factor that is important.[38,47] As explained in Chapters 6 and 10, good running economy involves a low submaximal VO_2, and therefore the ability to run faster at a given percent of the LT.

Running economy is determined by having the subject complete at least three exercise intensities known to be below the LT. The durations of each stage should be at least 4 minutes and data of VO_2 should be obtained continuously during the testing. The steady-state VO_2 values (y-axis) are graphed against intensity on the x-axis, and the linear regression line of best fit represents the efficiency of the subject (Figure 19.2).

This test sequence is also useful in research when specific running paces or cycle ergometer intensities (Watts) need to be determined. For this purpose the regression equation is used to calculate the intensity at a given VO_2. Thus, if a protocol was required to demand an exercise intensity of 60% VO_2max, the VO_2 at 60% VO_2max could be determined from an incremental exercise test, and the steady-state VO_2 versus exercise intensity relationship would need to be obtained from additional testing. A regression equation would be determined from the steady-state VO_2 data, and the exercise intensity at 60% VO_2max could be calculated.

VO_2 Kinetics

Another test to evaluate the cardiorespiratory condition of a subject is to measure the rate of change in VO_2 for a

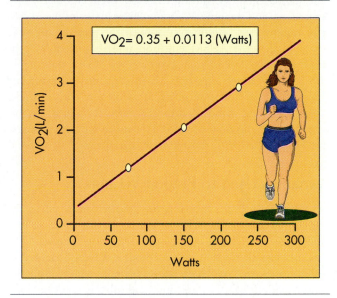

FIGURE 19.2

A subject's economy and efficiency during cycling can be determined by graphing at least three submaximal steady state VO_2 data points with exercise intensity (Watts). A linear fit of this data can be used to determine the VO_2 for a given intensity, as well as intensities that correspond to certain percentages of VO_2max.

$$VO_2 = 0.35 + 0.0113 \text{ (Watts)}$$

given increase in exercise intensity. The more rapid the increase in VO_2, the greater the cardiorespiratory and muscular endurance. This test requires the use of a breath-by-breath indirect calorimetry system as detailed in Chapter 7. Figures of breath-by-breath system data for VO_2 during increments in exercise intensity are presented in Chapter 10.

The rate of increase in VO_2 is typically expressed as a time constant (tVO_2) from a single exponential equation, such as $VO_2 = A + B[1-e^{(-t/t)}]$. Such an equation is derived from a computer curve-fitting program. However, care should be taken when statistically comparing rate constants because of their susceptibility for change from erroneous noise in data rather than from changes that have a physiologic cause.

prediction (pre-**dic**'shun)

the estimation of one variable from the measurement of others

criterion variable

the variable that is being predicted; also known as the "dependent variable"

multiple regression

the use of multiple variables (independent) in the prediction of a criterion variable; "Multiple regression" results in the formulation of an equation that contains variables that best combine to predict the criterion variable

Predicting Cardiorespiratory and Muscular Endurance

Submaximal VO$_2$

Typically the ACSM equations have been used to calculate submaximal VO$_2$ during treadmill, cycle ergometry, arm ergometry, and stepping. Recently the accuracy of the ACSM equation for cycle ergometry has been questioned. Lang et al. revealed that the ACSM equation underestimated VO$_2$ by approximately 260 ml/min across a range of VO$_2$ from 0.5 to 2.5 L/min.[44] A new equation was subsequently validated and shown to have better accuracy of prediction with a similar correlation and standard error of estimate.[45] It is recommended that this new equation be used to estimate submaximal steady-state VO$_2$ during cycle ergometry.

Variables Used to Predict VO$_2$max

Focus Box 19.1 explains the research involved in the development and validation of equations that estimate VO$_2$ and presents equations developed from this research. The research can be divided into methods involving maximal or submaximal exercise. The reasons for the presence of prediction equations based on maximal and submaximal exercise is that for many individuals the risks inherent in maximal exercise testing may be avoided when using a submaximal test. However, as indicated in Table 19.2, many of the submaximal prediction equations were formulated from apparently healthy and young individuals. It is unclear how this fact influences the generalizability of the equations to more elderly individuals or to individuals with degenerative diseases.

Prediction of VO$_2$max depends on measuring variables that are known to change proportionally with VO$_2$max. Thus heart rate, change in heart rate, and exercise duration for a given protocol have been used widely by different researchers (see Table 19.2). The heart rate response to exercise is an important variable for predicting VO$_2$max, since individuals with increased cardiorespiratory endurance have a lower heart rate for a given exercise intensity. However, since other variables besides VO$_2$ are known to influence heart rate (e.g., dehydration, arousal, the type of exercise), prediction of VO$_2$max based on heart rate alone is still associated with prediction error. Error of prediction is also associated with maximal exercise times resulting from differences between individuals in tolerance to intense exercise because of motivation, muscle strength and power, and anaerobic capacity.

Maximal Tests

Treadmill protocols. VO$_2$max can be predicted from maximal exercise duration during the Bruce or Balke treadmill protocols for specific populations and generally have moderate to high correlations between tests that measure VO$_2$ directly (see Table 19.2); however, the standard error of esti-

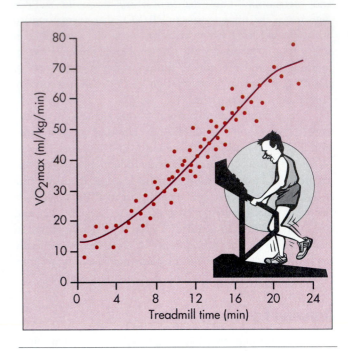

FIGURE 19.3

Curvilinear relationship between measured maximal oxygen uptake to treadmill performance of persons of varied abilities. (Based on Foster C et al: *Am Heart J* 107:1229-1234, 1984.)

mate is typically high.[11,27] For example, Figure 19.3 presents data for measured and estimated VO$_2$max versus exercise duration during the Bruce protocol. The resulting curve is sigmoidal and reveals that data were equally distributed above and below the line of identity throughout the range of exercise durations studied. However, the variation in data around the line of identity reveals that for individuals who exercised for 12 minutes, actual VO$_2$max values ranged from 36 to 50 ml/kg/min, a potential maximal error of ±16%.

Cycle ergometer protocols. The maximal cycle ergometer protocol by Storer et al. is the most accurate method and equation for estimating VO$_2$max during cycle ergometry.[67] After a warm-up of 4 minutes with zero load, subjects perform an incremental exercise test with a 15 Watt/min increment until volitional fatigue. The maximal Watts attained during the exercise is used in gender-specific multiple regression equations that also involve body weight and age (see Table 19.2).

Submaximal Tests

Treadmill protocols. VO$_2$max can also be estimated by equations that use the heart rate response to exercise at different submaximal intensities, accompanied by the ACSM equations for steady-state VO$_2$. For example, if a 35-year-old female completed steady-state treadmill running exercise at

FIGURE 19.4

The graphic template used for plotting heart rates during cycle ergometry for the estimation of maximal oxygen consumption (VO₂max) using the YMCA protocols. As illustrated, three submaximal heart rates are plotted against workload, and a straight line of best fit is drawn through the lines and extended to the subject's estimated maximal heart rate. The point along the x-axis that corresponds to this intersection is located and the estimated VO₂max is obtained. In this example, the subject's estimated VO₂max is 4.25 L/min. (Since this is a redrawn version, it is recommended that a copy of the original chart be used for data collection purposes. (Adapted from *The Y's way to physical fitness* with permission of the YMCA of the USA, 101 N. Wacker Drive, Chicago, IL 60606.)

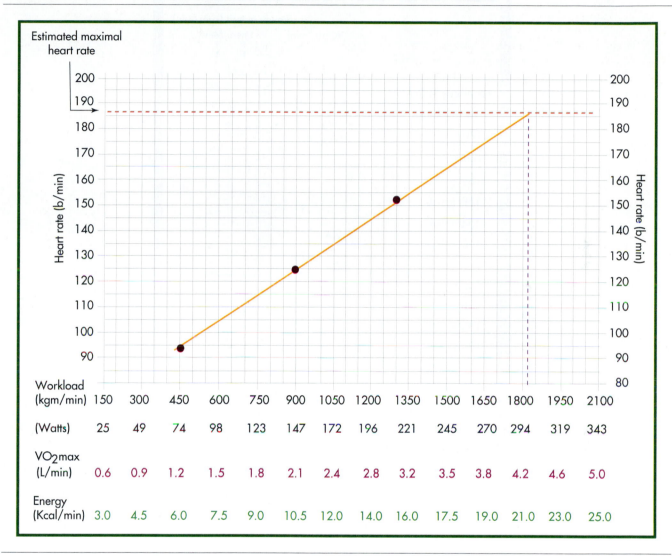

each of 6.7 kmh at 0% grade at a heart rate of 125 bpm, and 12.1 kmh at 2.5% grade at a heart rate of 155 bpm, VO_2 would be calculated by estimating VO_2 at each intensity from the ACSM equations and completing the following calculations:

19-1

$$2VO_2 = 48.3 \text{ ml/kg/min}$$
$$1VO_2 = 35.7 \text{ ml/kg/min}$$
$$b = (2VO_2 - 1VO_2) / (2HR - 1HR)$$
$$= (48.3 - 35.7) / (155 - 125)$$
$$= 12.6 / 30$$
$$= 0.42$$

19-2

$$VO_2max = 2VO_2 + [b(maxHR - 2HR)]$$
$$= 48.3 + [0.42((220 - 35) - 155))]$$
$$= 48.3 + [0.42(185 - 155)]$$
$$= 48.3 + 12.6$$
$$= 60.9$$

Other protocols exist for estimating VO_2max from treadmill walking protocols. Widrick et al. applied the Rockport walk test to a treadmill situation, in which subjects had to walk 1.61 km (1 mile) as fast as possible.[72] Walk time, heart rate during the last 2 minutes of walking, body mass, gender, and age were used to estimate VO_2max from gender-specific and general equations developed from multiple-regression analyses. Results indicated that predicted VO_2max was accurate for both men and women of low to moderate fitness, but VO_2max was underpredicted in highly fit males (VO_2max > 55 ml/kg/min).

Ebbeling et al. also developed a walking test on the treadmill, but unlike the Rockport walk, this test was based on an estimation of VO_2max from a single submaximal stage.[22] The test is conducted by having subjects perform a warm-up of 4 minutes of walking at a self-selected speed of 4 to 7.2 kmh (2 to 4.5 mph) at 0% grade, causing heart rate

FIGURE 19.5

Two nomograms used to predict VO₂max from submaximal steady state cycle ergometer exercise. **A,** The Åstrand-Rhyming nomogram for estimating VO₂max from a single submaximal exercise intensity. To use the nomogram for cycle ergometry exercise, a line is drawn connecting the gender specific submaximal steady state heart rate to the gender specific workload (kgm/min). Where this straight line intersects the diagonal VO₂max line represents the VO₂max value. (As this is a redrawn version, it is recommended that a copy of the original be used for data collection purposes. *Continued.*

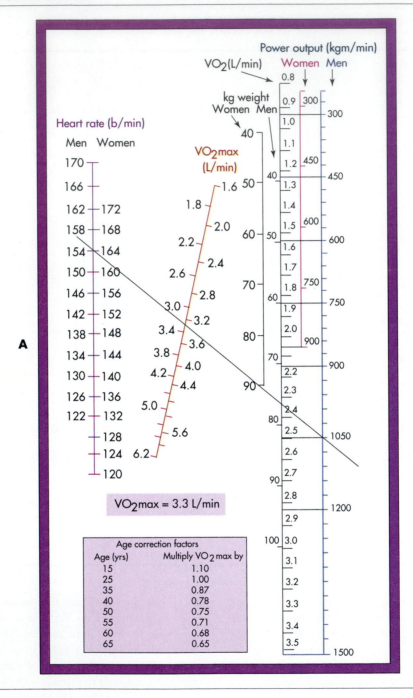

to be between 50% and 70% of age–predicted maximum. The grade is then increased to 5% for another 4 minutes, where heart rate is recorded during the final 30 seconds. Treadmill speed, final heart rate, age, and gender were used to estimate VO₂max expressed as ml/kg/min.

Cycle ergometer protocols. Bicycle ergometer tests are commonly used to measure and predict oxygen uptake. One of the most common submaximal cycle ergometer protocols

used to predict VO₂max was developed by the YMCA.[34] This protocol uses 3-minute stages. To calculate functional capacity, two HR and power output data points need to be obtained within a 110 to 150 beat/min HR range. Functional capacity can be predicted by plotting the last two heart rate–power output values obtained on a calibrated chart (Figure 19.4).

Another widely used protocol is that of the Åstrand-Rhyming test and nomogram (Figure 19.5, *A*). The original

FIGURE 19.5—Cont'd

B, The Bannister-Legge nomogram. The Åstrand-Rhyming nomogram has been the most validated of the two monomograms; however, research done in the development of the Bannister-Legge nomogram indicates that it may have significantly better accuracy in predicting VO_2max for untrained to moderately trained males. (Adapted from Åstrand I: *Acta Physiologica Scandinavica* 49(Suppl. 169), p. 51, 1960 and Legge BJ, Bannister EW: *J Appl Physiol* 61(3) 1203-1209, 1986.)

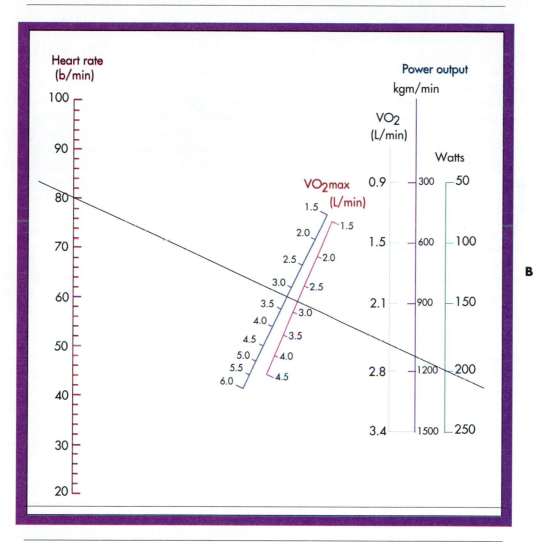

nomogram did not have an age adjustment, which decreased accuracy of the prediction because of the known reduction in maximal heart rate with increasing age.[3] The age-corrected factors were validated by Åstrand on 144 subjects.[4] However, because of the limited number of subjects in these early validation studies, research has produced varied results on the accuracy of the Åstrand-Rhyming nomogram and exercise protocol. Legge and Bennister modified the Åstrand-Rhyming nomogram (Figure 19.5, *B*) by using the change in heart rate after zero–loaded cycling rather than absolute heart rate during exercise.[46] Such a change decreased the error of prediction and improved the accuracy of prediction of VO_2max in small samples of trained and untrained males.

Because of the small numbers of subjects and limited populations used by Legge and Bannister, it is difficult to recommend this modified nomogram for widespread use in the prediction of VO_2max.[46] However, the modified nomogram does seem to have improved accuracy that needs to be validated on differing populations and larger numbers of subjects.

To perform the exercise suited for either nomogram, subjects perform cycle ergometry at 75, 100, or 125 Watts, depending on their endurance training status. Heart rates are recorded at minutes 5 and 6. If these heart rates do not differ by more than 5 bpm, they are averaged and their value determines the progression of exercise. If the average heart rate is less than 150 bpm, the intensity should be increased by 50

Watts and exercise continued. This is repeated until the average heart rate exceeds 130 bpm after 6 minutes. Data used in the Åstrand-Rhyming nomogram are the final power output (Watts) and final exercise heart rate. A line is drawn connecting the inner axis of the exercise intensity scale to the exercise heart rate. The intercept of the line across the VO_2max axis indicates the VO_2max.

For the Bannister-Legge nomogram, the procedure is similar to the Åstrand-Rhyming nomogram, but a delta heart rate (ΔHR) rather than absolute heart rate axis is used.

Siconolfi et al. modified each of the YMCA and Åstrand-Rhyming procedures. Exercise is performed similar to the YMCA procedure.[64] An estimated VO_2 from the Åstrand-Rhyming nomogram is obtained (not age corrected) and used with age in a gender-specific regression equation. This test had good accuracy and low error of prediction across a wide range of VO_2 (1 to 3 L/min) for individuals between the ages of 20 to 70 years.

Field Tests

Cooper's 1.5-mile run. The 1.5-mile test, originally developed by Kenneth Cooper, is a popular test used to predict cardiovascular fitness.[15] This test is conducted on a quarter-mile track. After subjects have warmed up, they walk, jog, or run as fast as they can six times around the track. Oxygen uptake is predicted by formula (Table 19.2).

Rockport walk test. The Rockport walking test is an excellent test used to predict cardiovascular fitness, especially for sedentary individuals. Individuals are instructed to walk as fast as they can for 1 mile and then record their heart rate at the end of the walk. VO_2max is predicted by using a multiple regression equation developed by Kline et al.[40]

Step tests. The 3-minute step test predicts oxygen uptake from the recovery heart rate after 3 minutes of stepping.[50] The test is conducted using a bench $16^{1}/_{4}$ inches high. A metronome should be set to 88 counts (22 step/min) for women and 96 counts (24 steps/min) for men. At the signal to start, subjects step to a four-step cadence (up-up-down-down). At the end of 3 minutes, the subject remains standing and a 15-second pulse rate is recorded between 5 to 20 seconds into recovery.

Lactate Threshold

During incremental exercise, heart rate has been shown to increase in a linear manner until a given submaximal exercise intensity (denoted fc) that corresponds to the LT.[17] However, results from different studies have produced conflicting findings over similarities and dissimilarities between the LT and fc.[39,62] It seems that the heart rate response to an incremental exercise test is protocol dependent, since the original study by Conconiti et al. was actually performed in the field during multiple bouts of track running, rather than the typical continuous incremental exercise performed in the laboratory.[17] Clearly, more research needs to be done on this topic, since a noninvasive and inexpensive method to estimate the LT would have considerable application to sports and athletics training.

Measuring Maximal Muscle Power and Anaerobic Capacity

During high-intensity exercise, muscle ATP regeneration must be provided at a high rate to prevent fatigue and continue muscle contraction. In many daily, sports, and athletic activities, intense muscle contraction is required and often completed before significant increases in mitochondrial respiration. For these activities a large capacity for ATP regeneration despite low oxygen consumption is essential for optimal performance. Research has had difficulty in measuring the capacity of nonmitochondrial ATP regeneration, or anaerobic capacity; however, several methods are available to estimate this component of fitness.

Maximal muscle power and anaerobic capacity depend largely on age, gender, morphologic characteristics, and training, all of which need to be taken into account during testing and when interpreting the results of a test.[9] Tests of maximal muscle power can be conducted in the field and in the laboratory. Simple tests of muscle power involve quantifying and comparing an athlete's performance during bouts of high-intensity exercise (e.g., stair climbing), whereas more sophisticated laboratory tests can involve isokinetic testing equipment or computer-integrated cycle ergometers.

Measuring Maximal Muscle Power

Tests of muscle power are categorized according to the length of the test. Short-term tests last 10 seconds or less, the intermediate-term anaerobic tests last between 20 to 60 seconds, and long-term anaerobic tests last 60 to 120 seconds. Each type of test indirectly reflects a measure of the subject's ability to regenerate ATP during that interval. As explained, additional factors, such as muscle fiber type proportions and muscle buffer capacity, also influence ATP regeneration.

Short-Term Tests of Muscle Power

Sargent's jump and reach test. The Sargent's jump and reach test measures the difference between standing reach height and the maximum jumping reach height. Although the Sargent's jump and reach test has been used for decades to evaluate leg power, its ability to assess an individual's anaerobic capacity or true muscle power is questionable. The test can produce erroneous results because of the brevity of the test and because the skill involved in performing the test is not factored into the nomogram equation. Muscle power is calculated from the vertical height as follows:

$$Power(Watts) = 21.67 \times mass(kg)$$
$$\times \text{ vertical displacement(m)}^{0.5}$$

Bosco developed a 60-second vertical jump test protocol.[10] The test consists of performing consecutive maximal vertical jumps during a 60-second period. The time in contact with the platform and time in the air are measured via a force plate and electrical timing device. Bosco reported a test-retest reliability of 0.95. Power is calculated as[10]:

$$W = (9.8 \times Tf \times 60) / 4N (60 - Tf)$$

where
W	=	mechanical power (W/kg)
Tf	=	sum of total flight time of all jumps
N	=	number of jumps during 60 seconds
9.8	=	acceleration of gravity (m/s²)

Margaria power test. The Margaria test was developed in the early 1960s, and was modified by Kalamen.[39,49] The Margaria-Kalamen protocol has subjects start 6 meters from a flight of stairs and run up the stairs taking two or three steps at a time for a total distance of 1.75 m. Because this distance can be spanned in less than 1 second, electronic timing mats are recommended at the first and last step.

Power is calculated from the following equation:

19.4   Power (Watts) = [(mass;kg)(vertical
displacement;m)(9.8)] / (time;s)

Intermediate-Term Tests of Muscle Power

Wingate test. The Wingate test (WT), developed in the early 1970s at the Wingate Institute in Israel, has become one of the most widely used protocols in exercise research for determining peak **muscle power** and indirectly reflecting anaerobic capacity.[6] The WT involves pedaling or arm cranking at maximal effort for 30 seconds against a constant load. Performance is expressed as mean power (mean work output over 30 seconds), peak power (highest power output during any one 5-second period), or fatigue index (difference between the peak power and the lowest 5-second power output divided by peak power).

The resistance setting equation for leg cycling for women is equal to (kp/kg BW = 0.075) and for men is (kp/kg BW = 0.083 to 0.092).[21,23]

Isokinetic tests. Isokinetic testing protocols for determining intermediate anaerobic power are popular because they can be designed to test specific muscle groups (Figure 19.6). The ability to generate peak force is indicative of an individual's anaerobic power, and this premise is supported by research documenting significant relationships between peak power and muscle fiber type proportions.

FIGURE 19.6

A Cybex isokinetic muscle testing program. (Courtesy, Cybex®, Bay Shore, New York.)

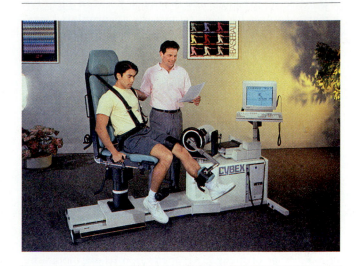

Anaerobic Capacity

The **anaerobic capacity** of an individual represents the ability to regenerate ATP from nonmitochondrial sources. Although the name reflects a capacity, and therefore a given amount of energy, such a capacity is difficult to measure, as discussed subsequently.

Muscle Metabolite Accumulation

The rate of ATP regeneration cannot be measured directly but is often estimated by sampling muscle tissue and assaying for key intermediates of glycogenolysis and glycolysis (see Chapter 10). It is assumed that during intense muscle contractions, when there is minimal muscle blood flow because of high intramuscular pressures, muscle contraction occurs in a closed system where the accumulation of glycolytic intermediates (including lactate) reflects glucose-6-phosphate flux through glycolysis, from which ATP regeneration can be estimated (e.g., three ATP from one glucose-6-phosphate flux to lactate when muscle glycogen is the carbohydrate source).

Accumulated Oxygen Deficit

An indirect and noninvasive method for determining anaerobic capacity is to estimate the total energy require-

muscle power
the mechanical power during dynamic by muscle contractions

anaerobic capacity
the capacity of skeletal muscle to regenerate ATP from nonmitochondrial respiration pathways

ments of exercise by calculating the theoretical VO_2 required for the exercise intensity and subtracting from this value the measured VO_2. Exercise is usually performed on a cycle ergometer or treadmill. The difference between these two integrated values has been termed the **accumulated oxygen deficit** (aO_2D) and has been argued to reflect anaerobic capacity.[51-53]

The aO_2D is maximal after intense exercise is performed that causes fatigue between 2 and 5 minutes.[51-53] Figure 19.7 illustrates values for aO_2D for different athletes and different testing conditions.

Strength

Defining Muscular Strength

Muscular strength is defined as the maximal force exerted by a muscle or muscle group at a specific velocity. Measurement of strength has application to the monitoring of improvement during a resistance training program. Given that resistance training programs are used by individuals of all ages and health statuses, correct evaluation of strength is a necessity. Muscular strength can be measured during each type of muscle contraction: isotonic, isometric, eccentric, and isokinetic; however, tests of dynamic muscle strength using isotonic contractions are most common.

FIGURE 19.7

The accumulated oxygen deficit (aO_2D) of different trained athletes, as well as for different conditions of exercise. The fact that the aO_2D increases during more intense exercise, as well as being larger in power trained individuals, provides some degree of validation of the measure and method.

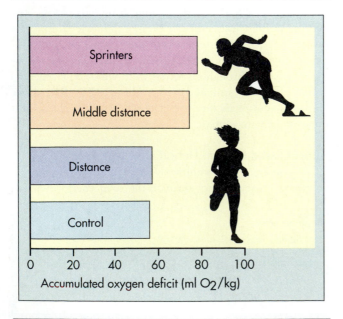

Muscular Strength Testing Equipment

Strength testing equipment can vary in price from several hundred dollars to thousands of dollars. A **dynamometer** is an inexpensive device used to measure static strength. Dynamometers typically have an adjustable handle to fit varying hand sizes. A common dynamometer measures forces between 0 and 100 kilograms. Larger dynamometers are also available to measure back and leg strength. Cable tensiometers are used in conjunction with special tables to measure static strength of up to 38 different muscle groups.

Strength can also be tested with free weights, variable resistance weight-lifting machines, and isokinetic systems. Isotonic or dynamic strength is typically measured by the maximum amount of weight that can be lifted in one repetition (**1 repetition maximum** [1 RM]), or in a given number of repetitions (e.g., 10 RM) using either free weights or a resistance machine. Since multiple joints and muscles are involved in muscle strength testing with free weights, free-weight testing may be better suited to specific sports or athletic movements. Conversely, resistance machines better isolate specific muscles and therefore can evaluate how specific muscles or muscle groups are responding to a given intervention.

Isokinetic measurements of strength can be performed at different velocities, with the velocity of contraction determining the time for force application and therefore muscular strength. Thus contractile velocity must be known before comparisons on strength can be made from isokinetic machines.

Interpreting the Results of Muscular Strength Tests

Muscular strength and endurance are specific to the muscle group being tested; therefore no single test is available to assess total body muscular strength and endurance. It is recommended that a variety of muscular strength tests be performed so that a fair assessment of upper and lower body strength is determined (see Tables 19.5 and 19.6). As with all previous comments on measuring physiologic capacities, the evaluation of strength changes requires that the same test be performed in as identical a manner as done previously.

TABLE 19.5

Norms for grip strength

RATING	LEFT GRIP (kg)		RIGHT GRIP (kg)	
	M	**F**	**M**	**F**
Excellent	>68	>37	>70	>41
Good	56-67	34-36	62-69	38-40
Average	43-55	22-33	48-61	25-37
Poor	39-42	18-21	41-47	22-24
Very poor	<39	<18	<41	<22

Adapted from Corbin CB, Dowell LJ, Lindsey R, Tolson H: *Concepts in physical education,* Dubuque, Iowa, 1978, WC Brown.

TABLE 19.6

Strength* norms expressed relative to body weight for 1 RM bench press

RATING	AGES 20-29	AGES 30-39	AGES 40-49	AGES 50-59	AGES 60+
MEN					
Excellent	>1.26	>1.08	>0.97	>0.86	>0.78
Good	1.17-1.25	1.01-1.07	0.91-0.96	0.81-0.85	0.74-0.77
Average	0.97-1.16	0.86-1.00	0.78-0.90	0.70-0.80	0.64-0.73
Fair	0.88-0.96	0.79-0.85	0.72-0.77	0.65-0.69	0.60-0.63
Poor	<0.87	<0.78	<0.71	<0.64	<0.59
WOMEN					
Excellent	>0.78	>0.66	>0.61	>0.54	>0.55
Good	0.72-0.77	0.62-0.65	0.57-0.60	0.51-0.53	0.51-0.54
Average	0.59-0.71	0.53-0.61	0.48-0.56	0.43-0.50	0.41-0.50
Fair	0.53-0.58	0.49-0.52	0.44-0.47	0.40-0.42	0.37-0.40
Poor	<0.52	<0.48	<0.43	<0.39	<0.36

Modified from Gettman LR: Fitness testing. In Blair S, Painter P, Pate R et al, editors: *Resource manual for guidelines for exercise testing and prescription,* Philadelphia, 1988, Lea & Febiger.
* Strength data = strength (lb) / body weight (lb).

accumulated oxygen deficit
the amount of energy able to be generated by contracting skeletal muscle that did not involve mitochondrial respiration

muscular strength
the maximal force generated by contracting skeletal muscle for a given contractile velocity

dynamometer (di-na-mom'e-ter)
an instrument for the measurement of muscle force application

1 repetition maximum (1RM)
the maximum strength from one contraction. Typically, the 1 RM is obtained during dynamic contractions. When the contraction is isometric, this strength measure is termed the **maximal voluntary contraction (MVC)**

SUMMARY

- Tests that measure or estimate cardiorespiratory endurance are used to evaluate an individual's capacity to acquire and transport oxygen in the blood to fuel muscle mitochondrial respiration. Conversely, tests that measure or estimate muscle power development evaluate the capacity for skeletal muscle ATP regeneration from creatine phosphate hydrolysis and glycolysis. Finally, tests that measure strength evaluate muscle mass and neuromuscular function.

- The choice of prediction versus measurement of a physiologic capacity is highly dependent on the purpose of the testing. Research and clinical evaluation require measurement of physiologic capacities; however, the determination of general fitness profiles for a large number of subjects may make prediction protocols the method of choice. Prediction methods have more validity when used for intraindividual comparisons.

- Tests used to measure cardiorespiratory and muscular endurance and the potential for endurance exercise performance are the test of VO_2max, the lactate or ventilatory threshold, running economy, and the kinetics of increase in VO_2. The measures of VO_2max and the LT combine to provide an accurate indication of cardiorespiratory and muscular endurance, as well as the potential for success in prolonged endurance events.

- The test of VO_2max should be between 8 and 12 minutes in length to obtain a true VO_2max. In addition, a plateau in VO_2 with increasing exercise intensity, an RER greater than 1.1, and the attainment of age predicted maximal heart rate (220-age) have been used as criteria to validate VO_2peak as VO_2max. However, individuals with cardiovascular diseases or chronic obstructive pulmonary disease prematurely terminate a maximal test because of clinical symptoms of exercise intolerance, such as angina, abnormal ECG, dyspnea (breathlessness), or leg fatigue resulting from claudication. For the more clinically determined maximal VO_2 values, the expressions *symptom-limited VO_2max* or **VO_2peak** are more appropriate.

- The need to tailor a protocol to the fitness and health status of an individual indicates that using predetermined protocols is inappropriate. However, the exercise testing of diseased individuals has been performed using standard protocols that allow comparison of data within and between populations. In addition, using a standard protocol allows the ability to estimate VO_2max from a prediction equation that has been validated for that protocol.

- The detection of LT is based on graphing blood lactate concentration (y-axis) versus some measure of exercise intensity (e.g., VO_2, Watts, running velocity) (x-axis). Thus there is increased precision in detecting the LT with more data points. Therefore it is recommended that at least eight blood samples be obtained during an incremental exercise test.

- The LT can be noninvasively determined by plotting ventilation and respiratory data obtained from an incremental exercise test to VO_2max. Caiozzeo et al. have determined that the most accurate variables to use are minute ventilation (VE), the ventilatory equivalent for oxygen (VE/VO_2), and the ventilatory equivalent for carbon dioxide (VE/V_{CO_2}).

- Running economy is determined by having the subject complete at least three exercise intensities known to be below the LT. The durations of each stage should be at least 4 minutes and data of VO_2 should be obtained continuously during the testing. The steady-state VO_2 values (y-axis) are graphed against intensity on the x-axis, and the linear regression line of best fit represents the efficiency of the subject.

- Another test to evaluate the cardiorespiratory condition of a subject is to measure the rate of change in VO_2 for a given increase in exercise intensity. The more rapid the increase in VO_2, the greater the cardiorespiratory and muscular endurance. This test requires the use of a breath-by-breath indirect calorimetry system. The rate of increase in VO_2 is typically expressed as a time constant (tVO_2) from a single exponential equation, such as $VO_2 = A + B[1-e^{(-t/t)}]$.

- **Prediction** of VO_2max, or any **criterion variable,** depends on measuring variables that are known to change proportionally with that variable. Thus heart rate, change in heart rate, and exercise duration for a given protocol have been used widely by different researchers. The heart rate response to exercise is an important variable for predicting VO_2max, since individuals with increased cardiorespiratory endurance have a lower heart rate for a given exercise intensity. Typically, prediction of VO_2max is done by using a statistical technique called **multiple regression.**

- VO_2max can be predicted from maximal exercise duration using the Bruce or Balke treadmill protocols for specific populations. The maximal cycle ergometer protocol by Storer et al. is the most accurate method and equation for estimating VO_2max during cycle ergometry.

- VO_2max can be estimated by equations that use the heart rate responses to submaximal exercise and demographic characteristics (e.g., age, gender, body weight). Since these tests avoid maximal exertion, they are safer to implement on more elderly or diseased populations.

- One of the most common submaximal cycle ergometer protocols used to predict VO_2max was developed by the YMCA.[34] This protocol uses 3-minute stages. Another widely used protocol is that of the Åstrand-Rhyming test and nomogram, which has been improved by Legge and Bannister by using the change in heart rate after zero-loaded cycling rather than absolute heart rate during exercise.

- Maximal **muscle power** and **anaerobic capacity** depend largely on age, gender, morphologic characteristics, and training, all of which need to be taken into account during testing and when interpreting the results of a test.[9] Simple tests of muscle power involve quantifying and comparing an athlete's performance during bouts of high-intensity exercise (e.g., stair climbing), whereas more sophisticated laboratory tests can involve isokinetic testing equipment or computer-integrated cycle ergometers.

- The Wingate test (WT) has become one of the most widely used protocols in exercise research for determining peak muscle power and indirectly reflecting anaerobic capacity. The WT involves pedaling or arm cranking at maximal effort for 30 seconds against a constant load. Performance is expressed as mean power (mean work output over 30 seconds), peak power (highest power output during any one 5-second period), or fatigue index (difference between the peak power and the lowest 5-second power output divided by peak power).

- An indirect and noninvasive method for determining anaerobic capacity is to estimate the total energy requirements of exercise by calculating the theoretical VO_2 required for the exercise intensity and subtracting from this value the measured VO_2. Exercise is usually performed on a cycle ergometer or treadmill. The difference between these two integrated values has been termed the **accumulated oxygen deficit** (aO_2D) and has been argued to reflect anaerobic capacity.[51-53]

- **Muscular strength** is defined as the maximal force exerted by a muscle or muscle group at a specific velocity. Muscular strength can be measured during each type of muscle contraction: isotonic, isometric, eccentric, and isokinetic; however, tests of dynamic muscle strength using isotonic contractions are most common.

- A **dynamometer** is an inexpensive device used to measure static strength. Dynamometers typically have an adjustable handle to fit varying hand sizes. A common dynamometer measures forces between 0 and 100 kilograms. Larger dynamometers are also available to measure back and leg strength. Cable tensiometers are used in conjunction with special tables to also measure static strength of up to 38 different muscle groups.

- Strength can also be tested with free weights, variable resistance weight-lifting machines, and isokinetic systems. Isotonic or dynamic strength is typically measured by the maximum amount of weight that can be lifted in one repetition (**1 repetition maximum** [-1 RM]), or in a given number of repetitions (e.g., 10 RM) using either free weights or a resistance machine. Isokinetic measurements of strength can be performed at different velocities, with the velocity of contraction determining the time for force application and therefore muscular strength.

REVIEW QUESTIONS

1. Explain the tests you would use to evaluate each of the metabolic pathways, and why: creatine phosphate, glycolytic, mitochondrial respiration.

2. Why do you think VO_2max does not predict endurance exercise performance well in a group of highly trained athletes?

3. Why are good running economy and rapid O_2 kinetics important for optimizing distance running performance?

4. Why is it more difficult to measure a person's anaerobic capacity than aerobic capacity?

5. What tests would you use to experimentally assess a person's ability to perform well during explosive events such as jumping? What test would you recommend for athletes involved in more prolonged sprinting, such as the 200-meter and 400-meter sprint and sprint cycling?

6. Explain the concept of the accumulated oxygen deficit. What are some potential problems that might prevent its accurate measurement?

7. What are the uses for a dynamometer and a cable tensiometer?

8. What are some typical assessment activities used to measure muscular strength?

APPLICATIONS

1. Can individuals with cardiovascular, pulmonary, or other chronic diseases attain a VO_2max during incremental exercise? How would you know if the highest VO_2 was a VO_2max?

2. Of the tests covered in this chapter, which have the most relevance to a physical therapy application? Explain these applications.

3. What are the benefits and drawbacks of isokinetic testing of muscle power and strength?

REFERENCES

1. Allen G, Freund BJ, Wilmore JH: Interaction of test protocol and horizontal run training on maximal oxygen uptake, *Med Sci Sports Exerc* 18(5):581-587, 1986.

2. American College of Sports Medicine: *Guidelines for exercise testing and prescription,* ed 4, Philadelphia, 1991, Lea & Febiger.

3. Åstrand PO, Rhyming I: A nomogram for calculation of aerobic capacity (physical fitness) from pulse rate during submaximal work, *J Appl Physiol* 7:218-221, 1954.

4. Åstrand PO: Aerobic work capacity in men and women with special reference to age, *Acta Physiol Scand* 49(Suppl 169):1-92, 1960.

5. Balke B, Ware R: An experimental study of Air Force personnel, *US Armed Forces Med J* 10:675-688, 1959.

6. Bar-Or O: The Wingate anaerobic test: an update on methodology, reliability and validity, *Sports Med* 4:381-394, 1987.

7. Beaver WL, Wasserman K, Whipp BJ: Improved detection of the lactate threshold during exercise using a log-log transformation, *J Appl Physiol* 59:1936-1940, 1985.

8. Bergh U, Sjodin B, Forsberg A, Svedenhag J: The relationship between body mass and oxygen uptake during running in humans, *Med Sci Sports Exerc* 23(2):205-211, 1991.

9. Bouchard C, Dionne FT, Simoneau J-A, Boulay MR: Genetics of aerobic and anaerobic performances. In Holloszy J, editor: *Exerc Sport Sci Rev* 20:27-58, 1992.

10. Bosco C, Luhtanen P, Komi PV: A simple method for measurement of mechanical power in jumping, *Eur J Appl Physiol* 50:273-282, 1983.

11. Bruce RL, Kusumi F, Hosmer D: Maximal oxygen intake and nomographic assessment of functional aerobic impairment in cardiovascular disease, *Am Heart J* 85:545-562, 1973.

REFERENCES—Cont'd

12. Buchfuhrer MJ, Hansen JE, Robinson TE et al: Optimizing the exercise protocol for cardiopulmonary assessment, *J Appl Physiol* 55:558-564, 1983.

13. Caiozzo VJ, Davis JA, Ellis JF et al: A comparison of gas exchange indices used to detect the anaerobic threshold, *J Appl Physiol* 53:1184-1189, 1982.

14. Consolazio CF, Johnson RE, Pecora LJ: *Physiological measurements of metabolic functions in man,* New York, 1963, McGraw-Hill.

15. Cooper KH: A means of assessing maximal oxygen intake, *JAMA* 203:201-204, 1968.

16. Coleman RJ, Wilkie S, Viscio L et al: Validation of 1-mile walk test for estimating VO$_2$max in 20-29 year olds, *Med Sci Sports Exerc* 19(2)(Abstract 171):S29, 1987.

17. Conconi F, Ferrari M, Ziglio PG et al: Determination of the anaerobic threshold by a noninvasive field test in runners, *J Appl Physiol* 52:869-873, 1982.

18. Corbin CB, Dowell LJ, Lindsey R, Tolson H: *Concepts in physical eduction,* Dubuque, Iowa, 1978, WC Brown.

19. Coyle EF, Coggan AR, Hopper MK, Walters TJ: Determinants of endurance in well trained cyclists, *J Appl Physiol* 64:2622-2630, 1988.

20. Davis JA, Caiozzo VJ, Lamarra N et al: Does the gas exchange anaerobic threshold occur at a fixed blood lactate concentration of 2 or 4 mM? *Int J Sports Med* 4:89-93, 1983.

21. Dotan R, Bar-Or O: Load optimization from the Wingate anaerobic test, *Eur J Appl Physiol* 51:409-417, 1983.

22. Ebbling CB, Ward A, Puleo EM et al: Development of single stage submaximal walking test, *Med Sci Sports Exerc* 23(8):966-973, 1991.

23. Evans JA, Quinney HA: Determination of resistance settings for anaerobic power testing, *Can J Appl Sports Sci* 6:53-56, 1981.

24. Farrell P, Wilmore JH, Coyle E et al: Plasma lactate accumulation and distance running performance, *Med Sci Sports Exerc* 11:338-344, 1979.

25. Forbes GB: The adult decline in lean body mass, *Human Biol* 48:161-173, 1979.

26. Foster C, Pollock ML, Rod JL et al: Evaluation of functional capacity during exercise radionuclide angiography, *Cardiology* 70:85-93, 1983.

27. Foster C, Jackson AS, Pollock ML et al: Generalized equations for predicting functional capacity from treadmill performance, *Am Heart J* 107:1229-1234, 1984.

28. Fox EL: A simple, accurate technique for predicting maximal aerobic power, *J Appl Physiol* 35(6):914-916, 1973.

29. Freund BJ, Allen D, Wilmore JH: Interaction of test protocol and inclined run training on maximal oxygen uptake, *Med Sci Sports Exerc* 18(5):588-592, 1986.

30. Froelicher VF, Lancaster MC: The prediction of maximal oxygen consumption from a continuous graded exercise protocol, *Am Heart J* 87:445-450, 1974.

31. Froelicher VF, Myers J, Follansbee WP, Labovitz AJ: *Exercise and the heart,* ed 3, St. Louis, 1993, Mosby.

32. Gettman LR: Fitness testing. In Blair S, Painter P, Pate R et al, editors: *Resource manual for guidelines for exercise testing and prescription,* Philadelphia, 1988, Lea & Febiger.

33. Glassford RG, Baycroft GHY, Sedgwick AW, MacNab RBJ: Comparison of maximal oxygen uptake values determined by predicted and actual methods, *J Appl Physiol* 20(3):509-513, 1965.

34. Golding LA, Meyers CR, Shinning WE: *Y's way to physical fitness: the complete guide to fitness testing and instruction,* ed 3, Champaign, Illinois, 1989, Human Kinetics.

35. Hoeger WWK, Hopkins DR, Button S, Palmer TA: Comparing of the sit and reach and the modified sit and reach flexibility tests, *Med Sci Sports Exerc* 22(2):S10, 1990.

36. Hoeger WWK, Hoeger SA: *Lifetime physical fitness and wellness,* ed 3, Englewood, Colorado, 1992, Morton.

37. Jones NL: Evaluation of a microprocessor controlled exercise testing system, *J Appl Physiol* 57:1312, 1984.

38. Joyner MJ: Modeling optimal marathon performance on the basis of physiological factors, *J Appl Physiol* 70(2):683-687, 1991.

39. Kalamen J: *Measurement of maximum muscular power in man,* Doctoral Dissertation, Ohio State University, 1968.

40. Kline GM, Porcari JP, Hintermeister R et al: Estimation of VO$_2$max from a one-mile track walk, gender, age, and body weight, *Med Sci Sports Exerc* 19:253-259, 1987.

41. Komi PV: *Strength and power in sport,* Cambridge, Massachusetts, 1992, Blackwell Scientific.

42. Kuipers H, Keizer HA, deVries T et al: Comparison of heart rate as a non-invasive determinant of the anaerobic threshold with the lactate threshold when cycling, *Eur J Appl Physiol* 58:303-306, 1988.

43. Kumagai S, Tanaka K, Matsuura V et al: Relationships of the anaerobic threshold with the 5km, 10km, and 20 mile races, *Eur J Appl Physiol* 49:13-23, 1982.

44. Lang PB, Latin RW, Berg KE, Mellion MB: The accuracy of the ACSM cycle ergometry equation, *Med Sci Sports Exerc* 24(2):272-276, 1992.

45. Latin RW, Berg KE, Smith P et al: Validation of a cycle ergometry equation for predicting steady-rate VO$_2$, *Med Sci Sports Exerc* 25(8):970-974, 1993.

REFERENCES—Cont'd

46. Legge BJ, Bannister EW: The Åstrand-Rhyming nomogram revisited, *J Appl Physiol* 61(3):1203-1209, 1986.

47. Londeree BR: The use of laboratory tests with long distance runners, *Sports Med* 3:201-213, 1986.

48. MacDougall JD, Wenger HA, Green HJ: Physiological testing of the high-performance athlete, ed 2, Champaign, Illinois, 1991, Human Kinetics.

49. Margaria R: Measurement of muscular power in man, *J Appl Physiol* 21:1662-1664, 1966.

50. McArdle WD, Katch FI, Pechar GS et al: Reliability and interrelationships between maximal oxygen intake, physical work capacity and step-test scores in college women, *Med Sci Sports Exerc* 4:182-186, 1972.

51. Medbo JI, Mohm AC, Tabata I et al: Anaerobic capacity determined by the accumulated O_2 deficit, *J Appl Physiol* 64:50-60, 1988.

52. Medbo JI, Tabata I: Relative importance of aerobic and anerobic energy release during shortlasting, exhausting bicycle exercise, *J Appl Physiol* 67:1881-1886, 1989.

53. Medbo JI, Burgers S: Effect of training on the anaerobic capacity, *Med Sci Sports Exerc* 22:501-507, 1990.

54. Naughton J, Balke B, Nagle F: Refinement in methods of evaluation and physical conditioning before and after myocardial infarction, *Am J Cardiol* 14:837, 1964.

55. Noakes TD: Implications of exercise testing for prediction of athletic performance: a contemporary perspective, *Med Sci Sports Exerc* 20:319-330, 1988.

56. Patton JF, Vogel JA, Mello RP: Evaluation of a maximal predictive cycle ergometer test of aerobic power, *Eur J Appl Physiol* 49:131-140, 1982.

57. Pollock ML, Bohannon RL, Cooper KH et al: A comparative analysis of four protocols for maximal treadmill stress testing, *Am Heart J* 92:39-46, 1976.

58. Pollock ML, Foster C, Schmidt D et al: Comparative analysis of physiological responses to three different maximal graded exercise protocols in healthy women, *Am Heart J* 103:363-373, 1982.

59. Pollock ML, Wilmore JH: *Exercise in health and disease,* ed 2, Philadelphia, 1990, Saunders.

60. Rhodes EC, McKenzie DC: Predicting marathon time from anaerobic threshold measurements, *Phys Sports Med* 12:95-98, 1984.

61. Robergs RA, Costill DL, Fink WJ et al: Blood lactate differences between arterialized and venous blood, *Int J Sports Med* 11(6):446-451, 1990.

62. Robergs RA: Predictors of marathon running performance. In Wood S, Roach R, editors: *Sports and exercise medicine.* Vol 76. *Lung biology in health and disease,* New York, 1994, Marcel Dekker.

63. Rowell LB, Taylor HL, Wang Y: Limitations to prediction of maximal oxygen intake, *J Sports Med* 19:919-927, 1964.

64. Siconolfi SF, Cullinane EM, Careton RA, Thompson PD: Assessing VO_2max in epidemiologic studies: modification of the Åstrand-Rhyming test, *Med Sci Sports Exerc* 14(50):335-338, 1982.

65. Sjodin B, Svedenhag J: Applied physiology of marathon running, *Sports Med* 2:83-99, 1985.

66. Stegman H, Kinderman W, Schnabel A: Lactate kinetics and individual anaerobic threshold, *Int J Sports Med* 3:105-110, 1982.

67. Storer TW, Davis JA, Caiozzo VJ: Accurate prediction of VO_2max in cycle ergometry, *Med Sci Sports Exerc* 22(5):704-712, 1990.

68. Tanaka K, Matsuura Y: Marathon performance, anaerobic threshold and onset of blood lactate accumulation, *J Appl Physiol* 57:640-643, 1984.

69. Tokmakidis SP, Leger LA: Comparison of mathematically determined blood lactate and heart rate "threshold" points and relationship with performance, *Eur J Appl Physiol* 64:309-317, 1992.

70. Wasserman K, Whipp BJ: Exercise physiology in health and disease, *Am Rev Respir Dis* 112:219-249, 1975.

71. Whipp BJ, Ward SA, Lamarra N et al: Parameters of ventilatory and gas exchange dynamics during exercise, *J Appl Physiol* 52:1506-1513, 1982.

72. Widrick J, Ward A, Ebbeling C et al: Treadmill validation of an over-ground walking test to predict peak oxygen consumption, *Eur J Appl Physiol* 64:304-308, 1992.

73. Williams T, Krahenbuhl GS, Morgan DW: Daily variation in running economy of moderately trained male runners, *Med Sci Sports Exerc* 23(8):944-948, 1991.

74. Wilmore JH, Costill DL: Semiautomated systems approach to the assessment of oxygen uptake during exercise, *J Appl Physiol* 36:618-620, 1974.

75. Wilmore JH, Davis JA, Norton AC: An automated system for assesssing metabolic and respiratory function during exercise, *J Appl Physiol* 40:619-624, 1976.

RECOMMENDED READINGS

■ American College of Sports Medicine: *Guidelines for exercise testing and prescription,* ed 5, Philadelphia, 1995, Lea & Febiger.

■ Beaver WL, Wasserman K, Whipp BJ: Improved detection of the lactate threshold during exercise using a log-log transformation, *J Appl Physiol* 59:1936-1940, 1985.

■ Bergh U, Sjodin B, Forsberg A, Svedenhag J: The relationship between body mass and oxygen uptake during running in humans, *Med Sci Sports Exerc* 23(2):205-211, 1991.

■ Bouchard C, Dionne FT, Simoneau J-A, Boulay MR: Genetics of aerobic and anaerobic performances. In Holloszy J, editor: *Exerc Sports Sci Rev* 20:27-58, 1992.

■ Caiozzo VJ, Davis JA, Ellis JF et al: A comparison of gas exchange indices used to detect the anaerobic threshold, *J Appl Physiol* 53:1184-1189, 1982.

■ Coyle EF, Coggan AR, Hopper MK, Walters TJ: Determinants of endurance in well trained cyclists, *J Appl Physiol* 64:2622-2630, 1988.

■ Kline GM, Porcari JP, Hintermeister R et al: Estimation of VO_2max from a one-mile track walk, gender, age, and body weight, *Med Sci Sports Exerc* 19:253-259, 1987.

■ Noakes TD: Implications of exercise testing for prediction of athletic performance: a contemporary perspective, *Med Sci Sports Exerc* 20:319-330, 1988.

■ Londeree BR: The use of laboratory tests with long distance runners, *Sports Med* 3:201-213, 1986.

■ Robergs RA: Predictors of marathon running performance. In Wood S, Roach R, editors: *Sports and exercise medicine.* Vol 76. *Lung biology in health and disease,* New York, 1994, Marcel Dekker.

■ Sjodin B, Svedenhag J: Applied physiology of marathon running, *Sports Med* 2:83-99, 1985.

■ Storer TW, Davis JA, Caiozzo VJ: Accurate prediction of VO_2max in cycle ergometry, *Med Sci Sports Exerc* 22(5):704-712, 1990.

CHAPTER **20**

Measuring Pulmonary Function and Ventilatory Control

OBJECTIVES

After studying this chapter you should be able to:

- Demonstrate a basic understanding of pulmonary function testing.

- Explain the procedures involved in spirometry testing.

- Explain the information gained from pulmonary function testing.

- Describe the special procedures and equipment used to determine residual lung volume.

- Describe the procedures for interpreting the results of pulmonary function tests.

- Calculate lung volumes from a spirometry tracing.

- Explain the principles of tests for quantifying sensitivity to chemical stimulants that control ventilation.

KEY TERMS

spirometry

kymograph

pneumotachometer

oximetry

residual volume

helium dilution

nitrogen washout

hypoxic ventilatory response (HVR)

hypercapnia

The structure and function of the lung and respiratory system were discussed in detail in previous chapters. By now, you should have a basic understanding of (1) the structure and function of the lung and respiratory system; (2) the process of ventilation, gas diffusion, and pulmonary blood flow; (3) ventilation-perfusion relationships; (4) the mechanics and control of breathing; and (5) acute and chronic adaptations of the lung to exercise. Measurement of lung volumes and function is important not only to sports physiology, but also to the diagnosis and evaluation of lung disorders, such as chronic obstructive lung diseases and asthma. This chapter introduces the principles of selected tests and procedures that measure lung volumes and capacities and the sensitivity to chemical stimuli that control breathing.

Overview of Pulmonary Function Testing

Table 20.1 lists some of the pulmonary function tests and the parameters they measure. Pulmonary function testing can be performed in a variety of settings and for many different reasons. For example, tests are done in hospitals and physician's offices to evaluate lung damage from cigarette smoke or other pollutants or to evaluate the severity of asthma or the effects of medications. Tests done in exercise physiology laboratories may be a component of a total fitness and health series of tests, which are performed in part to evaluate the function of the lungs relative to possible lung damage (e.g., emphysema) or as a part of body composition assessment in the measurement of residual volume. Pulmonary function tests can also be performed on individuals to assess the body's sensitivity to chemical stimulants to ventilation (e.g., increased partial pressure of arterial carbon dioxide [$PaCO_2$] or decreased partial pressure of arterial oxygen [PaO_2]), which has furthered our understanding of how individuals adapt to high altitude (see Chapter 26). Finally, pulmonary function tests are an important tool for evaluating lung function and detecting mild pulmonary edema during acute and chronic exposure to high altitude.

TABLE 20.1	
Examples of specific pulmonary function tests and their purpose	

TESTS	PURPOSE
LUNG VOLUMES AND CAPACITIES	
Vital capacity	Functional lung volume
Residual volume	Body composition assessment; evaluation of lung damage
LUNG MECHANICS	
Lung and chest compliance	Evaluation of airway damage
Airway resistance	Evaluation of airway damage
LUNG DYNAMICS	
Flow rates	Evaluation of lung damage and respiratory muscle power
Airway closure	Evaluation of integrity of small airways
GAS EXCHANGE	
Ventilation-perfusion relationships	Assessment of regional distributions of ventilation and perfusion of the lungs; estimation of physiologic dead space
Gas diffusion	Assessment of edema and lung damage
Blood gas measurement	Evaluation of functional gas exchange
REGULATION OF VENTILATION	
Hypoxia	Assessment of sensitivity of ventilation to hypoxia
Hypercapnia	Assessment of sensitivity of ventilation to hypercapnia
EXERCISE TOLERANCE	
Graded exercise test	Assessment of functional capabilities of cardiopulmonary function; when combined with other tests, allows for differentiation of cardiovascular insufficiency from pulmonary insufficiency

Modified from Chusid EL: Pulmonary function testing: an overview. In Chusid EL, editor: *The selective and comprehensive testing of adult pulmonary function*, Mount Kisco, New York, 1983, Futura.

Pulmonary Function Testing: Equipment and Methods

The equipment used in pulmonary function testing has become quite sophisticated in the past century. The cost can range from less than $100 for portable instruments that measure flow rates to thousands of dollars for whole-body plethysmographs. This chapter describes several important instruments used to test athletes, as well as routine clinical testing of patients.

Volume-Displaced Spirometer

In the early 1800s John Hutchinson[11] discovered that he could measure lung volumes accurately by having a person breathe into a system that recorded volume displacements on paper. John Hutchinson's early experiments led to the development of the technique now known as **spirometry**. Even

today, the spirometer remains one of the basic tools for evaluating pulmonary function.

A spirometer (Figure 20.1) consists of (1) an upright metal cylinder that is open at the top; (2) a second cylinder, approximately $1/2$ inch smaller in diameter, that is closed at the top except for two holes (exit holes for the tubes that run from the inside of the spirometer to the outside); and (3) a plastic cylinder (often called a *bell*), which is open at the bottom. The two metal cylinders create a space filled with water, and the bell sits in the water between them. When the bell rests in the water, an airtight seal is formed between the bell and the water, and when air is forced into or out of the spirometer, the bell moves up or down.

When a person breathes into the spirometer (exhales), the bell moves up because air is forced into the closed system. The

TABLE 20.2			
Pulmonary lung volumes and capacities measured by spirometry and their changes during exercise			
VOLUME/CAPACITY	**ABBREVIATION**	**DESCRIPTION**	**CHANGE DURING EXERCISE**
Residual volume	RV	Volume of air remaining in the lungs after maximum exhalation; cannot be determined with spirometery	Slight increase
Expiratory reserve volume	ERV	Maximum volume of air exhaled from end-expiratory level	Slight decrease
Functional residual capacity	FRC	Sum of RV and ERV; cannot be determined with spirometry	Slight increase
Tidal volume	V_T	Volume of air inhaled and exhaled with each breath during quiet breathing	Increase
Inspiratory reserve volume	IRV	Maximum volume of air inhaled from end-inspiratory level	Decrease
Inspiratory capacity	IC	Sum of IRV and V_T	Increase
Vital capacity	VC	Maximum volume of air exhaled from the point of maximum inspiration	Slight decrease
Total lung capacity	TLC	Sum of all volume compartments of the lung	Slight decrease
Forced vital capacity	FVC	Forced vital capacity performed with maximally forced expiratory effort	Decrease
Forced expiratory volume in 1 sec	FEV_1	Volume of air expired in 1 sec	
Maximum voluntary ventilation	MVV	Volume of air expired in a specified period during repetitive maximum respiratory effort	Slight decrease

air exhaled into the system is mixed throughout by a fan, and carbon dioxide (CO_2) is absorbed by soda lime contained in a canister inside the bell. When the person inhales, air is removed from the closed system, creating a vacuum-like effect because of the airtight seal, and the bell moves down. The oxygen removed from the air in the system by the body is replaced by an inflow of pure oxygen at a rate that equals oxygen consumption (VO_2). Thus spirometry is also a means to measure VO_2. However, because carbon dioxide is removed and not measured, carbon dioxide production (VCO_2) is not known, and therefore the respiratory exchange ratio (RER) and an accurate estimate of energy expenditure cannot be calculated.

The movement of the bell up and down represents the volume of air entering and exiting the lungs. When the bell is connected to a pen, its movements can be recorded on a rotating drum, called a **kymograph.** Once the volume conversion of the bell is known (ml/mm), volume can be calculated (ambient temperature and pressure, saturated [ATPS]). Various lung volumes and capacities at rest are illustrated in Figure 20.2; Table 20.2 shows which lung volumes change during exercise.

Bellows-Type Spirometer

Another type of volume displacement spirometer is the bellows spirometer, often called a *spirograph* or *vitalograph*. This device consists of a collapsible bellows that folds and unfolds in response to inhalation and exhalation. When a person exhales into the spirometer, the bellows expands and the volume of air is recorded on paper. The displacement of the bellows by a volume of air is transferred to either a mechanical or an electrical recording on a computer (Figure 20.3). Typically an individual exhales as hard and as fast as possible into a vitalograph, and vital capacity and expired flow rates can be computed from the calibrated paper used on the instrument.

spirometry (spi-rom'e-tri)
the measurement of lung volumes and functional capacities with a spirometer

kymograph (ki'mo-graf)
the rotating drum component of an instrument, such as a spirometer, that records wavelike modulations (e.g., ventilation)

FIGURE 20.1

A, A Collins spirometer used for quantifying lung volumes and capacities. (Courtesy, Warren E. Collins, Braintree, Massachusetts) **B,** Air is directed into and from the spirometer by pipes and low resistance tubing that connect the system to the outside air or the subject. Vertical displacement of the floating bell during inspiration and expiration is marked on paper on the kymograph (rotating bell). Each millimeter rise or fall of the bell represents a given volume of gas, which depends on the volume conversion factor for the bell expressed in ATPS conditions.

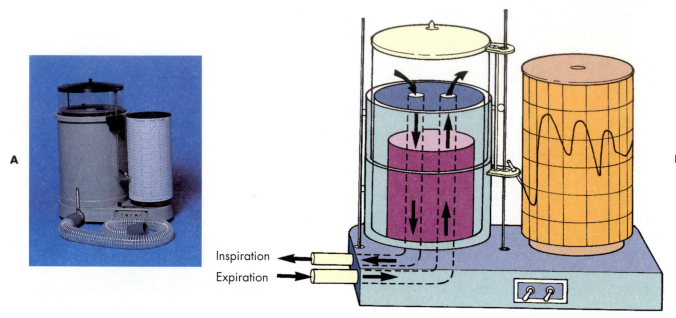

FIGURE 20.2

A standard trace from a spirometer showing lung volumes. A standard spirometer can also be used to measure lung capacities and flow rates by increasing the speed of the paper and recording forced maximal inspiratory and expiratory efforts.

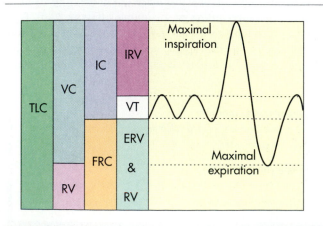

FIGURE 20.3

A bellows-type spirometer. The version illustrated has a bellow that expands during expiration and can be used to measure vital capacity.

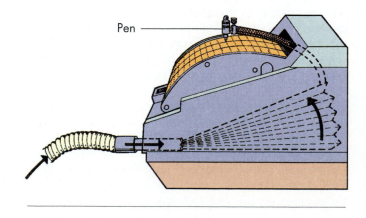

FIGURE 20.4

Advances in electronics have developed the pneumotach, which measures flow rates by sensing pressure differences between air before and after crossing a resistance membrane. Devices like the pneumotach can record air flow changes during inspiration and expiration. Computer processing of the signal can convert flow rates into ventilation volumes per unit time. (Courtesy, Warren E. Collins, Braintree, Massachusetts)

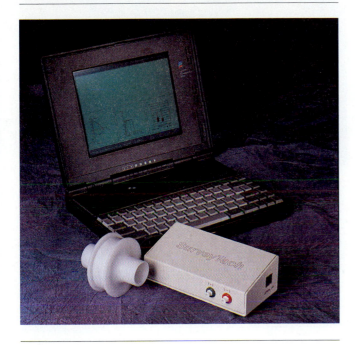

Flow-Sensing Spirometers

A more sophisticated type of spirometer calculates lung volumes by directly measuring the flow of air (Figure 20.4). A **pneumotachometer** measures the rate of airflow during inhalation and exhalation. Airflow during exhalation is based on the difference between the pressure of air entering the pneumotachometer against resistance (usually a small mesh screen) (P_1) and the pressure of air on the other side of the resistance (P_2). The greater the airflow into the pneumotachometer, the greater the resistance and the greater the pressure difference; therefore, the greater the volume of air moving through the instrument.

The pressure difference ($P_1 - P_2$) is measured continuously by a special pressure-sensing transducer, which transmits a signal to a computer, which in turn integrates the signal and transforms flow rates into volumes per unit time. Volumes can be calculated from the flow measurements because

$$\text{Volume (ml)} = \text{Flow (ml/sec)} \times \text{Time (sec)}$$

Pneumotachometers are being used more and more for cardiopulmonary testing because of their small size, high sensitivity, and accuracy.

Breathing Valves

Two types of breathing valves are commonly used in pulmonary function testing: free-breathing valves and multiple one-way directional valves (Figure 20.5). A free-breathing valve is commonly seen on a volume displacement spirometer because it allows the subject to be switched from breathing room air (open circuit) to breathing gas contained in the spirometer (closed circuit). The directional valve apparatus most often used in exercise testing is the Daniels valve. This device actually consists of two one-way valves, which direct inspired air into the mouth and expired air into a sampling hose.

The drawback to a valve apparatus that is placed in the mouth is the stimulus this gives to increase ventilation. Thus, when a mouthpiece valve is used to test ventilation, the subject must be given a familiarization period (usually 2 or 3 minutes of quiet breathing through the mouthpiece) before data collection begins. To avoid this hyperventilation, face masks are also available with multiple one-way valves to direct inspired and expired air.

Pulse Oximetry

Oximetry is a method of indirectly determining the percentage of hemoglobin (Hgb) that is combined with oxygen. Oximetry is a noninvasive technique often used in hospitals and exercise testing to assess blood oxygenation. One of the newer devices used during exercise testing is the pulse oximeter.[9] Pulse oximeters measure the change in transmission of infrared light through a finger or the earlobe to calculate arterial saturation. This principle is based on the color change that occurs in oxyhemoglobin at different oxygen saturations. The pulse oximeter has proved fairly accurate in exercise testing.[9,22] A drop in arterial oxygenation under normal barometric pressure indicates respiratory failure; as discussed in Chapter 12. When used during exercise, the pulse oximeter can detect inadequate pulmonary function indicated by exercise-induced hypoxemia.

Gas Analyzers

Chapter 6 discussed the need and use for oxygen and carbon dioxide analyzers during exercise. However, it must be emphasized that expired gas concentrations are important values in pulmonary function. The concentrations of oxygen and carbon dioxide in expired air vary, depending on the phase of tidal volume. At end-tidal volume, air represents alveolar air and therefore is very similar to true alveolar fractions of oxygen and carbon dioxide. Of course, rapid-

pneumotachometer (nu′mo-ta-kom′e-ter)
an instrument for measuring instantaneous flow during ventilation

oximetry (ok′sim′e-tri)
indirect measurement of the oxygen saturation of hemoglobin in the blood

FIGURE 20.5

A typical Daniel's valve, with two one-way valves that direct inspired air into the mouth via one valve and expired air away from the subject via a second valve. Typically, expired air is collected and analyzed for expired gas fractions and volume. (Equipment courtesy Warren E. Collins, Braintree, Massachusetts.)

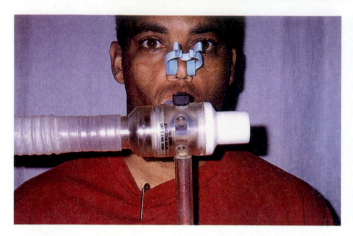
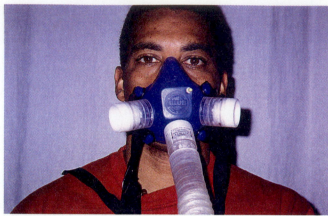

response analyzers are needed, and models are available that are based on standard electronic principles. Gas mass spectrometers have a response time measured in milliseconds, and these instruments are being used to evaluate both pulmonary function and exercise cardiorespiratory effects.

Pretest Scheduling Instructions

A few important conditions must be met to obtain valid results from pulmonary function tests. Research has shown that previous submaximal and maximal exercise reduces vital capacity and forced expiratory volume in 1 sec (FEV_1) within 30 minutes of recovery[16,21] and increases residual volume.[3,8] Therefore it has been recommended that the subject forgo exercise for up to 12 hours before pulmonary function testing.[7] A medical history should also be taken before each test to determine if the individual has an upper respiratory tract infection, asthma, or allergies. Finally, although no difference in lung volumes and functional capacities has been detected between the standing and seated positions, the posture used during testing should be recorded and used consistently.

Table 20.3 lists the normal values for lung volumes and gives equations suitable for estimating dynamic lung capacities. These values and equations should be used to compare measured results and thus detect abnormalities.

Minute Ventilation

The amount of air inspired and expired in 1 minute is referred to as *minute ventilation* (V_E). Minute ventilation is found by multiplying the rate of breathing, or breaths/min (f), by the tidal volume (V_T). At rest, a normal breathing rate is 12 breaths/min and a normal tidal volume is approximately 0.5 L/breath. Therefore:

20-1
$$V_E = f \times V_T$$
$$V_E = 12 \times 0.5$$
$$V_E = 6 \text{ L/min}$$

During exercise, V_E increases because the rate of breathing (f) and tidal volume (V_T) increase (Table 20.4). In endurance athletes, who are well conditioned, V_E during strenuous exercise can increase 27 times the resting value.[36]

Alveolar Ventilation

It is important to remember that not all inspired air reaches the alveoli (the site of gas exchange). *Alveolar ventilation* (V_A) is the portion of inspired air that reaches the alveoli and thus participates in gas exchange. The portion of inspired air that remains in the upper respiratory tract, and thus does not participate in gas exchange, is known as *anatomic dead space* (DS). Dead space averages about 30% of resting tidal volume. Alveolar ventilation can be estimated from spirometry by multiplying the difference of tidal volume (V_T) minus dead space (DS) by the rate of breathing (f). If normal resting values are used for V_T (0.5 L/breath), DS (30% of V_T, or 0.15 L/breath), and f(12 breaths/min), the equation becomes:

$$V_A = (V_T - DS) \times f$$
$$V_A = (0.5 - 0.15) \times 12$$
$$V_A = 4.2 \text{ L/min}$$

Changes in breathing patterns can affect alveolar ventilation, and thus the amount of air available for gas exchange (Table 20.5). An increase in breathing frequency (rapid, shallow breathing) causes a decrease in V_T and V_A. Slow, deep breathing causes an increase in V_T and V_A. During exercise, V_A is maintained by increases in both tidal volume and

TABLE 20.3

Lung volumes of healthy men and women and equations for predicting pulmonary capacities

VALUE	MEN	WOMEN
LUNG VOLUMES (ml, BTPS)		
V_T	400-500	350-450
IRV	3100	1900
ERV	1200	900
RV	1200	1000
TLC	6000	4200
PULMONARY CAPACITIES		
	< 25 yrs	20 yrs
FVC	$(0.05 \times H) + (0.078 \times A) - 5.508$	$(0.033 \times H) + (0.092 \times A) - 3.469$
FEV_1	$(0.046 \times H) + (0.045 \times A) - 4.808$	$(0.027 \times H) - (0.085 \times A) - 2.703$
$FEV_1\%$	$103.64 - (0.087 \times H) - (0.14 \times A)$	$107.38 - (0.111 \times H) - (0.109 \times A)$
	> 20 yrs	> 25 yrs
FVC	$(0.065 \times H) + (0.029 \times A) - 5.459$	$(0.037 \times H) + (0.022 \times A) - 1.774$
FEV_1	$(0.052 \times H) + (0.027 \times A) - 4.203$	$(0.027 \times H) - (0.021 \times A) - 0.794$
$FEV_1\%$	$103.64 - (0.087 \times H) - (0.14 \times A)$	$107.38 - (0.111 \times H) - (0.109 \times A)$
MVV	$(1.15 \times H) - (1.27 \times A) + 14$	$(0.55 \times H) - (0.72 \times A) + 50$

Data modified from 6, 12, and 29.

* *BTPS*, At body temperature and ambient pressure, and saturated with water vapor;

† *A*, Age; *H*, height (cm);

‡ $FEV_1\%$, Percentage of forced expiratory volume in 1 second.

TABLE 20.4

Pulmonary ventilation at rest and during exercise*

	V_E (L/MIN)	=	F (BREATHS/MIN)	×	V_T (L/BREATH)
Rest	6		12		0.5
Mild exercise	72		32		2.25
Maximal exercise	160		48		3.33

* Volumes in BTPS conditions.

breathing frequency. At the start of exercise, V_A is maintained more by an increase in V_T, with only a slight increase in breathing frequency. During intense exercise, V_T plateaus, and further increases in ventilation are the result of increased breathing frequency. Anatomic dead space also increases slightly during exercise.

Residual Volume

Residual volume (RV) is the volume of air remaining in the lungs after a maximal exhalation. Residual volume rep-

residual volume
the volume remaining in the lungs after a forced maximal exhalation

	V_T	F	V_E	V_A
TABLE 20.5				
Effect of breathing pattern changes on alveolar ventilation*				
TYPE OF BREATHING	(L/MIN)	(BREATHS/MIN)	(L/MIN)	(L/MIN)
Shallow, rapid	0.25	25	6	2.5
Normal resting	0.5	12	6	4.2
Slow, deep	1.25	6	6	6.6

* Ventilatory volumes in BTPS, assuming a constant DS (0.15 L).

resents the difference between total lung capacity (TLC) and vital capacity (VC). RV, a subdivision of functional residual capacity (FRC), is needed to accurately calculate body density as measured by hydrostatic weighing. In addition, in individuals with chronic obstructive lung disease, RV is increased because of premature airway closure.

A variety of methods can be used to measure RV indirectly. Most researchers use either the closed-circuit *helium dilution* method or the open-circuit *nitrogen washout* technique.

Closed-circuit multiple-breath helium dilution

Residual volume can be measured by two different **helium dilution** techniques, the single-breath and the multiple-breath equilibration methods. The multiple-breath equilibration method is explained here because the single-breath method, as with techniques such as nitrogen washout, requires rapid-response oxygen and carbon dioxide analyzers, which most laboratories do not have. Also, the single-breath helium method and the multiple-breath nitrogen washout method have a greater potential for measurement error and are known to be less accurate.[34] With the closed-circuit helium dilution procedure[15,20] (Figure 20.6), the subject breathes normally into a spirometer containing a known volume and concentration of helium. Oxygen is added to replace what is consumed metabolically, and carbon dioxide is absorbed chemically inside the spirometer. The individual is connected to the closed system at the end of a tidal volume end-expiration (at FRC), and oxygen inflow is matched to VO_2 as soon as possible. Breathing in the closed system continues for approximately 2 to 5 minutes until the helium equilibrates in concentration to the increased volume of the system (spirometer + subject's FRC). Because total volume increases after the subject is connected to the system, the helium concentration decreases, and the magnitude of the drop in helium is related to the subject's lung volume at FRC.

Calculating RV is relatively simple. The initial volume of the system is calculated by adding helium to the spirometer to obtain an initial helium concentration (C_1). V_1 is calculated by adding a known volume of air to the system and solving for V_2, as shown in equation 20.3.

20-3
$$V_2 \times C_2 = V_1 \times C_1$$
20-4
$$(V_1 + V_{air\ added}) \times C_2 = V_1 \times C_1$$

if $V_{air\ added}$ = 4 L; C_1 = 0.065; and C_2 = 0.035, then

$$(V_1 + 4) \times 0.035 = V_1 \times 0.065$$
$$0.035V_1 + 0.14 = 0.065V_1$$
$$0.14 = 0.065V_1 - 0.035V_1$$
$$0.14 = 0.03V_1$$
$$4.67\ L = V_1$$

therefore

$$V_2 = 4.67 + 4$$
$$V_2 = 8.67\ L$$

Once V_2 is known, the subject is connected to the system at FRC, thereby adding an FRC volume to V_2 and lowering the helium concentration to C_3; ERV is then measured by having the subject perform a maximal exhalation to RV. ERV can be calculated from the distance from end-expiration to the nadir of the maximal expiratory effort. FRC can then be calculated as for V_1 and V_2 above.

20-5
$$V_3 \times C_3 = V_2 \times C_2$$
$$(V_2 + FRC) \times C_3 = V_2 \times C_2$$

If FRC reduced C2 from 0.035 to 0.026, then

$$(8.67 + FRC) \times 0.026 = 8.67 \times 0.035$$
$$8.67 + FRC = 0.30345 \div 0.026$$
$$FRC = 11.6711 - 8.67$$
$$FRC = 3\ L$$

since

20-6
$$FRC = ERV + RV$$
$$RV = FRC - ERV$$

If ERV = 1 L, then

$$RV = 3 - 1$$
$$RV = 2\ L$$

These calculations can be done after data are collected by developing a computer program that contains all of the above mathematical equations. Some researchers adjust V_2 and C_2 to account for the small volume of helium that diffuses from the lungs into the blood. This is estimated as 0.1 L but varies with the subject's size, the helium concentrations used during rebreathing in the closed system, and the duration of the test. These additional unknowns make use of a correction factor questionable. Given the potential for helium loss from the system, the test should be done as

A common method for measurement of residual volume is by the multiple breath helium dilution procedure. Essentially, once a given amount of helium is known to exist in a system, addition of the subject while quietly breathing and at end-tidal expiratory volume increases the volume by an amount equal to the subjects FRC. Measuring the ERV from spirometry enables the calculation of RV (see text). (Adapted from West JB: *Respiratory physiology*, 3 ed, Philadelphia, 1985, Williams & Wilkins.)

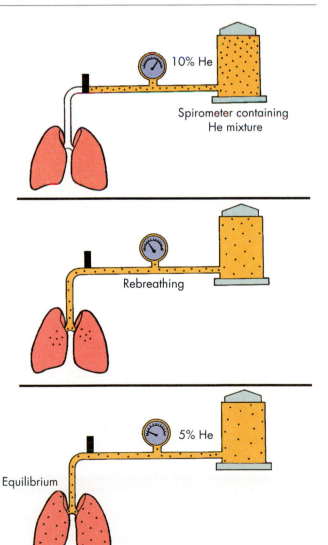

10% He

Spirometer containing
He mixture

Rebreathing

5% He

Equilibrium

quickly as possible. Assuming the subject has a consistent breathing pattern, skilled technicians can complete the rebreathing portion of the test in approximately 3 minutes.

Given that the standard error of measurement for this test is approximately 100 ml, the procedure should be repeated until two residual volumes are calculated that differ by no more than 100 ml. These values are averaged to provide the measure of RV.

Open-circuit nitrogen washout method

The open-circuit technique sometimes is called the "washout" method, because subjects breathe 100% oxygen for several minutes, which washes the nitrogen out of the lungs.[10] The **nitrogen washout** method is based on the fact that at the start of the test, the unknown FRC contains 80% nitrogen (N_2) and the unknown concentration of oxygen (O_2) (16% to 21%) and carbon dioxide (CO_2) (0.4% to 5%). By measuring the volume of N_2 in the FRC and applying a concentration dilution formula, the FRC volume can be determined.

Estimating residual lung volume

The equipment needed for open- and closed-system helium dilution tests is expensive and usually not available to most undergraduate or graduate students. When the equipment is not available to directly measure FRC, RV (in liters) can be estimated using the following equations:

Men: $RV = (A \times 0.0115) + (H \times 0.019) - 2.24$
Women: $RV = (A \times 0.03) + (H \times 0.0387) - (BSA \times 0.73) - 4.78$

where A is age (years), H is height (cm), and BSA is body surface area (mm^2). From respectively Boren et al[2] and O'Brien.[16]

Assessing the Chemosensitivity of Ventilation Control

The chemosensitivity of ventilation control is tested to evaluate the influence of central and peripheral chemoreceptor stimulation on increases in ventilation. As discussed in Chapter 12, the peripheral chemoreceptors consist of the carotid and aortic bodies, whereas the central chemoreceptors are found in the medullary region of the lower brain.

helium dilution

a method of measuring the functional residual capacity of the lung based on dilution of a known amount of helium

nitrogen washout

a method of measuring functional residual capacity based on dilution of the nitrogen fraction of air in the lung with pure oxygen

The peripheral chemoreceptors are sensitive to changes in arterial blood pH, Pa_{CO_2}, and Pa_{O_2}. Conversely, the central chemoreceptors are sensitive to cerebrospinal fluid (CSF) pH, which decreases with an increase in Pa_{CO_2}. The independent effects of hypoxia versus hypercapnia, and the roles of the peripheral versus central chemoreceptors, can be elucidated by independently altering the inspired partial pressures of oxygen and carbon dioxide.

To test the influence of hypoxia on increased ventilation, called the **hypoxic ventilatory response** (HVR), the subject rebreathes a hyperoxic gas mixture, causing the oxygen partial pressure of the air to gradually decrease and the nitrogen partial pressure to increase; as a result of the removal of carbon dioxide by an absorbent, the end-tidal partial pressure of carbon dioxide (PET_{CO_2}) is left to fall because of the hyperventilation (*poikilocapnic* HVR). Arterial hemoglobin saturation can be indirectly measured by an oximeter. The test can be modified by adding carbon dioxide to the inspired air at the mouthpiece to maintain a normal PET_{CO_2} (*isocapnic* HVR). Because the carotid bodies are sensitive to decreases in Pa_{O_2}; the tests of HVR essentially evaluate the carotid bodies' sensitivity to hypoxia.[24] Hyperventilation is greater during the isocapnic HVR test than during the poikilocapnic test because the alveolar partial pressure of carbon dioxide ($P_{A}CO_2$) and therefore Pa_{CO_2}, is maintained. Allowing $P_{A}CO_2$ and Pa_{CO_2} to decline removes the basal stimulus for ventilation by the aortic bodies and central chemoreceptors, which depresses the stimulation of ventilation, even during hypoxia. The poikilocapnic test best reflects exposure to hypobaric hypoxia (see Chapter 26).

Hypoxic ventilatory response is quantified by graphing ventilation against oxyhemoglobin saturation. The slope of a linear regression fit of the data represents the HVR and by convention is expressed as a positive value[13,24,27] (Figure 20.7).

Ventilatory response and chemosensitivity to carbon dioxide are assessed through the hypercapnic ventilatory response (HCVR) test. In this test, subjects rebreathe a volume of pure oxygen or a mix of oxygen (40%) and carbon dioxide (7%) in nitrogen.[27] The carbon dioxide content of the gas and $P_{ET}CO_2$ are continually measured by rapid-response analyzers. The slope of the relationship between ventilation and $P_{ET}CO_2$ quantifies HCVR. As with HVR, a positive slope is reported. As would be expected, HCVR is much greater than HVR, with values approximating 0.1 to 0.5 L/% for HVR and 3 to 11 L/mm Hg for HCVR.[27]

People differ in their ventilatory response to chemical stimuli such as decreases in Pa_{O_2} (hypoxia) or increases in P_{CO_2} **(hypercapnia)**.[24] For example, women differ in their ventilatory response to hypoxia depending on whether they

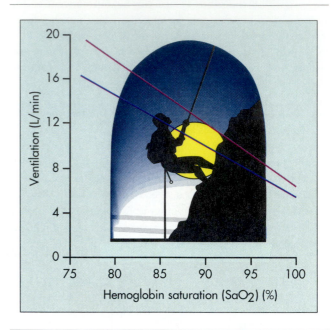

The hypoxic ventilatory response of two subjects. The more steep the slope, the greater the sensitivity of ventilation to hypoxia.

are in the luteal phase or the follicular phase of the menstrual cycle.[1,23,37] The relative increase in progesterone concentrations during the luteal phase acts as an added stimulant to ventilation and increases the ventilatory response.[23] Regardless of the phase of the menstrual cycle, women have a higher ventilatory response to hypoxia than men.[1] Acute and chronic exposure to hypobaric hypoxia increased HVR and HCVR.[22] Endurance-trained individuals tend to have a lower HVR.[4,15,20]

---

hypoxic ventilatory response (HVR)

the increase in ventilation for given changes in oxyhemoglobin saturation. HVR is expressed as the slope of this linear relationship and by convention is reported as a positive value

hypercapnia

increased arterial partial pressure of carbon dioxide (Pa_{CO_2}) above normal (40 mm Hg)

SUMMARY

- Pulmonary function tests can measure lung volumes and capacities, lung mechanics, ventilatory flow rates, adequacy of gas exchange, and chemosensitivity.

- Lung volumes are measured by having subjects breathe into a closed system, which records volume displacements on paper. This technique, called **spirometry,** dates back to the 19th century. Spirometry is still used today, aided by computer technology, to measure lung volumes.

- There are two types of spirometers: a bell vertical displacement system and a bellows-type system. With bell spirometry, movement of the bell up and down represents the volume of air entering and exiting the lungs; these movements are recorded on a rotating drum, called a **kymograph.** The bellows-type spirometer, often called a *spirograph* or *vitalograph,* can be used to measure vital capacity and expired flow rates.

- A **pneumotachometer** is a more sophisticated type of spirometer that calculates air volumes by measuring the rate of airflow. Two types of breathing valves are commonly used in pulmonary function testing: free-breathing and multiple one-way directional valves. To avoid hyperventilation from a mouthpiece, face masks are also available that have multiple one-way valves to direct inspired and expired air.

- **Oximetry** is the indirect determination of the percentage of oxygen saturation of hemoglobin. Pulse oximeters measure the change in transmission of infrared light through a finger or the earlobe to calculate arterial saturation. This technique is based on the color change in oxyhemoglobin at different oxygen saturations.

- Previous submaximal and maximal exercise reduces vital capacity and FEV_1 within 30 minutes of recovery and increases residual volume. It has been recommended that exercise not be performed for up to 12 hours before pulmonary function testing.

- The amount of air inspired and expired in 1 minute is referred to as *minute ventilation* (V_E). At rest, the normal minute ventilation equals approximately 6 L of air. During exercise, V_E increases as a result of a combination of an increase in breathing frequency (f) and tidal volume (V_T). *Alveolar ventilation* (V_A) is the portion of inspired air that reaches the alveoli and thus participates in gas exchange. A portion of inspired air remains in the upper respiratory tract and thus does not participate in gas exchange; this is referred to as *anatomic dead space* (DS). Dead space averages approximately 30% (150 ml) of resting tidal volume. Alveolar ventilation depends on the depth of respiration (V_T) minus dead space (DS) times the rate of breathing (f).

- **Residual volume** (RV) is the volume of air remaining in the lungs after maximal exhalation. Residual volume represents the difference between total lung capacity (TLC) and vital capacity (VC) and is a subdivision of functional residual capacity (FRC). FRC cannot be determined by spirometry and must be measured by other methods. Most researchers measure FRC by either closed-circuit **helium dilution** or open-circuit **nitrogen washout.**

- When equipment is not available to directly measure FRC, RV (in liters) can be estimated by using the equations of Boren et al.[2] and O'Brien et al.[21]

- The influence of hypoxia on increased ventilation, called **hypoxic ventilatory response** (HVR), can be tested by allowing the end tidal partial pressure of carbon dioxide ($P_{ET}CO_2$) to fall because of hyperventilation (*poikilocapnic* HVR), or when a normal $P_{ET}CO_2$ (*isocapnic* HVR) is maintained. Graphing ventilation against oxyhemoglobin saturation quantifies HVR. The slope of a linear regression fit of the data represents HVR and by convention is expressed as a positive value. The ventilatory response and chemosensitivity to increased partial pressure of carbon dioxide **(hypercapnia)** are assessed in the hypercapnic ventilatory response (HCVR). The slope of the relationship between ventilation and $P_{ET}CO_2$ quantifies HCVR. As with HVR, a positive slope is reported.

REVIEW QUESTIONS

1. From a spirogram tracing, calculate IRV, V_T, VC, ERV, and TLC.

2. If the FVC of a subject is 5.2 L (ATPS), the room and water temperature is 22.5°C, and P_B is 720 mm Hg, convert FVC (ATPS) to a BTPS volume. (see Appendix B).

3. Determine the FRC using values obtained from the closed–circuit multiple-breath equilibration helium dilution method.

   The test subject is a man who weighs 90 kg and is 185 cm tall. He complains of shortness of breath when exercising. He has smoked for 12 years and continues to smoke.

   A.
   $$V_2 \times C_2 = V_1 \times C_1$$
   $$(V_1 + V_{air\ added}) \times C_2 = V_1 \times C_1$$

   If $V_{air\ added}$ = 4.5 L; C_1 = 0.075; and C_2 = 0.041, then

   $$(V_1 + V_{air\ added}) \times 0.041 = V_1 \times 0.075$$

   Solve for V_1 and V_2 (volume of system before subject is connected).

   B.
   $$V_3 \times C_3 = V_2 \times C_2$$
   $$(V_2 + FRC) \times C_3 = V_2 \times C_2$$

   If FRC reduced C_2 from 0.041 to 0.029, then

   $$(V_2 + FRC) \times 0.029 = V_2 \times 0.041$$

   since

   $$FRC = ERV + RV$$
   $$RV = FRC - ERV$$

   If ERV = 1.2 L, solve for RV.

4. From the answer obtained in question 3, how does the calculated RV compare with the estimated RV? What might the RV and symptoms reveal about the condition of this person's lungs?

5. Why are lung volumes reported in BTPS conditions?

6. What are typical resting values for normal, healthy subject for
   (1) lung volumes (BTPS): IC, ERV, VC, RV, FRC, TLC;
   (2) ventilation (BTPS): V_T, f, V_E; and pulmonary dynamics: FVC, FEV_1, MVV

7. Compared with rest, which increases more during maximal exercise, minute ventilation (V_E) or alveolar ventilation (V_A)? Assume normal resting data, an exercise tidal volume (V_T) of 2.8 L, a maximal breathing frequency of 52 breaths/min, and an anatomic dead space of 150 ml. Explain why there is a difference.

APPLICATIONS

1. Why would lung damage (e.g., emphysema) increase residual volume?

2. Refer to Chapter 12. Individuals who suffer from exercise-induced bronchospasm have a reduced FEV_1 during recovery from exercise. Explain how FEV_1 is measured. What other pulmonary function tests would detect increased airway resistance?

3. Chapter 26 discusses the effect on pulmonary function of long-term, high-altitude exposure and the development of pulmonary edema. How would pulmonary edema alter vital capacity and FEV_1, and why?

4. Tests that measure lung compliance and elasticity were not covered in this chapter. Nevertheless, how would conditions of lung damage (e.g., emphysema) affect lung compliance, and what would be the functional consequences of this condition?

REFERENCES

1. Aitken ML, Franklin JL, Pierson DJ, Shoene RB: Influence of body size and gender on control of ventilation, *J Appl Physiol* 60(6):1894–1899, 1986.

2. Boren HG, Kory RC, Synder JC: The Veteran's Administration Army Cooperative Study of Pulmonary Function. II. The lung volume and its subdivisions in normal men, *Am J Med* 41:96–114, 1966.

3. Buono MJ, Constable SH, Morton AR et al: The effect of an acute bout of exercise on selected pulmonary function measurements, *Med Sci Sports Exerc* 13(5):290–293, 1981.

4. Byrne-Quinn E, Weil JV, Sodal IE et al: Ventilatory control in the athlete, *J Appl Physiol* 36(1):91–98, 1971.

5. Chusid EL: Pulmonary function testing: an overview. In Chusid EL, editor: *The selective and comprehensive testing of adult pulmonary function,* Mount Kisco, New York, 1983, Futura.

6. Comroe JH, Foster RE, Dubois AB et al: *The lung,* Chicago, 1962, Year Book.

7. Cordain L, Tucker A, Moon D, Stager JM: Lung volumes and maximal respiratory pressures in collegiate swimmers and runners, *Res Q Exerc Sport* 61(1):70–74, 1990.

8. Girandola R, Wiswell R, Mohler J et al: Effects of water immersion on lung volumes: implications for body compositional analysis, *J Appl Physiol* 43:276–279, 1977.

9. Hansen JE, Casaburi R: Validity of ear oximetry in clinical exercise testing, *Chest* 91:333–337, 1987.

10. Hickman JB, Blair E, Frayser R: An open-circuit helium method for measuring functional residual capacity and defective intrapulmonary gas mixing, *J Clin Invest* 33:1277-1282, 1954.

11. Hutchinson J: Lecture on vital statistics, embracing an account of a new instrument for detecting the presence of disease in the system, *Lancet* 1:567–594, 1844.

12. Knudsen RJ, Slatin RC, Lebowitz MD, Burrows B: The maximal expiratory flow-volume curve: normal standards, variability, and effects of age, *Am Rev Respir Dis* 113:587–600, 1976.

13. Levine BD, Friedman DB, Engfred K et al: The effect of normoxic or hypobaric hypoxic endurance training on the hypoxic ventilatory response, *Med Sci Sports Med* 24(7):769–775, 1992.

14. Lourenco RV: Clinical methods for the study of regulation of ventilation, *Chest* 70(suppl):109-195, 1976.

15. Mahler DA: Exercise-induced asthma, *Med Sci Sports Exerc* 25(5)554–561, 1993.

16. Maron M, Hamilton L, Maksud M: Alterations in pulmonary function consequent to competitive marathon running, *Med Sci Sports Exerc* 11(••):244-249, 1979.

17. Martin BJ, Sparks KE, Zwillich CW, Weil JV: Low exercise ventilation in endurance athletes, *Med Sci Sports Exerc* 11:181-185, 1979.

18. Martin BJ, Weil JV, Sparks KE et al: Exercise ventilation correlates positively with ventilatory chemoresponsiveness, *J Appl Physiol* 45:557-564, 1978.

19. Meneely GR, Ball COT, Kory RC: A simplified closed-circuit helium dilution method for the determination of the residual volume in the lungs, *Am J Med* 28:824-831, 1960.

20. Morris JF: Spirometry in the evaluation of pulmonary function, *West J Med* 125(2):110-118, 1976.

21. O'Brien RJ, Drizd TA: Roentgenographic determination of total lung capacity: normal values from a national population survey, *Am Rev Respir Dis* 128:949-952, 1983.

22. O'Krory JA, Loy RA, Coast JR: Pulmonary function changes following exercise, *Med Sci Sports Exerc* 24(12):1359-1364, 1992.

REFERENCES—Cont'd

23. Rebuk AS, Chapman KR, D'Urzo A: The accuracy and response characteristics of a simplified ear oximeter, *Chest* 83:860-864, 1983.

24. Regensteiner JG, McCullough RG, McCullough RE et al: Combined effects of female hormones and exercise on hypoxic ventilatory response, *Respir Physiol* 82:107-114, 1990.

25. Roach RC: Hypoxic ventilatory response and performance at high altitude. In Wood SC, Roach RC, editors: *Sports and exercise medicine.* Vol 76. *Lung biology in health and disease,* New York, 1994, Dekker.

26. Ruegg WR, Reynolds GP: A procedure for the measurement of lung volumes by helium dilution, *Analyzer* 10:18-22, 1980.

27. Ruppel G: *Manual of pulmonary function testing,* ed 6, St Louis, 1994, Mosby.

28. Schoene RB, Roach RC, Hackett PH et al: Operation Everest II: ventilatory adaptation during gradual decompression to extreme altitude, *Med Sci Sports Med* 22(6):804-810, 1990.

29. Taylor AE, Rehder K, Hyatt RE, Parker JC: *Clinical respiratory physiology,* Philadelphia, 1989, Saunders.

30. Wagner J: *Pulmonary function testing: a practical approach,* Philadelphia, 1992, Williams & Wilkins.

31. Wasserman K, Hansen JE, Sue DY, Whipp BJ: *Principles of exercise testing and interpretation,* Philadelphia, Lea & Febiger.

32. Weil JV, Zwillich CW: Assessment of ventilatory response to hypoxia: methods and interpretation, *Chest* 70:S124-S128, 1976.

33. Weil JV, Byrne-Quinn E, Sodal IE et al: Hypoxic ventilatory drive in normal man, *J Clin Invest* 49(6):1061-1072, 1970.

34. Welsh CH, Wagner PD, Reeves JT et al: Operation Everest II: Spirometric and radiographic changes in acclimatized humans at simulated high altitudes, *Am Rev Resp Dis* 147:1239-1244, 1993.

35. West JB: *Respiratory physiology: the essentials,* ed 3, Philadelphia, 1985, Williams & Wilkins.

36. Whipp BJ, Ward SA: Coupling of ventilation to pulmonary gas exchange during exercise. In Whipp BJ, Wasserman K, editors: *Exercise: pulmonary physiology and pathophysiology (lung biology in health and disease),* New York, 1991, Dekker.

37. White DP, Douglas NJ, Pickett CK et al: Sexual differences in the control of breathing, *J Appl Physiol* 54(4):874-879, 1983.

38. Wilmore JH: A simplified measurement for determination of residual lung volume, *J Appl Physiol* 27(1):96-100, 1969.

39. Wilmore JH, Vodak PA, Parr RB et al: Further simplification of a method for determination of residual lung volume, *Med Sci Sports Exerc* 12(30):216-218, 1980.

RECOMMENDED READINGS

▪ Bryne-Quinn E, Weil JV, Sodal IE et al: Ventilatory control in the athlete, *J Appl Physiol* 36(1):91-98, 1971.

▪ Martin BJ, Sparks KE, Zwillich CW, Weil JV: Low exercise ventilation in endurance athletes, *Med Sci Sports Exerc* 11:181-185, 1979.

▪ O'Krory JA, Loy RA, Coast JR: Pulmonary function changes following exercise, *Med Sci Sports Exerc* 24(12):1359-1364, 1992.

▪ Regensteiner JG, McCullough RG, McCullough RE et al: Combined effects of female hormones and exercise on hypoxic ventilatory response, *Respir Physiol* 82:107-114, 1990.

▪ Schoene RB, Roach RC, Hackett PH et al: Operation Everest II: ventilatory adaptation during gradual decompression to extreme altitude, *Med Sci Sports Med* 22(6):804-810, 1990.

▪ West JB: *Respiratory physiology: the essentials,* ed 3, Philadelphia, 1985, Williams & Wilkins.

▪ White DP, Douglas NJ, Pickett CK et al: Sexual differences in the control of breathing, *J Appl Physiol* 54(4):874-879, 1983.

▪ Wilmore JH, Vodak PA, Parr RB et al: Further simplification of a method for determination of residual lung volume, *Med Sci Sports Exerc* 12(30):216-218, 1980.

CHAPTER **21**

Estimating Body Composition

OBJECTIVES

After studying this chapter you should be able to:

■ Demonstrate a basic understanding of body composition, including the difference between overweight and overfat.

■ Describe the compartmentalization model of body composition.

■ Explain the purpose of body composition testing and how the data are applied.

■ Explain some of the procedures and equipment used to assess body composition.

KEY TERMS

body composition

overweight

overfat

essential fat

storage fat

fat-free body mass

lean body mass

body density

hydrodensitometry

bioelectrical impedance (BIA)

anthropometry

body mass index

The need to quantify the composition of the body has application to sports performance, to the assessment for risk of cardiovascular diseases and diabetes, and to body aesthetics. However, accurate assessment of body composition is difficult because of the varied composition of the body: water, protein, bone mineral, and fat. Most researchers' interest in the determination of body composition is in quantifying the fat mass, and this role of body composition is seen every day in advertisements in almost all forms of communications. Nevertheless, knowledge of the lean mass of the body has many applications in health and disease states, especially for those individuals who need to maintain or increase the nonfat components of the body. A variety of methods currently are used to assess body composition, varying from simple visual observation to techniques requiring sophisticated and expensive equipment. The purposes of this chapter are to identify and explain the different methods available to determine the composition of the body and to comment on the accuracy and recommended conditions for the use of each method.

Defining Body Composition Terminology

Body composition refers to the relative amounts of water, protein, mineral, and fat in the body; however, the majority of techniques for body composition assessment simply provide an estimate of lean (nonfat) and fat body masses. The details of the different methods and controversy over correct nomenclature are discussed later.

The assessment of body composition is generally performed to determine and monitor an individual's health and fitness status and to aid in planning training programs for athletes. It has been well established that a high percentage of body fat (low lean body weight) is associated with a higher risk of heart disease, diabetes, hypertension, cancer, hyperlipidemia, and a variety of other health problems.[46,69] On the other hand, a high percentage of lean body mass and low fat mass is associated with athletic prowess and good health.[71,72]

---

body composition
science of determining the absolute and relative contributions of specific components of the body

overweight (o'ver-wate)
a condition of excess weight based on a height-weight relationship or computed from body composition analysis

TABLE 21.1

1983 Metropolitan height and weight tables for men and women between the ages of 25 and 59.

HEIGHT		SMALL FRAME		MEDIUM FRAME		LARGE FRAME	
(ft:inch)	(cm)	(lb)	(kg)	(lb)	(kg)	(lb)	(kg)
MEN*							
5:2	157.5	128-134	57.6-60.3	131-141	59.0-63.5	138-150	62.1-67.5
5:3	160.0	130-136	58.5-61.2	133-143	59.9-64.4	140-153	63.0-68.9
5:4	162.6	132-138	59.4-62.1	135-145	60.8-65.3	142-156	63.9-70.2
5:5	165.1	134-140	60.3-63.0	137-148	61.7-66.6	144-160	64.8-72.0
5:6	167.6	136-142	61.2-63.9	139-151	62.6-68.0	146-164	65.7-73.8
5:7	170.2	138-145	62.1-65.3	142-154	63.9-69.3	149-168	67.1-75.6
5:8	172.7	140-148	63.0-66.6	145-157	65.3-70.7	152-172	68.4-77.4
5:9	175.3	142-151	63.9-68.0	148-160	66.6-72.0	155-176	69.8-79.2
5:10	177.8	144-154	64.8-69.3	151-163	68.0-73.4	158-180	71.1-81.0
5:11	180.3	146-157	65.7-70.7	154-166	69.3-74.7	161-184	72.5-82.8
6:0	182.9	149-160	67.1-72.0	157-170	70.7-76.5	164-188	73.8-84.6
6:1	185.4	152-164	68.4-73.8	160-174	72.0-78.3	168-192	75.6-86.4
6:2	188.0	155-168	69.8-75.6	164-178	73.8-80.1	172-197	77.4-88.7
6:3	190.5	158-172	75.6-77.4	167-182	75.2-81.9	176-202	79.2-90.9
6:4	193.0	162-176	72.9-79.2	171-187	77.0-84.2	182-207	81.9-93.2
WOMEN†							
4:10	147.3	102-111	45.9-50.0	109-121	49.1-54.5	118-131	53.1-59.0
4:11	149.9	103-113	46.4-50.9	111-123	50.0-55.4	120-134	54.0-60.3
5:0	152.4	104-115	46.8-51.8	113-126	50.9-56.7	122-137	54.9-61.7
5:1	154.9	106-118	47.7-53.1	115-129	51.8-58.1	125-140	56.3-63.0
5:2	157.5	108-121	48.6-54.5	118-132	53.1-59.4	128-143	57.6-64.4
5:3	160.0	111-124	50.0-55.8	121-135	54.5-60.8	131-147	59.0-66.2
5:4	162.6	114-127	51.3-57.2	124-138	55.8-62.1	134-151	60.3-68.0
5:5	165.1	117-130	52.7-58.5	127-141	57.2-63.5	137-155	61.7-69.8
5:6	167.6	120-133	54.0-59.9	130-144	58.5-64.8	140-159	63.0-71.6
5:7	170.2	123-136	55.4-61.2	133-147	59.9-66.2	143-163	64.4-73.4
5:8	172.7	126-139	56.7-62.6	136-150	61.2-67.5	146-167	65.7-75.2
5:9	175.3	129-142	58.1-63.9	139-153	62.6-68.9	149-170	67.1-76.5
5:10	177.8	132-145	59.4-65.3	142-156	63.9-70.2	152-173	68.4-77.9
5:11	180.3	135-148	60.8-66.6	145-159	65.3-71.6	155-176	69.8-79.2
6:0	182.9	138-151	62.1-68.0	148-162	66.6-72.9	158-179	71.1-80.6

Modified from Metropolitan Life Insurance Company: *1983 height and weight tables announced*, New York, 1983, Metropolitan Life Insurance Company.

* Indoor clothing weighing 2.3 kg.

† Indoor clothing weighing 1.4 kg.

TABLE 21.2					
Standard values for percent body fat					
			AGE (YRS)		
RATING	20-29	30-39	40-49	50-59	60+
MEN					
Excellent	<11	<12	<14	<15	<16
Good	11-13	12-14	14-16	15-17	16-18
Average	14-20	15-21	17-23	18-24	19-25
Fair	21-23	22-24	24-26	25-27	26-28
Poor	>23	>24	>26	>27	>28
WOMEN					
Excellent	<16	<17	<18	<19	<20
Good	16-19	17-20	18-21	19-22	20-23
Average	20-28	21-29	22-30	23-31	24-32
Fair	29-31	30-32	31-33	32-34	33-35
Poor	>31	>32	>33	>34	>35

Modified from Jackson AS, Pollack ML: *Br J Nutr* 40:497-504, 1978; Jackson AS, Pollack ML, Ward A: *Med Sci Sports Exerc* 12:175-812, 1980.

Overweight is defined as body weight in excess of a reference standard, generally the mean weight for a given height and skeletal frame size grouped by gender (Table 21.1). However, research has clearly shown the inadequacy of this approach in defining overweight since individuals with a large muscle mass and minimal fat can be classified as overweight, yet be less fat and more healthy than individuals with minimal muscle mass.[72] Consequently, height-weight tables should be avoided, and the concept of overweight should be replaced with the concept of being **overfat.**

Being overfat indicates an excess accumulation of body fat. Thus the prediction of body fat from body composition analysis is required before this term can be used.

Body composition is often expressed as the relative amounts of fat mass to fat-free mass (FFM). Fat mass (FM) includes both essential and storage fat. **Essential fat** is found in bone marrow, brain, spinal cord, muscles, and other internal organs and is essential to normal physiologic and biologic functioning. The level that essential fat should never go below is thought to be approximately 3% of the total body weight for men and 12% of total body weight for women. Women have a higher essential fat storage requirement because of gender-specific fat deposits in breast tissue and surrounding the uterus. When essential fat drops below these critical values, normal physiologic and biologic functioning may be impaired.

Storage fat is composed of two types of fat, yellow fat, which is approximately 99% of all storage fat, and brown fat, which is rich in mitochondria and can increase heat production by converting stored energy. Yellow fat is found in adipose tissue and serves three basic functions: (1) as an insulator to retain body heat, (2) as an energy substrate, and (3) as padding against trauma. The majority of adipose tissue is found directly beneath the skin. Subcutaneous fat distribution can vary between genders and with age.[43] Men tend to store more fat around the waist (android obesity), whereas women tend to store more fat around their hips and thighs (gynoid obesity). Older individuals tend to have less subcutaneous fat than younger individuals.

Fat-free body mass (FFBM), often referred to as *lean tissue* or *lean body mass* (LBM), includes muscle, bone, organs,

overfat (o′ver-fat)

a condition of excess body fat, as determined from body composition analysis

essential fat

fat and lipid component of the body that comprises, for example, cell membranes, bone marrow, and intramuscular fat

storage fat

fat and lipid stored in adipose tissue

fat free body mass

component of the body that is not storage and essential fat

lean body mass

component of the body that is not storage fat

TABLE 21.3

Body composition characteristics of athletes grouped by sports type

ATHLETIC/SPORT GROUP	GENDER	AGE	HEIGHT(cm)	WEIGHT(kg)	RELATIVE FAT (%)
Baseball	M	20.8	182.7	83.3	14.2
Basketball	M	26.8	193.6	91.2	9.7
	F	19.2	168.0	79.0	24.0
Gymnastics	M	20.3	178.5	69.2	4.6
	F	20.0	158.5	51.1	15.5
	F	19.4	163.0	57.9	23.8
Ice hockey	M	26.3	180.3	86.7	15.1
Horse jockeys	M	30.9	158.2	50.3	14.1
Swimming	M	21.8	182.3	79.1	8.5
	F	19.4	168.0	63.8	26.3
Track and field	M	21.3	180.6	71.6	3.7
Distance running	M	22-26	176.0	64.5	7.0
	M	40-59	180.7	71.6	11.2
	M	>60	175.5	67.0	13.0
	F	20.0	161.3	52.9	19.2
	F	32.4	169.4	57.2	15.2
Jumpers and hurdlers	F	20.3	165.9	59.0	20.7
Volleyball	F	19.4	266.0	59.8	25.3
Wrestling	M	15-18	172.3	66.3	6.9
	M	20-25	176.0	80.0	9.5
Weight lifting	M	24.9	166.4	59.8	25.3
Body builders	M	29.0	172.4	83.1	8.4

Modified from Wilmore JH, Bergfeld JA: A comparison of sports: physiological and medical aspects. In Strauss RJ, editor: *Sports medicine and physiology,* Philadelphia, 1979, Saunders.

from dual x-ray absorptiometry), protein (e.g., from body potassium), and fat. An ideal body composition technique would noninvasively measure all these components and therefore once again provide a reference value that is a true gold standard rather than a best prediction. These techniques are being developed at a fast rate, and once research has completed tests on different populations in multiple compartment models of body composition, prediction equations should improve. Understandably, the future of body composition research is exciting and is directed toward multiple-compartment validation of prediction equations from less expensive and more accessible methods.

Component System of Body Composition and Densitometry

The body can be divided into components that differ in composition. In the original body component system described by Benke (Figure 21.1), the body was divided into two simple components: lean and fat body mass.[3] Since then, **lean body mass** (LBM) has been identified as not being completely fat free because it contained lipid within, for example, muscle, cell membranes, and bone marrow. The term **fat-free body mass** (FFBM) therefore represents a large component of LBM.[10,63]

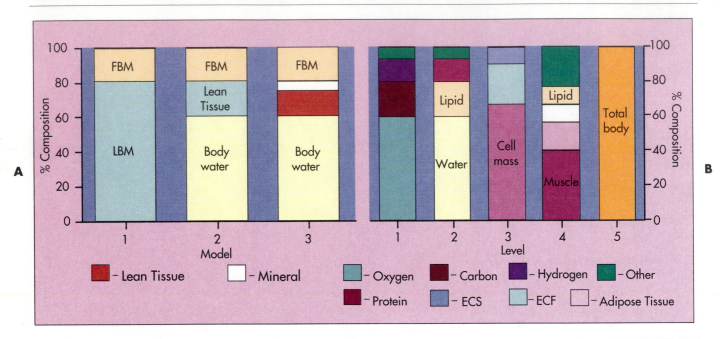

FIGURE 21.1

A, The compartmental models of body composition. The original two compartment model has been further subdivided based on chemical divisions of the body that are able to be quantified, either directly or indirectly. These multiple compartment models are used to modify the equation of Siri (see 46) to provide a more accurate conversion of body density to % body fat. **B,** The multi-compartment and multi-level model of body composition proposed by Wang et al. (Adapted from Lohman TG: *Advances in body composition assessment. Current issues in exercise science series—monograph number 3,* Champaign, Illinois, 1992, Human Kinetics; and Wang ZM et al: *Am J Clin Nutr* 56:19-28, 1992.)

Figure 21.1 also presents other component models of body composition. The body has been divided into chemical components, anatomic components, and tissue components that vary depending on the number of components that can be measured.[31,47,69] The concept of dividing the body into components suggests that if each of the components can be quantified and their respective density determined, their respective contribution to total body density from hydrodensitometry can be used to provide a specific equation for calculating percentage of body fat.

Two-Component Systems

Brozek, Siri, and Behnke developed the two-component system of body composition based on the following assumptions[3,10,63]:

1. The density of fat is 0.900 g/ml at 37° C.
2. The density of lean body mass is 1.100 g/ml at 37° C.
3. All individuals have the previously stated densities for fat and lean body mass.

Their second and third assumptions are invalid, since the density of the lean body mass is variable as a result of differences in bone mineral density among individuals of different races, ages, and certain disease states, and because of differences in total body water as an individual ages and among

races. Modified equations exist that improve the accuracy of the two-compartment approach to hydrodensitometry, but these are restricted to differences between genders and between African-Americans and Caucasians in the density of the LBM (see Focus Box 21.1).

Multiple (More Than Two) Component Systems

Body composition can be grouped into categories based on chemical characteristics. Thus because the body is composed mainly of water, lipid, protein, and mineral, these are the main categories evaluated to quantify body composition. Such a division of body mass is referred to as the *four-component model.* When only one of protein, mineral, or water can be measured, the traditional two-component model is improved to a three-component model (Figure 21.1).

The development of a standard compositional scheme for the body has placed increased importance on the chemical order of body structure. For example, researchers have questioned the biologic logic behind simply a two-, three-, or four-compartment model.[31,69] The main questions have been whether simply dividing the body into fat, protein, water, and mineral compartments is the most representative of different components of body composition or the most

TABLE 21.4

Current techniques used for the assessment of body composition compartments

METHOD	FAT AND FAT-FREE BODY	MUSCLE	BONE MINERAL
Densitometry	Yes	No	No
Hydrometry	Yes	No	No
Spectrometry (40K)	Yes	Yes	No
Ultrasonics	Yes	Yes	No
Radiographics	Yes	Yes	Yes
Electrical conductivity	Yes	No	No
Neutron activation	Yes	Yes	Yes
NMR	Yes	Yes	Yes
Creatinine excretion	No	Yes	No
Urinary 3-methylhistidine	No	Yes	No
Serum creatinine	No	Yes	No
Photon absorptiometry	No	No	Yes

Modified from Lohman TG: *Med Sci Sports Exerc* 16:596-603, 1984.

suitable for accurate measurement or estimation. Based on these concerns, Wang et al. have devised a multiple-component five-level classification of body composition (Figure 21.1, *B*).[69] The utility of the molecular components is that methods exist for the measurement of total body water, such as isotope dilution (e.g., deuterium dilution), and bone mineral can be quantified by total body dual energy x-ray absorptiometry (DEXA).[2] Protein requires indirect measurement (e.g., neutron activation). There is also validity in researching the cell-based components of body composition, since cell mass can be quantified by total body potassium, extracellular fluid can be measured by fluid compartment molecular dilution, and extracellular solids can be estimated by neutron activation analysis (Table 21.4).[17,69] However, because the molecular and tissue levels of body composition provide data only on the lipid and fat component of the body, these are obviously the approaches favored by body composition research applied to health and fitness.

Body Composition Testing Methods and Procedures

Body composition research has led to the development of new and sophisticated ways to assess body composition (see Table 21.4). At present, many of these new techniques remain research tools and have little practical or clinical application. Many of the newer body composition assessment techniques are limited in their use-

fulness because of poor reliability and validity, expense, and complexity. Nevertheless, as previously explained, a way to noninvasively determine accurate body composition from multiple components is needed to provide a better gold standard. It is for this reason that many of the following methods are being researched and applied to quantify human body composition.

Densitometry

Densitometry (density = mass per unit volume; ometry = measurement) is the study of the measurement of human **body density.** Body density has long been held as the gold standard for the measurement of body composition and is routinely measured using the procedure of hydrodensitometry.

Hydrodensitometry

Hydrodensitometry, or hydrostatic weighing, has been the standard by which all other methods of body composition assessment are validated. Despite the errors of hydrosta-

body density
density of the body when submerged in water, expressed in gm/ml

hydrodensitometry (hi'dro-den'si-tom'e-tri)
method of determining body density by underwater weighing

FOCUS BOX 21.1

Estimating body composition from hydrodensitometry

Once whole body density (D_b) is determined, a decision must be made about which equation to use to convert body density to percentage of body fat. As previously explained, the original equations of Brozek and Siri were based on a sample of male cadavers and violate known differences in the FFM among individuals of different gender, age, race, and specific illnesses.[10,63]

Siri	% body fat = $[(4.95/D_b) - 4.50] \times 100$
Brozek	% body fat = $[(4.57/D_b) - 4.142] \times 100$

Table 21.5 presents other equations that can be used and the populations they represent.

TABLE 21.5

Alternative equations to those of Siri and Brozek for estimating percentage of body fat

AGE	GENDER	PERCENTAGE OF BODY FAT	D_{FFB}
15-16	M	$[(5.03/D_b) - 4.59] \times 100$	1.096
	F	$[(5.07/D_b) - 4.64] \times 100$	1.094
17-19	M	$[(4.98/D_b) - 4.53] \times 100$	1.0985
	F	$[(5.05/D_b) - 4.62] \times 100$	1.095
20-50	M	$[(4.95/D_b) - 4.50] \times 100$	1.100
	F	$[(5.03/D_b) - 4.59] \times 100$	1.096

For African-Americans, subtract 1.9% (males) and 1% (females) from each percentage of body fat calculation. Modified from Lohman TG: *Exer Sports Sci Rev* 14:325-327, 1986.

FIGURE 21.2

An underwater system that can measure underwater weight by either the traditional autopsy scale method or by the more modern strain gauge method. Nevertheless, no matter how accurate the underwater weight is, problems with converting the body density calculation to % body fat remains the largest source of error in hydrodensitometry.

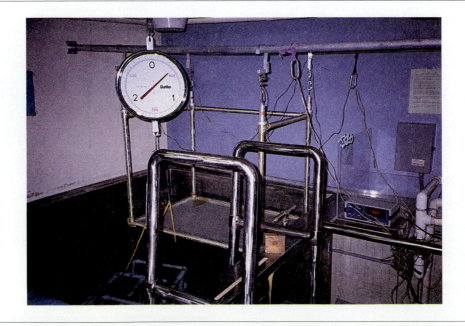

Focus Box 21.1—Cont'd

Estimating body composition from hydrodensitometry

Procedure for Measuring Underwater Weight

Underwater weight can be measured via suspension from an autopsy scale or by using a submerged seat or support that is connected to strain gauges (Figure 21.2).

Step 1: Complete pretesting requirements and the measurement of RV (see text).

Step 2: Obtain a dry-on-land body weight (kg).

Step 3: Determine tare weight of the weighing apparatus.

Step 4: Record the temperature of the water (in degrees C).

Step 5: Record D_w from Table 21.6.

Step 6: Determine the underwater weight of the subject (W_{uw}).

Step 7: Compute body density using equations 21.5 and 21.6.

Step 8: Convert body density to percent body fat using an appropriate formula (Siri, Brozek, or those in Table 21.5).

TABLE 21.6

Determining the density of water

WATER TEMP (°C)	D_w	WATER TEMP (°C)	D_w
23	0.997569	31	0.995372
24	0.997327	32	0.995057
25	0.997075	33	0.994734
26	0.996814	34	0.994403
27	0.996544	35	0.994063
28	0.996264	36	0.993716
29	0.995976	37	0.993360
30	0.995678		

For example, for a healthy male who weighs 84 kg, has a residual lung volume of 1.96 L, and obtains the following underwater weights in water at a density of 0.9937 g/ml:

Trial 1 - 4.47
Trial 2 - **4.65**
Trial 3 - **4.68**
Trial 4 - 4.52
Trial 5 - **4.68**
Average weight = (3.65 + 3.68 + 3.68) / 3 = 4.67 kg

Tare weight = 2.1 kg
Underwater weight = 4.67 − 2.1 = 2.57 kg

$$D_b = 84.0 / [((84.0 - 2.57) / 0.9937) - (1.96 + 0.10)]$$
$$= [84 / (81.9463 - 2.06)]$$
$$= 84 / 79.8863$$
$$= 1.0515$$

Using the Siri equation, percentage of body fat calculates to be:

$$\% \text{ fat} = [(4.95 / 1.0515) - 4.5] \times 100$$
$$= 20.76$$

tic weighing by anything other than a multicompartment model that includes each of water, fat, protein, and mineral or from chemical compartment models, hydrostatic weighing using a two–compartment model has remained a gold standard for composition analysis. Ironically, as early as 1961, Siri reported that differences between individuals in the density of the FFM would cause errors as large as 4% in percentage of body fat.[46,63]

Hydrostatic weighing is based on Archimedes' principle, which states that when an object is placed in water, it is buoyed up by a counterforce equal to the water it displaces. Thus there are two ways to measure body density; (1) by measuring the displaced water volume, or (2) by measuring the change in body weight underwater. The latter method is widely used and is the method suited to discussion in this section. Based on Archimedes' principle, body density can be calculated as follows:

21-5 $D_b = Mass_b / Volume_b$

21-6 $D_b = W_a / [([W_a - W_w] / D_w) - (RV + 100 \text{ ml})]$

Where: D_b = body density (g/ml)
            W_a = body weight out of water (kg)
            W_w = weight in water (kg)
            D_w = density of water (g/ml)
            RV = residual volume (ml)

The major disadvantages of hydrostatic weighing are as follows:

1. The cost and time to conduct a test
2. The need for subjects to tolerate water submersion at a residual lung volume
3. The constraints by limited population-specific equations that convert body density to percentage of body fat

In addition, subjects need to prepare themselves adequately before being tested. Such pretest requirements include the following:

1. A normal diet and fluid intake but with no ingestion of food or liquids for 3 hours before the test
2. Avoidance of foods that cause increased intestinal gas
3. Because of the need to expel lung air to residual volume, no smoking for 2 hours before the test
4. Avoidance of any condition that would alter the hydration of the body, such as physical activity, saunas, underhydration, or overhydration
5. For females avoidance of testing for 3 days before, during, and 3 days after menstruation
6. Bringing minimal swim clothing to decrease the risk for air trapping in the swim suit
7. A soap shower to remove excess body oils
8. The emptying of the bowel and bladder before testing
9. When in the tank, completely submerging the body and rubbing the skin and hair to remove air bubbles

Obtaining an accurate underwater weight is crucial to hydrodensitometry. Given the need for subjects to submerge themselves and maintain a still posture at residual volume, the accurate measurement of underwater weight is not a simple task. Early research indicated that there is a learning curve to the measurement of underwater weight, involving both the subject and technician.[39] Based on this fact, it was recommended that up to 10 recordings of underwater weight be required for acceptable accuracy.[39] However, subsequent research has shown that averaging three underwater weights that are within 100 g is equally accurate and therefore saves time and prevents undue stress on the subject.[6]

Residual volume (RV) of the subject can be determined before, during, or after the test with no significant difference in the estimation of percentage of body fat from either choice so long as measurement of RV outside the tank is done in a similar posture to the RV maneuver underwater.[5,7,19] Because of the added expense and equipment needs for RV determination while underwater, most laboratories perform the RV measurement either before or after the underwater weighing. If RV is estimated (see Chapter 20), errors of estimation of percentage of body fat can increase by as much as 3% body fat, which significantly reduces the accuracy of hydrodensitometry to the extent that body fat estimation should be done by less sophisticated and time-consuming methods (e.g., skinfold analysis).[54]

The procedures for conducting a test of hydrodensitometry are provided in Focus Box 21.1.

Skinfold Measurements

It is possible to measure the subcutaneous fat at selected sites with skinfold calipers and to predict the percentage of body fat by using various regression equations. Assessing body composition by measuring the thickness of selected skinfold sites is probably the most common and widely available technique in use today. It is important for fitness instructors and exercise physiology students to become proficient with this technique.

A variety of skinfold calipers are on the market, from expensive research calipers including the Harpenden, Lange, and Lafayette calipers, which generally cost in excess of $200, to less expensive (although not necessarily less accurate) calipers including the Slimguide, the Fat-O-Meter, and the Adipometer, which range in price from $10 to $50. The more expensive calipers maintain a constant jaw pressure of 10 g per square millimeter of surface area. Such precision is required for the accurate use of the skinfold technique to estimate percentage of body fat. Furthermore, evidence exists to indicate that skinfold calipers should be used that were used in the formulation of specific equations, since skinfold thicknesses can differ even among the expensive calipers.[44]

Before any skinfold measurements are taken, it is important to follow the guidelines listed in Focus Box 21.2.

Bioelectrical Impedance

Bioelectrical impedance (BIA) is a relatively new body composition assessment technique based on Hoffer's research, which demonstrated a high correlation between

bioelectrical impedance (BIA)
method of determining body fat, fat-free body mass, and total body water by measuring the resistance to current passed through the body

FOCUS BOX 21.2

Measurement of skinfolds and prediction equations for body fat percentage

Skinfold measurements

Research has provided many validated equations for estimating body fat from skinfolds. Some of these equations were developed from cadaver analyses, and the majority were validated against underwater weighing as the so-called gold standard.

1. It is important that the technician explain the following points to the subject:
   a. Why the test is being performed
   b. The technique involved
   c. Any risks or discomforts the subject might experience
   d. What the subject has to do to get prepared
   e. How the data will be used to predict the subject's percentage of body fat

The equation used should be predetermined based on the subject's personal demographics and health history.

2. Once the test and procedures have been thoroughly explained to the subject and all questions have been answered, the subject should be taken to a location where his or her privacy is protected.

3. All sites to be measured should be first marked with a water-soluble, felt-tip pen. All measurements should be taken on the right side of the body (Figures 21.3).

4. After all the sites have been marked, each fold is measured by grasping (drawing up) a layer of skin (skinfold) with the thumb and forefinger of the nondominant hand. For example, a right-handed examiner should hold the caliper in the right hand and grasp the skin with the left hand. The examiner should avoid "pinching" the subject. The proper technique is to pull the skin together and slightly away from the body but not so hard that the skinfold is compressed.

5. With the skinfold site isolated, the calipers should be placed perpendicular to the fold, approximately 1/2 inch below from the index finger and the thumb of the left hand. The pressure on the calipers and the skinfold grasp of the examiner's left hand should be released.

6. The calipers should have a chance to settle for 2 to 3 seconds, after which a measurment should be recorded in millimeters, and the calipers opened and removed completely.

7. Three measurements should be recorded to the nearest 0.1 to 0.5 mm. The average of the two closest readings should be recorded for the final value. All recordings should be taken as quickly as possible to avoid excessive compression of the skin.

8. For good reliability and validity, all repeat measurements should be taken at the same time of the day, preferably in the morning.

Skinfold sites

- Abdominal fold: A vertical fold taken at a distance of 2 cm to the right of the umbilicus

- Biceps fold: A vertical fold (taken 1 cm above the level used to mark the triceps) on the anterior aspect of the arm over the belly of the biceps muscle

- Chest or pectoral fold: A diagonal fold taken one half the distance between the anterior axillary line and the nipple for men and one third of the distance between the anterior axillary line and the nipple for women

FIGURE 21.3

A subject prepared for skinfold assessment.

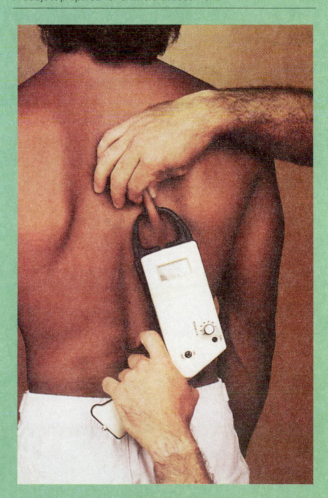

Continued.

FOCUS BOX 21.2—Cont'd

Measurement of skinfolds and prediction equations for body fat percentage

- Medial calf fold: A vertical fold at a level of the maximum circumference of the calf on the midline of the medial border

- Midaxillary fold: A vertical fold taken on the midaxillary line at the level of the xiphoid process of the sternum

- Subscapular fold: An angular fold taken at a 45-degree angle 1 to 2 cm below the inferior angle of the scapula

- Suprailium fold: An oblique fold in line with the natural angle of the iliac crest taken in the anterior axillary line immediately superior to the iliac crest

- Thigh fold: A vertical fold on the anterior midline of the thigh, midway between the proximal border of the patella and the inguinale crease (knee joint and the hip); the midpoint should be marked while the subject is seated

- Triceps fold: A vertical fold on the posterior midline of the upper right arm, halfway between the acromion and the ole-

cranon process tip of the shoulder to the tip of the elbow; the arm should be relaxed and fully extended

Equations for body fat percentage

Once the necessary final skinfold measurements have been recorded, the percentage of body fat can be obtained by using a variety of tables or formulas. For the highest reliability and validity, it is important to choose the right regression and prediction tables based on the population being tested. Regression equations, such as those listed in Table 21.7, estimate whole body density, which can then be used to predict the percentage of body fat (Table 21.5, Focus Box 21.1). The percentage of body fat can also be predicted from tables such as Table 21.8. The relationship between body density and skinfold thickness is presented in the section on skinfold sites.

TABLE 21.7

Regression equations to predict body density from skinfold measurements

EQUATION	r	SE	REFERENCE
NON-SPECIFIC			
$D_b = 1.0982 - 0.000815(\text{sum of 3}) + 0.00000084^2(\text{sum of 3})^2$ Where (sum of 3) = triceps, subscapula, and abdomen	—	—	46
MALES			
18-61 years			
$D_b = 1.1093800 - 0.0008267(\text{sum of 3}) + 0.0000016(\text{sum of 3})^2 - 0.0002574(\text{age})$ Where (sum of 3) = chest, abdomen, and thigh	0.91	0.0077	35
College athletes			
$D_b = 1.10647 - 0.00162(\text{subscapular}) - 0.00144(\text{abdominal}) - 0.00077(\text{triceps}) + 0.00071(\text{midaxillary})$	0.84	0.006	24
FEMALES			
18-55 years			
$D_b = 1.0994921 - 0.0009929(\text{sum of 3}) + 0.0000023(\text{sum of 3})^2 - 0.001392(\text{age})$ Where (sum of 3) = triceps, suprailiac, and thigh	0.84	0.0086	36
College athletes			
$D_b = 1.096095 - (0.0006952(\text{sum of 4}) + 0.0000011(\text{sum of 4})^2 - 0.0000714(\text{age})$ Where (sum of 4) = triceps, suprailiac, abdominal, and thigh	0.85	0.0084	36

Data modified from 35, 36, and 46.
r, Correlations coefficient; *SE*, standard error of estimate.

TABLE 21.8A

Percent fat estimate for women: sum of triceps, abdomen, and suprailium skinfolds

	PERCENT FAT AGE TO LAST YEAR								
SUM OF SKINFOLDS (mm)	18-22	23-27	28-32	33-37	38-42	43-47	48-52	53-57	OVER 57
8-12	8.8	9.0	9.2	9.4	9.5	9.7	9.9	10.1	10.3
13-17	10.8	10.9	11.1	11.3	11.5	11.7	11.8	12.0	12.2
18-22	12.6	12.8	13.0	13.2	13.4	13.5	13.7	13.9	14.1
23-27	14.5	14.6	14.8	15.0	15.2	15.4	15.6	15.7	15.9
28-32	16.2	16.4	16.6	16.8	17.0	17.1	17.3	17.5	17.7
33-37	17.9	18.1	18.3	18.5	18.7	18.9	19.0	19.2	19.4
38-42	19.6	19.8	20.0	20.2	20.3	20.5	20.7	20.9	21.1
43-47	21.2	21.4	21.6	21.8	21.9	22.1	22.3	22.5	22.7
48-52	22.8	22.9	23.1	23.3	23.5	23.7	23.8	24.0	24.2
53-57	24.2	24.4	24.6	24.8	25.0	25.2	25.3	25.5	25.7
58-62	25.7	25.9	26.0	26.2	26.4	26.6	26.8	27.0	27.1
63-67	27.1	27.2	27.4	27.6	27.8	28.0	28.2	28.3	28.5
68-72	28.4	28.6	28.7	28.9	29.1	29.3	29.5	29.7	29.8
73-77	29.6	29.8	30.0	30.2	30.4	30.6	30.7	30.9	31.1
78-82	30.9	31.0	31.2	31.4	31.6	31.8	31.9	32.1	32.3
83-87	32.0	32.2	32.4	32.6	32.7	32.9	33.1	33.3	33.5
88-92	33.1	33.3	33.5	33.7	33.8	34.0	34.2	34.4	34.6
93-97	34.1	34.3	34.5	34.7	34.9	35.1	35.2	35.4	35.6
98-102	35.1	35.3	35.5	35.7	35.9	36.0	36.2	36.4	36.6
103-107	36.1	36.2	36.4	36.6	36.8	37.0	37.2	37.3	37.5
108-112	36.9	37.1	37.3	37.5	37.7	37.9	38.0	38.2	38.4
113-117	37.8	37.9	38.1	38.3	39.2	39.4	39.6	39.8	39.2
118-122	38.5	38.7	38.9	39.1	39.4	39.6	39.8	40.0	40.0
123-127	39.2	39.4	39.6	39.8	40.0	40.1	40.3	40.5	40.7
128-132	39.9	40.1	40.2	40.4	40.6	40.8	41.0	41.2	41.3
133-137	40.5	40.7	40.8	41.0	41.2	41.4	41.6	41.7	41.9
138-142	41.0	41.2	41.4	41.6	41.7	41.9	42.1	42.3	42.5
143-147	41.5	41.7	41.9	42.0	42.2	42.4	42.6	42.8	43.0
148-152	41.9	42.1	42.3	42.8	42.6	42.8	43.0	43.2	43.4
153-157	42.3	42.5	42.6	42.8	43.0	43.2	43.4	43.6	43.7
158-162	42.6	42.8	43.0	43.1	43.3	43.5	43.7	43.9	44.1
163-167	42.9	43.0	43.2	43.4	43.6	43.8	44.0	44.1	44.3
168-172	43.1	43.2	43.4	43.6	43.8	44.0	44.2	44.3	44.5
173-177	43.2	43.4	43.6	43.8	43.9	44.1	44.3	44.5	44.7
178-182	43.3	43.5	43.7	43.8	44.0	44.2	44.4	44.6	44.8

From Jackson AS, Pollack ML: *Phys Sportsmed* 13:76-90, 1985.

TABLE 21.8B

Percent fat estimate for men: sum of triceps, chest, and subscapular skinfolds

SUM OF SKINFOLDS (mm)	PERCENT FAT AGE TO LAST YEAR UNDER 22	23-27	28-32	33-37	38-42	43-47	48-52	53-57	OVER 57
8-10	1.5	2.0	2.5	3.1	3.6	4.1	4.6	5.1	5.6
11-13	3.0	3.5	4.0	4.5	5.1	5.6	6.1	6.6	7.1
14-16	4.5	5.0	5.5	6.0	6.5	7.0	7.6	8.1	8.6
17-19	5.9	6.4	6.9	7.4	8.0	8.5	9.0	9.5	10.0
20-22	7.3	7.8	8.3	8.8	9.4	9.9	10.4	10.9	11.4
23-25	8.6	9.2	9.7	10.2	10.7	11.2	11.8	12.3	12.8
26-28	10.0	10.5	11.0	11.5	12.1	12.6	13.1	13.6	14.2
29-31	11.2	11.8	12.3	12.8	13.4	13.9	14.4	14.9	15.5
32-34	12.5	13.0	13.5	14.1	14.6	15.1	15.7	16.2	16.7
35-37	13.7	14.2	14.8	15.3	15.8	16.4	16.9	17.4	18.0
38-40	14.9	15.4	15.9	16.5	17.0	17.6	18.1	18.6	19.2
41-43	16.0	16.6	17.1	17.6	18.2	18.7	19.3	19.8	20.3
44-46	17.1	17.7	18.2	18.7	19.3	19.8	20.4	20.9	21.5
47-49	18.2	18.7	19.3	19.8	20.4	20.9	21.4	22.0	22.5
50-52	19.2	19.7	20.3	20.8	21.4	21.9	22.5	23.0	23.6
53-55	20.2	20.7	21.3	21.8	22.4	22.9	23.5	24.0	24.6
56-58	21.1	21.7	22.2	22.8	23.3	23.9	24.4	25.0	25.5
59-61	22.0	22.6	23.1	23.7	24.2	24.8	25.3	25.9	26.5
62-64	22.9	23.4	24.0	24.5	25.1	25.7	26.2	26.8	27.3
65-67	23.7	24.3	24.8	25.4	25.9	26.5	27.1	27.6	28.2
68-70	24.5	25.0	25.6	26.2	26.7	27.3	27.8	28.4	29.0
71-73	25.2	25.8	26.3	26.9	27.5	28.0	28.6	29.1	29.7
74-76	25.9	26.5	27.0	27.6	28.2	28.7	29.3	29.9	30.4
77-79	26.6	27.1	27.7	28.2	28.8	29.4	29.9	30.5	31.1
80-82	27.2	27.7	28.3	28.9	29.4	30.0	30.6	31.1	31.7
83-85	27.7	28.3	28.8	29.4	30.0	30.5	31.1	31.7	32.3
86-88	28.2	28.8	29.4	29.9	30.5	31.1	31.6	32.2	32.8
89-91	28.7	29.3	29.8	30.4	31.0	31.5	32.1	32.7	33.3
92-94	29.1	29.7	30.3	30.8	31.4	32.0	32.6	33.1	33.4
95-97	29.5	30.1	30.6	31.2	31.8	32.4	32.9	33.5	34.1
98-100	29.8	30.4	31.0	31.6	32.1	32.7	33.3	33.9	34.4
101-103	30.1	30.7	31.3	31.8	32.4	33.0	33.6	34.1	34.7
104-106	30.4	30.9	31.5	32.1	32.7	33.2	33.8	34.4	35.0
107-109	30.6	31.1	31.7	32.3	32.9	33.4	34.0	34.6	35.2
110-112	30.7	31.3	31.9	32.4	33.0	33.6	34.2	34.7	35.3
113-115	30.8	31.4	32.0	32.5	33.1	33.7	34.3	34.9	35.4
116-118	30.9	31.5	32.0	32.6	33.2	33.8	34.3	34.9	35.5

From Jackson AS, Pollack ML: *Phys Sportsmed* 13:76-90, 1985.

FIGURE 21.4

A subject prepared for body composition analysis by bioelectrical impedance (BIA), and a chart showing the data obtained from BIA analysis.

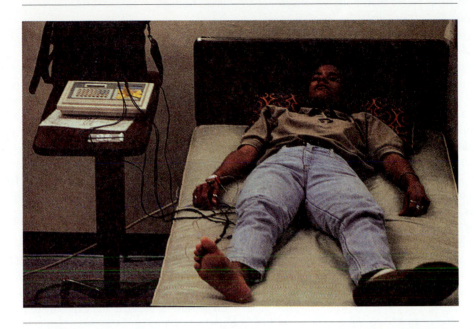

TABLE 21.9

Regression equations to predict fat-free body mass (kg) from bioelectrical impedance measurements

EQUATION*	r	SE	REFERENCE
MALE			
$[0.485(L^2 / R)] + [0.338(weight;kg)] + 5.32$	—	2.9	46
FEMALE			
$[0.475(L^2 / R)] + [0.295(weight;kg)] + 5.49$	—	2.9	46

r, Correlations coefficient; SE, standard error of estimate.

*Equations derived from combined data from multiple research studies; L^2 / R = resistive index = height^2 / Resistance modified from Lohman TG: *Advances in body composition assessment, Current Issues in Exercise Science Series,* Monograph number 3, Champaign, Illinois, 1992, Human Kinetics.

whole body electrical impedance and total body water (TBW).[33] Hoffer further demonstrated that TBW and LBM were strongly correlated with height^2/resistance, where body resistance or impedance was measured with a tetrapolar electrode configuration (Figure 21.4). The principle of BIA is based on electrical conductance and on the fact that fat-free mass, with its richer electrolyte content, has a much greater conductivity than does fat, allowing for the establishment of a relationship between conductance and fat-free mass. Once the electrical resistance has been determined, body composition estimates can be extrapolated from generalized prediction equations (Table 21.9).

Changes in electrolyte status of the body dramatically affect BIA measurements, which is one of the main limitations of the BIA technique. In addition, when BIA was first developed for body composition analysis, the prediction equations supplied by the manufacturers of BIA testing equipment often overestimated LBM in obese subjects. However, recent cross-validation studies have suggested that prediction of LBM can be enhanced by gender- and fatness-specific equations.[28]

Although BIA testing is a rapid, safe, and noninvasive method of estimating body composition, its accuracy can be questioned. Liang et al. revealed that percentage of body fat from BIA analysis was overestimated by approximately 3%; Eckerson et al. reported that BIA equations, even those improved from manufacturers recommendations, did not improve body fat prediction better than body weight alone; and percentage of body fat in lean males has been reported to be better predicted from visual observation than by BIA analysis.[21,22,42] Nevertheless, reports of the accuracy of BIA analysis exist, and Kushner and Van Loan have written excellent reviews on the use of BIA in body composition analysis.[41,67]

To improve the accuracy of BIA testing, it is important that subjects strictly follow guidelines before testing:

1. Urinate within 30 minutes of the test.
2. Consume no alcohol 48 hours before the test.
3. Do not exercise within 12 hours of the test.
4. Consume no food or fluid within 4 hours of the test.

These guidelines exist to avoid alterations in hydration of the body. As far as exercise is concerned, the recommendation of no exercise before the test is not entirely supported by research. Liang et al. performed BIA analyses before and immediately after 30 minutes of exercise at 83% of maximal heart rate and found that BIA analyses were unchanged.

Isotope Dilution

Total body water can be measured and used to predict LBM through an isotope dilution technique. Total body water can be measured by using either radioactive water (^3H_2O) or nonradioactive water (^2H_2O, $H_2{}^{18}O$). Subjects drink or are injected with a known amount of labeled water. After 3 to 4 hours the concentration of the isotope is determined in a sample of the subject's saliva, urine, or serum. The measurement of total body water and the prediction of LBM are based on LBM containing a relatively constant proportion (73.2%) of water. Body cell mass (an accurate estimate of LBM) can be estimated as intracellular water divided by 0.72 (the fraction of cell mass accounted for by water). The measurement of intracellular water is an excellent means to compare body cell mass between lean and obese individuals.

As previously explained, use of a measurement of total body water can also be incorporated into the original Siri equation for the development of a three-compartment model of percent fat estimation from total body density.[46]

Photo Absorptiometry

Dual-photo absorptiometry (DPA) and dual-energy x-ray absorptiometry (DEXA) are techniques used to measure bone mineral content (see Chapter 14). The basic principle for DEXA is the same as for DPA, except that DEXA uses an x-ray source instead of a gadolinium source. LBM and FM absorb the x-rays in different degrees, so that the percentage of each can be calculated. The DEXA method of assessing body composition appears to be very reliable compared with other body composition assessment techniques.[68]

The use of DEXA is increasing in the development of multicompartmental models of body composition, since it can provide a regional and total body measurement of bone mineral.

Potassium-40 Count

Potassium is a major intracellular component in lean tissue but is virtually absent in adipose tissue. Knowledge of total body potassium permits estimation of LBM. A small percentage of all naturally occurring potassium is the naturally radioactive isotope ^{40}K. By comparing the radioactive of isotope ^{40}K with known amounts of potassium, total body potassium and thus LBM can be calculated. Although considered valid and reliable, this technique has limited usefulness because of its expense.

Radiography

It is possible to measure the widths of fat, muscle, and bone with an x-ray film of a limb. Although this can be an accurate method to estimate regional body composition, it is impractical because of expense and exposure to high levels of radiation.

Ultrasound

Ultrasound has recently been used to measure the thickness of subcutaneous fat. If several ultrasound scans are taken at several different sites, total body adipose tissue can be estimated. The primary weakness of this technique is that it requires substantial extrapolation from just a few subcutaneous sites to estimate the total percentage of body fat. In this sense, ultrasound provides an alternative to skinfold measurement, yet it does not have the extensive research validation.

Computed Tomography and Nuclear Magnetic Resonance Imaging

Both computed tomography (CT) and magnetic resonance imaging (MRI) have been used to provide a visual image of LBM and FM. By scanning multiple sections of the body, and by summing the volume of adipose tissue in each section serially, it is possible to estimate the total volume of fat within the body.[62] Magnetic resonance imaging has been validated in animal models; however, the expense and the remaining need to estimate the density of the FFM decreases the application of this technique.[25]

Near-Infrared Interactance

Near-infrared interactance (NIR) is a relatively recent technique that involves the transmission of electromagnetic radiation through a probe into subcutaneous tissue and analysis of the reflected and scattered energy from the electromagnetic radiation to estimate tissue composition. The validity of a commercially available (NIR) testing device (Futrex-5000) has been cross-validated with other techniques.[51] It appears that NIR overestimates body fat in lean subjects with less than 8% body fat and underestimates it in subjects with greater than 30% body fat. As with the BIA method, many equations have been developed using this methodology; however, compared with the accuracy of underwater weighing or skinfold techniques, it is not a method of choice in the laboratory or in the field.

Total Body Electroconductivity

Total body electroconductivity (TOBEC) is a method of estimating body composition that relies on the properties of hydrated lean tissue and extracellular water to conduct electrical energy when subjected to appropriate radio frequencies. TOBEC works by surrounding the body with an electromagnetic field and measuring the rate at which the body conducts electrical energy. Subjects are placed in a chamber that generates an electrical current at a specific radio frequency. Measurement of the changes in the electromagnetic field lost because of the conductive mass of the body (lean tissue and body water conduct electricity more rapidly than fat) makes it possible to predict LBM.

Anthropometry

Anthropometry (anthropo=human; metry=measure) is a set of standardized techniques and measurements for determining the size, proportions, and shape of an individual's body. Basic anthropometric measurements include standing height, body weight, girths, bone widths, waist-to-hip ratio, and skinfold measurements. The ability to assess body composition depends greatly on the type of equipment used, type of prediction equation used, and technician reliability.

Anthropometric measurements are relatively accurate in estimating body composition profiles and in tracking changes in growth and development. Anthropomorphic measurements are placed in regression equations to estimate the FFM and percentage of body fat.

Body Mass Index

Body mass index (BMI) is the ratio of weight to height squared. A high BMI is associated with a high prevalence of mortality from heart disease, cancer, and diabetes (Figure 21.5). To calculate BMI divide body weight in kilograms by height in meters squared (kg/m^2). A BMI score less than 20 is considered underweight, 20 to 24.9 is considered desirable, 25 is considered overweight, and greater than 30 is considered obese.

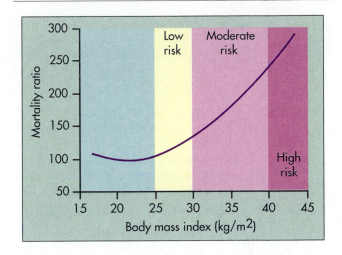

FIGURE 21.5

The increase in mortality with increases in body mass index.

Waist-to-Hip Ratio

Another simple technique to assess and monitor changes in body composition is by measuring an individual's waist-to-hip ratio. Waist-to-hip ratio measurements can help identify the distribution of body fat in both men and women. Body fat distribution is important because research has shown that android obesity is associated with greater morbidity and mortality than gynoid obesity.[61]

A waist-to-hip ratio greater than 1 for men and greater than 0.85 for women is considered high risk; moderately high risk for men is 0.90 to 1 and for women 0.80 to 0.85; lower risk for men is less than 0.90 and for women less than 0.80. For good health, it is recommended the waist-to-hip ratio be below 1 for both men and women.[61] A variety of other girth measurements can be measured and used in body composition prediction equations. The reader is referred to the suggested reading list for additional sources on anthropometric measurements.

---

anthropometry

study of body and body part dimensions

body mass index

ratio of body weight/height²

SUMMARY

▪ **Body composition** refers to the relative amounts of water, protein, mineral, and fat in the body. **Overweight** is defined as body weight in excess of a reference standard, generally mean weight for a given height and skeletal frame size grouped by gender. However, height-weight tables should be avoided, and the concept of being overweight should be replaced with the concept of being **overfat.** Being overfat indicates an excess accumulation of body fat.

▪ Body composition is often expressed as the relative amounts of fat mass to fat-free mass. *Fat mass* (FM) includes both essential and storage fat. **Essential fat** is found in bone marrow, brain, spinal cord, muscles, and other internal organs and is essential to normal physiologic and biologic functioning. **Storage fat** is composed of two types of fat: yellow fat, which is approximately 99% of all storage fat, and brown fat. **Lean body mass** (LBM) represents nonfat tissue plus essential fat stores, whereas **fat-free body mass** (FFBM) represents LBM minus essential fat.

▪ The original body component system described the body as divided into two simple components: lean and fat body mass. Since then, *lean body mass* (LBM) has been identified as not being completely fat free because it contained lipid within, for example, muscle, cell membranes, and bone marrow. The term *fat-free body mass* (FFBM) represents LBM minus essential fat stores. Brozek, Siri, and Behnke developed the two-component system of body composition based on the following assumptions:

1. The density of fat is 0.900 g/ml at 37° C

2. The density of lean body mass is 1.100 g/ml at 37° C

3. All individuals have the previously stated densities for fat and lean body mass

▪ The second and third assumptions are invalid, since the density of the lean body mass is variable because of differences in bone mineral density between individuals of different races, ages, and certain disease states, and because of differences in total body water as an individual ages and among races.

▪ Because the body is mainly composed of water, lipid, protein, and mineral, these are the main categories evaluated to quantify multiple compartments of body composition.

▪ Densitometry (density = mass per unit volume; ometry = measurement) is the study of the measurement of human **body density.** Body density has long been held as the gold standard for the measurement of body composition and is routinely measured using the procedure of **hydrodensitometry,** or hydrostatic weighing. Hydrodensitometry has been the standard by which all other methods of body composition assessment are validated. Hydrostatic weighing using a two-compartment model has remained a gold standard for composition analysis, despite the known errors that exist for individuals in the density of the FFM.

▪ Hydrostatic weighing can be performed by measuring the displaced water volume or by measuring the change in body weight underwater. The latter method is more widely used. Obtaining an accurate underwater weight is crucial to hydrodensitometry. Averaging three underwater weights that are within 100 g has been verified as a criterion for determining underwater weight.

▪ The determination of residual volume of the subject can be conducted before, during, or after the test with no significant difference in the measurement of RV and the estimation of percentage of body fat.

▪ It is possible to measure the subcutaneous fat at selected sites with skinfold calipers and to predict the percentage of body fat by using various regression equations. Once the necessary final skinfold measurements have been recorded, the percentage of body fat can be obtained by using a variety of tables or formulas. For the highest reliability and validity, it is important to choose the right regression and prediction tables based on the population being tested.

■ **Bioelectrical impedance** (BIA) is a relatively new body composition assessment technique based on research that has demonstrated a high correlation between whole body electrical impedance and total body water (TBW). The principle of BIA is based on electrical conductance and on the fact that fat-free mass, with its richer electrolyte content, has a much greater conductivity than does fat, allowing the establishment of a relationship between conductance and fat-free mass. Once the electrical resistance has been determined, body composition estimates can be extrapolated from generalized prediction equations.

■ Total body water can be measured and used to predict LBM through an isotope dilution technique. Total body water can be measured by using either radioactive water (^3H_2O) or nonradioactive water (^2H_2O, $H_2^{18}O$). The measurement of total body water and the prediction of LBM are based on LBM containing a relatively constant proportion (73.2%) of water. Body cell mass (an accurate estimate of LBM) can be estimated as intracellular water divided by 0.72 (the fraction of cell mass accounted for by water).

■ Dual-photo absorptiometry (DPA) and *dual energy x-ray absorptiometry* (DEXA) are techniques used to measure bone mineral content. The basic principle for DEXA is that LBM and FM absorb x-ray radiation differently, so that the percentage of each can be calculated by measuring x-ray penetration of the body.

■ A small percentage of all naturally occurring potassium is the naturally radioactive isotope ^{40}K. By a comparison of the radioactive of isotope ^{40}K with known amounts of potassium, total body potassium and thus LBM can be calculated.

■ Near-infrared interactance (NIR) involves the transmission of electromagnetic radiation through a probe into subcutaneous tissue and analysis of the reflected and scattered energy from the electromagnetic radiation to estimate tissue composition. It appears that NIR overestimates body fat in lean subjects with less than 8% and underestimates it in subjects with more than 30% body fat. As with the BIA method, many equations have been developed using this methodology.

■ **Anthropometry** (anthropo = human; metry = measure) is a set of standardized techniques and measurements for determining the size, proportion, and shape of an individual's body. Basic anthropometric measurements include: standing height, body weight, girths, bone widths, waist-to-hip ratio, and skinfold measurements. The ability to assess body composition is highly dependent on the type of equipment used, type of prediction equation used, and technician reliability.

■ **Body mass index** (BMI) is the ratio of weight to height squared. A high BMI is associated with a high prevalence of mortality from heart disease, cancer, and diabetes. BMI is calculated by dividing body weight in kilograms by height in meters squared (kg/m^2). A BMI score less than 20 is considered underweight, 20 to 24.9 is considered desirable, 25 is overweight, and greater than 30 is considered obese.

REVIEW QUESTIONS

1. Why are standard height and weight tables not a true representation of an individual's body composition?

2. Explain the differences between essential fat and storage fat.

3. Define the two-component system of body composition. What are some of the weaknesses of the model?

4. How were the Siri and Brozek equations derived?

5. How is anthropometry used in body composition analysis?

6. Is measurement of residual volume necessary for optimal accuracy of body composition determined by hydrodensitometry? Explain.

7. Define and list the benefits and limitations of bioelectrical impedance, infrared analysis, and dual x-ray absorptiometry.

8. Is there really a true gold standard to validate body composition methods? Explain how this fact detracts from research in body composition and the interpretation of the results.

9. Know the standard values of percent body fat for different age ranges and genders.

10. Sally is a 22-year-old female with a body fat of 29.5% and a weight of 150 lb. Determine her desirable weight if her goal is to have 18% body fat.

11. Calculate a BMI score with a weight of 185 pounds (84.1 kg) and a height of 5'11" (179 cm). Remember, BMI = (kg/m^2).

12. With the data listed below, calculate the percentage of body fat for a male using the appropriate regression equation of Table 21.7.

    Age = 25

    Gender = male

    Race = African-American

    Fitness = endurance-trained athlete

    Chest skinfolds = 13.25, 14.5, 13.5, 13.5, and 13.75 mm

    Abdomen skinfolds = 20.5, 20.25, 21, 20.5, and 22 mm

    Thigh skinfolds = 13.5, 14.0, 13.75, 14.5, 14.0, and 14.25 mm

13. Calculate the percentage of body fat based on the following data obtained during a hydrostatic weighing test:

    Age = 53

    Gender = female

    Subject height = 148 cm

    Subject weight = 67 kg

    Suit weight = 13.5 g

    RV = 1.58 L

    Weight of scale underwater = 2.85 kg

    Water temperature = 36.5° C

    Underwater weights = 4.81, 4.61, 4.92, 4.99, 4.78, 4.94 kg

APPLICATIONS

1. Measurement of the body composition of clinically ill individuals in a hospital setting presents several obstacles for the application of hydrodensitometry. What are some patient populations that should not be submerged in water? What alternative methods would you use for each population, and why?

2. How accurate should body composition analysis be? For example, is an error greater than ±3% body fat really unacceptable for application to clinical and general use? Explain.

REFERENCES

1. American Alliance for Health, Physical Education, Recreation & Dance: *Physical best manual,* Reston, Virginia, 1988, American Alliance for Health, Physical Education, Recreation & Dance.

2. Bartoli WP, Davis JM, Pate RR, et al: Weekly variability in total body water using ^2H_2O dilution in college-age males, *Med Sci Sports Exerc* 25(12):1422-1428, 1993.

3. Behnke AR, Feen BG, Welman WC: The specific gravity of healthy men: body weight/volume as an index of obesity, *JAMA* 118:495-498, 1942.

4. Behnke AR: The estimation of lean body weight from skeletal measurement, *Human Biol* 31:295-315, 1959.

5. Behnke AR, Wilmore JH: *Evaluation and regulation of body build and composition,* Englewood Cliffs, NJ, 1974, Prentice-Hall.

6. Bonge D, Donnelly JE: Trials to criteria for hydrostatic weighing at residual volume, *Res Q Exerc Sport* 60(2):176-179, 1989.

7. Bosch PR, Wells CL: Effect of immersion on residual lung volume of able-bodied and spinal cord injured males, *Med Sci Sports Exerc* 23(3):384-388, 1991.

8. Bouchard C: Heredity and the path to overweight and obesity, *Med Sci Sports Exerc* 23(3):285-291, 1991.

9. Bray GA: Obesity: definition, diagnosis and disadvantages, *Med J Aust* 142:S2-S8, 1982.

10. Brozek J, Grande F, Anderson JT, Keys A: Densiometric analysis of body composition: revision of some quantitative assumptions, *Ann NY Acad Sci* 110:113-140, 1963.

11. Bunt JC, Lohman TG, Boileau RA: Impact of total body water fluctuations on estimation of body fat from body density, *Med Sci Sports Exerc* 21(1):96-100, 1989.

12. Bunt JC, Going SB, Lohman TG et al: Variation in bone mineral content and estimated body fat in young adult females, *Med Sci Sports Exerc* 22(5):564-569, 1990.

13. Buskirk ER, Mendenz J: Sports science and body composition analysis: emphasis on cell and muscle mass, *Med Sci Sports Exerc* 16(6):584-593, 1984.

14. Casey VA, Dwyer JT, Coleman KA, Valadian I: Body mass index from childhood to middle age: a 50 yr follow-up, *Am J Clin Nutr* 56:14-18, 1992.

15. Cassady SL, Nielsen DH, Janz KF et al: Validity of near infrared body composition analysis in children and adolescents, *Med Sci Sports Med* 25(10):1185-1191, 1993.

16. Cohn SH, Abesamis C, Zanzi I et al: Body elemental composition: comparison between black and white adults, *Am J Physiol* 232(4):E419-E422, 1977.

17. Cohn SH, Vartsky D, Yasumura S et al: Indexes of body cell mass: nitrogen versus potassium, *Am J Physiol* 244(7):E305-E310, 1983.

18. Cote KD, Adams WC: Effect of bone density on body composition estimates in young adult black and white women, *Med Sci Sports Exerc* 25(2):290-296, 1993.

19. Craig AB, Kyle LH: Effect of immersion in water on vital capacity and residual volume of lungs, *J Appl Physiol* 23:423-425, 1967.

20. Dietz WH: Childhood obesity: susceptibility, cause, and management, *J Pediatr* 103:676-686, 1983.

21. Eckerson JM, Housh TJ, Johnson GO: The validity of visual estimations of percent body fat in lean males, *Med Sci Sports Exerc* 24(5):615-618, 1992.

22. Eckerson JM, Housh TJ, Johnson GO: Validity of bioelectrical impedance equations for estimating fat-free weight in lean males, *Med Sci Sports Exerc* 24(11):1298-1302, 1992.

23. Forbes GB, Simon W, Amatruda JM: Is bioimpedance a good predictor of body-composition change? *Am J Clin Nutr* 56:4-6, 1992.

fluid, and any other tissue excluding lipid and fat tissue. There is often argument about whether to use *LBM* or *FFBM*. One of the first definitions of LBM included a small amount of essential fat, approximately 2% to 3%.[4] Lohman has suggested researchers and clinicians use the term *LBM* in most applications and FFBM when conducting body-composition validation studies.[46]

Adult Norms for Body Fatness and Health and Fitness

Desirable body weight and percentage of body fat are important for three reasons: health, athletic performance, and aesthetic purposes. From a health perspective, excessive weight and body fat is a major concern in the United States.

Table 21.2 lists standard values for percent body fat for health and fitness purposes.

Some events require athletes to have an extremely low percentage of body fat to be successful. For example, some elite marathon runners have body fat percentages as low as 3% to 5%. Other sports allow for high percentages of body fat (Table 21.3).

Youth Norms for Body Fatness and Health and Fitness

Results from the National Children and Youth Fitness Study II indicate that subcutaneous fat levels have been increasing in children since the 1970s.[59] It has also been estimated that significant obesity affects from 10% to 25% of all children in the United States.[20] Thus it has become apparent that children's body composition should be evaluated early and be retested over time.

Determining Desirable Weight

Once an individual's body composition has been obtained, a desirable weight can be determined. An individual's desirable weight should be carefully chosen. Most people have an unrealistic expectation of their desirable weight. Desirable weight calculations should be used as a tool to help promote weight loss for good health and can be estimated as follows:

21.1 Fat weight =
current weight $\times$ (%fat / 100)

21.2 Lean body mass (LBM) =
current weight − fat weight

21.3 Desirable weight =
LBM / [1 − (%fat desired / 100)]

21.4 Desirable fat loss =
present weight − desirable body weight

Historical Development of Body Composition Analysis

The measurement of body composition was originally performed on cadavers, where the fat of the body was separated from the remaining components, and total body fat content was compared with hydrodensitometry to validate prediction equations of percentage of fat.[10,63] Based on these cadavers, average values were determined for the density of fat and lean mass, with these values being 0.901 g/ml and 1.1 g/ml, respectively. The cadavers used in this original research were Caucasian, middle-aged men, and the inability to obtain cadavers of different ages, genders, races, and medical history limited the inference of prediction from these equations. For example, it is now known that the density of lean body mass varies with age, between genders, during the menstrual cycle of the female, between different races, in individuals with osteoporosis, in individuals with spinal cord injury, and in exercise-trained individuals.[*] Most variation occurs in total body water, the largest component of body composition, however, additional variation occurs in body mineral (mainly bone mineral).[2,16,38,46] The science of body composition using hydrodensitometry is therefore based on a *prediction* of body composition rather than its measurement, and not surprisingly, the so-called gold standard of hydrodensitometry is associated with errors of prediction.

Since this original research, added research has been conducted to improve the original equations of Brozek and Siri. Modified age, gender, and ethnicity equations have been developed to adjust a given body density to provide a more accurate estimation of percentage of fat. These modified equations were developed by measuring water, protein, or mineral of the body, and when these differed from the original assumed values, the difference was used to modify the percentage of fat calculation from body density (see Hydrodensitometry).

Because not all settings or individuals are suited for hydrodensitometry, research in body composition techniques has also attempted to decrease the error of prediction for alternative methods of body composition assessment. For example, skinfold equations have been developed that are population specific and thereby have a decreased error of prediction. Equations from other techniques of body composition analysis, such as bioelectrical impedance or infrared analysis, have also been validated for use in field settings. However, of more importance has been the development of body composition models that quantify body water (e.g., from deuterium dilution of total body), body mineral (e.g.,

---

*References 7, 12, 16, 37, 43, 46, 50, 57, 60, 71, and 72.

REFERENCES—Cont'd

24. Forsyth JS, Sinning WE: The anthropometric estimation of body density and lean body weight of male athletes, *Med Sci Sports Exerc* 5:174-180, 1973.

25. Fowler PA, Fuller MF, Glasbey CA et al: Validation of the in vivo measurement of adipose tissue by magnetic resonance imaging of lean and obese pigs, *Am J Clin Nutr* 56:7-13, 1992.

26. Fulco CS, Hoyt RW, Baker-Fulco CJ et al: Use of bioelectrical impedance to assess body composition changes at altitude, *J Appl Physiol* 72(6):2181-2187, 1992.

27. Fuller NJ, Elia M: Potential use of bioelectrical impedance of the whole body and of body segments for the assessment of body composition: comparison with densitometry and anthropometry, *Eur J Clin Nutr* 43:779-791, 1988.

28. Gray DS, Brag GA, Gemayel N, Kaplan K: Effect of obesity on bioelectrical impedance, *Am J Clin Nutr* 50:255-260, 1989.

29. Hergenroeder AC, Fiorotto ML, Klish WJ: Body composition in ballet dancers measured by total body electrical conductivity, *Med Sci Sports Exerc* 23(5):528-533, 1991.

30. Hergenroeder AC, Wong WW, Fiorotto ML et al: Total body water and fat-free mass in ballet dancers: comparing isotope dilution and TOBEC, *Med Sci Sports Exerc* 23(5):534-541, 1991.

31. Heymsfield SB, Waki M: Body composition in humans: advances in the development of multicompartment chemical models, *Nutr Rev* 49(4):97-108, 1991.

32. Heyward VH, Jenkins KA, Cook KL et al: Validity of single site and multi-site models for estimating body composition of women using near-infrared interactance, *Am J Human Biol* 4:579-593, 1992.

33. Hoffer EC, Meador CK, Simpson DC: Correlation of whole-body impedance with total body water volume, *J Appl Physiol* 27:531-534, 1969.

34. Jackson AS, Pollock ML: Factor analysis and multivariate scaling of anthropometric variables for the assessment of body composition, *Med Sci Sports Exerc* 8(3):196-203, 1976.

35. Jackson AS, Pollock ML: Generalized equations for predicting body density of men, *Bri J Nutr* 40:497-504, 1978.

36. Jackson AS, Pollock ML, Ward A: Generalized equations for predicting body density of women, *Med Sci Sports Exerc* 12:175-182, 1980.

37. Janz KF, Nielsen DH, Cassidy SL et al: Cross-validation of the Slaughter skinfold equations for children and adolescents, *Med Sci Sports Exerc* 23(9):1070-1076, 1993.

38. Johansson AG, Forslund A, Sjodin A et al: Determination of body composition—a comparison of dual-energy x-ray absorptiometry and hydrodensitometry, *Am J Clin Nutr* 57:323-326, 1993.

39. Katch FI: Practice curves and errors of measurement in estimating underwater weight by hydrostatic weighing, *Med Sci Sports Exerc* 1(40):212-216, 1969.

40. Keys A, Brozek J: Body fat in adult men, *Physiol Rev* 33:245-325, 1953.

41. Kushner RF: Bioelectrical impedance analysis: a review of principles and applications, *J Am Coll Nutr* 11(2):199-209, 1992.

42. Liang MT, Norris S: Effects of skin blood flow and temperature on bioelectrical impedance after exercise, *Med Sci Sports Exerc* 25(11):1231-1239, 1993.

43. Lohman TG: Skinfolds and body density and their relation to body fatness: a review, *Human Biol* 53:181-225, 1981.

44. Lohman TG: Research progress in validation of laboratory methods of assessing body composition, *Med Sci Sports Exerc* 16:596-603, 1984.

45. Lohman TG: Applicability of body composition techniques and constants for children and youths, *Exerc Sports Sci Rev* 14:325-357, 1986.

46. Lohman TG: Advances in body composition assessment, *Current Issues in Exercise Science Series,* monograph number 3, Champaign, Illinois, 1992, Human Kinetics.

47. Lukaski HC, Mendez J, Cohn SH: A comparison of methods of assessment of body composition including neutron activation analysis of total body nitrogen, *Metabolism* 30(8):777-782, 1981.

48. Lukaski HC: Soft tissue composition and bone mineral status: evaluation by dual-energy x-ray absorptiometry, *J Nutr* 123:438-443, 1993.

REFERENCES—Cont'd

49. Marks C, Katch V: Biological and technological variability of residual lung volume and the effect on body fat calculations, *Med Sci Sports Exerc* 18(4):485-488, 1986.

50. Mazess RB, Barden HS, Ohlrich ES: Skeletal and body composition effects of anorexia nervosa, *Am J Clin Nutr* 52:438-441, 1990.

51. McLean KP, Skinner JS: Validity of Futrex-5000 for body composition determination, *Med Sci Sports Exerc* 24(2):253-258, 1992.

52. Meredith CN, Zackin MJ, Frontera WR, Evans WJ: Body composition and aerobic capacity in young and middle-aged endurance-trained men, *Med Sci Sports Exerc* 19(6):557-563, 1987.

53. Metropolitan Life Insurance Company: *1983 height and weight tables announced,* New York, 1983, Metropolitan Life Insurance Company.

54. Morrow JR, Jackson AS, Bradely PW, Hartung GH: Accuracy of measured and predicted residual lung volume on body density measurement, *Med Sci Sport Exerc* 18(6):647-652, 1986.

55. Ortiz O, Russell M, Daley TL et al: Differences in skeletal muscle and bone mineral mass between black and white females and their relevance to estimates of body composition, *Am J Clin Nutr* 55:8-13, 1992.

56. Pierson RN Jr, Wang J, Heymsfield SB et al: Measuring body fat: calibrating the rules: intermethod comparisons in 389 normal Caucasian subjects, *Am J Physiol* 261(24):E103-E108, 1991.

57. Plowman SA, Liu NY, Wells CL: Body composition and sexual maturation in premenarcheal athletes and nonathletes, *Med Sci Sports Exerc* 23(1):23-29, 1991.

58. Quatrochi JA, Hicks VL, Heyward VH et al: *Res Q Exerc Sport* 63(4):402-409, 1992.

59. Ross JG, Pate RR, Lohman TG, Christenson GM: The national children and youth fitness study II: a summary of the findings, *J Phys Educ Recr Dance* 58:51-56, 1987.

60. Schoeller DA: Changes in total body water with age, *Am J Clin Nutr* 50:1176-1181, 1989.

61. Shimokata H, Torbin JD, Muller DC et al: Studies in the distribution of body fat. I. effects of age, sex, and obesity, *J Gerontol* 44:M66-M73, 1989.

62. Sjostrom L, Kvist H, Cederbland A, Tylen U: Determination of total adipose tissue and body fat in women by computed tomography, ^{40}K, and tritium, *Am J Physiol* 250:E736-E745, 1986.

63. Siri WE: Body composition from fluid space and density. In Brozek J, Hanschel A, editors: *Techniques for measuring body composition,* Washington, DC, 1961, National Academy of Science.

64. Sloan AW: Estimation of body fat in young men, *J Appl Physiol* 23:311-315, 1967.

65. Snyder WS, Cook MJ, Nasset ES et al: *Report on the task group on reference man,* Oxford, 1984, Pergamon Press.

66. Timson BF, Coffman JL: Body composition by hydrostatic weighing at total lung capacity and residual volume, *Med Sci Sports Exerc* 16(4):411-414, 1984.

67. Van Loan MD: Bioelectrical impedance analysis to determine fat-free mass, total body water and body fat, *Sports Med* 10(4):205-217, 1990.

68. Van Loan MD, Mayclin PL: Body composition assessment: dual-energy X-ray absorptiometry (DEXA) compared to other methods, *Eur J Clin Nutr* 46:125-130, 1992.

69. Wang ZM, Pierson RN, Heymsfield SB: The five-level model: a new approach to organizing body-composition research, *Am J Clin Nutr* 56:19-28, 1992.

70. Ward DS, Bar-Or O: Role of the physician and physical educator teacher in the treatment of obesity at school, *Pediatrician* 13:44-51, 1986.

71. Wilmore JH, Bergfeld JA: A comparison of sports: physiological and medical aspects. In Strauss RJ, editor: *Sports Med Physiol,* Philadelphia, 1979, Saunders.

72. Wilmore JH, Haskell WL: Body composition and endurance capacity of professional football players, *J Appl Physiol* 33:564-567, 1972.

RECOMMENDED READINGS

■ Bartoli WP, Davis JM, Pate RR et al: Weekly variability in total body water using ^2H_2O dilution in college-age males, *Med Sci Sports Exerc* 25(12):1422-1428, 1993.

■ Bonge D, Donnelly JE: Trials to criteria for hydrostatic weighing at residual volume, *Res Quart Exer Sport* 60(2):176-179, 1989.

■ Bunt JC, Lohman TG, Boileau RA: Impact of total body water fluctuations on estimation of body fat from body density, *Med Sci Sports Exerc* 21(1):96-100, 1989.

■ Bunt JC, Going SB, Lohman TG et al: Variation in bone mineral content and estimated body fat in young adult females, *Med Sci Sports Exerc* 22(5):564-569, 1990.

■ Eckerson JM, Housh TJ, Johnson GO: The validity of visual estimations of percent body fat in lean males, *Med Sci Sports Exerc* 24(5):615-618, 1992.

■ Eckerson JM, Housh TJ, Johnson GO: Validity of bioelectrical impedance equations for estimating fat-free weight in lean males, *Med Sci Sports Exerc* 24(11):1298-1302, 1992.

■ Heymsfield SB, Waki M: Body composition in humans: advances in the development of multicompartment chemical models, *Nutr Rev* 49(4):97-108, 1991.

■ Jackson AS, Pollock ML, Ward A: Generalized equations for predicting body density of men, *Med Sci Sports Exerc* 12:175-182, 1980.

■ Kushner RF: Bioelectrical impedance analysis: a review of principles and applications, *J Am Coll Nutr* 11(2):199-209, 1992.

■ Lohman TG: Advances in body composition assessment. *Current issues in exercise science series,* monograph number 3, Champaign, Illinois, 1992, Human Kinetics.

■ Lukaski HC, Mendez J, Cohn SH: A comparison of methods of assessment of body composition including neutron activation analysis of total body nitrogen, *Metabolism* 30(8):777-782, 1981.

■ Morrow JR, Jackson AS, Bradely PW, Hartung GH: Accuracy of measured and predicted residual lung volume on body density measurement, *Med Sci Sport Exerc* 18(6):647-652, 1986.

■ Timson BF, Coffman JL: Body composition by hydrostatic weighing at total lung capacity and residual volume, *Med Sci Sports Exerc* 16(4):411-414, 1984.

■ Wang ZM, Pierson RN, Heymsfield SB: The five-level model: a new approach to organizing body-composition research, *Am J Clin Nutr* 56:19-28, 1992.

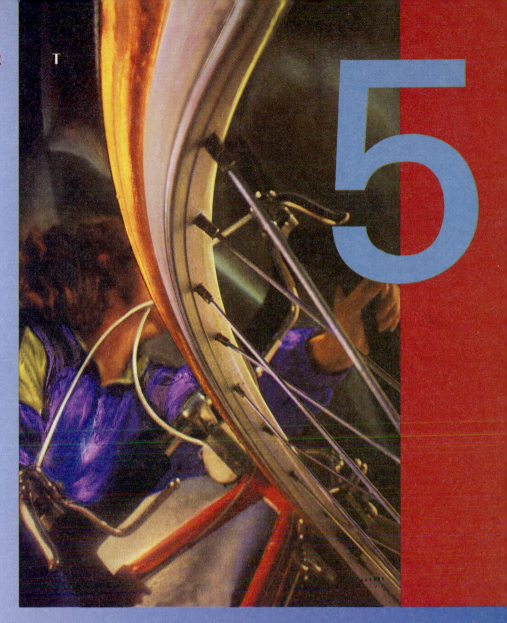

5

Special Topics

Within

Exercise

Physiology

CHAPTER 22

Factors Contributing to Fatigue During Exercise

OBJECTIVES

After studying this chapter you should be able to:

- Explain why fatigue is a general term that requires clarification of the type of exercise performed and the environmental conditions in which it is performed.

- List the different potential causes of fatigue during intense exercise.

- List the different potential causes of fatigue during prolonged exercise.

- Identify the central and peripheral limitations to maximal oxygen consumption.

- Discuss the value of the maximal oxygen consumption (VO_2max) measurement, given the research evidence that certain factors may limit this capacity.

- Identify potential central and peripheral causes of fatigue during prolonged endurance exercise and short-term intense exercise.

KEY TERMS

fatigue

ionization state

muscle fatigue

adenylate charge

phosphorylation potential

ammonia

inosine monophosphate (IMP)

central fatigue

peripheral limitations

central limitations

*J*ust about anyone who exercises has had the experience of reaching a point where he or she cannot continue exercising at a given intensity. The working muscles cannot perform as well, ventilation seems inadequate, and it takes more and more conscious effort simply to keep moving. Whether this occurs during intense exercise (e.g., mountain biking up a long, steep slope) or prolonged exercise (e.g., after 4 hours of hiking with minimal fluid and carbohydrate intake), the word fatigue is used to describe the decline in exercise tolerance. General use of the word *fatigue* is incorrect because the conditions that predispose an individual to the development of fatigue are specific to the exercise and environmental conditions and result in a specific set of circumstances that impair exercise tolerance. Thus many types of fatigue are possible during exercise. Because of this, the term "fatigue" must be qualified by the specific characteristics of the exercise stress. In addition, because fatigue develops over time, it is a process, not an endpoint.

Fatigue may be defined by anatomic site (e.g., neuromuscular fatigue, central nervous system [CNS] fatigue, or skeletal muscle fatigue) or by function (e.g., electrochemical fatigue, metabolic fatigue, fatigue of energy-contractile coupling, or fatigue resulting from hypoglycemia, substrate depletion, hyperthermia, or dehydration). This multiplicity of the types of fatigue that can occur under different exercise conditions requires a knowledge of muscle contraction and metabolism, systems physiology, and exercise nutrition to understand the causes, development, tolerance, and reversal of fatigue. This chapter demonstrates that fatigue is a process that develops over time, identifies the different types of fatigue that can arise during exercise, and presents the research findings that have attempted to explain the mechanisms causing fatigue.

Main Types of Fatigue During Exercise

*A*pplying muscle biochemistry to muscle energy metabolism during exercise (Chapters 4 and 10) reveals that both the intensity and the duration of exercise determine the reactions that predominantly regenerate adenosine triphosphate (ATP), and the metabolic and systemic events that may lead to fatigue (Table 22.1). For this reason the following sections are organized according to the type of exercise performed. In these sections special circumstances that can alter the development of fatigue are presented.

Short-Term, Intense Exercise

During short-term, intense exercise, continued muscle contraction relies on a high rate of ATP regeneration from the dephosphorylation of creatine phosphate (CrP) and an increased flux of glucose through glycolysis. Potential contributors to muscle fatigue during this type of exercise could be related to *muscle energy production,* such as a decline in the muscle ATP concentration, creatine phosphate depletion, or glycogen depletion. Fatigue could also be related to the *production and accumulation of metabolites,* such as lactate and acidosis, or it could be related to impaired functioning of the *electrochemical events of muscle contraction and relaxation.* Finally, there is evidence of a *central nervous system* contribution to fatigue during intense exercise.

---

fatigue (fa′**teeg**)

in relation to exercise, fatigue can be generally defined as the inability to continue to exercise at a given intensity

TABLE 22.1

Functional limitations and proposed causes of fatigue during different exercise intensities and durations

EXERCISE	FUNCTIONAL LIMITATIONS	CAUSES OF FATIGUE
Intense (< 30 sec)	CrP depletion; inadequate rate of ATP synthesis	↓ CrP, ↑ ADP
Intense (30 sec–10 min)	CrP depletion; inadequate rate of ATP synthesis; acidosis	↓ CrP, ↑ ADP, ↓ pH, ↑ ammonia, electrochemical disturbances
Low intensity (< 90 min)	Hyperthermia; muscle damage	
Low intensity (> 90 min)	Low muscle glycogen; hypoglycemia; muscle damage; low liver glycogen; dehydration; hyperthermia	Inadequate carbohydrate stores, electrochemical disturbances, CNS and cardiovascular impairment

Energy Production

Creatine phosphate and ATP depletion.

Chapters 4 and 10 detail muscle metabolic reactions and how they change to maintain the muscles' ATP concentration during repeated muscle contraction. Use of creatine phosphate in muscle is a means of regenerating ATP at high rates, thus preserving the muscle ATP concentration. What has research revealed about the relationship between decreasing concentrations of creatine phosphate and muscle ATP and the development of muscular fatigue during intense exercise? Numerous studies have reported decreases in exercise performance, or the force development of skeletal muscle, when creatine phosphate stores decrease.[*] These fatigue responses do not occur just for simple depletion of creatine phosphate but rather when the CrP concentration declines to less than half its original resting concentration (Figure 22.1). Logically, this would mean that:

1. The fatigue mechanism is not due to creatine phosphate reduction, since adequate creatine phosphate remains despite the symptoms of muscle fatigue.
2. The lowered creatine phosphate concentration may accompany a reduced capacity for ATP regeneration, which in turn may be associated with muscle fatigue.
3. Other metabolites produced during creatine phosphate use may be associated with muscle fatigue.

Data on muscle ATP concentrations during intense voluntary exercise indicate that these concentrations remain stable or decline only minimally during intense exercise to muscular fatigue (Figure 22.1). These results have been confirmed through phosphorus magnetic resonance sphehroscopy (^{31}P MRS).[4,6] In contrast, research involving artificial electrical stimulation of animal or human muscle has shown reductions in muscle ATP concentrations when creatine phosphate stores are low.[14]

Research into ATP concentrations during intense exercise indicates that factors besides the decrease in CrP concentrations must contribute to muscular fatigue.

Glycogen depletion.

Prolonged, intense exercise is associated with a high rate of glycogenolysis. Interestingly, this rate declines during continued intense exercise,[58-60] as explained in Chapter 9. Nevertheless, low muscle glycogen stores may limit the substrate available for glycolysis and impair muscle contraction. For example, research on muscle metabolites from single muscle fibers after intense exercise indicated that muscle fibers low in glycogen had greater concentrations of inosine monophosphate (IMP), which indicates increased metabolic strain when muscle glycogen was low.[6,47] However, it is not known whether extremely low muscle glycogen concentrations (<20 mmol/kg wet weight) impair intense exercise performance in humans, or whether fiber type–specific depletion of muscle glycogen occurs during intense exercise.

Production and Accumulation of Metabolites

As muscle metabolism increases, many by-products increase in concentration, and several of these have been implicated in the development of muscle fatigue. The most notable is lactate, but free protons also increase, as indicated by decreases in pH and increases in muscle free inorganic phosphate, adenosine diphosphate (ADP), and ammonia.[*]

Lactate production and muscle acidosis.

Large increases in carbohydrate flux through glycolysis increase the production of lactate.[65,67] Of course, if the oxygen supply to skeletal muscle is reduced, the production of lactate increases. During intense exercise, in which the forceful, frequent contraction of muscle constricts blood vessels and occludes blood flow, both an increased glycolytic rate and ischemic hypoxia are involved in increasing lactate production.[15]

The increase in lactate production and accumulation in muscle has been interpreted as a contributor to fatigue, independent of the increase in acidosis. The proposed mechanism is based on the theory that the negative charge of the lactate molecule changes the membrane potentials within the mus-

---

[*]References 4, 6, 14, 25, 33, 69.

[*]References 10, 15, 31, 33–35, 65, 67.

The change in creatine phosphate (CrP), ADP, free hydrogen ions ([H+]), and ATP during intense muscle contractions to muscular fatigue. The decrease in CrP serves to retain a consistent ATP concentration. The increase in each of ADP and [H+] coincide with the full range of the decrease in muscle force production or the increase in muscle fatigue.

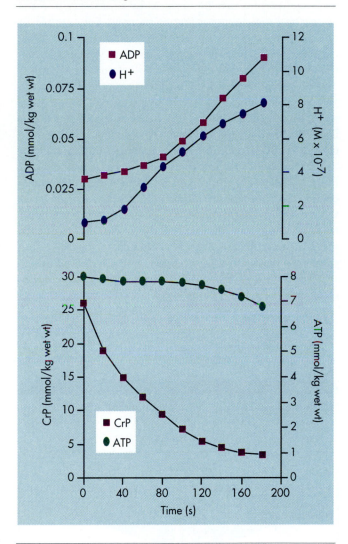

cle fibers and in the sarcolemma surrounding each muscle fiber. This explanation is discussed further in the section on electrochemical events.

The muscle acidosis that results from lactate production has been the main reason that researchers and students alike have misinterpreted data and designated lactate as the cause of muscle fatigue. However, as previously explained, the aspect of lactate production that most relates to muscle and systemic symptoms of fatigue is the acidosis and not lactate accumulation. During intense exercise, both lactate and pro-

tons leave the muscle fiber and are removed by the circulation.[31,35] During short bursts of high-intensity exercise, muscle lactate accumulates to higher concentrations than are present in the blood, which provides a concentration gradient from which lactate is facilitatively transported from the cell.[31,51] Free protons leave the cell, resulting in a blood acid-base disturbance. The blood bicarbonate–carbon dioxide system is the main buffer of these protons; however, plasma proteins and the movement of electrolytes between the vascular and extravascular spaces are also involved in establishing the magnitude of the blood acid-base disturbance.[35]

The increased intracellular acidity can impair muscle contraction through several processes. The myosin ATPase enzymes required to catalyze the reactions involved in the Na^+/K^+ pump, Ca^{++} pump, and muscle contraction can have an altered **ionization state** of their amino acid side chains. The location of these amino acids may influence the enzymes' catalytic rate. This effect has been reported in research on the in vitro regulation and function of phosphofructokinase, phosphorylase, and the ATPase enzymes.[16,39,48,54] Muscle biopsy research and studies using ^{31}P MRS have shown that muscle pH can drop to values below 6.4 during intense exercise.[12] In addition, other studies have shown increases in the ratio of fructose-6-phosphate to fructose-1,6-bisphosphate after intense exercise to exhaustion, as explained in Chapter 10, and this result is interpreted as an imbalance between the rates of glycogenolysis and glycolysis resulting from a pH inhibition of phosphofructokinase.[10,35,62,64]

Additional evidence of the important role of acidosis in fatigue during intense exercise is the fact that ingestion of sodium bicarbonate, which increases the buffering capacity of the blood, reduces perceived exertion and delays fatigue during intense, intermittent exercise.[72] (See Chapter 19.)

The increased acidosis of the blood during intense exercise elicits systemic responses (e.g., feelings of nausea and increased ventilation) and these complications may contribute to fatigue via central mechanisms during more prolonged bouts of intense exercise.

Increased ADP. In 1978, Dawson[14] applied ^{31}P MRS to the study of fatigue during repeated electrical stimulation of anaerobic frog muscle. As creatine phosphate declined, so did muscle contractile force. However, muscle force decrements continued despite a plateau in creatine phosphate at relatively low concentrations. Muscle ATP stores decreased marginally, and muscle ADP increased. In fact, the only metabolites that changed in concert with muscle fatigue to complete contractile failure were increases in muscle ADP and free hydrogen ions. These researchers interpreted the findings to indi-

ionization state

the charge characteristics of a molecule; usually used for amino acid molecules within proteins

cate that an increasing muscle ADP concentration may impair muscle metabolic and contractile functioning and therefore be the eventual cause of extreme **muscle fatigue** (see Figure 22.1).

Debate continues as to whether the ADP concentration alone, or the resultant decreases in the **adenylate charge** and **phosphorylation potential** of the cell, induces the development of muscle fatigue (see Chapter 4).[3]

Increased Pi.   An increase in the concentration of free inorganic phosphate (Pi) has been shown to induce muscle fatigue.[39,48,71] The mechanism of this effect is believed to be a decreased sensitivity of the contractile proteins to calcium.[48] However, because fatigue continues despite a return to normal Pi concentrations, the independent role of Pi in inducing muscle fatigue may be minor.

Increased ammonia and inosine monophosphate.   The increased activity of adenosine monophosphate (AMP) dehydrogenase during intracellular acidosis increases the production of **ammonia** and **inosine monophosphate (IMP)**. Ammonia is known to impair cellular function, but the exact mechanism is unclear. The increase in muscle IMP has been interpreted to reflect a decreasing adenine nucleotide pool, which in turn may reflect a decreasing adenylate charge.[3]

Electrochemical Events of Muscle Contraction and Relaxation

During repeated dynamic muscle contraction, the muscle fibers of recruited motor units must be able to restore the membrane potential of the sarcolemma and internal excitable membranes in less than 500 ms. For repeated intense and rapid (powerful) muscle contractions, this duration can be considerably less and can continue for several minutes. Evidence shows that under these stressful conditions, the sarcolemma's ability to depolarize and repolarize repeatedly is reduced. For example, electromyography (EMG) results indicate a reduced conduction velocity during muscle fatigue stemming from intense exercise.[37] These findings are interpreted to reflect an impairment in the response of the muscle fibers' excitable membranes to depolarization or repolarization, or both.

Factors that contribute to the reduced excitability of the skeletal muscle membranes are the efflux of potassium from the muscle during contraction,[26] which in turn disrupts the membrane potentials; the acidotic impairment of the ATPases necessary to restore concentrations of intracellular and sarcoplasmic reticulum Ca^{++} and the normal resting membrane potential[16]; the contribution of the negativity of lactate, which accumulates inside skeletal muscle; and diminished neuromuscular function.[30]

Central Nervous System

The role of the central nervous system in muscular fatigue during intense exercise was identified as early as the late 19th century.[39] Greater muscular force occurred when a muscle was electrically stimulated than from maximal voluntary contractions. However, subsequent research has contradicted these early findings; for intense exercise lasting less than 60 seconds, maximal force values have been shown to equal artificial electrically stimulated maximal muscle contractions.[30] Despite these findings, intense exercise performed for longer periods may be impaired by an inability to focus on maximal muscle motor unit recruitment. For example, in one study in which the subjects' level of motivation was varied, exercise was terminated earlier if there was no external motivation than if the subjects had an external motivation.[39] The mechanism of **central fatigue** lies somewhere in the processes of formulating movement patterns, transmitting them throughout the cortex, cerebellar, and midbrain nuclei involved in refinement, and finally synapsing with the specific efferent motor nerve cell bodies within the spinal cord.

There has been evidence of a reduced rate of motor unit firing at the level of the spinal cord during continued muscle contraction to fatigue.[30] However, additional evidence has shown that afferent output from muscle provides inhibitive feedback to the motor unit cell bodies within the spinal cord that matches recruitment and summation to the decreasing contractile potential of the muscle.[30]

The rating of perceived exertion (RPE) was initially based on a heart rate response to exercise. However, since the

---

FIGURE 22.2

The potential contributing factors to muscle fatigue during intense exercise.

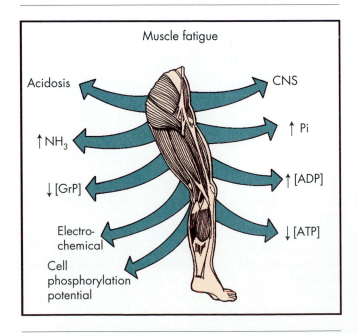

TABLE 22.2

Proposed biochemical mediators of muscle fatigue

MEDIATOR	CONSEQUENCES		
	ELECTRICAL	BIOCHEMICAL	MECHANICAL
↑ [H⁺] (hydrogen)	Prolonged repolarization	↓ Glycolytic flux	↓ Contractile force, impaired Ca^{++} pump, ↓ rate of relaxation
↓ CrP (creatine phosphate)		↓ Ca^{++} uptake into sarcoplasmic reticulum (SR)	↓ Rate of relaxation
↓ ATP (adenosine triphosphate)		↓ Rate of ATP supply	↓ Contractile force
↑ ADP (adenosine diphosphate)		↑ Glycolytic flux, ↑ respiration, ↓ adenylate charge	↓ Contractile force, ↓ rate of relaxation, ↑ mitochondrial relaxation
↑ Pi (inorganic phosphate)		↑ Glycolytic flux, ↑ mitochondrial respiration, ↑ mitochondrial Ca^{++}	↓ Contractile force, ↓ Ca^{++} sensitivity
↑ Na⁺ic (intracellular sodium)	↓ Membrane potential	↑ Na^+–K^+ ATPase activity	↓ Contractile tension
↑ K⁺ec (extracellular potassium)	Prolonged action potential		
↑ Ca^{++}ic (intracellular calcium)		↑ Mitochondrial respiration ↑ Uncoupling of oxidative phosphorylation	↑ Rate of contraction
↓ Muscle Po₂ (partial pressure of oxygen)		↓ Rate of mitochondrial respiration, ↑ glycolysis	
Muscle damage	???	↑ Ca^{++} leakage	↓ Contractile tension ?

Data from Vollestad NK, Sejersted OM: Biochemical correlates of fatigue, *Eur J Appl Physiol* 57:336-347, 1988.

RPE is a conscious rating of effort, it is based on the central processing of central and peripheral cues of fatigue. Modifying either central or peripheral factors affects the RPE independent of heart rate involvement. The evidence proving the role of the central nervous system in fatigue and the termination of exercise has made the science of sports psychology and the sports psychologist important ingredients in the success of many professional athletes involved in intense exercise.

Summary of Fatigue During Intense Exercise

The potential contributing factors to fatigue during intense exercise are presented in Figure 22.2 and Table 22.2. CNS, spinal cord, neuromuscular junction, and muscle membrane excitability; intracellular decreases in ATP regeneration capabilities; and metabolite accumulation all contribute to diminished exercise performance. The more intense and short-term the exercise, the greater the contribution from peripheral or muscle-based factors to the development of fatigue.

muscle fatigue
fatigue caused by changes in the functioning of skeletal muscle

adenylate charge
the ratio between the phosphate bound to adenylate molecules that can be used in chemical transfer, to the total adenylate phosphate molecule concentration

phosphorylation potential
the ratio of ATP to ADP

ammonia (a-mo'ni-ah)
a by-product of the AMP deaminase reaction in which IMP is formed

inosine monophosphate (IMP)
the product of the AMP deaminase reaction

central fatigue
fatigue caused by changes in the CNS processing and execution of motor patterns

Prolonged Submaximal Exercise

During prolonged exercise, fatigue can also be felt when muscle concentrations of metabolites produced from metabolism remain close to resting values. Under most circumstances the fatigue experienced during prolonged exercise arises from depletion of energy substrates. However, depending on environmental and nutritional considerations, the development of hyperthermia and dehydration can exacerbate the development of fatigue.

Substrate Supply

Research evidence on the importance of muscle glycogen stores to prolonged exercise was presented in Chapter 17. However, the mechanism or mechanisms that induce fatigue when muscle glycogen concentrations are reduced to low levels remains unclear. Data from the research on carbohydrate ingestion during exercise help clarify the cause of fatigue under low-carbohydrate conditions. Ironically, despite a person's inability to continue to exercise when hypoglycemic, the return of blood glucose concentrations to above normal values allows further exercise to be performed, yet fatigue still occurs 20 to 30 minutes later when blood glucose concentrations are normal. An initial interpretation of these findings was that the hypoglycemia that results during low muscle glycogen conditions is what causes fatigue during prolonged exercise. Additional metabolic factors in fatigue are implied by the evidence that when carbohydrate is ingested late in exercise, a time at which muscle glycogen stores are low, carbohydrate oxidation by the skeletal muscles increases and exercise can be continued for another 30 minutes.[11]

The total supply and availability of triglyceride stores in skeletal muscle are unknown. It is assumed that these stores would not be exhausted during prolonged exercise and therefore would not be involved in fatigue during prolonged exercise. Clearly, both central and peripheral metabolic factors contribute to fatigue when muscle glycogen and blood glucose concentrations are low.

Hyperthermia

The heat produced by the body's skeletal muscle mass at rest is less than 60 Kcal/hour[44]. During intense exercise (e.g., exercise close to or above the lactate threshold), the rate of heat production can increase to over 1000 Kcal/hour in highly trained endurance athletes. Of course, greater heat production can occur during extremely intense exercise, but these rates pose minimal danger in the development of hyperthermia because of the muscular fatigue that develops, resulting in short exercise duration. The more endurance-trained individual has a greater risk of hyperthermia, because this person can sustain a higher exercise intensity and therefore a higher rate of heat production for a long period.[46]

Dissipation of heat from muscle depends on increased perfusion of the muscle by blood. Despite rapid increases in muscle blood flow during exercise, heat is still stored in skeletal muscle, as indicated in Figure 22.3. Usually the body's thermoregulatory adaptations, which increase evaporative cooling, prevent continued increases in muscle and body core temperatures. However, when metabolic heat production is too great for the body's thermoregulatory responses, muscle and core temperatures can continue to rise resulting in core temperatures that can exceed 40° C (104° F). If exercise continues, muscle temperatures obviously climb higher still, although for ethical reasons human research has not been able to quantify these values.

FIGURE 22.3

The increase in muscle and core temperatures during intense short-term exercise and prolonged exercise.

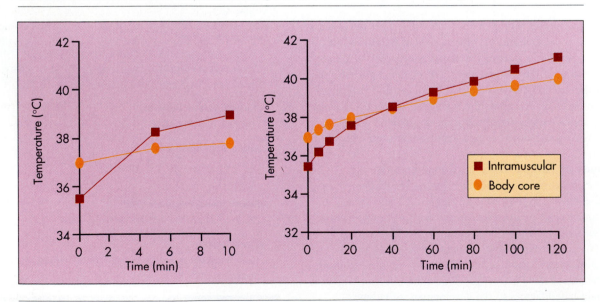

The dehydration-related aspects of fatigue during hyperthermia are presented in the next section. For now, our concerns are whether there is evidence that increased intramuscular temperature alone induces muscle fatigue, and whether increasing core temperature induces CNS fatigue.

In vitro research has demonstrated that increasing cellular temperatures can partly uncouple oxidative phosphorylation.[43] This is powerful evidence of a fatigue-causing mechanism, since it would reduce the rate of ATP regeneration from mitochondrial respiration for a given intensity, which in turn would increase dependence on glycolytic- and creatine phosphate–based ATP regeneration. Not surprisingly, evidence exists that an increasing body temperature increases the muscles' reliance on muscle glycogen as an energy substrate.[17] However, whether this increased reliance prematurely depletes muscle glycogen and contributes to fatigue is unknown.

Continued increases in the body's core temperature can lead to permanent damage to the hypothalamus. Because the hypothalamus is involved in integrating the body's peripheral endocrine and metabolic responses to CNS regulation, the involvement of the central nervous system in detecting hyperthermia and eliciting behavioral responses, such as terminating exercise, must also be considered in this fatigue response.

Dehydration

Figure 22.4 illustrates the change in heart rate, perceived exertion, and plasma volume during prolonged exercise to exhaustion when no fluid is ingested.[5] The increased temperature and dehydration caused premature exhaustion, which seemed to coincide with a heart rate close to maximal even though the oxygen demand of the exercise remained relatively low. These data, like other data published on this topic, indicate a central cardiovascular component to dehydration-induced fatigue.

Blood Flow and Oxygen Transport

Since the late 1980s, evidence has been mounting that blood flow may be limiting to skeletal muscle and may influence the metabolic function in skeletal muscle. For example, Brechue et al.[8] demonstrated that increasing blood flow to contracting skeletal muscle in a hind-limb animal model increased maximum oxygen consumption (VO_2max). In contrast, Lundgren et al.[38] have shown that increased blood flow delays fatigue without increasing oxygen consumption. The interpretation of these results in animal in vitro research is that increased blood flow can improve muscle function by oxygen-dependent and oxygen-independent mechanisms. The oxygen-independent mechanism is thought to involve the removal of metabolites that may influence muscle fatigue (e.g., hydrogen ions and ammonia).

Evidence also points to a blood flow limitation on human skeletal muscle during maximal exercise.[52,53] The details of cardiovascular limitations during exercise are discussed in Chapter 11. The important concerns for the development of fatigue are whether the compression of blood vessels during moderate to intense contractions contributes to peripheral markers of fatigue, and whether the body's cardiovascular regulation prevents maximal perfusion of contracting musculature.

Summary of Fatigue During Prolonged Submaximal Exercise

The factors that contribute to fatigue during prolonged exercise are illustrated in Figure 22.5. Skeletal muscle sub-

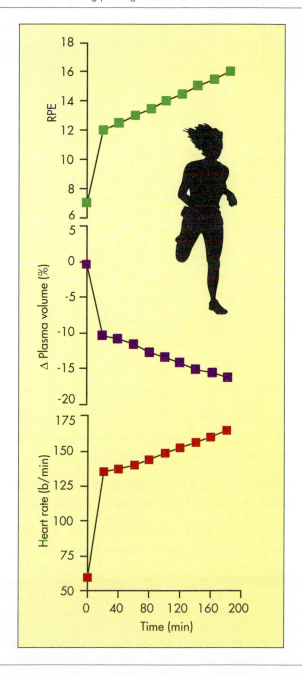

FIGURE 22.4

The change in heart rate, rate of perceived exertion (RPE), and plasma volume during prolonged exercise to exhaustion.

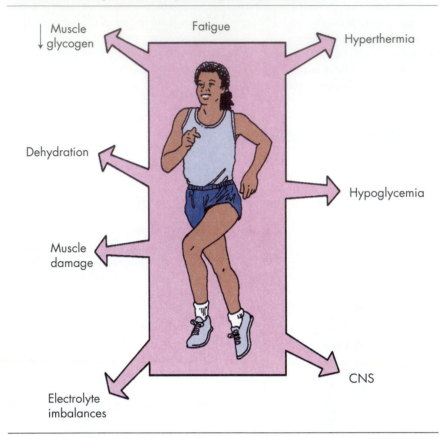

FIGURE 22.5

Potential contributing factors to fatigue during prolonged exercise.

strates, cardiovascular function, and the development of hyperthermia are involved in the fatigue experienced during prolonged exercise. Despite these factors, when carbohydrate is ingested to stabilize blood glucose and retard dehydration and hyperthermia, fatigue still occurs.[11] This is evidence that additional factors influence the development of fatigue, and it may indicate the importance of CNS, neuromuscular junction, or muscle electrochemical abnormalities in this process.

Limitations to Maximal Oxygen Consumption

Debate continues over the physiologic limitations on cellular and total body oxygen consumption during exercise.[20,58] The measure of VO_2max involves the body's ability to ventilate the lungs; exchange oxygen and carbon dioxide; transport oxygen and carbon dioxide; exchange these gases at the level of the tissues; and utilize the oxygen within the mitochondria of the contracting musculature (Figure 22.6). The measure of VO_2max dates back to 1923, when Hill and Lupton[24] measured oxygen consumption relative to blood lactate accumulation. Other researchers demonstrated that athletes have remarkably high VO_2max values,[51] and the measure was quickly accepted, even though no evidence was available for what determined VO_2max. Obviously, the need to understand this measure was recognized, and since the 1920s, research has produced two competing theories, **peripheral limitations** and **central limitations.** Furthermore, some researchers have questioned whether such a measure as maximal oxygen consumption really exists and whether interpretations of function relative to VO_2max have any meaning.[45] The following sections present the research evidence supporting the explanations of limitations to VO_2max, as well as arguments that question the meaning of this measurement. It will become obvious that the deductive reasoning used in interpreting the following research findings is that if one component of the total system can be modified and can change VO_2max, this factor must be limiting to VO_2max in

The physiologic and biochemic determinants of VO_2max, indicating peripheral and central components.

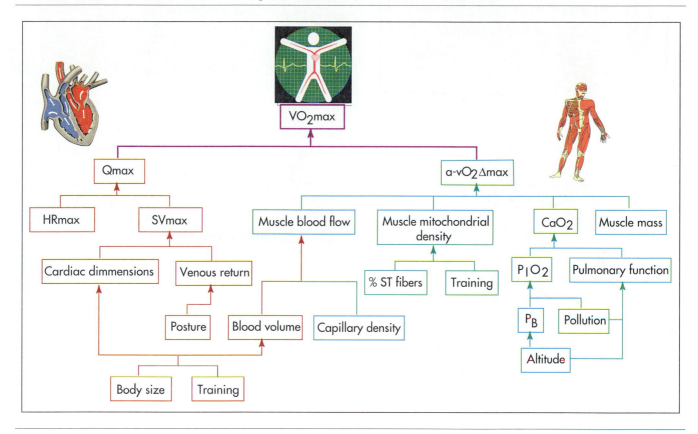

vivo. Although it is difficult to argue against this interpretation, similar evidence is reported to support both peripheral and central limitation.

Peripheral Limitations

The peripheral limitations on VO_2max involve factors at the muscle level, which include structural and functional issues such as capillarization, neuromuscular and sarcolemmal function, muscle fiber type, oxygen extraction capabilities, and oxygen utilization capacities of the mitochondria (see Figure 22.6).

Research done from the 1950s to the 1970s demonstrated the remarkable plasticity of human skeletal muscle in response to endurance training.[19] Peripheral adaptations such as increased mitochondrial density, increased capillarization, and increased fast-twitch oxidative muscle fibers were more numerous and greater in magnitude than the known central cardiovascular or neuromuscular adaptations to exercise. This general comparison, and the functional belief that if exercise were limited by the weakest link in a chain, this link would be improved the most from training, led scientists to specu-

late that peripheral function limited maximal rates of oxygen consumption in skeletal muscle.

In 1976 a classic study by Saltin et al.[59] involving one-legged cycle ergometer exercise and training revealed that oxygen consumption (VO_2) increased only after training in the trained leg (Figure 22.7). If central adaptations were the important determinants of VO_2max, improvements should have been seen in exercise tolerance, oxygen consumption, and delay in fatigue in the nontrained leg. The belief that peripheral factors limited maximal oxygen consumption predominated at this time.

More recent evidence of peripheral limitation has been obtained through electromyography.[20] During cycle ergome-

peripheral limitations
conditions in skeletal muscle that reduce the cells' ability to take up and use oxygen during exercise

central limitations
cardiorespiratory or CNS functions or conditions that limit skeletal muscles' ability to consume oxygen during exercise

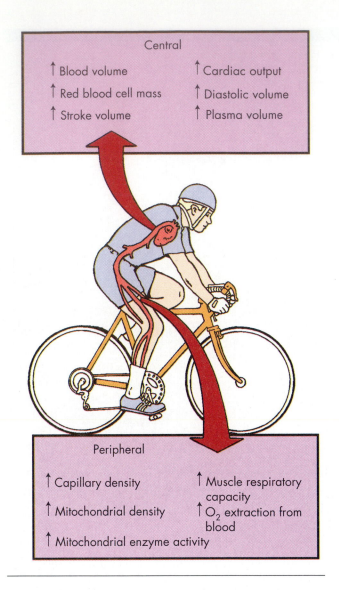

Central

↑ Blood volume   ↑ Cardiac output

↑ Red blood cell mass   ↑ Diastolic volume

↑ Stroke volume   ↑ Plasma volume

Peripheral

↑ Capillary density   ↑ Muscle respiratory capacity

↑ Mitochondrial density   ↑ O₂ extraction from blood

↑ Mitochondrial enzyme activity

FIGURE 22.7

Peripheral and central changes during single-leg cycle ergometry before and after endurance training.

try the muscles of the hip, thigh, and lower leg contribute differently to the movement of cycling as exercise intensity increases. Despite the involvement of several muscles, the overriding metabolic importance of the gluteus maximus during increasing exercise intensities may bias fatigue to metabolic factors within this muscle. Because muscle biopsy research is based on samples from the vastus lateralis, the metabolic state and level of fatigue in the gluteus maximus are unknown during incremental cycle ergometry.

Central Limitations

The central limitations on VO_2max include factors within the central nervous system and the systemic circulation, such as arousal, cardiac function, blood volume, and oxygen transport capacities (see Figure 22.7).

Early research supporting a central limitation on VO_2max dates back to the 1920s. Researchers observed the reduced heart rate in athletes compared with nonathletes for a given intensity of exercise and speculated that endurance-trained athletes had an increased stroke volume, increased maximal cardiac output, and increased heart mass. These speculations were supported by animal research, in which

FIGURE 22.8

The cardiovascular limitations during combined exercise of the upper and lower body musculature.

Problems

1. Active muscle mass is too large
2. Decreased muscle blood flow

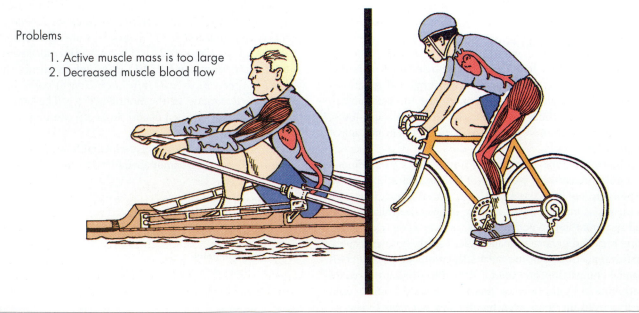

training rats increased the hypertrophy of the heart. In addition, research on the cardiovascular response to arm exercise combined with leg exercise[60] revealed the limitations of cardiac output and blood flow redistribution when an increased muscle mass was exercised (Figure 22.8). These findings have been replicated in more recent research.[70] The inability to maximally perfuse leg musculature alone has been theorized by Rowell[52] and experimentally documented.[53,70] For well-trained individuals the body cannot transport enough blood to a large working muscle mass without compromising systemic blood pressures and blood flow to the remainder of the body. Consequently, the vessels supplying the contracting muscle must become vasoconstricted, as explained in Chapter 11. Based on this research, the peripheral muscle metabolic markers of fatigue may result partly from the inability to maximally perfuse the tissue with blood.

Other evidence exists of a central limitation on VO_2max. The use of sophisticated methods to evaluate central cardiovascular function and systemic and peripheral limb blood flow (e.g., echocardiography and Doppler flowmetry) has shown positive relationships between heart size, ventricular volumes, and cardiorespiratory endurance (VO_2max). Similarly, endurance training increases ventricular volumes, blood volume, and erythrocyte mass.

The importance of red blood cell content and blood oxygen-carrying capacity in the measuring of VO_2max has been documented time and again by research involving reinfusion of red blood cells into the circulation *(erythrocythemia)*. For example, Spriet et al.[61] reinfused different volumes of red cells and demonstrated that VO_2max increased when more than 3 U of red cells was infused (Figure 22.9). Evidence also exists that infusing saline alone can increase central cardiovascular function and improve VO_2max.[13]

Summary of Peripheral and Central Limitations

The body's maximal ability to consume oxygen appears to be determined by the amount of oxygen delivered to contracting muscle. Increasing oxygen delivery by increasing maximal blood flow, or increasing the blood's oxygen-carrying capacity increases VO_2max. These results indicate that the muscles' ability to extract and utilize oxygen exceeds the body's ability to supply them with oxygen. This fact has been documented in research on the adaptability of human muscle to endurance exercise, which showed that muscle mitochondrial density continued to increase in trained skeletal muscle even though muscle VO_2max did not increase.[21]

The interpretation of muscle fatigue based on metabolic versus oxygen provision capacities is understandable when the kinetic principles used in the study of enzyme kinetics are applied. Both substrate (rate of oxygen delivery) and enzyme (muscle oxidative capacity) factors can alter VO_2. Increasing oxidative capacity increases VO_2max, as documented by the long history of exercise-training studies. Increasing oxygen delivery also increases VO_2. These two facts are logical, and neither argument can be used in isola-

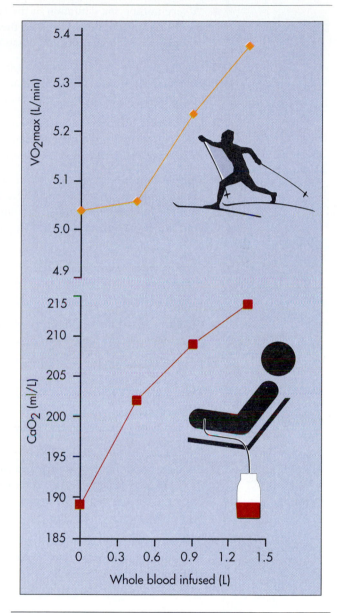

FIGURE 22.9

The changes in the blood oxygen carrying capacity and VO_2max during different quantities of erythrocythemia.

tion as evidence of a limitation on VO_2max. Thus the impressive evidence of a central limitation comes from the decreases in VO_2max that occur with large increases in the muscle mass exercised. The combination of several muscles and tissues demanding increased blood flow (muscle and skin) and the need to perform numerous functions of increased blood flow (oxygen delivery, thermoregulation, and blood pressure regulation) limits cardiovascular function during exhaustive exercise. This is especially true for endurance-trained individuals, who also show a decline in arterial oxygen saturation (see Chapter 12).

SUMMARY

- A very nonspecific definition of the term **fatigue** is development of the inability to continue to exercise at a given intensity. However, there are many causes of fatigue, and the main determinants differ depending on the intensity and duration of exercise, as well as environmental conditions.

- During intense exercise, creatine phosphate declines and the force development of skeletal muscle decreases, yet muscle ATP concentrations remain stable. Consequently, other factors besides the decrease in CrP and the rate of ATP regeneration must contribute to muscular fatigue.

- Low muscle glycogen stores may limit substrate available for glycolysis and impair muscle contraction. Although there is no research to support this theory, no study has evaluated whether extremely low muscle glycogen concentrations (<20 mmol/kg wet weight) impair intense exercise performance in humans.

- During intense exercise, in which forceful, frequent contraction of muscle constricts blood vessels and occludes blood flow, both an increased glycolytic rate and transient ischemic hypoxia are involved in increasing lactate production. The muscle acidosis that results from lactate production is more involved with the development of muscle fatigue than lactate itself.

- During intense exercise, increased intracellular acidity can impair muscle contraction by altering the **ionization state** of amino acid side chains, which in turn can influence the activity of enzymes involved in energy metabolism, muscle contraction, and calcium flux within the cell, and the electrolyte distributions of the excitable membranes of the muscle cell.

- Ingestion of sodium bicarbonate, which increases the buffering capacity of the blood, reduces perceived exertion and delays fatigue during intense intermittent exercise.

- Based on research using ^{31}P MRS, the only metabolites that increase in concert with muscle fatigue to complete contractile failure are muscle ADP and free hydrogen ions. Thus increased muscle ADP concentrations may impair muscle metabolic and contractile function and therefore may be the eventual cause of extreme **muscle fatigue.** Debate continues as to whether the ADP concentration alone or the resultant decreases in the **adenylate charge** and **phosphorylation potential** of the cell induce the fatigue.

- An increase in free inorganic phosphate (Pi) has been shown to induce muscle fatigue. The mechanism of this effect is believed to be a decreased sensitivity of the contractile proteins to calcium. However, since fatigue continues despite the return to normal Pi concentrations, the independent role of Pi in inducing muscle fatigue may be minor.

- The increased activity of AMP dehydrogenase during intracellular acidosis increases the production of **ammonia** and **inosine monophosphate (IMP).** Ammonia is known to impair cellular function, but it is unclear exactly how this mechanism works. The increase in muscle IMP has been interpreted to reflect a decreasing adenine nucleotide pool, which in turn may reflect a decreasing adenylate charge.

- Factors that contribute to the decreased excitability of skeletal muscle membranes are the efflux of K^+ from the muscle during contraction, the acidotic impairment to the ATPases necessary to restore intracellular and sarcoplasmic reticulum Ca^{++} concentrations and the normal resting membrane potential, and decreased neuromuscular function.

- Intense exercise that lasts less than 60 seconds has been shown to result in maximal force values that equal artificial electrically stimulated maximal muscle contractions, indicating no involvement of CNS limitations in intense muscle contractions. However, for more prolonged intense exercise, or when altering the level of subjects' motivation, exercise is terminated earlier without an external motivation than with external motivation, suggesting a role for **central fatigue.**

- During prolonged exercise, fatigue can also be experienced when muscle concentrations of metabolites produced by metabolism remain close to resting values. The fatigue experienced during prolonged exercise involves depletion of energy substrates and environmental and nutritional considerations.

■ Prolonged exercise performance declines when muscle glycogen concentrations are low. The mechanism for this fatigue is believed to be the hypoglycemia that accompanies low muscle and liver glycogen concentrations, and this theory is supported by research showing that fatigue is delayed when carbohydrate solutions are ingested during exercise.

■ In vitro research has demonstrated that increasing cellular temperatures can partly uncouple oxidative phosphorylation. This is powerful evidence of a fatigue-causing mechanism, since it would reduce the rate of ATP regeneration from mitochondrial respiration for a given intensity, which in turn would increase dependence on glycolytic- and creatine phosphate–based ATP regeneration.

■ Since the late 1980s, evidence has been mounting that blood flow may be limiting to skeletal muscle and may influence the metabolic function in skeletal muscle. This limitation involves the delivery of oxygen and an oxygen-independent role for perfusion in the removal of metabolites from the contracting muscle.

■ Two competing theories have been advanced to explain limitations on VO_2max, **peripheral limitations** and **central limitations.** Peripheral limitations include factors at the muscle level, including structural and functional elements such as capillarization, neuromuscular and sarcolemmal function, muscle fiber type, oxygen extraction capabilities, and oxygen utilization capacities of the mitochondria.

■ The central limitations on VO_2max include factors within the central nervous system and the systemic circulation, such as arousal, cardiac function, blood volume, and oxygen transport capacities. Cardiovascular research has documented that well-trained individuals cannot transport enough blood to a large working muscle mass without compromising systemic blood pressures and blood flow to the rest of the body. Consequently, the peripheral muscle metabolic markers of fatigue may result in part from the inability to maximally perfuse the tissue with blood.

REVIEW QUESTIONS

1. Define fatigue.

2. What factors influence fatigue during short-term intense exercise?

3. Explain the mechanisms by which an increase in muscle acidosis might cause muscle fatigue.

4. Why might an increase in ADP cause muscle fatigue?

5. Why are the main factors that contribute to fatigue different between short-term, intense exercise and prolonged submaximal exercise?

6. What are the connections between the development of dehydration, hyperthermia, and fatigue during prolonged exercise?

7. What evidence shows that glycogen depletion influences the development of fatigue during prolonged exercise? Why are the muscle and liver glycogen stores less important in the fatigue process during intense exercise?

8. Is blood flow, and therefore oxygen delivery, a limiting factor in prolonged exercise?

9. List the main peripheral and central limitations on VO_2max.

10. Explain whether central or peripheral factors are more important to VO_2max.

APPLICATIONS

1. Would a person who is taking a nonspecific ß-blocker be expected to have greater central or peripheral limitations to endurance exercise? Why?

2. Why do researchers have such a hard time separating the contributions of peripheral and central limitations to VO₂max? Try to devise a study method or model that might circumvent some of these problems.

3. Why is it difficult to isolate possible individual causes of muscle fatigue within skeletal muscle? Is it useful to try to pinpoint individual metabolic causes of muscle fatigue?

4. Using your knowledge of cardiovascular and neuroendocrine physiology, try to explain the mechanisms that result in fatigue symptoms of the CNS during exercise-induced dehydration and hypoglycemia.

REFERENCES

1. Armstrong RB, Laughlin MH: Muscle blood flow–fatigue relationships. In Saltin B, editor: *Biochemistry of Exercise VI,* 16:365-376, 1986.

2. Arthur PG, Hogan MC, Bebout DE et al: Modeling the effects of hypoxia on ATP turnover in exercising muscle, *J Appl Physiol* 73(2):737-742, 1992.

3. Atkinson DE: *Cellular energy metabolism and its regulation,* New York, 1977, Academic Press.

4. Baker AJ, Kostov KG, Miller RG, Weiner MW: Slow force recovery after long-duration exercise: metabolic and activation factors in muscle fatigue, *J Appl Physiol* 74(5):2294-2300, 1993.

5. Barr SI, Costill DL, Fink WJ et al: Six-hour cycling exercise in the heat: effects of fluid replacement with or without saline, *Med Sci Sports Exerc* 22(2):S118, 1990 (abstract 75).

6. Bertocci LA, Fleckenstein JL, Antonio J: Human muscle fatigue after glycogen depletion: a ³¹P magnetic resonance study, *J Appl Physiol* 73(1):75-81, 1992.

7. Bouchard C, Lesage R, Lortie G et al: Aerobic performance in brothers, dizygotic and monozygotic twins, *Med Sci Sports Exerc* 18(6):639-646, 1986.

8. Brechue WF, Ameredes BT, Andrew GM, Stainsby WN: Blood flow elevation increases VO₂ maximum during repetitive tetanic contraction of dog muscle in situ, *J Appl Physiol* 74(4):1499-1503, 1993.

9. Buse MW, Maassen N: Effect of consecutive exercise bouts on plasma potassium concentration during exercise and recovery, *Med Sci Sports Exerc* 21(5):489-493, 1989.

10. Cheetham ME, Boobis LH, Brooks S, Williams C: Human muscle metabolism during sprint running, *J Appl Physiol* 61(1):54-60, 1986.

11. Coggan AR, Coyle EF: Metabolism and performance following carbohydrate late in exercise, *Med Sci Sports Exerc* 21(1):59-65, 1989.

12. Costill DL, Sharp RL, Fink WJ, Katz A: Determination of human muscle pH in needle biopsy specimens, *J Appl Physiol* 53(5):1310-1313, 1982.

13. Coyle EF, Hemmert MK, Coggan AR: Effects of detraining on cardiovascular responses to exercise: role of blood volume, *J Appl Physiol* 60(1):95-99, 1986.

14. Dawson MJ, Gadian DG, Wilkie DR: Muscular fatigue investigated by phosphorus nuclear magnetic resonance, *Nature* 274:861-866, 1978.

15. Dodd SL, Powers SK, Brooks E, Crawford MP: Effects of reduced O₂ delivery with anemia, hypoxia, or ischemia on peak VO₂ and force in skeletal muscle, *J Appl Physiol* 74(1):186-191, 1993.

16. Donaldson SKB: Effect of acidosis on maximum force generation of peeled mammalian skeletal muscle fibers. In Knuttgen HG, Vogel JA, Poortmans JR, editors: *Biochemistry of Exercise* 13:126-133, 1983.

17. Fink WJ, Costill DL, Van Handel PJ: Leg muscle metabolism during exercise in the heat and cold, *Eur J Appl Physiol* 34:183-190, 1975.

18. Friden J, Lieber RL, Structural and mechanical basis of exercise-induced muscle injury, *Med Sci Sports Exerc* 24(5):521-530, 1992.

19. Gollnick PD: Metabolism of substrates: energy substrate metabolism during exercise and as modified by training, *Fed Proc* 44:353-357, 1985.

20. Green HJ, Patla AE: Maximal aerobic power: neuromuscular and metabolic considerations, *Med Sci Sports Exerc* 24(1):38-46, 1992.

REFERENCES—Cont'd

21. Green HJ, Jones S, Ball-Burnett ME et al: Adaptations in muscle metabolism to prolonged voluntary exercise and training, *J Appl Physiol* 78(1):138-145, 1995.

22. Hamel P, Simoneau J, Lortie G et al: Heredity and muscle adaptation to endurance training, *Med Sci Sports Exerc* 18(6):690-696, 1986.

23. Harris RC, Hultman E, Sahlin K: Glycolytic intermediates in human skeletal muscle after isometric contraction, *Pflugers Arch* 389:277-282, 1989.

24. Hill AV, Lupton H: Muscular exercise, lactic acid and the supply and utilization of oxygen, *Q J Med* 16:135-171, 1923.

25. Hirvonen J, Rehunen S, Rusko H, Harkonen M: Break-down of high-energy phosphate compounds and lactate accumulation during short supramaximal exercise, *Eur J Appl Physiol* 56:253-259, 1987.

26. Hink P, Vystocil F, Ujec E et al: Work-induced potassium loss from skeletal muscles and its physiological implications. In Saltin B, editor: *Biochemistry of Exercise VI,* 16:345-364, 1986.

27. Hogan MC, Welch HG: Effect of altered arterial O_2 tensions on muscle metabolism in dog skeletal muscle during fatiguing work, *Am J Physiol* 251(20):C216-C222, 1986.

28. Holloszy JO, Coyle EF: Adaptations of skeletal muscle to endurance training and their metabolic consequences, *J Appl Physiol* 56(4):831-838, 1984.

29. Honig CR, Connett RJ, Gayeski TEJ: O_2 transport and its interaction with metabolism; a systems view of aerobic capacity, *Med Sci Sports Exerc* 24(1):47-53, 1992.

30. Jones DA, Bigland-Ritchie B: Electrical and contractile changes in muscle fatigue. In Saltin B, editor: *Biochemistry of Exercise VI,* 16:377-392, 1986.

31. Jorfeldt L, Juhlin-Dannfelt A, Karlsson J: Lactate release in relation to tissue lactate in human skeletal muscle during exercise, *J Appl Physiol* 44:350-352, 1978.

32. Joyner MJ: Modeling: optimal marathon performance on the basis of physiological factors, *J Appl Physiol* 70(2):683-687, 1991.

33. Karlsson J, Nordesjo LO, Jorfeldt L, Saltin B: Muscle lactate, ATP, and CP levels during exercise after physical training in man, *J Appl Physiol* 33:199-203, 1972.

34. Katz A, Sahlin K: Role of oxygen in regulation of glycolysis and lactate production in human skeletal muscle, *Exerc Sport Sci Rev* 18:1-28, 1990.

35. Kowalchuk JM, Heigenhauser GJF, Lindinger MI: Role of lungs and inactive muscle in acid-base control after maximal exercise, *J Appl Physiol* 65(5):2090-2096, 1988.

36. Lewis SF, Haller RG: Skeletal muscle disorders and associated factors that limit exercise performance, *Exerc Sport Sci Rev* 17:67-114, 1989.

37. Lindstrom L, Petersen I: Electromyography in muscle fatigue studies: power spectrum analysis and signal theory aspects. In Knuttgen HG, Vogel JA, Poortmans JR, editors: *Biochemistry of Exercise* 13:187-196, 1983.

38. Lundgren F, Bennegard K, Elander A et al: Substrate exchange in human limb muscle during exercise at reduced flow, *Am J Physiol* 255(24):H1156-H1164, 1988.

39. MacLaren DP, Gibson H, Pary-Billings M, Edwards RHT: A review of metabolic and physiological factors in fatigue, *Exerc Sport Sci Rev* 17:29-66, 1989.

40. Miyachi M, Tabata I: Relationship between arterial oxygen desaturation and ventilation during maximal exercise, *J Appl Physiol* 73(6):2588-2591, 1992.

41. Moritani T, Takaishi T, Matsumoto T: Determination of maximal power output at neuromuscular fatigue threshold, *J Appl Physiol* 74(4):1729-1734, 1993.

42. Nadel ER: Effects of temperature on muscle metabolism. In Knuttgen HG, Vogel JA, Poortmans JR, editors: *Biochemistry of Exercise* 13:134-143, 1983.

43. Nadel ER: Limits imposed on exercise in a hot environment, *Sports Sci Exchange* 3(27):1-6, 1990.

44. Noakes TD: Implications of exercise testing for the prediction of athletic performance: a contemporary perspective, *Med Sci Sports Exerc* 20():319-330, 1988.

45. Noakes TD: Dehydration during exercise: what are the real dangers, *Clin J Sports Med* 5(2):123-128, 1995.

46. Norman B, Jansson E, Sollevi E, Kaijser L: IMP and muscle glycogen during exercise in man, *Acta Physiol Scand* 120:50A, 1984.

47. Poortmans JR: The intracellular environment in peripheral fatigue. In Knuttgen HG, Vogel JA, Poortmans JR, editors: *Biochemistry of Exercise* 13:113-115, 1983.

48. Ren JM, Henriksson J, Katz A, Sahlin K: NADH content in type I and type II human muscle fibers and after dynamic exercise, *Biochem J* 25:183-187, 1988.

49. Robinson S, Edwards HT, Dill DB: New records in human power, *Science* 85:409-410, 1937.

50. Roth DA: The sarcolemmal lactate transporter: transmembrane determinants of lactate flux, *Med Sci Sports Exerc* 23(8):925-934, 1991.

51. Rowell LB: *Human circulation: regulation during physical stress,* New York, 1986, Oxford University Press.

52. Rowel LB, Saltin B, Kiens B, Christensen NJ: Is peak quadriceps blood flow in humans even higher during exercise with hypoxemia? *Am J Physiol* 251(20):H1038-H1034, 1986.

53. Sahlin K: Effects of acidosis on energy metabolism and force generation in skeletal muscle. In Knuttgen HG, Vogel JA, Poortmans JR, editors: *Biochemistry of Exercise* 13:151-106, 1983.

REFERENCES—Cont'd

54. Sahlin K: NADH in human skeletal muscle during short-term intense exercise, *Pflugers Arch* 403:193-1986, 1985.

55. Sahlin K: Metabolic changes limiting muscle performance. In Saltin B, editor: *Biochemistry of Exercise VI.* 16:323-344, 1986.

56. Sahlin K, Katz A, Henriksson J: Redox state and lactate accumulation in human skeletal muscle during dynamic exercise, *Biochem J* 245:551-556, 1987.

57. Saltin B, Strange S: Maximal oxygen uptake: "old" and "new" arguments for a cardiovascular limitation, *Med Sci Sports Exerc* 24(1):30-37, 1992.

58. Saltin B, Nazar K, Costill DL, The nature of the training response: peripheral and central adaptations to one-legged cycling. *Acta Physiol Scand* 96:289-305, 1976.

59. Secher NH, Clausen JP, Klausen K et al: Central and regional circulatory effects of adding arm exercise to leg exercise, *Acta Physiol Scand* 100:288-297, 1977.

60. Spriet LL, Gledhill N, Froese AB, Wilkes DL: Effect of graded erythrocythemia on cardiovascular and metabolic responses to exercise, *J Appl Physiol* 61(5):1942-1948, 1986.

61. Spriet LL, Lindinger ML, McKelvie RS et al: Muscle glycogenolysis and H^+ concentration during maximal intermittent cycling, *J Appl Physiol* 66(1):8-13, 1988.

62. Spriet LL, Sonderland K, Bergstrom M, Hultman E: Anaerobic energy release in skeletal muscle during electrical stimulation, *J Appl Physiol* 62(2):611-615, 1987.

63. Spriet LL, Sonderlund K, Bergstrom M, Hultman E: Skeletal muscle glycogenolysis, glycolysis, and pH during electrical stimulation in men, *J Appl Physiol* 62(2):616-621, 1987.

64. Stainsby WN: Biochemical and physiological bases for lactate production, *Med Sci Sports Exerc* 18(3):341-343, 1986.

65. Stainsby WN, Brooks GA: Control of lactic acid metabolism in contracting muscles and during exercise, *Exerc Sport Sci Rev* 18:29-63, 1990.

66. Stainsby WN, Brechue WF, O'Drobinak DM: Regulation of muscle lactate production, *Med Sci Sports Exerc* 23(8):907-911, 1991.

67. Taylor CR: Structural and functional limits to oxidative metabolism: insights from scaling, *Annu Rev Physiol* 49:135-146, 1989.

68. Tesch PA, Thorsson A, Fujitsuka N: Creatine phosphate in fiber types of skeletal muscle before and after exhaustive exercise, *J Appl Physiol* 66(4):1756-1759, 1989.

69. Toner MM, Glickman EL, McArdle WD: Cardiovascular adjustments to exercise distributed between the upper and lower body, *Med Sci Sports Exerc* 22(6):773-778, 1990.

70. Vollestad NK, Sejersted OM: Biochemical correlates of fatigue, *Eur J Appl Physiol* 57:336-347, 1988.

71. Wagner PD: Gas exchange and peripheral diffusion limitation, *Med Sci Sports Exerc* 24:54-58, 1992.

72. Weibel ER: Scaling of structural and functional variables, *Annu Rev Physiol* 49:147-159, 1987.

73. Williams JH, Powers SK, Stewart MK: Hemoglobin desaturation in highly trained athletes during heavy exercise, *Med Sci Sports Exerc* 18(2):168-173, 1986.

74. Williams MH: Bicarbonate loading, *Sports Sci Exchange* 4(36):1-5, 1992.

RECOMMENDED READINGS

▪ Brechue WF, Ameredes BT, Andrew GM, Stainsby WN: Blood flow elevation increases VO_2 maximum during repetitive tetanic contraction of dog muscle in situ, *J Appl Physiol* 74(4):1499-1503, 1993.

▪ Dodd SL, Powers SK, Brooks E, Crawford MP: Effects of reduced O_2 delivery with anemia hypoxia, or ischemia on peak VO_2 and force in skeletal muscle, *J Appl Physiol* 74(1):186-191, 1993.

▪ Green HJ, Patla AE: Maximal aerobic power: neuromuscular and metabolic considerations, *Med Sci Sports Exerc* 24(1):38-46, 1992.

▪ Lundgren F, Bennegard K, Elander A et al: Substrate exchange in human limb muscle during exercise at reduced flow, *Am J Physiol* 255(24):H1156-H1164, 1988.

▪ MacLaren DP, Gibson H, Pary-Billings M, Edwards RHT: A review of metabolic and physiological factors in fatigue, *Exerc Sport Sci Rev* 17:29-66, 1989.

▪ Noakes TD: Implications of exercise testing for the prediction of athletic performance: a contemporary perspective, *Med Sci Sports Exerc* 20:319-330, 1988.

▪ Sahlin K: Metabolic changes limiting muscle performance. In Saltin B, editor: *Biochemistry of Exercise VI*, 16:323-344, 1986.

▪ Saltin B, Nazar K, Costill DL et al: The nature of the training response: peripheral and central adaptations to one-legged cycling, *Acta Physiol Scand* 96:289-305, 1976.

▪ Saltin B, Strange S: Maximal oxygen uptake: "old" and "new" arguments for a cardiovascular limitation, *Med Sci Sports Exerc* 24(1):30-37, 1992.

▪ Spriet LL, Gledhill N, Froese AB, Wilkes DL: Effect of graded erythrocythemia on cardiovascular and metabolic responses to exercise, *J Appl Physiol* 61(5):1942-1948, 1986.

▪ Stainsby WN: Biochemical and physiological bases for lactate production, *Med Sci Sports Exerc* 18(3):341-343, 1986.

▪ Toner MM, Glickman EL, McArdle WD: Cardiovascular adjustments to exercise distributed between the upper and lower body, *Med Sci Sports Exerc* 22(6):773-778, 1990.

▪ Vollestad NK, Sejersted OM: Biochemical correlates of fatigue, *Eur J Appl Physiol* 57:336-347, 1988.

CHAPTER **23** # Gender and Exercise Performance

OBJECTIVES

After studying this chapter you should be able to:

- Identify the main differences in structure and function between men and women.

- Explain why women have a limited cardiorespiratory capacity compared with men.

- Describe the importance of lean body mass to muscular strength and power.

- Describe the roles estradiol plays in women, and explain how the menstrual cycle is important to a woman's health.

- Explain the difficulty of doing research to further our understanding of the effects of exercise on pregnant women and their fetuses.

KEY TERMS

menstrual cycle

follicular phase

ovulatory phase

luteal phase

estradiol-17β

progesterone

athletic amenorrhea

Considerable research in exercise physiology has been devoted to the question of whether gender differences in body morphology, systems physiology, neuroendocrinology, and muscle metabolism influence acute and chronic adaptation to exercise. The original findings, that men had greater muscle mass and strength, as well as greater muscular and cardiorespiratory endurance, needed to be explored further. Other questions also needed to be answered. Some of the more important ones follow:

1. Are the differences in physique and function between men and women athletes based on differing functional capacities, or do they reflect socially enforced limitations on the development of women athletes?

2. Do men and women have different needs and concerns when training, or even when simply exercising?

3. Can women adapt to the same training stimuli as men?

4. What indices are best for comparing fitness components in men and women?

This chapter identifies the physiologic differences between men and women and assesses how these differences influence both acute and chronic responses to exercise. It also addresses specific considerations for women who exercise.

General Comparison of Male and Female Structure and Function

Figure 23.1 shows the external appearance of a postpubescent male and female and lists measurements pertinent to exercise performance. Because these pictures and data are average representations of men and women, ranges are given certain parameters. Also, some women will compare differently with men as indicated in Figure 23.1, and vice versa. However, for men and women of similar training and fitness, the relative differences between genders are valid.

The data in Figure 23.1 cover several main areas of functional difference between men and women. Body composition is known to influence both prolonged (endurance) exercise and short-term, intense exercise. It also may influence thermoregulatory capacities, which can be affected by the different sweat gland densities of men and women. The different capacities of the cardiovascular systems of men and women may amount to differences in oxygen transport capability. The hormonal differences produce female differences in substrate use during exercise and in ventilatory control at rest, during exercise, and when exposed to high altitude. Finally, these parameters combine to present different overall concerns for men and women participating in strenuous exercise training. The organization of this chapter is based on these general areas of structure and function.

Gender Differences in Cardiorespiratory Endurance

Cardiorespiratory endurance involves the functioning of the heart, lungs, vasculature, and skeletal muscle to exchange gases in the lung, transport gases and metabolites in the blood, and exchange gases and metabolites between the

FIGURE 23.1

An illustration and data table of the differences between males and females. These differences can be grouped based on structural and functional criteria. The female generally has a higher percentage of body fat that is distributed more around the hips and thighs, compared with the waist and stomach of the male. Males have a larger lean body mass, even when expressed relative to total body weight, and are taller than the average female. The male has a narrower pelvic region than the female. The female has fewer sweat glands than the male, a smaller heart, lower percentages of slow twitch motor units, a smaller blood volume, and a lower hemoglobin concentration and hematocrit. Females have ovaries that produce estrogen and progesterone, where males have testes that produce testosterone. These hormones exert different metabolic and regulatory functions on the body, especially during exercise.

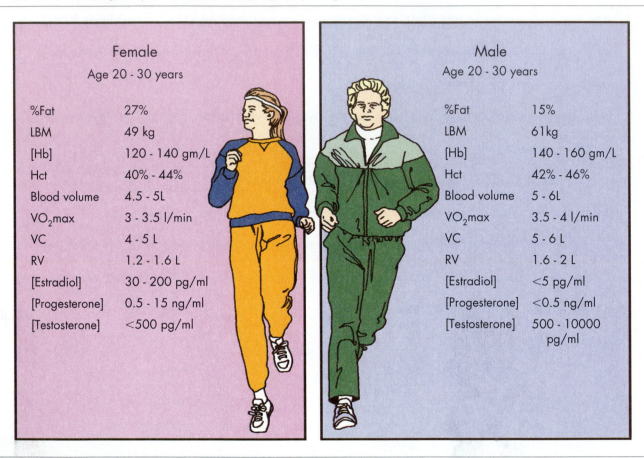

Female		Male	
Age 20 - 30 years		Age 20 - 30 years	
%Fat	27%	%Fat	15%
LBM	49 kg	LBM	61kg
[Hb]	120 - 140 gm/L	[Hb]	140 - 160 gm/L
Hct	40% - 44%	Hct	42% - 46%
Blood volume	4.5 - 5L	Blood volume	5 - 6L
VO$_2$max	3 - 3.5 l/min	VO$_2$max	3.5 - 4 l/min
VC	4 - 5 L	VC	5 - 6 L
RV	1.2 - 1.6 L	RV	1.6 - 2 L
[Estradiol]	30 - 200 pg/ml	[Estradiol]	<5 pg/ml
[Progesterone]	0.5 - 15 ng/ml	[Progesterone]	<0.5 ng/ml
[Testosterone]	<500 pg/ml	[Testosterone]	500 - 10000 pg/ml

blood and skeletal muscle. As explained in Chapter 10, the greater the body's capacity to perform these functions, the greater its cardiorespiratory endurance. These capacities involve central cardiovascular and pulmonary function, peripheral vascular function, and skeletal muscle fiber type and metabolic capacities.

Cardiovascular and Pulmonary Function

There is evidence of gender differences in pulmonary function. Women have a smaller lung volume and pulmonary capillary volume than men, resulting in lower maximal pulmonary ventilation.[36] However, as is explained later, it is unclear whether these differences simply reflect the composition of a smaller body mass. There is no evidence of a difference in the diffusion capacity of the lungs.[36]

Research on exercise-induced hypoxemia has been biased by predominantly male subject selection.[25,43] Whether this condition occurs more or less often in women is unknown, as is whether any potential gender differences in incidence are due to different cardiopulmonary function capacities.

Men and women have different cardiovascular capacities. Generally, women have smaller hearts, with a lower filling volume, maximal stroke volume, and cardiac output.[36,39] Because women also have a lower blood hemoglobin concentration, hematocrit, and total blood volume, they are at a definite disadvantage for transporting oxygen to skeletal muscles during exercise. The cardiovascular differences between men and women are best expressed by the relationship between cardiac output and oxygen consumption (VO$_2$) during exercise. For a given VO$_2$, women have a larger cardiac output than men because of their lower (a–vo₂Δ) secondary to reduced oxygen delivery.[15]

The fact that women have a lower cardiovascular capacity than men does not mean that women therefore are less able to adapt to endurance training. Pellicia et al.[39] reported that women also adapt to endurance training by improving the pumping effectiveness of the heart, as indicated by increased end-diastolic dimensions. These increases are similar to the adaptability found in men and indicate that gender differences in cardiovascular structure and function are due to genetic and related hormonal differences during the growth, development, and sexual maturity phases. In fact, when cardiovascular parameters are expressed relative to body surface area and mass, gender differences become less notable.[36]

Skeletal Muscle Structure and Function

Limited data are available that compare the fiber type proportions of men and women. The data that do exist pertain to elite athletes and, because of genetic bias and athletic selection, it is unclear how well these data reflect true gender differences.

Research on the proportions of muscle fiber type in women and men runners indicate that women tend to have a smaller amount of the slow-twitch fiber type in the gastrocnemius muscle.[10] Despite this difference in fiber type, there is no evidence of a gender difference in lactate threshold expressed relative to maximal oxygen consumption (VO₂max).

Maximal and Submaximal Oxygen Consumption

VO₂max is very different between equally trained men and women. Given the previously detailed roles of both central cardiovascular function and muscular endurance capacities in determining VO₂max (Chapters 10 and 11), this is not surprising. In comparably trained men and women, VO₂max is higher in the men, with the difference depending on the expression of VO₂ (Figure 23.2).* After adjusting for fat-free mass and training status, the gender difference in VO₂max is reduced to a margin of approximately 15%.[15,52] However, recent data indicate that well-trained men and women can have a similar VO₂max when expressed relative to lean body mass.[36]

In studies on submaximal running, numerous researchers have reported contradictory findings on submaximal VO₂ for a given running velocity.[2,14,34] However, in the most extensive study done on elite male and female long-distance runners, Daniels and Daniels[14] documented a significantly lower VO₂ for men at a given running velocity, giving them a 6% to 7% advantage. Thus, for a given running velocity, elite male runners are consuming 6% to 7% less oxygen while remaining at steady state. With their higher VO₂max (and therefore potentially higher relative intensity at the lactate threshold), men can remain at steady state while running faster. Using the averaged data from Daniels and Daniels[14] and assuming a

*References 9, 10, 14, 18, 34, 52, 56.

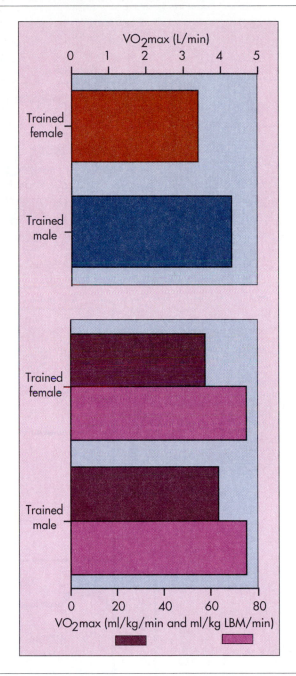

FIGURE 23.2

Differences in VO₂max between males and females when expressed in absolute and relative units.

lactate threshold of 85% VO₂max, the maximal steady state running speeds for the men and women athletes were 288.7 and 333.8 m/min, respectively. In a 10,000 m race, this amounts to a time difference of 4 minutes 42 seconds, or a 13% performance advantage for men.

FIGURE 23.3

The changing hormonal concentrations during the menstrual cycle. (Adapted from Griffin JE, Ojeda SR: *Textbook of endocrine physiology*, New York, 1988, Oxford University Press.)

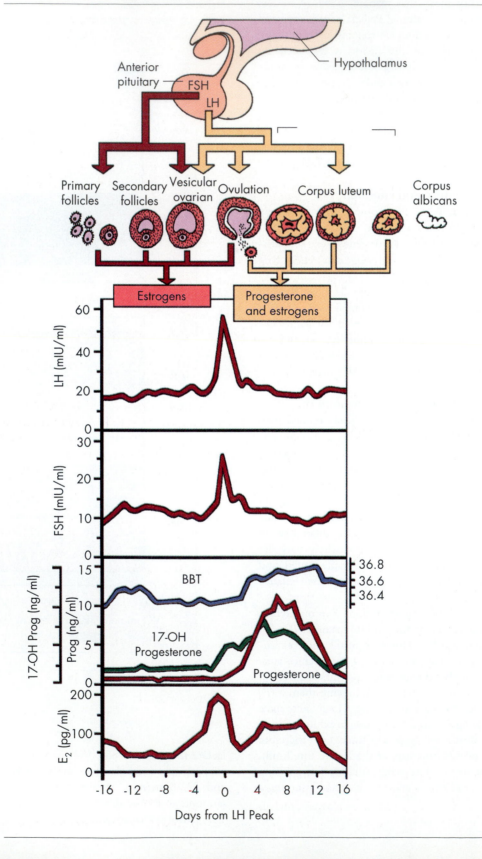

FIGURE 23.4

The decrease in muscle glycogen is less for females than males during equivalent relative exercise intensities. In addition, females are less dependent on amino acid oxidation during prolonged exercise. It is assumed that the difference in energy substrate utilization between males and females resides in the greater use of intramuscular stores of lipid.

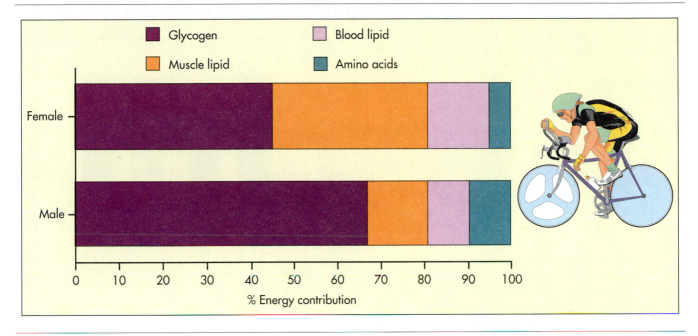

Gender Differences in Endocrine Function and Metabolism During Exercise

Because endurance fitness can alter metabolic responses to exercise, studies must control for endurance fitness to validly compare men's and women's metabolic responses to exercise. Because VO_2max is known to differ between genders, even when adjusted for training, age, and performance, it is not a good measure for standardizing fitness. For example, a woman athlete with a VO_2max similar to that of a male athlete has achieved a higher level of endurance training. In comparing men and women athletes, Tarnopolsky et al.[56] adjusted for training, age, and distance event and found that women had a 21% lower VO_2max (4.38 versus 3.42 L/min). However, when VO_2 was expressed relative to lean body mass (LBW), the ability to consume oxygen was similar (74.9 versus 74.7 ml/kg LBW/min).

Figure 23.3 illustrates and compares the changes in basal body temperature and circulating anterior pituitary and gonadal hormone concentrations in women relative to the **menstrual cycle.** These comparisons highlight the considerable endocrinologic differences between men and women and point to the dramatic variation in endocrine function during the menstrual cycle.

The menstrual cycle has three phases: the **follicular phase,** which begins with the onset of menstruation and varies in length from 9 to 23 days; the **ovulatory phase,** which results in the release of the ovum and may last 3 days;

and the **luteal phase,** which extends from the end of ovulation to the onset of menstrual bleeding. The luteal phase is generally more consistent in duration, lasting approximately 13 days. However, as is discussed in subsequent sections, the luteal phase is known to shorten in certain women athletes.[31,32]

menstrual cycle

the monthly variation in women's gonadal hormones, which results in the release of an ovum and, if fertilization does not occur, in eventual expulsion of the ovum and uterine lining, which is called menstruation

follicular phase

the phase of the menstrual cycle that begins with the onset of menstruation and ends with the start of ovulation; usually lasts 9 to 23 days

ovulatory phase

the phase of the menstrual cycle in which ovulation occurs; usually lasts 3 days

luteal phase

the phase of the menstrual cycle that starts with the end of ovulation and ends with the onset of menstruation; usually lasts 13 days

The distinct phases of the menstrual cycle are important because the differences in hormone concentrations during these phases are influential in regulating fuel mobilization during exercise. During the early to middle follicular phase, women have low concentrations of estrogen (specifically **estradiol-17β** or, simply, estradiol) and **progesterone.** Estradiol inhibits glucose uptake by tissues and indirectly favors lipid catabolism. Progesterone is a known stimulant to ventilation and has some effect in reducing the metabolic actions of estradiol. Consequently, during the early follicular phase the female is endocrinologically most like the male.

During the ovulatory and luteal phases the increased estradiol and progesterone concentrations may alter substrate use and ventilation at rest and during exercise. When exercising at a given percentage of VO_2max, women catabolize more fat than men[48,56] and rely less on muscle glycogen.[56] In a study of men and women running 15.5 km at 65% VO_2max, women used 25% less muscle glycogen than equally trained men and excreted 30% less urea nitrogen (less protein catabolism)[56] (Figure 23.4). Although regulation of the catabolism of endogenous lipids within skeletal muscle is unclear, data indicate that women may be able to use more of their intramuscular store of triacylglycerols for a given relative submaximal intensity. These differences are reduced for highly trained women because of their shortened luteal phase and lower circulating concentrations of estrogen.[48]

Given the endocrinologic potential for metabolic differences in women during the different phases of the menstrual cycle, the question becomes, what has research revealed on this topic? During the luteal phase, circulating free fatty acids (FFAs), glycerol, and blood lipoprotein lipase activity increase.[46] Insulin binding declines, compromising glucose uptake and eventually carbohydrate catabolism. Unfortunately, studies involving exercise have been less conclusive in identifying metabolic differences among phases of the menstrual cycle.[36,48] Kanaley et al[26] reported between no difference in the metabolic response to 90 minutes of running at 60% of VO_2max between the follicular phase and the luteal phase. These similarities existed despite large differences in circulating concentrations of estrogen and progesterone. The findings may be explained by the fact that progesterone has an antagonistic effect compared with estrogen, as well as the intrinsic (insulin-independent) increase in glucose uptake by contracting skeletal muscle. More research on this topic is needed before a definitive statement can be made about the need to control for the phase of the menstrual cycle when comparing men's and women's metabolic responses with exercise.

Gender Differences in Muscular Strength and Power

Men's greater lean body mass is a major determinant of their greater muscular strength. However, gender differences in strength and power are removed when either measure is

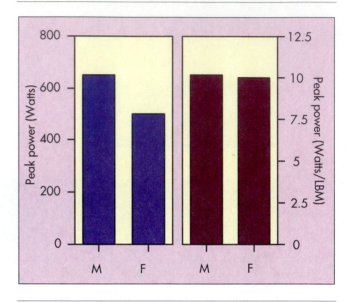

FIGURE 23.5

A comparison of muscular power between males and females, and how gender differences are removed when power is expressed relative to lean body mass.

expressed relative to lean body mass (Figure 23.5). This fact points to the importance of muscle mass on intense exercise performance, regardless of gender.

Although it has been widely accepted that women show less response to strength training than men, research does not support this claim. Cureton et al.[12] showed that men and women who participated in a 16-week weight-training program demonstrated equal muscle hypertrophy and muscular strength improvement when these results were expressed relative to pretraining values (Figure 23.6).

Gender Differences in Exercise in Extreme Environments

Exercise in climatic extremes (high temperature and humidity versus cold temperature) or high altitude demands additional physiologic adaptations, which research has shown to differ between genders.

Thermoregulation

It generally has been accepted that women sweat less than men and that this difference is due to a lower output from each sweat gland. However, research has not shown any difference in the change in sweat rate, core temperature, and cardiovascular responses between genders during exercise in a hot environment.[8,35] This is especially true when sweat rate is expressed relative to core temperature.[24]

Some evidence indicates that the electrolyte content of sweat (sodium [Na^+] and chloride [Cl^-]) is lower in women;

FIGURE 23.6

The increase in muscle strength for males and females in response to 16 weeks of weight training. Although the absolute changes are greater for the male, there are no gender differences in these changes relative to pretraining values.

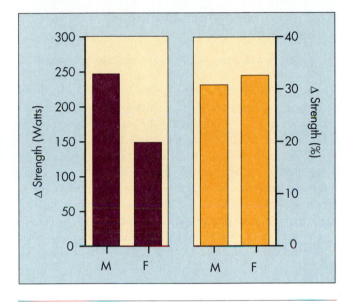

FIGURE 23.7

The gender difference in the maximal VE/VO_2 attained during graded exercise when breathing different hypoxic gas mixtures. The data indicate that females ventilate more during exercise at altitude than males.

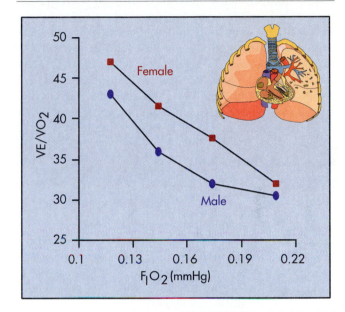

however, it is unclear whether these differences are due to a different aldosterone response, a real although not experimentally verified greater sweat rate in men, or some effect of estrogen on the rate of electrolyte reabsorption by the sweat glands.[35]

Regarding acclimatization to dry heat, research indicates that women may adapt better than similarly trained and fit men.[24] In one study, after 11 days of 120 minutes of exercise in dry heat (43° C), women (n = 4) showed a smaller increase in core temperature and could exercise longer than men (n = 6).[50] However, when men and women exercise at an equal absolute intensity in a hot environment, women have higher rectal temperatures and heart rates than men.[50] Thus, when referring to *relative exercise intensities,* women tolerate and adapt to heat stress better. When referring to *absolute intensities* and therefore an *absolute heat load,* men tolerate heat stress better.

Adaptation to High Altitude

Progesterone is a potent stimulant to ventilation, and it is well known that women have a greater hypoxic stimulus to ventilation than men because of their higher circulating concentrations of progesterone.[51] This increased sensitivity to ventilate during hypoxia should provide women with greater potential for increasing the alveolar partial pressure of oxygen ($P_{A}O_2$) and improving acute adaptation to high altitude. Conversely, women are known to retain water during the menstrual cycle, and becoming slightly edematous is recognized

as an increased risk for developing acute mountain sickness and the life-threatening conditions of pulmonary and cerebral edema.[20]

Given these physiologic differences between genders, do women adapt differently to high altitude then men do? Unfortunately, we do not know the answer to this question. The most thorough investigation of women at high altitude was completed in 1966.[21] This study, actually a series of studies done at Pike's Peak in Colorado (4300 m above sea level), revealed that women have a higher ventilation than men during exposure to high altitude and that iron supplementation was necessary for women to develop a polycythemic response to prolonged exposure to high altitude.

No data exist on gender comparisons of exercise performance at high altitude, or on susceptibility to acute mountain

estradiol-17β

the most biologically active estrogen steroid hormone that influences lipid metabolism, bone growth, and the development of female secondary sex characteristics. In women, estrogens are produced by the ovaries; in men, a smaller amount is produced by the adrenal cortex and testes

progesterone (pro-**jes**'ter-own)

a steroid hormone synthesized by the developing ovarian follicle and released during the luteal phase of the menstrual cycle

sickness and pulmonary or cerebral edema. However, studies have been done comparing men and women who were exercising while breathing hypoxic gas (17.39%, 14.4%, and 1.81% oxygen conditions).[38] Figure 23.7 shows the results of ventilation and oxygen consumption expressed as the ventilatory equivalent for oxygen (V_E/VO_2) (see Chapter 12). Women had a significantly larger ventilatory response for a given VO_2. In addition, although women's VO_2max values were lower than those for men, the relative decrement in VO_2max for women was significantly less than that for men (24% to 29.5%). Do women have a more effective adaptive response to hypoxia than men? Although the available data indicate that this may be true, the question seems to have been overlooked by altitude physiologists since the late 1980s.

Special Concerns for Women Who Exercise

*W*omen who exercise are more likely to improve their health and reduce their risk of degenerative disease (e.g., heart disease and osteo-porosis). However, because of the relative delicacy of the neuroendocrinologic regulation of the female hypothalamic-pituitary-ovarian axis, chronic exercise can lead to menstrual cycle irregularities. In addition, a pregnant woman and her fetus have special needs that exercise may impinge on.

Athletic Amenorrhea and Bone Mineral Status

A subgroup of women who exercise have been reported to have a shortened luteal phase of the menstrual cycle.[31,32] The degree to which the luteal phase is shortened has been shown to correspond to the intensity of training (duration and frequency); the more intense the training, the more the luteal phase is shortened (see Chapter 13).

If a women trains too hard, the luteal phase continues to shorten, and eventually the menstrual cycle disappears, a condition called **athletic amenorrhea.** The endocrinologic events believed to inhibit regulation of the menstrual cycle at the level of the hypothalamic-pituitary axis are explained in Chapter 13.

Loss of the menstrual cycle has ramifications for women other than a natural means of birth control. The absence of a

---

FIGURE 23.8

A summary of the potential risks to the fetus of a pregnant woman who exercises, as well as the potential benefits obtained.

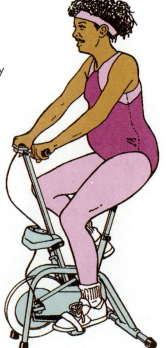

Exercise during pregnancy

Risks to Mother

Hypoglycemia

Hyperthermia

Musculo-skeletal injury

Risks to Fetus

Hypoglycemia

Hyperthermia

Decreased placental

blood flow

Physical shock

Benefits to Mother

Improved insulin sensitivity

Improved body fat control

Psychosocial interactions

Potential decreased birth

complications (???)

Potential decreased labor (???)

Benefits to Fetus

Potential decreased birth

complications (???)

Potential decreased labor (???)

surge in follicle-stimulating hormone (FSH) and luteinizing hormone (LH) prevents development of the ovarian follicle, which normally produces estradiol and progesterone. An inability to produce ovarian estradiol chronically lowers circulating concentrations of estradiol, increasing the rate of bone resorption from the skeleton and thereby increasing the risk of premature *osteoporosis*. Some evidence also connects menstrual irregularities with a higher incidence of musculoskeletal injury.[29]

An amenorrheic woman has a few alternatives that reduce the deleterious effects of this condition. First, she can reduce her training, which has been shown to reestablish the menstrual cycle. She could also maintain her training and seek medical advice on a suitable estradiol supplement. Estrogen patch treatment is more effective in increasing serum estradiol-17β than oral contraceptives.[48] Despite this fact, women are generally prescribed an oral birth control pill. Because of the time required to detect changes in bone mineral density, conclusive data are not available on the effectiveness of the birth control pill or the estrogen patch in retarding the development of osteoporosis.

Exercise During Pregnancy

The health benefits of exercise and women's increasing participation in exercise have raised concern about the effect of exercise on a mother and fetus during pregnancy. Initial inquiry into this topic concerned the effects of exercise on uterine and fetal blood flow, core and fetal temperature fluctuations, carbohydrate metabolism, and protection from the physical shock accompanying certain movements (e.g., running) (Figure 23.8).

One method used to assess fetal responses during exercise performed by the mother is to record changes in the fetal heart rate. Research done on sheep has documented increases in fetal heart rate; however, it is unclear whether similar responses in humans are a result of ischemic hypoxia or are simply a result of increased levels of catecholamines. The difficulty of using humans in research on pregnancy and exercise has resulted in similar vague findings for temperature changes and glucose metabolism.[8]

Despite the often publicized dangers of exercise during pregnancy, there is evidence of benefits. A pregnant woman who exercises may develop increased capacities for supporting the fetus, such as improved cardiovascular function and carbohydrate metabolism. Although some experts have said that exercise training may reduce the duration of labor and therefore the risk of childbirth, no experimental evidence exists to support this.[8,30]

According to a meta-analysis of the effects of exercise during pregnancy on the mother and fetus, no evidence arose that exercise performed three times a week for up to 45 minutes at a heart rate of 144 bpm was harmful.[30] The American College of Gynecology recommends a similar frequency and intensity but a duration of not longer than 15 minutes.[30] It is assumed that women who have symptoms of infection, cardiovascular disease, or other illness may not be suitable for the aforementioned recommendations. In addition, exercise performed for longer durations, at higher intensities, at high altitude, or during increased thermal stress (hot or humid conditions) may be unsafe. Because they pose less of a risk for trauma, non-weight-bearing exercises (cycling, swimming, or other water-based exercises) are most often recommend for pregnant women. However, because exercising in warm water poses a risk of hyperthermia, pregnant women should exercise in cool water (<29.4° C [85° F]).

---

athletic amenorrhea

the absence of a menstrual cycle as the result of endocrinologic responses, triggered by exercise training, that inhibit the release of follicle-stimulating hormone (FSH) from the anterior pituitary gland

---

SUMMARY

- Gender differences have been documented for body composition, cardiovascular function, energy metabolism, endocrine responses, muscle morphology, and exercise performance.

- Women have a smaller heart and a lower filling volume, maximal stroke volume, and cardiac output. Because they also have a lower blood hemoglobin concentration and hematocrit, women are at a definite disadvantage for transporting oxygen to their working muscles during exercise. Women adapt to endurance training by improving the pumping effectiveness of the heart, as indicated by increased end-diastolic dimensions. This is similar to the adaptability of men.

- Biopsy samples from the gastrocnemius muscle indicate that women tend to have a lower proportion slow-twitch fiber type. Despite this fiber type difference, there is no evidence of a gender difference in lactate threshold.

SUMMARY—Cont'd

■ Considerable endocrinologic differences between men and women relate to women's **menstrual cycle.** The menstrual cycle has three phases: the **follicular phase,** which begins with the onset of menstruation and varies in length from 9 to 23 days; the **ovulatory phase,** which results in the release of the ovum and may last 3 days; and the **luteal phase,** which extends from the end of ovulation to the onset of menstrual bleeding. The luteal phase is generally most consistent in duration, lasting approximately 13 days.

■ During the early to middle follicular phase, women have low concentrations of estrogen (specifically estradiol-17β or, simply, estradiol) and **progesterone.** Estradiol inhibits glucose uptake by tissues and indirectly favors lipid catabolism. Progesterone is a known stimulant to ventilation and has some effect in reducing the metabolic actions of estradiol. Consequently, during the early follicular phase, women are endocrinologically most like men.

■ When exercising at a given percentage of VO_2max, women catabolize more fat than men. This difference is reduced for highly trained women, but the change is due to the shortened luteal phase of highly trained women, and these results cannot be applied to the population of normally menstruating women who participate in moderate exercise training and sports. VO_2max is higher in comparably trained men than women, with differences approximating 15%. For elite athletes, VO_2max differences are explained by the lower lean body mass and relatively smaller cardiovascular capacities of women.

■ The greater lean body mass in men is a major determinant of their greater muscular strength. Muscular power also depends on muscle mass; however, differences in muscle power between the genders are removed when power is expressed relative to lean body mass. This fact points up the importance of muscle mass in intense exercise performance.

■ In women who train too hard, the luteal phase is likely to continue to shorten, and eventually the menstrual cycle is lost, a condition called **athletic amenorrhea.** The absence of a surge in FSH and LH prevents development of the ovarian follicle, from which estradiol and progesterone are produced. The inability to produce ovarian estradiol chronically lowers circulating concentrations of estradiol, increasing the rate of bone resorption from the skeleton and thereby increasing the risk of premature osteoporosis.

■ The American College of Gynecology states that exercise performed three times a week for no longer than 15 minutes at a heart rate of 144 bpm is not harmful to a pregnant woman or her fetus and may be beneficial. Research has indicated that exercise lasting up to 45 minutes may also be safe, but these recommendations may not be suitable for women with symptoms of infection, cardiovascular disease, or other illnesses.

REVIEW QUESTIONS

1. What are the differences in body composition between men and women? Explain how these differences influence exercise performance.

2. Explain why women have lower cardiovascular and oxygen transport capacities than men.

3. Why do normally menstruating women catabolize more lipid at a given submaximal exercise intensity than men do?

4. What are the phases of the menstrual cycle, how long do they last, and how do they differ endocrinologically?

5. If you were doing a study comparing the different metabolic responses of men and women with exercise, in what phase of the menstrual cycle should the women who participate be? Why?

APPLICATIONS

1. List the health benefits to women participating in a strength or endurance exercise training program.

2. Based on the material presented in this chapter, should women face different standards than men for certain vocations that involve life-threatening conditions (e.g., military, fire department, police force)?

3. What are the connections linking athletic amenorrhea, osteoporosis, and low circulating concentrations of estradiol?

4. What are some concerns for the pregnant woman who wants to exercise, and what are the current recommendations for pregnant women who do exercise?

REFERENCES

1. Bemben DA, Boileau RA, Bahr JM et al: Effects of oral contraceptives on hormonal and metabolic responses during exercise, *Med Sci Sports Exerc* 24(2):434-441, 1992.

2. Bhambani Y, Singh M: Metabolic and cinematographic analysis of walking and running in men and women, *Med Sci Sports Exerc* 17:131-137, 1985.

3. Bonen A, Campagna P, Gilchrist L et al: Substrate and endocrine responses during exercise at selected stages of pregnancy, *J Appl Physiol* 73(1):134-142, 1992.

4. Bunt JC: Metabolic actions of estradiol: significance for acute and chronic exercise responses, *Med Sci Sports Exerc* 22(3):286-290, 1990.

5. Bunt JC, Boileau RA, Bahr JM, Nelson RA: Sex and training differences in human growth hormone levels during prolonged exercise, *J Appl Physiol* 61(5):1796-1801, 1986.

6. Bunt JC, Going SB, Lohman TG et al: Variation in bone mineral content and estimated body fat in young adult females, *Med Sci Sports Exerc* 22(5):564-569, 1990.

7. Clapp JF III, Rokey R, Treadway JL et al: Exercise in pregnancy, *Med Sci Sports Exerc* 24(6):S294-S300, 1992.

8. Clapp JF III, Wesley M, Sleamaker RH: Thermoregulatory and metabolic responses to jogging prior to and during pregnancy, *Med Sci Sports Exerc* 19(2):1124-1130, 1987.

9. Costill DL, Fink WJ, Pollock ML: Muscle fiber composition and enzyme activities of elite distance runners, *Med Sci Sports Exerc* 8:96-100, 1976.

10. Costill DL, Fink WJ, Flynn M, Kirwan J: Muscle fiber composition and enzyme activities in elite female distance runners, *Int J Sports Med* 8:103-106, 1987.

11. Costill DL, Fink WJ, Getchell LH et al: Lipid metabolism in skeletal muscle of endurance-trained males and females, *J Appl Physiol* 47(4):787-791, 1979.

12. Cureton KJ, Collins MA, Hill DW, Mcelhannon FM Jr: Muscle hypertrophy in men and women, *Med Sci Sports Med* 20(4):338-344, 1988.

13. Dalsky GP: Effect of exercise on bone: permissive influence of estrogen and calcium, *Med Sci Sports Exerc* 22(3):281-285, 1990.

14. Daniels J, Daniels N: Running economy of elite male and elite female runners, *Med Sci Sports Exerc* 24(4):483-489, 1992.

15. Drinkwater BL: Women and exercise: physiological aspects, *Exerc Sport Sci Rev* 12:126-154, 1984.

16. Douglas PS, Clarkson TB, Flowers NC et al: Exercise and atherosclerotic heart disease, *Med Sci Sports Med* 24(6):S266-S276, 1992.

17. Fay L, Londeree BR, Lafontaine TP, Volek MR: Physiological parameters related to distance running performance in female athletes, *Med Sci Sports Exerc* 21(3):319-324, 1989.

18. Froberg K, Pedersen PK: Sex differences in endurance capacity and metabolic response to prolonged, heavy exercise, *Eur J Appl Physiol* 52:446-450, 1984.

19. Gauther JM, Theriault R, Theriault G et al: Electrical stimulation–induced changes in skeletal muscle enzymes of men and women, *Med Sci Sports Exerc* 24(11):1252-1256, 1992.

20. Hackett PH, Rennie RD, Hofmeidter SE et al: Fluid retention and relative hypoventilation in acute mountain sickness, *Respiration* 43:321-329, 1982.

21. Hannon JP, Shields JL, Harris CW: High altitude acclimatization in women. In Goddard RE, editor: *The effects of altitude on physical performance,* Chicago Athletic Institute 37-44, 1966.

22. Heinrich CH, Boing SB, Pamenter RW et al: Bone mineral content of cyclically menstruating female resistance and endurance trained athletes, *Med Sci Sports Exerc* 22(5):558-563, 1990.

REFERENCES—Cont'd

23. Herring JL, Mole PA, Meredith CN, Stern JS: Effect of suspending exercise training on resting metabolic rate in women, *Med Sci Sports Exerc* 24(1):59-65, 1992.

24. Horstman DH, Christensen E: Acclimatization to dry heat: active men vs. active women, *J Appl Physiol* 52(4):825-831, 1982.

25. Johnson BD, Saupe KW, Dempsey JA: Mechanical constraints on exercise hyperpnea in endurance trained athletes, *J Appl Physiol* 73(3):874-886, 1992.

26. Kanaley JA, Boileau RA, Bahr JA et al: Substrate oxidation and GH responses to exercise are independent of menstrual phase and status, *Med Sci Sports Exerc* 24(8):873-880, 1992.

27. Kohrt WM, Malley MT, Dalsky GP, Holloszy JO: Body composition of healthy sedentary and trained, young and older men and women, *Med Sci Sports Exerc* 24(7):832-837, 1992.

28. LaManca JL, Haymes EM: Effects of iron repletion on VO$_2$max, endurance, and blood lactate in women, *Med Sci Sports Exerc* 25(12):1386-1392, 1993.

29. Lloyd T, Triantafllou SJ, Baker ER et al: Women athletes with menstrual irregularity have increased musculoskeletal injuries, *Med Sci Sports Exerc* 18(4):374-379, 1986.

30. Lokey EA, Tran ZV, Wells CL et al: Effects of physical exercise on pregnancy outcomes: a meta-analytic review, *Med Sci Sports Exerc* 23(11):1234-1239, 1991.

31. Loucks AB: Effects of exercise training on the menstrual cycle: existence and mechanisms, *Med Sci Sports Exerc* 22(3):275-280, 1990.

32. Loucks AB, Vaitukaitis J, Cameron JL et al: The reproductive system and exercise in women, *Med Sci Sports Exerc* 24(6):S288-S293, 1992.

33. Marcus R, Drinkwater B, Dalsky G et al: Osteoporosis and exercise in women, *Med Sci Sports Exerc* 24(6):S301-S307, 1992.

34. Maughan R, Leiper L: Aerobic capacity and fractional utilization of aerobic capacity in elite and nonelite male and female marathon runners, *Eur J Appl Physiol* 52:80-87, 1983.

35. Meyer F, Bar-Or O, MacDougall D, Heigenhauser GJF: Sweat electrolyte loss during exercise in the heat: effects of gender and maturation, *Med Sci Sports Exerc* 24(7):776-781, 1992.

36. Mitchell JH, Tate C, Raven P et al: Acute response and chronic adaptation to exercise in women, *Med Sci Sports Exerc* 24(6):S258-S265, 1992.

37. Myburgh KH, Bachrach LK, Lewis B et al: Low bone mineral density at axial and appendicular sites in amenorrheic athletes, *Med Sci Sports Exerc* 24(11):1197-1202, 1993.

38. Paterson DJ, Pinnington H, Pearce AR, Morton AL: Maximal exercise cardiorespiratory responses of men and women during acute exposure to hypoxia, *Aviat Space Environ Med* 58:243-247, 1987.

39. Pellicia A, Maron BJ, Spataro A et al: The upper limit of physiologic cardiac hypertrophy in highly trained elite athletes, *N Eng J Med* 324(5):295-301, 1991.

40. Peterson SE, Peterson MD, Raymond G et al: Muscular strength and bone density with weight training in middle-aged women, *Med Sci Sports Exerc* 23(4):499-504, 1991.

41. Pivarnik JM, Lee W, Miller JF: Physiological and perceptual responses to cycle and treadmill exercise during pregnancy, *Med Sci Sports Exerc* 23(4):470-475, 1991.

42. Pivarnik JM, Lee W, Spillman T et at: Maternal respiration and blood gases during aerobic exercise performed at moderate altitude, *Med Sci Sports Exerc* 24(8):868-872, 1992.

43. Powers SK, Martin D, Dodd S: Exercise-induced hypoxemia in elite endurance athletes: incidence, causes, and impact on VO$_2$max, *Sports Med* 16(1):14-22, 1993.

44. Risser WL, Lee EJ, Leblanc A et al: Bone density in eumenorrheic female college athletes, *Med Sci Sports Exerc* 22(5):570-574, 1990.

45. Risser WL, Lee EJ, Poindexter HBW et al: Iron deficiency in female athletes: its prevalence and impact on performance, *Med Sci Sports Exerc* 20(2):116-121, 1988.

46. Ronkainen HRA, Pakarinen AJ, Kauppila AJI: Adrenocortical function of female endurance runners and joggers, *Med Sci Sports Exerc* 18(4):385-389, 1986.

47. Rowland TW, Green GM: Physiological responses to treadmill exercise in females: adult-child differences, *Med Sci Sports Exerc* 20(5):474-478, 1988.

48. Ruby BC, Robergs RA: Gender differences in substrate utilization during exercise, *Sports Med* 17(6):393-410, 1994.

49. Sawka MN, Young AJ, Pandolf KB et al: Erythrocyte, plasma, and blood volume of healthy young men, *Med Sci Sports Exerc* 24(4):447-453, 1992.

50. Shapiro Y, Pandolf KB, Avellini BA et al: Physiological responses of men and women to humid and dry heat, *J Appl Physiol* 40:786-796, 1980.

51. Shoene RB, Robertson HT, Peirson DJ, Peterson AP: Respiratory drives and exercise in menstrual cycles of athletic and nonathletic women, *J Appl Physiol* 50:1300-1305, 1981.

52. Sparling PB: A meta-analysis of studies comparing maximal oxygen uptake in men and women, *Res Q Exerc Sport* 51(3):542-552, 1980.

REFERENCES—Cont'd

53. Stillman RJ, Lohman TG, Slaughter MH, Massey BH: Physical activity and bone mineral content in women aged 30 to 85 years, *Med Sci Sports Exerc* 18(5):576-680, 1986.

54. Sullivan MJ, Cobb FR, Higginbotham MB: Stroke volume increases by similar mechanisms during upright exercise in normal men and women, *Am J Cardiol* 67:1405-1412, 1991.

55. Takano N: Changes of ventilation and ventilatory response to hypoxia during the menstrual cycle, *Pflugers Arch* 402:312-316, 1984.

56. Tarnopolsky IJ, MacDougall JD, Atkinson SA et al: Gender difference in substrate for endurance exercise, *J Appl Physiol* 68:302-308, 1990.

57. Telford RD, Cunningham RB: Sex, sport, and body-size dependency of hematology in highly trained athletes, *Med Sci Sports Exerc* 23(7):788-794, 1991.

58. Thorland WG, Johnson GO, Cisar CJ et al: Strength and anaerobic responses of elite young female sprint and distance runners, *Med Sci Sports Exerc* 19(1):56-61, 1987.

59. Walberg JL, Johnston CS: Menstrual function and eating behavior in female recreational weight lifters and competitive body builders, *Med Sci Sports Exerc* 23(1):30-36, 1991.

60. Wilmore J, Costill DL: *Physiology of exercise and sport,* Champaign, Illinois, 1994, Human Kinetics.

RECOMMENDED READINGS

■ Bunt JC: Metabolic actions of estradiol: significance for acute and chronic exercise responses, *Med Sci Sports Exerc* 22(3):286-290, 1990.

■ Bunt JC, Going SB, Lohman TG et al: Variation in bone mineral content and estimated body fat in young adult females, *Med Sci Sports Exerc* 22(5):564-569, 1990.

■ Clapp JF III, Rokey R, Treadway JL et al: Exercise in pregnancy, *Med Sci Sports Exerc* 24(6):S294-S300, 1992.

■ Fay L, Londeree BR, Lafontaine TP, Volek MR: Physiological parameters related to distance running performance in female athletes, *Med Sci Sports Exerc* 21(3):319-324, 1989.

■ Heinrich CH, Boing SB, Pamenter RW et al: Bone mineral content of cyclically menstruating female resistance and endurance trained athletes, *Med Sci Sports Exerc* 22(5):558-563, 1990.

■ Lokey EA, Tran ZV, Wells CL et al: Effects of physical exercise on pregnancy outcomes: a meta-analytic review, *Med Sci Sports Exerc* 23(11):1234-1239, 1991.

■ Loucks AB: Effects of exercise training on the menstrual cycle: existence and mechanisms, *Med Sci Sports Exerc* 22(3):275-280, 1990.

■ Loucks AB, Vaitukaitis J, Cameron JL et al: The reproductive system and exercise in women, *Med Sci Sports Exerc* 24(6):S288-S293, 1992.

■ Meyer F, Bar-Or O, MacDougall D, Heigenhauser GJF: Sweat electrolyte loss during exercise in the heat: effects of gender and maturation, *Med Sci Sports Exerc* 24(7):776-781, 1992.

■ Mitchell JH, Tate C, Raven P et al: Acute response and chronic adaptation to exercise in women, *Med Sci Sports Exerc* 24(6):S258-S265, 1992.

■ Telford RD, Cunningham RB: Sex, sport, and body-size dependency of hematology in highly trained athletes, *Med Sci Sports Exerc* 23(7):788-794, 1991.

CHAPTER 24 | Exercise and Aging

OBJECTIVES

After studying this chapter you should be able to:

- Define the following terms: aging, life expectancy, chronologic age, biologic age.

- Explain how normal aging affects physiologic systems.

- Explain how aging affects cardiorespiratory endurance and muscular strength.

- Document research evidence that indicates that elderly individuals can adapt to exercise training for strength and cardiorespiratory endurance.

- Describe some important health promotion strategies for elderly people.

- Identify special concerns while exercise testing and prescribing exercise for elderly individuals.

KEY TERMS

aging

life expectancy

chronologic age

biologic age

longevity

left ventricular hypertrophy

*I*t has been estimated that during the first decade of the twenty-first century the most rapid increase in the population will be among those over 85 years of age.[20] Furthermore, by the year 2030 over 20% of the population will be over the age of 65.[60] Consequently, the health, fitness, and well-being of an aging population are of increasing concern in today's society. The role of exercise and the preventive and rehabilitative strategies available for the aging population, as well as for all individuals, needs to be researched. Are there special concerns for aging individuals who exercise? For example, does the aging process decrease an individual's capabilities to adapt to exercise stress, both acutely and chronically? Are there any special concerns for the elderly during exercise? Are there any special reasons for exercising as one becomes older? Can exercise decrease or delay the aging process? The purpose of this chapter is to define aging, to document known detriments in human physiology during aging, to identify the benefits and risks of exercise by the elderly, and to summarize what research has shown regarding the trainability of the aging body.

Aging

*A*ging should not be viewed as a sickness but as a natural process that involves the gradual alteration of body appearance, function, and tolerance to stress. Aging has been defined as a progressive loss of physiologic capacities that culminates in death.[8] Aging encompasses the human life span, which starts at birth, and involves growth, development to maturity, and the apparent deterioration that we perceive from peak physical maturity during the third decade of life to the inevitable death that occurs from either accident or old age. Typical markers of progressive aging include loss of height, a reduction in lean body mass, graying of hair, wrinkling of skin, changes in eyesight, and to some extent slightly less coordination of movement (Focus Box 24.1).

Since premature death has been reduced in this century, an increasing proportion of the population lives through the natural life span, which is suggested to approximate the period from birth to the age of 85. **Life expectancy** is the average, statistically predicted length of life for an individual. Today the average life expectancy for the majority of men in developed countries is about 71 years and for women is about 78 years.

One of the most serious problems facing most developed countries is how to continue to provide quality health care to an increasingly elderly population. It has been estimated that

---

aging (a'jing)
the process of growing old, involving the inability to reverse the gradual deterioration of cells important to the life process

life expectancy
the average, statistically predicted length of life for an individual

FOCUS BOX 24.1

Changes during the aging process

Lists of common, natural, physiologic changes that occur with aging. It is important to note that there is great individual variance with respect to when, and to what expect, these changes occur in individuals.

Appearance

Graying of hair
Balding
Drying and wrinkling of skin

Nervous system

Impairment of near vision
Some loss of hearing
Reduced taste and smell
Reduced touch sensitivity
Slowed reactions (reflexes)
Slowed mental function
Mental confusion

Cardiovascular system

Increased blood pressure
Increased resting heart rate
Decreased functional capacity
Decreased maximal cardiac output

Body composition/metabolism

Increased body fat
Raised blood cholesterol
Slowed energy metabolism
    (↓ basal metabolic rate)

Other physical characteristics

Menopause (women)
Loss of fertility (men)
Joints (loss of flexibility)
Loss of teeth (gum disease)
↓ Bone mineral density

Proneness to accidents and disease

Accidents
Inherited diseases
Life-style diseases

Psychologic and other

Reduced self-esteem
Loss of sex drive
Loss of interest in work
Depression, loneliness
Reduced financial status

---

health care costs for the institutionalized elderly in 1990 were 75 billion dollars in the United States.[55] Will a more active and physically fit elderly population decrease this health care cost? At the moment it is difficult to answer this question; however, it is known that regular exercise, independent of other factors, increases the average life span and improves quality of life.[38,41]

Theories of Aging

Aging is a normal biologic process. All multicellular organisms undergo changes with time. The progression of development, reproductive maturity, and aging has been extensively investigated in the biologic sciences. Most physiologic functions do decline with age but to different extents, and there are several theories as to why the aging process occurs.

Basal Metabolic Rate

Different species of animals age at different rates. Smaller animals tend to age faster than larger animals. The correlation between body size and aging rate has been linked to the species basal metabolism. Small animals generally have high metabolic rates, whereas humans have a slower rate and thus a longer life span. Something associated with high basal metabolism may be the cause of aging.

Biologic Clock

It has been suggested that cells have "biologic clocks" under genetic control, in that they are preprogramed to grow and divide. For example, in vitro studies have shown that the greater the life span potential of a species, the greater the number of divisions a cell undergoes before growth ceases. The cellular theory of aging suggests that each species has a natural preprogramed life span, which can be interrupted by numerous disease processes. With aging, certain cellular functions and structures can be lost or diminished. If cells lose their ability to repair themselves, the aging process can be accelerated.

Genetic Error

Errors in transcription of DNA or alteration in the information carried by DNA may result in accelerated aging. For example, if damage occurs to DNA through mutation, macromolecular damage, or some sort of programed damage, degeneration of the DNA strands can cause possible abnormal or defective information to be passed along to the next set of cells. Similarly, errors in DNA transcription could result in an incorrect amino acid being inserted into a cellular protein, leading to the accumulation of abnormal proteins and the eventual death of the cell.

Free Radicals

The idea that free radicals are responsible for aging has increased in popularity in recent years. Free radicals are chemical species that contain an unpaired electron in an outer orbit, which makes them very reactive (see Chapter 17). Such radicals, which are produced transiently during metabolism, can attack DNA or proteins. Another effect of free radicals is to cause peroxidation of the membrane lipids, which can interfere with many cellular processes.

Over the past decade, there has been increasing scientific and public interest in the possibility that antioxidant vitamins, such as ß-carotene (provitamin A), vitamin C, and α-tocopherol (vitamin E) might prevent cancer and heart disease and slow the aging process. Antioxidants help remove free radicals before they have a chance to cause cell damage. Observational epidemiologic data from both case control and cohort studies have suggested that persons who take large amounts of antioxidant vitamins have somewhat lower than average risk of cancer and cardiovascular disease. Although the evidence is limited, consuming antioxidant vitamins might prevent some exercise-induced stress (e.g., lipid peroxidation).

Immune Dysfunction

When the body's immune system is affected (possibly resulting from external factors, such as chronic exposure to radiation), cancerous cells can proliferate, leading to a destruction of one or more body organs or systems. Excess accumulation of substances in inappropriate places, such as the increased deposition of calcium in the media or subendothelial layer of large arteries or collagen in myocardial cells, the lungs, and skin, is apparent with advancing age.

The causes of human aging remain unclear. It appears that aging results from both internal and external forces. In some organs, such as the brain, cells die and are not replaced. In other tissues, cell function changes. For example, cross-linkages develop between adjacent collagen fibrils, decreasing elasticity and facilitating mechanical injury of the affected tissue. Blood vessels become progressively affected by atherosclerosis and arteriosclerosis, thereby decreasing oxygen supply to all body organs. Regardless of the many different causes of aging, death occurs from an infection or environmental stress, which cannot be tolerated by an older individual. The challenge confronting the medical community is not necessarily how to delay aging but how to ensure optimal quality of life for as much of the human life span as pos-sible. As explained subsequently, exercise plays a major role in this endeavor.

Chronologic Age Versus Biologic Age

Chronologic age is best represented by a person's birthday but is generally divided into young, middle, and old age. **Biologic age** is assessed by such variables as maximal oxygen uptake, bone mineral content, muscle strength, or flexibility. A person who is 65 years of age may have a biologic age of 45, based on that person's fitness and health status. The importance of regular exercise and health promotion cannot be emphasized enough when comparing chronologic with biologic age.

Biologic age may be altered by maintaining a regular physical fitness program. Kasch et al. found that active middle-aged men who followed a regular endurance exercise program over a 10-year period were able to prevent the usual 9% to 15% decline in physical working capacity and maximal aerobic power, thus lowering their biologic age.[21] Nakurma et al. studied 12 elderly men who followed a regular exercise program and estimated that they had an average biologic age that was 4.7 years lower than their chronologic age based on variables collected from 18 physiologic tests and five physical fitness tests.[34] Individuals who maintain a regular physical fitness program over time may have quite different chronologic versus biologic ages, which may increase their potential for better health and **longevity.**

Longevity is defined in the *Random House Dictionary* as "a long duration of life." How long an individual lives depends on a variety of factors, including heredity, environmental factors, availability of good medical and health services, and individual responsibility for health maintenance. To date, a fountain of youth has not been discovered. Perhaps the only fountain of youth we can rely on at present is the research supporting the health-related benefits of proper nutrition, moderate use of alcohol, use of seat belts, avoiding drinking and driving, and regular exercise.

Aging is unfortunately associated with disease and disability. Most humans today ultimately die of cancer and heart disease. Approximately four of five people who die of a heart

---

chronologic age
  the age of a person expressed relative to time (usually years)

biologic age
  the functional age of an individual, based on physiologic conditioning

longevity (lon-jev'i-ti)
  the duration of a life beyond the norm

FIGURE 24.1

Rates of death from leading causes (1992). (Adapted from the National Center for Health Statistics and the American Heart Association.)

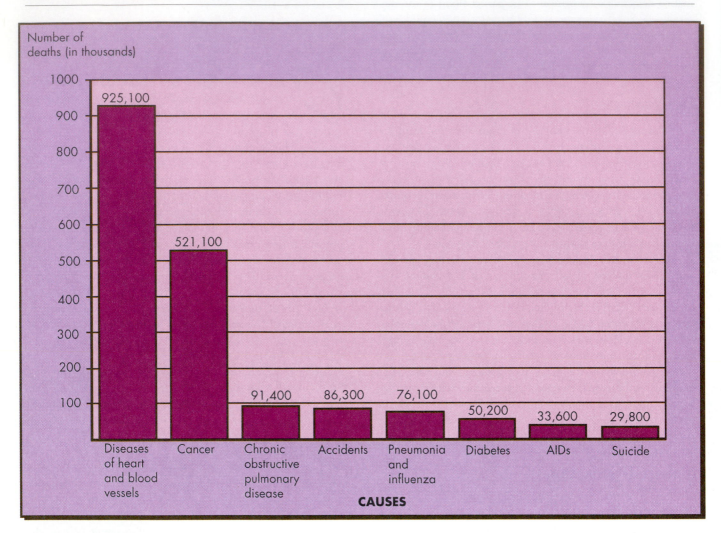

attack in the United States are over age 65 (Figure 24.1). For individuals over age 55, the incidence of stroke more than doubles in each successive decade. Of women age 55 to 64 in the United States, 53% have high blood pressure; for women over the age of 65 the figure rises to 68%.

The Framingham Study clearly established the link between age, gender, and risk of coronary heart disease (Figure 24.2). Even though certain physiologic changes are inevitable with aging, it appears that the rate of decline associated with the effects of aging can be reduced. Since the majority of people over 65 die from heart disease, cancer, and stroke, even preventive strategies initiated later in adult life may help improve the quality of elderly people's lives. It is becoming increasingly clear that regular, lifelong physical activity is an important component of preventive health strategies.

Normal Physiologic Changes With Aging

The study of physiologic changes with age comes from data collected from different cross-sectional and longitudinal studies. From approximately age 35, the effectiveness of various physiologic functions decreases. Changes occur in all organ systems with age. Nerve conduction velocity, cardiac index, maximum breathing capacity, and glomerular filtration rate show a considerable decline with age (Figure 24.3). To what extent these changes are affected by exercise is not completely understood. Table 24.1 lists some of the effects of exercise and aging on select body systems.

FIGURE 24.2

The increased risk for coronary heart disease with advancing age in both males and females. For a given age, risk is greater in males than females. (Adapted from Kannel WB, Gordon T: *Bull NY Acad Med* 54:579, 1978.)

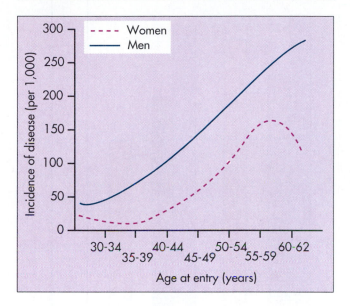

Cardiovascular Changes

It is difficult to pinpoint the effects of aging on the cardiovascular system. Deconditioning and disease also play significant roles in changes in the cardiovascular system over time. Both structural and functional changes occur to the cardiovascular system with increasing age. Functional and structural changes result in relatively minor changes in cardiovascular function at rest but significant differences in circulatory responses to exercise.

Structural Changes

Left ventricular hypertrophy is common in elderly people, probably resulting from long-term increases in afterload and arterial vascular stiffness.[14,27] There appears to be a decrease in the rate of ATP hydrolysis in contractile proteins isolated from myocardium of older versus younger animals.[4] In cardiac muscle isolated from senescent animals, contraction and relaxation times are prolonged. These changes are probably related to inhibition of calcium transport or alterations in calcium stores.

left ventricular hypertrophy

the increased mass of the myocardium of the left ventricle

TABLE 24.1

Effects of exercise training and aging on select body systems

BODY SYSTEM	EXERCISE TRAINING	AGING
CIRCULATORY		
CARDIOVASCULAR		
Maximal oxygen consumption	Increase	Decrease
Maximal heart rate	Increase	Decrease
Cardiac output	Increase	Decrease
Blood pressure	Same or decrease	Increase
Vascular resistance	Decrease	Increase
BLOOD COMPONENTS		
Total cholesterol	?	Increase
Triglycerides	Decrease	Increase
LDL cholesterol	?	Increase
HDL cholesterol	Increase	Decrease
IMMUNE SYSTEM	Increase	Decrease
MUSCULOSKELETAL		
MUSCLES		
Strength	Increase	Decrease
Endurance	Increase	Decrease
Flexibility	Increase	Decrease
BONY STRUCTURES		
Bone mineral content	Increase	Decrease
BODY COMPOSITION		
Lean body mass	Increase	Decrease
Adipose tissue	Decrease	Increase
REGULATORY SYSTEM		
METABOLIC		
Basal metabolic rate	Increase	Decrease
Heat gain	Increase	Decrease
Heat loss	Increase	Decrease
NERVOUS		
Sleep	Increase?	Decrease
Anxiety and depression	Decrease?	Increase?
Congnitive functioning	Increase	Decrease

?, Inconclusive or inadequate evidence.

Decreases in the function of several important physiologic functions with increasing age.

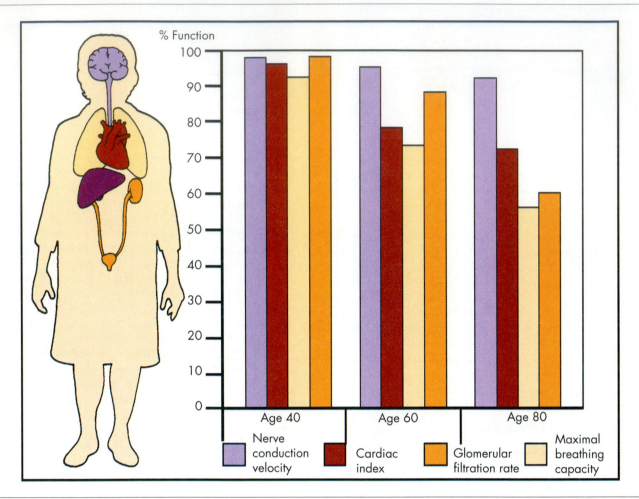

Older myocardial cells show increases in deposits of lipid and collagen, which cause myocardial changes, resulting in a stiffer and less compliant ventricle.[25] The cardiac valves become calcified with aging, leading to clinical manifestations, such as aortic stenosis and heart murmurs. Many elderly people require open heart surgery to replace or mend faulty heart valves (see the Clinical Application on p. 585). With age there is a progressive atrophy and fibrosis of the left bundle branches and a decrease in the number of SA node pacemaker cells. Changes in the electrical conduction system with age lead to the high rate of arrhythmias seen in elderly people and the increased need for artificial pacemaker implants.

Structural changes also occur to the vascular system with age. Arteriosclerosis is common in older people. Arteriosclerosis is defined as hardening and loss of elasticity of the arteries. Atherosclerosis is the buildup of fatty plaques in the arteries. With aging, blood vessels tend to increase in size and become dilated. Artery walls thicken with age, leading to a less compliant vascular system.

T A B L E   2 4 . 2

Age-related changes in cardiovascular function

FUNCTION	CHANGE
Resting heart rate	No change
Exercise heart rate	Slight decrease
Myocardial compliance	Moderate decrease
Systolic function	Slight decrease
Diastolic function	Moderate decrease
Stroke volume	Slight decrease
Cardiac output	Moderate decrease
Oxygen consumption	Moderate decrease
A-aO$_2$ difference	Slight increase

Exercise Testing and Training Guidelines for Valvular Heart Disease

The symptoms, limitations, and recommendations for physical activity in patients with valvular heart disease depend on the following:

- The valve(s) involved

- Whether the valve(s) are stenotic (do not open adequately) or regurgitate

- The severity of the valve lesions

- The presence of coronary artery disease, myocardial dysfunction, or other organ system disease

Exercise testing is not important in the diagnosis of most valvular diseases but can help quantify functional capacity. In general, exercise testing is relatively contraindicated in patients with critical aortic stenosis because of the risk of arrhythmia and death. For patients with pulmonic disease, exercise testing is carefully performed because of the risk of syncope.

Although not important for the diagnosis of mitral valve disease, exercise testing can provide important information regarding a patient's functional capacity. Exercise testing can be used to quantify the extent of hemodynamic impairment consequent to valvular heart disease. The results can be used to follow the progress of individuals and determine the appropriate time for intervention. Atrial arrhythmias may occur in patients with diagnosed mitral valve disease. In particular, atrial fibrillation eliminates the effective atrial contraction and worsens symptoms. A brief cardiac examination is usually performed before exercise testing in patients with aortic stenosis to determine if exercise testing is contraindicated. Exercise testing is not important in the diagnosis of tricuspid stenosis or regurgitation.

Patients with clinically significant mitral stenosis have marked limitation to exercise because cardiac output does not meet the demands of the exercising muscle. In general, if there is a significant limitation to activity, surgical correction is indicated. Otherwise, there is no therapeutic role for exercise training in mitral stenosis. Of course, improved skeletal muscle efficiency allows all patients to do more activity at the same cardiovascular workload. In addition, exercise may reduce other cardiovascular risk factors.

There is no specific therapeutic role for exercise training in mitral regurgitation. Patients with severe aortic stenosis should avoid vigorous physical activity because of the added risk of sudden death. Patients with cardiac dysfunction or limited cardiac reserve secondary to aortic insufficiency should refrain from vigorous exertion and sports.

With mitral valve disease, including mitral regurgitation, physical activity is limited mostly by the patient's symptoms. Before an exercise program begins, the upper training intensity and description of any symptoms should be documented using a diagnostic exercise test. Clearly the extent of the stenosis should be known. When symptoms of aortic stenosis, congestive heart failure, or syncope occur, valve replacement is generally pursued.

Functional changes

Heart rate, stroke volume, and cardiac output. Maximal heart rate is age related. With increasing age, maximal heart rate declines and is approximated by the following formula[18]:

24-1
$$HRmax = 220 - age$$

The decrease in maximal heart rate is probably related to a decreased chronotropic response to catecholamines. Because of the Fick equation ($VO_2 = HR \times SU \times [a-VO_2]$ Diff), a decrease in maximal heart rate decreases maximal cardiac output and thus contributes to a decreased maximal oxygen consumption.[32] Older sedentary individuals have achieved peak heart rates of 170 bpm or more during treadmill running and 160 bpm or more during cycle ergometry.[30]

Table 24.2 lists some of the physiologic age-related changes in cardiovascular function.

Maximal stroke volume also decreases during aging and can be a result of decreases in compliance, which limits ventricular filling, or an increase in vascular resistance. The presence of underlying heart or pulmonary disease can affect stroke volume performance, since certain diseases tend to increase preload and afterload, irrespective of aging or training. The increased impedance to ejection is largely responsible for the limiting increase in left ventricular stroke volume during exercise in elderly subjects. Elderly subjects rely heavily on the Frank-Starling mechanism (see Chapter 11) during exercise to overcome reduced responsiveness to catecholamines and decreased maximal heart rate.

CLINICAL APPLICATION

Exercise Testing and Training Guidelines for Individuals with Pacemakers and Intracardiac Defibrillators (ICDs)

Exercise testing can act as a diagnostic and a therapeutic tool in the adjustment of rate-responsive pacemakers. Once a permanent pacemaker with rate-responsive pacing capacity has been implanted, exercise testing is useful in the evaluation of pacemaker behavior, as well as optimizing the pacemaker response. Since most of the patients with pacemakers are older, the exercise protocol should use gradual increments in workload, such as modified Bruce, Balke, or Naughton protocol. It is important to remember that in patients with pacemaker dependence, ST segment changes do not reflect ischemic changes, and thus other diagnostic tests should be ordered (e.g., thallium).

Exercise testing is commonly used to evaluate the need for medical therapy in patients who survived an incidence of sudden death syndrome. Electrophysiologic testing can be used to evaluate underlying myocardial arrhythmias and the ability to generate and sustain reentry, the usual clinical mechanism for ventricular tachyarrhythmias. Clinically, the reentrant circuit is activated by some trigger that can include changes in heart rate.

Exercise Testing Guidelines

■ Indications for exercise testing in patients with implantable pacemakers or implantable cardioverter-defibrillators (ICDs) are the same for other populations, including diagnosis of coronary artery disease (CAD), evaluation of arrhythmias, and assessment of functional capacity. In addition, exercise testing is a useful tool to evaluate pacemaker function and to assist in pacer programing or reprograming.

■ Because of abnormalities in sinus node function, cardiac conduction, and neurohormonal systems, many patients with permanent pacemakers are unable to increase their intrinsic heart rate in response to exercise.

■ Before exercise testing the exercise technician and test supervisor should be familiar with the type and characteristics of the pacemaker or ICD.

■ Heart rate (HR), blood pressure (BP), and rating of perceived exertion (RPE) should all be closely monitored during the test and recovery period.

■ Since ST segment changes do not reflect ischemic changes in paced patients, if a test is being performed to evaluate CAD, other diagnostic tests should be performed, such as thallium scintography.

■ Low-increment treadmill protocols are preferred over the Bruce protocol in these patients.

Recent technologic advances have dramatically improved pacemaker function to the point at which they can nearly mimic normal cardiac function at rest and during exercise. Nevertheless, it is important that the exercise training upper heart rate limit be set below the patient's ischemic threshold.

Patients with ICDs are at risk of receiving inappropriate shocks during exercise. This can occur if the sinus heart rate exceeds the programed threshold rate or if the patient develops an exercise-induced supraventricular tachycardia. For this reason, patients with ICDs should be closely monitored during exercise to ensure that their heart rate does not approach the activation rate for the device. At least a 10% safety margin between exercise heart rate and rate cut-off for the device is advised.

Patients with ICDs and pacemakers can benefit from exercise training. In addition to improvements in functional capacity, exercise training can also reduce cardiac risk factors (e.g., cholesterol, hypertension) and improve psychosocial outcomes. Activities should be selected so that the intensity can be carefully regulated during exercise.

Both resting and maximal cardiac output are typically lower in older individuals. Resting cardiac output declines 1% per year after maturity, whereas resting stroke volume declines approximately 30% from the ages of 25 to 85. The drop in resting stroke volume, combined with the decrease in maximal heart rate, leads to a drop in maximal cardiac output in elderly individuals anywhere between 30% to 60%.[16] Specific concerns for exercise in individuals with implanted pacemakers are presented in the Clinical Application above.

Thomas et al. measured the response of cardiac output and left ventricular function to exercise in 96 men with an average age of 63.[56] Results indicated that cardiac output was approximately 10% lower in older individuals compared with younger subjects. During near-maximal exercise, cardiac out-

FIGURE 24.4

The changes in resting systolic and diastolic blood pressures with increasing age for both men and women. (Adapted from Kannel WB, Gordon T: *Bull NY Acad Med* 54:579, 1978.)

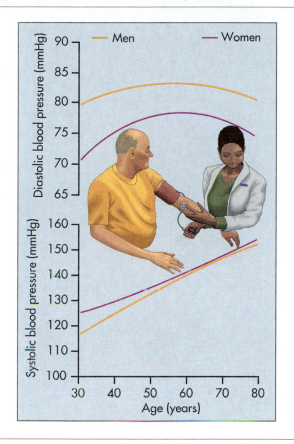

put reached 15 L/min and stroke volume was 95 ml. Peak a-$VO_2\Delta$ (150 ml/L) approached values of younger subjects. Ejection fraction increased from 66% at rest to 76% at peak exercise. Interestingly, the greatest limitation during exercise in the more elderly individual was a decreased central cardiovascular performance.

Blood pressure. One of the most obvious changes associated with age is resting blood pressure. Resting blood pressure increases with age (Figure 24.4). Systolic blood pressure seems to increase more with increasing age than diastolic blood pressure. The larger increase in systolic blood pressure may reflect the loss in elasticity of the vasculature with age. Compared with younger runners, older runners demonstrate a 15% to 20% higher vascular resistance, which results in higher blood pressure during submaximal and maximal exercise.[18] Endurance training can significantly reduce the mean blood pressure and the systemic vascular resistance in older individuals.[48]

Maximal oxygen uptake. With normal aging, maximal oxygen uptake (VO_2max) declines approximately 8% to 10% per decade after age 30.[45] Declines as great as 24% have been reported in the literature[10] (Figure 24.5). Kasch et al. performed serial measurements of cardiovascular function on 12 men, age 44 to 79 years of age and demonstrated that exercise training reduced the age-associated decline in VO_2max.[22]

The age-related decline in VO_2max has been associated with a decrease in maximal heart rate and stroke volume (thus

FIGURE 24.5

Schematic of the influence of age on cardiovascular function and exercise tolerance. As explained in the text, declining central cardiovascular functions are the main contributors to decreases in exercise performance in the elderly.

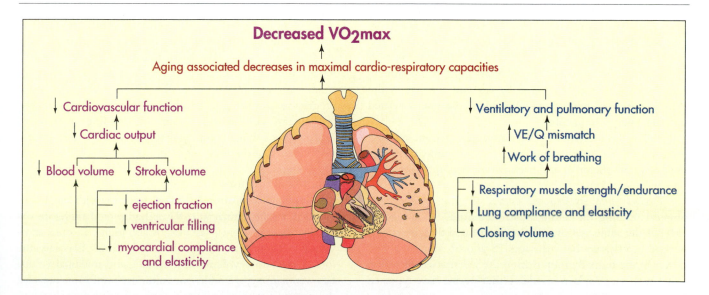

FIGURE 24.6

The age-related changes in lung volumes and pulmonary function. (Adapted from Shapiro BA, et al: *Clinical applications of blood gases*, 3 ed, Chicago, 1982, Year Book Medical.)

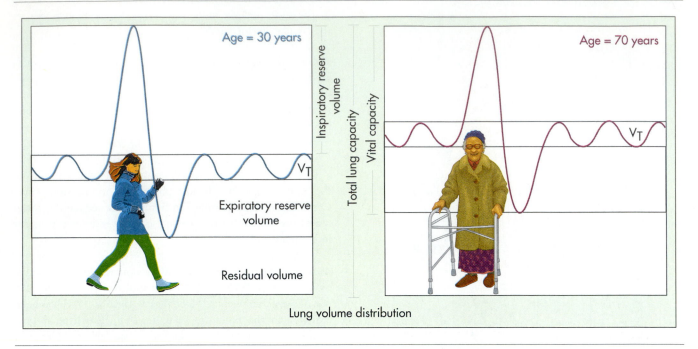

Lung volume distribution

a decrease in cardiac output), with only a slight decrease in a-$\dot{v}O_2\Delta$. Figure 24-6 shows the relation between aging changes in the cardiorespiratory system and reduced exercise capacity.

It is clear, however, that aerobic capacity can be improved at any age. Elderly women (mean age 73.6 years) who walked 5 days per week for 30 to 40 minutes per session at 60% of their heart rate reserve demonstrated a 12.6% increase in maximal oxygen uptake, compared with a matched control group.[22] A 6-month walking program (heart rate <120 bpm) increased VO_2max by an average of 12%, whereas high–intensity training (75% of heart rate reserve) improved VO_2max by 18% in 63-year-old.[48] Reduction in aerobic capacity can be altered by exercise training in the elderly, and more important, increasing age is not associated with declines in trainability.

Table 24.3 presents the effect of age, gender, and training status on cardiac output, heart rate, stroke volume, arteriovenous oxygen difference, and maximal oxygen uptake at maximal exercise.

Ogawa et al. studied the effects of aging, gender, and physical training on cardiovascular responses to training in 110 healthy subjects.[37] Researchers estimated that the rate of decline in VO_2max between ages 25 and 65 years was 40% slower in the trained group than in the sedentary male group (7.1% versus 11.3% per decade). Other studies have reported similar results.[18,45]

Pulmonary Changes

Aging causes significant changes in the structure and function of the pulmonary system, which in turn can limit participation of the elderly in moderate to strenuous physical activity.

Structural Changes

Some of the important structural changes that are a result of aging include a loss of alveolar elastic recoil, alterations in the chest wall structure, decreased respiratory muscle strength, a loss of alveolar surface area, and a loss of pulmonary blood volume. One of the most dramatic effects of aging is the progressive loss of elastic recoil, which leads to a progressive increase in residual lung volume. Changes in the pulmonary conduction system (excluding pathologic changes) are minimal and generally do not affect functional performance of the lung.

Functional Changes

Maximal ventilation (VEmax) decreases with age. However, for a submaximal VO_2, VE is higher and therefore the ventilatory equivalent (VE/VO_2) is also higher in older individuals.[37] There is a decrease in the expiratory flow rate, the forced expiratory volume in 1 second, and maximal voluntary ventilation.[24] In addition, pulmonary diffusion capacity, thoracic wall compliance, and vital capacity decrease with

TABLE 24.3

Effect of age, gender, and training status on cardiac output, heart rate, stroke volume, arteriovenous oxygen difference, and maximal oxygen uptake at maximal exercise

	SEDENTARY MEN		TRAINED MEN		SEDENTARY WOMEN		TRAINED WOMEN	
AGE (yr)	**23-31**	**60-68**	**21-31**	**59-72**	**20-27**	**60-72**	**18-30**	**51-63**
Cardiac output (L/min)	21.1	16.3	27.4	20.5	15.2	11.9	18.4	14.3
Heart rate (bpm)	185	163	178	165	189	162	181	167
Stroke volume (ml)	115	101	154	124	80	74	102	85
A-$\dot{v}O_2$ diff (ml/100 ml)	15.4	13.6	15.5	14.7	13.5	11.9	15.0	14.5
VO_2max (ml/kg/min)	45.9	27.2	63.5	47.6	37.0	22.2	52.1	35.3

TABLE 24.4

Age-related structural and functional changes in the pulmonary system

STRUCTURAL CHANGES	FUNCTIONAL CONSEQUENCES
THORAX	
Increased stiffness of costovertebral joints	Increased kyphosis
Decreased compliance of chest wall	Increased work of breathing
RESPIRATORY MUSCLES	
Decreased resting length	Decreased mouth occlusion pressures
	Decreased MVV
LUNG TISSUE	
Decreased size of alveoli and alveolar ducts	Less efficient mixing of alveolar and inspired air
	Decreased surface area for diffusion
Decreased number and thickness of elastic fibers	Increased resistance to flow in small airways
	Decreased $FEV_{1.0}$, FVC, $FEF_{200-1200ml}$, $FEF_{25\%-75\%}$
	Decreased elastic recoil
	Decreases VC, increased RV
	Change in resting length of respiratory muscles
	Increased closing volume, and redistribution of inspired air
VASCULATURE	
Decreased number of pulmonary capillaries	Decreased diffusing capacity
	Increased A-a O_2 gradient
	Decreased PaO_2, hemoglobin saturation
	VE/Q mismatch

MVV, maximal voluntary ventilation; $FEV_{1.0}$, forced expired volume in 1 s.; FVC, forced vital capacity; $FEF_{200-1200\,ml}$ forced expiratory flow; $FEF_{25\%-75\%}$, forced expiratory flow; VC, vital capacity; RV, residual volume.

FIGURE 24.7

The differences in cross-sectional area determined by computed tomography scans of the thigh in 12 men (mean age, 66 years) before and after 12 weeks of training. (Adapted from Frontera WR et al: *J Appl Physiol* 64(3):1038-1044, 1988.)

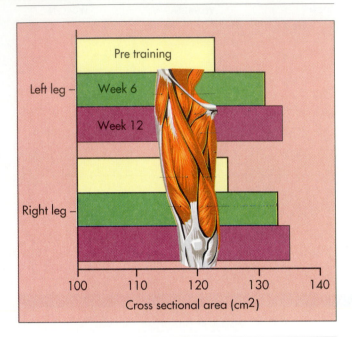

age, whereas residual volume increases.[3,11,58] The functional units of the lung, alveoli and alveolar ducts become smaller with aging.[40] Figure 24.6 shows the age-related changes in lung volumes, whereas Table 24.4 shows the age-related structural and functional changes in the pulmonary system.

The changes in lung function obviously make it harder for older individuals to move air in and out of the lung but do not impose any major problems in pulmonary gas exchange. During exercise, ventilation differs between young and old individuals. At low workloads, older persons tend to increase ventilation by increasing tidal volume, rather than via breathing frequency. In older individuals the increase in tidal volume may serve as a compensatory mechanism. High lung volumes decrease the resistance to inspiratory flow and improve elastic recoil. The increased elastic recoil improves expiratory flow. With aging, the ventilatory requirements during activities increase. A greater ventilation is needed for a given workload and for a given level of oxygen consumption.[40] Most age-related changes in respiratory capacity should not limit exercise capacity for generally healthy, active older individuals.

Musculoskeletal changes

Of perhaps greater concern to older individuals than age-related changes in cardiovascular and pulmonary func-

tion is the age-related changes that occur to the musculoskeletal system. The loss of bone and muscle strength often leads to serious and life-threatening injuries. Many of the age-related changes that occur to the musculoskeletal system are the result of physical inactivity.

Bones

With age, bones become more fragile because of osteoporosis. Serious and often debilitating fractures are common in the elderly. By the age of 90 as many as 32% of women and 17% of men will have sustained a hip fracture, and between 12% and 20% of this group will die of related complications. With age the loss of calcium results in a decrease in bone mass.[49] Bone mass decreases by approximately 10% at age 65 and by 20% at age 80. In women the loss is higher, amounting to approximately 20% by 65 and 30% by age 80. Osteoporosis, or a gradual loss or thinning of bone with aging, is a major concern to the elderly. Men tend to lose bone mass by about 1% per year after the age of 50, whereas women begin to lose bone mass in their early thirties with a 2% to 3% decline per year after menopause.[28] The causes of osteoporosis have been linked to hormonal, genetic, nutritional, and mechanical factors, in addition to immobilization and physical inactivity[7] (see Chapters 14, 17, and 23).

Regular exercise is known to help maintain bone mass. There is a significant correlation between muscle strength and bone mineral density.[50] The positive effect of exercise in preventing osteoporosis is based on extensive literature documenting the rapid onset and severe bone loss in immobilized individuals and the significant difference in bone density (bone strength) of physically active versus sedentary individuals.[52,53] Krolner et al. found that older women (50 to 73 years of age) who exercised for 1 hour twice weekly for 8 months increased their bone mineral content by 3.5%, whereas the sedentary controls of similar age lost 2.7% of bone mineral during the same period.[26] Regular physical activity, especially weight-bearing and resistance training, appears to have beneficial effects on the rate of age-related bone loss.

Skeletal Muscle

Muscle mass declines with age, resulting in decreased muscular strength and endurance. Muscular strength begins to decline around age 40 with an acceleration in decline after age 60. For each decade after the age of 25, 3% to 5% of muscle mass is lost. Muscle force and grip strength decrease significantly with age.[2,19] After age 74, 28% of men and 66% of women may not be able to lift objects weighing more than 4.5 kg.[15] The loss of muscle strength in elderly people can significantly affect the quality and length of life. Simple chores, such as taking out the trash or making the bed, can be terribly taxing in elderly individuals.

The loss of muscle mass has been attributed to changes in life-style and the decreased use of the neuromuscular system. Muscle cross-sectional area and the area of type II fibers

TABLE 24.5

Fiber type distribution and fiber areas in different age groups

AGE GROUP (YR)	N	MEAN AGE (YR)	FIBER TYPE DISTRIBUTION (%, TYPE II)	FIBER AREAS (μn_2) TYPE I	FIBER AREAS (μn_2) TYPE II
20-29	11	26.1 (0.8)	59.5 (3.9)	2944 (249)	3663 (224)
30-39	10	35.3 (1.0)	63.2 (1.5)	2854 (178)	3509 (282)
40-49	8	42.6 (0.8)	51.8 (5.1)	3133 (230)	3361 (296)
50-59	12	54.5 (0.6)	48.3 (3.0)	2877 (160)	2802 (125)
60-65	10	61.6 (0.6)	45.0 (4.5)	2264 (245)	2120 (174)

Data are means (±SD); adapted from Larson L, Grimby G, Karlsson J: *J Appl Physiol* 46:451-456, 1979.

decrease with advancing age.[9] The cross-sectional area of the quadriceps muscle has been shown to be reduced by 33%, resulting in a loss of strength of 35% in elderly women.[64] Other possible causes of the loss of muscle function and structure include deterioration of end-plate structures, impaired excitation-contraction coupling, and decrease in motor unit recruitment.[1] Muscle fiber type sizes and distributions change with age, which can lead to a decrease in muscle function (Table 24.5). Glenmark et al. recently found a gender-related fiber adaptation to increased age.[17] Glenmark found that type I fibers tend to increase in women and decrease in men, with fiber size remaining unchanged in both genders.

Significant strength gains are possible in the elderly. The results from a 1988 Tufts University study found that a group of 60- to 72-year-old untrained men, participating in 12 weeks of strength training (8 repetitions/set, 3 sets/day, 3 days/week at 80% of their 1 RM), showed a 107% increase in knee extensor strength and a 227% increase in knee flexor strength after 12 weeks of training.[15] Figure 24.7 shows the changes in thigh cross-sectional areas as quantified by CT scans of the right and left leg before, during, and 12 weeks after training in 12 men with a mean age of 66 years. This study demonstrated that strength gains do occur in older men, and these gains are associated with significant muscle hypertrophy and muscle protein turnover.

A low-intensity exercise program in 60- to 71-year-old men and women has been shown to significantly improve strength, balance, and flexibility.[6] Strength-trained athletes also tend to preserve their strength over time.[51] Rogers and Evans, in their excellent review of strength, aging, and training, noted that older individuals adapt to resistance training in a fashion similar to young people.[46]

Changes in Flexibility

With normal aging, connective tissue becomes stiffer and joints become less mobile. Loss of flexibility with age may be the result of underlying degenerative disease processes, such as arthritis. Flexibility does decrease with age, but there is no evidence that the biologic processes associated with aging are responsible for this loss. Loss of flexibility is more likely the result of diminishing physical activity. Flexibility can be improved at any age through exercises that promote the elasticity of the soft tissues. The degree to which flexibility can be improved in older individuals may be limited.[62] However, Rikli and Edwards recently demonstrated that flexibility can be significantly improved in 57- to 85-year-old women after an exercise program that included static stretching and range of motion exercises.[43]

Changes in Body Composition

With age, lean body weight declines and body fat increases. The changes in body composition resulting from age are primarily a result of a decrease in basal metabolic rate and declining physical activity habits. On average, there is a 10% reduction in basal metabolic rate between early adulthood and retirement age and a further 10% decrease after age 65.[35] The reduction in basal metabolic rate with age probably results from the decline in lean body mass, which has been estimated to be as high as 10% to 12% with advancing age.[5] The dramatic changes in body composition with age are also due to changes in overall body weight. A loss of 9 kg of muscle mass combined with an increase of 3.4 kg in body fat has been demonstrated in men in their eighth decade compared with men in their fifth decade.[59] By age 75 the typical composition of the body is 8% bone, 15% muscle, and 40% adipose tissue.[47]

Regular physical activity has been demonstrated to reverse the adverse changes in body composition typically experienced by elderly individuals. Exercise has been shown to preserve lean body mass, decrease fat stores, and stimulate protein synthesis.[31] Lean body mass has been shown to be maintained until age 65 in middle-aged and older athletes.[23] Poehlman et al. recently investigated the influence of age and endurance training on metabolic rate.[42] They found a higher resting metabolic rate (6%) and a normalized per kilogram measure of fat-free weight in endurance-trained older men than in untrained men.

Changes in Thermoregulation

Older individuals appear to have a less efficient thermal control system.[24] Both heat gain and heat loss mechanisms are less effective in older individuals. There are higher mortality and morbidity rates for heat-related illness in elderly, compared with younger, populations.[13] Older subjects tend to have higher rectal temperatures and heart rates when exercising in the heat compared with younger subjects.[61] In sedentary subjects the decreased thermoregulatory capacity in the heat is probably the result of a less-efficient sweating mechanism. However, trained elderly subjects tend not to display such discrepancy in thermoregulation versus their sedentary counterparts.[39] Pandolf et al. compared physically fit older subjects (46 to 68 years) with sedentary young subjects (19 to 30) and found that the older subjects did not differ significantly in their thermoregulation in the heat.[39]

Smolander et al. investigated the responses of young and older men during prolonged exercise in dry and humid heat.[54] Researchers found that there was not a significant difference in rectal or skin temperature, heart rate, thermal sensation, or RPE between the groups in any environmental

---

CLINICAL APPLICATION

Group Exercise Guidelines For Seniors

■ The pace of all movement should be slow to moderate. For choreographed routines, steps should be simple and repeated often. Fast transitions from one type of movement to another should be avoided to prevent postural hypotension and subsequent dizziness, falling, or fainting.

■ Several modes and positions of exercise should be used. Some positions include standing, sitting, standing with a chair for balance, and floor exercise using a mat. Before initiating floor exercise, feedback should be solicited from the group on whether the exercise is desirable. Some adults feel awkward or embarrassed if they have difficulty getting up from the floor in front of their peers. Instruction in how to get up from the floor may be necessary.

■ A variety of equipment should be used to achieve program objectives and sustain motivation. Examples include wands or dowels, surgical tubing, and towels or rubber strips for flexibility and range of motion; Frisbees and low walking beams for balance and coordination; and 1-pound weights for strength.

■ The pressor reflex should be avoided by keeping the overhead position of the arms to a minimum.

■ Special precautions should be taken for all participants who take medications. These include cardiovascular drugs, such as beta-blockers, calcium-channel blockers, and diuretics, which affect exercise tolerance. Hypotension may develop if a participant exercises soon after taking

nitroglycerin. The dose, type, and time of administration of insulin may need to be changed to prevent hypoglycemia. Medical approval and ongoing medical consultation for persons taking prescription drugs are recommended.

■ The exertion level of all participants should be continually monitored. Heart rate monitoring using the radial or carotid pulse should be taught. Permission to rest and get a drink of water should be given throughout the exercise class. Participants should be told frequently to progress at their own rate.

■ In addition to the instructor, one additional staff member should always be present to observe participants' physical reactions and to assist with any major or minor emergency.

■ The use of layered clothing should be suggested to prevent overheating or cooling. Older adults are less tolerant of the heat and cold.

■ A microphone should be used when conducting a program in a large area if the acoustics are poor. Lower tones can be more readily heard by the older adult.

■ For charts that will be viewed from a distance, such colors as yellow, orange, and red are seen more clearly.

■ The instructor should be certified in CPR, and a well-defined and routinely practiced procedure for emergencies should exist.

condition. The rectal temperatures and RPEs of the older subjects did continue to increase in the warm, humid environment. Thus researchers in this study concluded that age is not necessarily associated with a reduced ability to exercise in a hot environment and that functional capacity and physical activity habits may be more important in determining heat tolerance in the elderly.

Dehydration may also be a concern in older individuals, compared with younger subjects. Older persons generally have less body water and a reduced thirst mechanism, which increases their risk for dehydration during exercise.[12] Older individuals should be encouraged to gradually acclimatize to different environmental conditions, since the acclimatization process may take longer in elderly individuals. Furthermore, the need to ingest fluid during exercise is even more important in the elderly.

Exercise Prescription For The Elderly

Before starting an exercise program, elderly individuals should see their physician. Although many of the principles of prescribing exercise are the same for individuals of all ages, special care should be given when setting up a fitness program for older participants. A pre-exercise evaluation may involve a complete medical history, physical, and treadmill test because of the increased risk for cardiovascular disease in the elderly population. The results of the treadmill test can be used to develop the exercise prescription.

For most elderly patients, low-impact exercise is advisable. Exercise sessions should be tailored to combine endurance, muscle strength, and joint mobilization (Clinical Application, p. 592). Older individuals should be encouraged to become more physically active in all of their daily activities (e.g., use the stairs, walk to the store). Older individuals should be encouraged to bend, move, and stretch to keep joints flexible.

According to the American College of Sports Medicine, the goals for exercise in the elderly should include:

> maintenance of functional capacity for independent living, reduction in the risk of cardiovascular disease, retardation of the progression of chronic diseases, promotion of psychological well-being, and provision of opportunities for social interaction.

Intensity

The intensity of the exercise program should start out low, perhaps as low as 30% to 40% of VO_2max. Because low-intensity exercise is associated with a lower risk of injury and initial cardiorespiratory and thermoregulatory stress, it should be encouraged in the elderly population. Elderly individuals should know how to monitor their intensity level (i.e., breathing rate, heart rate, or rating of perceived exertion [RPE]). Elderly subjects may need a longer period of adjustment before exercising at higher intensity levels. Abrupt changes in exercise intensity are not recommended. Elderly people are more prone to exercise-related injuries, and they tend to need more time to recover between exercise sessions compared with younger participants.

Duration

The duration of an exercise program should start with short (10 to 15 minutes) periods and gradually progress from there. In addition to the duration of the exercise program itself, elderly people need additional warm-up and cool-down time, perhaps as much as 10 minutes or more. As the intensity of the exercise sessions gradually increases, the duration of the exercise sessions can also increase.

Frequency

In many cases, such as with individuals who have arthritis and peripheral vascular disease, the frequency of exercise training may be daily. Since many individuals can exercise for only short periods at a time because of structural and functional limitations, exercise training sessions have to be shorter, less intense, and thus more frequent. As functional capacity improves, the duration and intensity of the exercise training session can be increased and the frequency reduced.

Type

A comprehensive fitness program, including cardiorespiratory, flexibility, and strength training, is recommended. However, the type of exercise may need to be modified depending on pre-existing medical and health conditions. For example, for elderly individuals with degenerative joint disease, non–weight-bearing activities, such as stationary cycling, water exercises, and chair exercises, are recommended. Individuals with orthostatic hypotension benefit from sustained moderate activities with short rest intervals. Emphasis should be placed on movements that minimize changing body positions. The type of exercise should reflect the type and number of limitations they possess. Activities that involve a high degree of competition are discouraged initially.

Progression

The majority of elderly exercisers need to progress slowly. Changes in an exercise program need to be based on how well the individual is responding to the current regimen, the medical and health limitations of the individual, and individual goals. Exercise programs should be reviewed on a regular basis to ensure they are meeting the needs of the participant.

Special Precautions

Particular care should be given when prescribing weight-lifting exercises to those with high blood pressure, heart disease, or arthritis. Encourage an extended cool-down period of approximately 10 to 15 minutes. Elderly individuals often have a more difficult time when exercising in extreme environmental conditions. Physical activity should be planned for early morning or late evening during warm weather and midday during cold weather. Some elderly individuals with arthritis or poor joint mobility may have to participate in non–weight-bearing activities, such as cycling, swimming, and chair and floor exercises. Dehydration is a concern in the elderly; elderly exercisers should be encouraged to drink plenty of fluids before, during, and after exercise. Exercise adherence may be more difficult in the elderly population. Support and encouragement from physicians, spouses, and friends is highly recommended. Elderly exercisers should be instructed to report to their physician any unusual symptoms experienced before, during, or after exercise.

SUMMARY

- By the year 2030 more than 20% of our population will be over the age of 65. Currently, the **life expectancy** in developed countries is about 71 years for men and about 78 years for women.

- There are many theories of **aging,** including differences in basal metabolic rate, cellular preprogrammed life spans, errors in transcription of DNA, immune system dysfunction, free radicals, and excess accumulation of substances.

- A person might have a **chronologic age** of 65 yet have a **biologic age** of 45, based on that person's fitness and health status.

- Structural changes to the cardiovascular system with aging include **left ventricular hypertrophy,** increases in afterload and arterial vascular stiffness, decreases in the rate of ATP hydrolysis in contractile proteins isolated from myocardium, prolonged contraction and relaxation times, increases in deposits of lipid and collagen that cause myocardial changes, calcification of cardiac valves, progressive atrophy, and fibrosis of the left bundle branches.

- Functional changes to the cardiovascular system with aging include a decrease in maximal heart rate, an increase in blood pressure, vascular resistance, and myocardial oxygen consumption requirements, and a decrease in maximal stroke volume and cardiac output.

- With normal aging, VO_2max declines approximately 8% to 10% per decade after age 30. Declines as great as 24% have been reported in the literature. The age-related decline in VO_2max is more attributable to the decreases in central cardiovascular function than peripheral oxygen extraction (a-v$O_2\Delta$). Despite these decreases, VO_2max can be improved in the elderly, similar to young individuals, and may be evidence for improved **longevity** in elderly individuals who exercise.

- Some of the important structural changes to the pulmonary system that are a result of aging include a loss of alveolar elastic recoil, alterations in the chest wall structure, decreased respiratory muscle strength, a loss of alveolar surface area, and a loss of pulmonary blood volume.

- Functional changes to the pulmonary system that are a result of aging include a decrease in maximal ventilation (VEmax) and increases in the ventilatory equivalent for oxygen (V_E/VO_2). There are decreases in the expiratory flow rate, the forced expiratory volume in 1 second, and maximal voluntary ventilation. In addition, pulmonary diffusion, thoracic wall compliance, and vital capacity decrease with age and residual volume increases.

- With age, the loss of calcium results in a decrease in bone mineral content. Bone mass has decreased by approximately 10% at age 65 and by 20% at age 80. In women the loss is higher, amounting to approximately 20% by age 65 and 30% by age 80. Exercise, especially weight-bearing and resistance training, is known to help maintain bone mass.

- Muscle mass declines with age, resulting in decreased muscular strength and endurance. Muscular strength begins to decline around age 40 with an acceleration in the decline after age 60. For each decade after the age of 25, 3% to 5% of muscle mass is lost.

- With age, lean body weight declines and body fat increases. The changes in body composition resulting from age are due primarily to a decrease in the basal metabolic rate and physical activity habits of the elderly. On average, there is a 10% reduction in basal metabolic rate between early adulthood to retirement age.

- Older individuals appear to have a less efficient thermal control system. Trained elderly subjects tend not to display such large discrepancies in thermoregulation versus their sedentary counterparts. Older persons generally have less body water and a reduced thirst mechanism, which increases their risk for dehydration during exercise.

- Before starting an exercise program, elderly individuals should first see their physician. Although many of the principles of prescribing exercise to the elderly are the same for any group, special care should be given when setting up a fitness program for older participants.

REVIEW QUESTIONS

1. Define the term *aging*.

2. Why is there an increasing interest in the effects of exercise on elderly individuals?

3. List some of the physiologic changes that occur during aging.

4. Explain the aging processes and functions that exercise can potentially retard.

5. Why is it important to ensure that elderly individuals be concerned about fluid intake during exercise in a hot environment?

APPLICATIONS

1. What clinical conditions increase in incidence during aging?

2. What are some of the concerns for conducting exercise tests on elderly individuals?

3. Can an individual with an implanted pacemaker participate in regular physical activity? Explain.

4. Do the benefits of regular physical activity outweigh the risks in an elderly population? Explain.

REFERENCES

1. Aoyagi Y, Shephard RJ: Aging and muscle function, *Sports Med* 14:376-396, 1992.

2. Asmussen E, Fruensgaard K, Norgaard S: A follow-up longitudinal study of selected physiologic functions in former physical education students—after 4 years, *J Geriatr Soc* 23:442-450, 1975.

3. Belman MJ, Gasser GA: Ventilatory muscle training in the elderly, *J Appl Physiol* 64:899-905, 1988.

4. Bhatnagar GM, Walford GD, Beard ES: ATPase activity and force production in myofibrils and twitch characteristics in intact muscle from neonatal, adult, and senescent rat myocardium, *J Mol Cell Cardiol* 16:203-210, 1984.

5. Borkan GA, Hults DE, Gerzof AF et al: Age changes in body composition revealed by computed tomography, *J Gerontol* 38:673-677, 1983.

6. Brown M, Holloszy JO: Effects of a low intensity exercise program on selected physical performance characteristics of 60- to 71-year-olds, *Aging* 3(2):129-139, 1991.

7. Christiansen C: Consensus development conference on osteoporosis, *Am J Med* 95(5A), 1993.

8. Comfort A: *The biology of senescence,* London, 1973, Churchill Livingstone.

9. Davies CTM, White MJ: Contractile properties of the elderly human triceps surae, *Gerontology* 29:19-25, 1983.

10. Dehn M, Bruce R: Longitudinal variations in maximal oxygen uptake with age and activity, *J Appl Physiol* 33:805-807, 1972.

11. Donevan RE, Palmer WH, Varis CJ, Bates DV: Influence of age on pulmonary diffusing capacity, *J Appl Physiol* 14:483-492, 1959.

12. Eisenman PA: Hot weather, exercise, old age, and the kidneys, *Geriatr* 41:108-114, 1986.

13. Ellis FP: Mortality from heat illness and heat-aggravated illness in the United States, *Environ Res* 5:1, 1972.

14. Folkow B, Svanborg A: Physiology of cardiovascular aging, *Physiol Rev* 73(4):725-764, 1993.

15. Frontera WR, Meredith CN, O'Reilly KP et al: Strength conditioning in older men: skeletal muscle hypertrophy and improved function, *J Appl Physiol* 64:1038-1044, 1988.

16. Geokas MR, Lakatta EG, Makinodan T, Timiras PS: The aging process, *Ann Intern Med* 113:455-466, 1990.

17. Glenmark B, Hedberg G, Jasson E: Changes in muscle fiber type from adolescence to adulthood in women and men, *Acta Physiol Scand* 146(2):251-259, 1992.

18. Hagberg JM, Allen M, Seals DR et al: A hemodynamic comparison of young and older endurance athletes during exercise, *J Appl Physiol* 58:2041-2046, 1985.

19. Hagberg JM, Graves JE, Limacher M et al: Cardiovascular responses in 70- to 79-year-old men and women to exercise training, *J Appl Physiol* 66:2589-2594, 1989.

20. Institute of Medicine: *The second fifty years: promoting health and preventing disability,* Washington, DC, 1992, National Academy Press.

21. Kasch FW: The effects of exercise on the aging process, *Physiol Sports Med* 4:64-69, 1976.

22. Kasch FW, Boyer JL, Van Camp SP et al: Effect of exercise on cardiovascular aging, *Age and Aging* 22:5-10, 1993.

23. Kavanagh T, Shephard RJ: The effects of continued training on the aging process, *Ann NY Acad Sciences* 301:656-670, 1977.

24. Kenney R: Physiology of aging, *Clin Geriatr Med* 1:37-58, 1985.

25. Klausner SC, Schwartz AB: The aging heart, *Clin Geriatr Med* 1:119-141, 1985.

26. Krolner B, Toft B, Nielsin SP, Tondevold E: Physical exercise as prophylaxis against voluntary vertebral bone loss: a controlled study, *Clin Sci* 64:541-646, 1983.

27. Lakatta EG: Hemodynamic adaptations to stress with advancing age, *Acta Med Scand* 711(Suppl):39-52, 1985.

28. Landin RJ, Linnemeier TJ, Rothbaum DA et al: Exercise testing and training of the elderly patient, *Cardiovasc Clin* 15:201-218, 1985.

29. Larson L, Grimby G, Karlsson J: Muscle strength and speed of movement in relation to age and muscle morphology, *J Appl Physiol* 46:451-456, 1979.

30. Londeree BR, Moeschberger ML: Effect of age and other factors on maximal heart rate, *Res Quart* 53:297-304, 1982.

31. McMurray RC, Ben-Ezra V, Forsythe WA, Smith AT: Responses of endurance-trained subjects to caloric deficits induced by diet and exercise, *Med Sci Sports Exerc* 17:574-579, 1985.

32. Mann D, Denenberg BS, Gash AK et al: Effects of age on ventricular performance during graded supine exercise, *Am Heart J* 111:108-115, 1986.

33. Milne JS, Williamson J: Respiratory function tests in older people, *Clin Sci* 42:371-381, 1972.

34. Nakamura E, Moritani T, Kanetake A: Biological age versus physical fitness age, *Eur J Appl Physiol* 58:778-785, 1989.

35. National Academy of Sciences Committee on Dietary Allowances, Food and Nutrition Board: *Recommended dietary allowances,* Washington, DC, 1980, National Academy of Sciences.

36. National Center for Health Statistics: *Health, United States, 1989 and prevention profile,* DHHS Pub. No. (PHS) 90-1232, Hyattsville, Maryland, 1990, US Department of Health and Human Services.

REFERENCES—Cont'd

37. Ogawa T, Spina RJ, Martin WH et al: Effects of aging, sex, and physical training on cardiovascular responses to exercise, *Circulation* 86:494-503, 1992.

38. Paffenbarger RS, Hyde RT, Wing AL, Hsieh CC: Physical activity, all-cause mortality and longevity of college alumni, *N Engl J Med* 314:605-613, 1986.

39. Pandolf KB, Cadarette BS, Sawaka MN et al: Thermoregulatory responses of middle-aged and young men during dry-heat acclimation, *J Appl Physiol* 65:65-71, 1988.

40. Patrick JM, Bassey EJ, Fentem PH: The rising ventilatory cost of bicycle exercise in the seventh decade: a longitudinal study of nine healthy men, *Clin Sci* 65:521-526, 1983.

41. Pekkanen J, Marti B, Nissinen A et al: Reduction of premature mortality by high physical activity: 20-year follow-up of middle aged Finnish men, *Lancet* 1:1473-1477, 1987.

42. Poehlman ET, McAuliffe TL, Van Houten DR, Danforth E: Influence of age and endurance training on metabolic rate and hormones in healthy men, *Am J Physiol* 159:E66-E72, 1991.

43. Rikli RE, Edwards DJ: Effects of a three-year exercise program on motor function and cognitive speed in older women, *Res Quart Exer Sport* 62(1):61-67, 1991.

44. Robinson S, Dill DB, Tzankoff SP et al: Longitudinal studies of aging in 37 men, *J Appl Physiol* 38:263-267, 1975.

45. Rogers MA, Hagberg JM, Martin WH, et al: Decline in VO₂max with aging in master athletes and sedentary men, *J Appl Physiol* 68:2195-2199, 1990.

46. Rogers MA, Evans WJ: Changes in skeletal muscle with aging: effects of exercise training, *Exer Sport Sci Rev* 21:65-102, 1993.

47. Rudman D: Growth hormone, body composition, and aging, *J Geriatr Soc* 33:800-807, 1985.

48. Seals DR, Hagberg JM, Hurley BF et al: Endurance training in older men and women. I. Cardiovascular responses to exercise, *J Appl Physiol* 57:1024-1029, 1984.

49. Shephard RJ: *Body composition in biological anthropology,* London, 1991, Cambridge University Press.

50. Sinaki M: Exercise and osteoporosis, *Arch Phys Med Rehabil* 70(3):220-229, 1989.

51. Sipila S, Viitasalo J, Era P, Suominen H: Muscle strength in male athletes aged 70-81 years of age and a population sample, *Eru J Appl Physiol* 63(5):399-403, 1991.

52. Smith EL, Reddan W, Smith PE: Physical activity and calcium modalities for bone mineral increase in aged women, *Med Sci Sports Exerc* 13:60-64, 1981.

53. Smith EL: Exercise for prevention of osteoporosis: a review, *Phys Sports Med* 10(3):72-83, 1982.

54. Smolander J, Korhonen O, Ilmarinen R: Responses of young and older men during prolonged exercise in dry and humid heat, *Eur J Appl Physiol* 61:413-418, 1990.

55. Spirduso WW: Physical activity and aging: introduction. In American Academy of Physical Education Papers: *Physical activity and aging,* Champaign, Illinois, 1989, Human Kinetics Publishers.

56. Thomas SG, Paterson DH, Cunningham DA et al: Cardiac output and left ventricular function in response to exercise in older men, *Can J Physiol Pharmacol* 71:136-144, 1993.

57. Turlbeck WM, Anges GE: Growth and aging of the normal lung, *Chest* 67:35-75, 1975.

58. Turner JM, Mead J, Wohl ME: Elasticity of human lungs in relation to age, *J Appl Physiol* 25:664:671, 1968.

59. Tzankoff SP, Norris AH: Effect of muscle mass decrease on age-related BMR changes, *J Appl Physiol* 43:1001-1006, 1977.

60. US Dept of Health and Human Services: Healthy people 2000: national health promotion and disease prevention objectives, Washington, DC, 1991, US Government Printing Office.

61. Wagner JA, Robinson S, Tzankoff SP, Marino RP: Heat tolerance and acclimatization to work in the heat in relation to age, *J Appl Physiol* 33:616-622, 1972.

62. Walker JM, Sue D, Miles-Elkousy N et al: Active mobility of the extremities in older subjects, *Phys Ther* 64:919-923, 1984.

63. Warren BJ, Nieman DC, Dotson RG et al: Cardiorespiratory responses to exercise training in septuagenarian women, *Int J Sports Med* 14(2):60-65, 1993.

64. Young A, Stokes M, Crowe M: The size and strength of quadriceps muscles of old and young women, *Eur J Clin Invest* 14:282-287, 1984.

RECOMMENDED READINGS

■ Aoyagi Y, Shephard RJ: Aging and muscle function, *Sports Med* 14:376-396, 1992.

■ Borkan GA, Hults DE, Gerzof AF et al: Age changes in body composition revealed by computer tomography, *J Gerontol* 38:673-677, 1983.

■ Dehn M, Bruce R: Longitudinal variations in maximal oxygen uptake with age and activity, *J Appl Physiol* 33:805-807, 1972.

■ Frontera WR, Meredith CN, O'Reilly KP et al: Strength conditioning in older men: skeletal muscle hypertrophy and improved function, *J Appl Physiol* 64:1038-1044, 1988.

■ Hagberg JM, Allen M, Seals DR et al: A hemodynamic comparison of young and older endurance athletes during exercise, *J Appl Physiol* 58:2041-2046, 1985.

■ Landin RJ, Linnemeier TJ, Rothbaum DA et al: Exercise testing and training of the elderly patient, *Cardiovasc Clin* 15:201-218, 1985.

■ Ogawa T, Spina RJ, Martin WH et al: Effects of aging, sex, and physical training on cardiovascular responses to exercise, *Circulation* 86:494-503, 1992.

■ Patrick JM, Bassey EJ, Fentem PH: The rising ventilatory cost of bicycle exercise in the seventh decade: a longitudinal study of nine healthy men, *Clin Sci* 65:521-526, 1983.

■ Rogers MA, Hagberg JM, Martin WH et al: Decline in VO_2max with aging in master athletes and sedentary men, *J Appl Physiol* 68:2195-2199, 1990.

■ Rogers MA, Evans WJ: Changes in skeletal muscle with aging: effects of exercise training, *Exer Sport Sci Rev* 21:65-102, 1993.

■ Young A, Stokes M, Crowe M: The size and strength of quadriceps muscles of old and young women, *Eur J Clin Invest* 14:282-287, 1984.

CHAPTER **25**

Pediatric Exercise Science

OBJECTIVES

After reading this chapter you should be able to:

■ Describe the unique physiologic and anatomic aspects of children and adolescents.

■ List specific recommendations for exercise testing and training for children and adolescents.

■ Explain how children and youth respond and adapt to exercise compared with adults.

■ Describe the normal growth and development of children and how exercise affects growth and development.

■ Describe some important health promotion and disease prevention strategies for children and adolescents.

KEY TERMS

pediatric exercise science

pediatrician

criterion-referenced
  fitness standards

adolescence

puberty

peak height velocity

The term pediatric exercise science has evolved over time in an effort to include the diverse nature of exercise-related research being conducted on children and youth around the world. For example, youth fitness test norms have evolved from tests that could be conducted only in the field to tests using sophisticated laboratory equipment. Such tests have measured with greater accuracy the cardiorespiratory capacity of children of different ages or after growth, how skeletal muscle anaerobic capacity changes with growth and development, and how these capacities change with specific types of exercise training. Furthermore, we now know more about the effects of weight training on prepubertal children, the ability of children to tolerate exercise in hot or humid environments, and the role of exercise in promoting health and well-being through the reinforcement of appropriate behaviors and life-styles. The purpose of this chapter is to introduce the field of pediatric exercise physiology, explain how children of different ages respond acutely during exercise and chronically to exercise training, and identify areas of concern regarding children's participation in specific exercise conditions.

The Emerging Field of Pediatric Exercise Science

The field of **pediatric exercise science** has emerged as a powerful and influential subspecialty of the field of exercise physiology. Although still a young discipline, it boasts several national and international associations, including the European Group for Pediatric Work Physiology, formed in 1985, and has support from other organizations, including the American Academy of Pediatrics (AAP), the American Alliance of Health, Physical Education, Recreation and Dance (AAHPERD), and the American College of Sports Medicine (ACSM).

The first group of clinicians and physiologists to be established for the purpose of gathering and disseminating research on exercise and children was the International Group for Pediatric Work Physiology, formed in 1967. Since the early 1970s the International Group of Pediatric Work Physiology has been holding symposiums around the world. In 1985 the North American Society of Pediatric Exercise Medicine (NASPEM) was formed. NASPEM is the only American organization devoted solely to exercise and children. NASPEM's goals are to gather and disseminate research information on exercise as it affects health and fitness. The official journal of NASPEM is *Pediatric Exercise Science,* pub–

pediatric exercise science
a specialized sub-field of exercise physiology dealing with the unique aspects of the effects of exercise on children and adolescents

lished quarterly. Another group devoted to exercise and children is the Pediatric Exercise Forum, which is sponsored by the American College of Sports Medicine. The Pediatric Exercise Forum now sponsors pediatric exercise programs at ACSM annual meetings.

Such researchers as Bar-Or, Shephard, Rowland, Pate, Malina, Kuntzleman, Corbin, and Saris are some of today's leading pediatric exercise scientists. A dramatic increase in the number of topics focused on children can be seen by looking through any current exercise textbook or sports medicine journal. Between 1981 and 1982, journals of pediatric physiology and sports medicine published three to five times as many articles on the exercising child as had been published 10 years earlier.[2]

For many years, women and children were underrepresented in exercise research. Today, however, children are receiving more focus in exercise research (Figure 25.1). **Pediatricians** are currently performing routine exercise studies to diagnose and develop treatment strategies for a variety of health-related problems in children, such as asthma and congenital heart disease. In addition, physiologists are conducting pediatric research in an effort to plan health promotion strategies and exercise programs for children and youth. The next decade will likely witness an explosive growth in pediatric exercise research similar to that seen in the 1970s, 1980s, and 1990s for adult subjects.

Limitations of Research in Pediatric Exercise Physiology

Compared with adult exercise research, pediatric research has two distinct limitations—ethical and methodologic. Because children cannot freely give their consent to participate in research studies, is it really ethical to use children as subjects in research? The same reasoning and justification for allowing adults in exercise research can be used to answer this question. To use children in exercise studies, researchers must have sufficient justification (e.g., animal models cannot be used) and must be able to ensure their safety. The procedures and possible benefits of participating must be fully explained to subjects and their parents. It is important to note that pediatric exercise research has led to valuable insights in the prevention and treatment of such diseases as asthma, obesity, and cystic fibrosis.[12]

The other major problem associated with planning and conducting pediatric exercise research deals with methodology. For example, most exercise testing protocols and equipment are designed for adults. It is difficult to get young children to walk or run comfortably on a treadmill without a great deal of support and encouragement. When isokinetic testing is performed, the seats and resistance settings are often not adjustable to fit children accurately. Many of these

FIGURE 25.1

Completing an incremental exercise test on a treadmill.

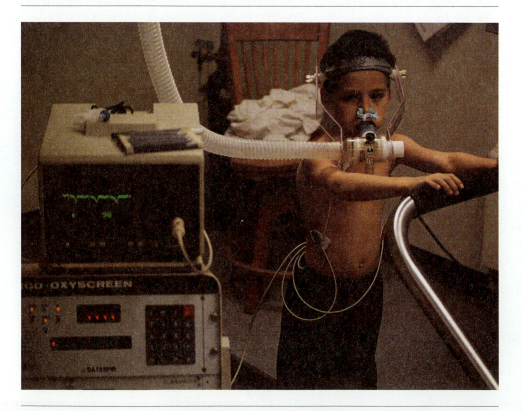

methodologic problems can be overcome with some creativity. All methodologic concerns and problems should be addressed in the discussion and conclusion of a research paper.

Other methodologic concerns regarding pediatric exercise research are how to correct physiologic data to individual or group changes in children's growth rates and how best to relate physiologic data in children to older children or adults. As children grow and develop, their absolute VO_2 increases linearly until the age of 18 in boys and 14 in girls, regardless of training. For example, if researchers claim that the exercise training increased VO_2max compared with pretraining, this brings forth the question of how much of the improvement in VO_2max was due to normal biologic development and how much to training. This is a good example of the need for a control group when studying physiologic responses of children, even in repeated measures designs. To further complicate the problem, there is tremendous individual and group variation in growth rates among children. Thus, if some of the children in the group receiving training were more mature at the start or matured at a faster rate during the study compared with a control group, the benefits of training on VO_2max in children would be exaggerated.

Another problem is how best to relate physiologic data in children to older children or adults. For example, VO_2max in adults is usually expressed as oxygen uptake per kilogram body weight. For years, researchers have been trying to establish norms for VO_2 based on height, age, body surface area, weight, and lean body mass. When VO_2 is compared between an 8-year-old child and an 18-year-old adult, in absolute terms (L/min) the child's aerobic capacity is lower, per kilogram of body weight (ml/kg/min) it is equal, per height squared (L/m^2) it is lower, and per height it is slightly lower.[13] Each method produces a different result. According to Rowland, "there is no clear cut means of equating oxygen uptake between individuals of varying sizes and functional maturity."[107]

Fitness and Health Status of American Children

Over the past two decades several large-scale youth fitness surveys have been conducted, and the results provide much of the evidence that is used to judge the past and current health and fitness status of American children and youth. The first youth fitness tests focused on skill related fitness, whereas more recent surveys have looked at health-related fitness. Some tests items, such as the softball throw, long jump, and 50-yard dash, have been replaced with items that measure body composition, flexibility, muscular strength, and endurance (Table 25.1). The initiative to change youth fitness tests to include more health-related variables has been based on the available literature linking improved cardiovascular fitness, muscle strength, flexibility, and body composition to reduced disease and disability.

In the late 1950s and early 1960s several organizations began surveying youth fitness in the United States. In 1957 AAHPERD developed a youth fitness test and established national fitness norms.[3] Since the first AAHPERD test, numerous other organizations, as well as AAHPERD, have conducted youth fitness tests.* How best to interpret the results of these tests continues to be a highly debated topic among physical educators and physiologists. Fitness test data are typically evaluated by comparing individual scores or group means with normative standards (percentile scores) or with previously collected data on the same population. The problem with this approach is that it is difficult to control for differences in test protocols, growth and development status of children, and genetic endowment, any of which could affect the accuracy of youth fitness tests. Review of secular trends in the fitness of children, such as comparisons between today's children and their counterparts from previous decades, has been used inaccurately to portray children today as fat, out of shape, and less fit than children from previous decades. Such reliance on the review of secular trends is unfortunate, since the only significant trend in American children is for a slight increase in subcutaneous fat, and American children compare favorably on most items with age-matched groups in Europe, Great Britain, Australia, and Canada.[40]

There is currently a movement among youth fitness experts to use criterion-referenced fitness standards that are based on established fitness and health relationships. **Criterion-referenced fitness standards** set minimal scores for selected variables that meet acceptable standards for good health.[32] Criterion-referenced standards for children have been developed by the Institute for Aerobic Research (Tables 25.2 and 25.3).[74] Based on these fitness standards, American children are reasonably fit. The only area in which children appear to be below the average fitness level is upper body strength.

Body Fat

The only secular trends in youth fitness that have been analyzed with a high degree of accuracy are skinfold data (see Focus Box 25.1). Skinfold data collected in the 1960s and 1970s have been compared with data collected in the National Children and Youth Fitness Survey II (Figure

---

*References 1, 4, 28, 54, 94, 103, and 104.

---

pediatrician (pe-di-a-trish´an)
a medical doctor who specializes in the care of children

criterion-referenced fitness standards
fitness standards that are based on an established fitness and health relationship

TABLE 25.1

Description of different youth fitness tests (1958 through 1988)

FITNESS COMPONENT	AAHPER YOUTH FITNESS TEST (1958)	AAHPER YOUTH FITNESS TEST (1965)	AAHPER YOUTH FITNESS TEST (1975)	AAHPERD HEALTH-RELATED PHYSICAL FITNESS TEST (1980)	AAHPERD PHYSICAL BEST (1988)
Cardiorespiratory endurance	600-yd (550-m) walk/run	600-yd (550-m) walk/run	600-yd (550-m) walk/run Options: 1-mile (1.6-km) or 9-min run (ages 10-12); 1.5-mile (2.4-km) or 12-min run (ages >13)	1-mile (1.6-km) or 9-min run Option: 1.5-mile (2.4-km) or 12-min run	1-mile (1.6-km) run/walk
Body composition	None	None	None	Sum of skinfolds (triceps and subscapular)	Sum of skinfolds (triceps and calf) Options: Sum of triceps and subscapular Triceps only Body mass index
Flexibility	None	None	None	Sit-and-reach	Sit-and-reach
Muscular strength and endurance Abdominal	Sit-ups: (straight leg, hands behind head; elbow touches opposite knee; maximum number)	Sit-ups (same as 1958)	Sit-ups: (bent knee; arms across chest; number in 1 min)	Sit-ups: (arms across chest; curl up to sitting position; elbows touch thighs; number in 1 min)	Sit-ups: (same as 1980)
Upper body	Pull-ups	Pull-ups (boys) Flexed arm hang (girls)	Pull-ups (boys) Flexed arm hang (girls)	None	Pull-ups
Anaerobic power	Standing long jump	Standing long jump	Standing long jump	None	None
Speed	50-yd (45.9) dash	50-yd (45.9) dash	50-yd (45.9) dash	None	None
Agility	Shuttle run	Shuttle run	Shuttle run	None	None
Motor skill	Softball throw for distance	Softball throw	None	None	None

From Pate RR, Shephard RJ: characteristics of physical fitness in youth. In Lamb DR, Gisolfi CV, editors: *Perspectives in exercise science and sports medicine, vol 2, youth, exercise, and sport,* 1989, Dubeque, Iowa, Times Mirror Higher Education Group.

25.2).[105] There appears to be a systematic increase in skinfold thickness among 6- to 9-year-old boys and girls from the 1960s and 1970s to the 1980s. Gortmaker et al. investigated the prevalence of obesity in children aged 6 to 17 using skinfold data obtained in the National Health Examination Survey (NHES) (1963-1970) and the National Health and Nutrition Examination Survey (1971-1974 and 1976-1980).[44] Obesity was defined as being above the eighty-fifth percentile for triceps skinfolds. Gortmaker et al. estimated that obesity in the 6-to-11 age group had increased from 17.6% between 1963 and 1965 to 27.1% between 1976 and 1980. Lohmann et al. compared NHES skinfold data from the 1960s with the National Children Youth Fitness Study (NCYFS) skinfold data from the mid-1980s.[64] Lohman's analysis revealed that obesity increased during this time period when 25% body fat for males and 32% body fat for

TABLE 25.2

The Prudential FITNESSGRAM: Standards for healthy fitness zone*

GIRLS

AGE	ONE-MILE min:sec		PACER # laps		VO$_2$max ml/kg/min		PERCENT FAT		BODY MASS INDEX		CURL-UP # completed	
5	Completion of		Participate in				32	17	21	16.2	2	10
6	distance. Time		run. Lap count				32	17	21	16.2	2	10
7	standards not		standards not				32	17	22	16.2	4	14
8	recommended.		recommended.				32	17	22	16.2	6	20
9							32	17	23	16.2	9	22
10	12:30	9:30	7	35	39	47	32	17	23.5	16.6	12	26
11	12:00	9:00	9	37	38	46	32	17	24	16.9	15	29
12	12:00	9:00	13	40	37	45	32	17	24.5	16.9	18	32
13	11:30	9:00	15	42	36	44	32	17	24.5	17.5	18	32
14	11:00	8:30	18	44	35	43	32	17	25	17.5	18	32
15	10:30	8:00	23	50	35	43	32	17	25	17.5	18	35
16	10:00	8:00	28	56	35	43	32	17	25	17.5	18	35
17	10:00	8:00	34	61	35	43	32	17	26	17.5	18	35
17+	10:00	8:00	34	61	35	43	32	17	27.3	18.0	18	35

AGE	TRUNK LIFT inches		PUSH-UP # completed		MODIFIED PULL-UP # completed		PULL-UP # completed		FLEXED ARM HANG seconds		BACK SAVER SIT & REACH† inches	SHOULDER STRETCH
5	6	12	3	8	2	7	1	2	2	8	9	
6	6	12	3	8	2	7	1	2	2	8	9	
7	6	12	4	10	3	9	1	2	3	8	9	
8	6	12	5	13	4	11	1	2	3	10	9	Passing = Touching the fingertips together behind the back.
9	6	12	6	15	4	11	1	2	4	10	9	
10	9	12	7	15	4	13	1	2	4	10	9	
11	9	12	7	15	4	13	1	2	6	12	10	
12	9	12	7	15	4	13	1	2	7	12	10	
13	9	12	7	15	4	13	1	2	8	12	10	
14	9	12	7	15	4	13	1	2	8	12	10	
15	9	12	7	15	4	13	1	2	8	12	12	
16	9	12	7	15	4	13	1	2	8	12	12	
17	9	12	7	15	4	13	1	2	8	12	12	
17+	9	12	7	15	4	13	1	2	8	12	12	

*Number on left is lower end of HFZ; number on right is upper end of HFZ
†Test scored Pass/Fail; must reach this distance to pass.

From The Cooper Institute for Aerobics Research, Dallas, Texas.

TABLE 25.3

The Prudential FITNESSGRAM: Standards for healthy fitness zone*

BOYS

AGE	ONE-MILE min:sec		PACER # laps		VO₂max ml/kg/min		PERCENT FAT		BODY MASS INDEX		CURL-UP # completed	
5	Completion of		Participate in				25	10	20	14.7	2	10
6	distance. Time		run. Lap count				25	10	20	14.7	2	10
7	standards not		standards not				25	10	20	14.9	4	14
8	recommended.		recommended.				25	10	20	15.1	6	20
9							25	10	20	15.2	9	24
10	11:30	9:00	17	55	42	52	25	10	21	15.3	12	24
11	11:00	8:30	23	61	42	52	25	10	21	15.8	15	28
12	10:30	8:00	29	68	42	52	25	10	22	16.0	18	36
13	10:00	7:30	35	74	42	52	25	10	23	16.6	21	40
14	9:30	7:00	41	80	42	52	25	10	24.5	17.5	24	45
15	9:00	7:00	46	85	42	52	25	10	25	18.1	24	47
16	8:30	7:00	52	90	42	52	25	10	26.5	18.5	24	47
17	8:30	7:00	57	94	42	52	25	10	27	18.8	24	47
17+	8:30	7:00	57	94	42	52	25	10	27.8	19.0	24	47

AGE	TRUNK LIFT inches		PUSH-UP # completed		MODIFIED PULL-UP # completed		PULL-UP # completed		FLEXED ARM HANG seconds		BACK SAVER SIT & REACH† inches	SHOULDER STRETCH
5	6	12	3	8	2	7	1	2	2	8	8	
6	6	12	3	8	2	7	1	2	2	8	8	
7	6	12	4	10	3	9	1	2	3	8	8	
8	6	12	5	13	4	11	1	2	3	10	8	
9	6	12	6	15	5	11	1	2	4	10	8	
10	9	12	7	20	5	15	1	2	4	10	8	
11	9	12	8	20	6	17	1	3	6	13	8	
12	9	12	10	20	7	20	1	3	10	15	8	
13	9	12	12	25	8	22	1	4	12	17	8	
14	9	12	14	30	9	25	2	5	15	20	8	
15	9	12	16	35	10	27	3	7	15	20	8	
16	9	12	18	35	12	30	5	8	15	20	8	
17	9	12	18	35	14	30	5	8	15	20	8	
17+	9	12	18	35	14	30	5	8	15	20	8	

Passing = Touching the fingertips together behind the back.

*Number on left is lower end of HFZ; number on right is upper end of HFZ.
†Test scored Pass/Fail; must reach this distance to pass.

From The Cooper Institute for Aerobics Research, Dallas, Texas.

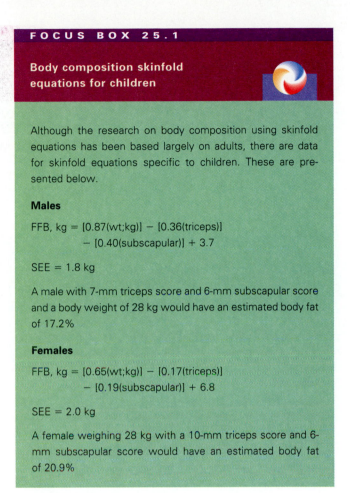

FOCUS BOX 25.1

Body composition skinfold equations for children

Although the research on body composition using skinfold equations has been based largely on adults, there are data for skinfold equations specific to children. These are presented below.

Males

FFB, kg = [0.87(wt;kg)] − [0.36(triceps)]
         − [0.40(subscapular)] + 3.7

SEE = 1.8 kg

A male with 7-mm triceps score and 6-mm subscapular score and a body weight of 28 kg would have an estimated body fat of 17.2%

Females

FFB, kg = [0.65(wt;kg)] − [0.17(triceps)]
         − [0.19(subscapular)] + 6.8

SEE = 2.0 kg

A female weighing 28 kg with a 10-mm triceps score and 6-mm subscapular score would have an estimated body fat of 20.9%

FIGURE 25.2

Comparison of the sum of median triceps and subscapular skinfold measurements taken during the 1960s with the data collected in the National Children and Youth Fitness Survey II of the 1980s. (Adapted from Ross JG et al: *JOPERD*, November/December, 1987.)

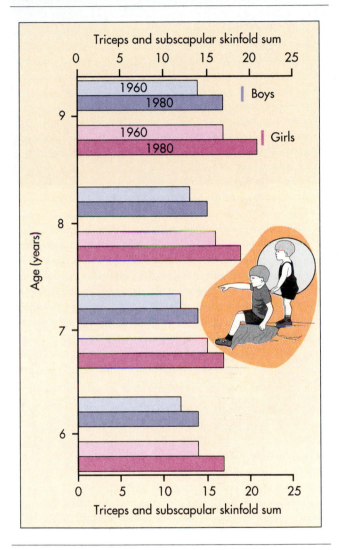

females were used as the criteria. The cause of the increase in body fat over the years has been related to decreased habitual physical activity and increased television viewing.[44,87,89,100]

Strength

Another particularly alarming statistic is the poor strength levels of American children, particularly upper body strength.[112] Field tests for upper body strength included the pull-up for boys and the flexed arm hang for girls. Although upper body strength for both boys and girls has long been a fitness concern, the validity of the pull-up and flexed arm hang tests has never been well established. Furthermore, the relationship between muscular strength and endurance field tests and poor health has not been clearly established in children.

The results of several large-scale fitness tests have shown that upper body strength among American children is poor. In part I of the National Children and Youth Fitness Study it was reported that over 30% of 10- to 11-year-old boys, and 60% of 10- to 18-year-old girls were unable to perform one chin-up.[103] In a 1985 study conducted by the President's Council on Physical Fitness and Sports, 18,857 American

schoolchildren aged 6 to 17 were tested.[97] The results of the strength tests included the following:

- 40% of the boys aged 6 to 12 could not do more than one pull-up. One in four could not do any.
- 70% of all girls tested could not do more than one pull-up and 55% could not do any.
- 45% of the boys aged 6 to 14 and 55% of all the girls tested could not hold their chin over a raised bar for more than 10 seconds.

A 1981-1982 test conducted by the Amateur Athletic Union found that 60% of the tested girls aged 6 to 17 could not perform one pull-up.[1] The mean number of pull-ups for boys did not exceed 10 for any age group between 6 and 17.

FIGURE 25.3

A modified pull-up test for the assessment of upper body strength.

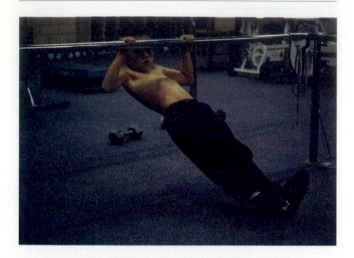

In 1986 part II of the NCYFS study, upper body strength was tested in 4678 children aged 6 to 9 using a modified pull-up test (Figure 25.3).[104] The rationale for the use of the modified pull-up test was that the traditional pull-up or flexed arm hang tests have traditionally provided poor measurement sensitivity for the range of children tested.[88] The median score for girls ranged from 6 to 9, and for boys the range was 6 to 10. Although there was an improvement in upper body strength compared with part I of the study, NCYFS II was the first large-scale test to use the modified pull-up, and further studies are needed to validate the results.

Recently Pate et al. determined the concurrent and construct validity of three common field tests of upper body muscular strength and endurance in children aged 9 and 10.[91] The field tests included the pull-up, the flexed arm hang, and the push-up. In addition, two modified pull-up tests were examined—the Vermont modified pull-up (VMPU) and the New York modified pull-up (NYMPU). The authors concluded that the most commonly used field tests for upper body strength and endurance do not correlate significantly with laboratory measures of absolute muscular strength and endurance. The authors state, "These field tests are, at best, moderately valid measures of weight-relative muscular strength."

As discussed previously, the rationale for the use of the modified pull-up test was that the traditional pull-up and flexed arm hang tests have provided poor measurement sensitivity for the range of children tested.[104] Pate et al. found that the pull-up, push-up, and NYMPU tests had the highest percentage of zero scores, meaning a large number of children could not even record one score.[12] Although the flexed arm hang yielded no zero scores in their study, many of the subjects could perform the test for only 1 to 2 seconds. By far the VMPU produced the best results. Only 7% of the subjects

tested with the VMPU scored zero, and it also correlated best with weight-relative strength. The authors concluded, "The VMPU is the most valid and appropriate test for application with 9 to 10 year old children."

Aerobic Capacity

Exercise capacity and maximal oxygen uptake (VO_2max) increase throughout childhood. The increase in endurance capacity is due to enhanced oxygen transport and enhanced metabolic capacities. In addition, as running economy improves, children are able to run at a lower percentage of VO_2max. The health-related reference standards for boys and girls for the 1-mile run/walk are listed in Table 25.2. One-mile run times for boys and girls have been compared with data collected in the Health-Related Physical Fitness Test (HRPFT) conducted in 1980 and the NCYFS published in 1985.[103] When the fiftieth percentile scores for the 1-mile run for boys and girls are compared with data collected in 1980 and 1985, the 1980 results are superior to the 1985 results. When American children are compared with children from other countries, foreign children appear to have better cardiovascular endurance. The reason for the discrepancy is not clear. One group of researchers has reported a 10% decline in aerobic fitness levels of children as measured by various distance runs since the 1980s.[62]

Coronary Artery Disease and Children

Serum cholesterol levels and obesity rates are high in American children. As many as 40% of children aged 5 to 8 show at least one heart disease risk factor (high cholesterol, physical inactivity, obesity, or high blood pressure) (Figure 25.4).[42] With the evidence linking the origins of coronary artery disease to childhood years, efforts should be made to reduce the potential for children maturing into high-risk adults by identifying children at highest risk.

Cardiovascular disease continues to be the leading cause of death in the United States. The natural progression of coronary artery disease is believed to be correlated strongly with the presence of the classic risk factors, such as hypertension, cigarette smoking, high serum cholesterol level, and physical inactivity. Coronary artery disease is now recognized as a pediatric disease with three basic periods of development.[56,71] The first stage, the incubation period, occurs between infancy and **adolescence.** During this period, mesenchymal cushions form on the inner layer of the arterial wall. Late in this period, fatty streaks begin to appear. Fatty streaks are found in the aorta during the first years of life and almost universally by the age of 3 years.[71] The second stage, the latent period, occurs between adolescence and early adulthood. During this period the fatty streaks are found in

The prevalence of risk factors for atherosclerotic coronary artery disease in children aged 7 to 12 years. (Adapted from Gilliam TB et al: *Med Sci Sports Exerc* 9(1):21-25, 1977.)

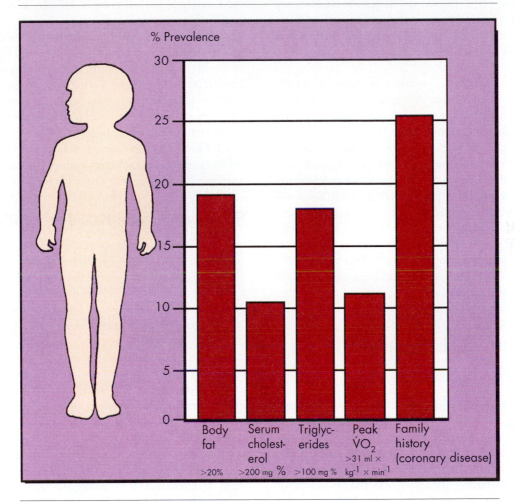

the coronary arteries. During the final stage, or clinical period, the clinical manifestations of the disease become apparent.

Further evidence that atherosclerosis has its beginnings in childhood was reported by Enos et al.[38] Enos found that 70% of autopsied American soldiers killed in the Korean War (average age was 22.1 years) already had at least moderately advanced coronary atherosclerosis. These soldiers had not demonstrated any early signs of coronary atherosclerosis. In a later study, McNamara et al. found evidence of atherosclerosis in 45% of Vietnam War casualties, with 5% demonstrating severe atherosclerosis.[72] A common theme throughout this paper was that cardiovascular disease begins at an early age and that prevention, which is preferable to rehabilitation, must begin at an early age.[81] Autopsy findings of children in the Bogalusa Heart Study have demonstrated that elevated risk factor levels accelerate the development of atherosclerotic fatty streaks and fibrous plaques in adolescence.[30]

Several large-scale epidemiologic studies have been conducted to assess cardiovascular disease risk factors in children. Of 5000 children examined, 24% had total cholesterol levels greater than 220 mg/dl, 20% were greater than 110% of relative body weight, and after the age of 9, 19% had diastolic blood pressures greater than 94 mm Hg. Wilmore and McNamara and Gilliam et al. also noted that more than 50% of the children they tested had one or more risk factors (e.g., elevated blood pressure, elevated total cholesterol level, elevated triglyceride concentrations, or elevated body fat).[42,124] Khoury et al. found the children they examined to be at high

adolescence (ad´o-les´ense)

the period when there is the most rapid growth and development of children

risk by virtue of their low-density lipoprotein cholesterol levels.[58] It appears that children who have risk factors at an early age remain at risk as they age, at least with lipoproteins and blood pressure.[70,125] Finally, the Bogalusa Heart Study demonstrated a relationship between early atherosclerotic lesions in the aorta and coronary arteries and high serum lipoprotein levels and systolic blood pressure measurements taken before death.[81]

The "Know Your Body" program is an organized health education program for children designed to encourage positive health behavior and discourage or interrupt behavioral patterns that are linked to illness, injury, disability, or death.[122] Components of the program included a 20-week curriculum; a survey of knowledge, attitudes, and behaviors; in-service training for elementary teachers; and a clinical screening. Clinical screenings included height, weight, body composition, serum cholesterol, pulse rate recovery after exercise, and blood pressure. Risk factors were combined into a summative index. These risk factors were obesity, a score of fair or poor on pulse rate recovery, greater than ninety-fifth percentile in diastolic or systolic blood pressure, and greater than 200 mg/dl of cholesterol. Results indicated that half the children had at least one risk factor and 20% had two or more.

Preventing Heart Disease in Children

*A*lthough no longitudinal studies have examined the question of whether early childhood control of coronary heart disease (CHD) risk factors will reduce the risk of fatal heart attacks or the incidence of heart disease in adult life, there is little doubt concerning the association of risk factors in adults and the incidence of cardiovascular disease. Since it is clear that atherosclerosis

begins in early childhood, screening and prevention strategies for cardiovascular risk should begin in childhood and continue throughout adulthood. These issues were identified in the recently published goals of Healthy People 2000 (Focus box 25.2).

Programs for primary prevention of cardiovascular disease in the adult population are widespread. Physicians, public health departments, hospitals, and government agencies have all assisted in implementing such programs, which have reduced the incidence of cardiovascular disease in the United States. Most of these prevention strategies focus on the adult population and thus begin late. Would even more lives be saved if preventive programs started earlier? If we accept the evidence that atherosclerosis begins in childhood, why do most preventive programs target adults?

School and Home-Based Prevention

In 1985 a cooperative heart health education and fitness program was developed by a team of clinicians from Pacific Presbyterian Medical Center, the San Francisco Chapter of the American Heart Association, and the San Francisco Unified School District's Central Health Committee. *Future Fit* was designed to be incorporated into existing after-school programs with minimal teacher training and nominal expenditures for equipment and supplies.[29] In the demonstration project, 55 third- and fourth-grade students enrolled in after-school programs at four sites were randomly assigned to experimental and control conditions.

The curriculum included anatomy and physiology of the cardiovascular system, attitude and decision-making skills, risk factors and prevention of heart disease, exercise physiology, heart healthy nutrition, the dangers of smoking, handling stress, and responding to emergency situations. The courses were taught twice a week for 12 weeks by regular after-school

---

FOCUS BOX 25.2

Healthy People 2000 Goals

- Increase to at least 30% the proportion of people aged 6 and older who engage regularly, preferably daily, in light to moderate physical activity for at least 30 minutes per day.

- Increase to at least 40% the proportion of people aged 6 and older who regularly perform physical activities that enhance and maintain muscular strength, muscular endurance, and flexibility.

- Reduce to no more than 15% the proportion of people aged 6 and older who engage in no leisure time physical activity.

- Increase to at least 50% the proportion of children and adolescents in first through twelfth grade who participate in daily school physical education.

- Increase to at least 50% the proportion of school physical education class time that students spend being physically active, preferably engaged in lifetime physical activities.

From Healthy People 2000: National Health Promotion and Disease Prevention Objectives, Department of Health and Human Services, Washington, DC, 1991.

teachers, after a brief in-service training. The fitness program consisted of three 45-minute exercise sessions each week. The aerobics classes were taught by a certified aerobics instructor.

Results indicated significant knowledge gains in prevention of heart disease for the experimental group compared with the control group. With regard to the exercise program, heart rates of participants did not, as a group, appear to have been maintained within the target heart zone for the necessary duration to produce a training effect. The authors conclude that health and fitness programing in the after-school setting can be an effective complement to the education provided within the school setting.

Heart Smart is a school-based cardiovascular health promotion program encompassing the total school environment, parents, school staff, and peers in grades kindergarten through six.[51] Four elementary schools in Jefferson Parish, Louisiana, were selected to participate in the study. The program encouraged children to adopt healthy life-styles by promoting personal abilities and self-esteem.

The success of the Heart Smart program was assessed by a variety of evaluative approaches. Measurement protocols were developed to detect biologic, behavioral, and cognitive effects of the intervention. Children were assigned to quartiles according to changes in risk factors (total cholesterol, weight/height[2], systolic and diastolic blood pressure.) The quartile showing the greatest reduction evidenced the largest number of healthy food choices. Similarly, the greatest improvement in body composition occurred in the quartile that selected three or more healthy foods per day. Physical fitness, as gauged by 1-mile run/walk times, significantly improved in the experimental group. Lastly, results of comparison between the intervention families and control families indicated that family health promotion activities were effective in increasing cardiovascular health knowledge, improving parent physical activity and child fitness levels, and changing dietary practices.

The *Know Your Body* (KYB) program was implemented in Washington, D.C.[25] The curriculum was designed to promote behavior changes that would reduce the risk of heart disease in students through value clarification, goal setting, modeling, rehearsal, feedback or screening results, and reinforcement. The study was conducted with students in grades four through six at nine public elementary schools. In 1985 a 5-year evaluation of the KYB program began among predominantly black children in grades four through six at nine elementary schools. The results indicated significant improvements in systolic blood pressure, HDL cholesterol, HDL/total cholesterol ratio, smoking reduction, and fitness at one or all four annual follow-up reexaminations. Favorable changes in diastolic blood pressure occurred at all reexaminations. Intervention students whose KYB teachers were judged to be the best showed significant reductions in serum cholesterol after 1 year.

Hearty Heart is a 5-week, 15-session curriculum designed for third-graders.[93] The program, derived from the social learning theory, targets changes in specific environmental, personality, and behavioral factors that are likely to influence children's health behavior. The school-based component, *Hearty Heart and Friends,* involves 15 sessions over 5 weeks. The home-based component, the *Home Team,* involves a 5-week correspondence course in which parental involvement is necessary to complete the activities. In a study of this program, participation rates for all aspects were high; 86% of the parents participated in the Home Team and 71% completed the 5-week course. Students in the school-based program gained more knowledge than students in the home-based program or controls. However, students in the home-based program reported more behavioral change, had reduced the total fat, saturated fat, and monounsaturated fat in their diets, and had more of the encouraged foods on their shelves. The authors concluded that parental involvement enhances eating pattern outcomes in children.

The 3-year project, *Go For Health* was designed to reduce cardiovascular risk factors in elementary school children.[84] The project goals were to implement changes in school policies and practices that would support increased aerobic physical activity and provide cardiovascular-healthful food and to increase daily aerobic physical activity and cardiovascular-healthful eating practices of third- and fourth-grade children. Evaluation of Go For Health focused on school and student outcomes. School lunch was assessed by chemical analysis of food item aliquots and by observation of children eating lunch. Observations were made of children's physical activity during physical education classes. Behavioral capability and self-efficacy were measured in the classroom. The average meal contained 31.4 grams of total fat and 1244 mg of sodium. Main dishes contributed 44.3% of total fat and 38.7% of sodium. Total fat provided 38.8% of total calories. The physical education class time taken up by different activities included 32.8% devoted to organization, 41% devoted to games, 17% devoted to fitness activities (of which only 6.1% were activities that were potentially aerobic), and 11.4% in other activities.

Prevention Programs in the Clinical Setting

There is controversy regarding the role of pediatricians in reducing risk factors for cardiovascular disease in children.[33] To determine the attitudes, current practices, and knowledge among primary care pediatricians regarding these risks, a national mail survey of 2000 pediatricians was conducted.[78] Responses indicated that a majority of pediatricians take a family history of cardiovascular diseases, assess blood pressure, recommend exercise to school-aged children, and advise patients and parents against smoking. Few pediatricians felt confident in their ability to effect change in patient life-style. There was a relativity low level of dietary advice given, and most pediatricians did not feel it was necessary to measure serum cholesterol levels, except in high-risk older children. Obesity was the topic most frequently chosen for con-

Recommendations for Cardiovascular Disease Prevention in Children

As discussed in the text, disease prevention should begin early in life. Some of the recommendations for disease prevention in children are listed below.

School and Home Prevention

- Family physicians and pediatricians should routinely screen for heart disease risk factors.

- School-site programs should be established to screen for risk factors, especially for those children who do not have access to health care services.

- Children in high-risk families should be carefully screened and monitored into adulthood.

- A combination of school- and home-site cardiovascular health education programs should be directed to children in the general population in an effort to encourage them to adopt healthy life-styles.

Clinical Prevention

- Courses in cardiovascular risk identification and treatment should be required for all medical school students.

- More continuing medical education in this area should be required for pediatricians.

- Strategies for pediatricians to prevent cardiovascular disease include the following:

  - During the child's annual physical examination the physician should do the following:

    - Take a family history.
    - Measure height, weight, and serum cholesterol.
    - Provide guidance for smoking cessation.
    - Advise parents about prudent diet and exercise habits.

  - For children tracking above height and weight and gender-specific ninety-fifth percentiles for blood pressure the physician should do the following:

    - Review history of sodium intake.
    - Exclude secondary causes of hypertension.
    - Obtain a urinalysis.
    - If a child is obese, encourage increased physical activity and restrict food intake.
    - If the child is unresponsive, begin antihypertensive medication therapy.

  - For children tracking above the age-specific ninety-fifth percentile for serum cholesterol the physician should do the following:

    - Review for steroid use, chronic renal disease, and hepatic disease.
    - Re-examine for xanthelasma.
    - Measure serum lipoprotein cholesterol.
    - If LDL is also high, advise a low-fat, low cholesterol diet.
    - If the child is unresponsive, begin antilipid medication.

Public Health Efforts

- Public health services should develop networks with schools in an effort to establish screening and education programs.

- Communities can develop cooperative programs among, for example, hospitals, physicians, and schools, in an effort to promote healthy life-styles.

- Nonprofit organizations, such as the American Heart Association, have excellent heart healthy programs for children (for little or no cost).

- Community awareness campaigns should be directed at adults as well as children.

- Population strategies to prevent cardiovascular disease include the following:

  - Elimination of cigarette smoking
  - Diagnosis and control of hypertension
  - Diagnosis and control of hyperlipidemia
  - Diagnosis and control of diabetes
  - Maintenance of ideal body weight
  - Participation in regular physical activity
  - Reduction in the intake of fat and sodium
  - Establishment of healthier life-style habits

Education Programs

- The curriculum should be broad and include training in nutrition, exercise, reduction in cigarette smoking and alcohol consumption, control of stress, and knowledge of cardiovascular risk factors.

- Programs should be geared to the specific age and developmental status of the child.

- Schools should be encouraged to incorporate health promotion and education programs into their curriculums.

- A variety of education resources are available for both home- and school-based programs (many at no cost to the user).

- A feedback and reward system should be set up ahead of time to instill long-term adherence to the program.

- If a program is used at home, the whole family should be encouraged to participate.

- The impact of these programs on health measures should be monitored and tracked on a regular basis.

tinuing medical education. Older pediatricians were the most likely to advocate and practice risk reduction in children.

Elevated cholesterol levels are associated with atherosclerotic disease in children. More than 10% of the children in the United States have a total blood cholesterol of 200 mg/dl or higher.[73] The degree of fatty arterial streaks in adolescents and young adults is highly correlated with blood cholesterol levels measured in school years.[81] Although most pediatricians routinely assess other cardiovascular risk factors, only a few currently perform blood cholesterol screening or offer dietary advice.[78] Blood cholesterol screening can be efficiently accomplished as a part of routine office visits for school-aged children.[73] An excellent review of the procedures for cholesterol testing of children in a clinical setting is provided by Davidson.[34]

Primary prevention of coronary artery disease in children and young adults is important and can be instituted through a family-oriented cardiac risk factor clinic (see the Clinical Application on p. 612).[102] The familial pattern of high cholesterol and other cardiac risk factors supports the need for family-oriented intervention.[31] In one study, children whose total cholesterol exceeded 200 mg/dl were referred by their primary care physician, along with their siblings and parents. The mean total cholesterol level was 258 mg/dl for index cases, 195 mg/dl for siblings, and 233 mg/dl for parents. Follow-up data obtained after therapy at a mean of 6 months showed a change in total cholesterol from 265 to 246 mg/dl. In 82% of the patients a decrease in total cholesterol was seen.[102]

It is clear that primary prevention of cardiovascular disease in children is a public health concern. Reducing cardiovascular risk factors and changing health behaviors in children require a cooperative effort among the school, parent, family physician, and public health office. Cardiovascular risk factors can be identified in children just as in adults, and these have a high correlation with the adult onset of the disease. Clinical risk factors tend to persist within a rank so that studies in childhood can be predictive of future levels.[18] Behavior and a life-style of unhealthy eating, cigarette smoking, alcohol intake, and use of oral contraceptives influence risk factors in children. The findings from the Bogalusa Heart Study and other epidemiologic studies of children show the need to begin prevention of adult heart disease in early life. Exercise can play an important role in prevention efforts, since it has been shown to reduce the risk of obesity, lower and control blood pressure, control diabetes, and cause favorable alterations in blood lipid levels in children and adolescents.*

Growth and Development

Children do not grow at a uniform rate throughout their development (Figure 25.5). There is a rapid increase in height, followed (particularly in boys) by a rapid increase in body mass over the period of **puberty** (the pubertal growth spurt). Further, there are substantial interindividual differences in biologic age at any given calendar age, with corresponding variations in the timing and magnitude of the pubertal growth spurt. These factors have implications for fitness professionals who are attempting to standardize fitness testing and programing.

Phases of Growth

There are four main phases of growth in humans (see Focus Box 25.3).[144] Growth is rapid in infancy and early childhood, remains relatively steady during middle childhood, increases rapidly during the adolescent period, and finally increases slowly until an eventual cessation with the

---

*References 35, 41, 47, 55, 63, 69, and 101.

FIGURE 25.5

The average growth (distance) curves for stature and body weight for American children from birth to 18 years of age. (From Malina RM, Bouchard C: *Growth, maturation, and physical activity*, 1991, Champaign, Illinois, Human Kinetics.)

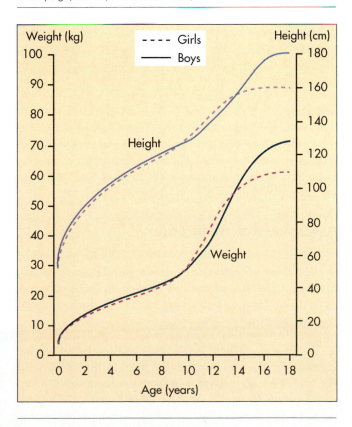

puberty (pu´ber-ti)

the period of growth and development in which the secondary sex characteristics that differentiate genders develop

FOCUS BOX 25.3

Basic growth and development terminology

The most common terms used in describing the growth and development of children are listed below.

■ Growth—Refers to the increase in total body size, or a particular body part, that occurs as a newborn goes from infancy through adolescence and beyond.

■ Development—Refers to the quantitative changes that occur through life, including physical growth and the qualitative changes that occur in organs and overall body function.

■ Maturation—Refers to the rate of progress toward maturity.

■ Childhood—The period of time from birth through adolescence.

■ Cephalocaudal—The head-to-toe developmental progression that occurs during childhood. For example, body control in children progresses from head to toe.

■ Proximodistal—The process of development occurs outward from the areas closest to the center of the body. For example, the child can control the trunk sooner than the arms and legs.

■ Differentiation—From fetal development through childhood, the body develops in a simple to complex mode. For example, the simple movements of the body (e.g., turning the head and trunk) occur before the more complex (e.g., holding a pencil and writing).

---

attainment of adulthood. The rate of growth is typically measured over time by changes in stature and body weight. The amount of growth depends on the time when the growth occurs and the speed of growth per unit of time. Measurements taken on individuals over time can be plotted to produce a graph. Growth curves are fairly linear over time, flattening out as sexual maturity is reached. Growth patterns are often measured at a pediatrician's office or at school. Figure 25.5 shows the average growth curves for stature and body weight for American Children from birth to 18 years of age This type of graph is referred to as a distance curve because it indicates the weight and height attained by children at any given age and thus the "distance" they have traveled toward adulthood.[67]

Another method commonly used to plot growth is to plot height or weight in time increments for a specified period (Figure 25.6). Velocity curves show the rate of growth. The velocity curve shows that the most rapid growth occurs before birth and begins to decelerate before delivery. During infancy and childhood there is a steady decline in the rate of growth. During adolescence there is a rapid increase in both height and weight. This rapid increase in growth has been termed the *adolescent growth spurt*. Girls generally reach their peak height velocity by 12, boys' growth continues until around 14. After the rapid spurt, growth dramatically slows. Girls reach 98% of their final height by the age of 16.5 and boys do the same at about 17.75 years.[114]

Figure 25.7 and 25.8 are reference growth charts. The National Center for Health Statistics has compiled these growth curves based on a very large sample of children. Pediatricians use these reference charts to plot growth patterns over time. Pediatricians often reference children's height and weight based on percentages of population norm (e.g., seventy-fifth percentile for age for weight and ninety-fifth percentile for height). Plotting growth over time can identify anomalies in growth and development, which often can be corrected with medical therapy.

Age and Gender Variation in Growth

A variety of biologic processes change with age. In addition, there are tremendous gender-related differences during growth (see Figures 25.5 and 25.6). There is a rapid rate of growth during the adolescent years, referred to as the **peak height velocity** (PHV). PHV usually occurs 2 years earlier for girls than boys. Girls tend to be slightly bigger and heavier than boys from 2 to 10 years old. Strength and body proportions of boys and girls are essentially equal until the beginning of the adolescent period. During puberty, hormonal changes begin to cause significant variation between the genders. Increased testosterone release in boys causes an increase in lean body mass, whereas in females an increase in estrogen causes increased body fat deposition, breast development, and widening of the hips (Figure 25.9).

Assessment of Maturation

The assessment of maturity is important for a variety of reasons. (The issues that arise from the rapid growth development of children are detailed in the Clinical Application on p. 619.) First, maturity assessment is important in the research process. Pediatric researchers try to match young subjects based on their maturity status. Even if two children are the same age, height, and weight, they may be at different stages of development, and thus the more mature child could be at an advantage. Second, maturity assessment is frequently used by pediatricians to evaluate growth and development patterns. Third, maturation assessment can help ensure that

FIGURE 25.6

The velocity growth curves for British males and females from birth to maturity. (Adapted from Tanner RH et al: *Arch Dis Child* 41:454-471.)

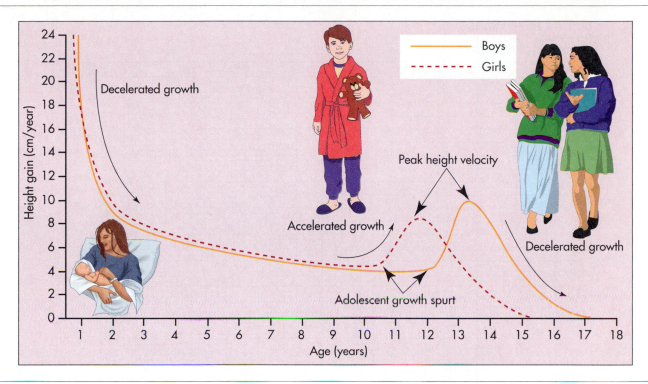

children are evenly matched for athletic competition. A variety of maturity assessment techniques exist, including skeletal age, sexual maturation, somatic maturation, and dental maturation. Pubertal stages of sexual maturity are outlined in Table 25.4. Sexual maturation is typically defined in a preparticipation physical examination.

The simplest method of adjusting data for individual differences in body size is to express findings as a ratio to body mass. For example, a subject's maximal aerobic power may be expressed in units of ml/kg/min. If a test score is to be used to assess a child's performance potential, this may be quite an effective tactic, since most vigorous athletic activities involve the displacement of body mass against gravity and the oxygen cost of a sustained physical task is usually roughly proportional to the individual's body mass. If the intent is to compare fitness scores from one age category with another, the choice of units becomes more controversial.

When aerobic power is expressed per kilogram of body mass, scores commonly decrease over much of childhood,

peak height velocity

the period of rapid growth during the adolescent period, usually occurring 2 years earlier for girls than boys.

TABLE 25.4

Tanner Stage of Sexual Maturation

STAGE	DESCRIPTION
1	Prepubertal stage of development. Absence of development of any secondary sexual characteristics.
2	Indicates the initial development of each secondary sexual characteristic. Initial elevation of breasts in girls and enlargement of the genitals in boys. For both sexes, pubic hair begins to appear.
3 & 4	Continued maturation of each secondary sexual characteristic. Pubic hair becomes coarser and begins to curl. Relative enlargement of larynx in boys. Increase in pelvic diameter begins in girls.
5	Indicates adult maturation. Mature spermatozoa are present in males. Full reproductivity in women. Axially hair is present and sweat and sebaceous glands are very active in both sexes.

Modified from: Tanner, JM: *Growth at adolescence*, Oxford, 1962, Blackwell Scientific.

FIGURE 25.7

Reference growth chart for boys, ages 2 to 18 years. (Courtesy, Ross Laboratories.)

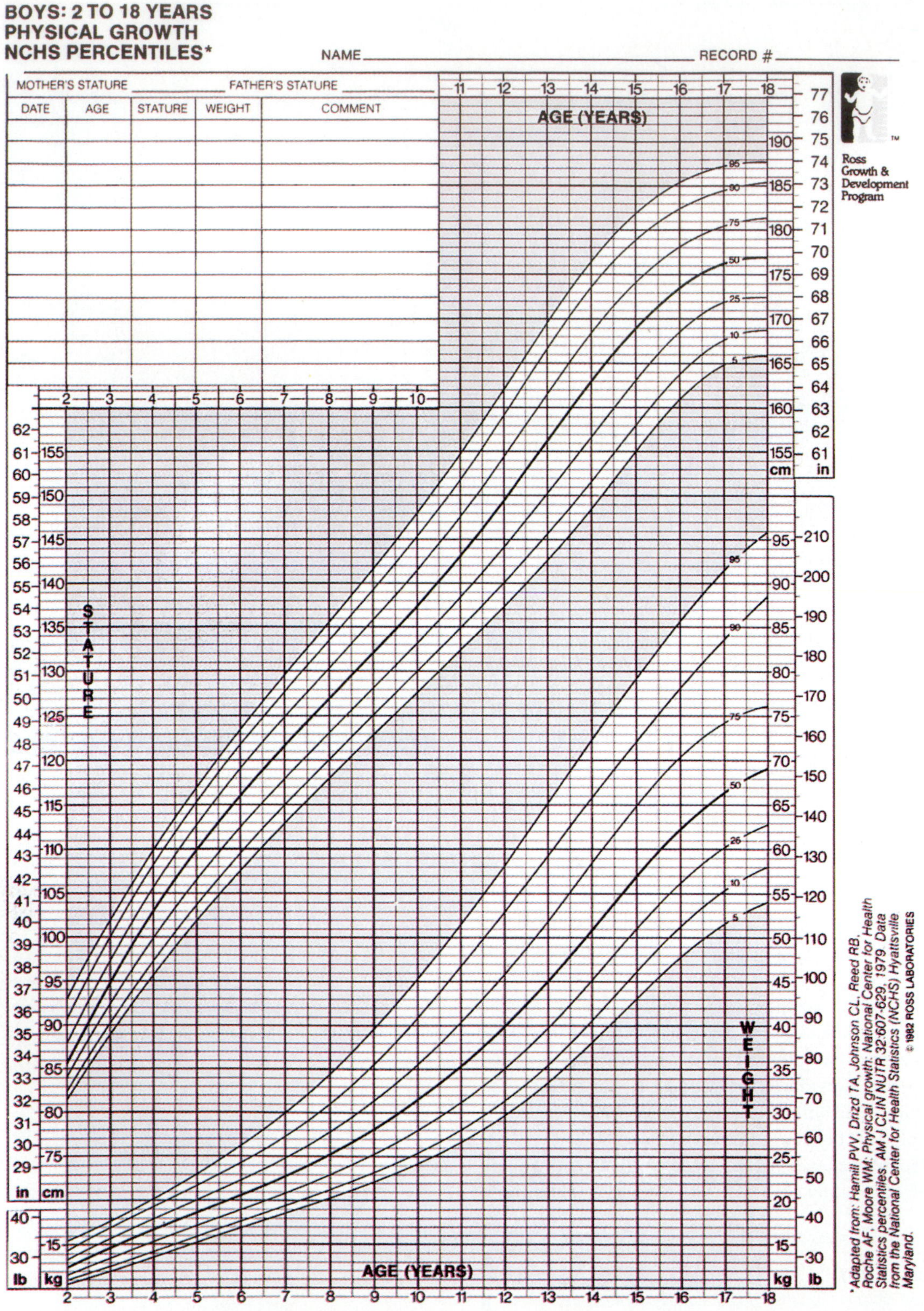

BOYS: 2 TO 18 YEARS PHYSICAL GROWTH NCHS PERCENTILES*

FIGURE 25.8

Reference growth chart for girls, ages 2 to 18 years. (Courtesy Ross Laboratories.)

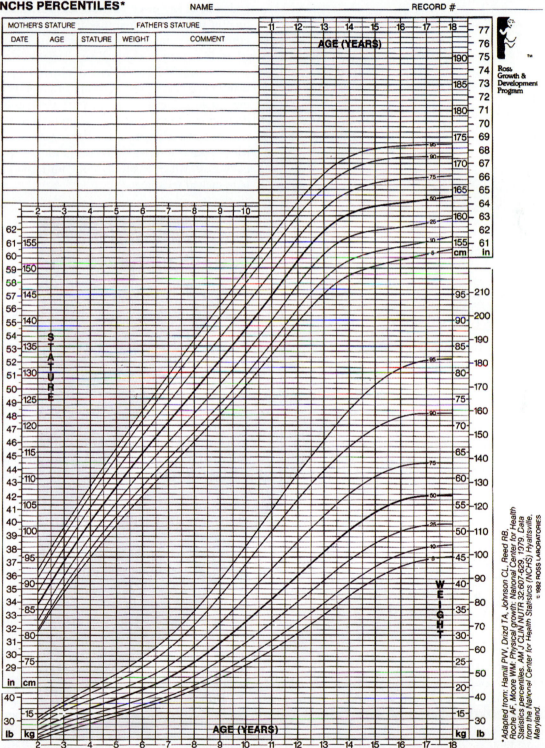

The effects of gender and age on changes in **A,** muscle mass and **B,** subcutaneous fat during development. (Adapted from Malina RM, Brouchard C: *Growth, maturation, and physical activity,* Champaign, Illinois, 1991, Human Kinetics.)

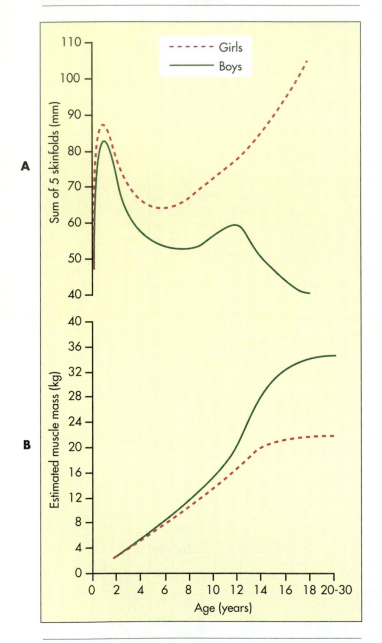

would no longer stand accused of causing a decrease in fitness among their pupils.

Team competition sports, such as football, are commonly classified by age-group. However, this is not a good approach, given that there are substantial interindividual differences in body size at any given calendar age. Particularly around the time of puberty, children may find they are playing against others who are much larger, stronger, and heavier than themselves. In consequence, small and late-maturing children are at a substantially increased risk of physical injury if they participate in contact sports. A combination of such hazards with the discouragement of unequal competition leads to a high dropout rate from age-category sports leagues, with selective retention of a minority of tall, heavy early maturers. An alternative option is to base the classification of players on their body mass, which is already done for some individual contests, such as wrestling.

Exercise, Growth, and Development

A variety of factors affect growth and development, including nutrition, socioeconomic status, disease, genetic control, and exercise. Growth and maturation are regulated primarily by genetics.[67] Regular training has no apparent effect on statural growth.[67] However, Figure 25.10 shows the effect of exercise training on fat-free mass and relative fatness in boys followed longitudinally and exposed to different levels of training.[86] Regular physical activity is also important for stimulating bone mineralization, which is obviously important to normal growth and development. Other factors, such as health and nutrition habits, also influence growth.[67]

Age-Appropriate Fitness Activities

Because there are great interindividual differences in growth and development patterns among children, the age-appropriate fitness activities should be based on a child's maturity and readiness to participate. Children should be given ample time to explore a variety of fitness activities, without pressure from peers or parents. As children mature and refine their skills, they will be able to learn more complicated skills and participate in more intense physical activities.

During early childhood, children should be encouraged to experience a variety of activities, structured games, and play. This is a period of rapid growth and development. The focus should be on the development of basic movement skills, such as running, balancing, jumping, kicking, throwing, and catching. Between the ages of 6 and 12, fitness programs should focus on refining skill development. Children should

Text continued on p. 624.

with the rate of loss accelerating at puberty; this has led to the inference that because of insufficient or inadequate school programs of physical education, aerobic fitness deteriorates once a child sits behind a classroom desk. However, there is no fundamental biologic reason why maximal oxygen intake should develop as a constant linear function of a child's body mass. A height^2 comparison would show that aerobic power remains relatively stable throughout childhood, and schools

Overview of Selected Developmental Periods and Their Relation to Fitness

Because the rate of growth in children can vary with age and between individuals, there can be both positive and negative influences on exercise and sports participation. Knowing when children are likely to experience high growth rates allows appropriate expectations of activity patterns. The issues concerning the complexities of the growth of children are presented in the following material.

Overview of the Toddler Period (1 to 3 years)
General Growth and Development Related to Fitness
■ Rate of growth depends on the individual child but should fall within the ranges identified in normal growth tables.

   ■ Major targets are as follows:
   By 2 years, a child generally should weigh 26 to 28 pounds and stand 32 to 33 inches.
   By 2½ years, a child should quadruple the birth weight.

■ Vital Signs:

   ■ Pulse should range from 80 to 120 beats per minute.
   ■ Respiration should range from 20 to 40/minute.
   ■ Temperature should normally range around 98.6° F.

■ Caloric needs are 1300 calories/day depending on height, weight, and build.

■ A complete set of baby teeth should develop by age 3.

■ The child will sleep through the night and may only need one nap during the day.

■ Generally, the child will have an exaggerated lumbar curve and a wide gait.

Age-Appropriate Activities
Curiosity is extensive during this period. Children want to touch, pick up, and feel everything in sight. Muscle coordination increases. Children tend to climb upward but not down. Children can typically jump in place at this point. Children can generally control blocks, cubes, and other objects with their hands. By the age of 2 to 3 years, children should be able to kick a ball, begin riding a tricycle, and begin swinging activities.

Fitness Promotion Activities
Proper nutritional habits, such as eating fruits and vegetables for snacks and water rather than juice intake, should be encouraged. Physical activities that encourage the development phase but do not push the next phase should also be encouraged. For instance, children need to learn first how to move, crawl, stand, then walk. Skipping phases can reduce the maturation necessary during that phase. Develop play activities that encourage movement, rather than sedentary play. Because of the short attention span during this phase, the types of physical activities should be changed frequently. Children enjoy musical and rhythm instruments, which can be used with physical activity, including the introduction of unstructured dance.

Overview of the Preschooler Period (3 to 6 years)
General Growth and Development Related to Fitness
■ Rate of growth continues to be individualized but falls within the following parameters:

   Child's height doubles birth height (length) by age 4.
   Height and weight are generally the same by age 5.

■ Vital Signs:

   ■ Pulse should range from 80 to 120 beats per minute.
   ■ Respirations should range from 23 to 30/minute.
   ■ Temperature should normally range around 98.6° F.

■ Caloric needs range from 1300 to 1700 calories/day depending on age, height, build, and activity level.

■ The child sleeps through the night, generally for 9 to 12 hours and may or may not require a nap.

■ Role models are imitated.

Fitness-Specific Development
■ Control of fine motor skills begins during this period.

■ The child will thin out (i.e., protruding abdomen begins to disappear, body proportions change as legs grow rapidly).

■ Posture is more erect.

■ An adult stride for walking develops.

■ The child can run, hop, and skip.

Adapted from Roberts SO, Robergs RA, Stolarczyk L et al: *Med Sci Sports Exerc* 26(5):583, 1994.

Continued.

Overview of Selected Developmental Periods and Their Relation to Fitness

■ The child can throw ball overhead with more control and increased precision.

■ The child can learn to swim side strokes.

Fitness Promotion Activities

Role modeling of proper nutritional habits by parents and other adults is important, since this age-group works to copy the behavior of those important to them. Children should be encouraged to participate in activities that develop muscle strength and coordination—including riding a tricycle, roller skating, ice skating, sledding, riding toys, running, skipping, and hopping. Upper body development can be encouraged through physical activities that require age-appropriate lifting, throwing, and swimming. Physical activity can be role modeled. In fact, children of this age can begin to participate in physical activities with parents and others. These include dancing, running short distances, hiking short distances, and going for walks. Children can understand short, clear, simple explanations of how proper eating habits, proper foods, adequate fluid intake, and rest can help them keep up their play energy. Children can generally understand and follow simple verbal directions and can be influenced by role modeling at this period.

Overview of the School-Age Period (6 to 12 years)
General Growth and Development Related to Fitness

■ Physical growth continues with weight gains averaging 5 to 7 pounds per year. Height increases at an average of 3 inches per year but growth may occur in spurts. Vision is 20/20 by age 7.

■ Vital Signs:

  ■ Pulse should range from 70 to 110 beats per minute.
  ■ Respiration should range from 18 to 30/minute.
  ■ Temperature will fall within normal adult ranges.
  ■ Blood Pressure should range from 100 to 110/60 to 70 mm Hg.

■ Caloric needs range from 2000 to 2400 calories/day, depending on age, height, build, and activity levels.

■ Sleeps from 8 to 12 hours a night.

■ A sense of the child's own ability to master physical activities is developed.

Fitness-Specific Development

■ Strength, physical ability, and coordination increase.

■ Hand-eye coordination is fully developed by age 9.

■ The child can learn to work in groups to achieve physical goals (i.e., team sports).

■ By age 12, boys surpass girls in strength, endurance, and agility.

■ By age 12, girls surpass boys in flexibility and graceful movement.

■ Throughout this period, children have high energy levels.

■ Balance and rhythm are refined.

■ Physical manipulation skills approximate the adult level.

■ The child will be influenced by his or her own physical ability and interests and by reactions of peers.

■ The child will be aware of his or her own developing body.

Fitness Promotion Activities

Teach, role model, and encourage proper fluid and food intake. Relate healthful eating to energy use, activity interests, and ability to compete successfully in team or individual sports. Encourage participation in physical activities at which the child can achieve success by using activities that interest the child. Focus activities on aerobic conditioning, strength, and endurance development.

Overview of the Adolescent Period (12 to 20 years)
General Growth and Development Related to Fitness

■ Physical growth continues and reaches adult levels by ages 17 to 20. Both girls and boys increase in height and weight.

■ Vital Signs:

  ■ Pulse should range from 50 to 100 beats per minute.
  ■ Respirations should range from 15 to 24/minute.
  ■ Temperature should be in the adult ranges.
  ■ Blood pressure should be 110 to 120/60 to 80 mm Hg.

- Caloric needs are based on build, activity level, and age, balanced with increased appetite:

  - Girls range from 1500 to 3000 calories/day.
  - Boys range from 2000 to 3700 calories/day.

- Primary gender characteristics develop:

  - Girls—size of genitals increase, ovulation, menarche occurs, and internal secretions begin.
  - Boys—testes, scrotum, and penis grow and mature; mature sperm is produced.

- Growth and hormonal changes create increased need for protein, calcium, iron, and zinc.

Fitness-Related Growth and Development

- Boys display an increase in shoulder width, basal metabolic rate, and bone growth.

- Girls display an increase in bone growth, basal metabolic rate, and fat deposits in the breasts, buttocks, and thighs, and the pelvis begins to widen.

- All physical activities are greatly influenced by peer pressure.

Fitness Promotion Activities

Relate physical activity to interests, such as music, clothing, socialization, and dance. Use peer pressure and support to promote proper eating habits and food choices. Use role models admired by youths to increase interest in physical activity. Involve youths in activities that promote muscular development and coordination.

FIGURE 25.10

The effects of exercise training on fat free mass and relative fatness in boys followed longitudinally and exposed to different levels of training. (Adapted from Malina RM, Brouchard C: *Growth, maturation, and physical activity,* Champaign, Illinois, 1991, Human Kinetics.)

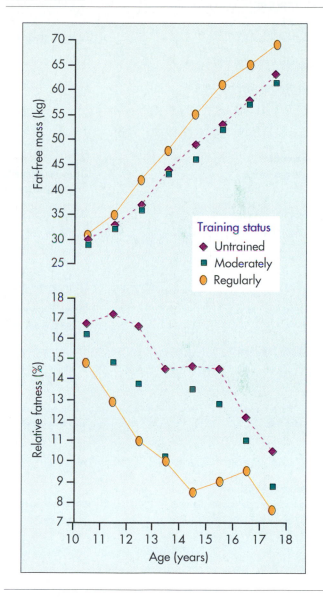

TABLE 25.5

Physiologic characteristics of the exercising child*

FUNCTION	COMPARISON WITH ADULTS	IMPLICATIONS FOR EXERCISE PRESCRIPTION
METABOLIC:		
Aerobic		
VO_2max (L/min)	Lower function of body mass	
VO_2max (ml/kg^{-1}/min)	Similar	Can perform endurance tasks reasonably well
Submaximal oxygen demand (economy)	Cycling: similar (18% to 30% mechanical efficiency); walking and running: higher metabolic cost	Greater fatigability in prolonged high-intensity tasks (running and walking); greater heat production in children at a given speed of walking or running
Anaerobic		
Glycogen stores	Lower concentration and rate of utilization of muscle glycogen	
Phosphofructokinase (PFK) activity)	Glycolysis limited because of low level of PFK	Ability of children to perform intense anaerobic tasks that last 10 to 90 seconds is distinctly lower than that of adults
LAmax	Lower maximal blood lactate levels	
Phosphagen stores	Stores and breakdown of ATP and CrP are the same	Same ability to deal metabolically with very brief intense exercise
Oxygen transient	Faster reaching of steady state than adults. Shorter half-time of oxygen increase in children	Children reach metabolic steady state faster. Children contract a lower oxygen deficit. Faster recovery. Children, therefore, are well suited to intermittent activities
LAsubmax	Lower at a given percent of VO_2max	May be reason why children perceive a given workload as easier
Heart rate at lactate threshold	Higher	
CARDIOVASCULAR:		
Maximal cardiac output (Qmax) Q at a given VO_2	Lower because of size difference Somewhat lower	Immature cardiovascular system means child is limited in bringing internal heat to surface for dissipation when exercising intensely in the heat
Maximal stroke volume (SVmax)	Lower because of size and heart volume difference	
Stroke volume at a given VO_2	Lower	
Maximal heart rate (HRmax)	Higher	Up to maturity HRmax is between 195 and 215 beats/min
Heart rate at submax work	At given power output and at relative metabolic load, child has higher heart rate	Higher heart rate compensates for lower stroke volume
Oxygen-carrying capacity	Blood volume, hemoglobin concentration, and total hemoglobin are lower in children	

TABLE 25.5—Cont'd

Physiologic characteristics of the exercising child*

FUNCTION	COMPARISON WITH ADULTS	IMPLICATIONS FOR EXERCISE PRESCRIPTION
Oxygen content in arterial and venous blood (CaO_2-CvO_2)	Somewhat higher	Potential deficiency of peripheral blood supply during maximal exertion in hot climates
Blood flow to active muscle	Higher	
Systolic and diastolic pressures	Lower maximal and submaximal	No known beneficial or detrimental effects on working capacity of child
CARDIOPULMONARY RESPONSE:		
Maximal minute ventilation $V_E$max (L/min)	Smaller	Early fatigability in tasks that require large respiratory minute volumes
VO_2max (ml/kg/min)	Same as adolescents and young adults	
VEsubmax; ventilatory equivalent	VE at any given VO_2 is higher in children	Less efficient ventilation would mean a greater oxygen cost of ventilation. May explain the relatively higher metabolic cost of submaximal exercise
Respiratory frequency and tidal volume	Marked by higher rate (tachypnea) and shallow breathing response	Children's physiologic dead space is smaller than that of adults; therefore alveolar ventilation is still adequate for gas exchange
PERCEPTION (rating of perceived exertion [RPE]):	Exercising at a given physiologic strain is perceived to be easier by children	Implications for initial phase of heat acclimatization
THERMOREGULATORY:		
Surface area	Per unit mass is approximately 36% greater in children (percentage is variable, depends on size of child, i.e., surface area per mass may be higher in younger children and lower in older ones)	Greater rate of heat exchange between skin and environment. In climatic extremes, children are at increased risk of stress
Sweating rate	Lower absolute amount and per unit of surface area. Greater increase in core temperature required to start sweating	Greater risk of heat-related illness on hot, humid days because of reduced capacity to evaporate sweat. Lower tolerance time in extreme heat
Acclimatization to heat	Slower physiologically, faster subjectively	Children require longer and more gradual program of acclimatization; special attention during early stages of acclimatization
Body cooling in water	Faster because of higher surface area per heat, producing unit mass; lower thickness of subcutaneous fat	Potential hypothermia
Body core heating during dehydration	Greater	Prolonged activity: hydrate well before and enforce fluid intake during activity

*Adapted from Bar-Or O: Exercise in childhood. In Walsh RP, Shephard RJ: *Current therapy in sport medicine, 1985-1986,* St Louis, 1985, Mosby. In Zwiren L, *ACSM resource manual for exercise testing and prescription,* 1993, Philadelphia, Lea & Febiger.

be encouraged to participate in a variety of sports. Fitness classes should focus on fun and variety. Fitness classes can be more structured during this period. After the age of 12, specialized training can begin for those individuals who have refined basic skills and are mature enough.

Trainability of Children

Trainability is the degree to which a tissue or a body system responds to a training stimulus with morphologic or functional changes. The degree to which children and adolescents can improve physiologic measures depends on growth and maturation rates and the exercise stimulus during the training program. In many ways, children respond to exercise much the same as adults do. Children may even have certain advantages over adults; for example, children seem to recover faster from exercise compared with adults.

Differences Between Children and Adults

There are major differences between children and adults with respect to physiologic responses and adaptations after exercise (Table 25.5). Most physiologic capacities depend on body and system dimensions. For example, both maximal stroke volume and cardiac output are lower in a child than in an adult because of the child's immature heart. In addition, children have a lower blood volume and a lower hemoglobin concentration than adults. These differences combine to reduce the oxygen transport capacity of the child; however, VO_2max relative to body weight is similar in children and adults. Children have a large surface-to-mass ratio, a higher metabolic rate, and an immature sweating capacity compared with adults. With normal growth and development, most of these dissimilarities disappear.

Aerobic Capacity In Children

In absolute terms the maximal oxygen uptake of children is much lower than that of adults, but when corrected for body weight the VO_2max of boys is similar to that found in young men. Young girls have a greater VO_2max per kilogram of body weight than young women but when the measurement is adjusted for height^2, they have lower capacities. Another measurement of aerobic power is peak oxygen uptake. Peak oxygen uptake is a more accurate measurement of aerobic power in children, since children have a difficult time reaching a true maximal effort because of local muscular fatigue, a limited attention span during testing, and a low threshold for discomfort.[15]

The accuracy of VO_2max for predicting cardiorespiratory fitness and endurance performance in children is not well established.[106] Maximal oxygen uptake is directly related to the maturity level of the individual (i.e., lean body mass,

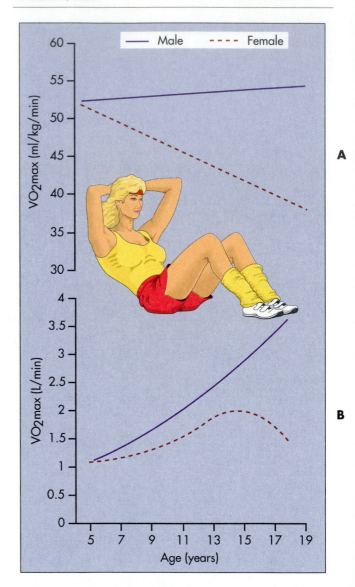

FIGURE 25.11

The relationships between VO_2max and chronologic age. **A,** VO_2max is expressed absolutely (L/min), and **B,** relative to body mass. (Adapted from Krahenbuhl GS et al: *Exerc Sport Sci Rev* 14:503-538, 1985.

height, and weight). As children mature, maximal oxygen uptake levels increase. Until maturity is reached, a relative rather than an absolute expression should be used to compare peak aerobic power (Figure 25.11). Values for VO_2max increase at about the same rate in both genders until age 12. After that age, boys continue to increase their maximal oxygen uptake until the age of 18, whereas girls show little improvement after age 14.

TABLE 25.6

Physiologic changes in children resulting from training and physical growth and maturation

CHARACTERISTIC	CHANGE
Heart rate, resting and submaximal	Decrease
Arterial blood pressure, maximal	Increase
Minute ventilation, submaximal	Decrease
Minute ventilation, maximal	Increase
Respiratory frequency, submaximal and maximal	Decrease
Ventilatory equivalent, submaximal and maximal	Decrease
Oxygen uptake, submaximal (per kilogram of body weight)	Decrease
Oxygen uptake, maximal (L/min)	Increase
Blood lactate, maximal	Increase
Muscle lactate, maximal	Increase
Lowest blood pH	Decrease
Muscle strength	Increase
Anaerobic power (in watts and per kilogram of body weight)	Increase
Muscle endurance* (in watts and per kilogram of body weight)	Increase

From Bar-Or O: The O_2 cost of child's movement in health and disease. In Russo P, Gass G, editors: *Exercise, nutrition and performances*, Sydney, Australia, 1985, Cumberland College.
*Represented by mean power in the Wingate Anaerobic Test.

Exercise capacity and maximal oxygen uptake increase throughout childhood. The increase in endurance capacity is due to enhanced oxygen transport and enhanced metabolic capacities. Several excellent reviews have been written on the effects of physical activity on the trainability of prepubescent children.[15,90,107,120] Some of the physiologic effects of training, growth, and maturation in children are listed in Table 25.6. In addition, numerous researchers have demonstrated improvements in VO2max after endurance training, with changes ranging from 5% to 18% depending on the mode of training, the intensity of the exercise, and the length of the study.*

Recently Payne and Morrow performed a meta-analysis on exercise and VO2max in children.[92] These authors found 69 training studies using children and used 28 of them in their analysis. In their review, Payne and Morrow found that the typical child in the studies they reviewed could be

expected to improve (before and after training) VO2max by only 2.07 ml/kg/min as a result of training. The researchers concluded by stating that "our work suggests the aerobic benefit of training is small-to-moderate for children and are a function of the experimental design."

Training Considerations

Sufficient evidence exists that children do adapt physiologically to endurance training. Lacking, however, is a general consensus on the quality and quantity of exercise required to improve and maintain a minimum level of fitness in children. Recommendations for adults have been published by the American College of Sports Medicine in their position stand, first published in 1978 and revised in 1990.[5,7] In 1988 the American College of Sports Medicine published an opinion statement on physical fitness in children and youth:[6]

The amount of exercise required for optimal functional capacity and health at various ages has not been precisely defined. Until more definitive evidence is available, current recommendations are that children and youth obtain 20-30 minutes of vigorous exercise each day. Physical education classes typically devote instructional time to physical fitness.

Several investigators have recommended that adult standards be used when establishing the intensity of exercise, as well as the frequency and duration of children's fitness programs.[12,107] These recommendations are supported by Rowland. He found that of eight studies reviewed, the six that used adult standards of aerobic training produced significant improvements in aerobic power, whereas no significant improvements were noted in the other two studies.[107]

Anaerobic Capacity In Children

Anaerobic power is defined as the maximal rate at which energy can be produced or work can be done without relying on any significant contribution of aerobic energy production. Anaerobic activities are those that are high in intensity and short in duration (see Chapter 19). Several tests are commonly used to assess anaerobic power. One of the most frequently used is the Wingate test, which is designed to determine both peak anaerobic power and mean power output during a 30-second test. The Wingate test has been used extensively when assessing the anaerobic capacities of children.[21,53,65]

Young children have distinctly lower anaerobic capacities when compared with adolescents and adults.[12] Some of the reasons for these differences may be related to low levels of male hormones, a lower glycolytic capacity, lower lactate production during exercise, a decreased capacity to buffer acidosis during exercise, lower rates of anaerobic use of glycogen during exercise, and lower lactate thresholds.[12,53,65] As children mature, their ability to increase their anaerobic power improves.[12,36,45]

*References 36, 37, 60, 68, 99, 106, and 118.

FIGURE 25.12

The increase in maximal anaerobic power in children as they age. (Adapted from Bar-Or O: *Pediatric sports medicine for the practitioner: from physiological principles to clinical applications*, New York, 1983, Springer-Verlag.)

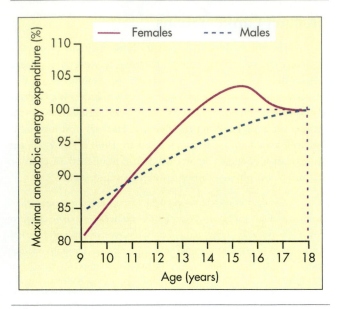

With maturation, responses to training also improve. Maximal oxygen uptake is strongly related to lean body mass, which increases throughout childhood. In addition, oxygen delivery to the working muscles, oxygen extraction, and oxygen use all improve with age and growth. Peak anaerobic power also increases with age and growth (Figure 25.12).

Muscular Strength and Endurance

The benefits of resistance, or strength training, in adults is well documented.[10] However, there is considerably less documentation of the benefits of resistance training in children. In fact, much of the research on the safety and efficacy of resistance training for children has been conducted only within the last 10 years. Early investigators concluded that strength gains were not possible in prepubertal children and that strength training could cause irreversible injury to the developing growth plates in bones.[119,123] The acceptance of children's participation in strength and resistance training has only recently gained acceptance. Although there are fewer resistance-training studies involving children than adults, the evidence demonstrating increases in strength after structured resistance training in children is mounting. The increases reported in the literature are similar to those observed in older age-groups, and the safety and efficacy of resistance training programs for children have been substantiated by research.

Importance of Adequate Strength

Adequate strength is considered an important part of health-related fitness and optimal physiologic function for both children and adults. It is also recognized as an important contributor to improved motor performance, self-image, and athletic performance. The National Strength and Conditioning Association, the American Orthopaedic Society for Sports Medicine, and the American Physical Therapy Association support supervised resistance training in children to reduce the chance of injury. Unfortunately, strength, specifically of the upper body, is poor among children.

Benefits of Resistance Training for Children

Numerous research studies and review articles published in the last decade have examined the effects of resistance training on prepubescent children. Some of the benefits of early resistance training have been discussed, but more research is needed to better understand other health- and performance-related benefits of resistance training for prepubescent children.

Improved Sports Performance

Several studies have evaluated the effects of resistance training on athletic performance.[82,95,121] After 14 weeks of supervised hydraulic resistance training, improvements in the vertical jump performance improved by 10.4% in the trained group versus a 3% decrease in performance in the control group from pretest values.[121] After isometric strength training, improvement in vertical jump scores for girls 7 to 19 years old was demonstrated.[82] Significant improvements in strength and performance have been demonstrated in prepubescent female gymnasts after 4 weeks of supervised resistance training.[95] Further research is needed to examine the effects of resistance training on performance in different sports.

Health Benefits

Numerous health-related benefits after resistance training have been reported in the literature. In addition to improvements in muscular strength, other fitness- and performance-related effects of resistance training include increased flexibility, improvements in body composition, reduction in serum lipids, reduction in blood pressure, and improvement in cardiorespiratory function.[47,97,113,121] With further research, additional benefits may be recognized.

Injury Prevention

Recent studies have also shown that a strength development program may help with injury prevention. A report by the American Physical Therapy Association concluded that poor physical conditioning may be the leading cause of injury in youth sports. Other data suggest that resistance training may help protect against injury in young children.[26,48,75] All sports place demands on the musculoskeletal system, and medical and sports medicine experts generally agree that increasing the strength of adult athletes enhances performance and decreases the chance of injury. Since it has been demonstrated that resistance training can increase both muscle and bone growth in children, encouraging them to participate in such training to reduce potential injuries appears justified.

Controversies in Youth Strength Training

For the majority of the twentieth century the idea of children's participation in strength- and resistance-training programs gained little support from physicians and physical educators, despite the evidence of poor strength levels in children. Much of the evidence in supporting the ban on prepubescent resistance training evolved from several early scientific reports, which concluded that young children could not gain strength before puberty and that they were more susceptible to injuries because of their developing musculoskeletal system. Fortunately, new information regarding the safety, effectiveness, and health benefits of resistance training for children is likely to reverse past skepticism.

Prepubescent Strength Training Research

There is substantial evidence demonstrating increases in strength after structured resistance training in children. These increases are similar to those observed in older age groups.

TABLE 25.7

Strength training studies in prepubescent children*

REFERENCE	AGE/GRADE	SEX	TRAINING MODE	TESTING MODE	DURATION (WEEKS)	FREQUENCY (PER WEEK)	CONTROL GROUP	STRENGTH INCREASE
Hetherington (1976)	Grade 5	M	Isometric	Isometric	6-8	2-5	Yes	No
Vrijens (1978)	10.4	M	Weights	Isometric	8	3	No	No
Nielson et al. (1980)	7-19	F	Isometric	Isometric	5	3	Yes	Yes
Baumgartner and Wood (1984)	Grades 3-6	M, F	Calisthenics	Calisthenics	12	3	Yes	Yes
Clarke et al. (1984)	7-9	M	Wrestling	Isometric; Calisthenics	12	3	Yes	Yes
McGovern (1984)[†]	Grades 4-6	M, F	Weights	Weights	12	3	Yes	Yes
Sevedio et al. (1985)[†]	11.9	M	Weights	Isokinetic	8	3	Yes	Yes
Pfeiffer and Francis (1986)	8-11	M	Weights	Isokinetic	8	3	Yes	Yes
Sewall and Micheli (1986)	10-11	M, F	Weights; Pneumatic	Isometric	9	3	Yes	Yes
Weltman et al. (1986)	6-11	M	Hydraulic	Isokinetic	14	3	Yes	Yes
Funato et al. (1987)	6-11	M, F	Isometric	Isometric; Isokinetic	12	3	Yes	Yes
Sailors and Berg (1987)	12.6	M	Weights	Weights	8	3	Yes	Yes
Siegal et al. (1988)	8.4	M, F	Weights; Calisthenics	Isometric Calisthenics	12	3	Yes	Yes
Ramsay et al. (1990)	9-11	M	Weights	Weights; Isokinetic; Isometric	20	3	Yes	Yes
Williams (1991)[†]	10.5	M	Weights	Isometric Calisthenics	8	3	Yes	Yes
Brown et al. (1992)[†]	Tanner 1-2[‡]	M, F	Weights	Weights	12	3	Yes	Yes
Westcott (1992)	10.5	M, F	Weights	Weights	7	3	No	Yes
Faigenbaum et al. (1993)	10.8	M, F	Weights	Weights	8	2	Yes	Yes
Stahle et al. (1995)	10-12	M	Weights	Weights	25	2-3	Yes	Yes

*Modified from Sale D: Strength training in children. In Gisolfi CV, Lamb DR, editors: *Youth exercise and sport,* vol 2, Dubeque, Iowa, 1989, Times Mirror Higher Education Group. In Faiaenbaum AD: Strength training: a guide for teachers and coaches, *NCSA J* (15) 5:20-30, 1993.

[†]Abstract

[‡]Refers to Tanner stages 1 and 2 of sexual maturation.

FIGURE 25.13

The known and theoretic factors contributing to increased strength gains in children during exercise training. (Adapted from Kraemer WJ: *Pediatr Exerc Sci* 1:336-350, 1989.)

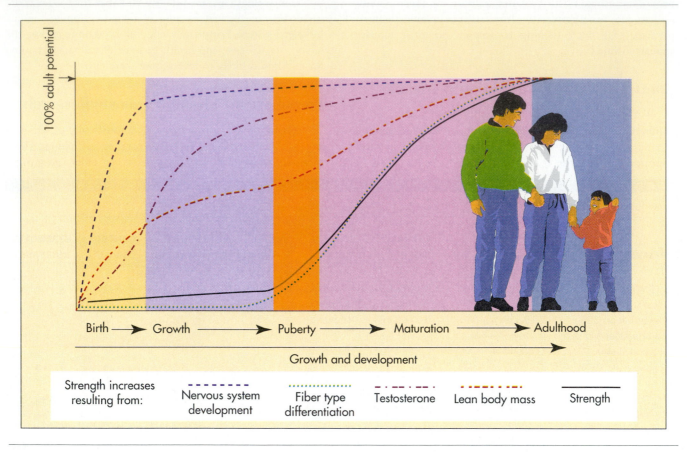

Furthermore, the safety and efficacy of resistance-training programs for prepubescent children have been well documented (Table 25.7).

Factors Influencing Strength Development in Prepubescent Children

The primary mechanisms responsible for strength gains in prepubescent children are neural adaptations and better coordination of agonist and antagonist muscle groups.[23] Several other mechanisms also influence strength development in prepubescent children (Figure 25.13).

- *Hormonal Influences*
  Up to the age of puberty in the male, the level of androgens is too low to promote muscle hypertrophy. Trainability increases rapidly during puberty as testosterone levels increase.
- *Increased Motor Unit Activation*
  Training-induced neural adaptations seem to be the primary means by which prepubescent children gain strength.
- *Increase in Lean Body Mass*
  Both aerobic capacity and strength are highly correlated to

lean body mass. Regular training results in a decrease in fatness and an increase in fat-free mass.
- *Fiber Type Differentiation*
  Muscle fiber types can influence skeletal muscle strength. Muscle fibers undergo a tremendous increase in size during childhood and adolescence. At the present time, there is little available data on the relationship between muscle fiber type distribution and strength development in children.

Safety of Resistance Training in Children

In the late 1970s and early 1980s, several scientific reports recommended that children not participate in weight training because the developing bones and musculature of young children are more susceptible to injuries than those of adults.[2,123] These recommendations were based primarily on the published report of growth-plate injuries that occurred in adolescent weightlifters.[46,109] The injuries in the earlier reports involved the wrist and occurred during excessive overhead lifts.[46,109] Growth-plate injuries do occur in young children. Some of the more common causes of growth-plate injuries

FOCUS BOX 25.4

Professional guidelines and recommendations for strength training of prepubescent children

The American Academy of Pediatrics, the National Strength and Conditioning Association, and the American Orthopaedic Society for Sports Medicine have published position stands on prepubescent strength training.

In 1990 the American Academy of Pediatrics (AAP) released an updated version of their 1983 report.[2] In this report the AAP recommended the following:

- Strength training programs for prepubescent, pubescent, and postpubescent athletes should be permitted only if conducted by well-trained adults. The adults should be qualified to plan programs appropriate to the athlete's stage of maturation, which should be assessed by medical personnel.

- Unless good medical data that demonstrate safety become available, children and adolescents should avoid the practice of weightlifting, power lifting, and body building, as well as the repetitive use of maximal amounts of weight in strength training programs, until they have reached Tanner stage 5 (adolescence) level of developmental maturity.

Because of concern over injury and the increased interest in strength training for youths, the National Strength and Conditioning Association (NSCA) developed a position stand on prepubescent strength training in 1985 (this position stand is currently under revision).[79] The NSCA believes that "when performed properly, strength training programs for the prepubescent athlete can improve strength, self-image, motor performance, and reduce injury."

In August 1985, eight sports medicine groups attended the American Orthopaedic Society for Sports Medicine (AOSSM) workshop in Indianapolis on strength training.[8] The major organizations present at that workshop included the AOSSM, AAP, NSCA, American College of Sports Medicine, National Athletic Trainers Association, President's Council on Physical Fitness and Sports, US Olympic Committee, and Society of Pediatric Orthopaedics. The consensus of these groups was that "strength training for prepubescent boys and girls is safe with proper program design, instruction, and supervision." In addition, the overall groups' position was that "the benefits of prepubescent strength training do outweigh the risks."

Resistance Training Principles for Young Athletes

Principle 1—Children should be encouraged to participate in regular exercise that involves repetitive movements against an opposing force. It is important to note that children can develop strength through a variety of activities, including partici-

pation in sports, weight training, manual resistance exercises, and simply playing.

Principle 2—Power lifting, or lifting in a competitive setting to determine the maximum amount of weight an individual can lift, is not recommended for children.

Principle 3—The primary focus of resistance training should, at least initially, be focused on developing proper technique, learning the exercises, and developing an interest in resistance training.

Principle 4—Before any resistance is used, proper technique should be demonstrated for each exercise. The next step is to apply resistance or weight gradually until the child can lift the weight for the repetition range (i.e., 8 to 12).

Principle 5—Children should perform 8 to 12 repetitions for upper body exercises and 15 to 20 in lower body exercises. Once children are able to perform an exercise for a predetermined maximum number of repetitions per set, the resistance or maximum number of repetitions should be increased.

Principle 6—One to three sets of each exercise should be performed, using 8 to 10 different exercises. In the early stages of training, one set of each exercise should be performed until such time as the child has demonstrated proper form and is used to resistance training.

Principle 7—Children should be encouraged to rest for 1 to 2 minutes between exercises.

Principle 8—Two to three exercise sessions per week is recommended, followed by at least 1 day of rest between workouts.

Principle 9—As children develop strength, the training stimulus should be adjusted. To maintain maximal stimulus, the resistance or number of repetitions (or both) must be increased.

Principle 10—Training programs should be designed with specific goals and objectives in mind. The exercises chosen should reflect the desired outcome. For the majority of children, specificity of training is less important than it will be in later years. Children should participate in a variety of activities to develop a wide range of skills.

Principle 11—A brief warm-up period should precede the exercise session and a brief cool-down should follow the session. Warm-up exercises increase the temperature and elasticity of the muscle, which improves the muscle's ability to perform work and reduces the risk of muscle and joint injury. Cool-down activities lower the muscle temperature and metabolic rate.

in children are accidents and participation in sports, such as baseball, skiing, football, gymnastics, and long-distance running.[27] There is, however, little if any evidence that supervised resistance training causes harm to the musculoskeletal system in children (See Focus Box 25.4).[98]

Weltman and his colleagues studied the safety and effectiveness of resistance training in 26 prepubescent children.[121] They found no evidence of damage to the epiphysis, bone, or muscle after a 14-week supervised strength-training program. Weltman concluded that "supervised strength training using hydraulic strength training equipment is safe and effective in pre-pubertal boys." In two other studies by Ramsay and Blimkie at McMaster University in Ontario, Canada, the safety and effectiveness of resistance training were evaluated in prepubescent boys.[22,96] In both studies, safety was monitored via physician evaluation before, during, and after training. Neither study found evidence of damage to the musculoskeletal system after resistance training. Furthermore, both studies reported significant strength gains in prepubescent children after the training programs.

Special Considerations

Thermoregulation

In normal or moderate climates, children are able to exercise and dissipate heat quite effectively. In very hot environments, however, children have a limited ability to dissipate heat. Children are not as efficient in dissipating heat as adults because they have a lower sweat rate at rest and at exercise, greater energy expenditure during exercise, and a lower cardiac output at any given metabolic level (see Chapter 26).[16] Araki compared the sweating rate and skin and rectal temperature of a 9-year-old boy and a 20-year-old man (Figure 25.14). The results reflect the lowered capacity for evaporative cooling in the prepubescent child.

During exercise, children produce large amounts of heat per kilogram of body weight, compared with adults.[16] Children have a low capacity for evaporative cooling and tend to rely more on convection and radiation to dissipate heat, rather than evaporation. Children can acclimatize to hot conditions, but the process takes considerably more time (repeated exposures) than with adults.[52] Special precautions should always be taken when children are exercising in extreme environmental conditions. Because of children's limited thermoregulatory capacities, the risk of thermal injury is much greater in children than in adults.

Asthma

Several investigations have demonstrated that children with asthma can improve their fitness level without adverse affects on their exercise-induced asthma (EIA).[59,83] Asthmatic children should be encouraged to participate in regular phys-

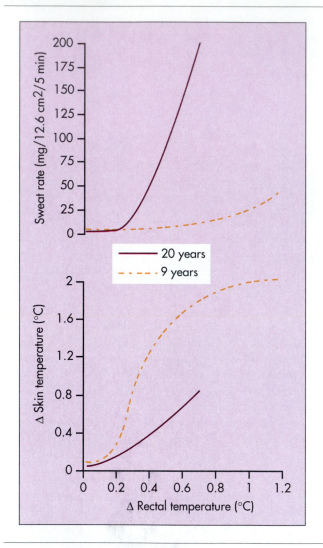

FIGURE 25.14

The change in sweat rate and skin temperature during exercise-induced increases in core temperature in a 9-year-old boy and a 20-year-old man. (Adapted from Araki T et al: *Jpn J Phys Fitness Sports Med* 28:239-248, 1979.)

ical activates at school and after school.[122] Such training may lower the intensity and frequency of EIA attacks.[17]

Diabetes

The benefits of exercise on diabetic control are well documented in adults.[19,57] However, there does appear to be controversy regarding the improvement of diabetic control in children who exercise.[17] Although nonexercising children with diabetes tend to be less fit than nonexercising children without diabetes, it is less evident that children with controlled diabetes should be encouraged to exercise in an effort to expend energy, reduce body fatness, and improve diabetic control.[39]

Obesity

Obesity is one of the most prevalent chronic diseases among adults and children. Numerous studies have demonstrated the beneficial effects of exercise alone or in combination with dieting on weight loss in children.[24,76,85] Other benefits of exercise in obese children include improved self-image, reductions in blood pressure, and reductions in serum lipids.[17]

SUMMARY

- The term **pediatric exercise science** has evolved over time in an effort to include the diverse nature of exercise-related research being conducted on children and youth around the world. Today, health promotion efforts are shifting focus from immunization against infectious diseases to reducing the risk factors associated with today's leading causes of death, such as heart disease and cancer. Medical doctors who specialize in children's medicine are termed **pediatricians.**

- Over the past two decades, several large-scale youth fitness surveys have been conducted, and the results provide much of the evidence that is used to judge the past and current health and fitness status of children and youth. There is currently a movement among youth fitness experts to use **criterion-referenced fitness standards** that are based on established fitness and health relationships.

- Childhood obesity has increased in the last decade. The cause of the increase in body fat over the years has been related to decreased habitual physical activity and increased television viewing. Strength, particularly upper body strength, of children in the United States is poor.

- As many as 40% of children ages 5 to 8 in the United States show at least one heart disease risk factor (i.e., high cholesterol, physical inactivity, obesity, high blood pressure). With the evidence linking the origins of coronary artery disease to childhood years, efforts should be made to identify children at the highest level of coronary heart disease risk and reduce the potential for these children maturing into high-risk adults.

- Children do not grow at a uniform rate throughout their development. There is a rapid increase in height, followed (particularly in boys) by a rapid increase in body mass over the period of **puberty** (the pubertal growth spurt). There are four main phases of growth in humans. Growth is rapid in infancy and early childhood, remains relatively steady during middle childhood, and again increases rapidly during **adolescence,** often referred to as **peak height velocity.** Finally, a slow increase and eventual cessation of growth occur with attainment of adulthood. There are tremendous gender differences during growth.

- The degree to which children and adolescents can improve physiologic measures depends on growth and maturation rates and the exercise stimulus during the training program. In many ways, children respond to exercise much the same as adults do. However, in absolute terms, the maximal oxygen uptake of children is much lower than adults, but when corrected for body weight the VO_2max of boys is similar to that found in young men. Young girls have a greater VO_2max per kg body weight than young women but when adjusted for height^2, they have lower capacities.

- Sufficient evidence exists that children do physiologically adapt to endurance training. Lacking, however, is a general consensus on the quality and quantity of exercise required to improve and maintain a minimum level of fitness in children. Several investigators have recommended that adult standards be used when establishing the intensity of exercise, as well as the frequency and duration of children's fitness programs.

- Young children have lower anaerobic capacities compared with adolescents and adults. As children mature, their ability to increase their anaerobic power improves. Structured resistance training can also increase muscle strength in children. These increases are similar to those observed in older age-groups. The primary mechanisms responsible for strength gains in prepubescent children are neural adaptations and better coordination of agonist and antagonist muscle groups.

- In normal or moderate climates, children are able to exercise and dissipate heat quite effectively. In very hot environments, however, children are quite limited in their ability to dissipate heat because of lower sweat rates and a reduced potential for evaporative cooling.

REVIEW QUESTIONS

1. Discuss two distinct limitations associated with pediatric exercise compared with adults, and give several examples.

2. How have youth fitness tests changed over the years, and what was the stimulus for such changes?

3. What are criterion-referenced fitness standards?

4. Do you think children are physically fit today? Provide specific documentation for your response.

5. Discuss the difference between growth and development and how exercise affects each.

6. Discuss some of the age and gender differences in growth.

7. Why is it important to assess for maturation in young athletes?

8. A coach comes up to you and asks, "are children as trainable as adults?" In several paragraphs give your response with specific documentation.

9. Is VO_2max an accurate predictor of fitness and performance in children? How should VO_2 be expressed?

10. List five benefits of resistance training in children and adolescents.

11. A concerned parent comes up to you and says, "I have heard that weight training is not safe for children, and that it will stunt their growth." How would you respond, giving specific examples?

12. What are the mechanisms associated with strength changes in prepubescent children?

13. Discuss some concerns regarding children exercising in hot or humid environments.

APPLICATIONS

1. Identify research supporting the need for early coronary artery disease prevention in children.

2. Describe a school- and home-based prevention program for children.

3. What are the roles of pediatrician in cardiovascular disease prevention in children? What are the roles of parents?

REFERENCES

1. Amateur Athletic Union: *Physical fitness program,* Indianapolis, 1981, AAU House.

2. American Academy of Pediatrics: Weight training and weightlifting: information for the pediatrician, *Phys Sportsmed* 11:157-161, 1983.

3. American Alliance for Health, Physical Education and Recreation: *AAHPER youth fitness test manual,* Washington, DC, 1965.

4. American Alliance for Health, Physical Education and Recreation: *Physical best: a physical fitness education and assessment program,* Reston, Virginia, 1988, Publisher.

5. American College of Sports Medicine: Position stand for the recommended quantity and quality of exercise for developing and maintaining cardiorespiratory and muscular fitness in healthy adults, *Med Sci Sports Exerc* 10:vii-x, 1978.

6. American College of Sports Medicine: Opinion statement on physical fitness in children and youth, *Med Sci Sports Exerc* 20:422-423, 1988.

7. American College of Sports Medicine: Position stand for the recommended quantity and quality of exercise for developing and maintaining cardiorespiratory and muscular fitness in healthy adults, *Med Sci Sports Exerc* 22:265-274, 1990.

8. American Orthopaedic Society for Sports Medicine: *Proceedings of the conference on strength training and the prepubescent,* Cahill B, editor, Chicago, 1988, Publisher.

9. Araki T, Toda Y, Matsushita K, Tsujino A: Age differences in sweating during muscular exercise, *Jap J Phys Fitness Sports Med* 28:239-248, 1979.

10. Atha J: Strengthening muscle, *Exer Sports Sci Rev* 91:1-73, 1981.

11. Bailey DA, Wedge JH, McCulloch RG et al: Epidemiology of fractures of the distal end of the radius in children associated with growth, *J Bone Joint Surg* 71-A(8):1225-1231, 1989.

12. Bar-Or O: *Pediatric sports medicine for the practitioner: from physiological principles to clinical applications,* New York, 1983, Springer-Verlag.

13. Bar-Or O: The growth and development of children's physiologic and perceptual responses to exercise. In Ilmarinen J, Valimaki J, editors: *Children and sport,* Berlin, 1984, Springer-Verlag.

14. Bar-Or O: The O_2 cost of child's movement in health and disease. In Russo P, Gass G, editors: *Exercise, nutrition and performances,* Sydney, Australia, 1985, Cumberland College.

15. Bar-Or O: Trainability of the prepubescent child, *Phys Sportsmed* 5:65-82, 1989.

16. Bar-Or O: Temperature regulation during exercise in children and adolescents. In Gisolfi CV, Lamb DR, editors: *Perspectives in exercise science and sports medicine,* Carmel, Indiana, 1989, Benchmark Press.

17. Bar-Or O: Disease-specific benefits of training in the child with a chronic disease: what is the evidence? *Pediatr Exer Sci* 2:384-394, 1990.

18. Berenson GS, Srinivasan SR, Hunter S et al: Risk factors in early life as predicators of adult heart disease: the Bogalusa heart study, *Am J Med Sci* 298(3):141-151, 1989.

19. Bjorntorp P, Krotkiewski M: Exercise treatment in diabetes mellitus, *Acta Med Scand* 217:3-7, 1985.

20. Blair SN, Clark DG, Cureton KJ, Powell KE: Exercise and fitness in childhood: implications for a lifetime of health. In Gisolfi CV, Lamb DR, editors: *Perspectives in exercise science and sports medicine,* Carmel, Indiana, 1991, Benchmark Press.

21. Blimkie CJ, Roche P, Bar-Or O: The anaerobic-to-aerobic power ratio in adolescent boys and girls. In Rutenfranz J, Mocellin R, Klimt F, editors: *Children and exercise XII,* Champaign, Illinois, 1986, Human Kinetics.

22. Blimkie CJR, Ramsay J, Sale D et al: Effects of 10 weeks of resistance training on strength development in prepubertal boys, In Oseid S, Carlsen KH, editors: *International series on sport sciences. Children and exercise XIII,* Champaign, Illinois, 1989, Human Kinetics.

23. Blimkie CJR: Resistance training during preadolescence, *Sports Med* 15(6):389-407, 1993.

24. Browell KD, Kelman JH, Stukard AJ: Treatment of obese children with and without their mothers: changes in weight and blood pressure, *Pediatrics* 71:515-522, 1983.

25. Bush PJ, Zuckerman AE, Taggart VS et al: Cardiovascular risk factor prevention in black school children: the "Know Your Body" evaluation project, *Health Educ Quart* 16(2)215-277, 1989.

26. Cahill BR, Griffith EH: Effect of preseason conditioning on the incidence and severity of high school football knee injuries, *Am J Sports Med* 4(6):180-184, 1978.

27. Caine DJ: Growth plate injury and bone growth: an update, *Pediatr Exer Sci* 2:209-229, 1990.

28. Canada Fitness Survey: *Fitness and lifestyles in Canada,* Ottawa, Ontario, Government of Canada, Fitness and Amateur Sport.

29. Connor MK, Smith G, Fryer A et al: Future fit: a cardiovascular health education and fitness project in an after-school setting, *J School Health* 56(8):329-333, 1986.

30. Cresanta JL, Hyg MS, Burke GL et al: Prevention of atherosclerosis in childhood, *Pediatr Clin N Am* 33(4):835-858, 1986.

REFERENCES—Cont'd

31. Croft JB, Cresanta JL, Webber LS et al: Cardiovascular risk in parents of children with extreme lipoprotein cholesterol levels: the Bogalusa Heart Study, *South Med J* 81:341-349, 1988.

32. Cureton KJ, Warren GL: Criterion-referenced standards for youth health-related fitness tests: a tutorial, *Res Quar Exer Sport* 61:7-19, 1990.

33. Davidson DM, Bradely BJ, Landry SM et al: School-based cholesterol screening, *J Pediatr Health Care* 3:3-8, 1989.

34. Davidson DM, Smith RM, Qaqunhad PY: Cholesterol screening in children during office visits, *J Pediatr Health Care* 4:11-17, 1990.

35. Dietz WH: Childhood obesity: susceptibility, cause, and management, *J Pediatr* 103:676-686, 1983.

36. Docherty D, Wenger HA, Collis ML: The effects of resistance training on aerobic and anaerobic power in young boys, *Med Sci Sports Exerc* 19:389-392, 1987.

37. Ekbolm B: Effect of physical training in adolescent boys, *J Appl Physiol* 27:350-355, 1969.

38. Enos WF, Holmes RH, Beyer J: Coronary artery disease among United States soldiers killed in action in Korea, *JAMA* 152:1090-1093, 1953.

39. Etkind EL, Cunningham L: Physical abilities in diabetic boys, *Isreal J Med Sci* 8:848,1972.

40. Falls HB, Pate RR: Status of physical fitness in U.S. children. In Leppo M, editor: *Healthy from the start: new perspectives on childhood fitness,* Washington, DC, 1993, ERIC Clearinghouse On Teacher Education.

41. Fraser GE, Phillips RL, Harris R: Physical fitness and blood pressure in school children, *Circulation* 67:405-412, 1983.

42. Gilliam TB, Katch VL, Thorland WG, Weltman AW: Prevalence of coronary heart disease risk factors in active children, 7 to 12 years of age, *Med Sci Sports Exerc* 9(1):21-25, 1977.

43. Gilliam TB, MacConnie SE: Coronary heart disease risk in children and their physical activity patterns. In Boileau RA, editor: *Advances in pediatric sport sciences,* Champaign, Illinois, 1984, Human Kinetics.

44. Gortmaker SL, Dietz WH, Sobol AM, Wehler CA: Increasing pediatric obesity in the United States, *Am J Dis Child* 141:535-540, 1987.

45. Grodjinovsky A, Inbar O, Dotan R, Bar-Or O: Training effect on the anaerobic performance of children as measured by the Wingate anaerobic test. In Berg K, Eriksson B, editors: *Children and exercise international series on sports science* 10:139-145, Baltimore, 1980, University Park Press.

46. Gumps VL, Segal D, Halligan JB, Lower G: Bilateral distal radius and ulnar fracture in weightlifting, *Am J Sports Med* 10:375-379, 1982.

47. Hagberg JM, Ehsani AA, Golding B et al: Effect of weight training on blood pressure and hemodynamics in hypertensive adolescents, *J Pediatr* 104(1):47-151, 1984.

48. Henjia WF, Rosenberg A, Buturusis DJ, Krieger A: Prevention of sports injuries in high school students through strength training, *NSCA J* 4(1):28-31, 1982.

49. Hertzel B, Berenson G: *Cardiovascular risk factors in childhood: epidemiology and prevention,* New York, 1987, Elsevier.

50. Hoffman A, Walter HJ, Connely PA, Vaughan RD: Blood pressure and physical fitness in school children, *Hypertension* 9:188-191,1987.

51. Hunter SM, Johnson CC, Little-Christian S et al: Heart smart: a multifaceted cardiovascular risk reduction program for grade school students, *Am J Health Promotion* 4(5):352-360, 1990.

52. Inbar O: *Acclimatization to dry and hot environments in young children 8-10 years old,* PhD dissertation, 1978, Columbia University, New York.

53. Inbar O, Bar-Or O: Anaerobic characteristics in male children and adolescents, *Med Sci Sports Exerc* 18:264-269, 1983.

54. Institute for Aerobic Research: *FITNESSGRAM,* Dallas, 1987, Publisher.

55. Jensen MD, Miles JM: The roles of diet and exercise in the management of patients with insulin dependent diabetes mellitus, *Mayo Clin Proc* 61:813-819, 1986.

56. Kannel WB, Dawber TR: Atherosclerosis as a pediatric problem, *J Pediatr* 80:544-554, 1972.

57. Kemmer FW, Berger M: Exercise in therapy and the life of diabetic patients, *Clin Sci* 67:279-283, 1984.

58. Khoury P, Morrison JA, Kelly K et al: Clustering and interrelationships of coronary heart disease risk factors in schoolchildren, ages 6-19, *Am J Epidemiol* 112(4):524-538, 1980.

59. King MJ, Noakes TD, Weinberg EG: Physiological effects of a training program in children with exercise-induced asthma, *Pediatr Exer Sci* 2:137-144, 1989.

60. Krahenbuhl GS, Skinner JS, Kohrt WM: Developmental aspects of maximal aerobic power in children, In Terjung RL, editor: *Exerc Sport Sci Rev* 14:503-538, 1985.

61. Kuntzleman CT: Childhood fitness: what is happening? What needs to be done? *Prevent Med* 22:521, 1993.

62. Lauer RM, Connor WE, Leaverton PE et al: Coronary heart disease risk factors in school children: the Muscatine study, *J Pediatr* 86(5):697-706, 1975.

REFERENCES—Cont'd

63. Linder CW, DuRant RH: Exercise, serum lipids, and cardiovascular disease-risk factors in children, *Pediatr Clin North Am* 29:1341-1354, 1982.

64. Lohman TG: *Advances in body composition assessment,* Champaign, Illinois, 1992, Human Kinetics.

65. Macek M: Aerobic and anaerobic energy output in children. In Rutenfranz J, Mocellin R, Klimt F, editors: *Children and exercise XII,* Champaign, Illinois, 1986, Human Kinetics.

66. Malina RM: Growth and maturation: normal variation and effect of training. In Gisolfi CV, Lamb DR, editors: Perspectives in exercise science and sports medicine, vol 2, *Youth, exercise, and sport,* Indianapolis, 1989, Benchmark Press.

67. Malina RM, Brouchard C: *Growth, maturation, and physical activity,* Champaign, Illinois, 1991, Human Kinetics.

68. Massicotte DR, MacNab RBJ: Cardiorespiratory adaptations to training at specified intensities in children, *Med Sci Sports Exerc* 6:242-246, 1974.

69. Mayer J, Bullen BA: Nutrition, weight control and exercise. In Johnson WR, Buskurk ER, editors: *Science and medicine of exercise and sport,* ed 2, New York, 1974, Harper & Row.

70. Mellies MJ, Laskarzewski PM, Tracy T, Glueck CJ: Tracking of high- and low-density-liproprotein cholesterol from childhood to young adulthood in a single large kindred with familial hypercholesterolemia, *Metabolism* 34:747-753, 1985.

71. McMillian GC: Development of arteriosclerosis, *Am J Cardiol* 31:542-546, 1973.

72. McNamara JJ, Molot MA, Stremple JF, Cutting RT: Coronary artery disease in combat casualties in Vietnam, *JAMA* 216,1185-1187, 1971.

73. McNamara DG: Can (should) the pediatrician wage preventive medicine war against coronary heart disease, *J Dis Child* 140:985-986, 1986.

74. Meredith MD: *FITNESSGRAM user's manual,* Dallas, 1987, Institute for Aerobics Research.

75. Micheli LJ: Strength training in the young athlete. In Brown EW, Crystal CF, editors: *Competitive sports for children and youth: an overview of research and issues,* Champaign, Illinois, 1988, Human Kinetics.

76. Moody DL, Wilmore JH, Girandola RN, Royce JP: The effects of a jogging program on the body composition of normal and obese high school girls, *Med Sci Sports Exerc* 4:210-213, 1972.

77. Morbidity and Mortality Weekly Report: Psychosocial predictors of smoking among adolescents, *Med Sci Sports Exerc* 36(Suppl 4):S1-S47, 1987.

78. Nader PR, Taras HL, Sallis JF, Patterson TL: Adult heart disease prevention in childhood: a national survey of pediatricians' practices and attitudes, *Pediatrics* 79(6):843-851, 1987.

79. National Strength and Conditioning Association: Position paper on prepubescent strength training, *Nat Strength Condition Assoc J* 7:27-29, 1985.

80. Newman WP, Strong JP: Natural history, geographic pathology, and pediatric aspects of atherosclerosis. In Strong WB, editor: *Atherosclerosis: its pediatric aspects,* New York, 1978, Grune & Stratton.

81. NewmanWP, Freedman DS, Voors AW et al: Relation of serum lipoprotein levels and systolic blood pressure to early atherosclerosis, *N Engl J Med* 314:138-144, 1986.

82. Nielsen B, Nielsen K, Brhrendt Hansen M, Asmussen A: Training of function muscular strength in girls 7-19 years old. In Berg K, Erikson BK, editors: *Children and exercise* 9:69-78, Baltimore, 1980, University Park Press.

83. Orenstein DM, Reed ME, Grogan FT, Crawford LV: Exercise conditioning in children with asthma, *J Pediatr* 106:556-561, 1985.

84. Parcel GS, Simmons-Morton BG, O'Hara NM et al: School promotion of healthful diet and exercise behavior: an integration of organizational change and social learning theory interventions, *J School Health* 57(4):150-156, 1987.

85. Parizkova J, Vamberova M: Body composition as a criterion of the suitability of reducing regimens in obese children, *Dev Med Child Neurol* 9:202-211, 1967.

86. Parikova J: Particularities of lean body mass and fat development in growing boys related to their motor activity, *Acta Paediatr Belgica Suppl* 28:233-242, 1974.

87. Pate RR, Ross JG: Factors associated with health related fitness, *J Phys Educ Rec Dance* 58(9):93-95, 1987.

88. Pate RR, Ross JG, Baumgartner TA, Sparks RE: The modified pull-up test, *J Phys Educ Rec Dance* November/December:72, 1987.

89. Pate RR, Shephard RJ: Characteristics of physical fitness in youth. In Gisolfi CV, Lamb DR, editors: *Perspectives in exercise science and sports medicine,* Carmel, Indiana, 1989, Benchmark Press.

90. Pate RR, Ward DS: Endurance exercise trainability in children and youth. In Grana WA, Lombarade JA, Sharkey BJ, Stone JA, editors: *Advances in sports medicine and fitness,* St Louis, 1990, Mosby.

91. Pate RR, Burgess ML, Woods JA et al: Validity of field tests of upper body muscular strength, *Res Quar Exerc Sport* 64(1):18, 1993.

REFERENCES—Cont'd

92. Payne GV, Morrow JR: Exercise and VO₂max in children: a meta-analysis, *Res Quar Exerc Sport* 64(3):305-313, 1993.

93. Perry CL, Luepker RV, Murray DM et al: Parent involvement with children's health promotion: the Minnesota home team, *Am J Public Health* 78(9):1157-1161, 1988.

94. President's Council on Physical Fitness and Sports: *The Presidential Physical Fitness Award Program: instructor's guide,* DHHS Publication No. HHS 396, Washington, DC, 1987, Government Printing Office.

95. Queary JL, Laubach LL: The effects of muscular strength endurance training, *Technique* 12:9-11, 1992.

96. Ramsay JA, Blimkie CJR, Smith K et al: Strength training effects in prepubescent boys, *Med Sci Sports Exerc* 22:605-614, 1990.

97. Reiff GG, Dixon WR, Jacoby D et al: *President's Council on Physical Fitness and Sports, national school population fitness survey,* Research project 282-84-0086, 1985, The University of Michigan.

98. Risser WL, Risser JMH, Preston D: Weight-training injuries in adolescents, *Am J Dis Child* 144(9):1015-1017, 1990.

99. Roberts SO, Roberrgs RA, Stolarczyk L et al: Effects of combined step aerobic and resistance training in children on cardiorespiratory endurance and strength, *Med Sci Sports Exerc* 26(5):S83, 1994.

100. Robinson TN, Hammer LD, Killen JD et al: Does television viewing increase obesity and reduce physical activity? Cross-sectional and longitudinal analysis among adolescent girls, *Pediatrics* 91(2):273-279, 1993.

101. Roccine AP, Katch V, Anderson J et al: Blood pressure in obese adolescents: effect of weight loss, *Pediatrics* 82:16-23, 1988.

102. Rogers LQ, Fincher R-ME, Strong WB: Primary prevention of coronary artery disease through a family-oriented cardiac risk factor clinic, *South Med J* 83(11):1270-1272, 1990.

103. Ross JG, Gilbert GG: The national children and youth fitness survey: a summary of the findings, *J Phys Educ Rec Dance* 56(1):45-50, 1985.

104. Ross JG, Pate RR: The national children and youth fitness survey II: a summary of the findings, *J Phys Educ Recr Dance* 58(9):51-56, 1987.

105. Ross JG, Pate RR, Lohman TG, Christenson GM: Changes in the body composition of children: summary of findings from the national children and youth fitness study II, *J Phys Educ Recr Dance* November/December, 1987.

106. Rotstein A, Dotan R, Bar-Or O: Effect of training on anaerobic threshold, maximal aerobic power and anaerobic performance of preadolescent boys, *Int J Sports Med* 7:281-286, 1986.

107. Rowland TW: Aerobic responses to endurance training in prepubescent children: a critical analysis, *Med Sci Sports Exerc* 17:493-497, 1985.

108. Rowland TW: Developmental aspects of physiological function relating to aerobic exercise in children, *Sports Med* 19(4):265, 1990.

109. Ryan JR, Salciccioli GG: Fracture of the distal radial epiphysis in adolescent weight lifters, *Am J Sports Med* 4:26-27, 1976.

110. Safrit MJ: Health-related fitness levels of american youth: effects of physical activity on children, *American Academy of Physical Education Papers No. 19,* Champaign, Illinois, 1986, Human Kinetics.

111. Shea S, Basch CE: A review of five major community-based cardiovascular disease prevention programs. Part I: rationale, design, and theoretical framework, *Am J Health Prom* 4(3):203-213, 1990.

112. Siegel J: Fitness in prepubescent children: implications for exercise training, *Natl Strength Condition Assoc J* 10(3):43-48, 1988.

113. Siegel JA, Camaione DN, Manfredi TG: The effects of upper body resistance training on prepubescent children, *Pediatr Exerc Sci* 1:145-154, 1989.

114. Sinclari D: *Human growth after birth,* ed 4, New York, 1985, Oxford University Press.

115. Spiegal PG, Cooperman DR, Laros GS: Epiphyseal fractures of the distal ends of the tibia and fibula: a retrospective study of 237 cases of children, *J Bone Joint Surg* 60A:1046-150, 1978.

116. Updyke W, Willett MS: Physical fitness trends in American youth 1980-1989, Bloomington, Indiana, 1989, AAU Physical Fitness Program.

117. US Department of Health and Human Services Public Health Service: *Healthy people 2000,* DHHS Publication No. (PHS) 91-50212. Washington, DC, Superintendent of Documents, 1991, US Government Printing Office.

118. Vaccaro P, Clarke DH: Cardiorespiratory alterations in 9- to 11-year-old children following a season of competitive swimming, *Med Sci Sports Exerc* 10:204-207, 1978.

119. Vrijens J: Muscle strength development in the pre- and postpubescent age, *Med Sport* 11:157-161, 1978.

120. Wells CL: The effects of physical activity on cardiorespiratory fitness in children. In Stull GA, Eckert HM, editors: *American academy of physical education papers,* Champaign, Illinois, 1986, Human Kinetics.

121. Weltman A, Janney C, Rians CB et al: The effects of hydraulic resistance strength training in prepubescent males, *Med Sci Sports Exerc* 18:629-638, 1986.

REFERENCES—Cont'd

122. Wheeler RC, Marcus AC, Cullen JW, Konugres E: Baseline chronic disease risk factors in a racially heterogeneous elementary school population: The "Know Your Body" program, Los Angeles, *Prevent Med* 12:569-587, 1983.

123. Wilkins KE: The uniqueness of the young athlete: musculoskeletal injuries, *Am J Sports Med* 8:377-382, 1980.

124. Wilmore JH, McNamara JJ: Prevalence of coronary disease risk factors in boys, 8 to 12 years of age, *J Pediatr* 84:527-533, 1974.

125. Woynarowska B, Mukherjee D, Roche AF, Siervogel RM: Blood pressure changes during adolescence and subsequent adult blood pressure levels, *Hypertension* 7:695-701, 1985.

RECOMMENDED READINGS

- Rowland TW: *Exercise and children's health,* Champaign, Illinois, 1990, Human Kinetics.

- Rowland TW: *Pediatric laboratory exercise testing,* Champaign, Illinois, 1993, Human Kinetics.

- Gisolfi CV, Lamb DR, editors: Perspectives in exercise science and sports medicine, vol 2, *Youth exercise, and sport,* Indianapolis, 1989, Benchmark Press.

- Bar-O O: *Pediatric sports medicine for the practitioner,* New York, 1983, Springer-Verlag.

- Leppo M: *Healthy from the start: new perspectives on childhood fitness,* Washington, DC, 1993, ERIC Clearinghouse On Teacher Education.

- Roberts SO, Weider B: *Strength and weight training for young athletes,* Chicago, 1994, Contemporary Books.

CHAPTER 26

Exercise in Extreme Environments

OBJECTIVES

After studying this chapter you should be able to:

■ Identify the different environmental conditions that can deleteriously affect the ability to tolerate the varied stressors experienced during exercise.

■ Describe in detail the detrimental affects of increasing altitude on human physiology at rest and during submaximal and maximal exercise.

■ Identify the differences between the body's chronic adaptations to endurance exercise training at sea level and during prolonged exposure to hypoxia.

■ Explain the risks to life, and their pathophysiology, when a person is exposed to high altitude.

■ Explain the risks to life, and their pathophysiology, when a person is exercising in a hot or humid environment.

■ Explain the importance of adequate hydration during prolonged exercise in a hot or humid environment.

■ Identify the complications of rehydration after thermal- and exercise-induced dehydration.

■ Explain the risks to life, and their pathophysiology, when a person is exercising in a cold or windy environment.

■ Explain the dangers of high-pressure environments.

■ Describe why exposure to microgravity is a unique stress to specific physiologic functions of the body.

■ Explain the cardiovascular problems that can develop during exposures of the body to increased gravitational forces.

KEY TERMS

acclimatization

acclimation

hypobaria

hypobaric hypoxia

normobaric hypoxia

acute mountain sickness

lactate paradox

dehydration

hyperthermia

heat exhaustion

heat stroke

voluntary dehydration

water intoxication

rehydration

wet bulb globe index (WBGI)

hypothermia

microgravity

orthostatic tolerance

hyperbaria

When exercise is performed in environmental conditions that deviate from temperate conditions at altitudes close to sea level, the body's physiologic responses are exaggerated or additional stresses exist. Extreme environments can consist of high or low temperatures; increased altitude and the associated decreases in barometric pressure and blood oxygen content; increased barometric pressures, such as during SCUBA diving; altered conditions of gravity, such as the increased gravitational force experienced by fighter pilots during severe maneuvers and the microgravity experienced by astronauts; and exposure to air pollution. Because of the increasing frequency of people becoming exposed to these conditions, there is a vital need to understand how the body responds to extreme environments and especially how exercise influences this exposure. The purpose of this chapter is to identify the stresses to the body that exist during exposure to different environments, investigate the physiology of the body's responses to these stresses, explain what research has revealed about the acute and chronic adaptations to these environments, and show how exercise influences these adaptations.

Overview of Extreme Environments

Exercise in abnormal environmental temperatures can stress the body's thermoregulatory capacities, compromise cardiovascular function, and alter the nutritional demands of the exercise. The low pressures that accompany high altitude decrease the oxygen content of a given volume of air and compromise the body's cardiorespiratory capacity to supply oxygen to the tissues. Exposure to high pressures, such as during SCUBA diving, increases risks for specific types of gas toxicity and increases the energy demands of movement. Exposure to conditions of increased gravitational force, which is best exemplified by fighter pilots during severe maneuvers, can compromise cardiovascular function. Human endeavors in space exploration have provided exposure to microgravity, which compromises the body's cardiovascular regulation, skeletal integrity, and muscle

metabolism. Finally, exercise in densely populated areas can occur during times of increased air pollution, which can impair lung function and exercise performance. Because of the increasing frequency with which people are becoming exposed to these conditions, there is a need to understand how the body responds to extreme environments and how exercise influences this exposure.

Acclimatization and Acclimation

Because repeated exposure to many environmental conditions can induce chronic adaptations of the body that are beneficial (e.g., altitude exposure, hot or humid conditions) or harmful (e.g., microgravity, air pollution), research is being performed to evaluate whether exercise training can increase the adaptability of the body to extreme environments and therefore decrease the stress of these exposures. When individuals are chronically exposed to an altered environment, adaptations occur as part of **acclimatization.** Depending on the extreme nature of the environmental change and the biologic response, this process may take several days to months. Intermittent exposure to artificial environmental conditions has been shown to stimulate adaptations similar to acclimatization. The adaptations resulting from these testing conditions exposures occur as part of a process known as **acclimation.** The details from research on acclimatization and acclimation to specific environmental changes are presented in the sections on chronic adaptation in this chapter.

Section I: Exercise at Increased Altitude

*T*he interest of humans in exposure to high altitude has a long history. Charles Houston noted that historical evidence of high-altitude exploration dates to before Christ, and written reports of the headache accompanying acute mountain sickness have a similarly long history.[69] In approximately AD 400, Chinese pilgrims provided the first known written record of the symptoms of pulmonary edema. Ironically, Houston was the physician to report this condition "first"—1500 years later.

In the 1968 Mexico City Summer Olympic Games the impact of altitude on exercise performance received considerable media attention and therefore was catapulted into public awareness. During preparation for the Mexico City Olympics, concerns existed about possible beneficial effects of the lower pressure and air resistance at the altitude of 2300 meters for events involving speed and power (e.g., jumping, throwing, and sprinting events) and about the possible detrimental affects of the reduced oxygen at this altitude for the endurance events (e.g., running distances greater than 1 mile). It has been argued ever since these Olympics that Bob Beaman's world record in the long jump is attributable to the decreased air resistance at the higher altitude. Conversely, the relatively impaired performance (based on winning times) for running distances in excess of 1 mile was attributed to reductions in arterial oxygen content. At 2300 meters the hemoglobin-oxygen saturation is approximately 96% (versus 98% at sea level), which clearly had a negative impact on endurance exercise performance. Scientists and the public were asking such questions as why is endurance exercise impaired at moderate altitude? At what altitude does endurance exercise become impaired? Can training at altitude improve endurance exercise performance at altitude? What are the acute physiologic responses to moderate altitude exposure? What are the adaptations that occur to prolonged altitude exposure? The answers to these and other questions are provided in this section of the chapter.

The study of athletic performance is not the only exercise-related science that has had an interest in human physiology at altitude. The sport of mountaineering has also been prominent in forcing the physiologic demands of high altitude into the scientific and public arenas. Mountaineering involves not only high altitude, but also extremes of cold temperature, exposure to solar radiation, and difficulty providing adequate intake of food and liquids.

In 1946, Houston organized and successfully implemented the first scientific study of the ascent to extreme artificial altitudes.[68] In 1985, he conducted another, more comprehensive study involving a 40-day simulated ascent in an altitude chamber, reaching a barometric pressure equivalent to 8840 meters above sea level, the altitude of the summit of Mt. Everest; not surprisingly, the title of the research project was Operation Everest II (OEII). Many of the findings from OEII have been published in internationally renowned scientific journals and the obtained data appear in many of the figures in this chapter.*

Altitude and Hypoxia

Before the influence of altitude on exercise performance is explained, the physiologic and biochemical changes that occur with an increase in altitude should be clarified. Figure 26.1 presents the decrease in barometric pressure as altitude increases from sea level (approximately 760 mm Hg) to 10,000 meters above sea level (approximately 215 mm Hg).

*References 37, 54, 55, 60, 117, 118, 119, 130, 154, and 155.

*References 37, 54, 55, 60, 117, 118, 119, 130, 154, and 155.

FIGURE 26.1

The decrease in barometric pressure with an increase in altitude above sea level. The pressure for a given altitude may vary by ±10 mm Hg as a result of extremes in climatic conditions. Between the altitudes of sea level and 3,000 meters the change in pressure with increasing altitude is close to linear, and can be approximated by an 8 mm Hg decrease in atmospheric pressure every 100 meters.

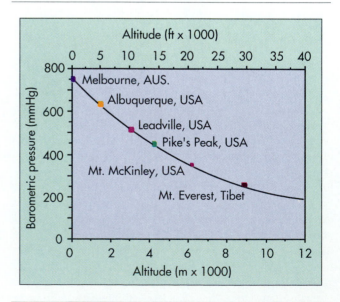

This decrease in pressure (**hypobaria**) with an increase in elevation above sea level results in pressures approximating 630 mm Hg at 1500 meters, and 520 mm Hg at 3000 meters. Many cities in the United States and around the world are located at altitudes between sea level and 4000 meters. Table 26.1 presents abbreviations used routinely when applying cardiorespiratory physiology to the understanding of the body's responses to altitude exposure.

The hypobaria associated with increases in altitude is potentially detrimental because of the direct proportional relationship between gas partial pressure and absolute barometric pressure.

26-1   Total pressure = $PO_2 + PCO_2 + PN_2 + P$ rare gases

As discussed in Appendix B, it is standard to ignore the rare gases in atmospheric air because of their small contribution (less than 1%). Thus, given the constant fractions of air that comprise oxygen, carbon dioxide, or nitrogen, an increase in altitude and the accompanied hypobaria will decrease the amount of oxygen, carbon dioxide, and nitrogen in the air.

Sea level

26-2 $P_IO_2 = 0.2093 \times 760$ mm Hg

           $= 159.1$ mm Hg

26-3 $P_AO_2 = (760 - 47) \times 0.1458$

           $= 104$ mm Hg

3000 meters

     $P_IO_2 = 0.2093 \times 520$ mm Hg

           $= 108.8$ mm Hg

     $P_AO_2 = (520 - 47) \times 0.1458$

           $= 69$ mm Hg

Use of the conversion factor (0.1458) to calculate P_AO_2 is an approximation. P_AO_2 values vary at a given barometric pressure with changes in the carbon dioxide content of the body. This relationship is best expressed by the alveolar gas equation.

26-4 $P_AO_2 = P_IO_2 - (P_AO_2/R)$

           $+ [P_AO_2 \times F_IO_2 \times [(1-R)/R]]$

and when simplified for conditions at sea level,
where $PA_{CO_2} = 40$ mm Hg, $FI_{O_2} = 0.2093$, RER $= 0.8$

26-5 $P_AO_2 = P_IO_2 - (P_ACO_2/R) + 2$

Based on material presented in Chapters 11 and 12, a reduction in P_IO_2 lowers the alveolar partial pressures of oxygen (P_AO_2) and carbon dioxide (P_ACO_2) and has the potential to lower the arterial pressures of oxygen (PaO_2) and carbon dioxide ($PaCO_2$). Of course, given the affinity between hemoglobin and oxygen and the shape of the oxygen–hemoglobin dissociation curve, the relationship between pressure and arterial content of oxygen (CaO_2) is not linear. Figure 26.2 presents the relationships between altitude and P_IO_2, P_AO_2, and CaO_2.

Based on the data in Figure 26.2, increases in altitude do not appear to cause significant reductions in CaO_2 until altitudes in excess of 2000 meters. Despite the small changes in CaO_2 with moderate altitude exposure, the following sections discuss research that has shown that these changes are enough to deleteriously affect maximal cardiorespiratory capacities at altitudes as low as 1070 meters.[111,138]

Qualifying Altitude: Low, Moderate, and High Altitude

Discussion on low, moderate, and high altitude has already been undertaken. These terms obviously need defining. Based on Figure 26.2, it is clear that the physiologic implications of altitude on human function is not a simple linear relationship with altitude. Lower altitudes cause minimal alterations in hemoglobin saturation, but when altitude is increased above 4000 meters where alveolar and arterial partial pressures of oxygen decrease to less than 60 mm Hg (90% SaO_2), blood oxygen transport capacity is dramatically

TABLE 26.1	
Terms and abbreviations for cardiorespiratory function in altitude exposure	
TERM	**ABBREVIATION**
Oxygen	O_2
Carbon dioxide	CO_2
Nitrogen	N_2
Alveolar partial pressure	P_A
Arterial partial pressure	Pa
Mixed venous partial pressure	Pv
Arterial content/concentration	Ca
Mixed venous content/concentration	Cv
Arterial hemoglobin-oxygen saturation	SaO_2
Respiratory exchange ratio	RER
Minute ventilation	V_E
Hypoxic ventilatory response	HVR
Ventilation-perfusion ratio	VE/Q

acclimatization (a′**kly**-ma-**ty**-za′shun)
the process of chronic adaptation to a given environmental stress

acclimation (a′**kli**-ma′shun)
the process of chronic adaptation to an artificially imposed environmental stress

hypobaria (hi-po-**bar**′i-ah)
decreased barometric pressure

FIGURE 26.2

As altitude increases and barometric pressure decreases, the inspired partial pressure of oxygen (P_IO_2), alveolar partial pressure of oxygen (P_AO_2), and arterial oxygen content (CaO_2) all decrease. The decreases in P_IO_2 and P_AO_2 reflect the decrease in barometric pressure. The decrease in CaO_2 reflects the sigmoidal shape of the oxygen-hemoglobin dissociation curve, (Chapter 11) which causes the apparent exponential decay of CaO_2 with increasing altitude. The data presented (solid line) are theoretic values, whereas the shaded area of each curve reflect chronic adaptation to increasing altitude. After acclimatization to altitude, there is less of a decrease in P_AO_2 because of a sustained hyperventilation, which raises hemoglobin saturation and P_AO_2 and effectively lowers the physiologic altitude. (Theoretic data were adapted from Jones[85]. Data from chronic adaptation were adapted from.[75,165,178])

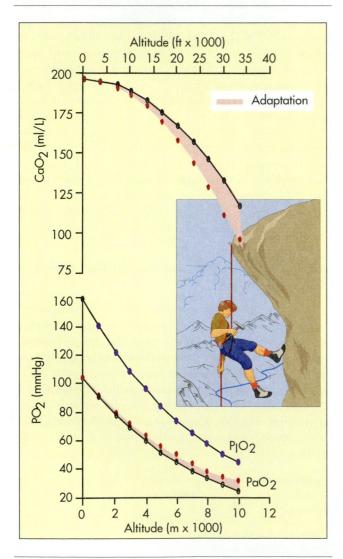

reduced. How do these changes relate to the rating of altitude as low, moderate, high, or extreme?

The data in Table 26.2 are grouped according to low, moderate, high, and extreme altitudes. These groupings are based on the changes in CaO_2 that occur with the reduced barometric pressures and changes in the oxygen-hemoglobin dissociation curve and on research documenting altitude-specific changes in physiology during acute and chronic exposure. Such altitude groups are referred to throughout this section of the chapter in the discussion of acute and chronic adaptations.

Acute Adaptations to Altitude Exposure

Research on human altitude exposure has been conducted using several different models, including on location at actual altitude, artificial altitude exposure in a hypobaric chamber, and breathing gas mixtures of below normal oxygen content without changing atmospheric pressure. When the hypoxia is produced by a reduction in barometric pressure, it is termed **hypobaric hypoxia** and applies to on-location and altitude chamber studies. Conversely, hypoxia induced by breathing hypoxic gas when at or near sea level is termed **normobaric hypoxia.** It is generally assumed that the hypobaria does not contribute to the physiologic effects of acute altitude exposure. However, the independent effects of hypobaria and hypoxia on human physiology during altitude exposure have not been clearly defined.

When the body is first exposed to increased altitude, certain physiologic functions change from normal when at rest or during exercise. The magnitude of these responses varies depending on the level of activity performed at altitude and on the magnitude of the altitude. Unfortunately, adequate research has not been completed to profile how many of the body's physiologic and biochemical functions during rest and exercise change with increments in altitude above sea level. Altitudes at which most published research has been conducted have been 4300 meters (Pike's Peak) and simulated altitudes used in research from Operation Everest II (greater than 5500 meters). However, it must be stated that by design, studies from OEII are neither purely acute nor purely chronic exposures for a given altitude. The gradual ascent to increased altitude did, however, provide an opportunity to perform noninvasive and invasive procedures for the evaluation of changes in human physiology and biochemistry during high- to severe-altitude exposure. Numerous studies have also used various hypoxic gas mixtures, but the majority of these gases equated to altitudes in excess of 2000 meters above sea level.

Changes at Rest

When the body is exposed to increasing altitude and the associated reductions in blood oxygen transport capacities, there are immediate changes in ventilation, cardiac function,

TABLE 26.2

The theroretic* changes in barometric pressure, inspired and alveolar partial pressures of oxygen, oxygen-hemoglobin saturation, and arterial blood oxygen content (CaO_2) for different altitudes above sea level

ALTITUDE		P_B	P_IO_2	P_AO_2	O_2-Hb sat[†]	CaO_2[‡]
METERS	FEET	(mm Hg)	(mm Hg)	(mm Hg)	(%)	(ml/L)
LOW						
0	0	760	159	104	98	197
500	1640	714	149	97	97	195
1000	3281	670	140	91	97	195
MODERATE (>1067 m [3500 FT])						
1524	5000	627	131	85	96	193
2134	7000	581	122	78	96	193
2500	8202	559	117	75	96	193
HIGH (>3048 m [10,000 FT])						
3048	10000	517	108	72	95	191
3500	11483	489	102	64	93	185
4000	13123	460	96	60	89	179
EXTREME (>4573 m [15,000 FT])						
5500	18045	380	80	49	84	169
7000	22966	314	66	39	72	145
8000	26247	277	58	34	65	131
10000	32808	215	45	25	49	131

*Data are theoretic because they do not take into consideration acute or chronic changes in ventilation and pulmonary function during altitude exposure, which can increase %Hb-O_2 and CaO_2 (see Figure 26.2).
†Based on arterial blood at a pH=7.4 and temperature=37° C.
‡Based on an arterial hemoglobin concentration of 150 gm/L and unimpaired alveolar-blood gas exchange.

and blood flow redistribution that function to oppose the hypoxic exposure.

Pulmonary Function. During exposure to altitudes in excess of 2000 meters, it is generally believed that the reductions in PaO_2 stimulate the peripheral chemoreceptors (see Chapter 12) and provide a hypoxic drive that increases ventilation. At 4300 meters above sea level, ventilation is increased by approximately 30%, which further reduces P_ACO_2 and $PaCO_2$ (Figure 26.3) and causes a temporary respiratory alkalosis that lasts for approximately 2 days because of a delayed renal compensation.[89,139] Hyperventilation is also important for raising P_AO_2 and PaO_2 above values calculated from barometric pressures (see Figure 26.2), thereby making the absolute altitude effectively much lower.

Data from studies measuring hypoxic ventilatory drive indicate that the increased ventilation to hypoxia occurs at a rate of 0.18 L/min for every percent decrease in SaO_2 saturation.[130] Thus, based on Table 26.2, at approximately 3000 meters resting ventilation would be increased relative to sea level by 1 L/min. The hyperventilation resulting from hypoxia is not large because of the resultant decreases in alveolar and arterial PCO_2. Reduced $PaCO_2$ decreases stimulation to the peripheral and central chemoreceptors, thereby decreasing the main chemical stimulation of increased ventilation. Nevertheless, as previously explained, even a small increase in ventilation that continues for hours, days, or even indefinitely results in a significant removal of carbon dioxide from the body.

Data from OEII revealed that as altitude increases, there is an increasing difference between P_AO_2 and PaO_2.[154] Fur-

hypobaric hypoxia

decreased oxygen availability because of decreased barometric pressure

normobaric hypoxia

decreased oxygen availability at normal barometric pressure because of a lowered oxygen fraction of inspired air

F I G U R E   2 6 . 3

During exposure to increased altitude, the increase in ventilation causes increased removal of carbon dioxide, thereby lowering the P_aCO_2. Further decreases in P_aCO_2 occur with acclimatization.

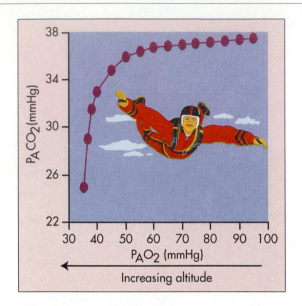

Increasing altitude

F I G U R E   2 6 . 4   (o p p o s i t e)

A, During exposure to altitudes between 3000 and 4300 m, research has documented near immediate changes in cardiovascular, respiratory, and metabolic parameters at rest and during submaximal and maximal exercise. Changes are expressed as a percent of prealtitude exposure. Positive values represent an increase, whereas negative values represent a decrease. **B,** During chronic exposure to altitudes between 3000 and 4300 m, many physiologic variables differ not only to sea level, but also to values during acute exposure. **C,** A barometric chamber used for research of hypobaric and hyperbaric human physiology. (Courtesy, Exercise Science Program, The University of New Mexico.)

thermore, with increasing altitude the contribution of diffusion limitation to this difference increases. Such a decreased diffusion capacity of the lung at low to moderate altitude is due predominantly to the decreased P_AO_2 to $P_{\bar{v}}O_2$ gradient and the position on the Hb-O_2 dissociation curve rather than structural limitations, such as lung damage or pulmonary edema. However, as altitude increases to high and extreme values, increased pulmonary edema also contributes to lung malfunction. Data from Wagner et al. suggest that a ventilation-perfusion inadequacy also contributes to lung malfunction at high altitude, accounting for 50% of the P_AO_2 to PaO_2 difference at 4000 meters but that this contribution decreases with further increases in altitude.[154]

Cardiovascular Function. Exposure to even low altitudes increases fluid loss via evaporative cooling because of the lower pressure and greater ease of water changing state from liquid to gas (i.e., water boils at lower temperatures at increasing altitudes) and renal diuresis. These responses increase with increased altitude and can cause a rapid development of dehydration. Such a loss of body fluid decreases blood volume, raises hematocrit and viscosity, and can compromise cardiovascular hemodynamics.

The hypoxia of moderate to extreme altitude is known to stimulate the release of erythropoietin (EPO) from special PO_2-sensitive cells within the kidney.[150] The altitude above which a hypoxic stimulus elicits EPO production and release is not known. However, it is known that the duration of exposure is important.[21,80] Knaupp et al. demonstrated that hypoxia sufficient to lower hemoglobin saturation to below

85% required 120 minutes of exposure before a detectable increase in EPO.[80] Under these circumstances an increased EPO was not evident until after approximately 120 minutes from the start of exposure, with significant differences not evident until after 240 minutes from the initiation of hypoxia. During continuous and more prolonged altitude exposure at 4300 m (Pike's Peak), peak EPO concentrations occurred after 2 days and then decreased to near preexposure levels by day 7.[1] The temporal relationship between the altitude-induced increases in EPO release and the known polycythemia of prolonged moderate to extreme altitude exposure remains obscure. Furthermore, studies that have attempted to measure altitude-induced polycythemia by changes in hemoglobin and hematocrit may be in question because of the known hemoconcentration from dehydration that occurs with altitude exposure.

Another hematologic response during hypoxia is an increased production of 2,3-bisphosphoglycerate (2,3-BPG) by erythrocytes.[83] Increases in whole blood 2,3-BPG concentrations lower the Hb-O_2 dissociation curve, thus increasing oxygen release at the tissues. This is a favorable adaptation at increased altitude because it partially offsets the lowered Ca-C$\dot{v}O_2$ difference (Ca-C$\dot{v}O_2\Delta$) that accompanies the lower CaO_2 during hypoxia.

During exposure to moderate to extreme altitudes, the reduced CaO_2 lowers the effective diffusion gradient for oxygen at the tissues, and despite increases in 2,3-BPG there is a decreased a-$\dot{v}O_2\Delta$. To maintain a given VO_2, heart rate increases. During exposure to high altitudes, cardiac stroke volume decreases in response to an increased peripheral vascular resistance and increased circulating catecholamines, which in turn further increases resting heart rate (Figure 26.4).[156] Based on the principles of the Fick equation, these developments cause resting cardiac output to increase at altitude.

Energy Metabolism. Unfortunately, minimal research has quantified resting metabolism during exposure to moderate to extreme altitudes. Brooks et al. indicated that at rest, acute exposure to 4300 meters did not increase carbohydrate

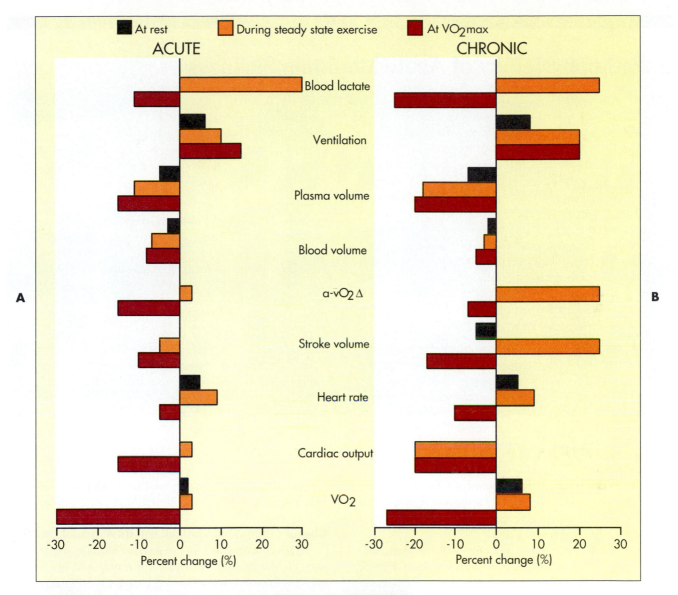

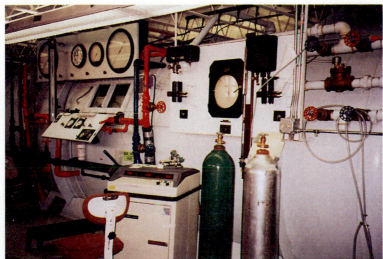

FIGURE 26.4

For legend see opposite page.

Pathophysiology of Acute Mountain Sickness

Exposure to moderate to extreme altitudes (Figure 26.5) can result in headache, lethargy, and nausea. The condition characterized by these symptoms on exposure to increased altitude is termed **acute mountain sickness** (AMS). The susceptibility for AMS is known to vary among individuals and is believed to be the result of multiple acute adaptations to the hypoxia and hypobaria of altitude. Of primary importance in AMS is a person's tolerance of hypoxia. There is evidence for an earlier and more severe onset of altitude illness in individuals who have an increased ventilation-perfusion mismatch, which induces more severe hypoxia.[119] It is believed that the hypoxia indirectly increases blood flow in the brain, which is thought to contribute to a mild cerebral edema and the development of headache.[143]

The two most prominent additional contributors to AMS are inadequate hyperventilation and inadequate diuresis, causing a relative fluid retention. Exercise is believed to exacerbate the development of AMS, and symptoms are alleviated with supplemental oxygen, pharmacologic stimulants to acid-base balance, and ventilation (e.g., acetazolamide), or relocation to lower altitudes.[143,146] The last strategy is the most successful treatment. There is no evidence that AMS is reduced in more highly endurance-trained individuals.

AMS should not be regarded as a clinically minor disorder. If not treated appropriately, AMS may develop into the more life-threatening conditions pulmonary edema or cerebral edema. Pulmonary edema results from sustained increases in pulmonary blood pressure, causing an increase in water flux from the pulmonary vasculature.[60,143] The etiology of cerebral edema is less clear but is believed to be a result of prolonged increases in cerebral blood flow. Figure 26.6 shows the operation of a portable hyperbaric chamber (Gamow bag) used to treat pulmonary edema on location. Increasing pressure on location can reduce symptoms of pulmonary edema and provide time to arrange for the transport of the patient to lower altitudes.

---

dependence, as measured by increased whole body blood glucose turnover and disposal.[16] Furthermore, data from OEII revealed that muscle glycogen stores are well preserved at moderate, high, and severe altitude.[54,55]

There is an immediate increase in basal metabolic rate (BMR) during the first days of moderate to high altitude exposure. BMR then decreases yet remains elevated compared with sea level after day 10.[20] Consequently, altitude exposure increases the demand for caloric intake. This change has been used to explain part of the increase in resting VO_2 and ventilation on acute ascent to increased altitude.[20]

Renal Function. As previously explained, the hyperventilation that accompanies moderate to extreme altitude exposure induces a respiratory alkalosis. This condition is compensated for by increased base (bicarbonate) secretion by the kidneys, termed *renal compensation for respiratory alkalosis*. This process requires at least 3 days to correct the blood acid–base disturbance but results in a lowered blood bicarbonate concentration and therefore a lowered blood acid-buffering capacity (see Chapter 12).

Monitoring body weight is an effective way to ensure correct fluid balance during altitude exposures. Fluid replacement is required to minimize the cardiovascular complications of dehydration. Similarly, ensuring that too much fluid intake does not occur is important to prevent overhydration,

which has a negative impact on the development of acute mountain sickness (see the Clinical Application above).

Changes during Submaximal and Incremental Exercise

The consequences of exercise at altitude depend not only on the altitude but also on the type and intensity of exercise. Research has measured changes in VO_2max at different altitudes, as well as various indices of exercise performance. Because of the impact of altitude on blood oxygen capacity and the known effects of these changes on cardiorespiratory endurance, researchers have predominantly investigated the effects of altitude on endurance exercise. However, comment will also be made on how acid–base responses to acute altitude exposure may influence intense exercise performance.

Submaximal Exercise
Respiratory Function. For a given submaximal exercise intensity at moderate to severe altitude, there is a larger ventilation response than at sea level (see Figure 26.4, *A*). This change is in response to the greater stimulation to ventilation at increased altitude, which is beneficial in raising P_AO_2 and SaO_2.

Despite the increased alveolar ventilation at altitude, diffusion in the lung decreases, causing a larger P_AO_2-$PaO_2\Delta$.[114,115] Unfortunately, the widening P_AO_2 to PaO_2

FIGURE 26.5

Hikers ascending from a base camp of 4200 m in the northwestern Himalayas of Ladakhh, India. At this location, the elevation is approximately 5,000 m above sea level.

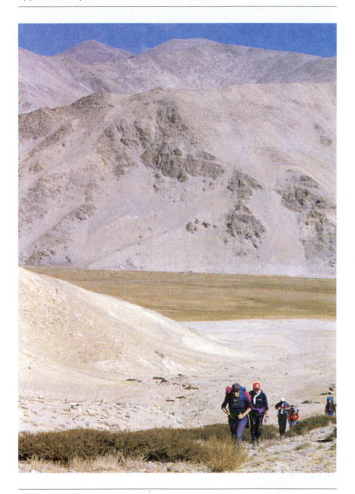

decreases the functional improvement resulting from increases in P_AO_2 or hematocrit.

Cardiovascular function. Figure 26.4, *A* presents data obtained during submaximal exercise at between 3000 to 4300 meters during the first 2 days of altitude exposure. During a given absolute submaximal exercise intensity approximating 50% VO_2max at sea level, VO_2 increased at altitude, cardiac output increased, heart rate increased, and stroke volume decreased compared with sea level values. The increase in VO_2 (worse economy) during exercise at moderate to high altitude is due to an increased work of breathing in combination with increased circulating catecholamines. Cardiac output increases during submaximal exercise at moderate to extreme altitude because of a lowered a-$\dot{v}O_2\Delta$ secondary to the low SaO_2, as is expected from the Fick equation (see Chapter 11).[140,156]

It is unclear at what altitude and exercise intensities changes in cardiac output first occur. For example, during OEII, cardiac output responses to submaximal exercise at

acute mountain sickness

the illness that accompanies acute altitude exposure, typically expressed by symptoms of headache and lethargy

FIGURE 26.6

A portable hyperbaric chamber used to treat high altitude pulmonary edema (HAPE). An individual suffering from the condition was inside the bag. After 1 hour of treatment, the subject had significantly less severe symptoms of HAPE and was safely driven to a lower altitude for medical treatment.

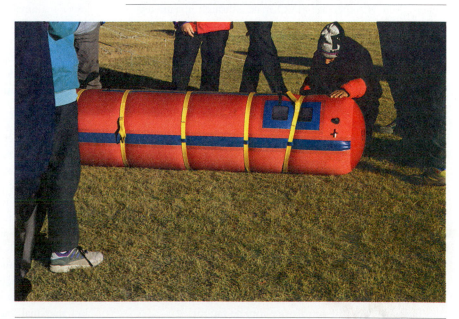

increased altitude did not appear to increase above sea level values until exercise at a VO_2 greater than 1.5 L/min at a simulated altitude of 6100 meters.[37,119] These data differ from those of acute altitude exposure (i.e., subjects of the OEII study were gradually exposed to increasing altitude), in which submaximal leg blood flow at 4300 meters is higher than sea level for exercise intensities less than 150 Watts, and cardiac output during exercise at 4300 meters is higher than at sea level for VO_2 values less than 2 L/min.[12,156]

Despite the relative hypoxia, muscle blood flow in working muscle during exercise at altitude is not greater than at sea level for given exercise intensities.[12,62,156] This response has been explained by the increased hematocrit during both acute (from a decreased plasma volume) and chronic exposure (from polycythemia), which appears to normalize oxygen provision for a given blood flow volume.

Energy metabolism. During the transition from rest to steady-state exercise at moderate to extreme altitudes there is a reduced rate of increase in VO_2, causing a larger oxygen deficit.[137] This response would also increase reliance on carbohydrate during exercise. In fact, Brooks et al. demonstrated that during exercise there is an increased reliance on blood glucose during acute exposure to 4300 meters, and that skeletal muscle was the primary tissue for increased disposal.[18] However, it remains unclear whether this response is insulin dependent or independent.

Research of the lactate threshold during high to severe altitude exposure has shown that when expressed as a percent of VO_2max, the lactate threshold (LT) does not change; however, for a given submaximal intensity (relative or absolute) blood lactate concentrations are higher.[144] Since there is a predictable decrease in VO_2max with increasing altitude exposure, the absolute intensity at the LT decreases. Thus the maximal steady-state intensity is also reduced at altitudes where there is a decrease in VO_2max, although it is unclear at what altitude such decreases first appear.

Given that the LT changes in concert with reductions in VO_2max at altitude, it is no surprise that exercise times to exhaustion for a given exercise intensity decrease at moderate to extreme altitudes. For example, Faulkner et al. reported that running time trials of 1 to 3 miles were approximately 2% to 13% slower at 2300 meters than at sea level.[46,47]

Incremental exercise

Pulmonary function. During moderate to severe altitude exposure, the exercise intensity attained during incremental exercise to exhaustion decreases and, as is explained in subsequent sections, VO_2max decreases. Nevertheless, for a given VO_2, ventilation is greater at altitude when expressed as either standard (STPD) or body temperature and pressure saturated (BTPS) volumes.[118,119,159] However, studies from OEII reveal that even during exposure to severe altitudes, at which ventilation is greatest, there are no signs of ventilation limitation because of ventilatory muscle fatigue.[154]

During exercise to VO_2max at moderate to severe altitude, there is an increase in VE/Q mismatch and diffusion is limited, which causes further reductions in PaO_2 and CaO_2.[148] Because of the decreasing P_AO_2 with increases in altitude, the absolute P_AO_2 to PaO_2 difference does not increase. In fact, the P_AO_2 to PaO_2 difference is largest at sea level during maximal exertion because of the high P_AO_2.[174,175] However, it is not the P_AO_2 to PaO_2 difference that is meaningful to peripheral metabolism but the absolute PaO_2 and SaO_2, and these are significantly lower during exercise at altitude compared with sea level. Thus even at moderate altitude the decreasing pulmonary function can significantly reduce SaO_2 and CaO_2 and compromise cardiorespiratory endurance.

Cardiovascular function. In 1968, Saltin observed that on arrival at 4300 meters, cardiac output at VO_2max decreased by approximately 2.8 L/min (13% of sea level value).[123] This decrease was almost entirely due to a decreased stroke volume. This early study provided evidence of a central cardiovascular limitation to exercise at high altitude in addition to the lowered CaO_2.

Saltin's findings were initially interpreted as evidence of a depressed cardiac function during hypoxia. However, more recent research from OEII has cast doubt on this interpretation.[119] For example, data from EOII indicated that relative to VO_2, maximal cardiac output and stroke volume were no different at altitude than at sea level.[117] Furthermore, studies using pharmacologic alteration of heart rate during altitude exposure revealed that VO_2max was not further compromised, which means that stroke volume must have increased to retain the maximal cardiac output. Thus cardiac function is well maintained during moderate to severe altitude exposure.[117]

Given the preceding data, the question remains, is the lower maximal cardiac output at altitude the cause or result of the lowered VO_2max? The results of OEII suggest that blood CaO_2 and a decreased muscle glycolytic capacity (see section on intense exercise) may be the cause of the lower VO_2max. The lowered cardiac output and stroke volume at altitude may simply reflect the lower exercise intensity at VO_2max.

VO_2max. Decreases in VO_2max are similar for simulated hypobaric hypoxia, acute exposure to high altitude locations, and breathing hypoxic gas.[24] Data from field studies, altitude chambers, and exercise laboratories at different altitudes using inspired air of lowered oxygen content have been used to derive a relationship between altitude and VO_2max. A compilation of data from studies published since the 1950s (Figure 26.7) reveals that VO_2max does not decrease on ascent to altitude until above approximately 1000 meters above sea level. The reduction in VO_2max at this moderate altitude is surprising given that there is only a minor decrease in SaO_2 and maximal cardiac output and that minimal increases in

The relative decrease in VO₂max during acute exposure to increased altitude. When data from research since the 1960s are combined, VO₂max expressed as a percent of sea level decreases linearly after approximately 1050 m above sea level. The decrement in VO₂max approximates 8.7% every 1,000 m increase in altitude (2.6% every 1,000 ft). (Data adapted from references 5, 11, 14, 22, 26, 42, 46, 52, 55, 75, 90, 91, 101, 125, 137, 158, 159, 165, 181.)

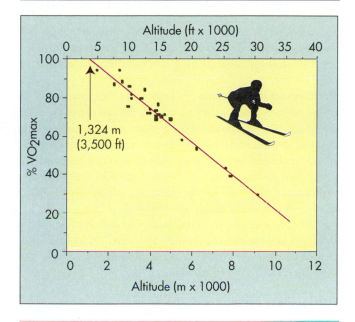

maximal muscle lactate concentrations were actually lower at moderate and high altitudes. These data indicate that at altitude the muscle's capacity for glycolysis is decreased or the stimulation of glycolysis is decreased.[119] The factor(s) responsible for this change is unknown.

Chronic Adaptations to Altitude Exposure

Researchers have not extensively studied chronic adaptation over a range of altitudes. Obviously, Pike's Peak at 4300 meters has been an important site for studies of chronic altitude exposure. In addition, the gradual ascent to the high and severe altitudes used in the OEII studies represents chronic adaptation to increased altitude, but it remains unclear whether results would be different if subjects remained at given altitudes for weeks rather than days.

Changes at Rest

Pulmonary function. Ventilation continues to increase during the first 2 weeks of exposure to an increased altitude, regardless of severity (see Figure 26.4, *B* and *C*).[130] This continued increase in ventilation is retained at altitude even when the person is breathing hyperoxic gas mixtures and is also retained for several days after a return to sea level.[130] Perhaps the main explanation for the continued hyperventilation during chronic altitude exposure is an increased isocapnic hypoxic ventilatory response (HVR) during chronic altitude exposure, as well as during increasing altitude exposure.[84,130] These findings indicate that the function of the carotid bodies is important to the hyperventilation of acute and chronic altitude exposure.

No data exist on the changes in alveolar ventilation perfusion (VE/Q) mismatch and diffusion limitation of the lung during chronic exposures at given altitudes. Nevertheless, data from OEII indicate that VE/Q mismatch would increase with chronic altitude exposure, especially to high and extreme altitudes. This inequality is proportional to increases in pulmonary blood pressure and the resultant increase in pulmonary edema.[154,155] The increasing pulmonary edema accompanying chronic exposure to 8848 meters during OEII not only decreases oxygen diffusion capacities, but also decreases forced vital capacity, although it does not decrease air flow rates because of the decreased air density at high altitude.[155]

Cardiovascular function. Chronic exposure to increased altitude is known to cause an increase in erythropoiesis because of the previously described acute increase in circulating EPO. The time duration for the stimulation of erythropoiesis and the appearance of mature erythrocytes is 7 days.[131] Thus at least 1 week is required for the polycythemia of altitude exposure to become meaningful. It is unknown whether the altitude exposure must be continuous or intermittent to cause a detectable increase in the erythrocyte content of the blood, but increased EPO concentrations have been shown after intermittent exposure to normobaric hypoxia.[80]

P$_A$O$_2$ to PaO$_2\Delta$ would be expected at these pressures (see Table 26.2). Nevertheless, it is clear from Figure 26.8 that few studies have evaluated exercise physiology at moderate altitude, and when interpretation is based on observation, there are numerous reports of lowered exercise tolerance from athletes within the altitude range of 1000 to 1500 meters. Recent data also indicate that the reduction in VO₂max with increasing altitude is worse in endurance-trained individuals because of a greater exercise-induced hypoxemia.[49,53]

The relationship between VO₂max and altitude may be different for females, as indicated in Chapter 23. Paterson et al. reported that females retain significantly more of their VO₂max with increases in altitude than do males.[111] Whether this response is due to the greater hyperventilation during hypoxia in females is unknown, and whether it applies to females of different ages and training status is equally uncertain.

Energy metabolism. Research has shown that exposure to moderate and high altitudes does not increase the degradation of muscle glycogen during exercise to exhaustion, and muscle lactate concentrations also do not increase compared with similar exercise performed at sea level.[6,54,55] In fact,

The polycythemia of altitude exposure in combination with altitude-induced reductions in plasma volume can increase hematocrit from approximately 46% at sea level to greater than 54% after 15 days of exposure at 4300 meters (see Figure 26.4, B).[65,156] Compared with acute altitude exposure, the chronic increase in hematocrit and the increased saturation of hemoglobin increased CaO_2 by 30 ml/L. Such adaptability of the blood oxygen transport is illustrated in Figure 26.2. These changes in blood composition occur without a change in total blood volume, since the increased red blood cell mass is offset by the reduced plasma volume.[156]

Muscle morphology and metabolic capacities. The hypoxia of moderate to severe altitude exposure raises the question of whether chronic exposure to hypoxia induces adaptations in skeletal muscle that improve oxygen diffusion or utilization. Such changes include increases in capillary density, smaller muscle fiber areas, increased myoglobin stores, and increased mitochondrial density.

Early research on muscle adaptation to high altitude revealed increased stores of myoglobin and increased muscle enzyme activities.[121] These findings were interpreted to indicate an improvement in skeletal muscle morphology and aerobic metabolism after altitude acclimatization. Unfortunately, more recent research has questioned the occurrence of beneficial muscle adaptation to high altitude. Green et al. reported a decrease in muscle fiber area and an increased muscle capillary density after the increasing altitude exposure of OEII.[55] However, these changes occurred with no increases in enzyme activity from the glycogenolytic, glycolytic, β-oxidative, or TCA cycle pathways.[54] In fact, after exposure to the extreme altitude of 7260 meters, muscle enzymatic activities actually decreased.

Energy metabolism. After 21 days of acclimatization to 4300 meters, individuals increased their dependence on blood glucose at rest.[16] However, despite an increased reliance on carbohydrate catabolism, resting muscle glycogen stores are not decreased.[54,55] Because the muscle glycogen data were obtained from the EOII studies, which involved forced inactivity between testing sessions, it remains unclear how daily physical activity at increased altitude may influence muscle glycogen synthesis and resting concentrations, especially when food intake is inadequate, which is typical for moderate to severe altitude exposure.[20] It is unknown whether lipid catabolism at rest changes during altitude exposure.

Body composition. Prolonged exposure to moderate to extreme altitudes is associated with a loss in lean body mass and total body weight.[20] This response has been explained in part by a reduced caloric intake, an increased basal metabolic rate, dehydration, and decreased gastrointestinal function (poor nutrient absorption).[20] Body weight during 21 days of exposure at 4300 meters can be better preserved when caloric intake is increased to account for the increase in basal

metabolic rate.[20] Such an increase in calories amounted to approximately 340 Kcal/day. Clearly, a person exposed to increased altitude should increase food and fluid intake.

Changes during Submaximal and Incremental Exercise

Pulmonary function. For a given VO_2, ventilation is increased further after acclimatization to increased altitude.[65,160] For example, after 15 days at 4300 meters maximal ventilation had increased to 205 L/min compared with 186 L/min during acute exposure.[65] Based on previous explanations, an increased ventilation relative to VO_2 increases P_AO_2. However, no data exist on whether this improvement is offset by continued deterioration in VE/Q mismatch and oxygen diffusion limitation during chronic altitude exposure.[154]

Cardiovascular function. Despite the improvements in blood oxygen transport from chronic altitude exposure, there is evidence that muscle blood flow and cardiac output decrease during submaximal exercise at 4300 meters because of an increased sympathetic stimulation and reduced leg blood flow during exercise[12,156] (see Figure 26.4, B). The data indicate that the body may preserve a given oxygen transport to contracting muscle for a given VO_2.[12]

During exercise to exhaustion, maximal cardiac output decreases during chronic altitude exposure.* Nevertheless, as described below, VO_2max values at moderate and high altitude increase after acclimatization.

VO_2max. The earlier research of Saltin et al. and Horstman et al. indicated that after as little as 14 days of altitude exposure to an altitude of 4300 meters VO_2max increases.[65,123] The reported increases are not large (approximately 10%), which is small compared with the reductions in VO_2max, which exceed 20% for altitudes greater than 3000 meters (Figure 26.4, B). Given the previously described reductions in cardiac output, decreased limb blood flow, and reduced CaO_2 experienced during moderate to severe altitude exposure, the inability for acclimatization to altitude to cause large changes in VO_2max is not surprising. In fact, the increase in VO_2max after moderate to high altitude acclimatization is remarkable considering the previously described decreases in pulmonary and cardiovascular function. Therefore the increase in VO_2max must be a result of the improvements in hematologic and muscle metabolic capacities that accompany prolonged moderate to high altitude exposure.

Energy metabolism. Acclimatization to moderate to extreme altitude decreases muscle glycogen degradation for a given submaximal intensity and increases the utilization of blood glucose.[16,17,56] Ironically, despite the hypoxia and increased reliance on carbohydrates during moderate to intense exercise at altitude after acclimatization, there is a decreased circulating blood lactate compared with exercise

---

*References 12, 37, 117, 118, 123, and 156.

during acute exposure[13,18,90] (Figure 26.4, *B*). This was initially an unexpected finding because of the known decreases in maximal cardiac output and peak muscle blood flow that exist at altitude after acclimatization.[12,156] Lower lactate release from skeletal muscle therefore could not be explained by increased oxygen delivery. Similarly, the known stability of muscle mitochondrial enzyme activity after altitude acclimatization indicated that some nonmetabolic explanation must exist for the lactate findings, which have been termed the **lactate paradox**.[13,18,56,90,118]

Research has indicated that the lowered lactate release is probably a result of an increased lactate uptake by active and inactive skeletal muscle, the heart, the kidney, and the liver during chronic exposure to hypoxia.[18] However, Kayser et al. have presented evidence for a central nervous system limitation to exhaustive exercise at moderate to severe altitude.[77] These researchers revealed that when compared with sea level, exhaustive cycling exercise at 5050 meters occurs with lower blood lactate accumulation and acid–base disturbance and without a continued increase in integrated electromyographic signal near maximal exertion. The inability to document an increased integrated electromyographic (IEMG) signal at maximal exertion was interpreted to indicate that peripheral fatigue was not occurring, since heightened neuromuscular activation and increased motor unit recruitment occur when skeletal muscle fatigue develops. Furthermore, increasing the P_IO_2 during exercise enabled subjects to continue to exercise and increase the IEMG activity of the quadriceps muscles. Unfortunately, blood lactate data were not reported after exercise with hyperoxic gas. The issue of a peripheral or central explanation for the lactate paradox requires further research.

Short-Term Intense Exercise Performance

The question of whether acute altitude exposure alters the capacity for short-term intense exercise has not received widespread research interest. However, the alkalosis accompanying even low to moderate altitude exposure and the resulting decreases in blood bicarbonate concentrations suggest that muscle metabolism during intense exercise could be impaired during increasing altitude exposure.

DiPrampero et al. studied the effects of simulated altitude on the ability to generate maximal power during 10 seconds of cycling.[40] Mechanical power output over time was no different for exercise at sea level, during normobaric hypoxia with a P_IO_2 equivalent to 3000 meters, and during hypobaric hypoxia at 4500 meters (Figure 26.8, *A*). Thus for very short-duration intense efforts the muscles' abilities to regenerate ATP at high rates are not impaired at moderate to high altitude.

For more prolonged intense exercise, when there is an increased contribution from glycolysis and lactate production, acclimatization of sea level Caucasian subjects to 5350 meters not only decreases maximal blood lactate accumulation, but also increases the blood acidosis experienced at given blood lactate values[23] (Figure 26.8, *B*). Such a reduced

FIGURE 26.8

A, The maximal power output during 10 s of "all out" effort during cycle ergometry performed at sea level and at 3,000 m above sea level.[47] **B,** During more prolonged intense exercise, individuals that have acclimatized to an altitude of 5350 m have a lower maximal blood lactate concentration, yet a lower blood buffering capacity as indicated by a greater decrease in blood pH relative to an increase in blood lactate. (Adapted from Di Prampero PE, Mognoni P, Veicsteinas A: The effects of hypoxia on maximal anaerobic alactic power in man. In Brendel W, Zink RA, editors: *High altitude physiology and medicine,* New York, 1982, Springer-Verlag.)

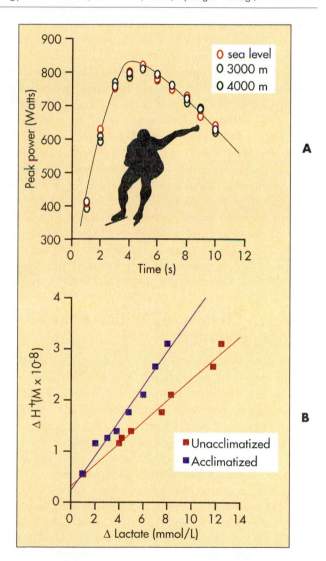

buffer capacity of the blood is directly related to the decreased blood bicarbonate concentration during acute and chronic altitude exposure.

lactate paradox

the decreased maximal lactate production by contracting skeletal muscle after chronic altitude exposure

Does Living at Altitude Improve Exercise Tolerance at Altitude?

A useful research design in altitude physiology has been to compare the physiology of moderate or high altitude exposure in higher altitude natives with sea level residents. Maresh et al. exposed moderate altitude natives (1830 to 2200 meters) and sea level residents (both groups citizens of the United States) who had similar cardiorespiratory fitness to a simulated altitude of 4270 meters. Moderate altitude natives reported fewer symptoms of acute mountain sickness, experienced half the decrement in each of VO_2max and maximal blood lactate accumulation, and had a larger maximal ventilation compared with sea level residents during maximal exercise testing at altitude. The lactate threshold was not different between groups at altitude. The results indicated that individuals who had lived at moderate altitude all their lives responded better to acute altitude exposure than did sea level residents. Because no measures of hematology, pulmonary function, or muscle metabolic capacities were completed, the reasons for these differences were not addressed.

Interestingly, similar evidence of improved acute adaptation to increased altitude exists for residents of altitudes as low as 1600 meters (Denver). Reeves indicated that when exposed to 4300 meters, residents of Denver have a lower resting P_ACO_2 and higher $Hb-O_2$ saturation and achieve stable P_ACO_2 and SaO_2 values earlier than sea level residents.[119] Clearly, living at altitudes that are low to moderate improves tolerance and responsiveness to increased altitude exposure.

Living and Training at Altitude to Improve Exercise Performance

Ever since the Mexico City Olympic Games, the potential for enhanced performance from high-altitude training has been a topic of widespread debate. Interest in this topic has focused on two issues: (1) whether altitude training can improve sea level performance, and (2) whether altitude training can improve performance at altitude.

Altitude Training and Altitude Performance

Before and after the Mexico City games, researchers demonstrated that training at high altitude was essential for improved endurance performance at altitude. For example, acclimatization to moderate altitudes was associated with 5% to 10% improvements in VO_2max compared with acute exposure.[46,47,115]

At the time of the Mexico City Olympics (1970s), the obvious question to why exercise performance in endurance events at altitude could be improved with prolonged altitude exposure. Findings of increased hematocrit and hemoglobin concentrations of blood after prolonged altitude exposure provided evidence for improved blood oxygen transport capacities, and the notion that altitude training may be beneficial for even sea level exercise performance was reinforced.

Altitude Training and Sea Level Performance

Scientific studies of changes in VO_2max and exercise performance at sea level after altitude acclimatization have produced results that both confirmed and negated the benefit of altitude training.* For example, exposure of athletes to altitudes between 2300 and 3300 meters above sea level for 2 weeks resulted in an increased VO_2max on return to sea level and improved performance in the 1500-meter and mile races.[10,38,46,47] Conversely, studies in which athletes were exposed to 4000 meters and 3100 meters for between 20 to 63 days revealed slower running times at sea level and reduced or unchanged VO_2max values.[2,19,59]

Sutton correctly pointed out that the difficulty with scientific research on this topic is the many flaws in research design.[145] For example, studies have included different quality athletes, different altitudes, different durations of exposure, and different training regimens at altitude. No "perfect" study of this topic has been conducted. Such a study would involve different altitudes, different combinations of residence and training at altitude or sea level, groups of subjects with different cardiorespiratory fitness, groups of both genders, and different durations of training and chronic altitude exposure. Clearly, this study would be difficult if not impossible.

Based on the previous explanations of acute and chronic adaptations to altitude, there is clear evidence that if living at altitude were to provide any potential benefit, it would accrue to those residing at moderate altitude. Living at high altitudes would be accompanied by reduced pulmonary function and capacities, reduced cardiovascular capacities, losses in muscle enzyme capacities, and decreases in lean body mass. These are all detrimental to the optimal development of cardiorespiratory endurance. In addition, to reap benefits from improved training quality at lower altitudes yet retain the chronic mild hypoxic stimulus of living at moderate altitude, athletes should live at moderate altitude and train at lower altitudes.[85]

A global statement concerning the scientific evaluation of exercise training at altitude would be that there is no consistent scientific evidence to support training at altitude to improve sea level performance. Conversely, training at altitude to improve altitude performance provides a definite advantage for cardiorespiratory endurance. The influence of altitude training for more intense exercise performance has not been adequately addressed by research. Despite these statements, Olympic class and professional athletes from around the world travel to moderate altitude because they believe that altitude training will improve sea level performance. Those who do so achieve world records and personal best times, which reinforces the practice of altitude training. There may be positive aspects of altitude training that science has not yet detected. For this reason, scientific interest in altitude training and athletic performance continues.

---

*References 10, 19, 38, 46, 47, and 59.

Qualifying Chronic Adaptation to Altitude: Acclimatization versus Acclimation

One of the most limiting factors for conducting altitude research and for athletes wanting to train at altitude is the need to relocate for training. Similar concerns exist for individuals who would benefit from altitude acclimatization to perform their duties at high altitude (e.g., fire fighters, emergency rescue staff, military personnel). An obvious question has been whether chronic altitude exposure is necessary to reap such benefits as reduced symptoms of acute mountain sickness and improved cardiorespiratory endurance.

An alternative to chronic altitude exposure is to provide intermittent exposure to hypoxia or hypobaric hypoxia. As previously described, Knaup et al. indicated that an erythropoietic response can result from intermittent breathing of hypoxic gas.[80] This finding indicates that intermittent exposure to hypoxia may induce an increased red blood cell mass. Furthermore, Klausen et al. transported endurance athletes from 1695 to 2700 meters daily for hours per day for altitude training.[78] These athletes experienced significant increases in EPO, immature and mature red blood cell counts, hematocrit, and hemoglobin concentrations, compared with baseline values. In animal studies, similar erythropoietic responses to intermittent altitude exposure have occurred.[131] Clearly, the topic of intermittent exposure to altitude, a form of altitude acclimation, needs to be researched to demonstrate the benefits it may provide for human performance during acute exposures to increased altitude.

Section II: Exercise in Hot or Humid Environments

Continuous or intermittent exercise performed for prolonged periods is associated with increased sweat rates and the development of **dehydration.** The

dehydration (de-hi-dra'shun)

decreased body water content

FIGURE 26.9

During exercise, heat loss to the surroundings can occur by radiation, convection, conduction, and evaporative cooling.

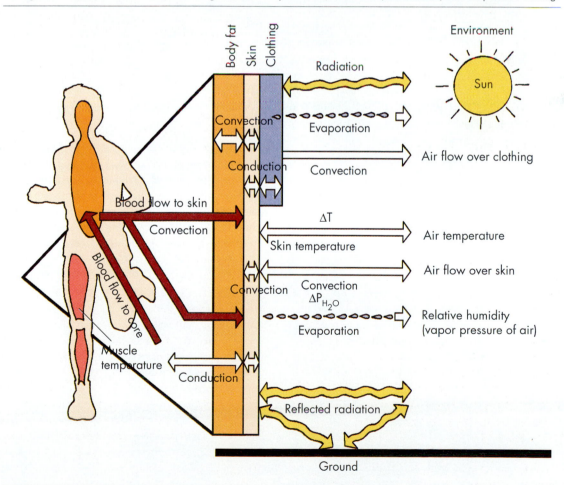

FOCUS BOX 26.1

Calculating body heat storage and evaporative heat loss during exercise

During exercise the body retains a portion of the heat released from energy metabolism and muscle contraction. Also, the body does not have a consistent temperature for all tissues. The temperature of the skin and subcutaneous tissue is lower than core temperature when environmental temperatures are lower than 37° C because of radiant and convective heat loss, as well as evaporative cooling from insensible perspiration. Conversely, when environmental temperatures are warmer than skin temperatures, there is a radiant heat gain to the body that adds to metabolic heat production unless compensated for by evaporative cooling of sweat from the skin. Also, the temperature within contracting muscles can exceed core temperature during exercise. It is this added heat generated during exercise that must be removed from the body to maintain thermal balance.

Researchers have studied how to best measure body temperatures, which include core, skin, and average body temperatures. Core temperatures can be measured at varied sites on and within the body—rectal, axillary, oral, inner ear (tympanic/auditory meatus), or esophageal methods. During exercise, rectal probe and esophageal methods are most commonly used. It is generally accepted that the esophageal temperature most accurately reflects core temperature.[126] More important, during conditions of changing heat load (e.g., exercise) the esophageal temperature is more sensitive to changes in the temperature of central venous and arterial blood than core temperature measured from the rectum.[126] This improved sensitivity is due to the low heat capacity of the esophagus and the proximity to the heart and pulmonary circulation. For a concise summary of the efficacy of different sites for the measurement of core temperature, see Sawka and Wenger.[126]

Skin temperatures vary depending on anatomy, the type of exercise motion, wind strength, and environmental temperature. Consequently, measures of skin temperatures from different parts of the body must be weighted according to their reflection of the mass and surface area of the body part, their specific contribution to the body's sweat response, and the specific thermal sensitivity of the body site.[96,97,116] For example, the back and chest have been shown to have the largest increase in sweat rate for an increase in core temperature, and it has been proposed that for a given skin temperature there can be different levels of neural input to the hypothalamus in different body regions.[96,97]

Average skin temperature can be estimated from weighted measurements of specific skin temperatures by either of the following equations:

26-6   Average skin temperature in °C =
[0.3 (chest + upper arm)] + [0.2 (thigh + calf)]
From Ramanathan[131]

or

26-7   Average skin temperature = (0.21 face)
+ 0.21[(chest + back)/2] + (0.17 abdomen)
+ (0.15 thigh) + (0.08 calf) + (0.12 upper arm)
+ (0.06 forearm)
From Nadel et al.[110]

The equations for average skin temperature presented above have been shown to produce similar results.[86]

A weighted sum of the core temperature and average skin temperature is used to estimate the average temperature of the body, which is a better measure of changes in total body heat storage.

26-8   Total body temperature ° C ≈
(0.33 Tskin) + (0.67 Tcore)

26-9   Body heat storage (Kcal) =
Body weight* × 0.83† × Total body temperature
*kilograms;
†the thermal capacity of the average of all
body tissues (Kcal/kg/°C)

Once these temperatures are known, they can be used to interpret the degree of heat stress imposed on the body. For example, if it is assumed that no effective heat loss from the body occurred during 60 minutes of exercise at a VO$_2$ of 2 L/min and an RER at 0.9, the heat produced from the exercise (2 L/min × 4.924 Kcal/L × 60 min × 0.7 = 413.7 Kcal) actually equals the increased body heat storage. If this were the case, and it were assumed that the average skin and core temperatures at rest were 25° and 37° C, respectively, there would be an increase in total body temperature from 33.04° to 40.2° C. Assuming an increased average skin temperature to 30° C during the exercise, core temperature would have increased to 45.2° C. Such an increase in core temperature is not conducive to life. Obviously, the ability to lose heat from the body by evaporative cooling enables the body to exercise for prolonged periods without accumulating excessive body heat and incurring the risk of death! For cool or even cold environmental temperatures there is a larger component of heat loss because of radiation, and the body heat storage is less. However, if environmental temperatures are warmer than skin temperature, there could be radiative heat gain, and body heat storage would be higher than estimated.

Physiologists interested in thermoregulation can measure sweat rates by adjusting the loss in body weight for respiratory water loss and ineffective sweating.

26-10   Sweat loss (ml) ≈ [(preweight* − post weight*) × 1000] − (0.11 × Kcal†) − (0.12 × Kcal)
*nude weight (kg),
†exercise caloric expenditure (total Kcal)

Sweat loss is not the only evaporative heat loss mechanism, since heat is lost through ventilation. Thus evaporative water loss is different to sweat loss, even when adjusting for ineffective sweat.

26-11   Evaporative water loss (EWL)(ml)
EWL ≈ [(preweight − postweight) × 1000] − (0.11 Kcal)

Given that 1 liter of sweat evaporated from the body requires 580 Kcal of heat energy, the calculation of evaporative water loss can be converted to evaporative heat loss.

26-12   Evaporative heat loss (Kcal)
= Evaporative water loss (L) × 580

For the previous calculation example, in which an individual exercised for 1 hour at a given intensity and caloric heat production (413.7 Kcal), if it is assumed that 0.7 kg body weight was lost during this exercise, evaporative water loss would have been 604.8 ml and the evaporative heat loss would have been 350.8 Kcal. Thus body heat storage would have increased by approximately 62.9 Kcal (413.7-350.8), total body temperature would have increased to 34.1° instead of 40.2° C, and given a slight increase in the average skin temperature to 27° C, core temperature would have increased to 37.6° C.

These calculations stress the importance of the evaporative cooling mechanism during exercise. Furthermore, they provide the ability to estimate changes in body heat storage for given environmental, heat production, and sweat rate conditions. As discussed in latter sections of this chapter, when sweating stops because of excessive dehydration and impaired thermoregulatory function of the hypothalamus, continued exercise can rapidly cause increases in body core and average temperatures and place a person in a life-threatening situation.

FIGURE 26.10

During exercise-induced dehydration, body water is lost from intracellular, interstitial, and vascular fluid compartments. As dehydration increases, a larger portion of water loss comes from cells. However, when expressed relative to the estimated total fluid volume in each compartment, the loss of fluid from plasma represents a significant portion of the available volume.

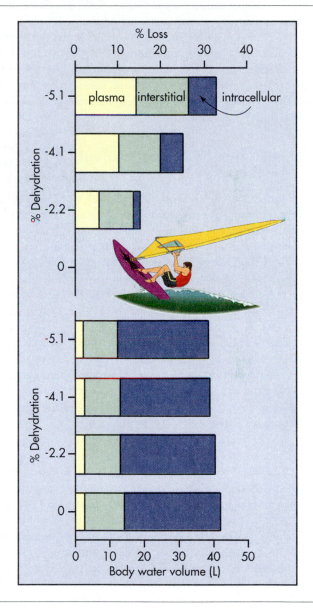

detrimental effects of exercise-induced dehydration on cardiovascular function are discussed in Chapter 11. When exercise is performed in hot or humid environments, the potential for body water losses through sweating is increased. In addition, the heat generation from exercise in combination with the heat stress from the environment can increase the risk of excessive body heat storage (hyperthermia) and result in cardiovascular complications, central nervous system and motor function impairment, and death.

It is important to understand how and why body functions deteriorate during exercise-induced dehydration and hyperthermia, how these deteriorations influence exercise performance, how to prevent them or reduce their severity, and how to recover from them. These issues are presented in this section.

Mechanism of Body Heat Storage and Heat Loss

During exercise the body is producing free energy and heat according to the laws of thermodynamics (Chapter 2). Heat production amounts to 70% to 75% of the total caloric expenditure during exercise. Thus, when a person is exercising at a VO_2 of 2 L/min and an RER of 0.9, the rate of heat production is 6.9 Kcal/min (2 L/min $\times$ 4.924 Kcal/L $\times$ 0.7). This added heat production must be dissipated to the environment if normal body temperatures are to be maintained (see Focus Box 26.1).

The body can lose heat to the surroundings by several processes (Figure 26.9). Conduction, convection, evaporative cooling, and radiation can contribute to body heat losses. However, the mechanism that has the greatest capacity for heat loss and is the main method of heat loss during exercise is evaporative cooling.

When exercise intensity increases or the capacity for effective evaporative cooling diminishes (e.g., humid conditions), there can be far greater heat production than heat loss. As discussed in Focus Box 26.1, if there was no evaporative cooling and no other mechanism for heat loss, even this mild exercise example (VO_2 of 2 L/min for 1 hour) would cause intolerable increases in core and body temperatures. Because of the importance of evaporative cooling during exercise and the consequence of a fluid loss from sweating, where does the fluid from sweat come from within the body, and what are the physiologic consequences of the fluid loss?

Acute Adaptations during Exercise

Changes in Body Temperatures

The change in core temperature during exercise is influenced by the metabolic rate (exercise intensity), the environmental temperature, and an individual's effectiveness for increasing evaporative heat loss.[87,101,105,126] For a range of environmental heat stress conditions, the change in core temperature is not influenced by the environment but mostly by the metabolic heat load of the exercise. However, as exercise intensity increases, core temperature increases more abruptly.[87] In addition, the actual core temperature response for an individual is influenced by that individual's cardiorespiratory fitness and therefore the degree of acclimatization to heat exposure.[126]

The rise in skin temperature during exercise depends on the environmental temperature, the rate of evaporative cooling, the degree of dehydration, and the rate of cutaneous blood flow. All of these factors are related during exercise-induced dehydration, as explained in the following material.

Exercise-Induced Evaporative Heat Loss and Dehydration

During prolonged submaximal exercise in a hot or humid environment, a person's sweat rate can increase to between 2 and 3 L/hr. Depending on gender and body size, the total blood volume may be 5 L, the plasma volume may be 2.75 L, and the total body water may be 35 L. Obviously, compared with the total body water the blood cannot lose a large volume of water during exercise. Figure 26.10 illustrates the sources of fluid lost during exercise-induced dehydration. Initially, the largest volume of water is lost from interstitial fluid. As dehydration increases, there is an increasing contribution from intracellular fluid. Although the relative loss (to total loss) of fluid from the plasma remains constant during dehydration, more severe dehydration represents a larger volume of fluid loss and therefore a larger volume reduction in each compartment. Because plasma volume represents the smallest fluid compartment, a given volume change in plasma is a large fluid loss relative to the small absolute plasma volume. A 4% decrease in body weight for a person weighing 70 kg approximates 7 kg fluid loss. A 10% volume of this loss equals 700 ml, or 25% of the plasma volume. Fluid losses from plasma of this magnitude have detrimental cardiovascular repercussions.

Despite the large fluid volume losses during exercise at high sweat rates, the electrolyte losses are not physiologically significant, as presented in Chapter 17.[32-36] Some researchers have hypothesized that different degrees of dehydration and different relative losses of water from the cellular compartment would result from thermal-induced dehydration, diuretic-induced dehydration, and exercise-induced dehydration.[129] However, research on this topic has found no difference in physiologic responses during exercise among the methods of dehydration.[24,30] However, diuretic-induced dehydration results in a greater decrease in plasma volume.[129]

The decreasing fluid volumes of the body also have detrimental effects on sweating and therefore evaporative cooling. As the body becomes dehydrated, sweat rates actually decrease and body core temperature increases. In fact, when dehydration becomes severe, the sweat response can dramatically decrease, increasing risk for heat injury (see the Clinical Application on p. 657). Such a decreased sweat response occurs from the fatigue of the sweat gland, rather

CLINICAL APPLICATION

Pathophysiology of Heat Illness: Heat Exhaustion and Heat Stroke

The increasing hyperthermia that accompanies exercise, regardless of the state of dehydration, can lead to a series of system and cellular changes that increase risk for exhaustion, organ failure (especially the kidney and liver), and death.[70-72] Although hyperthermia can occur without severe dehydration, dehydration exacerbates the condition. What are the symptoms that reveal the more clinically serious conditions of hyperthermia? What are these conditions called and what are the physiologic mechanisms for their development?

When a person is dehydrated and hyperthermic, the compromised cardiovascular function because of a decreased plasma and total blood volume in combination with the increased core temperature, produces symptoms of central nervous system disturbances, such as lethargy, dizziness, and lack of coordination. These symptoms mark the condition commonly referred to as **heat exhaustion.** Although there is hyperthermia, it is not usually extreme during heat exhaustion; the compromised cardiovascular system is the main cause of the symptoms.[73]

If dehydration and body heat storage continue beyond heat exhaustion, as is often the case during exercise, the increasing hyperthermia (more than 39.5° C) causes the development of disorientation, confusion, psychoses, and coma, along with elevated serum enzyme levels.[135] These symptoms mark the phase of the heat illness spectrum termed **heatstroke.**

Individuals vary in their tolerance of a hot environment; however, research has not been able to define accurate predic-tors of susceptibility to heat illness other than being sedentary, overweight, dehydrated, and unacclimatized to the heat. The completion of a heat tolerance test (exercise in a controlled temperature and humidity environment) is the most accurate method to evaluate a predisposition to heat injury. However, such procedures are not cost effective when large numbers of individuals are being evaluated for their heat tolerance. Research has shown that an individual who has previously had heatstroke is more susceptible to another bout of heat illness. This observation has been explained by residual or permanent damage to the hypothalamus.[42,70]

The symptoms of heat illness are multifaceted. The severe symptoms of heatstroke are explained by cellular changes caused by high core temperatures between 40° and 44° C (Figure 26.12).[70] The rising core temperature increases the rates of metabolic reactions, increases ion fluxes across membranes, and decreases the efficiency of mitochondrial respiration. Accompanying changes are an increase in lactate production and acidosis, decreased excitability and contractility of skeletal and cardiac muscle, and increased leakage from skeletal muscle of K^+, Ca^{++}, and the enzymes creatine kinase and lactate dehydrogenase.[70-72,132] During severe cases of heatstroke, cell leakage is so severe that large proteins circulate in the blood and eventually cause damage to the liver and kidneys. During these conditions, muscle cells swell and become necrotic. This symptom of severe heat injury is termed *rhabdomyolysis*.

---

than from an altered central nervous regulation of sweat gland function.[149] Given the decreasing fluid volume in each of the body's fluid compartments and the increasing core temperature, how do these losses influence cardiovascular function, muscle metabolism, and exercise performance?

Cardiovascular Adaptations

Figure 26.11 presents the changes in body weight and cardiovascular function during progressive dehydration while exercising in a hot and humid environment. Increasing dehydration causes a continued increase in core temperature, increases in heart rate because of reductions in venous return

hyperthermia (hi'per-ther-mi'ah)
a body core temperature above 37° C

heat exhaustion
decreased exercise tolerance because of a combination of dehydration, a reduced plasma volume and cardiovascular compromise, and hyperthermia

heatstroke
the progression from heat exhaustion when body core temperature increases to values that impair central nervous system and damages peripheral tissues

FIGURE 26.11

The changes in body weight, stroke volume, heart rate, and rectal temperatures during exercise in a hot environment. When acclimated to the heat, exercise can be performed for longer before each of the measures changes to the extent observed before acclimation.

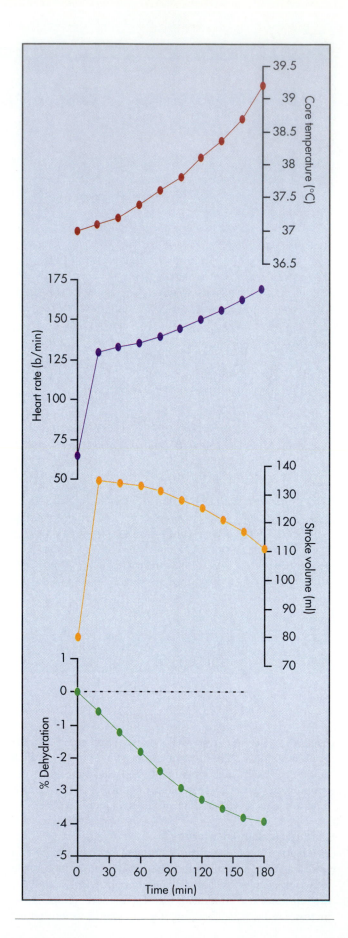

and stroke volume, decreases in cardiac output, and increases in a-vO$_2\Delta$.[126] Nadel et al. have reported a strong association between stroke volume and the percent decrease in plasma volume (reflecting dehydration).[100]

The decreased central cardiovascular function during dehydration is accompanied by alterations in peripheral blood flow to the skin and to the contracting skeletal muscle. For example, an important cardiovascular response to exercise in neutral and hot environments is to increase cutaneous blood flow. This response improves both radiative and evaporative heat loss from the body; radiative heat loss improves most during cool environments, and evaporative heat loss improves most in hot environments with increased air flow (i.e., wind).[2] The increased skin blood flow is not uniform over the entire body, with largest changes being detected in the forearm.[103] With increasing dehydration, neural reflexes respond to a decreasing blood volume and systemic blood pressure and induce an increasing splanchnic and cutaneous vasoconstriction, which increases the central blood volume at the expense of a decreased capacity for heat transport to the skin.[152] Consequently, if exercise is continued, skin temperatures may decrease because of evaporative, convective, and radiative cooling despite an increasing core temperature and increasing average body temperature.

Skeletal Muscle Adaptations

Because dehydration and core temperatures increase during exercise in a hot environment, the increased heat load, altered redistribution of the cardiac output, and increased catecholamine release have the potential to alter muscle metabolism. Fink et al. demonstrated that during cycling in a hot or cold environment, greater muscle glycogen degradation occurred in the hot environment, as well as greater blood lactate accumulation.[48] These authors hypothesized that the altered muscle metabolism was due to a reduced muscle blood flow and accompanied hypoxia. More recent research has shown that muscle blood flow does not decrease during exercise in the heat and that muscle glycogen does not decrease more during exercise in a hot environment than in neutral thermal conditions.[102,124,161] The increased blood lactate accumulation has been a consistent research finding and may relate to an increased fast twitch motor unit recruitment in combination with decreased blood lactate removal.[126]

Effects on Exercise Performance

Cardiovascular indications of dehydration occur with as little as 1% dehydration, but more severe dehydration to 3% is required before detriments in VO_2max are detected.[129] This statement is based on a review of research that measured VO_2max in neutral and hot environments. However, the decrements in VO_2max reported by different studies have been extremely variable. The variability in research results is probably the result of differences in environmental heat stress among studies, since heat stress during exercise in adequately hydrated individuals has been reported to decrease VO_2max by 7%.[126,127] The added fatigue during exercise in the heat when a person is dehydrated is related to the decreased maximal cardiac output and a central nervous system impairment because of the increased core temperature.[129]

Submaximal exercise performance is also impaired in a hot environment. Exhaustion occurs at a reduced exercise time and at a lower core temperature when a person is dehydrated during exercise in a hot environment compared with neutral thermal stress.[129] These responses are understandable, given the previously described acute cardiovascular adaptations during prolonged exercise in the heat.

Improving Exercise Tolerance during Exposure to Hot or Humid Environments

Because of the devastating results of dehydration on exercise tolerance in both neutral and hot environments, fluid ingestion during exercise is vital to decrease the rate of exercise-induced dehydration and its physiologic consequences. Numerous research studies have shown the benefit of fluid ingestion during exercise in a hot environment. In addition, the body can acclimatize to hot or humid environments or be acclimated to tolerate exercise in a hot or humid environment.

Fluid Intake

Numerous studies have shown the benefits of fluid ingestion during exercise in hot environments.[*] In fact, research on this topic was conducted as early as 1944 using military personnel, and this study has been a classic reference for the importance of hydration during exercise.[113] Basically, ingesting fluid retards the development of dehydration (however, it is not totally prevented), dampens the increase in heart rate, improves venous return and cardiac output, retains an increased cutaneous blood flow, lessens the increase in core temperatures, and delays the onset of fatigue.[†]

As with the topics of fluid, electrolyte, and carbohydrate intake during exercise that are detailed in Chapter 17, questions have been raised regarding the best type of fluid to ingest during exercise in a hot environment. Based on the work of Gisolfi et al., the ability for carbohydrate-electrolyte

solutions to increase intestinal water absorption should indicate the superiority of carbohydrate-electrolyte drinks above water alone during exercise in the heat.[51] Despite this evidence, research has shown a similar benefit between carbohydrate drinks and water and between electrolyte drinks and water for the changes in sweating, core temperatures, and cardiovascular responses to exercise in the heat.[*] However, carbohydrate intake during exercise did increase blood glucose concentrations and cause improved exercise performance as would be expected from the findings presented in Chapter 17.[39,92,93]

A possible explanation for the similar physiologic benefits of the ingestion of water and carbohydrate solutions during exercise in the heat is an impairment of either gastric emptying or intestinal absorption of carbohydrate solutions during heat stress, which in turn would minimize hydration effects differences compared with water alone. Ryan et al. measured the gastric emptying of water and drinks with different carbohydrate concentrations during 3 hours of cycling at 60% VO_2max in the heat.[138] The results revealed that all drinks emptied at similar rates over the total duration of exercise. However, using a more sensitive gastric emptying technique (double sampling to provide gastric emptying rates in 10-minute intervals), Rehrer et al. reported that when a person is dehydrated during exercise in the heat there is increased gastric distress causing a reduced gastric emptying of a 7% carbohydrate solution compared with when the person is normally hydrated.[120] No comparison to plain water was made. Clearly, the known benefit of ingesting carbohydrate solutions to improved fluid delivery to the body has not been verified during dehydration.

An important research finding of studies evaluating fluid intake during exercise in hot environments is that ad libitum fluid intake is less effective than forced drinking for replacing fluid lost through sweating.[57,113] This developing dehydration despite the availability of fluid has been termed **voluntary dehydration**. However, there have also been cases where individuals have ingested too much water, causing **water intoxication** and the development of *hyponatremia* (decreased serum sodium less than 130 mEq/L).[57,64]

---

[*]References 11, 22, 39, 92, 93, 107, and 122.

---

voluntary dehydration
the progressive development of dehydration despite the availability of fluid to drink ad libitum

water intoxication
excess drinking of fluid (typically plain water) that lowers the concentration of serum sodium, increasing the risk for developing hyponatremia

---

[*]References 11, 32, 35, 39, 57, 92–94, 107, 113, 120, 122, and 128.
[†]References 7, 11, 12, 30, 34, 35, 39, 107, 128, and 147.

Heat Acclimation and Acclimatization

The reproducibility of the cardiovascular compromise during prolonged exercise in the heat has enabled researchers to use these responses to evaluate individual tolerance of exercise in hot environments, as well as adaptations to exercise in hot environments that occur after acclimatization or acclimation. Standard heat tolerance tests (HTTs) have been developed to provide a reference protocol from which to compare physiologic responses with exercise in the heat under different conditions. For example, Houmard et al. reported that HTTs have generally involved low-intensity exercise (less than 40% to 50% VO_2max) in a hot and dry environment (~ 40° C and 30% RH) for between 60 to 100 minutes. Individuals with a greater increase in core temperature and heart rate are less tolerant of exercise in a hot environment.

The utility of HTTs has also been demonstrated in determining acclimatization or acclimation to exercise in a hot environment. Typically, subjects demonstrate improved heat tolerance after endurance training in a hot environment for 60 to 100 minutes for between 4 and 10 days[67] (see Figure 26.12). In addition, evidence indicates that even endurance-trained athletes who live in cool or temperate climates have experienced partial heat acclimation. However, even when these individuals are artificially heat acclimated, improvements are detected.[7,50,108] The more intense the exercise training, and therefore the more extreme the heat load, the greater the apparent benefit for heat acclimation. Consequently, highly endurance-trained individuals have near maximal heat acclimation regardless of their environmental climatic conditions.[7,50,108] However, research by Avellini et al. revealed that endurance training will improve heat acclimation only if there is training-induced hyperthermia.[9] Swimmers who improved VO_2max by training in cold water did not have improved heat acclimation compared with athletes trained in warm water or on land. For individuals who train in a hot environment, exercise training does not need to be intense, since the added heat stress seems to be adequate to maximally stimulate the adaptive mechanisms of heat accli-

---

FIGURE 26.12

Exercise in a hot or humid environment can increase the risk for heat illness. Initially, heat illness is manifested through the fatigue resulting from a compromised cardiovascular system. If exercise or another heat stress is continued, the sweat response can decrease, resulting in increased heat storage, and the development of heat stroke with potential heat damage occurring to body tissue. (Adapted from O'Donnell TF: *Orthop Clin North Am* 11:841-855, 1980.)

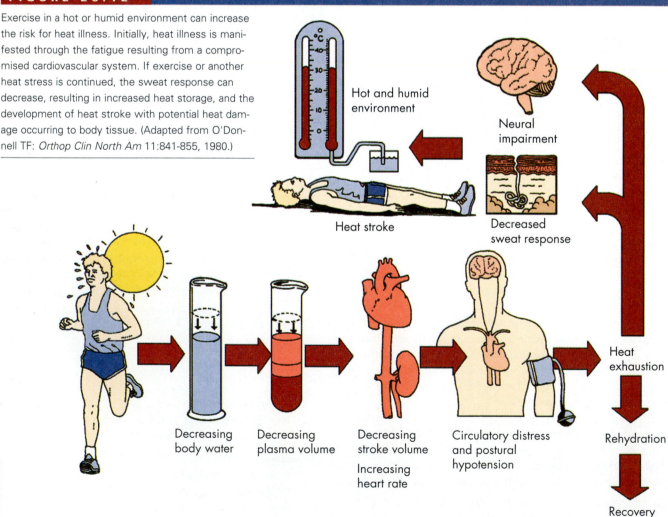

Hot and humid environment

Neural impairment

Heat stroke

Decreased sweat response

Decreasing body water

Decreasing plasma volume

Decreasing stroke volume

Increasing heart rate

Circulatory distress and postural hypotension

Heat exhaustion

Rehydration

Recovery

T A B L E 2 6 . 3	
Chronic adaptations to exercise and exercise in a hot environment that improve acclimation to exercise in the heat	
ACCLIMATION ADAPTATION	**PHYSIOLOGIC BENEFIT**
↑ Plasma volume	↑ Blood volume
	↑ Venous return
	↑ Cardiac output
	↓ Submaximal heart rate
	More sustained sweat response
	↑ Capacity for evaporative cooling
Earlier onset of sweating	Improved evaporative cooling
↓ Osmolality of sweat	Electrolyte conservation (mainly sodium)
↓ Muscle glycogen degradation	↓ Likelihood for muscle fatigue during prolonged exercise

mation.[67] Thus a person's VO_2max is a poor reflection of heat acclimation, since cardiorespiratory endurance is not the causal factor that stimulates heat acclimation.

Chronic adaptations. The adaptations associated with heat acclimation are similar to those of standard endurance training that stresses thermoregulation and consist of an increased plasma volume, earlier onset of sweating during exercise, an increased submaximal exercise stroke volume, more dilute sweat electrolyte composition, and decreased muscle glycogen degradation (see Table 26.3). As previously explained, these adaptations have implications for thermoregulation, cardiovascular function, and muscle metabolism during prolonged exercise.

Rehydration from Dehydration

Given that maximal sweat rates exceed the maximal ability of the body to absorb water (see Chapter 17), prolonged exercise or exercise in a hot or humid environment will always lead to some degree of dehydration. Ideally, this dehydration should be small if preventive strategies are adhered to, such as frequent ingestion of fluids.

The condition of dehydration is accompanied by increased serum concentrations of the hormones ADH and aldosterone (see Chapter 13). The hormones increase fluid conservation by decreasing urine volumes and ADH along with angiotensin II raise peripheral vascular resistance to maintain systemic blood pressures. A fluid loss from the body amounting to 4% body weight, or 3 L for a euhydrated 75-kg adult, must be replaced as rapidly as possible for optimal **rehydration.** Early research on the topic of rehydration revealed that this process was not simple because rehydration was incomplete after 4 hours of recovery even when ingested volumes during rehydration equaled the volume of water lost during dehydration.[30] Furthermore, rehydration was more effective when a carbohydrate electrolyte solution was used, rather than distilled water.[30]

More recent research has combined neuroendocrine physiology, renal physiology, cardiovascular physiology, and muscle metabolism to determine the optimal procedure for rehydration from exercise-induced dehydration.[51] Nose et al. reported that sodium replacement with water increased fluid replacement during rehydration compared with water alone.[106] Similarly, the addition of carbohydrate to solutions for purposes of rehydration increases drink osmolality and, based on the research of Costill and Sparks, should also improve fluid replacement.[30] However, more recent research using carbonated and noncarbonated solutions indicated that neither carbonation nor carbohydrate improved rehydration compared with water.[81] Additional research is required to determine how best to rehydrate the body during the recovery from exercise. An optimal drink would be one that retains a high percentage of the initial volume within the vascular space without being removed by the kidney and lost as urine.

Evaluating Environmental Conditions for Risks for Heat Injury

When the risks of exercise in a hot environment are combined with the development of dehydration and the occurrence of heat illness, prevention of dehydration and hyperthermia is of primary importance. The American College of Sports Medicine has devised a scoring system derived from weighted temperatures that reflect the environmental thermal conditions of dry heat, radiative heat, and the potential for evaporative cooling.[4] This index of risk to thermal injury is based on the following temperatures:

Dry bulb temperature: measure of air temperature

Black bulb temperature: measure of the potential for radiative heat gain

Wet bulb temperature: measure of the potential for evaporative cooling

The index developed by ACSM places greatest importance on the wet bulb temperature, because of the overwhelming influence of evaporative cooling on body heat gain, with next highest importance placed in radiative heat gain and then air temperature. The adjusted temperature is termed the *wet bulb globe temperature* (WBGT).

rehydration (re-hi-dra′shun)
the process of returning fluids to the body

TABLE 26.4

Relative risks for heat injury at different ranges of the WBGI

WBGI	RECOMMENDATIONS
23-28	High Risk for Heat Injury — Red Flag Make runners aware that heat injury is possible, especially for those with a history of susceptibility to heat illness.
18-23	Moderate Risk for Heat Injury — Amber Flag Make runners aware that the risk for heat injury will increase during the race.
<18	Low Risk for Heat Injury — Green Flag Make runners aware that although risk is low, there is still a possibility for heat injury to occur.
<10	Possible Risk for Hypothermia — White Flag Make individuals aware that conditions may cause excessive heat loss from the body, especially for individuals who will have slow race times, and when conditions are wet and windy.

Adapted from American College of Sports Medicine: *Med Sci Sports Exerc* 10(5):ix-xiv, 1985.

26-13

$$WBGT = (0.7 \times Tw) + (0.2 \times Tb) + (0.1 \times Td)$$
$$Tw = \text{wet bulb temperature (°C)}$$
$$Tb = \text{black bulb temperature (°C)}$$
$$Td = \text{dry bulb temperature (°C)}$$

Since the WBGT is not really a temperature, expression of the rating as a temperature can lead to confusion. Rather, the WBGT is an index of the risk to heat illness for a given environmental condition and therefore should really be termed the **wet bulb globe index (WBGI).** Table 26.4 lists the range of WBGI values that are associated with different risks for heat injury.

Section III: Exercise in Cold Environments

*T*he thought of being exposed to cold temperatures conjures images and feelings of discomfort. Typically we dress ourselves to decrease sensations of cold when exposed to a cold environment. We do this even before exercising, and therefore the actual exposure to cold is minimized and the potential impact of exercise in the cold is reduced. Furthermore, because dressing the body for insulation during exercise actually minimizes the potential for heat loss from evaporative cooling, radiation, and convection, exercise in cold environments can actually lead to exercise-induced hyper-

thermia, exercise-induced dehydration, and therefore the symptoms that accompany heatstroke. These events can occur even when environmental temperatures are below freezing.

Acute Adaptations to Cold Exposure

When a person is not prepared for exposure to cold, skin and core temperatures decrease, which in turn stimulates peripheral temperature receptors and the central receptors of the hypothalamus. The neural response to cold involves the stimulation of shivering, which induces involuntary skeletal muscle twitches that can increase basal metabolic rate, and therefore heat production, several-fold.[110] The peripheral response to cold involves vasoconstriction of the cutaneous and skeletal muscle circulations, which of course decreases blood flow and therefore heat transfer from the core to the periphery. This latter response essentially increases the insulative properties of the dermal and skeletal muscle layers of the body. However, since vasoconstriction does not occur in the cerebral circulation, there is a large potential for heat loss from the head, which can amount to 25% of the total heat loss from the body.[110] The rate of heat loss increases when a person is submerged in cold water, since water has up to four times the thermal conductivity of air at the same temperature. Further increases in heat loss occur in water when there is water movement over the body because of the increased contribution of convective heat loss.

Heat loss from an individual will be less if there is more subcutaneous body fat. This relationship is more accurate when in water than air.[136] Similarly, the critical water and air temperatures below which the body increases basal metabolic rate are lower in individuals with more subcutaneous fat.[136,151]

Exercise during Cold Exposure

If submaximal exercise is performed and heat production is inadequate to match heat loss from the body, the increased VO_2 resulting from shivering increases submaximal VO_2.[110] However, as previously explained, typically when humans exercise in the cold, increased clothing prevents excessive heat loss and there is a net body heat gain. Unfortunately, the extent of body heat gain, sweating, and dehydration has not been extensively researched under the more realistic conditions of exercise in the cold when over-dressed. However, as indicated in Figure 26.13, it is known that the amount of clothing required to maintain thermal balance decreases with an increase in exercise intensity. Thus individuals should dress in layers during exercise in the cold and be able to remove layers once warm, causing a decrease in clothing insulation that matches the required insulative needs for the exercise condition.[110]

During water immersion conditions that lower the body core temperature, incremental exercise swimming performed to exhaustion results in a lower VO_2max.[98,99] Performance is also decreased during intense dynamic exercise

FIGURE 26.13

During exercise in a cold environment, there is a need to increase the insulative properties of the clothing. However, the insulation required in clothing decreases as exercise intensity increases. The unit of thermal insulation (clo) is defined from equations of heat flow. *Black,* sleep; *orange,* rest; *green,* very light work; *purple,* light work; *blue,* moderate work; *red,* heavy work. (Adapted from Burton AC, Edholm OG: *Monograph of the Physiological Society,* No, 2, Bethesda, 1955.)

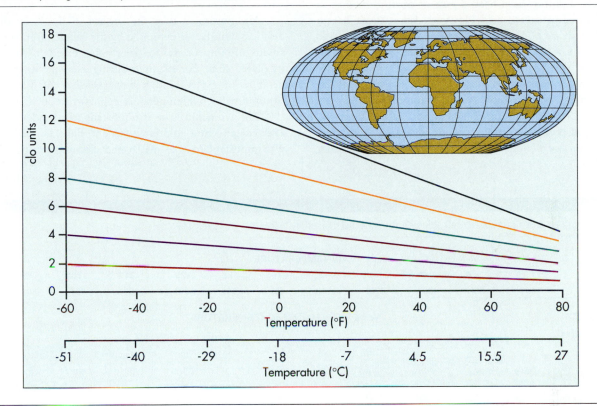

when muscle is cooled. Bergh et al. reported a decrease in maximal strength and power output after muscle cooling, with explanations of this phenomenon based on increased tissue viscosity, decreased speed of ATP breakdown, regeneration, and contraction cycling, and perhaps impaired eletrochemical function.[14]

Can Humans Adapt to Chronic Cold Exposure?

Unlike human adaptations to chronic exposure to altitude or heat, there is minimal adaptation to chronic cold exposure. Research on this topic has compared responses from individuals from different cultures and geographic location, as well as individuals from warm environments forced to live in a cold environment for an extended period.

Some of the earliest research on cold acclimatization was performed on Australian aborigines.[63] Although central Australian aborigines at the time of these studies lived outdoors in a desert environment where day temperatures could exceed 40° C, night temperatures dropped below freezing. Despite these temperature fluctuations the aborigine people wore no clothing and slept on the ground with minimal

structural protection from the elements. During exposure to cold, they did not shiver and their basal metabolic rate did not increase. Rather, they had an increased vasoconstriction of the cutaneous and skeletal muscle circulations and experienced larger decreases in temperatures of the skin and core than European subjects exposed to the same conditions.[61] These responses, although initially appearing to be maladaptations because of the larger decrease in core temperature and conserved energy, may have been an important adaptation for survival.

A similar total body response to cold exposure in Australian aborigines occurs in Korean pearl divers. In these women, core temperatures decrease to approximately 35° C during repeat dives, yet they have a higher shivering threshold than Europeans. It seems that shivering is really a poor response to total body cold exposure because it increases

wet bulb globe index WBGI

an abbreviation for the wet bulb globe index, used to rate the relative risk of heat injury associated with given environmental conditions

blood flow to the more active skeletal muscle and actually increases the rate of heat loss. Shivering is therefore counter-productive when the total body is exposed to the cold, especially cold water, which has a greater thermal conductance than air.[158]

Arctic Eskimos have been a race of obvious interest in research of adaptation to cold. However, data indicate that no unusual body responses are evident in Eskimos compared with Europeans.[158] However, Eskimos, like other races and Europeans who routinely expose body parts to cold water immersion, demonstrate a decreased vasoconstriction and warmer finger temperatures during exposure of the bare hand to cold.[158] In addition, there is a lesser increase in systemic blood pressure during hand immersion in cold water (cold pressor test). These responses do not occur when other body parts are exposed to cold water immersion. Thus this evidence indicates a potential adaptation to cold exposure in the body part routinely exposed to cold.

Wind Chill

Air movement over the surface of the body increases heat loss. This fact is expressed by the windchill index, which adjusts air temperatures to lower values based on wind velocity (Table 26.5). For example, during exposure to an air temperature of 10° C and a wind velocity of 32 kmh, the adjusted windchill temperature approximates 0° C (freezing).

The windchill issue is important to consider, especially after exercise in a cold environment. For example, just as it was important to take off layered clothing during exercise,

TABLE 26.5

Air temperatures and air temperatures adjusted for windchill caused by increased wind velocity

		AIR TEMPERATURE										
°C	10	4	-1	-7	-12	-18	-23	-29	-34	-40	-45	-51
(°F)	(50)	(40)	(30)	(20)	(10)	(0)	(-10)	(-20)	(-30)	(-40)	(-50)	(-60)

WIND SPEED		WINDCHILL ADJUSTED TEMPERATURE										
KMH	MPH											
0	0	10 (50)	4 (40)	-1 (30)	-7 (20)	-12 (10)	-18 (0)	-23 (-10)	-29 (-20)	-34 (-30)	-40 (-40)	-45 (-50)	-51 (-60)
8.0	5	9 (48)	3 (37)	-3 (27)	-9 (16)	-14 (6)	-21 (-5)	-26 (-15)	-32 (-26)	-38 (-36)	-44 (-47)	-49 (-57)	-56 (-68)
16.1	10	4 (40)	-2 (28)	-9 (16)	-16 (4)	-23 (-9)	-29 (-21)	-36 (-33)	-43 (-46)	-50 (-58)	-57 (-70)	-64 (-83)	-71 (-95)
9.3	15	2 (36)	-6 (22)	-13 (9)	-21 (-5)	-28 (-18)	-38 (-36)	-43 (-45)	-50 (-58)	-58 (-72)	-65 (-85)	-73 (-99)	-80 (-112)
32.2	20	0 (32)	-8 (18)	-16 (4)	-23 (-10)	-32 (-25)	-39 (-39)	-47 (-53)	-55 (-67)	-63 (-82)	-71 (-96)	79 (-110)	-87 (-124)
40.2	25	-1 (30)	-9 (16)	-18 (0)	-26 (-15)	-34 (-29)	-42 (-44)	-51 (-59)	-59 (-74)	-67 (-88)	-76 (-104)	-83 (-118)	-92 (-133)
48.3	30	-2 (28)	-11 (13)	-19 (-2)	-28 (-18)	-36 (-33)	-44 (-48)	-53 (-63)	-62 (-79)	-70 (-94)	-78 (-109)	-87 (-125)	-96 (-140)
56.4	35	-3 (27)	-12 (11)	-20 (-4)	-29 (-20)	-37 (-35)	-45 (-49)	-55 (-67)	-63 (-82)	-72 (-98)	-81 (-113)	-89 (-129)	98 (-145)
64.4	40	-3 (26)	-12 (10)	-21 (-6)	-29 (-21)	-38 (-37)	-47 (-53)	-56 (-69)	-65 (-85)	-73 (-100)	-82 (-116)	-91 (-132)	-100 (-148)

Little risk	Increasing risk	Greatest risk
(for properly clothed person)	(cover up fully)	(exercise indoors)

Adapted from Sharkey B: *Physiology of Fitness*, ed 3, Champaign, Illinois, 1990, Human Kinetics.

the need to add layered clothing after exercise is vital. After exercise the moistened clothing and skin can cause a rapid heat loss, which would be increased in windy conditions. The development of hypothermia after exercise is a definite risk and can be prevented by replacing wet clothes with dry clothes of even greater insulative properties.

Hypothermia and Frostbite

Decreases in core temperature, or **hypothermia,** are potentially life threatening. As previously explained, body core temperatures can decline during exposure to cold water and cold air, with increased risk as wind velocity increases. Symptoms of developing hypothermia are weakness, fatigue, decreased shivering, incoherency, and loss of communication skills. These initial symptoms should signal to other individuals the need to remove the person from the cold and start to reheat the person as soon as possible. Once unconsciousness occurs (the next symptom of hypothermia), the chances for successful treatment in the field decrease dramatically. Obviously, the risk for hypothermia on land increases during moist and windy conditions. The risk for hypothermia when submerged in water increases exponentially with decreases in water temperatures.[151]

Based on Table 26.5, the risk for frostbite increases when skin is exposed to extremely cold temperatures. Appropriate clothing needs to be worn to protect the areas most prone to frostbite:—the fingers, toes, ears, and nose.

Section IV: Human Function and Performance during Gravitational Challenge

*H*uman exercise performed in outer space is a modern example of exercise in an extreme environment. The earth has a gravitational force (g) that can be used as a standard force of 1 g. Astronauts are exposed to gravitational forces less than 1 g. For example, the moon has a gravitational force equal to 0.17 g, whereas a space craft and the objects within it (e.g., the space shuttle of NASA) are exposed to zero gravity (0 g) when outside a planetary orbit. Ever since the first human space exploration, when astronauts returned to earth unable to walk after leaving the space craft, it was evident that prolonged exposure to **microgravity** was detrimental to human function. It was obvious that science had to determine what functions of the body were compromised in microgravity and why. These were difficult challenges because it is expensive to generate microgravity conditions on earth and therefore conduct research in microgravity. However, researchers have devised methods that are used to mimic the stresses placed on the body during microgravity. The most common method is head-down bed rest for prolonged periods. Research results using these methods have supplemented knowledge obtained from spaceflight research.

Physiologic Effects of Exposure to Microgravity

The condition of microgravity unloads the work done by the body's muscles that maintain posture against the force of gravity. Similarly, microgravity environments unload the stress of weight bearing on bones and decrease the demands placed on the cardiovascular system during periods of muscle activity. For example, there is less need for physiologic adjustments to supply nutrients and remove waste products. Exposure to microgravity for extended periods may cause atrophy of muscle and bone, decreases function of skeletal muscle (biochemical capacities and contractile function), compromises cardiovascular function, and alters body composition.

The muscle atrophy accompanying exposure to microgravity closely resembles the atrophy from disuse or immobilization.[15,150] Muscle strength measures decrease and muscle fiber areas decrease, causing a reduced ability to perform work. Not surprisingly, the declining muscle function also occurs with increased bone mineral loss in bones that are weight bearing. Such mineral losses approximate 4% and are similar again to studies of bed rest.[157]

Extensive changes occur in cardiovascular function during exposure to microgravity. The decreased gravitational force decreases resistance to blood flow from the lower limbs and periphery to the heart, which decreases venous volume, increases arterial volume, increases systemic blood pressures, and stimulates the right atrium to release atrial natriuretic peptides that inhibit ADH release (see Chapter 13). These factors combine to result in a renal diuresis, decreasing plasma and blood volume.

During the prolonged space flights of Salyut-1 (23 days), Salyut-4 (63 days), and Salyut-6 (140 days), resting stroke volumes and heart rates did not change from preflight values. However, during exercise, heart rates increased after 41 days and stroke volumes decreased after 62 days of exposure, yet these changes were small, only 10% and 12%, respectively.[28] Clearly, the renal diuresis accompanying microgravity does not pose drastic limitations to rest or exercise conditions when a person remains in microgravity, even for extended periods. Interestingly, astronauts of the Skylab 4 mission who exercised daily did not show any decreases in cardiovascular function during exercise throughout their 84-day exposure to zero gravity.[125] This difference may indicate the ben-

hypothermia (hi'po-**ther**-mi'ah)
a decreased body temperature below 37° C

microgravity (mi-kro-**grav**'i-ti)
conditions of decreased gravitational force

eficial role of exercise in microgravity for preserving cardio-vascular function.

The detriment of chronic adaptations of the body to microgravity is not seen until return to earth and therefore to gravity. Astronauts have "detrained" their tolerance and regu-lation of venous return to the heart against gravity, and episodes of syncope are common during the initial days after their return to earth. The muscle atrophy and reduced strength confound their functional abilities, and because of the difficulty in measuring short-term changes in bone min-eral density, it remains unclear how exposure to microgravity will influence bone mineral homeostasis in the decades after exposure to microgravity.

Orthostatic Challenge: Cardiovascular Responses to Increased Gravitational Forces

Exposing the lower body to negative pressures mimics conditions to which many fighter pilots become exposed during aerial maneuvers that increase the gravitational forces on the body. As the pilots are seated, rapid turning of a plane can effectively increase the gravitational forces that retard blood flow to the heart and brain. If venous return is too compromised, pilots can experience syncope and therefore risk their lives and those of the rear co-pilots. This risk is so real that fighter pilots are rated on their g-tolerance; the

higher the g-tolerance, the more extreme the maneuvers that can be performed before syncope and therefore the more effective the pilot should be in air combat.

To decrease the risk of syncope, pilots wear a special suit (a g-suit) with bladders that inflate around the legs and waist to assist in pumping blood back to the heart (Figure 26.14). Pilots also perform a modified form of breathing that inter-mittently increases systemic blood pressures and intrathoracic pressure, which in turn improves the pumping of blood back to the right atrium.

Interestingly, research has shown that aerobic fitness does not improve a person's tolerance of a challenged venous return to the heart (**orthostatic tolerance**).[27,134,135] In fact, endurance training decreases orthostatic tolerance, whereas resistance training may actually improve orthostatic toler-ance.[134,142] The reasons for these findings have been explained by a reduced capacity for reflex vasoconstriction when a per-son is endurance trained. Possible causes of this difference are a resetting of the baroreceptors because of an increased total blood volume, an increased venous capacitance, or a depressed sympathetic nervous system and neuroendocrine response to cardiovascular challenge.[142] The functional importance of these variables was confirmed in a multivariate research study, in which variables reflecting leg venous compliance, increased leg volumes during lower body negative pressure, and total blood volume achieved significance for inclusion in

A pilot in a g-suit, designed to compress the lower limbs and abdomen in flight to improve venous return to the heart during severe flight maneuvers. (Photo courtesy of the New Mexico Air National Guard.)

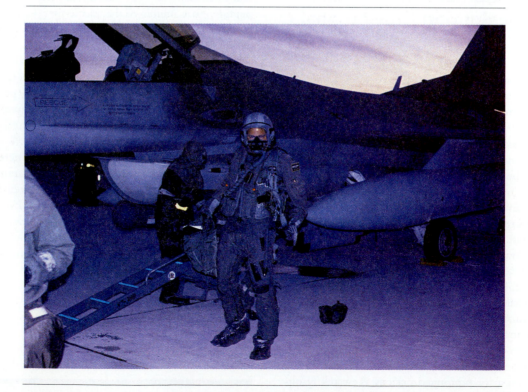

a regression equation to predict the tolerance to lower body negative pressure.[27]

The understanding of how the body responds acutely and chronically to altered gravitational stress has provided a unique condition for furthering our understanding of cardiovascular function and regulation. Given the beneficial roles of exercise training in combating the deconditioning of exposure in microgravity, the future applications of exercise physiology to life and function in and on return from outer space will require continued research. Conversely, the role of exercise training remains unclear in its effects on cardiovascular function during orthostatic challenges. Future research is needed to improve tolerance to orthostatic challenge and to determine what role, if any, exercise training has in this process.

Section V: Exercise in Hyperbaric Environments

Exposure of the body to increased pressure, or **hyperbaria,** can be accomplished when submerged in water or placed in a hyperbaric chamber. When the body is submerged in seawater, the pressure increases one atmosphere (ATM) (760 mm Hg) every 10 meters. In fresh water the pressure increase is not as great because of the different water density; it approximates 1 ATM every 10.4 m of depth.[95] Exposure to hyperbaria is evident for individuals who work beneath the surface of the ocean, toil beneath the ground in deep mines, or conduct experimental clinical or applied research in hyperbaric chambers. Obviously, the development of the self-contained underwater breathing apparatus (SCUBA) in 1943 and its widespread recreational use allowed large numbers of individuals to become exposed to the inherent risks of hyperbaric exposure. The physical, physiologic, and medical concerns about exposure to hyperbaria, especially when applied to SCUBA, are therefore worthy of inclusion in a text that focuses on the physiology of exercise.

When the body is submerged in water to the level of the neck, acute cardiovascular adaptations occur in response to the increased compressive forces exerted on the skin, resulting in decreased cutaneous blood flow, increased central blood volume, increased venous return, and a lowered heart rate. During immersion of the face in water an additional neurologic reflex (diving reflex) is excited that also lowers heart rate. Consequently, immersion of the body in water can be argued to improve cardiovascular function. However, this statement may be premature because when immersion from 15 minutes to 3 hours is followed by incremental exercise on land, there is a decrease in VO_2max.[75] It is theorized that prolonged water immersion decreases plasma volume because of an increased urine volume, and this may be detrimental to exercise performance when returning to dry land.[75]

When exercise in water is compared with exercise on land, the increased resistance provided by the water causes a higher VO_2 for a given amount of physical power output, yet for a given VO_2, heart rate is lower when under water.

The need to remain under water for extended periods requires the use of SCUBA or modifications of SCUBA that provide a continual supply of air. During these conditions, knowledge of the gas laws (Appendix B) is vital to understanding how the pulmonary and cardiovascular systems respond to hyperbaria. For example, Boyle's law concerns the inverse relationship between pressure and volume for a constant gas temperature, Charles' law concerns the direct proportionality between gas volume and temperature, and Dalton's law concerns how the total pressure of a gas volume represents the sum of the individual pressures of each gas. Boyle's and Dalton's laws are important to hyperbaric exposures. For example, when a person is submerged, the increasing pressure decreases gas volume in all body cavities (Boyle's law). In addition, the increasing pressure increases the total gas pressures in the lung in proportion to their fraction in the air (Charles' law). Thus lung volumes decrease during descent, but alveolar gas partial pressures increase during descent.

Breath-Holding during Submersion

During breath-holding (Figure 26.15), P_AO_2 increases and P_AO_2 decreases, as would be expected from the body's continual production of CO_2 and consumption of O_2.[82] Since the most potent ventilatory stimulant is an increasing $PaCO_2$, breath-holding is accompanied by an increasing chemical drive to ventilate. It is this drive that is sensed by the brain and causes what is normally an intolerable need to breathe. Although hyperventilating immediately before breath-hold can lower P_ACO_2 and therefore prolong the time that $PaCO_2$ increases to stimulate ventilation, this maneuver is dangerous because PaO_2 continues to decline and can cause a reduced oxygen supply to the brain and unconsciousness. This is a life-threatening occurrence when a person is submerged in water and especially when performing breath-hold diving where PaO_2 can decrease dramatically on ascent (see Figure 26.16).

With descent to greater depths during breath-hold, the increasing compressive forces decrease volumes in the lungs, as well as other body cavities. Thus body cavity pressures need to be equalized to the increasing pressure of the environment to prevent the rupture of vessels during excessive constriction (termed *squeeze*). Usually this is most noticeable for the inner ear and eustachian tube.

---

orthostatic tolerance

the ability to withstand gravitational force in opposing blood flow back to the heart

hyperbaria (hi-per-bar′i-ah)

increased barometric pressure

During breath-holding the $P_{A}O_2$ decreases and the $P_{A}CO_2$ increases, as would be expected from metabolism. During breath-holding when diving to increased depths, the increasing water pressure actually increases $P_{A}O_2$ despite continued metabolic activity of the body. However, on return to the surface, the decreasing pressure can rapidly decrease $P_{A}O_2$ to dangerous levels, increasing the risk for syncope. (Adapted from Young AJ, Young PM: Human acclimatization to high terrestrial altitude. In Pandolf KB et al (editors): *Human physiology and environmental medicine at terrestrial extremes,* Carmel, California, 1986, Cooper Publishing Group.)

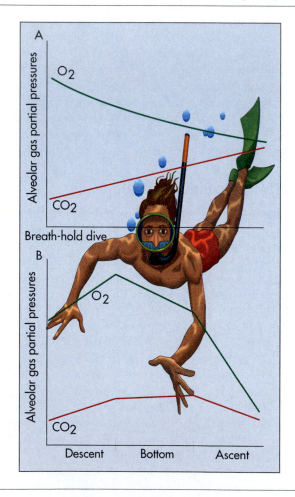

During diving to increased pressures, decreases in lung volumes can be tolerated to the point at which lung volume equals residual volume. Thereafter, continued increases in pressure are exerted on what is now a closed lung volume, which in turn risks the eventual rupturing of the alveoli. Thus the depth limit for breath-hold diving depends on the residual volume relative to total lung capacity. Generally, individuals have a lung capacity to residual volume of 4:1 to 5:1, which can be calculated from the known increase in pressure at increased depths and Boyle's law, to limit the depth of breath-hold dives to between 30 to 40 meters.[95]

SCUBA Diving

The use of SCUBA when submerged under water decreases risk for squeeze in body cavities that are "open" to the respiratory passages, as well as stabilizing alveolar gas partial pressures by providing a continual supply of oxygen and allowing removal of carbon dioxide. However, depending on the depth and duration of the dive, added problems arise that can impair exercise performance.

When a person breathes self-contained air through a regulator that equilibrates air pressure to that of the environment, the increasing depth increases the pressure of the air inhaled. This phenomenon increases the density of the gas, which in turn increases the work of breathing. This change causes divers to hypoventilate, which can cause altered acid-base balance, headache, and impaired cognitive function. Thus at depths causing pressures to exceed 6 ATM, air mixtures should be altered by including helium and less nitrogen, which lowers the density of the gas.

Another reason for lowering the nitrogen content of SCUBA compressed gas is to decrease the health risks of excess nitrogen retention by the body. Such risks include neurologic impairment (i.e., raptures of the deep), as well as increased risk for decompression sickness. Decompression sickness occurs when nitrogen dissolved in body fluids and tissues is forced to escape as bubbles of gas rather than as dissolved gas. This occurs because of a too-rapid decrease in pressure that causes nitrogen from tissues having a slow rate of desaturation to oversaturate and therefore force nitrogen to form gas bubbles. Although the general cause of decompression sickness is a too-rapid ascent, a rapid ascent is more severe if the dive duration was long (allows more time for nitrogen to saturate tissues) or the dive depth was great (decreases the time required for tissue saturation). Because some tissues (e.g., fat), desaturate slowly, the longer and deeper the dive, the more time required for safe desaturation of nitrogen. For these reasons, dive tables have been developed for recommended durations spent at certain depths during ascent after specific diving depths and times.

Another issue of concern for SCUBA divers who dive to depths in excess of 2 ATM for more than 5 hours is the development of oxygen toxicity.[95] These conditions do not apply for recreational divers, who do not have the equipment to allow such long dive times.

Section VI: Exercise and Air Pollution

Research and observation combine to indicate the potential for air pollution to adversely affect exercise performance.[112] This fact is important given the increasing urbanization and potential for air pollution in the major cities of most developed and developing countries. The potential negative effects of air pollution depend on the type of pollutant, its particulate size, water sol-

TABLE 26.6

Examples of air pollutants that can impair exercise performance

POLLUTANT	UPPER HEALTHY LIMIT*	DETRIMENT
Carbon monoxide (CO)	9 ppm	Greater affinity for hemoglobin than oxygen
Carbon dioxide (CO_2)	—	Hyperventilation, acid-base disturbance, headache
Ozone (O_3)	0.12 ppm	Decreased lung function, headache
Sulfuric acid (H_2SO_4)	—	Irritates upper-respiratory tract
Sulfur oxide (SO_2)	0.14 ppm	↑ Exercise-induced bronchospasm
Nitrogen dioxide (NO_2)	—	Lung irritant
Suspended particles	150 µg/m³	Aggravation of asthma and obstructive lung diseases

*Determined by the National Average Air Quality Standards of the United States of America.
Adapted from Pandolf KB: Air quality and human performance. In Pandolf KB, Sawka MN, Gonzalez RR: *Human Physiology and environmental medicine at terrestrial extremes*, Carmel, California,1986, Cooper Publishing Group; Pierson WE, Covert DE, Koenig JQ, et al: *Med Sci Sports Exer* 18(3):322-327, 1986.

ubility, effects on pulmonary function, and concentration relative to dose-response characteristics. Examples of common air pollutants are listed in Table 26.6.

Of the known air pollutants, carbon monoxide (CO) is the most abundant and because it has 200 times the affinity for hemoglobin (Hb) than oxygen, has high potential for being detrimental to health and exercise performance.[105] However, despite this fact, CO inhalation resulting in up to 20% COHb does not impair submaximal exercise performance. Conversely, CO inhalation causing 4% COHb has been shown to decrease VO_2max. The detrimental effects of CO inhalation are greater when exposed to increased altitudes, as would be expected based on the material presented in this chapter.[109]

The inhalation of air containing ozone at concentrations greater than the NAAQS recommendations (Table 26.6) has not been shown to impair submaximal exercise performance yet induces increased discomfort and decreased lung function.[109] During exercise performed to VO_2max, there is evidence for a detriment when breathing air with ozone as high as 0.75 ppm; however, this was an extremely high ozone concentration and lacks application to exercise outdoors.[109]

Sulfur dioxide is released into the atmosphere during the combustion of fossil fuels. Sulfur dioxide is highly water soluble and can be converted to sulfuric acid. Together, the sulfur oxides and their derivatives exert their negative functions by irritating the lung, thereby decreasing ventilatory flow rates.[109] Nitrogen dioxide is also produced from the combustion of fossil fuels, as well as being increased when one handles fertilizers. The effects of nitrogen dioxide on exercise performance have not been extensively researched.

SUMMARY

- Chronic exposure to environmental stress can cause alterations in many aspects of human physiology **acclimatization.** Exposure of the body to an artificial condition that mimics the environmental stress causes similar changes, and this adaptation process is termed **acclimation.**

- A decrease in barometric pressure **(hypobaria)** with an increase in elevation above sea level causes a reduction in P_IO_2, P_AO_2 and P_ACO_2, and has the potential to lower PaO_2 and $PaCO_2$ and cause the condition hypoxia. Given the affinity between hemoglobin and oxygen and the shape of oxygen–hemoglobin dissociation curve, the relationship between PaO_2 and CaO_2 is not linear.

- When hypoxia occurs by a reduction in barometric pressure, it is termed **hypobaric hypoxia** and therefore applies to on-location and altitude-chamber studies. Conversely, hypoxia induced by breathing hypoxic gas when at or near sea level is termed **normobaric hypoxia.** It is generally assumed that the hypobaria does not contribute to the physiologic effects of acute altitude exposure.

- During acute exposure to increased altitude, hyperventilation raises P_AO_2 and PaO_2, making the absolute altitude effectively much lower. The hyperventilation lowers P_ACO_2 and $PaCO_2$, causing a mild respiratory alkalosis. As altitude is increased, there is an increasing difference between P_AO_2 and PaO_2 caused by a combination of diffusion limitation from pulmonary edema and VE/Q mismatch.

- During exposure to moderate to extreme altitudes, the reduced CaO_2 lowers the effective diffusion gradient for oxygen at the tissues, causing a decreased a-$\dot{v}O_2\Delta$. To maintain a given VO_2, cardiac output increases because of an increased heart rate despite a decreased cardiac stroke volume.

- For a given submaximal exercise intensity at moderate to severe altitude, there is a larger ventilation response than when compared with sea level. There is an increased diffusion limitation in the lung, causing a larger P_AO_2 to PaO_2 difference that decreases the functional improvement resulting from increases in P_AO_2 or hematocrit. The increase in VO_2 (worse economy) during exercise at moderate to high altitude is due to an increased work of breathing in combination with increased circulating catecholamines. Cardiac output increases during submaximal exercise at moderate to extreme altitude because of a lowered a-$\dot{v}O_2$ Δ secondary to the low CaO_2 as expected from the Fick equation.

- During the transition from rest to steady-state exercise at moderate to extreme altitudes, there is a reduced rate of increase in VO_2, causing a larger oxygen deficit. This response increases reliance on carbohydrate during exercise, as has also been shown during steady-state exercise.

- For a given VO_2, ventilation is greater at altitude when expressed as either STPD or BTPS volumes. However, cardiac output at VO_2max decreases during moderate to severe altitude exposure. The lowered cardiac output and stroke volume at altitude reflect the lower exercise intensity at VO_2max, rather than impaired cardiac function.

- VO_2max does not decrease on ascent to altitude until approximately 1000 meters above sea level. For every 1000 meters of additional elevation, VO_2 max decreases by approximately 8.7%. Maximal muscle lactate concentrations are actually lower at moderate and high altitudes. These data indicate either that the muscle's capacity for glycolysis is decreased or that the stimulation of glycolysis is decreased at altitude.

- There is a continued hyperventilation during chronic altitude exposure that has been explained by an increased isocapnic hypoxic ventilatory response (HVR). VE/Q mismatch increases with chronic altitude exposure, especially to high and extreme altitudes, because of increases in pulmonary blood pressure and the resultant increase in pulmonary edema.

- Exposure to moderate to extreme altitudes can also result in symptoms of headache, lethargy, and nausea. The condition characterized by these symptoms in a person exposed to increased altitude is termed **acute mountain sickness** (AMS). The susceptibility for AMS is varies among individuals and is related to an abnormally low ventilatory response to hypobaric hypoxia, an increased ventilation-perfusion mismatch, an inadequate diuresis causing a relative fluid retention, and exertion during ascent.

■ The polycythemia of altitude exposure in combination with altitude-induced reductions in plasma volume can increase hematocrit from approximately 45% at sea level to over 54% after 15 days of exposure at 4300 meters. Compared with acute altitude exposure, the chronic increase in hematocrit and the increased saturation of hemoglobin can increase CaO_2 by 30 ml/L. These changes in blood composition occur without a change in total blood volume, since the increased red blood cell mass is offset by the reduced plasma volume.

■ Muscle blood flow and cardiac output decrease during submaximal exercise at 4300 meters because of an increased sympathetic stimulation and reduced leg blood flow during exercise. The data indicate that the body may preserve a given oxygen transport to contracting muscle for a given VO_2. During exercise to exhaustion, maximal cardiac output decreases during chronic moderate to high altitude exposure. Nevertheless, VO_2max increases by approximately 10%.

■ Despite the hypoxia and increased reliance on carbohydrates during moderate to intense exercise at altitude after acclimatization, there is a decreased circulating blood lactate level compared with exercise during acute exposure. This condition has been termed the **lactate paradox.** The lowered lactate may be a result of an increased lactate uptake by active and inactive skeletal muscle or of a central nervous system limitation to exhaustive exercise at moderate to severe altitude.

■ Maximal mechanical power output during short-term (less than 10 seconds) exercise is no different for exercise at altitude than it is at sea level. After acclimatization to altitude there is a decreased maximal blood lactate accumulation but an increased blood acidosis. Such a reduced buffer capacity of the blood is directly related to the decreased blood bicarbonate concentration during acute and chronic altitude exposure.

■ Individuals who have lived at moderate altitude all their lives respond better to acute altitude exposure than do sea level residents. Evidence of improved acute adaptation to increased altitude exists for residents of altitudes as low as 1600 meters (Denver). Clearly, living at altitudes that are low to moderate provides improved tolerance and responsiveness to increased altitude exposure.

■ Acclimatization to moderate altitudes is associated with 5% to 10% improvements in VO_2max compared with acute exposure and improved athletic performance in endurance events. Scientific studies of changes in VO_2max and exercise performance at sea level after altitude acclimatization have produced results that both confirmed and negated the benefit of altitude training. If living at altitude were to provide any potential benefit, it would be for residing at moderate altitude. It has been recommended that athletes live at moderate altitude and train at lower altitudes.

■ The body can lose heat to the surroundings by conduction, convection, evaporative cooling, and radiation. However, the mechanism that has the greatest capacity for heat loss is evaporative cooling, the main mechanism of heat loss during exercise. The rise in skin and core temperatures during exercise depends on the environmental temperature, the rate of evaporative cooling, the degree of dehydration, and the rate of cutaneous blood flow.

■ During prolonged submaximal exercise in a hot or humid environment, a person's sweat rate can increase to between 2 and 3 L/hr. Despite the large fluid volume losses **(dehydration)** during exercise at high sweat rates, the electrolyte losses are not physiologically significant. Increasing dehydration causes a continued increase in core temperature **(hyperthermia),** increases in heart rate because of reductions in venous return and stroke volume, decreases in cardiac output, and increases in a-vO_2 Δ.

■ An increased cutaneous blood flow during exercise in the heat improves both radiative and evaporative heat loss from the body. However, with increasing dehydration, neural reflexes respond to a decreasing blood volume and systemic blood pressure and induce an increasing splanchnic and cutaneous vasoconstriction, which increases the central blood volume at the expense of a decreased capacity for heat transport to the skin.

■ When a person is dehydrated and hyperthermic, symptoms of central nervous system disturbances occur, such as lethargy, dizziness, and lack of coordination. These symptoms mark the condition referred to as **heat exhaustion.** If dehydration and body heat storage continue beyond heat exhaustion, the increasing hyperthermia (greater than 39.5° C) causes disorientation, confusion, psychoses, and coma, along with elevated serum enzyme levels. These symptoms mark the phase of the heat illness spectrum termed **heatstroke.** The American College of Sports Medicine has developed an index of the likelihood for heat injury based on the environmental conditions, called the Wet bulb globe temperature (WBGT), or more correctly termed the **wet bulb globe index (WBGI).**

■ Cardiovascular indications of dehydration occur with as little as 1% dehydration; however, dehydration of at least 3% is required before detriments in VO_2max are detected. The added fatigue during exercise in the heat when a person is dehydrated is related to the decreased maximal cardiac output and a central nervous system impairment caused by the increased core temperature.

■ Ingesting fluid during exercise in the heat retards the development of dehydration (i.e., it is not totally prevented), dampens the increase in heart rate, improves venous return and cardiac output, retains an increased cutaneous blood flow, lessens the increase in core temperatures, and delays the onset of fatigue. Research has shown that carbohydrate drinks and water, as well as electrolyte drinks and water, have similar beneficial effects on changes in sweating, core temperatures, and cardiovascular responses to exercise in heat.

■ Ad libitum fluid intake is less effective than forced drinking for replacing fluid lost through sweating. Developing dehydration despite the availability of fluid has been termed **voluntary dehydration.** However, there have also been cases in which individuals have ingested too much water, causing **water intoxication,** and the development of hyponatremia (decreased serum sodium less than 130 mEq/L). The process of returning fluid to the body **(rehydration)** may take up to 24 hours.

■ Subjects demonstrate improved heat tolerance after endurance training in a hot environment for 60 to 100 minutes for between 4 to 10 days. Endurance-trained athletes who live in cool or temperate climates experience partial heat acclimation; however, further improvements are detected during training in the heat. For individuals who train in a hot environment, exercise training does not need to be intense, since the added heat stress seems to be adequate to maximally stimulate the adaptive mechanisms of heat acclimation.

■ The adaptations associated with heat acclimation consist of an increased plasma volume, earlier onset of sweating during exercise, an increased submaximal exercise stroke volume, more dilute sweat electrolyte composition, and decreased muscle glycogen degradation. As previously explained, these adaptations have implications to thermoregulation, cardiovascular function, and muscle metabolism during prolonged exercise.

■ When the body is not adequately prepared for exposure to cold, skin and core temperatures decrease, which in turn stimulates peripheral temperature receptors and the central receptors of the hypothalamus. The neural response to cold involves the stimulation of shivering, which can increase basal metabolic rate and heat production severalfold and the vasoconstriction of the cutaneous and skeletal muscle circulations, which decreases blood flow and therefore heat transfer from the core to the periphery. The rate of heat loss increases when the body is submerged in cold water, since water has up to four times the thermal conductivity of air at the same temperature.

■ The amount of clothing required to maintain thermal balance decreases with an increase in exercise intensity. Thus individuals should dress in layers during exercise in the cold and be able to remove layers once warm, causing a decrease in clothing insulation that matches the required insulative needs for the exercise condition. During conditions that lower body core temperature **(hypothermia),** VO_2max decreases, as do maximal muscle strength and power output.

SUMMARY—Cont'd

■ The condition of **microgravity** unloads the work done by the body's muscles that maintain posture against the force of gravity. Similarly, microgravity environments unload the stress of weight bearing on bones and decrease the demands placed on the cardiovascular system during periods of muscle activity. Exposure to microgravity for extended periods leads to atrophy of muscle and bone, decreases function of skeletal muscle (biochemical capacities and contractile function), compromises cardiovascular function, and alters body composition.

■ The detriment of the chronic adaptations of the body to microgravity is not seen until return to earth and therefore return to gravity. Astronauts have "detrained" their tolerance and regulation of venous return to the heart against gravity, and episodes of syncope are common during the intial days after their return to earth. The muscle atrophy and reduced strength confound their functional abilities. Because of the difficulty in measuring short-term changes in bone mineral density, it remains unclear how exposure to microgravity will influence bone mineral homeostasis in the decades afterward.

■ Exposing the lower body to negative pressures (LBNP) mimics conditions to which many fighter pilots become exposed during aerial maneuvers that increase the gravitational forces on the body. To decrease the risk of syncope, pilots wear a special suit (a g-suit) that has bladders that inflate around the legs and waist, effectively assisting in the pumping of blood back to the heart. Pilots also perform a modified form of breathing that intermittently increases systemic blood pressures and intrathoracic pressure, which improves the pumping of blood back to the right atrium.

■ Aerobic fitness does not improve a person's tolerance of a challenged venous return to the heart **(orthostatic tolerance).** In fact, endurance training decreases orthostatic tolerance, whereas resistance training may actually improve it.

■ When the body is submerged in water to the level of the neck, acute cardiovascular adaptations occur in response to the increased compressive forces that are exerted on the skin, resulting in decreased cutaneous blood flow, increased central blood volume, increased venous return, and a lowered heart rate. During immersion of the face in water an additional neurologic reflex *(diving reflex)* is excited that also lowers heart rate. When exercise is performed in water, VO_2 is higher than on land for a given amount of physical power output, yet for a given VO_2, heart rate is lower when under water.

■ During breath-holding P_ACO_2 increases and P_AO_2 decreases, as would be expected from the body's continual production of CO_2 and consumption of O_2. Although hyperventilating immediately before breath-hold can lower P_ACO_2 and therefore prolong the time that $PaCO_2$ increases to stimulate ventilation, this maneuver is dangerous because PaO_2 continues to decline and can cause a reduced oxygen supply to the brain and unconsciousness.

■ During diving to increased pressures **(hyperbaria),** decreases in lung volumes can be tolerated to the point at which lung volume equals residual volume. Thereafter, continued increases in pressure are exerted on what is now a closed lung volume, which may lead to the eventual rupturing of the alveoli. Thus the depth limit for breath-hold diving depends on the residual volume relative to total lung capacity. Generally, individuals have a lung capacity to residual volume of 4:1 to 5:1, which limits the depth of breath-hold dives to between 30 and 40 meters.

■ During SCUBA diving the increasing depth increases the density of the inspired gas, which increases the work of breathing. Thus at depths causing pressures to exceed 6 ATM, air mixtures should be altered to include helium and less nitrogen, which lowers the density of the gas. Another reason for lowering the nitrogen content of SCUBA compressed gas is to decrease the health risks of excess nitrogen retention by the body.

SUMMARY—Cont'd

- The potential negative effects of air pollution depend on the type of pollutant, its particulate size, water solubility, effects on pulmonary function, and concentration relative to dose-response characteristics.

- Of the known air pollutants, carbon monoxide is the most abundant and has 200 times the affinity for hemoglobin than oxygen. CO inhalation resulting in up to 20% COHb does not impair submaximal exercise performance. Conversely, CO inhalation causing 4% COHb has been shown to decrease VO_2max. The detrimental effects of carbon monoxide inhalation are greater when a person is exposed to increased altitudes, as would be expected based on the material presented in this chapter.

REVIEW QUESTIONS

1. Why do the physiologic responses to increasing altitude differ depending on the absolute altitude above sea level? What are some of these physiologic responses?

2. Explain the terms hypobaria, hypoxia, hypobaric hypoxia, and normobaric hypoxia.

3. Describe the change in barometric pressure with increasing altitude. How does the change in CaO_2 compare with this change, and if they are different, why is this so?

4. Why does the P_AO_2 to PaO_2 difference increase during exercise at altitude compared with rest conditions?

5. Describe the decrease in VO_2max with increasing altitude, and provide a physiologic justification for the decrease.

6. Whether VO_2max increases after chronic altitude exposure is a controversial topic. What chronic adaptations to high-altitude exposure would support an increase in VO_2max, and what chronic adaptations would oppose an increase in VO_2max?

7. Explain the "lactate paradox."

8. Is short-term intense exercise impaired at moderate to high altitudes? Explain.

9. You have been challenged by an elite athlete to disprove the widely accepted fact that altitude training will improve sea level endurance exercise performance. Basing your answer solely on published research, what would you tell this athlete?

10. Explain the relationships among body weight loss, dehydration, and increasing core temperature during exercise.

11. Most individuals cannot avoid dehydration when exercising in a hot environment. How should an individual best prepare himself or herself to limit dehydration during exercise?

12. Is exercise an adequate heat stress to optimize heat acclimation adaptations? Explain.

13. Explain the importance of cutaneous vasodilation to improved evaporative heat loss.

14. Is there an easy way to rehydrate the body? Explain.

15. Why is the issue of exercise in a cold environment of limited relevance to most individuals?

REVIEW QUESTIONS—Cont'd

16. Is the shivering response to cold exposure an appropriate mechanism for retaining body heat, regardless of whether on land or in water? Explain.

17. Is there evidence of human adaptation to cold environments? Explain.

18. Why is exposure to microgravity detrimental to human physiology on return to gravity?

19. What is an orthostatic challenge, and how does the body respond during such challenges?

20. Explain the dangers of breath-holding during underwater exercise.

21. Using both Boyle's and Charles' laws, explain the dangers of SCUBA diving.

22. What has research revealed about the effects of carbon monoxide and ozone on exercise performance?

APPLICATIONS

1. Describe the condition acute mountain sickness. What have researchers discovered regarding potential causes for this condition?

2. What is high-altitude pulmonary edema, and what simple measures of lung function can be used to detect its development on location at high altitude?

3. Explain the differences and similarities between heat exhaustion and heatstroke.

4. Should all people who are forced to work in a hot or humid environment be forced to perform endurance type exercise regularly (three times per week)? Why?

5. Explain why submersion of the body in cold water poses a far greater risk of developing hypothermia than exposure to cold air.

6. What is the rationale for using hyperbaric conditions to treat carbon monoxide poisoning?

REFERENCES

1. Abbrecht PH, Littell JK: Plasma erythropoietin in men and mice during acclimatization to different altitudes, *J Appl Physiol* 32(1):54-58, 1972.

2. Adams WC, Mack GW, Langhans GW, Nadel ER: Effects of equivalent sea-level and altitude training on VO₂max and running performance, *J Appl Physiol* 39:262, 1975.

3. Adams WC, Mack GW, Langhans GW, Nadel ER: Effects of varied air velocity on sweating and evaporative rates during exercise, *J Appl Physiol* 73(6):2668-2674, 1992.

4. American College of Sports Medicine: Position stand on the prevention of thermal injuries during distance running, *Med Sci Sports Exerc* 16(5)ix-xiv, 1984.

5. Anderson HT, Smeland EB, Owe JO, Myhre K: Analyses of maximum cardiopulmonary performance during exposure acute hypoxia at simulated altitude-sea level to 5000 meters (760-404 mm Hg), *Aviat Space Environ Med* 56:1192-1197, 1985.

6. Arbeille P, Pavy-Le Traon A, Fomina G et al: Femoral flow responses to lower body negative pressure: an orthostatic tolerance test, *Aviat Space Environ Med* 66:131-136, 1995.

7. Armstrong LE, Pandolf KB: Physical training, cardiorespiratory physical fitness and exercise-heat tolerance. In Pandolf KB, Sawka MN, Gonzalez RR: *Human physiology and environmental medicine at terrestrial extremes,* Carmel, California, 1986, Cooper Publishing Group.

8. Armstrong LE, Hubbard RW, DeLuca JP, Christensen EL: Heat acclimatization during summer running in the United States, *Med Sci Sports Exerc* 19(2):131-136, 1987.

9. Avellini BA, Shapiro Y, Fortney SM et al: Effects on heat tolerance of physical training in water and on land, *J Appl Physiol* 53:1291-1298, 1982.

10. Balke B: Effects of altitude acclimatization on work capacity, *Fed Proc* 15:7, 1966.

11. Barr SI, Costill DL, Fink WJ: Fluid replacement during prolonged exercise: effects of water, saline, or no fluid, *Med Sci Sports Exerc* 23(7):811-817, 1991.

12. Bender PR, Groves BM, McCullough RE et al: Oxygen transport to exercising leg in chronic hypoxia, *J Appl Physiol* 65(6):2592-2597, 1988.

13. Bender PR, Groves BM, McCullough RE et al: Decreased exercise muscle lactate release after high altitude acclimatization, *J Appl Physiol* 67(2):1456-1462, 1989.

14. Bergh U, Ekblom B: Influence of muscle temperature on maximal muscle strength and power output in human skeletal muscle, *Acta Physiol Scand* 107:33-37, 1979.

15. Booth FW: Effects of limb immobilization on skeletal muscle, *J Appl Physiol* 52:1113-1118, 1982.

16. Brooks GA, Butterfield GE, Wolfe RR et al: Increased dependence on blood glucose after acclimatization to 4,300 m, *J Appl Physiol* 70(2):919-927, 1991.

17. Brooks GA, Butterfield GE, Wolfe RR et al: Decreased reliance on lactate during exercise after acclimatization to 4,300 m, *J Appl Physiol* 71:333-341, 1991.

18. Brooks GA, Wolfel EE, Groves BM et al: Muscle accounts for glucose disposal but not blood lactate appearance during exercise after acclimatization to 4,300 m, *J Appl Physiol* 72(60):2435-2445, 1992.

19. Buskirk ER, Kollias J, Akers RF et al: Maximal performance at altitude and on return from altitude in conditioned runners, *J Appl Physiol* 23:259-266, 1967.

20. Butterfield GE, Gates J, Fleming S et al: Increased energy intake minimizes weight loss in men at high altitude, *J Appl Physiol* 72(5):1741-1748, 1992.

21. Cahan C, Hoekje PL, Goldwasser E et al: Assessing the characteristics between length of hypoxic exposure and serum erythropoietin levels, *Am J Physiol* 258(27):R1016-1021, 1990.

22. Carter JE, Gisolfi CV: Fluid replacement during and after exercise in the heat, *Med Sci Sports Exerc* 21(5):532-539, 1989.

23. Cerretelli P, Veicsteinas A, Marconi C: Anaerobic metabolism at high altitude: the lactacid mechanism. In Brendel W, Zink RA, editors: *High altitude physiology and medicine,* New York, 1982, Springer-Verlag.

24. Cerretelli P: O₂ breathing at altitude: effects on maximal performance. In Brendel W, Zink RA, editors: *High altitude physiology and medicine,* New York, 1982, Springer-Verlag.

25. Claremont AD, Costill DL, Fink WJ, Van Handel P: Heat tolerance following diuretic induced dehydration, *Med Sci Sports Exerc* 8(4):239-243, 1976.

26. Clark JM, Gelfand R, Lambertsen CJ et al: Human tolerance and physiological responses to exercise while breathing oxygen at 2.0 ATA, *Aviat Space Environ Med* 66:336-345, 1995.

27. Convertino VA, Sather TM, Goldwater DJ, Alford WR: Aerobic fitness does not contribute to prediction of orthostatic tolerance, *Med Sci Sports Exerc* 18(5):551-556, 1986.

28. Convertino VA: Potential benefits of maximal exercise just prior to return from weightlessness, *Aviat Space Environ Med* 58:568-572, 1987.

29. Convertino VA: Physiological adaptations to weightlessness: effects of exercise and work performance, *Exer Sport Sci Rev* 18:119-166, 1990.

30. Costill DL, Sparks KE: Rapid fluid replacement following thermal dehydration, *J Appl Physiol* 34(3):299-303, 1973.

REFERENCES—Cont'd

31. Costill DL, Fink WJ: Plasma volume changes following exercise and thermal dehydration, *J Appl Physiol* 37(4):521-525, 1974.

32. Costill DL, Cote R, Miller T, Wynder S: Water and electrolyte replacement during repeated days of work in the heat, *Aviat Space Environ Med* 46(6):795-800, 1975.

33. Costill DL, Cote R, Fink WJ: Muscle water and electrolytes following varied levels of dehydration in man, *J Appl Physiol* 40:6-11, 1976.

34. Costill DL: Sweating: its composition and effects on body fluids, *Ann NY Acad Sci* 301:160-174, 1977.

35. Costill DL: Water and electrolyte requirements during exercise, *Clin Sports Med* 3(3):639-648, 1984.

36. Costill DL: Muscle metabolism and electrolyte balance during heat acclimation, *Acta Physiol Scand* 128(Suppl 556):111-118, 1986.

37. Cymerman A, Reeves JT, Sutton JR et al: Operation Everest II: maximal oxygen uptake at extreme altitude, *J Appl Physiol* 66:2446-2453, 1989.

38. Daniels J, Oldridge N: The effects of alternate exposure to altitude and sea level on world-class middle distance runners, *Med Sci Sports Exerc* 2:107-112, 1970.

39. Davis JM, Lamb DR, Pate RR et al: Carbohydrate-electrolyte drinks: effects on endurance cycling in the heat, *Am J Clin Nutr* 48:1023-1030, 1988.

40. Di Prampero PE, Mognoni P, Veicsteinas A: The effects of hypoxia on maximal anaerobic alactic power in man. In Brendel W, Zink RA, editors: *High altitude physiology and medicine,* New York, 1982, Springer-Verlag.

41. Eckardt K, Boutellier U, Kurtz A et al: Rate of erythropoietin formation in humans in response to acute hypobaric hypoxia, *J Appl Physiol* 66(4):1785-1788, 1989.

42. Epstein Y: Heat intolerance: predisposing factor or residual injury? *Med Sci Sports Exerc* 22(1):29-35, 1990.

43. Evans WO, Robinson SM, Hortsman DH et al: Amelioration of the symptoms of acute mountain sickness by staging and acetazolamide, *Aviat Space Environ Med* 47(5):512-516, 1976.

44. Fagraeus L, Karlsson J, Linnarson D, Saltin B: Oxygen uptake during maximal work at lowered and raised ambient air pressures, *Acta Physiol Scand* 87:411-421, 1973.

45. Falk B, Bar-Or O, Calvert R, MacDougall JD: Sweat gland response to exercise in the heat among pre-, mid-, and late-pubertal boys, *Med Sci Sports Exerc* 24(3):313-319, 1992.

46. Faulkner JA: Effects of training at moderate altitude on physical performance capacity, *J Appl Physiol* 23:85, 1967.

47. Faulkner JA, Kollias J, Favour CB et al: Maximal aerobic capacity and running performance at altitude, *J Appl Physiol* 24:685-691, 1968.

48. Fink WJ, Costill DL, Van Handel PJ: Leg muscle metabolism during exercise in the heat and cold, *Eur J Appl Physiol* 34:183-190, 1975.

49. Gavin TP, Stager JM, Derchak PA: Mechanisms for the decrease in maximal oxygen uptake during acute hypoxia, *Med Sci Sports Exerc* 27(5)(Abstract 625):S110, 1995.

50. Gisolfi CV, Cohen JS: Relationships among training, heat acclimation, and heat tolerance in men and women: the controversy revisited, *Med Sci Sports Med* 11:56-59, 1979.

51. Gisolfi CV, Duchman SM: Guidelines for optimal replacement beverages for different athletic events, *Med Sci Sports Exerc* 24(6):679-687, 1992.

52. Geelan G, Greenleaf JE: Orthostasis: exercise and exercise training, *Exerc Sport Sci Rev* 21:201-230, 1993.

53. Gore CJ, Hahn AG, Watson DB et al: VO_2max and arterial O_2 saturation at sea level and 610 m, *Med Sci Sports Exerc* 27(5)(Abstract 42):S7, 1995.

54. Green HJ, Sutton JR, Young PM et al: Operation Everest II: muscle energetics during maximal exhaustive exercise, *J Appl Physiol* 66:142-150, 1989.

55. Green HJ, Sutton JR, Cymerman A et al: Operation Everest II: adaptations in human skeletal muscle, *J Appl Physiol* 66:2454-2461, 1989.

56. Green HJ, Sutton JR, Wolfel EE et al: Altitude acclimitization and energy metabolic adaptations in skeletal muscle during exercise, *J Appl Physiol* 73(6):2701-2708, 1992.

57. Greenleaf JE: Problem: thirst, drinking behavior, and involuntary dehydration, *Med Sci Sports Exerc* 24(6):645-656, 1992.

58. Grissom CK, Roach RC, Sarnquist FH, Hackett PH: Acetazolamide in the treatment of acute mountain sickness: clinical efficacy and effect on gas exchange, *Ann Intern Med* 116:461-465, 1992.

59. Grover RF, Weil JV, Reeves JT: Cardiovascular adaptations to exercise at high altitude, *Exerc Sport Sci Rev* 14:269-302, 1986.

60. Groves BM, Reeves JT, Sutton JR et al: Operation Everest II: elevated high-altitude pulmonary resistance unresponsive to oxygen, *J Appl Physiol* 63(2):521-530, 1987.

61. Hammel HT, Elsner RW, LeMessurier DH et al: Thermal and metabolic responses of the Australian aborigine exposed to moderate cold in summer, *J Appl Physiol* 14:605-615, 1959.

62. Hartley LH, Vogel JA, Landowne M: Central, femoral, and brachial circulation during exercise in hypoxia, *J Appl Physiol* 34(1):87-90, 1973.

63. Hicks CS: Terrestrial animals in cold: exploratory studies of primitive man. In Dill DB, Adolph EF, Wilber CG, editors: *Handbook of physiology, Section 4: adaptation to the environment.* Washington, DC, 1964, American Physiological Society.

REFERENCES—Cont'd

64. Hiller WDB: Dehydration and hyponatremia during triathlons, *Med Sci Sports Exer* 21(5):S219-S221, 1989.

65. Horstman DH, Weiskopf R, Jackson RE: Work capacity during 3-week sojourn at 4,300 m: effects of relative polycythemia, *J Appl Physiol* 49:311-318, 1980.

66. Horstman DH, Christensen E: Acclimatization to dry heat: active men vs women, *J Appl Physiol* 52(4):825-831, 1982.

67. Houmard JA, Costill DL, Davis JA et al: The influence of exercise intensity on heat acclimation in trained subjects, *Med Sci Sports Exerc* 22(5):615-620, 1990.

68. Houston CS, Riley RL: Respiratory and circulatory changes during acclimatization to high altitude, *Am J Physiol* 140:565-588, 1947.

69. Houston CS: High adventure: the romance between medicine and mountaineering, *Exerc Sports Sci Rev* 22:1-22, 1994.

70. Hubbard RW, Armstrong LE: The heat illnesses: biochemical, ultrastructural and fluid-electrolyte considerations. In Pandolf KB, Sawka MN, Gonzalez RR: *Human physiology and environmental medicine at terrestrial extremes,* Carmel, California, 1986, Cooper Publishing Group.

71. Hubbard RW: Heatstroke pathophysiology: the energy depletion model, *Med Sci Sports Exerc* 22(1):19-28, 1990.

72. Hubbard RW: An introduction: the role of exercise in the etiology of exertional heatstroke, *Med Sci Sports Exerc* 22(1):2-5, 1990.

73. Hughes RL, Clode M, Edwards RHT et al: Effects of inspired O_2 on cardio-pulmonary and metabolic responses to exercise in man, *J Appl Physiol* 24:366, 1968.

74. Jacobs I, Martineau L, Vallerand AL: Thermoregulatory thermogenesis in humans during cold stress, *Exerc Sports Sci Rev* 22:221-250, 1994.

75. Kame VD, Pendergast DR: Effects of short term and prolonged immersion on the cardiovascular responses to exercise, *Aviat Space Environ Med* 66:20-25, 1995.

76. Karvonen J, Saarela J: The effect of sprint training performed in a hypoxic environment on specific performance capacity, *J Sports Med* 26:219-224, 1986.

77. Kayser B, Narici M, Binzoni T et al: Fatigue and exhaustion in chronic hypobaria: influence of exercising muscle mass, *J Appl Physiol* 76(2):634-640, 1994.

78. Klausen K, Dill DB, Horvath SM: Exercise at ambient and high oxygen pressure at high altitude and at sea level, *J Appl Physiol* 24:336, 1970.

79. Klausen T, Mohr T, Ghisler U, Nelson OJ: Maximal oxygen uptake and erythropoietic responses after altitude training at moderate altitude, *Eur J Appl Physiol* 62:376-379, 1991.

80. Knaupp W, Khilnani S, Sherwood J et al: Erythropoietin response to acute normobaric hypoxia in humans, *J Appl Physiol* 73(3):837-840, 1992.

81. Lambert CP, Costill DL, McConell GK et al: Fluid replacement after dehydration: influence of beverage carbonation and carbohydrate content, *Int J Sports Med* 13(4):285-292, 1992.

82. Lanphier EH, Rahn H: Alveolar gas exchange during breath-hold diving, *J Appl Physiol* 18:478-482, 1963.

83. Lenfant CP: Effect of chronic hypoxic hypoxia on the O_2-Hb dissociation curve and respiratory gas transport in man, *Respir Physiol* 7:7, 1969.

84. Levine BD, Friedman DB, Engfred K et al: The effect of normoxic and hypobaric hypoxic endurance training on the hypoxic ventilatory response, *Med Sci Sports Exerc* 24(7):769-775, 1992.

85. Levine BD, Stray-Gunderson J: A practical approach to altitude training: where to live and train for optimal performance enhancement, *Int J Sports Med* 13:S209-S212, 1992.

86. Libert JP, Candas V, Sagot JC et al: Contribution of skin thermal sensitivities of large body areas to sweating response, *Jpn J Physiol* 34:75-88, 1984.

87. Lind AR: A physiological criterion for setting thermal environmental limits for everyday work, *J Appl Physiol* 16:51-56, 1963.

88. Margaria R, Camporesi E, Aghemo P, Sassi G: The effect of O_2 breathing on maximal aerobic power, *Pflugers Arch* 336:225-230, 1972.

89. Maresh CM, Noble BJ, Robertson KL, Sime WE: Maximal exercise during hypobaric hypoxia (447 Torr) in moderate-altitude natives, *Med Sci Sports Exerc* 15:360-365, 1983.

90. Mazzeo RS, Brooks GA, Butterfield GE et al: ß-Adrenergic blockade does not prevent the lactate response to exercise after acclimatization to high altitude, *J Appl Physiol* 76(2):610-615, 1994.

91. McLellan T, Jacobs I, Lewis W: Acute altitude exposure and altered acid-base balance, *Eur J Appl Physiol* 57:445-451, 1988.

92. Millard-Stafford M, Sparling PB, Rosskopf LB et al: Carbohydrate-electrolyte replacement during a simulated triathlon in the heat, *Med Sci Sports Exerc* 22(5):621-628, 1990.

93. Millard-Stafford M, Sparling PB, Rosskopf LB, Dicarlo LJ: Carbohydrate-electrolyte replacement improves distance running performance in the heat, *Med Sci Sports Exerc* 24(8):934-940, 1992.

94. Montain SJ, Coyle EF: Fluid ingestion during exercise increases skin blood flow independent of increases in blood volume, *J Appl Physiol* 73(3):903-910, 1992.

REFERENCES—Cont'd

95. Muza SR: Hyperbaric physiology and human performance. In Pandolf KB, Sawka MN, Gonzalez RR: *Human physiology and environmental medicine at terrestrial extremes,* Carmel, California, 1986, Cooper Publishing Group.

96. Nadel ER, Bullard RW, Stolwijk JAJ: Importance of skin temperature in the regulation of sweating, *J Appl Physiol* 31:80-87, 1971.

97. Nadel ER, Mitchell JW, Stolwijk JAJ: Differential thermal sensitivity in the human skin, *Pflugers Arch* 340:71-76, 1973.

98. Nadel ER, Pandolf KB, Roberts MF, Stolwijk JAJ: Mechanism of thermal activation to exercise and heat, *J Appl Physiol* 37:515-520, 1974.

99. Nadel ER, Holmer E, Bergh U et al: Energy exchanges of swimming man, *J Appl Physiol* 36:465-471, 1974.

100. Nadel ER, Fortney SF, Wenger CB: Circulatory and thermal regulations during exercise, *Fed Proc* 39:1491-1497, 1980.

101. Nielsen B, Nielsen M: Body temperature during work at different environmental temperatures, *Acta Physiol Scand* 56:120-129, 1962.

102. Nielsen B, Savard G, Richter EA et al: Muscle blood flow and muscle metabolism during exercise and heat stress, *J Appl Physiol* 69(3):1040-1046, 1990.

103. Nishiyasu T, Shi X, Gillen CM et al: Comparison of the forearm and calf blood flow response to thermal stress during dynamic exercise, *Med Sci Sports Exerc* 24(2):213-217, 1992.

104. Noakes TD: Fluid replacement during exercise, *Exerc Sport Sci Rev* 21:297-330, 1993.

105. Noakes TD, Myburgh KH, DuPlessis J et al: Metabolic rate, not percent dehydration, predicts rectal temperature in marathon runners, *Med Sci Sports Exerc* 23(4):443-449, 1991.

106. Nose H, Mack GW, Shi X, Nadel ER: Role of osmolality and plasma volume during rehydration in humans, *J Appl Physiol* 65:325-331, 1988.

107. Owen MD, Kregel KC, Wall PT, Gisolfi CV: Effects of ingesting carbohydrate beverages during exercise in the heat, *Med Sci Sports Exerc* 18(5):568-575, 1986.

108. Pandolf KB: Effects of physical training and cardiorespiratory fitness on exercise-heat tolerance: recent observations, *Med Sci Sports Exerc* 11:60-65, 1979.

109. Pandolf KB: Air quality and human performance. In Pandolf KB, Sawka MN, Gonzalez RR: *Human physiology and environmental medicine at terrestrial extremes,* Carmel, California, 1986, Cooper Publishing Group.

110. Pate RR: Special considerations for exercise in cold weather, *Gatorade Sports Sci Exchange* 10(1):1-5, 1988.

111. Paterson DJ, Pinnington H, Pearce AR, Morton AL: Maximal exercise cardiorespiratory responses of men and women during acute exposure to hypoxia, *Aviat Space Environ Med* 58:243-247, 1987.

112. Pierson WE, Covert DS, Koenig JQ et al: Implications of air pollution effects on athletic performance, *Med Sci Sports Exerc* 18(3):322-327, 1986.

113. Pitts GC, Johnson RE, Consolazio FC: Work in the heat as affected by intake of water, salt and glucose, *Am J Physiol* 142:253-259, 1944.

114. Pivarnik JM, Grafner TR, Elkins ES: Metabolic thermoregulatory, and psychological responses during arm and leg exercise, *Med Sci Sports Exerc* 20(1):1-5, 1988.

115. Pugh LGCE, Gill MB, Lahirim S: Muscular exercise at great altitudes, *J Appl Physiol* 19:431-440, 1964.

116. Ramanathan NL: A new weighting system for mean surface temperature of the human body, *J Appl Physiol* 19:531-533, 1964.

117. Reeves JT, Groves BM, Sutton JR et al: Operation Everest II: preservation of cardiac function at extreme altitude, *J Appl Physiol* 63:531-539, 1987.

118. Reeves JT, Wolfel EE, Green HJ et al: Oxygen transport during exercise at altitude and the lactate paradox: lessons from Operation Everest II and Pike's Peak, *Exerc Sport Sci Rev* 20:275-296, 1992.

119. Reeves JT, Groves BM, Sutton JR et al: Adaptations to hypoxia: lessons from Operation Everest II. In Simmons editor: St. Louis, 1991, Mosby.

120. Rehrer NJ, Beckers EJ, Brouns F et al: Effects of dehydration on gastric emptying and gastrointestinal distress while running, *Med Sci Sports Exerc* 22(6):790-795, 1990.

121. Reynafarje C: Myoglobin content and enzymatic activity of muscle and altitude adaptation, *J Appl Physiol* 17:301, 1962.

122. Ryan AJ, Bleiler TL, Carter JE, Gisolfi CV: Gastric emptying during prolonged cycling exercise in the heat, *Med Sci Sports Exerc* 21(1):51-58, 1989.

123. Saltin B, Grover RF, Blomqvist CG, et al: Maximal oxygen uptake and cardiac output after 2 weeks at 4,300 m, *J Appl Physiol* 25(4):400-409, 1968.

124. Savard GK, Nielsen B, Laszcynska I, et al: Muscle blood flow is not reduced in humans during moderate exercise and heat stress, *J Appl Physiol* 64:649-657, 1988.

125. Sawin CF, Rummel JA, Michel EL: Instrumented personal exercise during long-duration space flights, *Aviat Space Environ Med* 46:394-400, 1975.

REFERENCES—Cont'd

126. Sawka MN, Wenger CB: Physiological responses to acute exercise-heat stress. In Pandolf KB, Sawka MN, Gonzalez RR: *Human physiology and environmental medicine at terrestrial extremes,* Carmel, California, !986, Cooper Publishing Group.

127. Sawka MN: Body fluid responses and hypohydration during exercise-heat stress. In Pandolf KB, Sawka MN, Gonzalez RR: *Human physiology and environmental medicine at terrestrial extremes,* Carmel, California, !986, Cooper Publishing Group.

128. Sawka MN, Young AJ, Latzka WA et al: Human tolerance to heat strain during exercise: influence of hydration, *J Appl Physiol* 73(1):368-375, 1992.

129. Sawka MN: Physiological consequences of hypohydration: exercise performance and thermoregulation, *Med Sci Sports Exerc* 24(6):657-670, 1992.

130. Schoene RB, Roach RC, Hackett PH et al: Operation Everest II: ventilatory adaptation during gradual decompression to extreme altitude, *Med Sci Sports Exerc* 22(6):804-810, 1990.

131. Schooley JC, Mahlmann LJ: Hypoxia and the initiation of erythropoietin production, *Blood Cells* 1:429-448, 1975.

132. Shapiro Y, Seidman DS: Field and clinical observations of exertional heat stroke patients, *Med Sci Sports Exerc* 22(1):6-14, 1990.

133. Sharkey B: *Physiology of fitness,* ed 3, Champaign, Illinois, 1990, Human Kinetics.

134. Smith ML, Raven PB: Cardiovascular responses to lower body negative pressure in endurance and static exercise–trained men, *Med Sci Sports Exerc* 18(5):545-550, 1986.

135. Smith ML, Hudson DL, Raven PB: Effects of muscle tension on the cardiovascular responses to lower body negative pressure in man, *Med Sci Sports Exerc* 19(5):436-442, 1987.

136. Smith RM, Hanna JM: Skinfolds and resting heat loss in cold air and water: temperature equivalence, *J Appl Physiol* 39:93-102, 1975.

137. Springer C, Barstow TJ, Wasserman K, Cooper DM: Oxygen uptake and heart rate responses during exercise in children and adults, *Med Sci Sports Exerc* 23(1):71-79, 1991.

138. Squires RW, Buskirk ER: Aerobic capacity during acute exposure to simulated altitude, 914-2,286 meters, *Med Sci Sports Exerc* 14:36, 1982.

139. Stager JM, Tucker A, Cordain L et al: Normoxic and acute hypoxic exercise tolerance in man following acetazolamide, *Med Sci Sports Exerc* 22(2):178-184, 1990.

140. Stenberg J: Hemodynamic response to work at simulated altitude 4000m, *J Appl Physiol* 21:1589, 1966.

141. Stephensen LA, Kolka MA: Thermoregulation in women, *Exerc Sports Sci Rev* 21:231-262, 1993.

142. Stevens GHJ, Foresman BH, Shi X et al: Reduction in LBNP tolerance following prolonged endurance exercise training, *Med Sci Sports Exerc* 24(11):1235-1244, 1992.

143. Sutton JR, Coates G: Pathophysiology of high-altitude illnesses, *Exerc Sports Sci Rev* 111:210-231, 1983.

144. Sutton JR, Reeves JT, Wagner PD et al: Operation Everest II: oxygen transport during exercise at extreme simulated altitude, *J Appl Physiol* 64(4):1309-1321, 1988.

145. Sutton JR: Exercise training at high altitude: does it improve endurance performance at sea level? *Gatorade Sports Sci Exchange* 6(4):1-4, 1993.

146. Swenson ER, Highes JMB: Effects of acute and chronic acetozolamide on resting ventilation and ventilatory responses in men, *J Appl Physiol* 74(1):230-237, 1993.

147. Terrados N, Melichna J, Sylven C et al: Effects of training at simulated altitude on performance and muscle metabolic capacity in competitive road cyclists, *Eur J Appl Physiol* 57:203-209, 1988.

148. Terrados N, Jansson E, Sylven C, Kaijser L: Is hypoxia a stimulus for synthesis of oxidative enzymes and myoglobin? *J Appl Physiol* 68:2369-2372, 1990.

149. Thaysen JH, Schwartz IL: Fatigue of the sweat glands, *Clin Sci* 1719-1725, 1955.

150. Thornton WE, Rummel JA: Muscular deconditioning and its prevention in space flight. In Johnson RS, Dietlen SF, editors: *Biomedical results from Skylab.* Washington, DC, 1977, National Aeronautics and Space Administration.

151. Toner MM, McArdle WD: Physiological adjustments of man to the cold. In Pandolf KB, Sawka MN, Gonzalez RR: *Human physiology and environmental medicine at terrestrial extremes,* Carmel, California, 1986, Cooper Publishing Group.

152. Tripathi A, Mack GW, Nadel ER: Cutaneous vascular reflexes during exercise in the heat, *Med Sci Sports Exerc* 22(6):796-803, 1990.

153. Wagner PD, Gale GE, Moon RE et al: Pulmonary gas exchange in humans exercising at sea level and simulated altitude, *J Appl Physiol* 61:260-270, 1986.

154. Wagner PD, Sutton JR, Reeves JT et al: Operation Everest II: pulmonary gas exchange during a simulated ascent of Mt. Everest, *J Appl Physiol* 63(6):2348-2359, 1987.

155. Welsh CH, Wagner PD, Reeves JT et al: Operation Everest II: spirometric and radiographic changes in acclimatized humans at simulated high altitudes, *Am Rev Respir Dis* 147:1239-1244, 1993.

156. Wolfel EE, Groves BM, Brooks GA et al: Oxygen transport during steady state submaximal exercise in chronic hypoxia, *J Appl Physiol* 70(3):1129-1136, 1991.

REFERENCES—Cont'd

157. Wronski TJ, Morey ER: Alterations in calcium homeostasis and bone during actual and simulated space flight, *Med Sci Sports Exerc* 15:410-414, 1983.

158. Young AJ: Human adaptation to cold. In Pandolf KB, Sawka MN, Gonzalez RR: *Human physiology and environmental medicine at terrestrial extremes,* Carmel, California, 1986, Cooper Publishing Group.

159. Young AJ, Young PM: Human acclimatization to high terrestrial altitude. In Pandolf KB, Sawka MN, Gonzalez RR, editors: *Human physiology and environmental medicine at terrestrial extremes,* Carmel, California, 1986, Cooper Publishing Group.

160. Young AJ, Young PM: Human acclimatization to high terrestrial altitude. In Pandolf KB, Sawka MN, Gonzalez RR, editors: *Human performance physiology and environmental medicine at terrestrial extremes,* Indianapolis, 1988, Benchmark Press.

161. Young AJ: Energy substrate utilization during exercise in extreme environments, *Exerc Sports Sci Rev* 18:65-117, 1990.

RECOMMENDED READINGS

■ Adams WC, Mack GW, Langhans GW, Nadel ER: Effects of equivalent sea-level and altitude training on VO_2max and running performance, *J Appl Physiol* 39:262, 1975.

■ Anderson HT, Smeland EB, Owe JO, Myhre K: Analyses of maximum cardiopulmonary performance during exposure to acute hypoxia at simulated altitude-sea level to 5000 meters (760-404 mm Hg), *Aviat Space Environ Med* 56:1192-1197, 1985.

■ Armstrong LE, Hubbard RW, DeLuca JP, Christensen EL: Heat acclimatization during summer running in the United States, *Med Sci Sports Exerc* 19(2):131-136, 1987.

■ Barr SI, Costill DL, Fink WJ: Fluid replacement during prolonged exercise: effects of water, saline, or no fluid, *Med Sci Sports Exerc* 23(7):811-817, 1991.

■ Bender PR, Groves BM, McCullough RE et al: Oxygen transport to exercising leg in chronic hypoxia, *J Appl Physiol* 65(6):2592-2597, 1988.

■ Convertino VA: Physiological adaptations to weightless: effects of exercise and work performance, *Exer Sports Sci Rev* 18:119-166, 1990.

■ Cymerman A, Reeves JT, Sutton JR et al: Operation Everest II: maximal oxygen uptake at extreme altitude, *J Appl Physiol* 66:2446-2453, 1989.

■ Fagraeus L, Karlsson J, Linnarson D, Saltin B: Oxygen uptake during maximal work at lowered and raised ambient air pressures, *Acta Physiol Scand* 87:411-421, 1973.

■ Gisolfi CV, Duchman SM: Guidelines for optimal replacement beverages for different athletic events, *Med Sci Sports Exerc* 24(6):679-687, 1992.

■ Green HJ, Sutton JR, Wolfel EE et al: Altitude acclimatization and energy metabolic adaptations in skeletal muscle during exercise, *J Appl Physiol* 73(6):2701-2708, 1992.

■ Horstman DH, Weiskopf R, Jackson RE: Work capacity during 3-week sojourn at 4,300 m: effects of relative polycythemia, *J Appl Physiol* 49:311-318, 1980.

■ Klausen T, Mohr T, Ghisler U, Nelson OJ: Maximal oxygen uptake and erythropoietic responses after altitude training at moderate altitude, *Eur J Appl Physiol* 62:376-379, 1991.

■ Levine BD, Stray-Gunderson J: A practical approach to altitude training: where to live and train for optimal performance enhancement, *Int J Sports Med* 13:S209-S212, 1992.

■ Maresh CM, Noble BJ, Robertson KL, Sime WE: Maximal exercise during hypobaric hypoxia (447 Torr) in moderate-altitude natives, *Med Sci Sports Exerc* 15:360-365, 1983.

■ Muza SR: Hyperbaric physiology and human performance. In Pandolf KB, Sawka MN, Gonzalez RR: *Human physiology and environmental medicine at terrestrial extremes,* Carmel, California, 1986, Cooper Publishing Group.

■ Nadel ER, Fortney SF, Wenger CB: Circulatory and thermal regulations during exercise, *Fed Proc* 39:1491-1497, 1980.

■ Noakes TD: Fluid replacement during exercise, *Exerc Sports Sci Rev* 21:297-330, 1993.

■ Noakes TD, Myburgh KH, Du Plessis J et al: Metabolic rate, not percent dehydration, predicts rectal temperature in marathon runners, *Med Sci Sports Exerc* 23(4):443-449, 1991.

RECOMMENDED READINGS—Cont'd

■ Nose H, Mack GW, Shi X, Nadel ER: Role of osmolality and plasma volume during rehydration in humans, *J Appl Physiol* 65:325-331, 1988.

■ Pandolf KB: Effects of physical training and cardiorespiratory fitness on exercise-heat tolerance: recent observations, *Med Sci Sports Exerc* 11:60-65, 1979.

■ Pierson WE, Covert DS, Koenig JQ et al: Implications of air pollution effects on athletic performance, *Med Sci Sports Exerc* 18(3):322-327, 1986.

■ Pitts GC, Johnson RE, Consolazio FC: Work in the heat as affected by intake of water, salt and glucose, *Am J Physiol* 142:253-259, 1944.

■ Reeves JT, Wolfel EE, Green HJ et al: Oxygen transport during exercise at altitude and the lactate paradox: lessons from Operation Everest II and Pike's Peak, *Exer Sports Sci Rev* 20:275-296, 1992.

■ Saltin B, Grover RF, Blomqvist CG et al: Maximal oxygen uptake and cardiac output after 2 weeks at 4,300 m, *J Appl Physiol* 45:400-409, 1968.

■ Sawin CF, Rummel JA, Michel EL: Instrumented personal exercise during long-duration space flights, *Aviat Space Environ Med* 46:394-400, 1975.

■ Sawka MN, Young AJ, Latzka WA et al: Human tolerance to heat strain during exercise: influence of hydration, *J Appl Physiol* 73(1):368-375, 1992.

■ Schoene RB, Roach RC, Hackett PH et al: Operation Everest II: ventilatory adaptation during gradual decompression to extreme altitude, *Med Sci Sports Exerc* 22(6):804-810, 1990.

■ Wagner PD, Gale GE, Moon RE et al: Pulmonary gas exchange in humans exercising at sea level and stimulated altitude, *J Appl Physiol* 61:260-270, 1986.

■ Wolfel EE, Groves BM, Brooks GA et al: Oxygen transport during steady state submaximal exercise in chronic hypoxia, *J Appl Physiol* 70(3):1129-1136, 1991.

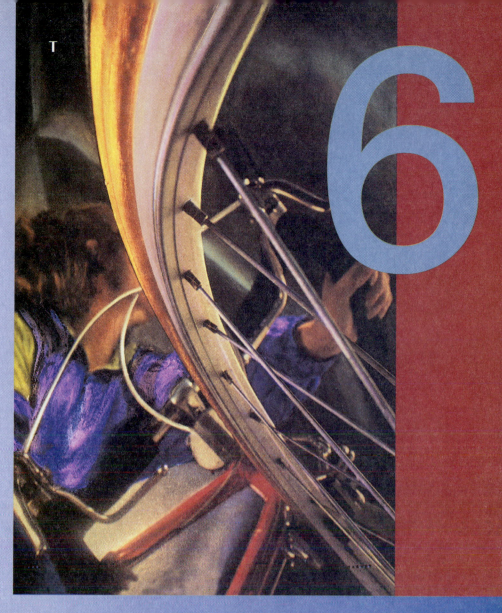

6

Exercise
and Health

CHAPTER 27

Exercise, Health, and Disease

OBJECTIVES

After studying this chapter you should be able to:

- Explain the role of exercise in the treatment and prevention of selected chronic diseases.

- List specific recommendations for exercise training for selected chronic diseases.

- Explain the epidemiology of atherosclerosis.

- Describe the current understanding of the possibility of reversing heart disease.

- Identify some important health promotion and disease prevention strategies for adults.

KEY TERMS

epidemiology

mortality

all-cause mortality

cause-specific mortality

coronary artery disease (CAD)

atherosclerosis

primary risk factors

secondary risk factors

angina pectoris

coronary artery bypass grafting (CABG)

percutaneous transluminal coronary angioplasty (PTCA)

cardiac rehabilitation

stroke

cerebrovascular accidents (CVAs)

transient ischemic attacks (TIAs)

peripheral vascular disease (PVD)

bronchitis

emphysema

chronic obstructive pulmonary disease (COPD)

osteoarthritis

rheumatoid arthritis

The benefits of regular physical activity and exercise have been the subject of provocative thoughts and intellectual curiosity for hundreds of years, as evidenced by the following quotes:

Parts of the body unused and left idle
become liable to disease, defective in
growth, and age quickly.—Hippocrates

Anyone contemplating an inactive lifestyle
should have a through physical exam to
see if his body can withstand it.—P-O Åstrand

Today, few would debate the benefits of physical activity to personal health. With the plethora of literature available, it appears that individuals who choose to be more physically active, in both their leisure and work activities, lower their risk for developing certain degenerative diseases, such as osteoporosis, diabetes, obesity, and cardiovascular diseases. Many organizations have realized the importance of regular exercise and have published major policy statements. In 1989 the United States Preventive Services Task Force concluded that the evidence linking exercise and health was strong enough to issue recommendations so that physicians could better counsel their patients.[29] Other major policy statements are presented in earlier chapters. The purpose of this chapter is to summarize the research that has established the important connections between exercise and prevention of some diseases, identify these diseases, and highlight why exercise is so beneficial for optimizing health.

Physical Activity, Health, and Disease

The **epidemiology** of the study of physical activity and morbidity and mortality had its origins in London, England. In the 1950s and 1960s, Jeremy Morris studied the association between physical activity during work and the rate of cardiovascular disease. Morris began by comparing the rate and severity of cardiovascular disease of London bus conductors, who had to walk up and down the stairs and aisles of double-decker buses collecting tickets, with bus drivers who sat most of day. Morris found that the conductors were more physically fit and had a lower incidence of coronary heart disease than the drivers. In addition, the conductors had a reduced fatality rate and a lower rate of early mortality from the disease.[41] Morris found similar findings when comparing the leisure-time exercise habits of civil servants.[42] Based on his early findings, Morris concluded the following:

Physical activity of work provides protection against ischaemic heart disease. Men in physically active jobs have less ischaemic heart disease during middle age, what disease they have is less severe, and they tend to develop it later than similar men in physically inactive jobs.[43]

Between 1951 and 1972, Paffenbarger et al. followed the work activity levels and coronary heart disease records of San Francisco longshoremen.[47] Paffenbarger et al. found that the men who expended 8500 or more kilocalories per week at

epidemiology (ep-i-de-mi-ol'o-ji)
the study of the presence and spread of disease in a community.

work had significantly less risk of fatal coronary heart disease risk at any age than men whose jobs required less energy expenditure. These authors later looked at leisure-time physical activity versus work-related physical activity and risk for coronary heart disease. Paffenbarger et al. compared the levels of habitual and leisure-time physical activity of 16,936 Harvard University alumni between the years 1962 and 1972. Once again a clear pattern of age-specific decreased rates of coronary heart disease and **mortality** was seen with an increase in energy expenditure, especially in the group expending more than 2000 kilocalories per week.[48]

Since the studies of London bus conductors in the early 1950s and the work of Paffenbarger in the 1960s and 1970s, the epidemiology of leisure and occupational activity, health, and disease has been investigated in hundreds of locations and occupations around the world. The consensus of the evidence from these studies is that physical activity has a protective effect against disease. More recently, Blair et al. studied the

association between physical fitness and risk of **all-cause** and **cause-specific mortality** in 10,224 men and 3120 women.[11] After an 8-year follow-up, higher levels of physical fitness delayed all-cause mortality, primarily because of lowered rates of cardiovascular disease and cancer (Figure 27.1).

The study of the association between regular physical activity and health and disease has continued to grow in recent years to include various chronic diseases, in addition to cardiovascular disease and cancer. There currently exists substantial evidence demonstrating the protective effect of exercise against various chronic diseases (Table 27.1).[37] The promotion of regular physical activity, including exercise, has truly become a national public health priority. An increase in the number of individuals who are habitually physically active could have a staggering impact on disease reduction and prevention, savings in health care costs, and reduced morbidity and mortality from chronic diseases.

FIGURE 27.1

Age-adjusted cause-specific death rates per 10,000 person-years of follow-up (1970 to 1985) by physical fitness levels. (Data from Blair SN et al: *JAMA* 262:2395, 1989.)

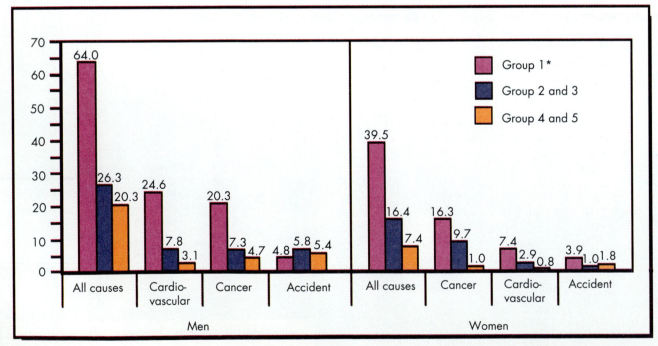

Group 1* = least fit Group and
Group 5   = most fit Group

TABLE 27.1

Summary of results of studies investigating the relationship between physical activity or physical fitness and incidences of selected chronic diseases*

DISEASE OR CONDITION	NUMBER OF STUDIES	TRENDS ACROSS ACTIVITY OR FITNESS CATEGORIES AND STRENGTH OF EVIDENCE
All-cause mortality	***	↓↓↓
Coronary artery disease	***	↓↓↓
Hypertension	**	↓↓
Obesity	***	↓↓
Stroke	**	↓
Peripheral vascular disease	*	→
Cancer		
Colon	***	↓↓
Rectal	***	→
Stomach	*	→
Breast	*	↓
Prostate	**	↓
Lung	*	↓
Pancreatic	*	→
Non-insulin dependent diabetes	*	↓↓
Osteoarthritis	*	→
Osteoporosis	**	↓↓

From Kenney WL, editor: *ACSM's guidelines for exercise testing and prescription,* ed 5, Philadelphia, 1995, Williams & Wilkins.

*Few studies, probably <5; ** approximately 5-10 studies; *** >10 studies.

→ No apparent difference in disease rates across activity or fitness categories; ↓ some evidence of reduced disease rates across activity or fitness categories; ↓↓ good evidence of reduced disease rates across activity or fitness categories, control of potential confounders, good methods, some evidence of biological mechanisms; ↓↓↓ excellent evidence of reduced disease rates across activity or fitness categories, good control of potential confounders, excellent methods, extensive evidence of biological mechanisms, relationship is considered causal.

Exercise and Cardiovascular Disorders

> A man is only as old as his arteries.—William Osler

Cardiovascular disease continues to be the leading cause of death in the Western world (see Figure 24.1).[3] In 1990, diseases of the heart and blood vessels killed 930,000 individuals in the United States, equal to more than two of every five deaths.

The good news is that cardiovascular disease is one of the most preventable diseases, and death rates from cardiovas-

mortality (mor-**tal'**i-ti)
death rate

all-cause mortality
the rate of death from all causes

cause-specific mortality
the rate of death from specific causes

cular disease have been on the decline. From 1980 to 1990, death rates from cardiovascular disease have decreased 26.7% in the United States; the decline has been explained by lifestyle changes among Americans and advances in medical treatments.[3]

Although there are a variety of cardiovascular diseases, including hypertension, stroke, and congestive heart failure, the majority of cardiovascular deaths are attributed to coronary artery disease. **Coronary artery disease (CAD)** results from a condition termed **atherosclerosis.** Atherosclerosis is caused by the narrowing of coronary arteries, which supply the myocardium with blood and oxygen. The narrowing is thought to be caused by several factors that are initiated by injury to the inner lining of the arteries (caused by high blood pressure, high levels of LDL cholesterol, or chemical agents, such as from cigarette smoking). Once the inner lining has been damaged, plaques (consisting of calcified cholesterol and fat deposits) begin to develop and reduce the inner (lumen) diameter of the coronary artery.

Epidemiology of Atherosclerosis and the Detection of Risk Factors

*T*he study of the epidemiology of CAD in the United States began in a small town in Massachusetts. In the late 1940s screening of residents of Framingham began in an effort to determine common patterns or risk factors of cardiovascular disease.[18] Since the start of the Framingham study, hundreds of studies have investigated specific causes of coronary artery disease, and several risk factors for the disease have been conclusively identified.

The risk factors for CAD can be grouped into those that can be prevented or modified and those that cannot be modified. The risk factors that research has proved to directly cause atherosclerosis are termed **primary risk factors**, whereas the risk factors that contribute to the severity of atherosclerosis and CAD are termed **secondary risk factors** (Focus Box 27.1).

Cigarette Smoking

The primary mechanism by which smoking increases CAD risk is through the toxic nature of the smoke, which can injure the inner lining of the artery. In addition, cigarette smoking decreases the oxygen-carrying capacity of the blood and elevates blood pressure, heart rate, and myocardial oxygen consumption. Cigarette smoke has undesirable effects on platelet adhesiveness and clotting factors, resulting in increased clotting potential. Cigarette smokers are at greater risk for developing CAD, as well as for recurrent events with continued smoking. The risk for a heart attack increases with the number of cigarettes smoked per day. There is now evidence linking passive smoke and development of heart disease in nonsmokers.[69] The good news for smokers is that

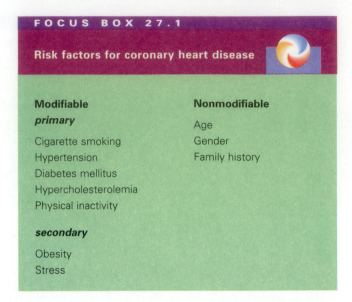

FOCUS BOX 27.1

Risk factors for coronary heart disease

Modifiable	Nonmodifiable
primary	
Cigarette smoking	Age
Hypertension	Gender
Diabetes mellitus	Family history
Hypercholesterolemia	
Physical inactivity	
secondary	
Obesity	
Stress	

within a few years of quitting their risk is reduced to the level of a nonsmoker.[31]

Cholesterol

The association between cholesterol and CAD has been well researched (Focus Box 27.2 and Figure 27.2). In fact, cholesterol abnormalities continue to be the major preventable risk factor for CAD. Early investigations of the association between CAD and cholesterol began with the Framingham Study. Since the beginning of the Framingham Study, numerous observational epidemiologic studies have confirmed that cholesterol is one of the strongest predictors of CAD, and data from the Multiple Risk Factor Intervention Trial (MRFIT) provide strong support for the association among hypercholesterolemia, coronary heart disease, and mortality.[59]

coronary artery disease (CAD)
a common disease resulting from a process known as atherosclerosis

atherosclerosis (ath′er-o-skle-ro′sis)
the condition of irregularly distributed lipid deposits in the intima of large- and medium-sized arteries

primary risk factors
those proved by research to be direct causes of atherosclerosis, including cigarette smoking, hyperlipidemias, inactivity, hypertension, and diabetes

secondary risk factors
those not yet proved to be direct causes of atherosclerosis but that are known to contribute to the disease, including obesity, gender, family history, and age

FOCUS BOX 27.2

Evidence linking lipid abnormalities to CAD

A large body of evidence links hypercholesterolemia to the development of atherosclerosis. The strength of the association is based on research from experimental, epidemiologic, and clinical trails.

Experimental

- Cholesterol present in atherosclerotic plaques

- High dietary cholesterol intake induces atherosclerosis

- Reduction in dietary fat intake causes regression of atherosclerosis

Epidemiologic

- Prevalence of coronary artery disease correlates with dietary cholesterol intake and serum cholesterol levels

- Incidence of coronary disease is low in patients exposed to dietary deprivation or wasting illness

Clinical Trials

- Reduction in dietary fat causes regression of atherosclerosis and slow progression

- Surgical lipid lowering causes regression of atherosclerosis and slows progression

- Pharmacologic lipid modification causes regression of atherosclerosis and reduces incidence of cardiovascular events

FIGURE 27.2

Relation between screening total cholesterol levels and CHD mortality (MRFIT). (Adapted from Stamler JD et al: *JAMA* 322:1700-1707, 1986.)

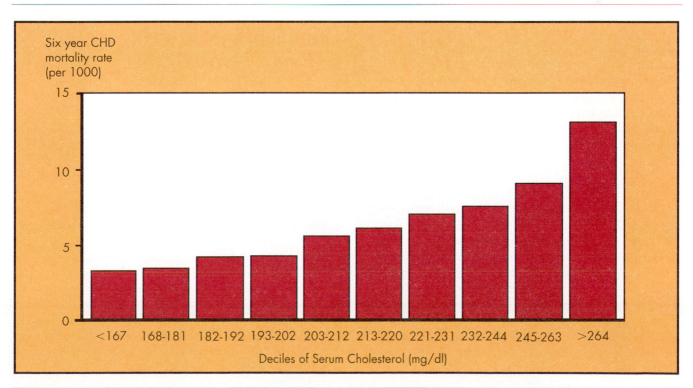

TABLE 27.2	
National Cholesterol Education Guidelines Goals for Cholesterol	
TOTAL CHOLESTEROL	
Desirable cholesterol	<200 mg/dl
Borderline-high cholesterol	200-239 mg/dl
High cholesterol	>240 mg/dl
HDL CHOLESTEROL	
Desirable HDL cholesterol	>35 mg/dl
Low HDL cholesterol	<35 mg/dl
LDL CHOLESTEROL	
Desirable LDL cholesterol	<130 mg/dl
Borderline-high LDL cholesterol	130-159 mg/dl
High LDL cholesterol	>160 mg/dl
Optimal LDL cholesterol	<100 mg/dl

From American Heart Association *J Am Med Assoc* 269:3015-3023, 1993.

The Lipid Research Clinics Coronary Primary Prevention Trial concluded that a 1% decrease in total serum cholesterol level correlated with a 2% decrease in CAD risk, and for each 1 mg/dl increase in HDL there is a 2% decrease in CAD risk for men and 3% for women.[63] It has been clearly established that HDL cholesterol has a protective effect against the development of CAD and that aerobic exercise raises the level of HDL.[60,63] Recent studies have also shown that the detection of lipoprotein particles that contain specific apolipoprotein antigens may prove useful in evaluating CAD risk, although routine testing is not economical at this point. The schedule for cholesterol testing and follow-up has been developed by the National Cholesterol Education Program (NCEP II) and is presented in Table 27.2.

Physical Inactivity

Powell et al. reviewed 43 epidemiologic studies involving physical activity and CAD and found that two thirds of the studies had a significant inverse relationship.[52] As Morris, Paffenbarger, Blair, and others have discovered in their studies, the greater the level of physical activity, expressed by total kilocalories expended per week, the less the risk for CAD. The exact mechanisms relating to a decreased CAD morbidity and mortality with exercise are not entirely clear but are probably related to the favorable effects exercise has on blood pressure, obesity, diabetes, hypercholesterolemia, and fibrinolytic activity.

Diabetes

Diabetes mellitus, especially type II or adult–onset diabetes, is often associated with obesity, hypercholesterolemia, hypertension, elevated LDL levels, and depressed HDL cholesterol levels. Coronary artery disease is the most common underlying cause of death in diabetic adults in the United States.[38] The risk of various heart diseases is twofold for diabetic men and threefold for diabetic women.

Blood Pressure

Hypertension is a major risk factor for CAD. Chronically elevated blood pressures are believed to alter blood flow patterns, which affects endothelial surfaces and may eventually cause an injury to the inner lining, beginning the atherosclerotic process. There is a continuous and direct association between risk of morbidity and mortality from coronary heart disease and increasing levels of blood pressure.[40] Hypertension is also a major risk factor for stroke.

Obesity

Although not a primary risk factor for CAD, obesity is now recognized as an independent risk factor. Fat distribution is another predictor of CAD risk. The ratio of waist–to–hip circumference correlates more closely with increased risk than do other parameters of obesity. In addition, individuals who carry excessive amounts of fat on their trunks (android obesity) have greater risk for CAD than individuals who carry fat lower on their body (gynoid obesity).

Pathophysiology of Atherosclerosis

Atherosclerosis develops as a result of adverse alterations in the arterial vasculature system (mainly in the majority of medium and larger arteries). Such adverse alterations may eventually lead to an inability of the arterial system to meet local and regional metabolic demands. When atherosclerosis affects the coronary arteries, clinical manifestations of this imbalance include ischemia, angina, and myocardial ischemia (heart attack). Other areas commonly affected by atherosclerosis include the carotid arteries, resulting in peripheral claudication.

Certain risk factors (e.g., hyperlipidemia, smoking) are directly related to the development of atherosclerotic plaques. When one or more risk factors are present, a cascade of events is triggered that eventually leads to plaque formation (Figure 27.3). Atherosclerotic plaques form as a response to injury of the inner lining of the arterial wall. The endothelial injury can be the result of hypertension, hypercholesterolemia, circulating vasoactive amines, viral infections, or

FIGURE 27.3

Response-to-injury hypothesis. (From Ross R, Glomset JA: The pathogenisis of atherosclerosis, *N Engl J Med* 295:369-377, 420-425, 1976.)

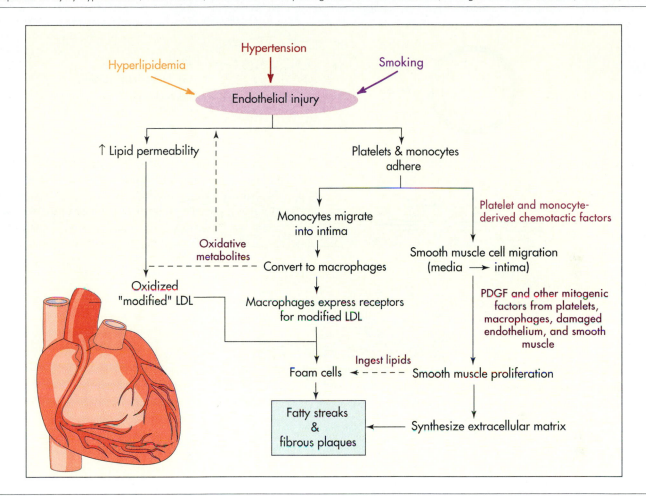

chemical irritants in tobacco smoke. If the injury is transient (an individual is identified with high cholesterol, but it is discovered early in life and decreased with diet therapy), the lesion will regress and not evolve into a plaque. However, if the injury is chronic (25-year history of smoking), the endothelial lining begins to respond to the chronic insult in an effort to repair the lesion.

The response-to-injury hypothesis best describes the events that lead to plaque formation (Figure 27.4).[56] Vascular injury to the endothelial lining of the artery triggers the repair process that eventually promotes deposition and adherence of monocytes and platelets. In response to injury and chronically elevated levels of LDL, monocytes cross the endothelium and accumulate in the subendothelial space, where they are transformed into macrophages and foam cells. Foam cells release toxic substances known as free radicals, which cause further injury to the endothelial lining. The presence of monocytes in the intima is considered the earliest event in experimental atherosclerosis.[56] Monocytes and

macrophages release enzymes that promote LDL oxidation, which leads to further endothelial injury.

The next step in plaque formation involves the release of platelet-derived growth factor (PDGF) from monocytes and platelets. Circulating platelets seem to adhere to the lesion, after which they stimulate migration and proliferation of smooth muscle cells (SMCs) through the release of PDGF. The migration of smooth muscle cells to the injury site is unfortunate, since SMCs have the ability to proliferate and synthesize large amounts of collagen, elastin, and proteoglycans. These substances assist with the development of the complex matrix that is the mature plaque.

The final stage of plaque formation is the development of the extracellular matrix. With increased synthesis of PDGF and SMCs, the plaque evolves into a complex matrix of fat, cholesterol crystals, degenerating cells, and lipoproteins. Rupture of complex atherosclerotic plaques causes occlusive thrombi, which eventually cut off blood supply to the myocardium and cause a myocardial infarction.

FIGURE 27.4

Changes (in order of progression) in the arterial wall with injury, illustrating the disruption of the endothelium and the subsequent alterations. (From Pollock ML, Wilmore JH: *Exercise in health and disease,* Philadelphia, 1990, Saunders.)

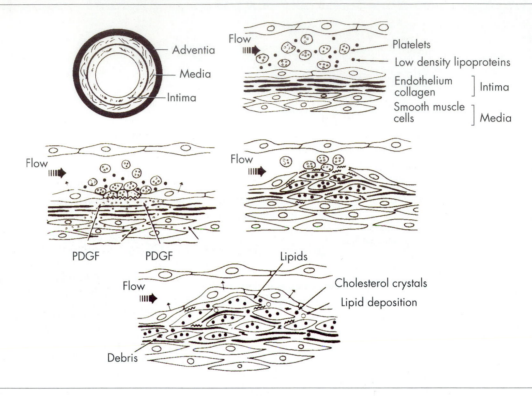

Treatment of Coronary Artery Disease

When coronary blood flow cannot meet the heart's demand for oxygen, an individual typically feels chest pressure or chest pain. Chest pain caused by lack of blood flow to the heart, termed *ischemia,* is intense or dull and sometimes radiates into the neck, jaw, left shoulder, or left arm. The transient symptoms of inadequate blood flow to the heart are referred to as **angina pectoris.** Angina pectoris can be caused by a temporary blockage or permanent blockage. A permanent blockage is dangerous because clots can form at these narrowed sections and result in a myocardial infarction.

If a permanent blockage is detected in one or more coronary arteries, the typical treatments include medical management; **coronary artery bypass grafting (CABG); percutaneous transluminal coronary angioplasty (PTCA);** other new forms of plaque removal, such as coronary laser (burning the plaque) and high-speed rotational

angina pectoris

severe pain about the heart, usually radiating to the left shoulder and down the left arm. Angina pectoris is caused by ischemia resulting from a temporary blockage or permanent blockage in one or more coronary arteries

coronary artery bypass grafting (CABG)

a major surgical procedure in which grafts of veins are harvested from the leg or arm and grafted from the aorta to a point past the blockage of one or more of the coronary arteries

percutaneous transluminal coronary angioplasty (PTCA)

an invasive procedure in which a specialized catheter is advanced through an artery (usually femoral) into a coronary artery to the atherosclerotic plaque. Once placed correctly, a small balloon is inflated until the plaque is compressed against the walls of the artery atherectomy (cutting and removing the plaque); and to a lesser degree, prescription of life-style modifications.

CABG (a procedure in which veins are harvested from a patient's leg and sewn from the aorta to the coronary artery to bypass the blockage) appears to prolong life in patients with severe three-vessel disease, but in comparison with medical therapy, it does not seem to prolong life in patients with less severe disease. However, total relief of angina typically occurs in 60% to 75% of patients during the 5 years after a CABG.

Percutaneous transluminal coronary angioplasty (PCTA), a procedure that uses a small balloon at the tip of a heart catheter to push open plaques, is on the rise. Unfortunately, approximately 30% of patients receiving a successful PTCA have a reocclusion within 3 to 6 months. Less severe cases of coronary artery disease are typically treated with life-style modification and medical therapy.

Can Coronary Atherosclerosis Be Reversed?

For decades physicians denied that coronary heart disease could be cured, let alone reversed. However, evidence is accumulating that human atherosclerosis is not only preventable, but to some extent reversible; at least the progression can be delayed.[13,34,39,46,68] Typically, regression or lack of progression is defined via coronary angiography, before and after some type of intervention. The most common interventions include surgery, life-style modification (e.g., diet, exercise, stress reduction), diet alone, and lipid-lowering medication.

Probably the first published article reporting reversal of atherosclerosis came from retrospective study of postmortem examinations of World War I casualties killed in battle and dying after spending time in prisoner of war camps.[7] The soldiers who spent time in war camps had significantly less coronary artery disease, thought to be the result of the semi-starvation conditions. Less severe coronary artery disease has been demonstrated in persons who have lost significant weight before they died compared with persons without such weight loss; animals who were fed a high-fat diet but exercised compared with animals that ate a high-fat diet without exercising; and persons who followed structured lifestyle or received pharmacologic interventions versus those who did not.*

The STARS trial was a prospective randomized trial of diet and cholestyramine (blood cholesterol–lowering medication) with angiography to assess coronary artery lesions at baseline and again 3 years later.[68] Progression of coronary narrowing was observed in 46% of the patients in the conventional care group only (no formal dietary counseling) and only 15% in the lipid-lowering diet group (fat intake decreased more than 27% and total cholesterol 100 mg/1000 kcal). In the lipid-lowering group, cholesterol level fell from 277 to 238 mg/dl versus 273 to 267 mg/dl in the conventional care group. The mean absolute width of arterial narrowing decreased by 0.2 mm. This study concluded that a diet low in saturated fat and cholesterol reduces serum cholesterol and retards the progression of coronary artery disease.

Lichtlen used coronary angiography to evaluate the progression of coronary artery disease over a 3-year period in 230 patients.[39] At baseline, 838 of the patients tested had coronary narrowing and 135 had total coronary occlusions. Average serum cholesterol level was 261 mg/dl. About 80% of the patients were smokers.[184] At follow-up evaluation, 82 patients with preexisting coronary narrowing showed increased progression to complete occlusion, 144 had newly formed narrowing, and 10 had new total occlusions. Altogether 129 (56.1%) of the patients had definite progression of coronary artery disease during the 3-year study. Risk factor analysis revealed a strong correlation between formation of new lesions and smoking and between progression of existing lesions and total cholesterol level.

Haskell et al. recently reported the results of a 4-year angiographic follow-up study involving 246 patients with documented CAD. Of the 246 patients, 119 received intervention consisting of a prescribed diet (23.8% fat, 6.8% saturated fat, and cholesterol intake of 143 mg/day), regular physical activity, and behavioral modification training, plus hypolipidemic drugs as necessary. The rest of the group received standard treatment for CAD. At follow-up, LDL cholesterol concentration fell by 20% in the intervention group versus 4% in the control group. The rate of progression of CAD in the intervention group was 58% less in the intervention group compared with the control group. Finally, 20% of intervention patients demonstrated regression compared with 10% in the control group.

Schuler et al. reported the results of a 1-year randomized follow-up in patients with documented CAD.[57] Fifty-six patients received an intervention consisting of a prescribed diet (less than 20% fat and less than 200 mg/day cholesterol) and 3 to 5 hours of moderate exercise training, whereas the control group received usual care for CAD. After 1 year, total cholesterol fell by 10%, triglycerides by 24%, and LDL by 8%, whereas HDL increased by 5% in the intervention group. In the intervention group, 90% showed no change or reversal of CAD compared with only 55% in the control group.

It appears from the results of recent research that aggressively modifying lipid levels in individuals who have established CAD can delay and even reverse atherosclerosis. Lowering of low-density lipoprotein (LDL) cholesterol levels to 100 mg/dl or less appears to be a threshold at which atherosclerotic disease can be delayed or reversed. Further research is needed to identify other variables besides cholesterol that may help retard atherosclerosis.

---

*References 13, 34, 39, 46, 68, 70 and 72.

Programs for Reversing Heart Disease

Hellerstein, in his book *Healing Your Heart: A Proven Program for Reversing Heart Disease,* shares the findings of his 58-year career. Hellerstein believes that coronary heart disease can be reversed through life-style modification. He recommends a seven-item program of sensible life-style changes that people can easily make and live with (Figure 27.5). Hellerstein's recommendations are based on his own research, as well as other major research projects.

Goals for reversing coronary heart disease

1. Reduce total cholesterol to below 200 mg/dl and LDL to below 130 mg/dl, with a total cholesterol/HDL ratio of 3.5. Diet recommendations—1500 to 2500 calories per day, with saturated fat content under 10% and total fat less than 30% of total calories, and 50 to 100 mg cholesterol per day.

2. Achieve a resting blood pressure of 140/90 mm Hg or better.

3. Burn at least 150 to 300 calories per day through aerobic exercise.

4. Maintain a normal body weight.

5. Reduce the stress in your life.

6. Do not use tobacco.

7. Maintain normal blood sugar levels.

Ornish claims that he is the first to prove scientifically that heart disease is reversible. In his Lifestyle Heart Trial, Ornish set out to determine the effects of life-style modification on coronary heart disease.[46] Ornish placed 28 patients on a comprehensive life-style modification program. Another group of 20 received standard medical care. Both groups had an initial coronary angiogram to assess the amount of blockage and

another angiogram 1 year later. After 1 year the group that followed the life-style modification program showed a significant overall regression of coronary atherosclerosis (40% to 37.8%) as measured by coronary angiography. The group that was following a less stringent life-style modification program showed significant overall progression of coronary artery blockage (42.7% to 46.1%).

Ornish's program for reversing coronary heart disease.

1. The Ornish diet recommendations include:

   a. Low-fat (10% of daily calories)

   b. Low cholesterol (5 mg/day)

   c. No animal products, except egg whites and 1 cup of nonfat milk or yogurt

   d. High intake of complex carbohydrates (70% to 75% of daily calories)

   e. No caffeine and no more than two units of alcohol per day

2. No smoking

3. Moderate exercise (3 hours/week for a minimum of 30 minutes per session at an intensity of 50% to 80% of the training heart rate)

4. About 1 hour per day of stress management techniques, including:

   a. Stretching

   b. Meditation

   c. Progressive relaxation exercises

   d. Deep-breathing exercises

Role of Exercise and Coronary Artery Disease

Clearly, regular physical activity reduces the risk of CAD. How effective is exercise at treating CAD? Initially, extended bed rest was recommended for patients recovering from a myocardial infarction. The thinking was that the heart takes approximately 6 weeks to heal after a heart attack and that any undue stress might compro-

mise the healing process. However, bed rest results in a decrease in work capacity, a decreased cardiovascular adaptability to changes in posture, a decrease in blood volume, a decrease in muscle mass, an increase in risk for thromboembolism, and a decrease in respiratory and pulmonary function (Figure 27.5).

In the early 1940s, physicians began experimenting with early mobilization after a cardiac event and the results were favorable. Early mobilization of cardiac patients resulted in

FIGURE 27.5

Changes in maximal oxygen uptake with bed rest and training. (Adapted from Saltin B et al: *Circulation 37-38*, Suppl 7: 1, 1968.)

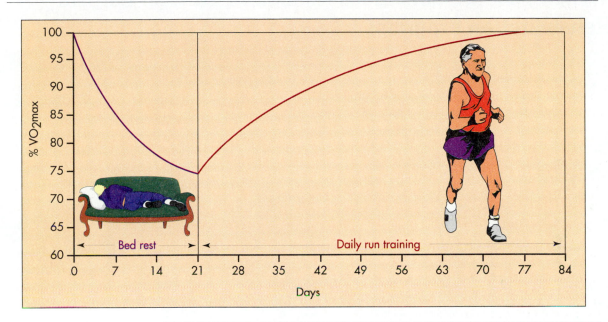

fewer complications, a faster recovery, and a reduction in many of the other previously listed complications of bed rest. Today, exercise is a standard therapeutic modality in the treatment of cardiac disease. In almost all cases, individuals recovering from a myocardial infarction, cardiac surgery, or other cardiac procedure benefit from a supervised cardiac rehabilitation program.

Overview of Cardiac Rehabilitation

The comprehensive rehabilitation of patients with cardiac disease is collectively referred to as **cardiac rehabilitation.** Cardiac rehabilitation is defined as the process by which persons with cardiovascular disease, including but not limited to patients with coronary heart disease, are restored to and maintained at their optimal physiologic, psychological, social, vocational, and emotional status.[1] It is typically divided into three or four phases.

Phase 1 is the period from the event until the patient leaves the hospital. During this period the focus is on overcoming deconditioning from bed rest; in addition, there is some education and recovery from the open heart surgery or other event or procedure. During *Phase 2* the patient attends regular exercise and education classes. During exercise the patient usually is continually monitored via ECG telemeter. *Phases 3* and *4* are maintenance phases.

The Clinical Application on p. 696 identifies the training and qualifications needed to work in cardiac rehabilitation programs.

Exercise Guidelines and Recommendations

Exercise guidelines are based on the clinical status of the patient. The reader is referred to more detailed descriptions of developing an exercise program for all levels of cardiac patients.[37] Low-risk cardiac patients should have established stable cardiovascular and physiologic responses to exercise. Low risk is generally classified as having had an uncomplicated clinical course in the hospital, having no evidence of resting or exercise-induced ischemia (ST segment depression), having functional capacities greater than 6 to 8 metabolic equivalents (METs) 3 weeks after the clinical event, having normal ventricular function (ejection fraction [EF] greater than 50%), and not having any significant resting or exercise-induced ventricular arrhythmias.

Individuals with identified cardiac risk factors need to have a physician release and referral before exercising. Ideally, low-risk patients with cardiac disease should have a treadmill test to determine their functional capacity and cardiovascular status. The treadmill results can then be used to establish a safe exercise prescription. The exact exercise prescription should be based on the medical history, clinical status, and symptoms.

cardiac rehabilitation

restoring and maintaining the person with cardiovascular disease to optimal physiologic, psychological, social, vocational, and emotional status

Training and Qualifications Needed to Work in Cardiac Rehabilitation Programs

The American Association of Cardiovascular and Pulmonary Rehabilitation (AACVPR) has developed minimum and preferred qualifications for exercise physiologists who desire to work in a cardiac or pulmonary rehabilitation setting. The minimum qualifications include the following:

- At least a BS degree in exercise physiology or related field

- Certification, experience, and training equivalent to those specified for an Exercise Specialist by the American College of Sports Medicine

- Experience in exercise program planning, supervision, and counseling with cardiovascular rehabilitation patients

- Certification in Basic Life Support (BLS)

Preferred qualifications include the following:

- An MS degree in rehabilitative exercise physiology or related field

- Certification in Advanced Cardiac Life Support (ACLS)

Today many universities in the United States, such as Wake Forest University and the University of Wisconsin–La Crosse, offer degrees and direct experience in cardiac rehabilitation. Hands-on experience can also be arranged through internship programs that are advertised in the American College of Sports Medicine's Job Guide.

Cardiac rehabilitation programs are available in most major cities and hospitals. Such programs are generally staffed by a physician, nurse, and exercise physiologist. Cardiac rehabilitation programs have been shown to reduce the incidence of further cardiac events in patients with CAD and to reduce health care expenses. Cardiac rehabilitation is an excellent career opportunity for an exercise physiologist.

General guidelines for patients with cardiac disease have been developed by the American College of Sports Medicine.[37]

Intensity: Rating of perceived exertion (RPE) less than 13 (6 to 20 scale)

After myocardial infarction: Heart rate less than 120 bpm or HR_{rest} + 20 bpm

After surgery: HR_{rest} + 30 bpm

To tolerance if asymptomatic

Duration: Intermittent bouts lasting 3 to 5 minutes

Rest periods at patient's discretion, lasting 1 to 2 minutes, shorter than exercise bout duration

Total duration up to 20 minutes

Frequency: Early mobilization: three to four times per day (days 1 to 3)

Later mobilization: two times per day (starting day 4)

Progression: Initially increase duration to 10 to 15 minutes of continuous exercise, then increase intensity

Hypertension

Hypertension is one of the most prevalent chronic diseases in the United States. Hypertensive individuals are those with chronically elevated blood pressures greater than 140/90 mm Hg. As many as 50 million individuals in the United States have chronically elevated blood pressure or are taking antihypertensive medication. Hypertension is related to the development of CAD, increased severity of atherosclerosis, stroke, congestive heart failure, left ventricular hypertrophy, aortic aneurysms, and peripheral vascular disease. Incidence is higher in blacks, Puerto Ricans, Cuban–Americans, and Mexican–Americans, as well as individuals with lower educational and income levels.[3]

The majority of hypertensive persons are not receiving any therapy to control their blood pressure and do not even know they have a problem. The cause of 90% to 95% of the cases of high blood pressure is not known, but once detected the condition can be controlled. Hypertension is a serious medical problem if left untreated. Hypertensive individuals

FOCUS BOX 27.3

Position statement on exercise and hypertension from the American College of Sports Medicine

The available evidence indicates that endurance training by individuals at high risk for developing hypertension will reduce the rise in blood pressure that occurs with time. Thus, it is the position of the American College of Sports Medicine that endurance exercise training is recommended as a nonpharmacological strategy to reduce the incidence of hypertension in susceptible individuals. The exercise recommendations to achieve this effect are generally the same as those prescribed for developing and maintaining cardiovascular fitness in healthy adults. However, exercise training at somewhat lower intensities appears to lower blood pressure as much or more than exercise at higher intensities, which may be more important in specific hypertensive populations.

Adapted from The American College of Sports Medicine: *Med Sci Sports Exerc* 25(10): i-x, 1993.

FOCUS BOX 27.4

Exercise guidelines for individuals with hypertension

- All hypertensive persons should be instructed to avoid holding their breath and straining during exercise (Valsalva's maneuver).

- Weight training should be used as a supplement to endurance training, not as the primary exercise. Circuit training is preferred over free weights. The resistance should be kept low and the repetitions high.

- It may be necessary to monitor exercise intensity by the rating of perceived exertion scale, since medications can alter the accuracy of the training heart rate during exercise.

- Any changes in medications and any abnormal signs or symptoms before, during, or immediately after exercise should be reported to the exercise leader immediately.

- Physicians often have patients with documented hypertension record their blood pressures before and after exercise.

- Individuals with hypertension should be instructed to move slowly when rising from the floor to standing, since they are more susceptible to orthostatic hypotension if taking antihypertensive medication.

- Individuals with severe hypertension need to be carefully monitored during exercise initially and possibly for the long term. Such individuals are likely to be taking one or more hypertensive medications that can affect their response to exercise. A detailed treatment plan, including specific exercise guidelines and blood pressure cut-off points, should be developed with the patient's physician and exercise staff so that the exercise training is both safe and effective.

- Individuals with hypertension may have multiple CAD risk factors, which should be considered when developing the exercise prescription.

Sample Exercise Prescription

Mode: The overall exercise training recommendations for persons with mild to moderate hypertension is basically the same as for apparently healthy individuals. Endurance exercise, such as low-impact aerobics, walking, and swimming, should be the primary exercise mode. Exercises with an isometric component should be avoided. Weight training can be prescribed, using low resistance and high repetitions.

Intensity: Low-intensity dynamic exercise. The exercise intensity level should be near the lower end of the heart rate range (40% to 65%).

Frequency: Persons with hypertension should be encouraged to exercise at least four times per week. Daily exercise may be appropriate for certain individuals with an initial low functional capacity.

Duration: A longer and more gradual warm-up and cool-down period (greater than 5 minutes) is recommended. Total exercise duration should be gradually increased, possibly to as much as 30 to 60 minutes per session, depending on the medical history and clinical status of the individual.

have three to four times greater risk of developing coronary artery disease and up to seven times greater risk of having a stroke.[3]

Role of Exercise in Controlling Hypertension

Exercise training is now recognized as an important part of therapy for controlling hypertension, although the antihypertensive effects of exercise have yielded conflicting results.[26] Regular aerobic exercise appears to reduce both systolic and diastolic blood pressure by an average of 10 mm Hg.[2,33,73] Although the mechanisms responsible for the reduction in blood pressure after endurance training are not completely understood, it appears that an exercise training–induced reduction in blood pressure can be caused by a reduction in cardiac output and total peripheral resistance at rest or by reduced sympathetic activity via a reduced plasma norepinephrine secretion.[20,33,64] Thus exercise training appears to have an antihypertensive effect via a combination of reduced total resting plasma catecholamine levels and a reduction in cardiac output and total peripheral resistance (through resetting baroreceptors, altering blood volume distribution, changing the renin-angiotensin axis, and reducing sympathetic nervous system activity).[26]

Hagberg reviewed 33 exercise training studies involving individuals with hypertension.[27] Approximately two thirds of these studies showed an average reduction in resting systolic blood pressure of about 10 mm Hg, and 70% of the studies reported a similar drop in diastolic blood pressure. Based on the available literature, the American College of Sports Medicine has recently released a position statement on exercise and hypertension (Focus Box 27.3).

Exercise Guidelines and Recommendations

Since many hypertensive persons have several CAD risk factors, including obesity, nondrug therapy is usually the first line of treatment. A combination of weight reduction, salt restriction, and increased physical activity has been recommended for reducing and controlling high blood pressure (Focus Box 27.4).[65] Factors to be considered when recommending exercise for hypertensive persons include clinical status; medications; frequency, duration, intensity, and mode of exercise in which the individual is currently participating; and how well the individual manages the hypertension.

In addition to regular aerobic exercise, Focus Box 27.5 presents recommendations of the Joint National Committee on Detection, Evaluation, and Treatment of High Blood Pressure.

Stroke

Stroke-related events were the third leading cause of death in the United States in 1990.[9] Strokes are also referred to as **cerebrovascular accidents (CVAs).** Similar to a myocardial infarction, a stroke affects the arteries of the nervous system, instead of the heart. When deprived of oxygen because of a blockage or rupture of a blood vessel supplying blood to the brain, nerve cells die within minutes. The results of a stroke can be devastating. Strokes can affect speech, thought patterns and memory, behavioral patterns, sight, and sometimes paralyze a part of the body. The risk factors for stroke include high blood pressure, heart disease, cigarette smoking, high red blood cell count, and presence of **transient ischemic attacks** (TIAs) (Focus Box 27.6).

Role of Exercise and Stroke

Data on the role of exercise and stroke are limited. Most of the studies looking at exercise and stroke showed equivocal findings.[12] In general, since the risk factors for stroke are the same as CAD, exercise may help reduce overall CAD risk and thus lessen the risk for stroke. Since hypertension is the major modifiable risk factor for preventing strokes, exercise should be recommended for hypertensive individuals at risk

---

FOCUS BOX 27.5

Life-style modification for hypertension control and cardiovascular risk reduction

- Lose weight if overweight.

- Limit alcohol intake to less than 1 oz/day of ethanol (24 oz of beer, 8 oz of wine, or 2 oz of 100-proof whiskey).

- Exercise (aerobic) regularly.

- Reduce sodium intake to less than 100 mmol/day (less than 2.3 g of sodium or approximately 6 g of sodium chloride).

- Maintain adequate dietary potassium, calcium, and magnesium intake.

- Stop smoking and reduce dietary saturated fat and cholesterol intake for overall cardiovascular health. Reducing fat intake also helps reduce caloric intake, which is important for control of weight and type II diabetes.

Adapted from the fifth Report of the Joint National Committee on Detection, Evaluation, and Treatment of High Blood Pressure, 1993.

Warning signs of stroke

- Sudden weakness or numbness of the face, arm, or leg on one side of the body.
- Sudden dimness or loss of vision, particularly in only one eye.
- Loss of speech or trouble talking or understanding speech.
- Sudden severe, unexplained headaches.
- Unexplained dizziness, unsteadiness, or sudden falls, especially in combination with any of the previous symptoms.

Adapted from the American Heart Association: *1993 heart and stroke facts statistics*, Dallas, 1992, American Heart Association.

Claudication pain scale

Grade I—definite discomfort or pain but only of a modest level (established but minimal)

Grade II—moderate discomfort or pain from which the patient's attention can be diverted, for example, by conversation

Grade III—intense pain (short of grade IV) from which the patient's attention cannot be diverted

Grade IV—excruciating and unbearable pain

---

for stroke or those recovering from a stroke. About 70% to 80% of strokes are caused by a thrombosis. Exercise may also reduce blood clots through enhanced fibrinolytic activity.[62]

Peripheral Vascular Disease

Peripheral vascular disease (PVD) is caused by atherosclerotic lesions in one or more peripheral (usually in the legs) arterial or venous blood vessels. Most patients with PVD are older and have long-established CAD risk factors. Common sites for atherosclerotic lesions include the iliac, femoral, and popliteal arteries. PVD is 20 times more common in diabetic individuals than in nondiabetic individuals.[9] PVD is a painful and often debilitating disease.

The major symptom of PVD is muscular pain caused by ischemia of the working muscles. This type of ischemia is referred to as claudication. The ischemic pain caused by PVD can result from spasms of the arteries or from occlusive blockages. Some patients with PVD experience chronic claudication and pain even at rest. When pain results from physical activity, such as walking, cycling, or stair climbing, it is referred to as intermittent claudication. Intermittent claudication is usually relieved by immediate rest. Most patients with PVD describe claudication as a dull aching, cramping pain. The claudication pain scale (Focus Box 27.7) is a sub-

jective rating of discomfort that can be used to regulate exercise intensity or duration and frequency.[37]

Role of Exercise and Peripheral Vascular Disease

Treatment for PVD usually includes a combination of medication (vasodilating agents), exercise (to improve blood flow and functional capacity), medical procedures (angioplasty, atheroectomy, stents), or surgery (arterial bypass). One

stroke
a condition caused by an embolus or thrombus that occludes one or more arteries leading to the brain

cerebrovascular accidents (CVAs)
a general term used to describe cerebrovascular symptoms caused by an ischemic or hemorrhagic lesion

transient ischemic attacks (TIAs)
temporary disruption of blood flow to the brain

peripheral vascular disease (PVD)
a condition caused by atherosclerotic lesions in one or more peripheral (usually in the legs) arterial or venous blood vessels

of the primary benefits of exercise for PVD is to lower overall CAD risk (e.g., hypertension, hypercholesterolemia). The other principal benefit of exercise for PVD appears to be improved blood flow and overall cardiovascular endurance. Exercise training studies have been shown to improve peak work capacity on exercise testing and walking duration in individuals with PVD.[32,53]

Exercise Guidelines and Recommendations

Individuals with PVD should undergo a complete medical evaluation before embarking on an exercise program. Initially, low-intensity, non–weight-bearing activities should be stressed. Individuals with PVD often have a high anxiety level when starting because they expect chronic pain. As confidence builds with gradual progress, additional activities can be added. Most individuals with PVD do not particularly want to be able to run a marathon, but merely wish to go shopping, climb stairs, and take a walk without experiencing pain. In addition to exercise, other life-style modifications should be stressed in an effort to lower overall CAD risk.

Diabetes

Diabetes mellitus is characterized by diminished secretion of insulin by the pancreatic β-cells and reduced sensitivity of insulin's target cells to insulin. Diabetes mellitus causes abnormalities in the metabolism of carbohydrates, protein, and fat.

Diabetics are at greater risk for numerous health problems, including kidney failure, nerve disorders, eye problems, and heart disease.[4] Prolonged and frequent elevation of blood glucose can lead to *microangiopathy,* a term that refers to damaged capillaries, which leads to poor circulation. In addition, diabetics are at greater risk for *neuropathy,* a term referring to damaged nerves, which can lead to permanent nerve damage.

There are four types of diabetes: insulin-dependent diabetes mellitus (IDDM), non–insulin-dependent diabetes mellitus (NIDDM), gestational diabetes mellitus (GDM), and impaired glucose tolerance (IGT). Insulin-dependent diabetes mellitus (IDDM) is caused by destruction of the insulin-producing β-cells in the pancreas, which leads to a reduction or cessation of insulin secretion. IDDM generally occurs in childhood, and regular insulin injections are required to regulate blood glucose levels. The typical symptoms of IDDM include excessive thirst and hunger, frequent urination, weight loss, blurred vision, and recurrent infections. During periods of insulin deficiency a higher than normal level of glucose remains in the blood because of decreased uptake and storage. A portion of the excess glucose is excreted in the urine, which leads to increased thirst, weight loss, and increased appetite.

Non–insulin-dependent diabetes mellitus (NIDDM) is the most common form of diabetes, affecting 90% of diabetic patients. NIDDM typically occurs in overly fat adults. It is characterized by a reduced sensitivity of insulin target cells to available insulin. Treatment of NIDDM varies and may include dietary changes, medication, and exercise therapy. Like IDDM, NIDDM is characterized by frequent states of

---

TABLE 27.3

Comparison of type I and type II diabetes

CHARACTERISTIC	TYPE I	TYPE II
Level of insulin	None or almost none	May be normal or exceed normal secretion
Term	Insulin-dependent (childhood onset)	Non-insulin dependent (adult onset)
Age at onset	Under 20 years old	Over 40 years
Basic defect	Destruction of β-cells	Reduced sensitivity of insulin's target cells
Associated with obesity	Very uncommon	Frequent
Family history	Infrequent	Frequent
Percent of diabetics	10% to 20%	80% to 90%
Use of insulin	Always	Infrequent
Onset of symptoms	Rapid	Slow
Treatment	Insulin injections; dietary management	Dietary control and weight reduction; occasionally oral hypoglycemic drugs

hyperglycemia, but without the increased catabolism of fats and protein. The typical individual with NIDDM is over 30 years of age, is obese, and has few, if any, classic symptoms of diabetes. Because 75% of individuals with NIDDM are obese, or have a history of obesity, NIDDM is often reversible with permanent weight loss. Table 27.3 lists the differences between IDDM and NIDDM.

Gestational diabetes mellitus (GDM) is a metabolic disorder that occurs in approximately 3% of pregnancies and disappears after delivery. Hyperglycemia associated with GDM can cause serious injury to the developing fetus. Women with GDM are at higher risk for developing diabetes at a later date.

Impaired glucose tolerance (IGT) occurs in persons who have hyperglycemia, but at a level lower than that which qualifies as a diagnosis of diabetes, and who do not have symptoms of diabetes. Individuals with IGT usually have additional risk factors for coronary heart disease, such as hypertension, obesity, and hypercholesterolemia.

Effective Diabetic Control

Effective diabetic control is based on long-term regulation of blood glucose levels. Glucose regulation in IDDM is achieved through regular glucose assessment, proper diet, exercise, and appropriate insulin medication.[5] For NIDDM, glucose regulation is achieved through a change in life-style centered on proper diet, weight loss and control, exercise, and insulin or oral agents if needed.[5] A combined diet and exercise

regimen results in improved weight control, and cardiorespiratory fitness, reduced need for insulin, improved self-image, and better ability to deal with stress (Focus Box 27-8).

Role of Exercise and IDDM

The benefits of exercise training for individuals with IDDM are not fully understood. Although it has been shown that individuals with IDDM can improve their functional capacity, reduce their risk for CAD, and improve insulin receptor sensitivity and receptor number, the role of exercise in improving glucose control has not been well demonstrated.[67] The American Diabetes Association's 1993 position on exercise for IDDM states the following:

> Exercise programs have not been exclusively shown to improve glycemic control in people with IDDM. However, IDDM individuals should be encouraged to exercise because of the potential to improve cardiovascular fitness and psychological well-being, and for social interaction and recreation.

Role of Exercise and NIDDM

Exercise plays an important role in diabetic control for NIDDM. The primary benefit of exercise for NIDDM is the effect it has on reducing blood cholesterol and triacylglycerol levels and body fat. The American Diabetes Association's 1993 statement on exercise for NIDDM includes the following:

> An appropriate exercise program should be an adjunct to diet or drug therapy to improve glycemic control, reduce certain cardiovascular risk factors, and increase psychological well-being in individuals with NIDDM. Patients who are most likely to respond favorably are those with mildly to moderately impaired glucose tol-

---

FOCUS BOX 27.8

Exercise guidelines for individuals with diabetes

- Do not inject insulin into primary muscle groups that will be used during exercise. This regimen can cause the insulin to be absorbed too quickly, resulting in hypoglycemia.

- Check blood glucose levels frequently. Determine the right insulin dosage, based in part on the blood glucose levels before and after exercise.

- Always carry a rapid-acting (high glycemic index) carbohydrate (such as juice or candy) to correct for hypoglycemia.

- Exercise at the same time each day for better control.

- Exercise should be avoided during peak insulin activity.

- Carbohydrate snacks should be consumed before and during prolonged exercise.

- Take very good care of the feet. Check regularly for any cuts, blisters, or signs of infection. Good-quality exercise shoes are also very important.

Sample Exercise Prescription

- **Mode:** Endurance activities, such as walking, swimming, and cycling.

- **Intensity:** 50% to 60% VO_2max gradually working up to 60% to 70% VO_2max

- **Frequency:** 5 to 7 days a week for IDDM, and 4 to 5 days a week for NIDDM. May need to start out with several daily sessions.

- **Duration:** Persons with IDDM should gradually work up to 20 to 30 minutes per session. For those with NIDDM, 40 to 60 minutes is recommended.

erance and hyperinsulinemia. This recommendation is based on the premise the benefits of exercise outweigh the risks.

Exercise Prescription Considerations

Before beginning an exercise program, persons with diabetes should speak with their physicians or diabetes educators to develop a program of diet, exercise, and medications. The primary goals of exercise for IDDM should be better glucose regulation and reduced heart disease risk. For persons with IDDM the timing of exercise, the amount of insulin injected, and the injection site are important considerations before exercising. Exercise should be performed daily so that a regular pattern of diet and insulin dosage can be maintained. Since the frequency and duration of exercise recommended are lower for those with IDDM than for those with NIDDM, the intensity can be slightly higher (Focus Box 27.8).

The primary goal of exercise for the person with NIDDM is weight (body fat) loss and control. About 80% of NIDDM diabetics are overweight. By losing weight through the combined effect of diet and exercise, NIDDM diabetics reduce the amount of oral insulin medication needed. The primary objective during exercise for the NIDDM diabetic is developing a caloric deficit. Since the recommended frequency and duration of exercise are high for NIDDM diabetics, the intensity of exercise should be kept low.

Asthma

*A*sthma is a reactive airway disease characterized by shortness of breath, coughing, and wheezing. The symptoms are caused by constriction of the smooth muscle around the airways, swelling of the mucosal cells, and increased secretion of mucus. Asthma can result from an allergic reaction, exercise, infection, emotion, or environmental irritants, such as pollens, inhalants, cigarette smoke, and air pollution. Asthma is one of the most common respiratory disorders, affecting as many as 1% to 2% of adults and 5% to 7% of children.[66]

The two main classes of asthma are *extrinsic asthma* and *intrinsic asthma*. Extrinsic asthma is caused by an external irritant or allergen (a substance that incites acquired sensitivity), such as ragweed, cigarette smoke, or air pollution. Intrinsic asthma is caused by internal factors, such as a bacterial respiratory tract infection. The pathophysiology of asthma is not completely understood, but it is believed that certain chemical mediators bind with the immunoglobulin IgE on the surfaces of mast cells. Mast cells are located within the airways and are coated with different IgE antibodies, which can bind with one or more different antigens. When released after exposure to a particular antigen the bronchostimulant mediators located within the mast cells cause the predictable changes in the airways leading to an asthma attack. Such bronchostimulant mediators include histamine, leukotrienes, and prostaglandins. Signs and symptoms of asthma include wheezing, dyspnea, and a nonproductive cough. The release of mediators from mast cells in response to a particular allergen is thought to be caused by altered levels of cyclic adenosine monophosphate (cAMP) and guanosine monophosphate (GMP), which normally prevent the release of chemical mediators that lead to bronchial spasms.[16]

Approximately 80% of persons with asthma experience asthma attacks during exercise testing, an occurrence referred to as *exercise-induced asthma* (EIA).[6] EIA is defined as 15% or greater postexercise reduction of either forced expiratory volume in 1 second (FEV_1) or peak expiratory flow rate on preexercise values after exercise testing.[45] EIA attacks are characterized by moderate obstruction and are not life threatening. The severity of an EIA attack is related to the intensity of exercise and the ventilatory requirement of the task, as well as the environmental conditions. Breathing in cold dry air rather than warm moist air seems to cause greater airway obstruction.

The exact cause of EIA is not well understood but is believed to be drying of the airways as moisture is absorbed from air passing through the conducting zone of the lung. As the airways become dryer, the osmolarity of the periciliary fluid increases, causing a release of broncho-active mediators.[28] Asthma is not a contraindication to exercise; however, before starting an exercise program, persons with asthma should develop a plan for exercise with their physicians. (See Focus Box 27.9.) Several studies have shown that regular exercise can reduce the number and severity of asthma attacks during exercise.[23,24]

Role of Exercise and Asthma

Although persons with asthma are more likely to experience breathlessness during exercise, this should not stop them from exercising. Exercise training may help to reduce the ventilatory requirement for various tasks, making it easier for individuals with asthma to participate in normal daily activities with less shortness of breath and possibly fewer asthma attacks.

Bronchitis and Emphysema

*B*ronchitis is a form of obstructive pulmonary disease. Chronic bronchitis is a chronic inflammation of the bronchial tubes. The major cause is cigarette smoking, although air pollution and occupational exposure play a lesser role. Acute bronchitis involves the additional inflammation of the mucous membranes or the bronchial tubes. However, an acute bout of bronchitis can develop after a cold or after exposure to certain dust particles or fumes and will resolve in several days or weeks. Chronic bronchitis persists for a lifetime in most cases.

Emphysema is another form of chronic pulmonary disease caused by overinflation of the alveoli. The overinfla-

FOCUS BOX 27.9

Exercise guidelines for individuals with asthma

- Before commencing exercise, have a medication and treatment plan to prevent or treat EIA attacks.

- Have a bronchodilating inhaler at all times and use it at the first sign of wheezing.

- Keep the exercise intensity low at first and gradually increase over time. Intensity of exercise is directly linked to the severity and frequency of EIA.

- Reduce exercise intensity if asthma symptoms occur.

- Use an inhaler several minutes before exercise to reduce the possibility of an EIA attack.

- The results of pulmonary exercise testing should be used to design the appropriate exercise prescription.

- Drink plenty of fluids before and during exercise.

- Take an extended time for warm-up and cool-down.

- More symptoms of respiratory distress will be experienced when exercising in extreme environmental conditions (high or low temperature, high pollen count, and heavy air pollution).

- Only persons whose asthma is stabilized should exercise.

- If an asthma attack is not relieved by medication, arrange transport to a medical facility immediately.

- Wearing a face mask during exercise helps in maintaining warmer and moister inspired air and can minimize EIA.

Sample Exercise Prescription

- **Mode:** Perform dynamic exercise, such as walking, cycling, and swimming. Upper body exercises, such as arm cranking, rowing, and cross-country skiing, may not be appropriate because of the higher ventilation demands. Swimming may be particularly beneficial because it allows persons with asthma to inhale moist air.

- **Intensity:** Low-intensity dynamic exercise rather than high-intensity, high-impact exercise is recommended. The exercise intensity should be prescribed based on the client's fitness status and limitations.

- **Frequency:** Exercise at least three to four times per week. Asthmatic persons who have low functional capacities or experience shortness of breath during prolonged exercise may benefit from intermittent exercise (two 10-minute sessions).

- **Duration:** Include a longer and more gradual warm-up and cool-down (more than 10 minutes). Total exercise duration should be increased gradually to 20 to 45 minutes.

---

tion results from a breakdown of the walls of the alveoli, which causes a significant decrease in respiratory function. The classic signs of emphysema are chronic breathlessness and coughing. Bronchitis and emphysema are collectively referred to as **chronic obstructive pulmonary disease** (COPD).

Role of Exercise and COPD

Individuals with chronic bronchitis and emphysema may benefit from mild exercise training. However, individuals with COPD may not receive any benefits from aerobic exercise because of the severity of their disease. Persons with COPD need to be carefully screened and followed by a physician. Most do not improve their pulmonary function with exercise. However, other benefits such as reduced anxiety, decreased body weight, lowered perceived stress, and an improved ability to perform in normal daily activities can be realized through exercise. The primary goals of exercise training for individuals with COPD are increased functional capacity, increased functional status, decreased severity of dyspnea, and improved quality of life.[54]

Individuals with COPD whose condition is stable and who have obtained all the potential benefits from a medically supervised exercise program should benefit from participating in non–medically supervised exercise. Individuals with COPD should be encouraged to "do the best they can," because every little bit of exercise they do may have health benefits.

---

bronchitis (brong-ki'tis)
a form of obstructive pulmonary disease involving an inflammation of the mucous membranes of the bronchial tubes

emphysema (em-fi-se'mah)
another form of chronic pulmonary disease caused by overinflation and damage of the alveoli

chronic obstructive pulmonary disease (COPD)
a term used to classify and group chronic respiratory disorders that obstruct airflow

Cancer

Cancer affects one of every four people in the United States. In 1990 cancer was diagnosed in more than 1 million Americans and about half that number of cancer deaths were recorded. It has been estimated that 80% of cancers may be avoided by life-style choices and changes. For example, regular exercise; a low-fat, high-fiber diet; and the avoidance of smoking reduce the risk of cancer.

The roles of diet and exercise appear to be particularly important in reducing the risk for cancer. Dietary changes can reduce the risk of bowel cancer, the second most common type of cancer overall. The leading cause of lung cancer in the United States is cigarette smoking. Thus it appears that many types of cancer are highly preventable. Focus Box 27.10 lists the seven warning signs of cancer.

Role of Exercise and Cancer

In general, physically inactive people have greater rates of cancer. Paffenbarger found in his Harvard alumni study that cancer mortality was the highest in those who exercised least, even after age and cigarette smoking were considered.[49] Sternfeld recently found that of the twelve studies he reviewed, seven demonstrated an inverse relationship between physical activity and all-cause mortality.[61] A recent study by Blair revealed a reduced relative risk for all cancer mortality in individuals who exercised.[11]

Bartram and Wynder recently reviewed the evidence linking physical activity and colon cancer.[8] Physical activity decreases the transit time in the colon, thus possibly decreasing the exposure of the colon to potential carcinogens. Physical activity has also been shown to increase secretion of prostaglandins that have a protective effect against colon cancer. There is also evidence that cancers of the breast and reproductive system in women are inversely related to physical activity. Another mechanism by which exercise may have a protective effect against cancer is through strengthening of the immune system. Several studies have shown an improvement in immune function after exercise.[21,55,58]

Exercise Guidelines and Recommendations

No specific guidelines for exercise and cancer are available. The reader is directed to the guidelines and recommendations for training for health and fitness in Chapter 16. Winningham recommends asking six questions before designing an exercise program for cancer patients[71]:

- Are there limitations to activity based on preexisting conditions?
- Are there limitations to activity based on medical procedures undergone by the patient?
- Are there limitations in mobility as a result of disease or treatment?
- Are there limitations in oxygen delivery as a result of disease or treatment?
- Are there limitations in activity as a result of nutritional and fluid deficits?
- Are there limitations based on risk for anemia, bleeding, or infections?

If individuals have any limitations based on the conditions listed previously, the exercise prescription should be adjusted accordingly.

Osteoporosis

Osteoporosis is characterized by decreased bone mineral density and increased susceptibility to fractures. Fractures occur more commonly in men than women before 45 years of age and more commonly in women than men after 45 years of age.[35] Osteoporosis affects between 15 to 20 million Americans at an estimated cost of $3.8 billion a year, primarily resulting from hip fractures.[15]

Osteoporosis is caused primarily by decreased bone mass, which increases the susceptibility of individuals to fractures (see Chapter 14). After reaching its peak, bone mass declines throughout life because of an imbalance of remodeling of the bone. Remodeling refers to the replacement of old bone with new bone. Bone remodeling serves to keep the skeletal system in peak form and helps maintain Ca^{++} homeostasis. Mechanical and electrolyte factors, hormones, and local regulatory factors influence remodeling (see Chapter 14).

Role of Exercise in the Treatment of Osteoporosis

The treatment for osteoporosis tries to prevent or retard bone mineral loss. Estrogen replacement is highly effective in delaying osteoporosis in women. Estrogen reduces bone

---

FOCUS BOX 27.10

Cancer's seven warning signals

- Change in bowel or bladder habits
- A sore that does not heal
- An unusual bleeding or discharge
- A thickening or lump in the breast or elsewhere
- Indigestion or difficulty in swallowing
- An obvious change in a wart or mole
- A nagging cough or persistent hoarseness

FIGURE 27.6

Effect of exercise on percent difference in lumbar bone mineral density.

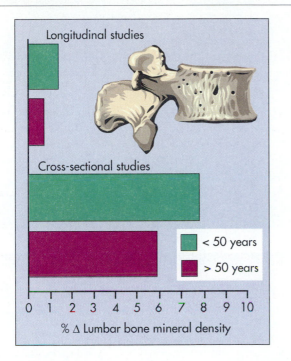

FIGURE 27.7

Example of the neutral spine.

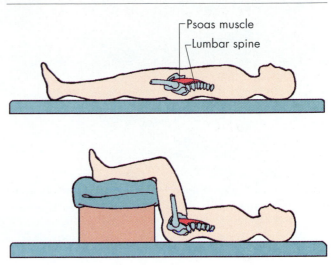

resorption and retards or halts postmenopausal bone loss. Premenopausal women should consume 1000 to 1500 mg of calcium each day. High dietary calcium intake suppresses age-related bone loss. Since physical inactivity is a known risk factor for osteoporosis, exercise is recommended for the prevention and treatment of osteoporosis (see Chapter 14) (Figure 27.6).

Low-Back Pain

Back injuries, including sprains and strains, are the number one disability for people under age 45. It has been estimated that 80% of the population will experience an episode of low-back pain at some time in their lives. Of the 80%, 5% will go on to develop chronic low-back pain.[25] Low-back pain accounts for 10% of all chronic health conditions in the United States and 25% of days lost from work. Medical experts have called it the most expensive benign health condition in America.[51]

Back injuries translate into millions of lost workdays every year and cost billions for medical care, disability payments, and legal payments. Reducing back injury rates is a top priority for employers. In fact, back strain or sprain is the most common type of workers' compensation claim, accounting for up to 25% of all claims and representing annual payments of $2.5 to $7 billion, or one half of all dis-

ability compensation payments annually. In addition, nearly 2% of the U.S. work force files back compensation claims.

The cause of low-back pain is often elusive, but four common causes are herniated disk (rupture of the outer layers of fibers that surround the gelatinous portion of the disk), spondylolisthesis (forward sliding of the body of one vertebra on the vertebral disc below it), trauma to the back (accident), and degenerative disk disease (progressive structural degeneration of the intervertebral disk). Lower back problems are often associated with an imbalance of strength and flexibility of the lower back and abdominal muscle groups. Poor flexibility of the hamstring and hip flexor muscles has also been linked to low-back pain.

Role of Exercise in Preventing Low-Back Pain

Physical fitness combined with a healthy life style may help prevent low-back pain. In fact, many physicians believe that the major cause of chronic low-back pain is simply physical deconditioning. More specifically, low endurance of large muscle groups, particularly the back extensor and abdominal muscles, seems to increase the risk of developing low-back pain. Exercises for the low back should be performed on a regular basis to gain maximal benefits. Aerobic conditioning is also important in the treatment and prevention of low-back pain.[14] In addition, strong correlations exist between body weight, smoking, and decreased physical activity and low-back pain.[19]

Exercise participants should be screened for low-back risk factors (Focus Box 27.11). Prevention is the key to avoiding low-back pain. Anyone who has experienced a recent low-back strain or injury should be cleared by a physi-

Risk factors for lower-back pain

- The incidence of low-back pain increases with age.

- Poor exercise tolerance, weakness, imbalance of the abdominal and extensor muscles, and being overweight or extremely tall correlate with a greater risk for low-back pain.

- Postural or structural abnormalities can be identified by physical examination and spinal radiology.

- One of the most powerful potential risk factors for low-back pain is lifting. Other occupational risk factors for low-back pain include twisting, bending, stooping, and floor surface conditions. Prolonged sitting, particularly without proper arm and spinal support, is associated with low-back pain.

- Cigarette smoking is a risk factor for low-back pain. Chronic coughing may also be associated with intravertebral disk pressure.

- A range of psychologic factors (including depression and anxiety) and social problems (especially stressful job environments) are associated with an increased incidence of disabling low-back pain.

- Golfing and tennis have been slightly associated with an increased risk of disk herniation, possibly because they involve twisting movements. Only a minimally significant statistical association has been found between low-back pain and jogging or cross-country skiing.

- Multiple pregnancies have been associated with an increase in low-back pain, probably because of loss of abdominal tone after pregnancy, the strain of lifting children, and various hormonal effects.

Exercise guidelines for individuals with low-back pain

- Be aware of proper form and postural alignment.

- Maintain pelvic neutral alignment and an erect torso during any lifting movements.

- Avoid head-forward positions in which the chin is tilted up.

- When leaning forward, lifting, or lowering an object, bend at the knees.

- Avoid hyperextending the spine in an unsupported position.

- Allow for an adequate warm-up and cool-down period during exercise classes.

- Most low-back pain is caused by muscle weaknesses and imbalances, including tight hamstring and lower back muscle groups, tight hip flexor muscles, and weak abdominal and lower back muscles. Exercises to improve muscle strength and flexibility should be routinely performed.

- Individuals who experience low-back pain or have a history of chronic low-back pain should consult a physician and obtain specific recommendations for exercises.

- If someone complains of low-back pain after an exercise class, have him or her sit or lie down in a comfortable position and apply ice to the affected area. After a mild back strain, individuals should be encouraged to take several days off from exercise.

Exercises For The Low Back

Position 1: Supine with knees bent.
Activity: Slowly pull one knee to chest and hold for 5 seconds, then do the same with the other knee.

Position 2: Supine with knees bent and legs together.
Activity: Slowly rotate knees from side to side while keeping them together.

Position 3: Hands and knees.
Activity: Arch your back up like a cat, hold 5 seconds, and relax.

Position 4: Hands and knees.
Activity: Slowly sit back between your knees and then return to hands and knees.

Position 5: Hands and knees.
Activity: Slowly bring one knee to the chest then extend the leg straight out behind you. Repeat on the other side.

Position 6: Standing against the wall.
Activity: Squat down so that your lower back is pressed against the wall. Move your feet out from the wall, bend your legs to a half-squat, and hold. Gradually straighten legs out and repeat.

Position 7: Lie on your stomach with legs and arms straight out.
Activity: Lift one arm, hold, and relax. Alternate arms. Lift one leg, hold, and relax. Alternate legs.
Lift one arm and one leg on opposite sides, hold, and relax. Alternate sides.

Position 8: Supine with knees slightly bent.
Activity: Flatten your back against the floor by contracting your stomach muscles and rotating your hips backward.

Additional activities: Side stretch, sit-ups, modified push-ups, lateral leg raises, groin stretch, hamstring stretch, calf stretch, and quadriceps stretch.

Classification of functional capacity for arthritis

Class 1: Complete ability to carry on all usual duties without disability.

Class 2: Adequate ability for normal activities despite disability, discomfort, or limited motion in one or more joints.

Class 3: Ability limited to little or none of the duties of usual occupation or to self-care.

Class 4: Incapacitated, largely or wholly. Bedridden or confined to a wheelchair; little or no self-care.

---

cian before starting an exercise program. Each exercise participant should be taught the neutral position (Figure 27.7). In addition, basic back exercise, in addition to aerobic and resistance training, should be performed on a regular basis. Focus Box 27.12 provides exercise guidelines for individuals with low-back pain.

Arthritis

The most common forms of arthritis are rheumatoid arthritis and osteoarthritis. **Osteoarthritis,** also referred to as *degenerative joint disease,* is an degenerative process caused by the wearing away of cartilage, leaving two surfaces of bone in contact with each other. Osteoarthritis is common in older individuals, affecting 85% of people in the United States over the age of 70. **Rheumatoid arthritis** is caused by an inflammation of the membrane surrounding joints. It is often associated with pain and swelling in one or more joints. Rheumatoid arthritis affects about 3% of women and 1% of men in the United States.

The treatment of arthritis depends on the severity and specific form of arthritis. Individuals with arthritis can be classified into four categories of functional capacity (see Focus Box 27.13). Class 1 and 2 arthritic individuals often can carry on their normal activities of daily living (ADLs) with little discomfort, whereas those in classes 3 and 4 typically are limited in what they can do.

The treatment for arthritis often involves medicine (gold-based drugs, such as penicillamine, and steroids, such as corticosteroids), physical therapy, physiotherapy (transcutaneous electrical nerve stimulation [TENS] and hot packs), occupational therapy to improve ADLs, and surgery (joint replacement). The benefits of exercise include stronger muscles and bones, improved cardiorespiratory fitness, and improved psychosocial well-being.[50] Exercise is contraindicated during inflammatory periods because it can worsen the inflammation.

Role of Exercise in the Treatment of Arthritis

Exercise is recommended for individuals with arthritis to help preserve muscle strength and joint mobility, improve functional capabilities, relieve pain and stiffness, prevent further deformities, improve overall physical conditioning, reestablish neuromuscular coordination, and mobilize stiff or contracted joints. Improvement of function and relief from pain are the ultimate goals.

Fitness programs should be carefully designed by the physician or physical therapist. The exercise prescription needs to be developed based on the functional status of the individual. For example, someone in functional class 1 should be able to perform most activities that a typical healthy person can. For those in functional class 2, non-weight-bearing activities are initially recommended, such as cycling, heated pool exercise, and eventually walking.[17,22,36,44] Individuals in functional class 3 should benefit from a cycling or swimming program. Exercise should be avoided during an arthritic flare-up. Arthritic individuals often report fatigue and some discomfort after exercise. A balance of rest, immobilization of affected joints, and exercise is needed to reduce the severity of the inflammatory joint disease.

osteoarthritis (os-te-o-ar-thri′tis)
also referred to as degenerative joint disease; a degenerative process caused by the wearing away of cartilage, leaving two surfaces of bone in contact with each other

rheumatoid arthritis
caused by an inflammation of the membrane surrounding joints

S U M M A R Y

■ The **epidemiology** of the study of physical activity and morbidity and mortality had its origins in a study comparing the rate and severity of cardiovascular disease of London bus conductors with bus drivers. Additional research was performed on San Francisco longshoremen, revealing age-specific decreased rates of coronary heart disease and **mortality** in those with greater energy expenditure.

■ The consensus of the research evidence is that physical activity has a protective effect against disease, decreasing the risk of **all-cause** and **cause-specific mortality.**

■ The majority of cardiovascular deaths are attributed to **coronary artery disease,** which results from the condition **atherosclerosis.** The risk factors that are directly associated with atherosclerosis are termed **primary risk factors,** whereas the risk factors that contribute to the severity of atherosclerosis and CAD are termed **secondary risk factors.**

■ Primary risk factors include cigarette smoking, hypercholesterolemia, diabetes, inactivity, and hypertension. Secondary risk factors include obesity, gender, age, and family history. All but gender, age, and family history are modifiable risk factors in the majority of individuals.

■ Chest pain caused by lack of blood flow to the heart is termed *ischemia*. The transient symptoms of inadequate blood flow to the heart are referred to as **angina pectoris.** The typical treatments for CAD include medical management; **coronary artery bypass grafting (CABG); percutaneous transluminal coronary angioplasty (PTCA)** or other new forms of plaque removal, such as coronary laser (burning the plaque) and high-speed rotational atherectomy (cutting and removing the plaque); and to a lesser degree, prescription of life-style modifications.

■ Human atherosclerosis is not only preventable but to some extent reversible (or at least the progression can be delayed). Aggressively modifying lipid levels to reduce LDL cholesterol levels to below 100 mg/dl in individuals with established CAD can delay and even reverse the disease.

■ The comprehensive rehabilitation of cardiac patients is collectively referred to as **cardiac rehabilitation.** Cardiac rehabilitation is defined as the process by which persons with cardiovascular disease, including but not limited to patients with coronary heart disease, are restored to and maintained at their optimal physiologic, psychological, social, vocational, and emotional status. It is typically divided into three or four phases.

■ Hypertension is one of the most prevalent chronic diseases in the United States. Hypertensive individuals are those with chronically elevated blood pressures (greater than 140/90 mm Hg). As many as 50 million individuals in the United States have chronically elevated blood pressure or are taking antihypertensive medication. Hypertension is related to the development of CAD, increased severity of atherosclerosis, stroke, congestive heart failure, left ventricular hypertrophy, aortic aneurysms, and PVD.

■ **Stroke**-related events were the third leading cause of death in the United States in 1990. Strokes are also referred to as **cerebrovascular accidents (CVAs).** The risk factors for stroke include high blood pressure, heart disease, cigarette smoking, high red blood cell count, and presence of **transient ischemic attacks (TIAs)**.

■ **Peripheral vascular disease (PVD)** is caused by atherosclerotic lesions in one or more peripheral arterial or venous blood vessels (usually in the legs). The major symptom of PVD is muscular pain caused by ischemia of the working muscles. This type of ischemia is referred to as claudication.

■ Persons with diabetes are at risk for numerous health problems, including kidney failure, nerve disorders, eye problems, heart disease, and peripheral neuropathy. Glucose regulation in individuals with diabetes is achieved through regular glucose assessment, proper diet, exercise, and appropriate insulin medication.

SUMMARY—Cont'd

■ **Bronchitis** is a form of obstructive pulmonary disease. Chronic bronchitis is a chronic inflammation of the bronchial tubes. The major cause is cigarette smoking, although air pollution and occupational exposure play a lesser role. **Emphysema** is another form of chronic pulmonary disease caused by overinflation and structural damage of the alveoli. Bronchitis and emphysema are collectively referred to as **chronic obstructive pulmonary disease** (COPD).

■ Although there are different forms of arthritis, the most common forms are **osteoarthritis** and **rheumatoid arthritis.** The treatment for arthritis often involves medicine (gold-based drugs, such as penicillamine, and steroids, such as corticosteroids), physical therapy, physiotherapy (TENS and hot packs), occupational therapy to improve ADLs, and surgery (joint replacement). The benefits of exercise include stronger muscles and bones, greater cardiorespiratory fitness, and improved psychosocial well-being.

REVIEW QUESTIONS

1. List some of the important early studies in the epidemiology of atherosclerosis and coronary artery disease.

2. Describe in detail how the major modifiable coronary risk factors lead to atherosclerosis.

3. What are the desirable levels for total, LDL, and HDL cholesterol?

4. Describe the processes that lead to formation of atherosclerotic plaques.

5. If someone asked you, "Is atherosclerosis reversible?" how would you answer the question?

6. Outline a heart disease prevention and reversal program.

7. Outline a rehabilitation exercise program for a low-risk cardiac rehabilitation patient.

8. How does exercise help lower hypertension?

9. Detail the differences between type I and type II diabetes and the specific exercise concerns for each population.

10. Outline an exercise program for someone with low-back pain.

11. In one page or less, provide an argument for the health-related benefits of exercise.

APPLICATIONS

1. Many physicians believe that despite the research evidence of exercise-related improvements in risk factors for CAD, cardiac rehabilitation is not effective. This decision is based on statistics that reveal similar rates of second events and mortality between patients who were placed in cardiac rehabilitation and those who were not.

   a. Why is it so difficult to increase longevity in individuals with CAD?

   b. Is mortality a suitable statistic to evaluate the efficacy of cardiac rehabilitation?

   c. Given the preventability of most risk factors for CAD, develop an argument for insurance companies to fund employee cardiac prevention programs rather than cardiac rehabilitation programs.

2. Use your knowledge of energy metabolism in skeletal muscle, the liver, and adipose tissue to explain why blood lipids are increased in persons with diabetes despite the excess availability of blood glucose.

3. How would your exercise prescription differ for the following individuals (assume a similar health status except for the following):

   a. An individual who experiences exercise-induced asthma

   b. An individual with type II diabetes

   c. A 55-year-old woman in phase 2 cardiac rehabilitation 5 weeks after an anterior wall myocardial infarction

REFERENCES

1. American Association of Cardiovascular and Pulmonary Rehabilitation: *Guidelines for cardiac rehabilitation programs,* ed 2, Champaign, Illinois, 1995, Human Kinetics.

2. American College of Sports Medicine Position Stand: Physical activity, physical fitness, and hypertension, *Med Sci Sports Exerc* 25(10):i-x, 1993.

3. American Heart Association: *1993 heart and stroke facts statistics,* Dallas, 1992, American Heart Association.

4. American Diabetes Association: *Physician's guide to non–insulin-dependent (type II) diabetes: diagnosis and treatment,* Alexandria, Virginia, 1988, American Diabetes Association.

5. American Diabetes Association: *Standards of medical care for patients with diabetes mellitus. 1992-93 clinical practice recommendations,* Alexandria, Virginia, 1993, American Diabetes Association.

6. Anderson SD, Silverman M, Konig P, Godfrey S: Exercise-induced asthma: a review, *Br J Dis Chest* 69:1-45, 1975.

7. Aschoff L: Atherosclerosis. In *Lectures in pathology,* New York, 1924, Hoeber.

8. Bartram HP, Wynder EL: Physical activity and colon cancer risk? Physiological consideration, *Am J Gastroenterol* 84:109-114, 1989.

9. Beach KW, Bedford GR, Berlin RO et al: Progression of lower extremity arterial occlusion disease in type II diabetes mellitus, *Diabetes Care* 11:464-472, 1988.

10. Benditt EP: The origin of atherosclerosis, *Sci Am* 2:76, 1977.

11. Blair SN, Kohl HW, Paffenbarger RS et al: Physical fitness and all-causes mortality: a prospective study of healthy men and women, *JAMA* 262:2395, 1989.

12. Blair SN, Kohl HW, Gordon NF, Paffenbarger RS: How much physical activity is good for health? *Annu Rev Pub Health* 13:99-123, 1992.

13. Brown G, Albers JJ, Fisher LD et al: Regression of coronary artery disease as a result of intensive lipid-lowering therapy in men with high levels of apolipoprotein B, *N Engl J Med* 323(19):1289-1298, 1990.

14. Cady LD, Bishcoff DP, O'Connell ER et al: Strength and fitness and subsequent back injuries in fire-fighters, *J Occ Med* 21:269-275, 1979.

15. Christiansen C: Consensus development conference on osteoporosis, *Am J Med* 95(5A):77-85, 1993.

16. Dail DH, Hammar SP, editors: *Pulmonary pathology,* New York, 1988, Springer-Verlag.

REFERENCES—Cont'd

17. Danneskiold-Samsoe B, Lyngberg K, Risum T, Telling M: The effect of water exercise therapy given to patients with rheumatoid arthritis, *Scand J Rehab Med* 19:31-35, 1987.

18. Dawber TR, Meadors GF, Moore FE: Epidemiological approaches to heart disease: the Framingham study, *Am J Public Health* 41:279-286, 1951.

19. Deyo RA, Bass JE: Lifestyle and low back pain: the influence of smoking, exercise and obesity, *Clin Res* 35:577A, 1987.

20. Duncan JJ, Farr JE, Upton J et al: The effects of aerobic exercise on plasma catecholamines and blood pressure in patients with mild hypertension, *JAMA* 254:2609-2613, 1985.

21. Edwards AJ, Bacon TH, Elms CA et al: Changes in the populations of lymphoid cells in human peripheral blood following physical exercise, *Clin Exp Immunol* 58:420-425, 1984.

22. Ekdahl C, Andersson SI, Mortiz U, Svensson B: Dynamic versus static training in patients with rheumatoid arthritis, *Scand J Rheumatol* 19:17-26, 1990.

23. Fitch KD: Effect of swimming training on children with asthma, *Arch Disabled Child* 51:190-198, 1976.

24. Fitch KD: The effect of running training on exercise-induced asthma, *Ann Allergy* 57:90-96, 1986.

25. Frymoyer JW, Pope MH, Contanza MC et al: Epidemiologic studies of low back pain, *Spine* 5:419-423, 1980.

26. Gordon NF, Scott CB: Exercise and mild essential hypertension. In Boone JL, editor: *Primary care: hypertension,* Philadelphia, 1991, Saunders.

27. Hagberg JM: Exercise, fitness and hypertension. In Bouchard C, Shepard RJ, Stephens T, et al, editors: *Exercise, fitness and health: a consensus of current knowledge,* Champaign, Illinois, 1991, Human Kinetics.

28. Hahn A, Anderson SP, Morton AR et al: A re-interpretation of the effect of temperature and water content of the inspired air in exercise-induced asthma, *Am Rev Respir Dis* 130:575-581, 1984.

29. Harris SS, Casperson CJ, DeFriese GH, Estes H: Physical activity counseling for healthy adults as a primary prevention intervention in the clinical setting: report for the U.S. preventive services task force, *JAMA* 261:3590-3608, 1989.

30. Haskell WL, Alderman EL, Fair JM et al: Effects of intensive risk factor reduction on coronary atherosclerosis and clinical events in men and women with coronary artery disease, *Circulation* 89:975-990, 1994.

31. Hennekens CH, Buring JE: Smoking and coronary heart disease in women, *JAMA* 253:3003-3004, 1985.

32. Hiatt WR, Regensteiner JG, Hargerten ME et al: Benefit of exercise conditioning for patients with peripheral arterial disease, *Circulation* 81:602-609, 1990.

33. Jennings G, Nelson L, Nestel P: The effects of changes in physical activity on major cardiovascular risk factors, hemodynamics, sympathetic function, and glucose utilization in man: a controlled study of four levels of activity, *Circulation* 73(1):30-40, 1986.

34. Kane JP, Malloy MJ, Ports TA et al: Regression of coronary atherosclerosis during treatment of familial hypercholesterolemia with combined drug regimes, *JAMA* 264(23):3007-3012, 1990.

35. Kanis JA, Pitt FA: Epidemiology of osteoporosis, *Bone* 13:S7-S15, 1992.

36. Karper WB, Evans BW: Cycling program effects on one rheumatoid arthritic, *Am J Phys Med* 65:167-172, 1986.

37. Kenney WL: *ACSM's* guidelines for exercise testing and prescription, ed 5, Philadelphia, 1995, Williams & Wilkins.

38. Kleinman JC, Donahue RP, Harris MI et al: Mortality among diabetics in a national sample, *Am J Epidemiol* 128:389-401, 1988.

39. Lichtlen PR, Nikutta P, Joss S et al: Anatomical progression of coronary artery disease in humans as seen by prospective, repeated, quantitated coronary angiography: relation to clinical events and risk factors: the INTACT study group, *Circulation* 86(3):828-838, 1992.

40. MacMahon S, Petro R, Cutler J et al: Blood pressure, stroke, and coronary artery disease. I. Prolonged differences in blood pressure—prospective observational studies corrected for the regression dilution bias, *Lancet* 335:765-774, 1990.

41. Morris JN, Heady J, Raffle PA et al: Coronary heart disease and physical activity of work, *Lancet* 2:1053-1057:1111-1210, 1953.

42. Morris JN, Clave SPW, Adam C et al: Vigorous exercise in leisure-time and the incidence of coronary heart-disease, *Lancet* 1:333-339, 1973.

43. Morris JN: *Uses of epidemiology,* ed 3, New York, 1975, Churchill Livingstone.

44. Nordemar R, Ekblom B, Zachrisson L et al: Physical training in rheumatoid arthritis—a controlled long-term study, *Scand J Rheumatol* 10:17-23, 1981.

45. Orenstein DM, Reed ME, Grogan FT, Crawford LV: Exercise conditioning in children with asthma, *J Pediatr* 106:556-561, 1985.

46. Ornish D, Brown SE, Scherwitz LW et al: Can lifestyle changes reverse coronary heart disease? The lifestyle heart trial, *Lancet* 336:129-133, 1990.

47. Paffenbarger RS, Gima AS, Laughlin ME: Characteristics of longshoremen related to fatal coronary heart disease and stroke, *Am J Public Health* 61:1362-1370, 1971.

REFERENCES—Cont'd

48. Paffenbarger RS, Wing AL: Chronic disease in former college students. XVI. Physical activity as an index of heart attack risk in college alumni, *Am J Epidemiol* 108:161-175, 1978.

49. Paffenbarger RS, Hyde RT, Wing AL et al: A natural history of athleticism and cardiovascular health, *JAMA* 252:491-499, 1984.

50. Panush RS, Brown DG: Exercise, the musculoskeletal system, and arthritis, *Postgrad Adv Rheumatol* 2:1-20, 1987.

51. Pope MH: Risk indicators in low back pain, *Ann Med* 21(5):387-392, 1989.

52. Powell KE, Thompson PD, Caspersen CJ, Kendrick JS: Physical activity and the incidence of heart disease, *Annu Rev Public Health* 8:253, 1987.

53. Regensteiner JG, Steiner JF, Panzer RJ, Hiatt WR: Evaluation of walking impairment by questionnaire in patients with peripheral arterial disease, *J Vasc Med Biol* 2:142-147, 1990.

54. Report of the European Respiratory Society Rehabilitation and Chronic Care Scientific Group: Pulmonary rehabilitation in chronic obstruction pulmonary disease (COPD) with recommendations for its use, *Eur Respir J* 5:266-275, 1992.

55. Robertson AJ, Ramesar KC, Potts RC et al: The effect of strenuous physical exercise on circulating blood lymphocytes and serum cortisol levels, *J Clin Lab Immunol* 5:53-63, 1981.

56. Ross R: The pathogenesis of atherosclerosis—an update, *N Engl J Med* 314:488-500, 1986.

57. Schuler G, Hambecht R, Schlierf G et al: Regular physical exercise and low fat diet: effects on progression of coronary artery disease, *Circulation* 86:1-11, 1992.

58. Soppie E, Varjo P, Eskola J, Laitinen LA: Effect of strenuous physical stress on circulating lymphocyte number and function before and after training, *J Clin Lab Immunol* 8:43-52, 1982.

59. Stamler J, Wentworth D, Neaton JD: Is relationship between serum cholesterol and risk of premature death from coronary heart disease continuous and graded? Findings from 356,222 primary screenings of the Multiple Risk Factor Intervention Trial (MRFIT), *JAMA* 322:1700-1707, 1986.

60. Stein RA, Michielli DW, Glantz MD et al: Effects of different exercise intensities on lipoprotein cholesterol fractions in healthy middle-aged men, *Am Heart J* 119:277-283, 1990.

61. Sternfeld B: Cancer and the protective effect of physical activity: the epidemiological evidence, *Med Sci Sports Exerc* 24:1195-2002, 1992.

62. Stratton JR, Chandler WL, Schwartz RS et al: Effects of physical conditioning of fibrinolytic variables and fibrinogen in young and old healthy adults, *Circulation* 83:1692-1698, 1991.

63. The Lipid Research Clinics Program: The Lipid Research Clinics Coronary Prevention Primary Prevention Trial results. I. Reduction in incidence of coronary heart disease, *JAMA* 251:351-364, 1984.

64. Tipton CM: Exercise, training, and hypertension: an update. In Hollozy JO, editor: *Exercise and sport science reviews,* vol 19, Baltimore, 1991, Williams & Wilkins.

65. Trials of Hypertension Prevention Collaborative Research Group: The effects of nonpharmacologic interventions of blood pressure of persons with high normal levels: results of the Trials of Hypertension Prevention, Phase I, *JAMA* 267:1213-1220, 1992.

66. US Department of Health and Human Services: *Asthma statistics,* Washington, DC, 1989, US Government Printing Office.

67. Vitug A, Schneider SH, Ruderman NB: Exercise and type I diabetes mellitus. In Pandolf K, editor: *Exerc Sports Sci Rev* 16:285-304, 1988.

68. Watts GF, Lewis B, Brunt JN et al: Effects on coronary artery disease of lipid-lowering diet, or diet plus cholestyramine, in the St. Thomas' Atherosclerosis Regression Study (STARS), *Lancet* 339:563-569, 1992.

69. Wells A: An estimate of adult mortality in the United States from passive smoking, *Environ Int* 14:249-265, 1988.

70. Wilens SL: Resorption of arterial atheromatous deposits in wasting disease, *Am J Pathol* 36:748, 1947.

71. Winningham ML: The role of exercise in cancer therapy. In Watson RR, Eisinger M, editor: *Exercise and disease,* Boca Raton, Florida, 1992, CRC Press.

72. Wissler RW, Vesselinovitch D: Regression of atherosclerosis in experimental animals and man, *Mod Conc Cardiovasc Dis* 26:27-36, 1977.

73. World Hypertension League: Physical exercise in the management of hypertension: a consensus statement by the World Hypertension League, *J Hypertension* 9:283-287, 1991.

RECOMMENDED READINGS

■ Blair SN, Kohl HW, Paffenbarger RS et al: Physical fitness and all–causes mortality: a prospective study of healthy men and women, *JAMA* 262:2395, 1989.

■ Blair SN, Kohl HW, Gordon NF, Paffenbarger RS: How much physical activity is good for health? *Annu Rev Public Health* 13:99-123, 1992.

■ Bouchard C, Shepard RJ, Stephens T et al, editors: *Exercise, fitness and health. A consensus of current knowledge,* Champaign, Illinois, 1990, Human Kinetics.

■ Watson RR, Eisinger M, editors: *Exercise and disease,* Boca Raton, Florida, 1992, CRC Press.

■ Durstine L, Moore G, Painter P et al, editors: ACSM's guide to exercise management for persons with chronic diseases and disabilities, Champaign, Illinois, Human Kinetics (in press).

■ Ockene I, Ockene J: *Prevention of coronary heart disease,* Boston, 1992, Little, Brown.

■ Ornish D, Brown SE, Scherwitz LW et al: Can lifestyle changes reverse coronary heart disease? The Lifestyle Heart Trial, *Lancet* 336:129-133, 1990.

■ Paffenbarger RS, Gima AS, Laughlin ME: Characteristics of longshoremen related to fatal coronary heart disease and stroke, *Am J Public Health* 61:1362-1370, 1971.

CHAPTER 28

Clinical Evaluation of Exercise Tolerance

OBJECTIVES

After studying this chapter, you should be able to:

■ Describe the indications, contraindications, and uses of clinical exercise testing.

■ List the guidelines for testing healthy individuals, individuals at high risk, and individuals with known disease(s).

■ Demonstrate a basic understanding of electrocardiography and interpretation of the 12-lead exercise electrocardiogram.

■ Explain normal and abnormal responses to clinical exercise testing.

■ Describe the predictive value (Bayes' theorem) of clinical exercise testing.

■ Explain the procedures involved in conducting an exercise test.

■ Describe the procedures for interpreting the results of an exercise test.

KEY TERMS

clinical

diagnostic

contraindication

collaterals

electrocardiograph

electrocardiogram

lead

bipolar

Einthoven's triangle

augmented

tachycardia

bradycardia

cardiac rhythm

arrhythmia

electrical axis

myocardial infarction

ST-segment depression

J point

Mason-Likar lead system

myocardial ischemia

predictive value

echocardiography

thallium-201 stress test

cardiac catheterization

coronary angiogram

This chapter introduces the fundamental principles of clinical exercise testing. The term *clinical* implies that the exercise test is medically oriented. Previous chapters discussed the principles of exercise testing to measure and estimate VO_2max and cardiorespiratory function. How then does clinical exercise testing differ from fitness or performance exercise testing? First, unlike general fitness tests, which are conducted to measure or predict aerobic or anaerobic power in apparently healthy individuals, clinical exercise tests are typically ordered by physicians to screen for coronary heart disease, to evaluate the severity of coronary heart disease, and to assess the status of the cardiovascular system after a myocardial infarction or medical procedure, such as coronary bypass surgery. Second, clinical exercise testing generally requires that personnel conducting the test have advanced training in emergency procedures, electrocardiography, stress testing principles, and basic and advanced principles of cardiovascular medicine. Third, clinical exercise testing requires different equipment, including emergency equipment and an electrocardiogram machine. Fourth, clinical exercise tests are generally performed in a hospital or physician's office, whereas fitness tests are commonly performed in health clubs, YMCAs, or exercise physiology laboratories at colleges and universities. The purpose of this chapter is to introduce the student to the fundamental principles of clinical exercise testing and to provide the foundation for more advanced training and education.

Indications and Uses of Clinical Exercise Testing

Clinical exercise testing has the following three main uses: (1) to diagnose the presence or severity of disease, (2) to establish the functional capacity of an individual, and (3) to evaluate medical therapy (Focus Box 28.1).[13] **Diagnostic** and prognostic evaluation of suspected or established cardiovascular disease is perhaps the most common clinical application of clinical exercise testing. The exercise test is probably the best test of the heart because exercise is the most common everyday stress that humans undertake.

Before ordering a clinical exercise test, a physician must have sufficient evidence and documentation that the test is needed. One of the most common reasons for ordering a clinical exercise test is to diagnose and evaluate the status of suspected or known cardiovascular disease. One situation in which clinical exercise testing is indicated is when a patient comes to a physician's office for a regular checkup so that he or she can start an exercise program. The physician discovers that the patient is sedentary and overweight, smokes a pack of cigarettes per day, has high cholesterol, and has recently complained of several episodes of chest pain during physical exertion. Because the patient in question is at high risk for coro-

clinical (klin′i-kl)
  pertaining to a medical issue

diagnostic (di-ag-nos′tik)
  having a value in diagnosing or detecting a medical condition

FOCUS BOX 28.1

Uses of clinical exercise testing

Exercise Testing of Apparently Healthy Individuals

Determine functional capacity

Screen for disease

Provide motivation

Develop an exercise prescription

Exercise Testing of High-Risk Individuals

Diagnostic tool

  Evaluate suspected heart disease

  Evaluate asymptomatic individuals with risk of coronary heart disease

  Assess patient after myocardial infarction

  Assess patient after coronary angioplasty

  Evaluate dysrhythmias

Identify peripheral vascular disease

Evaluate medical therapy

Exercise Testing of Individuals with a Known Disease

Determine functional capacity

  Assess patient after myocardial infarction

  Assess patient after heart surgery

  Assess patient after repair of heart valves or defects

  Evaluate chronic pulmonary disease

  Evaluate chronic renal disease

  Evaluate diabetes

Evaluate medical therapy

---

nary artery disease, the physician feels comfortable in ordering a clinical exercise evaluation. Clinical exercise testing is an effective way of evaluating the cardiovascular system's response to controlled physiologic stress (exercise). Regardless of whether the patient passes or fails the test, both physician and patient can be better assured of the patient's ability or inability to participate in an exercise program. Thus clinical exercise testing is useful in diagnosing or quantifying heart and other chronic disease conditions (diagnostic testing).

Clinical exercise testing is also commonly used to determine the functional capacity of healthy, sedentary, and asymptomatic individuals (functional testing). For example, when an individual has suffered a heart attack or is recovering from a coronary bypass operation, clinical exercise testing is useful in developing an exercise prescription. Exercise testing can be used to develop a safe and effective level of exercise for individuals with or without disease. The results of a graded exercise test can be used to set the initial intensity, duration, and frequency of exercise. Follow-up testing can be used to modify an earlier exercise prescription. Another indication for ordering a clinical exercise test is when various medical therapies must be assessed (therapeutic testing). Physicians often order a diagnostic exercise test to aid in diagnosing and quantifying heart and lung disease and to assess the patient's response to selected medications.

Risk Stratification

The American College of Sports Medicine defines an apparently healthy individual as someone who has no symptoms or signs of cardiopulmonary or metabolic disease (Focus Box 28.2), seems to be healthy, and has no more than one major coronary risk factor.[1] To help determine whether the patient meets these criteria for apparent health, he or she must complete *a medical health history questionnaire*. Such a questionnaire can be used to evaluate the patient's apparent risk for cardiovascular disease. Routine testing for coronary artery disease in asymptomatic low-risk individuals remains controversial because of the limited predictive capacity for detection of disease in this group.[2,8,11]

An individual classified as a high-risk individual has symptoms suggestive of possible cardiopulmonary or metabolic disease or who has two or more major coronary risk factors.[1] Obviously, testing high-risk individuals is more "risky" than testing apparently healthy individuals. A physician may or may not have to be present when high-risk individuals are tested, depending on the medical history of the individual.

An individual with a known disease is one who has documented evidence of cardiovascular, pulmonary, or metabolic disease.[1] A physician should always be present when an individual with a known disease is tested.

FOCUS BOX 28.2

Major symptoms or signs suggestive of cardiopulmonary or metabolic disease

- Pain or discomfort in the chest or surrounding areas that appears to be ischemic (lack of blood supply to the heart)

- Shortness of breath at rest

- Shortness of breath with mild physical activity

- Dizziness or syncope (syncope is a transient loss of consciousness caused by inadequate blood flow to the brain [fainting])

- Water retention in the lower extremities (edema)

- Skipped heart beats (palpitations) or a racing heart rate (tachycardia)

- Cramping pain in the lower extremities (claudication)

- A diagnosed heart murmur (a murmur is an abnormal heart sound resulting from a valve deformity)

FOCUS BOX 28.3

Contraindications to exercise testing

Major Contraindications

1. Recent acute myocardial infarction

2. Unstable angina (not controlled by medication)

3. Uncontrolled ventricular arrhythmias

4. Uncontrolled atrial arrhythmias that compromise cardiac function

5. Congestive heart failure (CHR) (a condition characterized by extreme weakness, edema [water retention] in the lower extremities and breathlessness because of a reduced pumping ability of the heart)

6. Severe aortic stenosis (a narrowing of the aorta)

7. Suspected or known dissecting aneurysm (the blood makes its way between the layers of a blood vessel wall, separating them in the process)

8. Active or suspected myocarditis (an inflammation of the myocardium)

9. Thrombophlebitis or intercardiac thrombi (an inflammation of a vein in conjunction with the formation of a thrombus [blood clot])

10. Recent systemic or pulmonary embolus (a mass of undissolved matter [solid, liquid, or gaseous] in the blood)

11. Acute infection

12. Third-degree heart block

13. Significant emotional distress

14. A recent significant change in the resting ECG

15. Acute pericarditis (an inflammation of the membrane surrounding the heart muscle)

Relative Contraindications

1. Resting diastolic blood pressure over 120 mm Hg or resting systolic blood pressure over 200 mm Hg

2. Moderate valvular heart disease

3. Digitalis or other drug effect (some medications, such as digitalis, can produce nonspecific ST-T wave changes and ST segment depression)

4. Electrolyte abnormalities (e.g., hypokalemia, hypomagnesemia)

5. Fixed-rate artificial pacemaker (rarely used since 1980s)

6. Frequent or complex ventricular irritability (PVCs)

7. Ventricular aneurysm (an abnormal dilation of a blood vessel, which weakens the artery)

8. Uncontrolled metabolic diseases (e.g., diabetes)

9. Any serious infectious disease (e.g., AIDS, hepatitis)

10. Neuromuscular, musculoskeletal, or rheumatoid disorders that make exercise difficult

11. Advanced or complicated pregnancy

*Adapted from American College of Sports Medicine: *Guidelines for exercise testing and prescription,* ed 5, Philadelphia, 1995, Lea & Febiger.

Contraindications to Clinical Exercise Testing

A variety of benefits can be derived from exercise testing, but the procedure is not without risks. Conditions that significantly increase the risks of such a test are collectively termed **contraindications**. Ideally, the benefits of the test and the results obtained should outweigh the potential risks of performing the test. The risk of death during an exercise test is approximately 0.5 per 10,000 tests.[20] Based on pooled data from several different studies, it has been determined that the risk of death after exercise testing is 1 per 10,000 tests, the risk of myocardial infarctions is 4 per 10,000 tests, and approximately 5 hospital admissions (including infarctions) occur per 10,000 tests.[4,20,22,23] Thus the test is extremely safe as long as the personnel administering it follow the recommended safety procedures and the patient is properly screened beforehand for potential contraindications (Focus Box 28.3).

For individuals with absolute contraindications the risks of the test may not outweigh the potential benefits. Other forms of diagnostic testing may be more appropriate in these situations (see section on other cardiovascular tests). The contraindications to exercise testing imply that patients should have a stable medical status before undergoing any form of exercise testing. Patients with stable medical conditions are at less risk for complications during and after exercise testing. Thus all patients scheduled to undergo exercise testing should have a complete medical history, a physical examination, and selected laboratory tests. In addition to the contraindications listed in Focus Box 28.3, the reliability of the diagnostic exercise test is reduced in individuals with certain clinical conditions, such as left bundle branch block, heart pacemakers, left ventricular hypertrophy, and anterior myocardial infarctions. Understanding of these contraindications is increased by knowing the arterial vasculature of the heart (see Focus Box 28.4).

FOCUS BOX 28.4

Coronary circulation

Because one of the main purposes of exercise testing is to identify poor circulation in the coronary arteries, a brief review of the coronary circulation is helpful. Remember that the heart has its own blood supply (Figure 28.1). The coronary arteries originate from the aorta at two main sites, the right and left coronary arteries. The left main artery divides into two main divisions, the left anterior descending and the left circumflex. The coronary arteries can be thought of as branches of a tree. Consider the aorta as the trunk, the right and left main coronary arteries, the posterior descending, anterior descending, and the circumflex as the main branches, and the other arteries as smaller branches. New branches form because of chronic ischemia, and are referred to as **collaterals.** Coronary collateral circulation becomes an important supply of blood to the heart muscle after a myocardial infarction. Because the heart muscle cells are highly aerobic $(a - vO_2 \Delta = 70\%$ to $80\%)$ and have a poor anaerobic capacity, the only way the heart can get additional ATP regeneration during periods of increased demand is by an increase in coronary blood supply. When coronary arteries become blocked because of coronary heart disease or have a spasm, coronary artery blood supply is compromised, resulting in a mismatch between supply and demand. This mismatch in supply and demand, if severe enough, can be detected on the ECG as ST segment depression or ST segment elevation in more extreme cases.

Electrocardiography

One of the essential tools used in clinical exercise testing is the **electrocardiograph**. There are two common abbreviations for electrocardiograph. *EKG* is an abbreviation for the German language, in which cardiograph is written as kardiograph, and ironically is used more frequently than the English abbreviation *ECG*. Both abbreviations are correct, and the English abbreviation is used in this chapter. The ECG is the instrument that provides an **electrocardiogram,** which is a recording of the electrical activity of the heart. The abbreviation ECG is often used interchangeably between the instrument and the tracing. An ECG is able to detect and record small changes in electrical activity on the surface of the skin that originate in the heart. When electrodes are placed at specific locations on the body and connected to an ECG, a reproducible tracing of the electrical activity of the heart can be recorded (electrocardiograph) (Figure 28.2). One complete cardiac cycle (heartbeat) recorded on the ECG represents the spread of electrical activity from the SA node all the way to the Purkinje fibers of the ventricular myocardium.

The ECG records the differences in voltage between a positive and a negative electrode. The voltage difference between two electrodes is termed a **lead**. As a wave of electricity or depolarization reaches a positive electrode, an

FIGURE 28.1

Coronary circulation from an **A,** anterior and **B,** posterior perspective. From an anterior perspective, the major coronary arteries seen are the left and right coronary arteries, circumflex artery, and left anterior descending artery. From the posterior perspective, the major arteries seen are the circumflex artery, right coronary artery, posterior descending artery, and the nodal artery. (From Thibodeau GA, Patton KT: *Anatomy and physiology,* 3 ed, St. Louis, 1996, Mosby. Art by Network Graphics.)

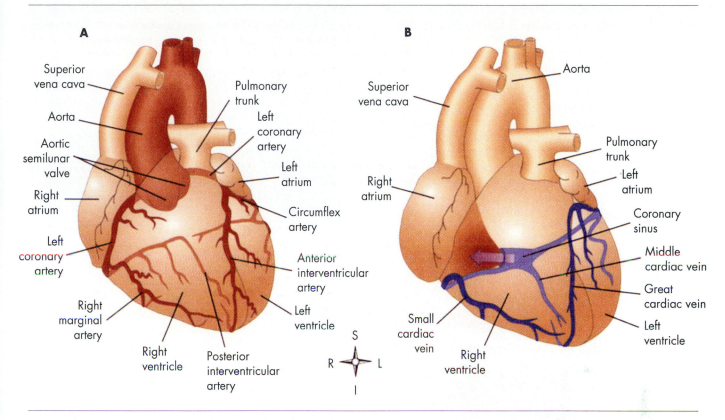

upward deflection occurs on the ECG paper (see Figure 28.2). As a wave of depolarization moves away from the positive electrode, a downward deflection occurs.

The ECG is recorded on ruled paper (Figure 28.3). The smallest divisions are 1 millimeter squares. There are five small squares between the heavy black lines. The height and depth of waves (measured in millimeters) are a measure of voltage. Upward deflections are called *positive deflections.* Downward deflections are called *negative deflections.* The horizontal axis of the ECG paper represents time and is measured in seconds. One millimeter square represents 0.04 second. If there are five small (1 millimeter) squares between two heavy black lines, (0.04 × 5) is equal to 0.2 second. The standard paper speed on an ECG is 25 mm/second, and the standard deflection calibration is 1 mV equaling a deflection of 10 mm or 1 cm.

Characteristics of the ECG

Five key waves and intervals make up the standard ECG trace. Each wave or interval represents a particular electrochemical phase of the cardiac cycle (see Chapter 11). A wave represents depolarization or repolarization, whereas an inter-val represents time during which the electrical signal is traveling away from the SA node and there is no depolarization of the myocardium. The height, width, and shape of the wave and the length and shape of the interval can indicate a variety of pathologic and medical conditions.

contraindication (kon-tra-**in**'di-ka'shun)
a condition that prevents the use or application of something

collaterals (co-**lat**'er'als)
coronary blood vessels that grow because of chronic exposure of a region to ischemia

electrocardiograph (ECG) (e'lek'tro-**kar**-di'o-graf)
the equipment used to detect and record the electrical activity of the heart

electrocardiogram (e'lek'tro-**kar**-di'o-gram)
the recording from an electrocardiograph

lead (leed)
the electrical arrangement of specific electrodes when placed on the body during electrocardiography

FIGURE 28.2

Top, The standard electrocardiograph showing repeated waves and segments. *Bottom,* The electrical changes during the cardiac cycle cause the changes seen on a standard electrocardiograph. Depolarization of the atrium causes the P-wave, depolarization of the ventricular myocardium causes the QRS complex, and repolarization of the ventricular myocardium causes the T-wave.

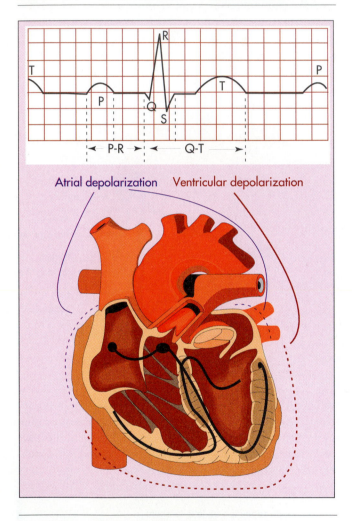

FIGURE 28.3

Paper used for the electrocardiograph (ECG) is precision graphed to reveal small and large grid-like boxes. When the paper is fed at a rate of 25 mm/s, each small box grid represents a time of 0.04 s, and each large box grid represents 0.2 s. The ECG is also calibrated to produce 1 mv of signal in 10 mm of vertical displacement (5 large box grids). (Adapted from Conover MB: *Understanding electrocardiography*, 6 ed, St. Louis, 1992, Mosby.)

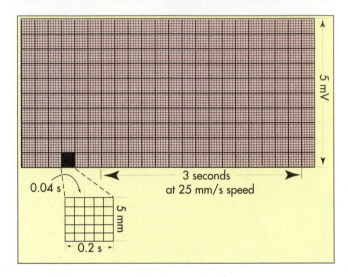

- **S wave**—the S wave results from ventricular depolarization.
  - **ST segment**—extends between the end of the S wave (J Point) and the beginning of the next T wave. The ST segment coincides with ventricular repolarization.
  - **T wave**—the T wave represents the repolarization of the ventricles.

The cellular membrane events of depolarization and repolarization are detailed in Chapters 7 and 8.

Standard 12-Lead Electrocardiograph

The standard 12-lead electrocardiograph is composed of three limb leads—I, II, III; three augmented limb leads—aVR, aVL, aVF; and six chest leads—V_{1-6}. The limb leads all lie in a plane that can be visualized over the patient's chest (frontal plane or top to bottom). The chest leads circle the heart and form the horizontal plane (front to back). Each lead provides a different angle or picture of the heart (Figure 28.4). It is possible to obtain an anterior view of the heart by looking at leads V_1 through V_4, a lateral view of the heart by looking at leads I, aVL, V_5, and V_6, and an inferior view of the heart by looking at leads II, III, and aVF.

The standard limb lead electrodes that are attached to the left arm (LA), left leg (LL), and right arm (RA) comprise

- **P wave**—the P wave represents right and left atrial depolarization.
- **PR segment**—extends between the end of the P wave and the onset of either the Q wave or the R wave if the Q wave is not present. The PR segment represents arrival and delay of the electrical impulse at the AV node and transmission through the bundle of His, bundle branches, and Purkinje fibers.
- **QRS complex**—the QRS complex represents ventricular depolarization.
- **Q wave**—the Q wave represents left-to-right septal depolarization.
- **R wave**—the R wave results from ventricular depolarization.

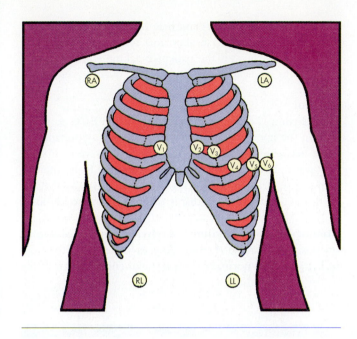

FIGURE 28.4

The location of electrodes for the 12-lead electrocardiograph. Traditionally, the limb leads (I, II, III) and their electrodes (RA, LA, RL, LL) were placed peripherally with arm electrodes on the wrists and leg electrodes on the ankles. However, as this arrangement is not conducive to exercise testing, the Mason-Likar lead system is used. As shown, the arm and leg electrodes are moved to the shoulders and lower torso regions, respectively. The chest electrodes are placed so that V_1 and V_2 occur in the 4th intercostal space, V_4 in the 5th intercostal space at the level of the mid-clavicle, V_3 mid-way between V_2 and V_4, and V_5 and V_6 in the fifth intercostal space evenly spread to the mid-auxillary region. (Source: Froelicher VF et al: *Exercise and the heart,* 3 ed, St. Louis, 1993, Mosby.)

the three bipolar leads. **Bipolar** means that the standard limb leads are recording the difference between two points. Lead I records the voltage difference between the LA and the RA, lead II records the voltage difference between the LL and the RA, and lead III records the voltage difference between the LL and the LA. The three leads form a triangle named **Einthoven's triangle**. Einthoven's triangle assumes that the human torso is a sphere of conducting ability and that the heart is a point at its center. Einthoven's law states that lead II is equal to the sum of the complexes in leads I and III. The **augmented** limb leads are *unipolar*, meaning that they measure electrical activity at one point or one electrode. The aVR measures the electrical activity at the RA, and all other limb leads act as grounds. The aVL measures the electrical activity at the LA, and aVF measures the electrical activity at the LL. The precordial (or chest leads) are also unipolar leads, so they also measure the electrical activity at one location.

Interpretation of the 12-Lead Electrocardiogram

Learning to interpret an ECG recording takes years of experience. The purpose of this chapter is to introduce the fundamental principles of ECG interpretation. The basic rule in ECG interpretation is to use the same approach or system every time you evaluate an ECG. There are three key steps to follow when evaluating any ECG. These steps include determining the rate, rhythm, and axis. Eventually you will learn to analyze all of the different waves, segments, and intervals to determine any abnormalities in the ECG. Because many exercise physiology students are finding employment opportunities in clinical settings, such as working in a hospital as a

cardiovascular technologist, it is highly recommended that students eventually take an advanced class in electrocardiography. These classes are often held at local hospitals, and frequently students are welcome to attend.

Rate

The first measurement to calculate when looking at the electrocardiogram is the heart rate. The rate is measured as cycles per minute or beats per minute (bpm). The PQRST waves represent one complete cardiac cycle. The first way to determine heart rate from the ECG is to find an R wave that falls on a heavy black line. Count off 300, 150, 75, 60 for each heavy black line that follows. Where the next R wave falls determines the rate. Another way uses small marks at the top of the ECG paper that indicate 3-second intervals with a paper speed of 25 mm/s. Count the number of cycles in a 6-second strip and multiply by 10. The last way to determine heart rate is simply to divide 1500 by the number of small squares (1 mm) between any two R waves. It is important to determine heart rate accurately and quickly in order to assess whether any abnormalities are present.

---

bipolar (bi-pole'ar)

a description of the leads that compare the electrical difference between two electrodes

Einthoven's triangle

the law that equates the limb leads of the 12-lead ECG, in which the average electrical potential of lead II equals the sum of leads I and III

augmented (awg'men'ted)

a description of the leads that measure the electrical activity at one electrode

Abnormalities in heart rate. A heart rate over 100 bpm is referred to as **tachycardia**. A heart rate below 60 bpm is referred to as **bradycardia**. A variety of factors affect heart rate, including age (declines with age), gender (females generally have higher resting heart rates), physical stature (small animals have higher heart rates), emotion (stress can elevate heart rate), type of food consumed (caffeine increases heart rate), body temperature (as body temperature rises, so does heart rate), environmental factors (smoking increases heart rate), medication, and exercise. Highly trained endurance athletes tend to have extremely low resting rates (35 to 50 bpm) as a result of greater parasympathetic tone at rest. It is important to recognize that some abnormalities in resting heart rate occur naturally (e.g., are brought on by exercise training) and may be perfectly fine for an individual, whereas other abnormalities are pathogenic in nature (e.g., sick sinus syndrome and bundle branch block) and may require medical therapy. Furthermore, causes of an abnormal resting heart rate may not be natural (e.g., if the patient is taking stimulants) and may lead to medical problems, especially during exercise.

Rhythm

Rhythm is the most difficult part of the ECG to interpret. In the normal **cardiac rhythm** there is a constant distance between similar waves (R wave to R wave or P wave to P wave). To determine rhythm, measure the R-R intervals across the entire strip. A constant R-R interval means that the rhythm is regular, or sinus, that is, originating in the SA node.

Abnormalities in rhythm. **Arrhythmias** are abnormal (inconsistent) cardiac rhythms. Any variation from the normal rhythm and normal electrical conduction pattern of the

---

FIGURE 28.5

Common arrythmias detected by the electrocardiograph: **A,** unifocal premature ventricular contractions (PVCs). **B,** Atrial fibrillation. **C,** Premature atrial contractions (PACs). (From Conover MB: *Understanding electrocardiography,* 6 ed, St. Louis, 1992, Mosby.)

A
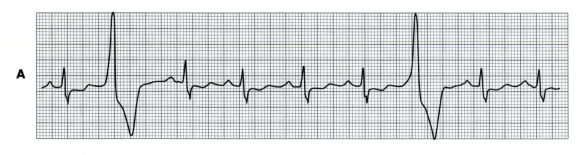

B
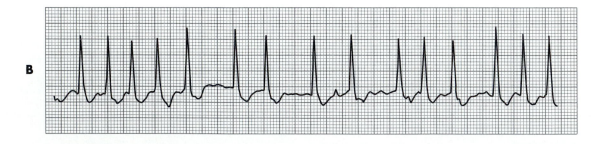

C
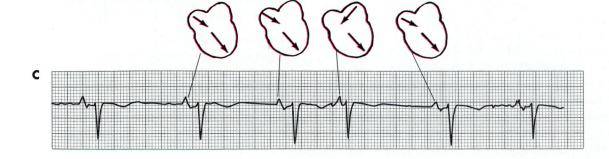

heart is referred to as an arrhythmia. Arrhythmias are determined by comparing a suspect ECG strip with a static 12-lead ECG from the same individual or with a memorized appearance of each lead of the normal 12-lead ECG. Arrhythmias are generally categorized based on the location of the ECG problem in relation to the electrical conduction system. Some common arrhythmias are described below and shown in Figure 28.5.

Normal sinus rhythm (NSR)
Rate—60 to 100 bpm
Rhythm—regular
P waves—upright in leads I, II, and aVF

Atrial fibrillation: results from multiple areas of reentry within the atria or from multiple ectopic foci.

---

tachycardia (tak-i-**kar**′di-ah)
a heart rate above 100 bpm

bradycardia (brad-i-**kar**′di-ah)
a heart rate below 60 bpm

cardiac rhythm
the electrical pattern of the electrocardiograph. The rhythm can be normal or abnormal. When normal, it is usually described as normal sinus rhythm.

arrhythmia (a-**rith**′mi-ah)
abnormal cardiac rhythm. There are many different cardiac arrhythmias.

CLINICAL APPLICATION

Treatment of Life-Threatening Arrhythmias

Anyone involved in clinical exercise testing needs to be able to provide basic cardiac life support (CPR) in an emergency situation. In addition, training and certification in advance cardiac life support (ACLS) also is highly desirable. When an emergency situation arises, all personnel must follow their individual emergency medical system (EMS) plan. Essential to the survival of a patient in cardiac arrest is to perform the ABCD's of emergency life support. *A* stands for airway, *B* stands for breathing, *C* stands for circulation, and *D* stands for defibrillation.

ABCD's of emergency life support*
Airway: *Open the airway.
Breathing: *Provide positive pressure ventilation.
Circulation: *Give chest compressions.
Defibrillation: *Shock VF/pulseless VT.

CPR is the most important emergency procedure when someone stops breathing and/or his or her heart stops. In a situation where ventricular fibrillation (VF) or pulseless ventricular tachycardia (VT) can be verified, the patient needs to be defibrillated immediately. Defibrillation only can be performed by trained personnel. Following is a list of essential medical equipment and supplies that need to be present during clinical exercise testing.

Essential medical equipment and supplies for clinical exercise testing†

EQUIPMENT
Defibrillator-monitor

Airway equipment
Oxygen
AMBU bag with pressure release valve
Suction equipment
Intravenous sets and stand
Intravenous fluids
Syringes and needles in multiple sizes
Adhesive tape

DRUGS (IV form unless otherwise indicated)
Lidocaine
Epinephrine
Atropine
Isoproterenol
Procainamide
Sodium bicarbonate
Bretylium
Verapamil
Propranolol or Esmolol
Diazepam
Dopamine
Nitroglycerine
Furosemide
Nitroglycerine tablets or oral spray

Figure 28.6 is an example of the advanced cardiac life support universal algorithm for adults. If VT or VF is present, then rescuers follow a different algorithm. For more information on advance cardiac care, see the American Heart Association's Textbook on Advanced Cardiac Life Support.

---

*Adapted from Cummins RO, ed.: *Textbook of advanced cardiac life support*, Dallas, 1994, American Heart Association.
†Adapted: American College of Sports Medicine: *Guidelines for exercise testing and prescription*, ed 5, Philadelphia, 1995, Lea & Febiger.

FIGURE 28.6

The leads of the 12-lead electrocardiograph (ECG) can be viewed radially, so that each passes through an identical central location. Such an hexaxial arrangement of the leads allows the 12-lead ECG to evaluate electrical axis and assist in relating one lead to another. (Source: Conover MB: *Understanding electrocardiography*, 6 ed, St. Louis, 1992, Mosby.)

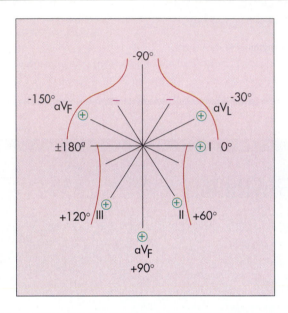

Rate—atrial rate (400 to 700 bpm) but cannot be counted with accuracy. Ventricular rate (160 to 180 bpm)

Rhythm—irregular

P waves—organized atrial activity is absent. This rhythm can be described as chaotic.

FIGURE 28.7

Universal algorithm for adult emergency cardiac care. (Adapted from Cummins RO (editor): *Textbook on advanced cardiac life support*, 1994, American Heart Association.)

Premature ventricular contraction (PVC): PVCs are caused by depolarization that arises in either ventricle before the next expected beat.

> Rate—varies
>
> Rhythm—irregular
>
> P waves—may be obscured by the QRS, ST segment, or T wave of the PVC.

The Clinical Application on p. 723 provides an overview to the basic and advance treatment of life threatening arrhythmias.

Axis

The **electrical axis** is referred to as the mean QRS vector and represents the mean direction of depolarization from the SA node to the AV node and ventricular myocardium. For example, if an imaginary circle is drawn over the chest, the center of the circle lies over the AV node. The circle is divided into a vertical plane and a horizontal plane. The vertical plane runs from the head (−90 degrees on the circle) to the feet (90 degrees on the circle). The horizontal plane runs from the right side of the body (180 degrees on the circle) to the left side of the body is equal (0 degrees on the circle). The normal QRS vector is located between −30 and +120 degrees, which correspond to leads aVL and II of the hexaxial lead configuration, respectively (Figure 28.7). When the left ventrical is hypertrophied (either from exercise or disease), the electrical axis shifts toward it to numbers more negative than −30 degrees (left axis deviation). In cases of necrosis of the left ventricular myocardium caused by a heart attack, the electrical axis shifts away from the left ventrical to numbers more positive than 120 degrees (right axis deviation). Determining axis assists in the overall interpretation of the ECG.

Determining axis. Electrical axis system is determined from the limb leads. For a given lead:

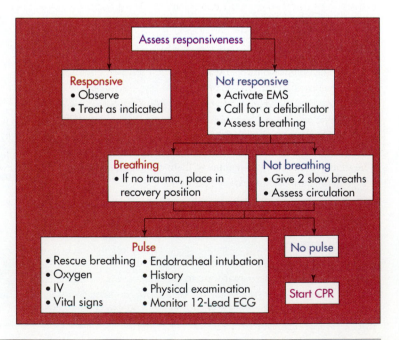

Positive QRS deflection occurs when the height of the R wave exceeds the combined deflection of the Q and S waves. Negative QRS deflection occurs when the combined deflection of the Q and S waves exceeds the height of the R wave. Zero mean QRS deflection occurs when the height of the R wave equals the combined deflection of the Q and S waves.

Step 1—Look at lead I and determine if the mean QRS deflection is positive or negative.

Step 2—Look at lead aVF and determine if the mean QRS deflection is positive or negative.

1. If the mean QRS deflection activity is upright in both leads, the axis is in the normal quadrant (0 to 90 degrees).
2. If the mean QRS deflection activity is positive in lead I but negative in lead aVF, the axis is in the left axis quadrant (0 to −90 degrees).
3. If the mean QRS deflection activity is positive in lead aVF but negative in lead I, the axis is in the right axis quadrant (90 to 180 degrees).
4. If the mean QRS deflection activity is negative in both leads, the axis is in the northwest axis quadrant (−90 to −180 degrees).

For refining the determination of axis within the normal, left, and right axis quadrants, check the remaining leads within that quadrant and ascertain which lead has the more positive R wave. If two leads have a similar R-wave magnitude, the axis is located between these two leads.

Myocardial Infarction

When the delivery of blood supply to the heart muscle is compromised for an extended period because of a spasm or a blood clot, the inner lining of the heart (subendocardial) or the entire thickness of the heart (transmural) can be affected. If the ischemia is severe or prolonged, the tissue being affected is injured, cell functions cease, and irreversible cell death occurs. This condition is termed **myocardial infarction**. The majority of myocardial infarctions (more than 87%) result from a portion of a plaque in the coronary arteries breaking loose and lodging at a site of narrowing farther down the artery, forming a clot. The affected muscle tissue is no longer able to contract. The extent of myocardial damage can be determined later through echocardiography and a thallium-201 exercise test. The changes in the ECG resulting from myocardial ischemia are presented in the Clinical Application on p. 726.

Exercise-Induced Arrhythmias

Exercise-induced arrhythmias occur as a result of enhanced sympathetic tone, increased myocardial oxygen demand, or both. The increased sympathetic tone in the myocardium may stimulate foci in the Purkinje fibers, initiating spontaneous discharge and leading to

increased automaticity. Some arrhythmias, such as premature ventricular contractions (PVCs) or premature atrial contractions, are common during exercise testing, occurring in as many as 40% of subjects who do not have cardiovascular disease.[18]

Since exercise increases myocardial oxygen demand, ectopic activity may develop in individuals with coronary artery disease. The immediate period after exercise is especially dangerous because of high catecholamine levels and generalized vasodilation. Peripheral arteriole vasodilation induced by exercise can reduce venous return, decrease cardiac output, and diminish coronary artery perfusion. Exercise may also induce cardiac arrhythmias under conditions including digitalis or diuretic therapy and recent ingestion of alcohol, caffeine, or other stimulants. Metabolic acidosis can also potentiate cardiac arrhythmias.

Sinus arrhythmias with sinus bradycardia and wandering atrial pacemaker are fairly common during exercise and recovery. First-degree AV block may occur in the late exercise phase and recovery phase in those who are predisposed by condition or drug therapy. This may include persons taking digitalis or beta blockers. The occurrence of second-degree AV block in the form of Wenckebach Mobitz type I AV block and Mobitz type II AV block is relatively rare, and the clinical significance is uncertain. The occurrence of complete or third-degree AV block at rest or with exercise is considered a contraindication to exercise testing.[1]

The occurrence of intraventricular blocks with exercise is relatively rare. Left or right bundle branch blocks and hemiblocks may occur with exercise and usually precede the appearance of chronic block at rest. Exercise may provoke, suppress, or not affect anomalous AV conduction in persons with known Wolff-Parkinson-White (WPW) syndrome. When anomalous AV conduction is present, ST segment depression may occur with exercise testing; it may be secondary to ischemia but is most likely a false-positive response. Exercise is considered a stimulus for tachyarrhythmias in WPW syndrome, although their occurrence is not common. Between 20% and 50% of individuals with anomalous AV conduction present on the ECG will have normal conduction during exercise.[5]

Exercise-induced atrial premature beats and nonsustained supraventricular tachycardia may occur in normal or diseased hearts. Exercise-induced atrial flutter or atrial fibrillation that is transient may occur in those with normal hearts or in conditions including ischemic heart disease, pulmonary

electrical axis
the average direction of depolarization, expressed as a degree based on the hexaxial arrangement of the leads

myocardial infarction
injury to myocardium because of lack of oxygen caused by ischemia

ST Segment Depression and Myocardial Infarction

ST segment depression

ST segment depression on the ECG is the hallmark of myocardial ischemia. ST segment depression is the principal abnormality during exercise that should concern individuals supervising a treadmill test. When the delivery of blood supply to the heart muscle is inadequate, the inner lining of the heart (subendocardium), which is under the greatest pressure contraction, suffers first. At the onset of ischemia the reduction of blood supply alters the normal cellular action potential, causing the ST segment to be displaced below the baseline. ST segment depression resulting from exercise is usually subendocardial ischemia.

ST segment depression occurs in three general varieties: horizontal, downsloping, or upsloping (Figure 28.8). The **J point** (end of QRS) serves as a reference point for the analysis of the ST segment. Upsloping ST segment depression is defined as an ST segment that is depressed from the baseline greater than 0.7 mm but less than 1.5 mm by 80 msec past the J point. In this case the ST segment depression may be suggestive of myocardial ischemia. Where it is greater than 1.5 mm, the response is suggestive of myocardial ischemia.[10]

Horizontal ST depression is defined as 1 mm or more of depression at the J point when ST depression continues for 80 msec after the J point. Because of motion artifact during exercise, this depression should be seen in three consecutive beats with a reasonably stable baseline.

Downsloping ST depression occurs when the ST segment measured 80 msec from the J point is greater than 1 mm, resulting in a negative slope of the ST segment. With a normal, isoelectric ST segment at baseline, the presence of either horizontal or downsloping ST depression is abnormal and suggests exercise-induced myocardial ischemia. With worsening ischemia the depth of ST depression may increase; occasionally it worsens during the recovery phase, and in about 10% of patients the ST depression occurs only during the recovery phase.[15]

ST segment depression occurs with ischemia because under normal conditions the ST segment is isoelectric at baseline. During exercise-induced ischemia the ischemic tissue produces an injury current that generates an electric dipole. This dipole results in an ST segment shift that consists mainly of ST depression relative to the ECG baseline. The lead location of this ST depression does not indicate the anatomic site of ischemia, nor does it identify which coronary artery is involved.[16] However, the severity of ST depression (greater than 2 mm), a downsloping character, early time of onset, the number of ECG leads involved, and persistence of the ST depression late into recovery are all associated with the severity of myocardial ischemia and the extent of the coronary artery disease.

Diagnostic ST segment criteria for myocardial ischemia

* Horizontal or downsloping ST segment depression that is equal to or greater than 1 mm at 80 msec past the J point

* ST segment elevation of greater than or equal to 1 mm at 80 msec past the J point

* Upsloping ST depression that is equal to or greater than 1.5 mm at 80 msec past the J point

Although J point depression is a normal finding during exercise, it is often seen with either a rapid or slow upsloping ST depression after the J point. A rapid upsloping ST segment (more than 1 mV/sec with less than 1.5 mm ST depression) is likely to be normal, whereas a slow upsloping ST segment (more than 1.5 mm ST depression 80 msec from the J point) is more likely to be abnormal in individuals with a high pretest likelihood of coronary artery disease. In other words, the probability and severity of coronary artery disease are inversely related to the slope of the ST segment.

ST segment elevation

Exercise-induced ST segment elevation is a relatively rare finding during treadmill testing. ST segment elevation is defined as 1 mm or more of J point elevation that persists during the ST segment for 80 msec in three consecutive beats. This finding is usually considered to represent cardiac pathology. The nature of this pathology depends on the clinical setting in which the treadmill test is performed. In evaluation of the significance of ST elevation, it is important to determine if Q waves are present in the same or adjacent leads. Without prior Q wave myocardial infarction, ST elevation and its location (inferior, anterior, lateral) identify a site of severe transient ischemia, often involving a proximal coronary artery stenosis in the territory surrounded by the lead changes.

In subjects with a prior Q wave myocardial infarction, the ST segment elevation may represent abnormal wall motion (e.g., left ventricular aneurysm), preinfarction ischemia, or both.[12] Several retrospective studies have suggested that patients having ST segment elevation with associated Q waves on a resting ECG have multivessel disease, whereas ST segment elevation in the absence of Q waves is associated with single-vessel disease at catheterization.[3,21]

FIGURE 28.8

The three types of st-segment depression: **A,** Down sloping, **B,** horizontal, and **C,** up sloping.

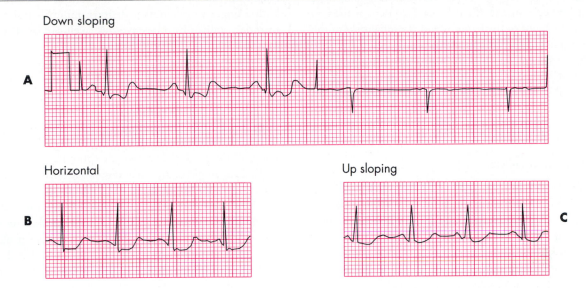

disease, rheumatic heart disease, hyperthyroidism, WPW syndrome, cardiomyopathy, or recent caffeine or alcohol ingestion. The occurrence of exercise-induced supraventricular arrhythmias is not diagnostic for ischemic heart disease.[6]

In approximately one third of subjects, ventricular ectopy develops in response to exercise testing. The appearance of premature ventricular complexes and three to six beats of nonsustained ventricular tachycardia is not diagnostic for ischemic or other forms of heart disease in the absence of ischemic ECG changes. Approximately 50% of subjects with coronary artery disease have ventricular arrhythmias during exercise. The prognostic significance of exercise-induced ventricular arrhythmias in persons with coronary artery disease remains controversial. Suppression of ventricular ectopy with exercise is a nonspecific finding and can occur in normal subjects, as well as those with coronary artery disease.

Using the exercise test to evaluate subjects with arrhythmias is an important part of the total evaluation, along with ambulatory monitoring and electrophysiologic studies. Exercise testing provokes repetitive ventricular beats in most subjects with a history of sustained ventricular arrhythmia. In subjects with a recent myocardial infarction, the presence of exercise-induced repetitive ventricular beats is associated with an increased risk of future cardiac events, including sudden death.

The exercise test is also valuable in the assessment of the effects of antiarrhythmic medications and in the management of subjects with chronic atrial fibrillation. Exercise testing can be indicated in subjects who have symptoms consistent with arrhythmias (e.g., syncope, palpitations). The testing may be used to reveal complex ventricular arrhythmias, to provoke supraventricular arrhythmias, to determine the relationship between arrhythmias and activity, to aid in determining optimal antiarrhythmic therapy, and to reveal proarrhythmic responses to antiarrhythmic drugs.

Conducting the Clinical Exercise Test

Pretest Data Collection and Informed Consent

Before an exercise test is administered for diagnostic purposes, certain medical information is needed from the patient. The following data should be obtained and tests conducted before the exercise test:

- Recent medical history
- Coronary heart disease risk factor assessment
- A brief physical examination conducted by a trained medical professional

ST segment depression
the lowering of the ST segment, usually because of myocardial ischemia. Pharmacologic and ventilation conditions can also lower the ST segment.

J point
the end of the QRS complex and the beginning of the baseline portion of the ST segment

• Laboratory tests, including total cholesterol, HDL cholesterol, and possibly triglycerides and blood glucose

Before a patient is allowed to exercise, he or she must sign an informed consent. An informed consent is used to "inform" the patient of the benefits and potential risks of the test. It does not remove any of the patient's right to receive responsible treatment, and this fact should be communicated to the patient.

When all of these data are collected, the physician can determine whether there are any absolute or relative contraindications to testing.

Patient Instructions

Instructions should always be given to patients before the day of the test. General pretest instructions include the following:
• Patients should abstain from food, tobacco, alcohol, and caffeine for at least 3 hours before the test.
• Patients should wear comfortable clothing, including sports or athletic shoes.
• Women patients should wear a jogging bra if they have one.
• Patients should continue to take their prescribed medication unless their physician has instructed otherwise (Focus Box 28.5).

On arrival at the clinic the patient should be made as comfortable as possible. Patients are often anxious before a diagnostic exercise test. To help make the patient feel more relaxed, the exercise test technologist should do the following:
• Explain the purpose of the test and the various procedures that are to follow.
• Explain each procedure before starting.
• Ensure that the patient's privacy is protected at all times.
• Explain the types of measurements and how often they will be taken.

Preparing the Patient

After all the preliminary data have been collected and the testing is approved, the exercise test technologist can start preparing the patient for the test. These procedures generally include obtaining the patient's weight (kg) and height (cm) and placing the ECG electrodes (see Figure 28.7).

Disposable electrodes with gel-filled caps and a silver chloride element are recommended to decrease motion artifact and to improve the accuracy of the recording.[12] The importance of skin preparation before electrode placement cannot be overemphasized. All of the sophisticated computerized equipment in use today is of little value if a clear recording with minimal artifact is not maintained during the stress test. Good electrode contact is the key to a high-quality recording. Skin oils should be removed with alcohol or acetone at the sites of electrode placement. Male patients may have to have hair shaved off in the appropriate locations. This is followed by removal of the superficial layer of skin with light abrasion using a fine-grain emery paper or other abra-

sive pad. Dead skin cells act as an insulator, increasing the skin resistance. The goal is to reduce skin resistance to less than 5000 ohms. After placement, each electrode should be tapped with a finger to ensure that there is minimal "noise" on the recorder with this maneuver. A well-prepared electrode should display no artifacts.

Lead Systems

During electrocardiographic analysis of exercise the use of multiple-lead systems has been shown to more accurately detect evidence of coronary artery disease than single-lead systems.[7] Optimal lead systems are those with 12 leads. Bipolar leads in single or multiple combination (CM5, CC5) are less sensitive for diagnostic testing but may be useful for routine ECG monitoring during testing of functional capacity.

During exercise, because of significant limb movement, a 12-lead ECG cannot be obtained accurately if electrodes are placed on wrists and ankles. Mason and Likar developed a 12-lead system in which limb leads were placed at the base of the limbs on the torso, thereby avoiding placement of electrodes on exercising limbs.[17] The Mason-Likar simulated standard 12-lead ECG electrode placement is presented in Figure 28.7. The ankle and wrist electrodes are replaced by electrodes mounted on the torso at the base of the limbs. The standard precordial leads use as their negative reference Wilson's central terminal, which is formed by connecting the right arm, left arm, and left leg. The triangular configuration around the heart results in a zero-voltage reference through the cardiac cycle.

The **Mason-Likar lead system** is the most commonly used electrode system for exercise testing. There is evidence that the Mason-Likar placement of electrodes causes amplitude changes and axis shifts when compared with standard placement of ECG electrodes. Therefore the Mason-Likar system should not be used for recording a resting ECG. Changes seen using modified lead placement with the Mason-Likar system can be limited by keeping the arm electrodes on the shoulders instead of the chest. A baseline ECG recording with the subject supine or standing and with standard electrode placement will provide an accurate baseline recording before the exercise test.

Standing and hyperventilation can change the configuration of the baseline ECG. Axis shifts, Q wave formation, and ST and T wave changes may occur as a result of these maneuvers. It is important to record a standing and hyperventilation ECG before beginning the exercise test. If standing or hyperventilation produces significant changes, especially in the ST segment, the specificity of the test can be reduced.

A study by Miranda et al. demonstrated that monitoring the inferior leads alone during exercise is of little value.[19] It was demonstrated, with angiographic data of coronary arteries, that ST segment depression in the inferior leads alone was a poor marker for coronary artery disease. It was also demonstrated that lead V_5 was markedly superior to lead II in reliably identifying true ischemia.[19] Approximately 70% to 89% of abnormal ST segment changes can be picked up by V_5 alone.[14]

Choosing the Test Protocol

A variety of graded exercise test protocols are available. The exercise testing protocol should be individually selected, based on the clinical and functional status of the patient. All protocols should have a gradual warm-up period and a progressive increase in workload. The Bruce protocol is popular in clinical settings. Most deconditioned patients can complete only one to three stages of the Bruce protocol, and thus the test ends quickly. Cardiac patients and extremely deconditioned individuals ask to stop because of musculoskeletal pain and fatigue resulting from the abrupt workload changes; therefore the Bruce protocol is generally not recommended for these individuals. Additional details of protocol selection are presented in Chapter 19.

> **Mason-Likar lead system**
>
> *the location of the limb electrodes on the torso, rather than wrists and ankles, during the 12-lead ECG*

FOCUS BOX 28.5

Brief description of selected cardiovascular medications and their effect during exercise

Below are descriptions of the main medications used to alter cardiovascular function. The effects of these medications at rest and during exercise are summarized in Table 28.1.

Beta Blockers

Description—Block or inhibit beta₁ receptors in the heart, thereby decreasing heart rate, blood pressure, myocardial contractility, and oxygen demand.

Purpose—Beta blockers remain one of the most commonly prescribed medications for heart disease. Beta-blocking agents are prescribed for angina pectoris, hypertension, previous myocardial infarctions, and cardiac arrhythmias.

Nitrates

Description—Provide nitric oxide to the vascular cells of arteries, thereby promoting coronary artery vasodilation, as well as decreasing systemic peripheral vascular resistance.
Purpose—To increase blood flow to the myocardium and reduce afterload and preload of the heart.

Calcium Channel Blockers

Description—Block the entry of calcium through calcium channels in smooth muscle and myocardium.
Purpose—To cause a coronary artery vasodilation and decrease myocardial contractility, thereby decreasing angina and supraventricular tachycardia arrhythmias.

Angiotensin-Converting Enzyme (ACE) Inhibitors

Description—Diminish the formation of angiotensin II, which reduces the opening of receptor-operated calcium channels of vascular smooth muscle and decreases the release of norepinephrine from sympathetic synapses.
Purpose—To decrease peripheral vascular resistance and therefore the preload and afterload of the heart.

Digitalis

Description—Inhibits the sodium pump of myocardial fibers.
Purpose—To lower heart rate, which in turn increases ventricular filling, increases preload, and increases inotropic function of the heart.

TABLE 28.1

Cardiovascular medications and their physiologic effects during exercise

	HEART RATE		BLOOD PRESSURE		ECG		EXERCISE CAPACITY
MEDICATIONS	Rest	Exercise	Rest	Exercise	Rest	Exercise	
BETA BLOCKERS							
Examples: propranolol* (Inderal), atenolol (Tenormin), metoprolol (Lopressor), nadolol (Corgard)							
	↓	↓	↓	↓	↓HR	↓ ischemia	↑ in patients with angina
NITRATES							
Examples: nitroglycerin (sublingual tablets, skin patches, ointment) (Nitrostat, Transderm), isosorbide (Isordil)							
	↑	↑	↓	↓	↑HR ↓ ischemia	↓ ischemia	↑ in patients with angina

Continued.

TABLE 28.1—Cont'd

Cardiovascular medications and their physiologic effects during exercise

MEDICATIONS	HEART RATE Rest	HEART RATE Exercise	BLOOD PRESSURE Rest	BLOOD PRESSURE Exercise	ECG Rest	ECG Exercise	EXERCISE CAPACITY
CALCIUM CHANNEL BLOCKERS Examples: nifedipine (Procardia), verapamil (Calan), diltiazem (Cardizem)	↓ (for verapamil)	↓	↓	↓	—	↓ ischemia	↑ in patients with angina
ANGIOTENSIN CONVERTING ENZYME INHIBITORS Examples: captopril (Capoten), enalapril (Vasotec), lisinopril (Prinivil, Zestril)	—	—	↓	↓	—	—	May ↑ in patients with congestive heart failure (CHF)
DIURETICS Examples: furosemide (Lasix)	—	—	—	—	May cause PVCs and false-positive test with hypokalemia		May ↑ in patients with CHF
DIGITALIS Examples: digoxin (Lanoxin)	↓ (for patients with CHF or atrial fibrillation)	↓	—	—	May produce nonspecific ST-T wave changes; may produce ST-segment depression		May ↑ in patients with CHF or atrial fibrillation

*Nonspecific beta blocker.

Exercise Test Sequence

Pretest Sequence

After the patient has been hooked up to the ECG machine, a standard 12-lead ECG should be obtained while the patient is in the supine position. A standard 12-lead ECG is obtained by placing the limb leads on the inside of the wrists and the inside of the ankles. After the standard 12-lead ECG is obtained, the ECG limb lead cables are placed in the modified position. A 12-lead with the modified hook-up should then be obtained. All ECGs should be clearly marked (standard supine or modified supine). A resting supine blood pressure should be recorded. Next, the patient should be asked to stand so that a standing ECG and blood pressure (on the arm to be used during the exercise test) can be recorded.

Baseline ECG Analysis

Six conditions can prevent reliable diagnostic ECG analysis during exercise testing. These include left bundle branch block, Wolff-Parkinson-White syndrome, physiologic rate-responsive pacing, left ventricular hypertrophy, extensive anterior wall infarction, and resting ST or T wave abnormalities caused by drug effects (e.g., digoxin) or electrolyte abnormalities. In the presence of these conditions, exercise testing can provide information about hemodynamic response to exercise and aerobic capacity, but electrocardiographic analysis will most likely be unreliable. All exercise subjects should be screened for these conditions with a resting ECG before the exercise test.

FOCUS BOX 28.6

Indications for stopping an exercise test

1. Progressive angina during the exercise test
   On a scale of 1 to 4 with 1 being barely noticeable and 4 being the most severe pain ever experienced, a test should be stopped at a rating of 3 or greater.
2. Ventricular tachycardia (VT)
   VT is defined as three or more successive PVCs. Sustained VT is a medical emergency.
3. Any significant drop (20 mm Hg) of systolic blood pressure or a failure of the systolic blood pressure to rise with an increase in exercise load
4. Lightheadedness, confusion, a loss of muscular coordination, nausea, or change of skin color to a pale complexion
5. Greater than 4 mm horizontal or downsloping ST segment depression
6. Onset of second- or third-degree heart block
7. An increase in ventricular arrhythmias
8. An excessive rise in blood pressure (systolic greater than 250 mm Hg; diastolic greater than 120 mm Hg)
9. Failure of heart rate to increase with increasing workloads or a sudden drop in heart rate during the exercise test
10. Sustained supraventricular tachycardia
11. Exercise-induced left bundle branch block
12. Subject requests to stop
13. Failure of the monitoring system

*Adapted from American College of Sports Medicine: *Guidelines for exercise testing and prescription,* ed 5, Philadelphia, 1995, Lea & Febiger.

Test Sequence

After the patient is given a detailed explanation of the testing procedures, the test can start. A blood pressure recording should be obtained once during every stage and additionally when necessary. The ECG should be monitored at all times during the test, and recordings should be obtained every minute. A rate of perceived exertion reading should be obtained once during each stage.

Recovery Sequence

Once the test has stopped, blood pressure and ECG recordings should continue for 4 to 6 minutes or until the heart rate and blood pressure are close to resting values. Some physicians like to have patients lie down immediately after the end of the test (static-supine protocol). A static-supine protocol may help in detecting ischemic ECG changes. Unless a static-supine protocol is requested, the patient should continue to walk or cycle at a low intensity to cool-down.

Test End Points

Either the patient or physician will decide when to stop the test. The patient may decide to stop because of pain, fatigue, or other symptoms, or the physician or the exercise test technologist (ETT) may choose to stop the test because of some abnormal findings or because a predetermined end point was reached (patient reached 85% of his or her age-adjusted heart rate) (Focus Box 28.6).

Interpretation of Exercise Test Results

Normal Responses to Dynamic Exercise

During dynamic exercise in the healthy, normal, or nondiseased heart, the following physiologic adjustments occur during exercise:

Cardiac output—increases in a linear fashion, much like VO$_2$. Increases in cardiac output result from systematic increases in stroke volume and heart rate.

Stroke volume—for the untrained individual, stroke volume increases in a linear fashion up to approximately 40% of VO$_2$max. After the plateau of stroke volume, increases in cardiac output are due to increases in heart rate alone.

Heart rate—increases in a curvilinear fashion with increases in workload.

Systolic blood pressure (SBP)—increases in a linear fashion with increased work; however, increases in SBP above 220 mm Hg during near-maximal exercise are unusual.

Diastolic blood pressure—may remain stable or drop or rise slightly (±5 to 10 mm Hg).

Total peripheral resistance—decreases during exercise as a result of peripheral vascular vasodilation.

Oxygen utilization—increases during exercise to meet increased metabolic demands.

ECG Changes

The following electrocardiographic responses are considered normal during exercise:

P wave—increases in amplitude above resting level

PR interval—becomes shorter

QT interval—becomes shorter

J point—becomes depressed below the baseline

ST segment—depression of the early part of the segment, turning into upsloping ST segment

T wave—amplitude decreases above resting level

R wave—amplitude decreases above resting level

Q wave—increases in amplitude above resting level

Axis—may shift to the right

Arrhythmias—ectopic beats are common, especially at peak exercise

Abnormal Responses to Dynamic Exercise

When the heart muscle is damaged (because of an infection or myocardial infarction), its ability to respond to the increased demands of exercise are reduced. The diseased heart has less reserve to respond to an increased demand, so cardiac output and stroke volume may not increase in a normal fashion. Another sign of heart failure is a drop in or failure of heart rate to increase during exercise. A drop in or a failure of systolic blood pressure to rise during incremental exercise is also a sign of a failing heart.

ECG Changes

ST segment depression below the baseline is the classic ECG response to coronary insufficiency or **myocardial ischemia**. Myocardial ischemia results from an imbalance between myocardial oxygen supply and demand. This imbalance is almost always the result of atherosclerotic plaques that narrow the vessels and sometimes completely block the blood supply to the heart.

Predictive Value of Clinical Exercise Testing

*T*he **predictive value** of exercise testing is a measure of how accurately an exercise test identifies an individual with coronary artery disease (positive test) or without coronary artery disease (negative test). Establishing the predictive value of exercise testing is based on *Bayes' theorem*, which is a mathematical rule relating the interpretation of present observations in light of past experience.[25] Bayes' theorem helps to increase the correlation between prediction of coronary artery disease (pretest probability) before the test and probability of disease after the test (post-test probability). The use of ischemic ST changes during treadmill testing to diagnose coronary artery disease is based on studies that compared exercise electrocardiography data with coronary angiography findings. Coronary artery angiography is the "gold standard" for detecting the extent and severity of coronary artery disease.

The probability of a subject having coronary artery disease is determined from the test result, the diagnostic features of the test, and the pretest likelihood of the patient having disease. Bayes' theorem determines that the probability of disease after a test is performed is the product of disease probability before the test and the probability that the test was a true positive.[1,10,13] More simply stated:

Past experience + present observations = future interpretation

With Bayes theorem it is easy to understand that the ability of a given test result to predict the presence or absence of disease is related to the presence of disease in the population of subjects being tested. For example, a teenage female with a positive ST segment depression during a stress testing has a low posttest likelihood of coronary disease compared with a 65-year-old man with typical chest pain and multiple risk factors, who would have a very high posttest likelihood of coronary artery disease. This difference is due to the significant difference in the pretest likelihood of disease in these two different populations, in spite of similar ST segment displacement during exercise.

Sensitivity

The predictive accuracy of exercise testing is determined by the sensitivity and specificity of the test and the prevalence of coronary artery disease in the population tested. Sensitivity refers to the percentage of individuals being tested who will have an abnormal test.

28.1   Sensitivity =
(True-positive tests* / True-positive + False-negatives tests†) × 100
where:
*True-positive test = individuals who had both an abnormal stress test and abnormal angiogram.
†False-negative test = individuals who had normal stress test but abnormal angiogram.

The sensitivity of clinical exercise testing is approximately 71% (varies from 50% to 90%).[26] Therefore there is a 71% pretest likelihood of correctly identifying an individual

---

myocardial ischemia

decreased blood flow to the myocardium

predictive value

a measure of how accurately an exercise test correctly identifies an individual with coronary artery disease (positive test) or without it (negative test)

with coronary artery disease, based on a true–positive exercise test (ST depression of at least 1 mm at 0.08 second past the J point). The sensitivity of exercise testing can be enhanced (increase in the likelihood of a true-positive test) by administering a true maximal exercise test, using multiple-lead ECG monitoring, and monitoring additional data, such as abnormal blood pressure responses. Test sensitivity can be decreased (increase in the likelihood of a false-negative test) by administration of a submaximal exercise test, insufficient ECG monitoring, and unrecognized use of certain cardiac drugs (beta blockers and nitrates).

Specificity

Specificity refers to the percentage of individuals being tested who will have a normal exercise stress test. Thus a true-negative stress test correctly identifies a person without coronary artery disease. The specificity of clinical exercise testing is approximately 73% (varies from 60% to 98%).[1,10,13]

28.2   Specificity =
(True-negative tests* / True-negative + False-positive tests†) × 100
where:
*True-negative test = individuals with normal a stress test who have a normal angiogram.
†False-positive test = individuals with an abnormal stress test who have a normal angiogram.

The specificity of exercise testing (increase in the likelihood of a false–positive test) is reduced by preexisting abnormal resting ECG abnormalities, hypertrophy of the left ventricle, certain medications (e.g., digitalis), mitral valve prolapse, and anemia.

Predictive Value

The predictive value of exercise stress testing is a measure of how accurately the results from an exercise stress test identify the presence or absence of coronary artery disease in individuals being tested (positive test means disease, negative test means no disease).

28.3   Predictive value (positive test) =
(True-positive tests / true-positive + false-positive tests) × 100

28.4   Predictive value (negative test) =
(True-negative tests / true-negative + false-negative tests) × 100

When an individual comes to a physician's office to have an exercise stress test and has several risk factors and symptoms of cardiovascular disease, the pretest likelihood of dis-

ease is high (predictive value for a positive test is high). On the other hand, if a young, active, healthy individual with only one or two CAD risk factors has an exercise stress test, the pretest likelihood of disease is low (predictive value for a positive test is low). In addition to ECG recordings, the predictive value of exercise stress testing is enhanced by recording additional data such as the total exercise time, maximal metabolic equivalent (MET) obtained, blood pressure responses before, during, and after exercise, and symptoms of angina or shortness of breath.

The risk ratio is the relative rate of occurrence of coronary heart disease in a group that has abnormal tests compared with a group that has normal tests; in other words, the relative chance of having disease if the test shows abnormal results as compared with the chance of having disease if the test shows normal results. If 1% of the population has disease, with 60% sensitivity and 90% specificity, the predictive value of exercise testing will be 5.7% and the risk ratio 14:25. If 10% of the population has disease, with 60% sensitivity and 90% specificity, the predictive value of exercise testing will be 40% and the risk ratio 8:5. From these examples, the accuracy of exercise testing is defined by sensitivity and specificity, and the results, when applied to the individual, depend on the prevalence of disease in the population to which the individual belongs.

Other Diagnostic Cardiovascular Testing Procedures

Echocardiography

Echocardiography is a safe and painless diagnostic procedure that uses high-frequency sound waves (ultrasound) to take dynamic pictures of the heart (Figure 28.9). Sound waves, emitted from a transducer, penetrate the patient's chest wall and rebound off and from within the heart so that various cardiac structures can be observed. From the echocardiogram recordings, it is possible to measure the size of the chambers of the heart, how well the heart valves are working, and how forcefully the heart muscle is contracting. Doppler echocardiography is a form of echocardiography that uses sound waves to measure the speed, velocity, and direction of blood flow. With Doppler echocardiography, accurate measurements allowing the calculations of cardiac output and stroke volume can be obtained.

echocardiography (ek'o-**kar**-di-og'ra-fi)
the process of recording the movement and dimensions of the heart and its structures by rebounding high-frequency (nonaudible) sound waves

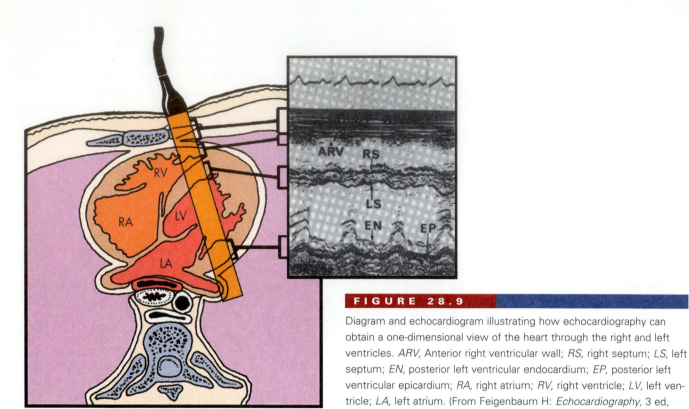

FIGURE 28.9

Diagram and echocardiogram illustrating how echocardiography can obtain a one-dimensional view of the heart through the right and left ventricles. *ARV,* Anterior right ventricular wall; *RS,* right septum; *LS,* left septum; *EN,* posterior left ventricular endocardium; *EP,* posterior left ventricular epicardium; *RA,* right atrium; *RV,* right ventricle; *LV,* left ventricle; *LA,* left atrium. (From Feigenbaum H: *Echocardiography,* 3 ed, Philadelphia, 1981, Lea & Febiger.)

Exercise Echocardiography

In exercise echocardiography a resting echocardiogram is taken just before the start of an exercise test to assess resting ventricular function. Immediately after a graded exercise test, another echocardiogram is repeated. Any differences between the resting and postexercise echocardiograms tell how well the left ventricle functions during exercise. If part of the heart muscle is damaged or compromised in any way, the echocardiogram records the abnormal activity. Some of the problems that are commonly reported in diseased hearts include the following:

Akinetic activity—literally means no motion. This means that part of the heart muscle is not contracting.

Dyskinetic activity—means that part of the myocardium is moving in the opposite direction from normal. Instead of the myocardium contracting inward to pump blood out of the ventricle, a portion of the myocardium is contracting outward.

Hypokinetic activity—means that part of the heart muscle is not contracting as well as it should be.

Thallium-201 Stress Testing

The **thallium–201 stress test** is a diagnostic examination used to evaluate the adequacy of blood supply to the heart. Before the start of an exercise test, an intravenous (IV) line is inserted into the patient's arm. At peak exercise, thal-

lium–201 radioisotope is injected into the IV line. The radioisotope is then carried to the heart via the blood. Immediately after the patient stops exercise, a special camera that can detect radiation visualizes the thallium–201 as it flows throughout the heart. If the coronary arteries are clear, thallium–201 is absorbed evenly throughout the myocardium within a matter of minutes. The first set of pictures, taken immediately after exercise, determines the adequacy of blood supply to the heart during stress. If the coronary arteries are normal, the entire myocardium will receive approximately the same amount of the radioactive isotope and the pictures taken will have a uniform appearance (Figure 28.10). If one or more of the coronary arteries is blocked, a portion of the myocardium will not receive the isotope and the pictures will show a spot of nonabsorption, sometimes referred to as a cold spot (see Figure 28.11). After a period of time the isotope is absorbed into the tissue and the cold spot disappears. The second set of pictures, taken several hours after exercise, helps to differentiate between exercise-induced ischemia and an area of nonabsorbing tissue (usually resulting from a heart attack).

thallium-201 stress test

the procedure of injecting an isotope into the circulation immediately after exhausting exercise to determine whether there are any blockages to coronary arteries

FIGURE 28.10

Thallium scintigrams in relation to cardiac anatomy and coronary artery distribution. (From Froelicher VF et al: *Exercise and the heart,* 3 ed, St. Louis, 1993, Mosby.)

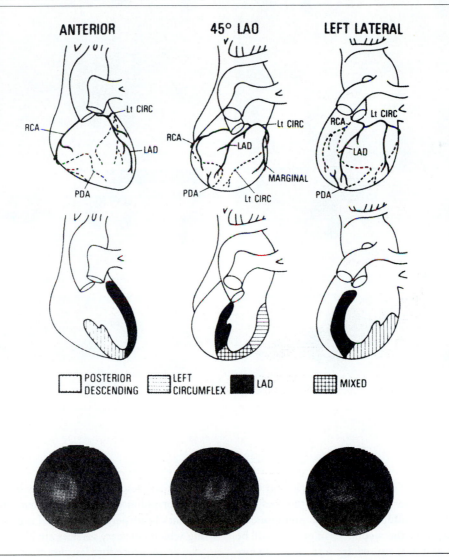

FIGURE 28.11

Thallium images immediately after exercise (top) and during redistribution phase 4 hours later (bottom). The arrow shows anteroseptal defect during exercise stress that exhibits redistribution, signifying viable but transient ischemic myocardium. (From Franklin BA et al: Additional diagnostic tests: special populations. In Durstine JL (editor): *ACSM resource manual for guidelines for exercise testing and prescription*, 2 ed, Philadelphia, Lea & Febiger.)

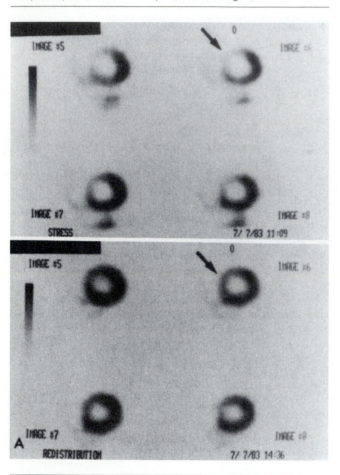

FIGURE 28.12

Thallium stress (top) and redistribution (bottom) images are shown in a patient with a previous myocardial infarction in the inferior wall *A*, with ischemia in the anteroseptal wall *B*. (From Franklin BA et al: Additional diagnostic tests: special populations. In Durstine JL (editor): *ACSM resource manual for guidelines for exercise testing and prescription*, 2 ed, Philadelphia, Lea & Febiger.)

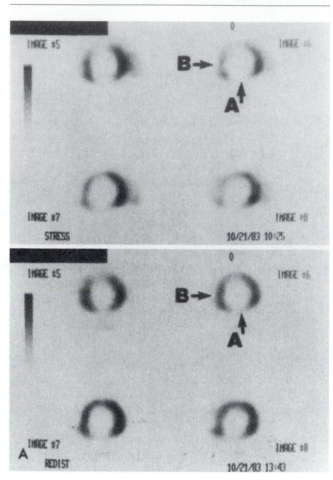

Old heart attacks leave a scar on the heart muscle, and these scars or injuries will not absorb the isotope. If the cold spot was caused by exercise-induced ischemia (temporarily reduced isotope absorption), the second set of pictures will be normal. If the cold spot was caused by scar tissue (Figure 28.12), the second set of pictures will be abnormal as well. The location of the absorption defects can be used to predict which coronary artery is blocked.

Cardiac Catheterization

Cardiac catheterization is an invasive procedure, meaning that the body is entered in some way, whereas the other tests described so far have been noninvasive. Cardiac catheterization is the most accurate method of measuring a patient's heart performance and is the only way of determining which coronary arteries are blocked and to what degree. The entire procedure lasts less than an hour. During the procedure a narrow, flexible tube (catheter) is inserted through the brachial or femoral artery (Figure 28.13). After the catheter has been inserted into the artery, it is slowly advanced toward the heart while the physician watches its progress on a television screen. During a *left ventricular angiogram* the catheter is advanced into the left ventricle. Dye is then injected and a series of pictures is obtained during contraction. During a **coronary angiogram** a catheter is

FIGURE 28.13

The cardiac catherization procedure involves the passage of a catheter into the junction of the aorta artery and the main coronary artery, or directly into the left ventricle.

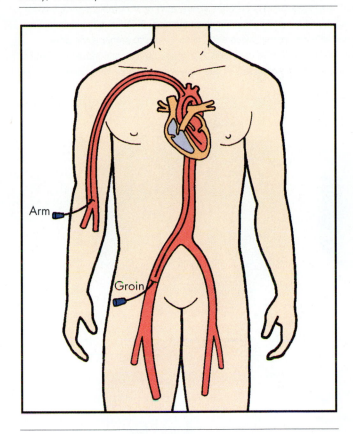

inserted into the opening of the left and then the right main coronary artery. Dye is injected through the catheter into each coronary artery, and an x-ray camera takes a series of pictures of the coronary arteries. These pictures show areas of narrowing (blockages) and indicate their severity (Figure 28.14).

Becoming Certified as an Exercise Test Technologist

Administering exercise stress tests in a clinical, or even a nonclinical, setting requires a great deal of skill, knowledge, and experience. It often takes years of hard work and training to become a highly skilled cardiovascular exercise technologist. Before attempting to become certified in this specialty, candidates should take courses in basic and advanced electrocardiography, exercise stress testing, exercise physiology, exercise laboratory procedures, and exercise prescription. In addition to class experi-

ence, practical experience is important. No amount of knowledge can replace practical experience, especially in the medical setting. Hospitals often allow students to observe, and sometimes offer training in, a variety of cardiovascular procedures.

The American College of Sports Medicine describes the responsibilities of an exercise test technologist (ETT).[1] The primary responsibility of the ETT is to administer exercise tests safely to individuals in various states of illness and health to obtain reliable and valid data. In addition, the ETT should demonstrate appropriate knowledge of functional anatomy, exercise physiology, pathophysiology, electrocardiography, and psychology to perform such tasks as preparing the exercise test station for administration of the exercise tests, screening the participant preliminarily for the exercise test, administering tests and recording data, implementing emergency procedures when necessary, summarizing test data, and communicating test results to the exercise specialists, program directors, and physicians. The ETT may administer an exercise test without a physician present based on the health status and age of the individual or if the physician has provided clearance for the test. The technologist must be able to recognize contraindications to exercise testing found in preliminary screening, recognize abnormal responses during the exercise test and recovery, respond appropriately, and provide a summary of results.

For more information on becoming certified in clinical exercise testing and other areas of cardiovascular technology, contact the following organizations: The American College of Sports Medicine; Certification Department; PO Box 1440; Indianapolis, IN 46206-1440; (317) 637-9200. Cardiovascular Credentialing International; PO Box 611; Dayton, Ohio 45409-0611; (800) 326-0268.

Stress Testing Case Studies

The case studies presented in this section will help you apply the information in this chapter. These are actual results from diagnostic exercise tests performed in a hospital setting. Practice developing a systematic approach for analyzing the results of an exercise test. Here are some points to consider when looking at the case studies:

- What was (were) the reason(s) for the test?
- Was the selection of the protocol appropriate for the patient being tested?

cardiac catheterization

the procedure in which a catheter is passed into the heart (ventricle or coronary artery) and dye is infused to visualize coronary blood vessels and the presence of any coronary occlusions

coronary angiogram

the image of the coronary artery network created by dye infusion during cardiac catheterization

FIGURE 28.14

Dye injected into the coronary artery allows the contrasting of coronary arteries to be seen, as well as to detect arteries that are either occluded or partially occluded. **A,** A right anterior oblique projection angiogram of a normal right coronary artery. **B,** A diseased artery having 95% occlusion in the distal $^2/_3$ of the artery. **C,** An angiogram of normal left main, circumflex, and left anterior descending (LAD) arteries. The branches diverging from the circumflex are termed *obtuse marginal arteries*. The branches diverging from the LAD are termed *diagonals*. **D,** A left coronary angiogram showing a diseased LAD with a 99% occlusion, and a diseased circumflex artery with near complete occlusion. Note the increased flow through an obtuse marginal artery. The circular shadows are gas bubbles in the stomach. **E,** A left ventricular angiogram at diastole in a patient who had previously had bypass surgery. Note the sternal wires and "clips" used to stabilize the artery graft. **F,** A left ventricular angiogram at systole for the same subject as E. Note that in each of E, and F, there is abnormal contrast outline of the ventricle in the inferior sternal portion. (Coronary artery and ventricular angiograms provided by the University of New Mexico Health Sciences Center, University Hospital Cardiac Catheterization Laboratory.)

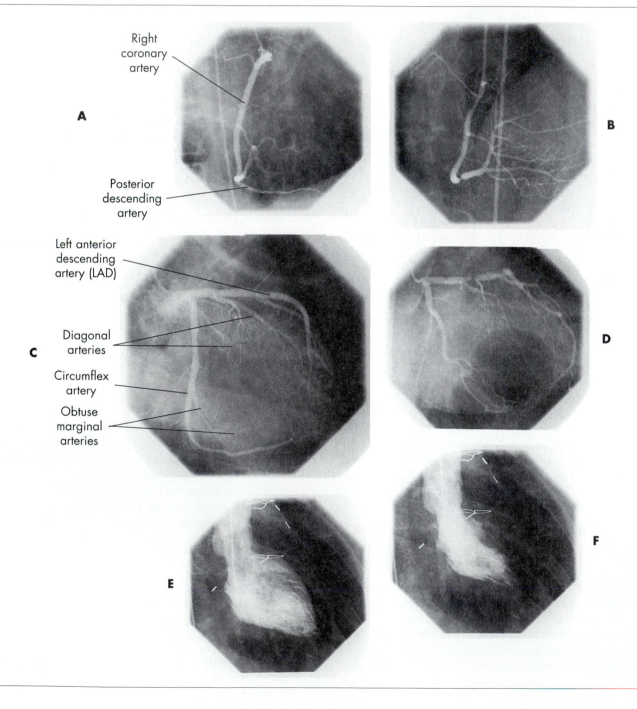

- What medications was the patient taking, and what effects would the medications have on the results of the test?
- Was there anything unusual about the resting patient data?
- What was the patient's physiologic response to the exercise?
- Were the heart rate and blood pressure responses appropriate?

- Why was the test stopped? Were there any arrhythmias?
- Did the ST segment change during or after the test?
- What were the physician's impressions?
- Was the exercise prescription appropriate for the patient based on the test results?

CASE HISTORY 1

DOB: 8/16/34　　　　　　　　　　　Baseline ECG: Normal
Gender: F　　　　　　　　　　　　Resting HR: 73
Reason for referral: Chest pain, angina　　Resting BP: 150/90
Current Medications: Synthroid, Cardizem, NTG-PRN　　Testing Protocol: Bruce

Stage:	Stage time:	HR(bpm)	BP	METs (calculate yourself)
Supine		73	150/90	
Standing		75		
Post-hyperventilation		72		
I	1	108		
	2	111	140/90	
	3	118		
II	4	122		
Recovery	1	94		
	2	83	175/90	

Treadmill Results

Total Exercise Time: 3.55 min. Total METS: 5.7
Max HR: 124　Max BP: 175/90
Max HR achieved/Max HR predicted: 68%
Predicted Max HR/Target HR: 180/153
Double product: 21.7 (thousands)
Predicted age/gender exercise duration (minutes): 5.5

Physiologic Response to Exercise

Functional Aerobic Impairment: 40%
Normal heart rate and blood pressure response

Test Stopped for:

Fatigue, 2+ angina noted

Arrhythmias

Rare premature ventricular complexes

ST Segment Response

Resting ECG—Nonspecific ST change(s)
Hyperventilation ECG—No change from baseline
Exercise ECG—1 to 2 mm ST segment in anteroseptal leads

Impression

Indeterminate for ischemia because of low maximal workload achieved
Aerobic capacity is decreased

Exercise Prescription for Case Study 1

Exercise Prescription
Name: Case Study 1　Gender: F　Age: 59　Date:
HT (in): 66　WT (Kg): 100 (lb-220)
Diagnosis: Several episodes of chest pain, obesity, physical inactivity, hypertension
Medications: Synthroid, Cardizem, NTG-PRN
Comments:
GXT Data:　Date Performed:　Where: Hospital
Rest HR: 73　Protocol: Bruce
Max HR: 124　Max METs: 5.7
Reevaluation Scheduled: 3 months
Target METs:　= 50% to 85% of max METs
　　　　　= 2.85 to 4.85
Target HR (bpm): = (max HR - rest HR) (65% to 90%) + (rest HR)
　　　　　= (124 - 73) (33 or 46) + 73
　　　　　= THR = 106 to 119

Type of exercise: The goal is to increase caloric expenditure and minimize angina episodes during exercise. Non–weight-bearing exercises, such as cycling, swimming and water exercises, are recommended. However, easy walking is appropriate.

Duration of exercise: 15 to 20 minutes to start gradually increasing to 30 to 45 minutes per exercise session. The duration of the exercise session should result in a caloric expenditure of 200 to 300 kilocalories per session.

Frequency: Because the goal is to increase caloric expenditure, more frequent exercise session may be necessary (five to six times per week).

Warm-up and cool-down activities: Stretch the calf, hamstring, quads, hip flexors (hold for 10 seconds, progress to 30 seconds).

Other activities: This patient has been referred for nutrition education and weight-reduction counseling.

Patient instructions: The patient has been instructed on how and when to take nitroglycerine. If angina occurs during exercise, the exercise intensity needs to be lowered.

Body composition data: Percentage of body fat: 40% Desirable: 25%

Body weight: 100 kg. Desired range: 54 to 60 kg.

CASE HISTORY 2

DOB: 12/14/25

Gender: M

Reason for referral: S/P CABG, CAD

Current Medications: Inderal, Questran, BASA, Pepsid

Baseline ECG: Normal

Resting HR: 74

Resting BP: 142/92

Testing Protocol: Bruce

Stage:	Stage time:	HR(bpm)	BP	METs (calculate yourself)
Supine		77		
Standing		90		
Post-hyperventilation		103		
I		105		
		112	150/80	
		114		
II		118		
		124	180/80	
		128		
III		128		
		151	190/80	
		159		
Max		160		
Recovery		145		
		129	202/80	
		117	190/80	
		108		
		100	172/80	
		101		
		94		

Treadmill Results

Total Exercise Time: 9.09 min. Total METs: 10.2

Max HR: 165 Max BP: 202/80

Max HR achieved/Max HR predicted: 92%

Predicted Max HR/Target HR: 178/151

Double product: 33.3 (thousands)

Predicted age/gender exercise duration (minutes):7.5

Physiologic Response to Exercise

The exercise duration exceeds the predicted duration

Normal heart rate and blood pressure response

Test Stopped for

Leg pain/fatigue

Arrhythmias

Premature ventricular complexes including couplets with peak exercise and early recovery

ST Segment Response

Resting ECG—Nonspecific ST change(s). T-wave abnormality in inferolateral leads

Hyperventilation ECG—ST abnormalities in inferolateral leads

Exercise ECG—No increase over baseline ST changes

Impression

TMT: Negative for ischemic ECG changes

Specificity reduced because of resting and/or hyperventilation ECG changes

Aerobic capacity is normal

Compared with previous TMT: 3/13/91

The exercise performance has deteriorated by 1 minute

The ECG response has improved

The BP/HR response has deteriorated

Exercise Prescription for Case Study 2

Exercise Prescription

Name: Case Study 2   Gender: M   Age: 68   Date:

HT (In): 74   WT (Kg): 79.5 (lb-175)

Diagnosis: This patient had CABG surgery 6 months ago

Current Medications: Inderal, Questran, BASA, Pepsid, and Motrin

Comments: This patient is being referred into cardiac rehabilitation. He has a history of hypercholesterolemia, which is still being treated for with Questran. He has mild arthritis and an ulcer. This patient is quite active. He and his wife play golf and travel a great deal.

GXT Data: Date Performed: Where: Hospital

Rest HR: 74 Protocol: Bruce

Max HR: 165 Max METs: 10.2

Reevaluation Scheduled: 3 months

Target METs: = 50% to 85% of max METs

= 5.1 to 8.7

Target HR (bpm): = (max HR - rest HR) (65% to 90%) + (rest HR)

= (165 - 74) (59 to 82) + 74

= THR = 133 to 156

Type of exercise: Aerobic exercise, with mild resistance training

Duration of exercise: Up to 45 minutes

Frequency: Three to four sessions per week

Warm-up and cool-down activities: Brisk walking (5 minutes), followed by stretching the calf, hamstring, quads, hip flexors (hold for 10 seconds, progress to 30 seconds).

Other activities: Since the patient enjoys golf, and does not use a golf cart, 3 to 4 days of aerobic conditioning should be sufficient.

Patient instructions: None at the present time.

Body composition data: Percentage of body fat: 16.5% Desirable: 15%

Body weight: 79.5 kg. Desired range: 77 to 80 kg.

SUMMARY

■ This chapter introduces the student to the fundamental principles of clinical exercise testing. The term **clinical** implies that the exercise test is medically oriented. The clinical exercise test is probably the best test of the heart because exercise is the most common everyday stress that humans undertake.

■ The most common reasons for ordering a clinical exercise test are for **diagnostic** purposes and for evaluating the status of suspected or known cardiovascular disease. Individuals who have developed cardiovascular disease of the heart usually have a compensated blood flow to a diseased region that results from the presence of **collaterals**. The benefits of the test and the subsequent results obtained should outweigh the potential risks of performing the test. Some individuals possess characteristics that preclude them from undertaking such a test. These conditions are known as **contraindications** to exercise testing.

■ The **electrocardiogram** (ECG) is an instrument that detects and displays electrical activity of the heart. The trace obtained from an ECG is an **electrocardiograph**. Five key waves and intervals make up the ECG. A wave represents depolarization or repolarization, whereas an interval represents time during which there is no myocardial depolarization or repolarization.

■ The standard 12-lead ECG is composed of three **bipolar** limb **leads**—I, II, III; three **augmented** limb leads—aVR, aVL, aVF; and six chest leads, V_{1-6}. The standard limb lead electrodes are attached to the left arm (LA), left leg (LL), and right arm (RA) and comprise leads I, II, and III.

Continued.

SUMMARY—Cont'd

■ **Einthoven's triangle** assumes that the human torso is a sphere of conducting ability and that the heart is a point at its center. Einthoven's law states that lead II is equal to the sum of the complexes in leads I and III.

■ A heart rate over 100 bpm is referred to as **tachycardia**. A heart rate below 60 bpm is referred to as **bradycardia**. **Cardiac rhythm** is determined by comparing a continuous ECG strip with a static 12-lead ECG. To determine rhythm, measure the R–R intervals across the entire strip. A constant R–R interval indicates that the rhythm is regular, or sinus, meaning that the rhythm originates in the SA node.

■ Any variation from the normal rhythm and normal electrical conduction pattern of the heart is referred to as an **arrhythmia**. The **electrical axis** is referred to as the mean QRS vector and represents the mean direction of depolarization from the SA to the AV node and ventricular myocardium node. **ST segment depression** on the ECG is the hallmark of myocardial ischemia and occurs in three general varieties—horizontal, downsloping, or upsloping. The **J point** serves as a reference for the analysis of the ST segment. Some arrhythmias such as premature ventricular contractions (PVCs) or premature atrial contractions occur in as many as 40% of normal subjects. When ischemia is severe and the death of myocardial tissue occurs, this event is termed a **myocardial infarction**.

■ The **Mason–Likar lead system** is the most commonly used electrode system for exercise testing. It differs from the standard lead system by the placement of the limb lead electrodes from the feet and wrists to the lower and upper torso.

■ Six conditions can prevent reliable diagnostic ECG analysis during exercise testing. These include left bundle branch block, Wolff-Parkinson-White syndrome, physiologic rate-responsive pacing, left ventricular hypertrophy, extensive anterior wall infarction, and resting ST or T wave abnormalities secondary to drug effects (e.g., digoxin) or electrode abnormalities. ST segment depression below the baseline is the classic ECG response to coronary insufficiency or **myocardial ischemia**.

■ The sensitivity of clinical exercise testing approximates 71%, and the specificity of clinical exercise stress testing approximates 73%. The **predictive value** of exercise stress testing is a measure of how accurately the results from an exercise stress test identify the presence or absence of coronary artery disease in individuals being tested (positive test means disease, negative test means no disease).

■ **Echocardiography** uses high-frequency sound waves (ultrasound) to take dynamic pictures of the heart. The **thallium-201 stress test** is a diagnostic examination used to evaluate the adequacy of blood supply to the heart. **Cardiac catheterization** is the most accurate method of measuring a patient's heart performance and is the only way of determining which coronary arteries are blocked and to what degree. The image of coronary blood vessels obtained by injecting dye during cardiac catheterization is termed a **coronary angiogram**.

REVIEW QUESTIONS

1. List five indications for and contraindications to clinical exercise testing.

2. Describe the difference between a diagnostic and functional capacity exercise test.

3. Explain the difference between someone who is apparently healthy and someone who is at high risk.

4. Discuss the safety of exercise testing.

5. Discuss how the heart receives its blood supply.

6. What do the markings on the ECG paper represent?

7. Define and discuss the common waves and segments on the ECG.

8. Define axis, rate, and rhythm of an ECG.

9. What is the clinical significance of ST segment depression?

10. What arrhythmias are common and considered normal during exercise testing?

11. What information has to be obtained before an exercise test can be performed and why?

12. What is the Mason-Likar system of electrode placement?

13. What pretest ECGs are performed and why?

14. What are some normal and abnormal hemodynamic and ECG responses to exercise testing?

15. Define the sensitivity, specificity, and predictive value of clinical exercise testing.

APPLICATIONS

1. What are the benefits and drawbacks of incorporating measurements of indirect calorimetry to clinical exercise testing?

2. What results from a standard clinical exercise test reflect each of the following: cardiorespiratory endurance, pulmonary function, hypertension, ventricular myocardial ischemia, ventricular myocardial failure or compromise, and angina?

3. Explain the importance of knowing the pharmacology of medication before exercise testing of individuals who are at high risk or have known disease.

REFERENCES

1. American College of Sports Medicine: *Guidelines for exercise testing and prescription,* ed 5, Philadelphia, 1995, Lea & Febiger.

2. Allen WH et al: Five-year follow-up of maximal treadmill stress test in asymptomatic men and women, *Circulation* 62:522-531, 1980.

3. Arora R, Ioachim L, Matza D, Horowitz SF: The role of ischemia and ventricular asynergy in the genesis of exercise-induced ST elevation, *Clin Cardiol* 11:127-131, 1988.

4. Atterhog J-H, Jonsson B, Sammuelsson R: Exercise testing: a prospective study of complication rates, *Am Heart J* 98:572-580, 1979.

5. Braunwald E: *Heart disease: a textbook of cardiovascular medicine,* ed 4, Philadelphia, 1992, Saunders.

6. Bruce RA, Cohn PF: Exercise testing. In Cohn PF, editor: *Diagnosis and therapy of coronary artery disease,* Boston, 1985, Martinus Nijhoff.

7. Chung EK: *Principles of cardiac arrhythmias,* Baltimore, 1989, Williams & Wilkins.

8. Cumming GR, Samm J, Borysyk L et al: Electrocardiographic changes during exercise in asymptomatic men: 3-year follow-up, *Can Med Assoc J* 112:578-595, 1975.

9. Dunn RF, Freedman B, Bailey IK et al: Localization of coronary artery disease with exercise electrocardiography: correlation with thallium-20 myocardial perfusion scanning, *Am J Cardiol* 48:837-843, 1981.

10. Ellested MH: *Stress-testing, principles and practice,* ed 3, Philadelphia, 1986, FA Davis.

11. Froelicher VF et al: An epidemiological study of asymptomatic men screened with exercise testing for latent coronary heart disease, *Am J Cardiol* 34:770-779, 1975.

12. Froelicher VF, Myers J, Follansbee WP, Labovitz AJ: *Exercise and the heart,* ed 3, St Louis, 1993, Mosby.

13. Froelicher VF: *Manual of exercise testing,* ed 2, St Louis, 1994, Mosby.

14. Koppes G, McKierman T, Bassan M, Froelicher VF: Treadmill exercise testing, *Curr Probl Cardiol* 7:1-44, 1977.

15. Lachterman B, Lehmann KG, Abrahamson D, Froelicher VF: "Recovery only" ST-segment depression and predictive accuracy of the exercise test, *Ann Intern Med* 112:11, 1990.

16. Mark DB, Hlatky MA, Lee KL et al: Localizing coronary artery obstructions with the exercise treadmill test, *Ann Intern Med* 106:53, 1987.

17. Mason RE, Likar I: A new system of multiple-lead exercise electrocardiography, *Am Heart J* 71:196-205, 1966.

18. McHenry PL, Morris SN, Kavalier M: Exercise-induced arrhythmias—recognition, classification and clinical significance, *Cardiovasc Clin* 6:245, 1974.

19. Miranda CP, Liu J, Kadar A et al: Usefulness of exercise-induced ST segment depression in the inferior leads during exercise testing as a marker for coronary artery disease, *Am J Cardiol* 69:303-307, 1992.

20. Rochmis P, Blackburn H: Exercise tests: a survey of procedures, safety, and litigation experience in approximately 170,000 tests, *JAMA* 217:1061, 1971.

21. Sriwattanakomen S, Ticzon AR, Zubritsky SA, et al: ST segment elevation during exercise: electrocardiographic and arteriographic correlation in 38 patients, *Am J Cardiol* 45:762-768, 1980.

22. Stuart RJ, Ellestad MH: National survey of exercise stress testing facilities, *Chest* 77:94-102, 1980.

23. Thompson PD: The safety of exercise testing and participation. In Blair SN, Painter P, Pate RR et al, editors: American college of sports medicine—resource manual or guidelines for exercise testing and prescription, Philadelphia, 1993, Lea & Febiger.

RECOMMENDED READINGS

- American College of Sports Medicine: *Guidelines for exercise testing and prescription,* ed 5, Philadelphia, 1995, Lea & Febiger.

- Blair SN, Painter P, Pate RR et al: *American College of Sports Medicine—resource manual or guidelines for exercise testing and prescription,* Philadelphia, 1993, Lea & Febiger.

- Roberts SO, Robergs RA, Hanson P: *Clinical exercise testing and prescription: theory and application,* Boca Raton, Florida, CRC Press, (in press).

- Durstine L, Moore J, Painter P et al, editors: *Exercise management for persons with chronic diseases and disabilities,* Champaign, Illinois, 1990, Human Kinetics.

- Conover MB: *Understanding electrocardiography: arrhythmias and the 12-lead ECG,* St. Louis, 1992, Mosby.

- Froelicher VF: *Manual of exercise testing,* ed 2, St Louis, 1994, Mosby.

CHAPTER 29

Exercise, Diet, and Weight Control

OBJECTIVES

After studying this chapter you should be able to:

- Explain the role of exercise in treating and preventing weight loss and weight maintenance.

- List specific recommendations for exercise training for obese individuals.

- Identify the causes of obesity.

- Explain basic nutrition principles.

- Describe the health implications of obesity and overweight.

KEY TERMS

overweight

body mass index (BMI)

obesity

gynoid obesity

android obesity

waist to hip ratio

hyperplastic obesity

hypertrophic obesity

thermogenesis

weight cycling

set point theory

Most people in developed countries are obsessed with their weight. At any given time, 20% of the population in the United States is taking part in some form of weight-loss program.[42] Americans spend more than $30 billion a year on various weight-loss methods, most of which fail. Excess body weight is associated with numerous health problems, including diabetes, hyperlipidemia, and an increased risk of coronary artery disease. However, the primary reason most people are not happy with their weight is appearance. Even so, 95% of dieters are unsuccessful at keeping weight off after dieting. Repeated weight loss and weight gain, called the "yo-yo effect," can lead to long-term detrimental changes in metabolism. In addition, an obsession with weight and weight loss can lead to self-imposed starvation (anorexia nervosa) or binge eating followed by emaciation caused by purging (bulimia), which are both serious medical problems. This chapter presents information on how to incorporate exercise into a regimen designed to reduce body fat.

Essential Principles of Nutrition

Proper nutrition is essential to good health. Good nutrition promotes normal growth and development and can help prevent disease. Today, in most developed countries, good nutritional habits have helped prevent a variety of diseases and health problems. For example, rickets, scurvy, and goiter, which are caused by a lack of certain vitamins and minerals, were once common but now are quite rare. However, living in a developed country does not guarantee a healthy diet. Many Americans are undernourished as a result of poverty, medical problems, or self-imposed regimens, and malnourishment can result in growth retardation, anemia, and other serious health problems. However, far more people are overnourished than undernourished. Even with our modern increased awareness of and education in nutrition and exercise, most people find it hard to eat suitable quantities of nutritionally balanced food and to exercise regularly. Focus Box 29.1 lists some common dietary guidelines.

The three basic foods—carbohydrates, fats, and proteins—provide the energy for every function of the human body. A healthy diet is composed of 55% to 60% carbohydrates, 25% to 30% fat, and 10% to 15% protein. The best way to achieve a balanced diet is to eat a variety of foods. The U.S. Department of Agriculture's food guide pyramid (see Chapter 17) was developed to help individuals make the right nutritional choices.

Carbohydrates

Carbohydrates are often referred to as the body's primary source of fuel for energy systems. Carbohydrates are found almost exclusively in plant sources. The name "carbohydrate" comes from the chemical structure: carbon (C), hydrogen (H), and oxygen (O); thus CHO. Carbohydrates are classified as simple or complex. Some simple carbohydrates are table sugar, glucose, fructose, honey, and molasses. Some complex carbohydrates are grains, beans, potatoes, vegetables, and rice. Starches (e.g., rice, potatoes, cereal grains, and vegetables) supply energy, vitamins, minerals, fiber, and water. A healthy diet should be high in complex carbohydrates and low in simple carbohydrates; at least 50% to 60% of calories should come from complex carbohydrates. Excess consumption of carbohydrates results in conversion of carbohydrate to fat in the liver and therefore can be equated with increasing body fat. Carbohydrates supply only 4 kilocalories (Kcals) per gram consumed, whereas fats have 9 Kcal/g. Table 29.1 lists the different classes of carbohydrates.

Proteins

Proteins are often called the building blocks of the body. They make up approximately 18% to 20% of the human body. Protein is composed of compounds known as amino acids, which are joined in unique chains to form specific proteins. Protein is broken down into amino acids during the digestive process. There are 22 common amino acids, 11 of which the body does not produce and which therefore must be supplied by the diet; these are called essential amino acids.

The main functions of protein are growth and repair. Protein is the structural basis for all body tissues and can also be used for energy in some cases. When protein is used for energy, it can supply 4 Kcal/g. Proteins are categorized into complete and incomplete proteins. Complete proteins, (e.g.,

---

TABLE 29.1

Classes of carbohydrate

CHEMICAL NAME	MEMBERS	SOURCE
Polysaccharides (multiple sugars, complex carbohydrates)	Starch	Grains and grain products: cereal, bread, crackers, other baked goods; pasta; rice, corn, bulgur; legumes; potatoes and other vegetables
	Glycogen	Animal tissues; liver and muscle meats
	Dietary fiber	Whole grains; fruits; vegetables; seeds, nuts, skins of fruits
Disaccharides (double sugars, simple carbohydrates)	Sucrose	"Table" sugar: sugar cane, sugar beets; molasses
	Lactose	Milk
	Maltose	Starch digestion; intermediate sweetener in food products; starch digestion, final
Monosaccharides (simple sugars, simple carbohydrates)	Glucose (dextrose)	Corn syrup (extensively used in processed foods)
	Fructose	Fruits, honey
	Galactose	Lactose (milk)

eggs, milk, cheese, and meat) contain all the essential amino acids. Incomplete proteins (e.g., grains, nuts, vegetables, and fruits) must be combined with complementary protein sources to achieve all the essential amino acids. Thus vegetarians need to make sure they eat a balanced diet to get all of the essential amino acids. One way to do this is to mix foods such as grains, legumes, and milk products.

According to the Recommended Daily Allowance (RDA), the daily protein requirement for active, healthy adults is approximately 0.8 g/kg body weight. Certain individuals (e.g., growing athletes, people recovering from illness, or athletes involved in strenuous resistance-training programs) can consume up to 1.3 to 1.6 g/kg body weight/day. However, eating large amounts of protein will not lead to greater gains in strength. According to a recent report by the National Research Council, no one should eat more than twice the RDA because of the convincing evidence that high protein intake is associated with certain types of cancers and heart disease. Furthermore, a high protein intake places a heavy burden on the liver and kidneys to metabolize and excrete excess nitrogen, and it may even damage those organs.

Sources of protein include meat, fish, poultry, eggs, milk, cheese, nuts, dried peas, beans, bread, cereals, and vegetables. The best foods to choose are those that are both high in protein and low in fat, such as fish, chicken, turkey, lean beef and pork, low-fat cheese, skim milk, and egg whites (see Table 29.2). Because the average individual living in the United States already eats twice the RDA for protein, expensive protein supplements are unnecessary.

Fats

Fat is a very concentrated source of energy. Fats contain twice as many calories (9 kcal/g) as carbohydrates (4 kcal/g). The true chemical name for fats is *lipids*. The main building blocks of lipids are fatty acids. Fatty acids have two classifications, saturated and unsaturated. Saturated fatty acids come from animal sources. Unsaturated fatty acids are less dense and are found predominantly in grains, seeds, and legumes.

According to the American Heart Association, a diet should derive no more than 30% of total daily kilocalories from lipids. Individuals should strive to cut back on the amount of saturated fat they consume because it is associated with greater health risks.

Vitamins

Vitamins are noncaloric, organic substances essential for building the body's cells, digestion, tissue building, and energy release. Vitamins are present in small quantities in the body and function to promote many naturally occurring chemical reactions. Vitamins are classified according to their solubility in fat or water. The fat-soluble vitamins are A, D, E, and K. The water-soluble vitamins are C and all of the B vitamins. Vitamins play a vital role as control agents in cell metabolism

TABLE 29.2	
Grams of protein per serving for basic food exchanges	
MILK—8 g/serving	
One Serving	*Kilocalories*
1 cup skim milk	90
1 cup plain low-fat yogurt	90
LEAN MEAT—7 g/serving	
One Serving	*Kilocalories*
1 ounce lean beef or pork	55
1 ounce chicken or turkey (no skin)	45
1 ounce fish, shrimp, lobster, or tuna	40
1 ounce low-fat cheese	55
2 large egg whites	35
STARCHY VEGETABLES, BREADS, AND CEREALS—3 g/serving	
One Serving	*Kilocalories*
$1/2$ cup cooked or dry cereal	80
$1/2$ cup cooked pasta	80
$1/3$ cup cooked rice	80
$1/2$ bagel	80
1 slice of bread	80
1 small baked potato	80
$1/4$ cup baked beans	80
VEGETABLES—2 g/serving	
One Serving	*Kilocalories*
$1/2$ cup cooked vegetables	25
1 cup raw vegetables	25
FRUITS—≤1 g/serving	
One Serving	*Kilocalories*
1 small apple	60

Adapted from American Dietetic Association and American Diabetes Association.

(enzymes and coenzymes), as components of body tissue construction, and in preventing damage to body tissues (see Focus Box 29.2).

RDAs have been established for most vitamins (see inside cover). There is no need to take large quantities of supplemental vitamins, and in fact, this practice can be dangerous. The preferred source of vitamins is a balanced diet. Fat-soluble vitamins can be toxic when taken in large amounts.

A standard over-the-counter multivitamin can be taken to help supplement a healthy diet. Taking large doses, called "megadoses," can be extremely harmful. Some people may need additional vitamin supplementation, such as pregnant or lactating women, women taking oral contraceptives, the elderly and individuals who smoke. The decision to take additional vitamin supplementation should be discussed with a physician first.

Minerals

Minerals are inorganic substances that exist freely in nature. They are necessary for the growth and repair of bones and teeth, metabolic activity, and functioning of body fluids and secretions. Minerals maintain or regulate such physiologic processes as muscle contraction, normal heart rhythm, and nerve impulse conduction. As with vitamins, mineral intake can be abused. People who are especially active and who sweat profusely for prolonged periods may need to add salt and potassium to the diet. Both minerals can easily be replaced by drinking a commercially available sports drink or by adding a little extra salt to food. However, a well-balanced diet provides a far greater amount of minerals, especially sodium and potassium, than is lost during exercise. Other important minerals are calcium (found in milk, cheese, egg yolk, and green vegetables), iron (liver), iodine (seafood and iodized salt), and phosphorus (milk and cheeses).

Water

Approximately 70% of total body weight is water. Water is the most important nutrient, involved in almost every vital body process. It is essential for maintaining body temperature, transporting materials, and assisting with chemical reactions. A person should consume 2 to 3 quarts of water a day by drinking fluids and through the water contained in fruits and vegetables. With excess sweating (e.g., during exercise and in hot, humid weather), a large amount of water is lost. In such cases it is important to consume large quantities of water to remain hydrated.

Body Weight Control

Excess weight is a serious medical, health, and social issue. Since the evolution of industrialized societies, the incidence of obesity has risen dramatically. We no longer need to hunt or pick our food, we just drive by a fast-food window or go to a supermarket. The ease of obtaining food, combined with the fact that most people today work in sedentary professions, has led to an epidemic of obesity in the United States and other developed nations. Today it takes a conscious effort to increase one's physical activity level and choose healthy foods. Even most well-educated people feel they do not have the time or knowledge to plan healthy meals and get enough exercise.

Weight Categories

Most of the data on the U.S. national height and weight measurements comes from the Second National Health and Nutrition Examination Survey (NHANES II)[30], which was conducted between 1976 and 1980.[30] NHANES II provided an insight into the weight, height, and nutritional status of Americans 18 to 74 years of age. NHANES III, which provides more current data, has been compiled, but the results of the data have only begun to be disseminated and for the most part are not yet available. Table 29.3 provides an overview of some of the weight data from NHANES II, and the Clinical Application on p. 751 provides simple methods for indirectly evaluation body composition.

The two terms often used to classify excess weight are *overweight* and *obesity*. The National Center for Health Statistics has defined **overweight** as having a **body mass index (BMI)** of 27.8 or higher for men and 27.3 or higher for

overweight
a body mass index ≥27.8 in men and ≥27.3 in women.

body mass index (BMI)
body weight expressed in relation to height; BMI = weight (kg) ÷ height² (m).

TABLE 29.3

Mean body mass index and percentage of overweight and severely overweight U.S. adults*

	MEN			WOMEN		
	MEAN BMI	**OVERWEIGHT (N = 15.4 MILLION)**	**SEVERE OVERWEIGHT (N = 5.1 MILLION)**	**MEAN BMI**	**OVERWEIGHT (N = 18.6 MILLION)**	**SEVERE OVERWEIGHT (N = 7.4 MILLION)**
AGE						
20-24	23.5	12.1	4.2	22.6	11.4	3.5
25-34	25.2	20.4	6.7	24.1	20	8.8
35-44	26	28.9	8.9	25.3	27	12.1
45-54	26.3	31	10.7	26.1	32.5	12.9
55-64	26.1	28.1	9.2	26.5	37	14.2
All ages	25.3	24.2	8	25	27.1	10.6
ETHNICITY						
White	25.4	24.4	7.8	24.8	24.6	9.6
Black	25.3	26.3	10.4	27.1	45.1	19.7
Mexican	25.9	31.2	10.8	26.6	41.5	16.7
Cuban	26	28.5	10.3	25.8	31.9	6.9
Puerto Rican	25.5	25.7	7.9	26.1	39.8	15.2

*Adapted from Najjar MF, Rowland M: Anthropometric reference data and prevalence of overweight, United States, 1976-80. Vital and Health Statistics, series 11, no 238, DHHS pub no (PHS) 87-1688, Public Health Service, Washington, DC, 1987, U.S. Government Printing Office.

CLINICAL APPLICATION

Simple Methods of Quantifying Body Weight and Composition

Most people either have minimal access to advanced body composition analysis or do not want to invest the time and money needed for these tests. The following simple methods of evaluating body size, mass, and appearance can be used to indirectly evaluate body composition.

Weight tables: Weight tables, although convenient, are limited in their ability to provide accurate estimates of ideal weight for the entire population. Traditionally, a weight 20% or more above the table weight defines obesity, whereas a weight 10% or more below the table weight defines underweight (see Chapter 21).

Body mass index (BMI): A convenient, accurate method of quantifying body weight is to express it relative to stature (BMI = weight [kg] ÷ height² [m]). BMI relates fairly well to total body fatness. The National Center for Health Statistics has defined overweight as a BMI ⩾27.8 in men and ⩾27.3 in women. Severe overweight is defined as a BMI ⩾31.1 in men and ⩾32.3 in women.

Waist to hip ratio: Waist measurement divided by hip measurement provides another measure of weight status. A waist to hip ration >1 for men and >0.85 for women is an indication of overweight.

Pinch test: Remember the pinch test: "If you can pinch more than an inch, you're fat."

Belt test: A good sign that you're losing body weight, and thus probably fat, is finding yourself having to tighten your belt. Of course, the reverse is also true for gaining weight!

women.[30] A normal BMI has been classified as 20 for men and 25 for women. These classifications of overweight are based on BMI measurements corresponding to approximately 20% or more above the 1983 Metropolitan Life Insurance Company Tables (see Chapter 17). **Obesity** is excess fat relative to body weight. An ideal body fat percentage for good health is 10% to 15% for young men and 20% to 25% for young women. A body fat percentage over 20% for men or 30% for women is considered an indication of obesity.

The terms overweight and obesity should not be used interchangeably. The dissociation between being overweight and being obese was demonstrated as far back as the 1940s, when researchers studied a group of professional football players. When they compared the players' weights to early actuary weight tables, most of the players were considered seriously overweight. But when they tested the players' body compositions, most had a body fat percentage under 20%, meaning that they simply did not fit the normal standards for the weight charts.[47]

Health Implications of Obesity

Among the most alarming statistics in NHANES II was the increasing rate of obesity. Of Americans age 18 to 74 years surveyed from 1976 through 1980, one fourth had a BMI of 27.5 or higher, meaning that they were 24% or more above desirable weight. Approximately 10% of men and 15% of women had a BMI of 30.4 or higher, equating to 36% or more above desirable weight. Thus obesity has been described as an epidemic in the United States. Obesity rates are high at every age for both men and women, including children.

It is estimated that obesity affects one in three people in the United States, and some authorities consider it this country's number 1 health problem. Obesity is associated with a higher risk of diabetes mellitus and with hypertriglyceridemia, diminished levels of high-density lipoprotein (HDL) cholesterol, and increased levels of low-density lipoprotein (LDL) cholesterol, gallbladder disease, chronic hypoxia, some forms of cancer, sleep apnea, and degenerative joint disease.[50] Obesity is also a major contributor to such illnesses as hypertension, hypercholesterolemia, and diabetes[31] and is an independent risk factor for cardiovascular disease.[18] In 1985 the National Institutes of Health (NIH) held a consensus development conference on the health implications of obesity.[31] Three main questions were addressed: what is obesity, what is the evidence that obesity adversely affects health, and what is the evidence that obesity affects longevity. The panel of medical experts concluded the following:

The evidence is now overwhelming that obesity, defined as excessive storage of energy in the form of fat, has adverse effects on health and longevity. Obesity is clearly associated with hypertension, hypercholesterolemia, NIDDM [non–insulin-dependent diabetes mellitus], and excess of certain cancers and other medical problems.

NHANES II found that hypertension was 2.9 times more common in overweight adults than in nonoverweight

adults. The Framingham Study found that in men, for every 10% increase in relative weight, blood pressure increased by 6.5 mm Hg; a 15% gain resulted in an 18% increase in systolic blood pressure.[19] It is estimated that approximately one third of all cases of hypertension stem from obesity.[28]

A recent study by Denke[6] found that excess body weight is associated with high lipoprotein levels. For all ages, the higher the BMI, the higher the lipoprotein levels. The overall risk of coronary heart disease is higher in obese individuals, primarily because of the alterations in lipoprotein levels and blood sugar and hypertension.[18] Obesity is also associated with an increased prevalence of diabetes mellitus[46]; gallbladder disease[27]; respiratory problems, especially hypercapnic and hypoxic respiratory drives; irregular breathing patterns and frequent periods of apnea[23]; cancer[8]; gout; and arthritis.[35]

Fat Distribution

Obesity is clearly associated with an increase in medical and health risks. However, exactly where the excess fat is stored is also related to overall mortality and increased risk of cardiovascular disease. In general, women tend to store fat on the lower half of the body, around the hips and thighs **(gynoid obesity),** whereas men tend to store fat on the upper part of the body, around the abdomen **(android obesity).** A simple method that partly reflects body structure and fat distribution is the **waist to hip ratio.** Compared with gynoid obesity, android obesity is associated with a greater risk of diabetes, hypertension, and heart disease.[7]

Causes of Obesity

A number of factors contribute to the development of obesity. The diagnosis and treatment of obesity, although a daily occurrence for many physicians, is difficult. The frustrations of obesity are usually evident in both the patient and the physician. A detailed medical and dietary history is required before a physician can begin to determine the cause or causes of obesity. In many cases, obesity is caused by complex psychosocial issues that require referral to a psychologist or psychiatrist. Many people still feel that obesity is simply caused by eating too much. Although caloric consumption and physical activity habits are directly related to increased prevalence of excess weight, these are not the only causes of obesity.

Fat Cell Hypothesis

One theory of obesity deals with the amount of lipid stored in fat cells and the number of fat cells an individual has.[22] As children grow and develop, their fat stores steadily increase throughout childhood, reaching a peak around 7 years of age. Fat deposition also increases during adolescence. It is during these key periods that fat cells proliferate. An individual with more fat cells is at greater risk of becoming obese. Parents and pediatricians need to take great care to prevent childhood and adolescent obesity.

Hyperplastic obesity is a classification of obesity in which a person has a greater than normal number of fat cells, which are also larger than normal. This type of obesity begins at an early age and results in severe obesity. In **hypertrophic obesity,** the most common form, the person has a normal number of fat cells, but they have increased in size. Most severely obese individuals have both types.

Genetics

There is a high correlation between being overweight and having overweight parents. The family can be a powerful influence on a child's health and weight status. Within families, if one parent is obese, a child has a 40% chance of becoming obese. If both parents are obese, a child has an 80% chance of becoming obese. Serdula et al.[38] recently examined epidemiologic literature published between 1970 and 1992. They found that approximately one third of preschool children who had been obese were obese as adults, and about 50% of school-age children who were obese grew up to be obese adults. For all studies and ages, the risk of adult obesity was twice as high for obese children as for non-obese ones.

Metabolic Rate

Obesity can be caused by altered metabolic rates. The thermic effect of food represents approximately 10% of total energy needs. It appears that some individuals may not be as efficient in the way they utilize food when it is digested. One theory that may help explain this imbalance involves brown fat. Brown adipose tissue (BAT) is composed of highly specialized adipocytes whose main function is to produce heat. The distinctive characteristics of BAT cause greater uncoupling of oxidative phosphorylation, so that increased heat is generated at a given rate of adenosine triphosphate (ATP) regeneration. It has been shown that in rodents, stimulating BAT by exposure to cold can account for 30% to 80% non-shivering heat production, or **thermogenesis.** Thus lean individuals may have a higher percentage of brown fat compared with obese individuals, although the exact role of BAT in human metabolism is not yet known.

Diet Composition

Compared with lean individuals, most obese people tend not only to eat more, but also to eat foods higher in fat and lower in complex carbohydrates. In comparing a group of lean people with a group of obese individuals, Miller et al.[29] found that the lean group derived 29% of energy from fat and 53% from carbohydrates, versus 35% and 46%, respectively, for the obese group, even though there was no difference between the two groups in the number of calories consumed (Figure 29.1). These researchers also found that as the percentage of body fat increased, the percentage of energy derived from fat increased and calories from carbohydrates decreased.

Physical Inactivity

Substantial evidence points to physical inactivity, rather than overeating, as the cause of most obesity. In a number of randomized, controlled trials, sedentary men who took up jogging lost body fat even though they increased their caloric intake.[49] People who are habitually physically inactive tend to be at greater risk of obesity. With normal aging, the metabolic rate declines approximately 3% a year. Combining physical inactivity, aging, and a high-fat diet makes it inevitable that a person will gain weight and body fat. At least one study has shown that obese individuals tend to exercise less than lean people.[29]

Environmental Factors

One factor that has been associated with childhood obesity is the amount of time children and adults spend watching television. In one study, metabolic rate was found to be lower in obese children while they were watching TV and overall during the day, compared with normal-weight children.[23] Another study, which focused on adults, found that women who watched 3 to 4 hours of TV a day showed twice the prevalence of obesity, and when TV viewing rose above 4 hours, the prevalence of obesity more than doubled again, compared with the reference group (<1 hour/day).[44] The results were similar for adult men. Men who watched TV more than 3 hours a day were twice as likely to be obese as those who watched television less than 1 hour a day.[44]

---

obesity
the condition of having excess fat relative to body weight; men with body fat >20% and women with body fat >30% are considered obese.

gynoid obesity
storage of fat in the lower half of the body, in the hip and thigh area, primarily seen in women.

android obesity
storage of fat in the upper part of the body, in the abdominal area, a common tendency in men.

waist to hip ratio
waist circumference divided by hip circumference; this is another method used to assess excess body weight.

hyperplastic obesity
a type of obesity in which an individual has a greater than normal number of fat cells, which also are larger than normal, this type begins at an early age and results in severe obesity.

hypertrophic obesity
a type of obesity in which an individual has a normal number of fat cells, but they have increased in size.

thermogenesis
energy expenditure.

FIGURE 29.1

The components of energy intake and expenditures in lean and obese subjects. (Adapted from James WPT, Trayburn P: *Br Med Bull* 37:43-48, 1981.)

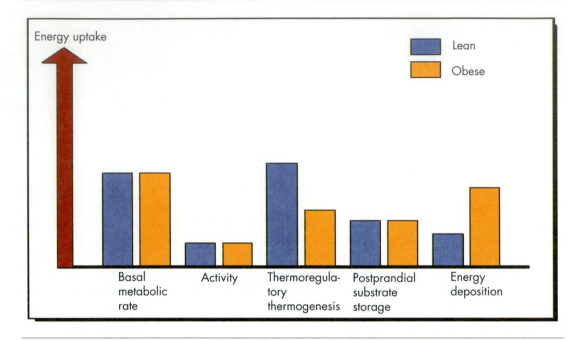

Dieting

Caloric restriction without exercise has detrimental effects on the metabolic rate. When the body senses a reduction in calories being consumed, it automatically slows the metabolic rate in an effort to conserve energy (Figure 29.2). Therefore if a person is trying to lose weight, dieting alone is one of the worst ways to go about it. That is why diets do not work. Frequent dieting, also called "yo-yo dieting" or **weight cycling,** has actually been shown to increase the prevalence of obesity.[3] After each diet cycle the rate of weight loss is slower and the rate of weight gain is faster.

Set Point Theory

The **set point theory,** a popular theoretical model for explaining obesity, maintains that an individual's weight is regulated through biologic signals to the hypothalamus.[20] In the set point model, blood glucose, lipid stores, and body weight routinely send signals to the hypothalamus to regulate appetite. If the hypothalamus senses a decrease in blood glucose or fatty acids, appetite is stimulated to reestablish energy stores. If the set point theory is correct, it is obvious why dieting does not work. Once the hypothalamus senses a decrease in energy stores, appetite is stimulated to regain the energy stores lost from dieting. As a person gets older, it appears that the set point gradually rises. If the set point could be lowered, a lower body weight could be maintained. One of the most effective ways to lower the body's set point is to exercise more, which appears to depress appetite and increase both resting and total energy expenditure through an increased metabolic rate.

FIGURE 29.2

Reduction in daily energy expenditure in obese individuals during severe caloric restriction. (Adapted from Bray GA: *Lancet* 2:397-398, 1969.)

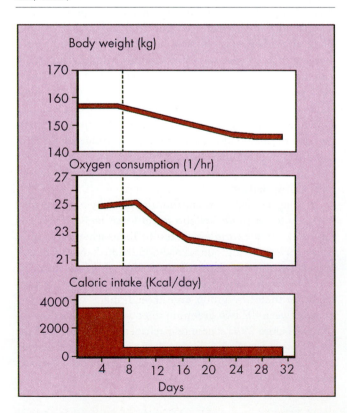

Weight Loss

Dieting has become a national pastime for Americans. Even though most people know that dieting alone is ineffective in achieving long-term success, it is still the method of choice for most overweight individuals. It has been estimated that as many as 40% of adult women and 20% of adult men are trying to lose weight at any one time.[41]

In 1992 the U.S. Food and Drug Administration (FDA) and the National Heart, Lung, and Blood Institute (NHLBI) set out to determine the weight loss practices of U.S. adults.[25] This survey found that adult Americans participate in a wide range of weight loss methods, from diet and exercise to appetite suppressant pills. Frequently reported weight-loss practices included weighing oneself regularly (71% of women and 70% of men), walking (58% and 44%), using diet soft drinks (52% and 45%), taking vitamins and minerals (33% and 26%), counting calories (25% and 17%), skipping meals (21% and 20%), using commercial meal replacements (15% and 13%), taking diet pills (14% and 7%), and participating in organized weight-loss programs (13% and 5%). On the bright side, two thirds of the respondents combined diet and exercise in their weight loss plan. Unfortunately, 20% of the respondents were engaged in such weight loss practices as taking weight-loss pills and appetite suppressants, fasting, and vomiting after eating. Thirty percent had been on a diet for longer than 1 year.

Energy Balance Equation

Weight loss or gain can be represented simply by the first law of thermodynamics, as presented in Chapter 2. This law clearly defines the basic principles and limitations of weight loss:

Caloric balance (loss or gain) = calories ingested − calories expended

The only way to lose excess body fat is to reduce the minuend (eat less) and increase the subtrahend (exercise more) (Figure 29.3) (See Focus Box 29.3). This process is aided by knowledge of the caloric energy in stored body fat.

To maintain an ideal body weight, energy intake (food consumed daily) must equal energy output (daily physical activity). When these two factors are equal, a person is said to be in energy balance. To gain or lose weight, either or both of these factors must be adjusted. To lose weight, energy (caloric) intake must be reduced and energy output (activity) must be increased. Either a caloric decrease of 1000 Kcal or an increase in energy expenditure of 1000 Kcal (or a combination of a decrease in energy expenditure of 500 Kcal and an increase in energy expenditure of 500 Kcal) is needed to lose approximately 2 pounds per week, the maximum recommended weight loss.

Unlike weight loss through dieting alone, losing weight through exercise and diet conserves BMR by preserving lean body mass. It has been estimated that as much as 25% of the weight lost through dieting alone is lean body mass. Because

The energy balance equation is based on the balance between caloric intake and caloric expenditure. Caloric expenditure is composed of basal metabolic rate, dietary thermogenesis, and physical activity.

- Calories from food
- Basal metabolism
- Thermic effect of digestion
- Activity

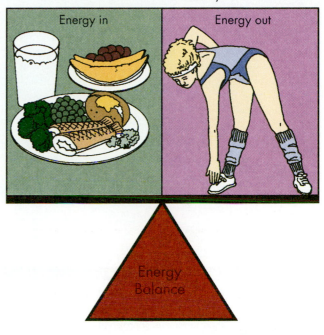

Energy in

Energy out

Energy Balance

lean body mass consists of tissues that are most metabolically active, any loss in this component will affect the resting metabolic rate (RMR) and weight loss.[32]

Role of Exercise in Weight Loss and Weight Control

Exercise appears to play a critical role in losing and maintaining body weight.[2] It is clear that neither diet nor exercise alone is effective in achieving long-term weight loss compared with when diet and exercise are combined. Saris[37] conducted a study in which two groups followed a 12-week weight-management program. One group simply followed a very low calorie diet (470 Kcal/day); the second group followed the same diet but added an exercise program (walking,

weight cycling

the increase and decrease in body weight experienced by individuals who try to lose weight by dieting alone.

set point theory

the theory that body fat is based on a genetically predetermined regulation of food intake linked to several physiologic stimuli (e.g., blood glucose, fatty acids, and the size and number of adipocytes).

FOCUS BOX 29.3

Components of caloric expenditure

Basal metabolic rate (BMR)

The minimum energy expenditure required to carry on normal biologic reactions such as circulation, respiration, and creation and conduction of nerve signals. BMR is different from resting metabolic rate (RMR) because true BMR is measured in a laboratory setting after complete bed rest, whereas RMR can be measured any time of day. In adults, BMR is approximately 20 to 25 kcal/kg body weight (1 to 1.2 kcal/min) and requires an oxygen consumption (VO_2) of approximately 200 to 250 ml/min. BMR can be estimated from the equation presented in Figure 29.4.

Diet-induced thermogenesis

Ingestion, digestion, storage, absorption, and transportation of food require energy. During eating, BMR increases slightly.

Facultative thermogenesis

Facultative thermogenesis, or nonshivering thermogenesis, is an increase in BMR during periods of exposure to cold or prolonged exposure to caloric excess.

Physical activity

Energy is expended during periods of physical labor or exercise. Increasing physical activity is a primary means of expending energy and changing the energy balance equation.

For the average sedentary adult with a BMR requirement of 2300 Kcal, BMR accounts for 75% of average daily expenditure (1725 Kcal); dietary thermogenesis, 7% (161 Kcal); and physical activity, 18% (414 Kcal).

FIGURE 29.4

Basal metabolic rate (BMR) can be estimated for men and women based on gender specific alterations of body weight. Physical activity can be approximated as a percentage of BMR, and dietary thermogenesis approximates 10% of ingested calories. (From Williams SR: *Basic nutrition and diet therapy,* St. Louis, 1995, Mosby.)

Estimate Your Own Daily Energy Requirement

• **Basal metabolism (BMR)**
Use general formula: Women—0.9 kcal/kg body weight/hr
　　　　　　　　　　　Men—1.0 kcal/kg body weight/hr
Convert weight (pounds) to kg: 1 kg = 2.2 pounds
Multiply according to formula: 1 (or 0.9) × (hours in day)

• **Physical activity**
Estimate your general average level of physical (muscular) activity. Find energy cost of activity (% of BMR) and add it to BMR.

Average activity level	Energy cost: % of BMR
Sedentary	20%
Very light	30%
Moderate	40%
Heavy	50%

For example, if you are sedentary (mostly sitting): BMR (step 1) + (.20 × BMR).

• **Specific dynamic action (SDA) of food**
Record food intake for day and calculate approximate energy (kcal) value.
Find energy cost of food effect (10% of kcal in food consumed).

• **Total energy output**
BMR 1 physical activity 1 SDA

FOCUS BOX 29.4

Kilocalorie adjustment required for weight loss

To lose 454 g (1 lb) a week through a 500 Kcal/day caloric deficit   454 g × 9 Kcal/g = 4086 Kcal (pure fat)
1 lb body fat = 454 g   454 g × 7.7 Kcal/g = 3496 Kcal (or 3500 kcal)
1 g pure fat = 9 Kcal   500 Kcal × 7 days = 3500 Kcal = 454 g body fat = 1 lb body fat
1 g body fat = 7.7 Kcal

From Williams SR: *Basic nutrition and diet therapy*, ed 10, St Louis, 1992, Mosby.

cycling, running, or swimming). Weight loss was more successful in the second group, and at a 24-week follow-up, that group also showed better weight maintenance, regaining an average of only 0.4 kg compared with the diet-only group's 1.8 kg.

The metabolic mechanisms by which exercise contributes to weight loss and weight maintenance are the following[1]:

- Increased energy expenditure
- Enhanced fat mobilization by increasing the activity of adipose tissue
- Slight increase in postexercise RMR
- Increased thermogenic response to food if exercise is done in close proximity to a meal
- Maintenance of or increase in lean body mass
- Dampened decrease, maintenance, or increase in BMR
- Improved psychologic states
- Improved appetite control

Exercise in combination with a sensible diet produces the best long-term weight-loss results. Exercise can contribute a 300 to 400 Kcal deficit per exercise bout (Focus Box 29.4). Keeping food intake constant, an exercise regimen done three times a week (at an intensity and duration eliciting 300 to 400 Kcal/session) could result in a 7.3 kg (16 pound) weight loss in 1 year. Despite the relatively long timeframe, especially compared with the rapidity of weight and body fat gain, this weight loss is remarkable and would occur even faster with added dietary restriction. Exercise is important because it helps maintain RMR by maintaining the fat-free mass. Regular exercise may also help control appetite and improve psychologic outlook.

A recent study by Hinkleman and Nieman[17] revealed that after 15 weeks of brisk walking five times a week for 45 minutes, overweight women showed a decrease in overall body weight, but not body fat, indicating that moderate exercise alone may not be enough to affect body composition. It appears that overweight women may not respond to exercise the same way men do. A recent review of the literature by Gleim[11] revealed that exercise alone can stimulate weight loss, but not in women. Women are at a disadvantage compared with men when it comes to elevating and maintaining their RMR because of their smaller body size, differences in

body fat distribution, and lower aerobic capacity. When obese young women were subjected to a negative energy balance of 3500 Kcal/week, either through exercise or dieting, over a 12-week period, weight loss was nearly identical by either method; however, the rate of body fat loss in the exercise group was significantly greater, suggesting a gain in lean body mass and loss of body fat.[40] Other studies have shown similar results.[2,14,26,34]

Special Considerations for Obese Exercisers

The timing of exercise may be important when designing exercise programs for obese individuals. In a recent study on the thermogenic effects of preprandial and postprandial exercise in obese women, investigators found that obese women who exercise after a meal produce the greatest thermogenic response, compared with not eating before exercise or after exercise.[5]

Before an obese individual begins an exercise program, he or she must have a complete medical examination and probably a diagnostic exercise test. Obese individuals are at greater risk for a variety of medical and health problems compared with nonobese individuals (Focus Box 29.5). Once an individual is cleared for exercise, it is important to discuss previous exercise experiences and what types of activities the person is interested in. Initially, exercise intensity should be kept low; the emphasis should be on duration rather than intensity. Walking is probably the single best activity for obese individuals. It involves fewer musculoskeletal problems, calls for minimal skill, is highly accessible, can easily be varied in intensity, and does not require expensive equipment or clothing. Other activities include swimming, water exercise classes, and stationary cycling.

Designing an Exercise Program

Before an exercise program is designed for an obese client, several factors must be considered. First and foremost is whether the client has any physical or medical problems, besides obesity, that would place him or her at risk during exercise. Second, fitness testing may provide valuable information that can be used to set specific goals and training limits. Third, an interview with the client will help establish clear goals and objectives for the exercise program. Neglecting any

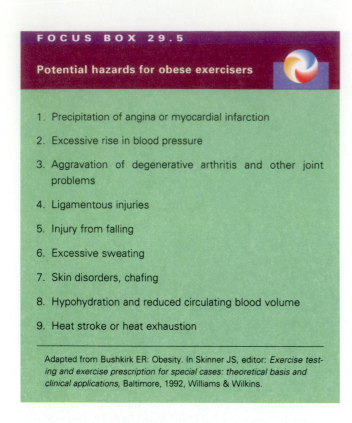

Adapted from Bushkirk ER: Obesity. In Skinner JS, editor: *Exercise testing and exercise prescription for special cases: theoretical basis and clinical applications*, Baltimore, 1992, Williams & Wilkins.

one of these three components can affect the safety and effectiveness of an exercise program.

The examiner should be considerate and conservative when performing any fitness tests on an obese client. For an extremely obese individual, the best body composition measurements to take are BMI, waist to hip ratio, and scale weight. Once the client loses some weight, a more accurate body composition test can be performed. Muscular strength, endurance, and flexibility are poor in most obese clients. A cardiovascular test, possibly with a resting metabolic rate test, would be helpful. Ideally, a diagnostic exercise test should be conducted in a medical setting. Unfortunately, many treadmills have a 300-pound weight limit. Extremely obese clients need to be examined by a physician to determine whether there are any contraindications to exercise.

Exercise intensity. The exercise training should be planned and conducted so that the obese client can exercise for a relatively long period with as little discomfort as possible. Initially the intensity should be low, possibly as low as 40% to 50% of maximal heart rate. As fitness improves, the intensity level will need to be increased. With obese clients the Borg scale rather than heart rate is a better gauge of intensity. Signs that an obese client is working at too high an intensity level are excessive sweating, higher than normal rate of breathing, joint pain, excessive fatigue, inability to complete an exercise session, and a flushed color. If these or other stressful signs and symptoms appear, exercise intensity should be reduced and the client should progress more slowly.

Exercise duration. Since most obese clients cannot exercise at a high intensity level, duration is the essential exercise variable, especially at the start of a program. Generally, for individuals with low cardiorespiratory endurance, the longer the duration, the greater the caloric expenditure. However, not all individuals have large blocks of time available for exercise.

There is controversy over the appropriate exercise prescription with regard to intensity and duration. The lower the exercise intensity, the longer the exercise can be performed. In addition, the lower the exercise intensity, the greater the contribution from fat to energy metabolism. For these reasons, many people, including so-called exercise experts, claim that low-intensity exercise is the best way to optimize fat loss. Unfortunately, there is no research evidence to support this claim. Although it seems to "make sense," it could be in error because low-intensity, long-duration exercise results in a low VO_2, and absolute VO_2 is the most important component of energy expenditure during exercise. The two examples below present conditions that differ in exercise duration and intensity:

Condition 1

VO_2	= 1 L/min
(RER)	= 0.75 = 4.739 Kcal/L VO_2
Duration	= 90 min

Kcal expended = 1 × 4.379 × 90 = 426.51

Condition 2

VO_2	= 2.5 L/min
RER	= 0.95 = 4.985 Kcal/L VO_2
Duration	= 45 min

Kcal expended = 2.5 × 4.985 × 45 = 560.81

The examples above indicate that exercising at a higher intensity for half the time actually would expend more calories and for a given calorie intake would generate a higher caloric deficit. According to the first law of thermodynamics, this condition would result in greater fat loss. Clearly, the recommendation that low-intensity exercise is best for fat loss is oversimplistic and is correct only for individuals, such as obese people or individuals with physical disabilities, who cannot exercise at moderate absolute exercise intensities. Furthermore, exercise training at higher absolute intensities induces greater muscular adaptations, which increase a person's ability to catabolize fat during exercise—which in turn leads to greater potential for fat combustion during exercise. Of course, the added cardiorespiratory adaptations would add to the health benefits of the exercise.

Frequency. Training frequency is an important consideration in prescribing exercise for weight loss. Basically, any additional amount of exercise adds to the caloric expenditure. It is important for overweight individuals to make exer-

FOCUS BOX 29.6

Characteristics of an obese individual most likely to benefit from an exercise program

1. Slightly or moderately obese

2. Became obese as an adult

3. Has not previously tried to lose weight

4. Sincerely desires weight reduction

5. Psychologically adjusted to pursuit of weight reduction goal

6. Can intelligently follow directions

7. Has no complicating disease or disability

Adapted from Bushkirk ER: Obesity. In Skinner JS, editor: *Exercise testing and exercise prescription for special cases: theoretical basis and clinical applications,* Baltimore, 1992, Williams & Wilkins.

cise a habit. For the obese client, 7 days of exercise a week would be ideal; at least 5 days a week should be recommended. Obese clients may need to start out with as few as 2 or 3 days a week. Consistency is the important variable leading to exercise adherence.

Rate of progression. The rate of progression for an obese client must be slow. Initially these clients are more than likely to experience a great deal of fatigue and muscle soreness. Compliance with the exercise program can be affected if the program is started or progresses too abruptly. The rate of progression is modified by changing three variables: intensity, duration, and frequency. The initial conditioning stage might last several months. Once the obese client has lost his or her desired weight, a maintenance exercise program should be devised.

Mode. Studies have demonstrated that walking is a highly effective form of exercise for losing and controlling weight. Walking, cycling, and aerobic dance have shown better results than swimming because evidence indicates that swimming may protect against subcutaneous fat loss to regulate temperature and prevent heat loss.

Aerobic dance. Aerobic dance exercise can be an effective, safe, and fun form of exercise for individuals who want to lose weight. The speed of movement should be slow and progress gradually. Low-impact classes are better than high-impact ones. If steps are used, the step should be as low as possible, with as great a base of support as possible. One of the most important things to stress to the obese client is the need to know where his or her center of gravity is. Obese clients will have to take some time to explore how far they can move in different directions and still maintain their center of gravity. It is extremely important that obese clients maintain their center of gravity during all exercise movements.

The characteristics of obese individuals that will influence their involvement in an exercise program are listed in Focus Box 29.6.

SUMMARY

- At any given time, 20% of the U.S. population is taking part in some form of weight-loss program. Americans spend more than $30 billion a year on various weight-loss methods, most of which fail. Excess body weight is associated with numerous health problems, including diabetes, hyperlipidemia, and an increased risk of coronary artery disease.

- Excess body weight is a serious medical, health, and social issue. The National Center for Health Statistics has defined **overweight** as having a **body mass index (BMI)** ≥27.8 for men and ≥27.3 for women. A normal BMI values is 20 for men and 25 for women. The **waist to hip ratio** is also used to assess excess body weight.

- **Obesity** is the condition of having excess body fat relative to body weight. For good health the ideal body fat percentage is 10% to 15% for men and 20% to 25% for women. Obesity is a body fat percentage >20% for men and >30% for women. In general, women tend to store fat in the lower half of the body, around the hips and thighs **(gynoid obesity),** whereas men tend to store fat on the upper part of the body, around the abdomen **(android obesity).** Android obesity is associated with a greater risk of diabetes, hypertension, and heart disease.

- Obesity has been linked to the amount of lipid stored in fat cells **(hypertrophic obesity)** and to the number of fat cells a person has **(hyperplastic obesity),** as well as to genetics, low basal metabolic rate, poor diet, physical inactivity, and environmental factors, such as the amount of time spent watching TV and excessive dieting.

- To maintain an ideal body weight, energy consumed (i.e., food eaten daily) must equal energy expended (through basal metabolic rate, dietary **thermogenesis,** and daily physical activity). When these factors are equal, a person is said to be in energy balance.

- Frequent dieting, also called "yo-yo dieting" or **weight cycling,** increases the prevalence of obesity. After each diet cycle, the rate of weight loss is slower and the rate of weight gain is faster. The **set point theory,** a popular theoretical model for explaining obesity, maintains that weight is regulated through biologic signals to the hypothalamus.

REVIEW QUESTIONS

1. Briefly describe the characteristics of a healthy diet.

2. Define the terms obesity, overweight, weight cycling, and thermogenesis.

3. Explain why obesity is a health risk.

4. Which is the best way to lose body fat and maintain the loss: dieting alone, exercise alone, or a combination of dieting and exercise? Why?

5. How much exercise equates to the loss of 15 pounds of body fat? What exercise and diet regimen would you recommend for losing 15 pounds safely?

6. What is the best way to exercise to lose body fat? Explain.

APPLICATIONS

1. What obstacles do severely obese individuals face in exercising? How would these obstacles influence their motivation to exercise?

2. What are the health risks of exercise for severely obese individuals?

REFERENCES

1. Brownell KD, Grilo CM: Weight management. In Durstine JL et al, editors: *American College of Sports Medicine's resource manual for guidelines for exercise testing and prescription, ed 2,* Philadelphia, 1993, Lea & Febiger.

2. Brownell KD, Stunkard AJ: Physical activity in the development and control of obesity. In Stunkard AJ, editor: *Obesity,* Philadelphia, 1980, Saunders.

3. Brownell KD, Greenwood MRC, Stellar E, Sharger EE: The effects of repeated cycles of weight loss and regain in rats, *Physiol Behav* 38:459-464, 1986.

4. Danford DE, Stephenson MG: Healthy People 2000: development of nutrition objectives, *J Am Diet Assoc* 91:1517-1519, 1991.

5. Davis JM, Sargent RG, Brayboy TD, Bartoli WP: Thermogenic effects of preprandial and postprandial exercise in obese females, *Addict Behav* 17(2):185-190, 1992.

6. Denke MA, Sempos CT, Grundy SM: Excess body weight: an underrecognized contributor to high blood cholesterol levels in white American men, *Arch Intern Med* 153:1093-1103, 1993.

7. Ducimetiere P, Richard JL: The relationship between subsets of anthropometric upper versus lower body measurements and coronary heart disease risk in middle-aged men: the Paris Prospective Study, *Int J Obes Relat Metab Disord* 13:111-112, 1989.

8. Garfinkel L: Overweight and cancer, *Ann Intern Med* 103:1034-1036, 1985.

9. Garrow JS: Treatment of obesity, *Lancet* 340:409-413, 1992.

10. Gaziano JM, Manson JE, Buring JE, Hennekens CH: Dietary antioxidants and cardiovascular disease, *Ann NY Acad Sci* 669:249-259, 1992.

11. Gleim GW: Exercise is not an effective weight loss modality in women, *J Am Coll Nutr* 12(4):363-367, 1993.

12. Goldfarb AH: Antioxidants: role of supplementation to prevent exercise-induced oxidative stress, *Med Sci Sports Exerc* 25(2):232-236, 1992.

13. Hahn DB, Payne WA: *Focus on health,* St Louis, 1994, Mosby.

14. Hagan RD, Upton SJ, Wong L, Whittam J: The effects of aerobic conditioning and/or caloric restriction in overweight men and women, *Med Sci Sport Exer* 18:87-94, 1986.

15. Foster WR, Burton BT: Health implications of obesity, *Ann Intern Med* 103:981-1077, 1985.

16. Hennekens CH: Micronutrients and cancer prevention, *N Engl J Med* 315:1288-1289, 1986.

17. Hinkleman LL, Nieman DC: The effects of a walking program on body composition and serum lipids and lipoproteins in overweight women, *J Sports Med Phys Fitness* 33(1):49-58, 1993.

18. Hubert HB, Feinleib M, McNamara PM et al: Obesity as an independent risk factor for cardiovascular disease: 26-year follow-up of participants in the Framingham Study, *Circulation* 67:968-977, 1983.

19. Kannel WB, Brand N, Skinner JJ et al: The relation of adiposity to blood pressure and development of hypertension: the Framingham Study, *Ann Intern Med* 67:48-59, 1967.

20. Keesey RE: A set point theory of obesity. In Brownell KD, Foreyt JP, editors: *Handbook of eating disorders: physiology, psychology, and treatment of obesity, anorexia and bulimia,* New York, 1986, Basic Books.

21. Klesges RC, Shelton ML, Klesges LM: Effects of television on metabolic rate: potential implication for children obesity, *Pediatrics* 91(2):281-285, 1993.

22. Knittle JL: Obesity in childhood: a problem in adipose tissue cellular development, *J Pediatr* 81:1048-1059, 1972.

23. Kopelman PG, Apps MC, Cope DA et al: Nocturnal hypoxia and sleep apnea in asymptomatic obese men, *Int J Obes Relat Metab Disord* 10:211-217, 1986.

24. Leach RE, Baumgard S, Broom J: Obesity: its relationship to osteoarthritis of the knee, *Clin Orthop* 93:271-273, 1973.

25. Levy AS, Heaton AW: Weight control practices of U.S. adults trying to lose weight, *Ann Intern Med* 119(7 pt 2):661-666, 1993.

26. Lewis S, Haskell WL, Wood PD et al: Effects of physical activity on weight reduction in obese middle-aged women, *Am J Clin Nutr* 29:151-156, 1976.

27. Maclure KM, Hayes KC, Colditz GA et al: Weight, diet, and the risk of symptomatic gallstones in middle-aged women, *N Engl J Med* 321:563-569, 1989.

28. MacMahon SW, Blacket RB, Macdonald GJ, Hall W: Obesity, alcohol consumption, and blood pressure in Australian men and women: the National Heart Foundation of Australia Risk Factor Prevalence Study, *J Hypertens* 2:85-91, 1984.

29. Miller WC, Lindeman AK, Wallace J, Niederpruem M: Diet composition, energy intake, and exercise in relation to body fat in men and women, *Am J Clin Nutr* 52:426-430, 1990.

30. Najjar MF, Rowland M: Anthropometric reference data and prevalence of overweight, United States, 1976-80. Vital and Health Statistics, series 11, no 238, DHHS pub no (PHS) 87-1688, Public Health Service, Washington, DC, 1987, U.S. Government Printing Office.

31. National Institutes of Health Consensus Development Conference Statement: *Health implications of obesity.* National Institutes of Health Consensus Development Conference Statement, vol 5(9), 1985.

32. Nieman DC, Onasch LM, Lee JW: The effects of moderate exercise training on nutrient intake in mildly obese women, *J Am Diet Assoc* 90(11):1557-1562, 1990.

REFERENCES—Cont'd

33. Nutrition science policy: an evaluation of dietary guidance graphic alternatives: the evolution of the eating right pyramid, *Nutr Rev* 50(9):275-282, 1992.

34. Pavlov K, Steffee WP, Lerman RH, Burrows BA: Effects of dieting and exercise on lean body mass, oxygen uptake, and strength, *Med Sci Sports Exer* 17:466-471, 1985.

35. Rimm AA, Werner LH, Yserloo BV, Bernstein RA: Relationship of obesity and disease in 73,532 weight-conscious women, *Public Health Rep* 90:44-54,1975.

36. Robinson TN, Hammer LD, Killen JD et al: Does television viewing increase obesity and reduce physical activity?: cross-sectional and longitudinal analysis among adolescent girls, *Pediatrics* 91(2):273-279, 1993.

37. Deleted in proofs.

38. Serdula MK, Ivery D, Coates RJ et al: Do obese children become obese adults?: a review of the literature, *Prev Med* 22:167-177, 1993.

39. Spielman AB, Kanders B, Kienholz M, Blackburn GL: The cost of losing: an analysis of commercial weight-loss programs in a metropolitan area, *J Am Coll Nutr* 11(1):36-41, 1992.

40. Deleted in proofs.

41. Stephenson MG, Levy AS, Sass NL, McGarvey WE: 1985 NHIS findings: nutrition knowledge and baseline data for the weight-loss objectives, *Public Health Rep* 102:61-67, 1987.

42. Storlie J, Jordan HA editors: *Nutrition and exercise in obesity management: LaCrosse Health and Sports Science Symposium,* New York, 1984, SP Medical Science Books.

43. Tucker LA, Bagwell M: Television viewing and obesity in adult females, *Am J Public Health* 81(7):908-910, 1991.

44. Tucker LA, Freidman GM: Television viewing and obesity in adult males, *Am J Public Health* 79(4):516-518, 1989.

45. Our vitamin prescription: the Big Four, *University of California at Berkeley Wellness Letter,* 10(4):1992.

46. Van Itallie TB: Health implications of overweight and obesity in the United States, *Ann Intern Med* 103:983-988, 1985.

47. Welham WC, Behnke AR: The specific gravity of healthy men: body weight divided by volume and other physical characteristics of exceptional athletes and of naval personnel, *JAMA* 118:498-501, 1942.

48. Williams SR: *Basic nutrition and diet therapy,* St Louis, 1995, Mosby.

49. Wood PD: Impact of experimental manipulation of energy intake and expenditure on body composition, *Crit Rev Food Sci Nutr* 33(4):369-373, 1993.

50. Xavier Pi-Sunyer F: Medical hazards of obesity, *Ann Intern Med* 119(7):655-660, 1993.

RECOMMENDED READINGS

▪ Stunkard AJ, editor: *Obesity,* Philadelphia, 1980, Saunders.

▪ Health implications of obesity, *Ann Intern Med* 103:981-1077, 1985.

▪ Brownell KD, Foreyt JP, editors: *Handbook of eating disorders: physiology, psychology, and treatment of obesity, anorexia, and bulimia,* New York, 1986, Basic Books.

▪ Methods for voluntary weight loss and control, *Ann Intern Med* 119(7 pt 2):661-666, 1993.

▪ National Institutes of Health Consensus Development Conference Statement: *Health implications of obesity,* National Institutes of Health Concensus Development Conference Statement, vol 5(9), 1985.

▪ Stefanick ML: Exercise and weight control, *Exerc Sports Sci Rev* 21:363-398,1993.

CHAPTER 30

Training for Health and Fitness

OBJECTIVES

After reading this chapter you should be able to:

- Explain the principles involved in designing a comprehensive exercise program for healthy individuals.

- Describe the key components involved in the design of an exercise program.

- Outline a conditioning program for general muscular strength and endurance.

- Outline a detailed walking program for health and fitness.

- Describe some of the important health-related benefits of exercise for healthy individuals.

KEY TERMS

health-related fitness

medical history

rating of perceived exertion

static stretching

proprioceptive neuromuscular facilitation (PNF)

ballistic stretching

The benefits of regular physical activity and exercise are becoming increasingly clear. Individuals who choose to be more physically active, in both their leisure and work activities, can lower their risk for developing certain degenerative diseases, such as osteoporosis, diabetes, obesity, and cardiovascular disease. Despite the mounting evidence of the benefits of regular exercise, only 22% of adults engage in leisure-time activities at or above the level recommended for health benefits in the U.S. Public Health Service's health and disease prevention goals and objectives for the nation (Clinical Application p.767).[7] This finding suggests an epidemic of nonparticipation in exercise. The term *epidemic* at first appears harsh, but lack of exercise increases one's risk for the development of many disease processes. The purpose of this chapter is to present information on how regular exercise can improve health and well-being.

Health-Related Fitness

Research has shown that there are many health-related benefits of regular exercise participation. These are summarized in Focus Box 30.1. The term **health-related fitness** appears frequently in exercise literature to describe the health benefits of exercise. The simplest definition of health-related fitness is the ability of the body's systems (heart, lungs, blood vessels, and muscles) to function efficiently, to resist disease, and be able to participate in a variety of activities without undue fatigue. The five components of health-related physical fitness are the same as those of general fitness and include muscular strength, muscular endurance, cardiorespiratory endurance, flexibility, and body composi-

tion. A comprehensive fitness program should have activities that develop and maintain each of the five components.

In designing an exercise program, several things need to be considered. First and foremost, individuals need to know if there are any physical or medical problems that would place them at risk if they exercise. Second, fitness testing may provide valuable information that can be used to set specific goals and training limits. Finally, an interview with a client helps establish clear goals and objectives for the exercise pro-

---

health-related fitness
fitness that provides benefits to health and well-being

FOCUS BOX 30.1

A summary of the selected health benefits associated with regular exercise

The health benefits of exercise can combine to prevent disease processes and rehabilitate patients who have them. Listed below are conditions and behaviors that result from regular physical activity and that are known to increase health and well-being.

- Increases HDL-cholesterol (HDL-C)

- Decreases LDL-cholesterol (LDL-C)

- Favorably changes the ratios between total cholesterol and HDL-C and between LDL-C and HDL-C

- Decreases triglyceride levels

- Promotes relaxation; relieves stress and tension

- Decreases body fat and favorably changes body composition

- Reduces blood pressure, especially if it is high

- Causes blood platelets to be less sticky

- Reduces number of cardiac arrhythmias

- Increases myocardial efficiency by lowering resting heart rate and increasing stroke volume

- Increases oxygen-carrying capacity of the blood

- Helps control diabetes by increasing the sensitivity of cells to insulin and decreasing body fat

- Develops stronger bones that are less susceptible to injury

- Promotes joint stability by increasing muscular strength and the strength of ligaments, tendons, and cartilage

- Contributes to fewer low-back problems

- Acts as a stimulus for other life-style changes

- Improves self-concept

---

gram. Neglecting any one of the three components can affect the safety and effectiveness of an exercise program.

Program Design for Apparently Healthy Individuals

This chapter deals with designing fitness programs for apparently healthy people. Program design considerations for individuals with medical and health concerns is covered in earlier chapters. The American College of Sports Medicine defines an apparently healthy individual as asymptomatic, with no more than one major coronary risk factor.[1] Individuals who have symptoms suggestive of cardiac, pulmonary, or metabolic disease, who have two or more coronary risk factors, or who have known disease should have a complete medical evaluation with a diagnostic exercise test before exercise. Safety should always be the primary factor dictating the readiness of an individual to exercise.

The American College of Sports Medicine (ACSM), in conjunction with the Centers for Disease Control and Prevention (CDC) and the President's Council on Physical Fitness and Sports, recently issued a new recommendation on increased physical activity for Americans.[1] The recommendation states the following:

Every American adult should accumulate 30 minutes or more of moderate-intensity physical activity over the course of most days. Incorporating more activity into the daily routine is an effective way to improve health. Activities that can contribute to the 30-minute total include walking up stairs (instead of taking the elevator), gardening, raking leaves, dancing,

and walking part or all of the way to or from work. The recommended 30 minutes of physical activity may also come from planned exercise or recreation such as jogging, playing tennis, swimming, and cycling. One specific way to meet the standard is to walk 2 miles briskly.

Because most adult Americans fail to meet this recommended level of moderate-intensity physical activity, almost all should strive to increase their participation in moderate or vigorous physical activity. Persons who currently do not engage in regular physical activity should begin by incorporating a few minutes of increased activity into their day, building up to 30 minutes of additional physical activity. Those who are irregularly active should strive to adopt a more consistent pattern of activity. Regular participation in physical activities that develop and maintain muscular strength and joint flexibility is also recommended.

The ACSM/CDC position statement on exercise means that multiple short durations of physical activity that occur each day can accumulate and result in health-related benefits. Individuals should strive to participate in activities to improve and maintain key components of health-related fitness.

The importance of exercise to health was also stressed in the Healthy People 2000 report of the health promotion and disease prevention objectives for the nation. Although these objectives were not stated in order of importance, the immediate attention given to both exercise and nutrition reflects their current inadequacy in today's society, as well as their importance to preventive medicine (Clinical Application p. 767).

Designing an Exercise Program

The term *exercise prescription* is frequently used when discussing the design of an exercise program. Actually, unless you

Healthy People 2000—National Health Promotion and Disease Prevention Objectives for the Nation

Objective 1.3—Increase to at least 30% the proportion of people aged 6 and older who engage regularly, preferably daily, in light to moderate physical activity for at least 30 minutes. (Baseline: 22% of people aged 18 and older were active for at least 30 minutes, five or more times per week, and 12% were active seven or more times per week in 1985.)

Objective 1.4—Increase to at least 20% the proportion of people aged 18 and older and to at least 75% the proportion of children and adolescents aged 6 through 17 who engage in vigorous physical activity that promotes the development and maintenance of cardiorespiratory fitness three or more days per week for 20 or more minutes per occasion. (Baseline: 12% for people aged 18 and older in 1985; 66% for youth aged 10 through 17 in 1984.)

Objective 1.5—Reduce to no more than 15% the proportion of people aged 6 and older who engage in no leisure-time physical activity. (Baseline: 24% for people aged 18 and older in 1985.)

Objective 1.6—Increase to at least 40% the proportion of people aged 6 and older who regularly perform physical activ-

ities that enhance and maintain muscular strength, muscular endurance, and flexibility. (Baseline data available in 1991.)

Objective 1.7—Increase to at least 50% the proportion of overweight people aged 12 and older who have adopted sound dietary practices combined with regular physical activity to attain an appropriate body weight. (Baseline: 30% of overweight women and 25% of overweight men aged 18 and older in 1985.)

Objective 1.10—Increase the proportion of work sites offering employer-sponsored physical activity and fitness programs.

Objective 1.11—Increase community availability of and accessibility to physical activity and fitness facilities.

Objective 1.12—Increase to at least 50% the proportion of primary care providers who routinely assess and counsel their patients regarding the frequency, duration, type, and intensity of each patient's physical activity practices. (Baseline: Physicians provided exercise counseling for about 30% of sedentary patients in 1988.)

Adapted from *Healthy People 2000: National Health Promotion and Disease Prevention Objectives*, Department of Health and Human Services, Washington, DC, 1991.

are a medical doctor or perhaps a nurse, no one actually prescribes an exercise program. Rather, educated professionals make recommendations based on accepted standards. In most situations, fitness instructors or personal trainers should not recommend exercise to clients requiring special needs. Ideally, the exercise recommendation for someone with a medical or health problem should come from a physician, nurse, or other allied-health professional. However, fitness instructors can and should monitor the client's response to exercise and should be able to provide sound advice that will make exercise safer and more effective. For example, fitness instructors can assist clients with their exercise programs by: (1) helping them monitor their progress or lack of progress, (2) providing encouragement and support, (3) offering suggestions for safer exercises or exercise moves, (4) making sure clients follow the exercise prescription for maximum safety and benefit, and (5) working with the medical practitioner to formulate the clinical exercise prescription. Safety should be the first priority when designing and leading an exercise class.

Components of the Exercise Program

An exercise program is based on five key principles. These include screening, warm-up, exercise session, cooldown, and rest.

Preexercise Health Screening

The potential benefits of exercise must outweigh the potential risks for an individual. For most healthy individuals the risks associated with exercise are extremely low. It is estimated that death occurs in 1 in 15,000 to 20,000 adult exercisers as a result of vigorous exercise. In individuals with a known or unknown medical condition, exercise may cause serious injury or even death. Thus an individual's health status needs to be evaluated before his or her exercise program is designed.

A preexercise health screening should include the following:

- A self-administered questionnaire, such as the PAR-Q (Figure 30.1)
- A complete physical examination by a physician

FIGURE 30.1

The Physical Activity Readiness Questionnaire (PAR-Q).

Physical Activity Readiness
Questionnaire - PAR-Q
(revised 1994)

PAR - Q & YOU

(A Questionnaire for People Aged 15 to 69)

Regular physical activity is fun and healthy, and increasingly more people are starting to become more active every day. Being more active is very safe for most people. However, some people should check with their doctor before they start becoming much more physically active.

If you are planning to become much more physically active than you are now, start by answering the seven questions in the box below. If you are between the ages of 15 and 69, the PAR-Q will tell you if you should check with your doctor before you start. If you are over 69 years of age, and you are not used to being very active, check with your doctor.

Common sense is your best guide when you answer these questions. Please read the questions carefully and answer each one honestly: check YES or NO.

YES	NO		
☐	☐	1.	Has your doctor ever said that you have a heart condition <u>and</u> that you should only do physical activity recommended by a doctor?
☐	☐	2.	Do you feel pain in your chest when you do physical activity?
☐	☐	3.	In the past month, have you had chest pain when you were not doing physical activity?
☐	☐	4.	Do you lose your balance because of dizziness or do you ever lose consciousness?
☐	☐	5.	Do you have a bone or joint problem that could be made worse by a change in your physical activity?
☐	☐	6.	Is your doctor currently prescribing drugs (for example, water pills) for your blood pressure or heart condition?
☐	☐	7.	Do you know of <u>any other reason</u> why you should not do physical activity?

If you answered

YES to one or more questions

Talk with your doctor by phone or in person BEFORE you start becoming much more physically active or BEFORE you have a fitness appraisal. Tell your doctor about the PAR-Q and which questions you answered YES.

- You may be able to do any activity you want—as long as you start slowly and build up gradually. Or, you may need to restrict your activities to those which are safe for you. Talk with your doctor about the kinds of activities you wish to participate in and follow his/her advice.
- Find out which community programs are safe and helpful for you.

NO to all questions

If you answered NO honestly to all PAR-Q questions, you can be reasonably sure that you can:

- start becoming much more physically active—begin slowly and build up gradually. This is the safest and easiest way to go.
- take part in a fitness appraisal—this is an excellent way to determine your basic fitness so that you can plan the best way for you to live actively.

DELAY BECOMING MUCH MORE ACTIVE:

- if you are not feeling well because of a temporary illness such as a cold or a fever—wait until you feel better; or
- if you are or may be pregnant—talk to your doctor before you start becoming more active.

Please note: If your health changes so that you then answer YES to any of the above questions, tell your fitness or health professional. Ask whether you should change your physical activity plan.

<u>Informed Use of the PAR-Q</u>: The Canadian Society for Exercise Physiology, Health Canada, and their agents assume no liability for persons who undertake physical activity, and if in doubt after completing this questionnaire, consult your doctor prior to physical activity.

You are encouraged to copy the PAR-Q but only if you use the entire form

NOTE: If the PAR-Q is being given to a person before he or she participates in a physical activity program or a fitness appraisal, this section may be used for legal or administrative purposes.

I have read, understood and completed this questionnaire. Any questions I had were answered to my full satisfaction.

NAME _____

SIGNATURE _____   DATE _____

SIGNATURE OF PARENT _____   WITNESS _____
or GUARDIAN (for participants under the age of majority)

© *Canadian Society for Exercise Physiology*
Société canadienne de physiologie de l'exercice

Supported by: 🍁 Health   Santé
Canada   Canada

- A diagnostic exercise test
- Some combination of the above three

Deciding on which health screening procedure to use depends on the age, gender, and health status of the individual, the desired starting level of exercise intensity an individual wants, and the resources and trained personnel available.

Client interview. Goals of the client should be thoroughly explored before an exercise program is designed. The most thorough health screening and fitness test will mean little if the client's needs are not discussed. A preexercise interview should include such topics as:

- Past exercise experiences
- Specific health goals (i.e., "I want to lose weight")
- Time constraints (i.e., "I can exercise only for $1/2$ hour between 5:30 and 6:00 AM")
- Equipment needs (i.e., "I love to swim but the closest pool is a $1/2$-hour drive from my house"), and
- Personal reasons for exercising (i.e., "I really just want to look and feel better!").

Individuals generally adhere to an exercise program better, if clear, measurable, and concise goals have been identified.

A health appraisal can provide valuable information that can be used to detect risk factors and improve the safety and appropriateness of the exercise program. More specific medical information regarding a client's past and present medical status can be obtained by reviewing a **medical history**. A medical history is generally obtained from a physician or nurse and in most cases can be made available on request. The purpose of the health appraisal is to establish the current health status of an individual and provide fitness professionals with baseline information that will be used to design an exercise program; it is not intended to screen for all health conditions that could affect the safety and effectiveness of an exercise program. A good motto to follow is "when in doubt about an individual's readiness to exercise, have them consult a physician."

Fitness Testing/Assessment

Fitness testing generally falls into two categories—field tests and laboratory tests. There are simple field tests and sophisticated laboratory tests that are used to measure the five components of physical fitness. Baseline data collected from fitness tests can be used to plan safe and effective exercise, motivate a client, and change or modify an exercise program. An initial fitness evaluation should be used to establish baseline measurements of body composition, muscular strength, aerobic capacity, flexibility, and muscular endurance.

Warm-up. The purpose of the warm-up period is to prepare the body for more vigorous activity and to reduce the chance of injury (see Chapter 18). Typically the warm-up period consists of a light aerobic period, followed by some flexibility exercises. The light aerobic period might consist of some light calisthenics, jogging in place, or 5 to 10 minutes on stationary aerobic exercise equipment. Flexibility exercises described later in this chapter are appropriate during the warm-up period but only after a brief aerobic exercise period. An adequate warm-up period should last at least 10 minutes.

Exercise program

Mode. Mode refers to the type of activity performed during the exercise session. Various modes of exercise can affect the components of fitness differently. For example, aerobic exercise affects aerobic capacity and body composition but has little effect on muscular strength, flexibility, and muscular endurance. Choosing the correct mode of exercise is important because it has a direct effect on the outcome. Activities that improve cardiorespiratory endurance must use large muscle groups, rhythmically, for a continuous period (e.g., running, swimming, cycling). Activities that develop muscular strength must work large and small muscle groups for brief periods (i.e., weight training).

Intensity. Intensity refers to the level of stress achieved during the exercise period. Exercise sessions can be low intensity or high intensity. Intensity is best determined by measuring oxygen consumption, but indirect methods are heart rate, breathing rate, or the **rating of perceived exertion** (RPE) (Table 30.1).[3] To determine a training heart rate range, an individual's maximal heart rate (HR_{max}) must be determined. An individual's maximal heart rate can be directly determined from a submaximal or maximal exercise test, or it can be estimated by subtracting one's age from 220. For example, an estimated maximal heart rate for a 20-year-old is 200.

Low-intensity exercise would be equal or 50% to 60% of an individual's maximal heart rate, whereas 85% to 90% would relate to high-intensity exercise (Table 30.2). Although it is assumed that the VO_2-heart rate relationship is linear, it really is not and best fits a sigmoid curve (see Chapter 11). This deviation from linearity is partly responsible for the error in estimating submaximal and maximal VO_2 from heart rate (see Chapter 19).

It is best to begin an exercise program at a low intensity and gradually increase the intensity over time. The heart rate to reach during training can be determined as a direct percentage of the maximal heart rate obtained from an exercise

medical history
the medical records of an individual.

rating of perceived exertion (RPE)
a rating based on an individual's perception of exercise intensity.

TABLE 30.1

RPE Scales

CATEGORY RPE SCALE		CATEGORY-RATIO RPE SCALE	
6		0	Nothing at all
7	Very, very light	0.5	Very, very weak
8		1	Very weak
9	Very light	2	Weak
10		3	Moderate
11	Fairly light	4	Somewhat strong
12		5	Strong
13	Somewhat hard	6	
14		7	Very strong
15	Hard	8	
16		9	
17	Very hard	10	Very, very strong
18		•	Maximal
19	Very, very hard		
20			

Original scale (6 to 20) on left and revised scale (1 to 10) on right. (Adapted from Borg GA: *Med Sci Sports Exerc* 14:377-387, 1982.)

TABLE 30.2

Relationships between maximal heart rate, Karvonen heart rate range, and VO$_2$max expressions of exercise intensity

PERCENT HR$_{max}$	% HRR*	PERCENT VO$_2$max
50	33	28
60	47	42
70	60	56
80	73	70
90	87	83
100	100	100

HR$_{max}$, Maximal heart rate; *HRR*, heart rate reserve.
*Assumes HR$_{max}$ is 200 and resting heart rate is 50.

test or can be estimated by taking a percentage of an individual's heart rate reserve (HRR) using the Karvonen method.

$$
\begin{aligned}
HR_{max} &= 220 - age \\
HR_{max} &= 220 - 40 = 180 \\
HR_{rest} &= 60 \\
HRR &= 180 - 60 = 120 \\
lower\ HR &= HR_{rest} + (HRR \times 0.6) \\
&= 132 \\
higher\ HR &= HR_{rest} + (HRR \times 0.85) \\
&= 162
\end{aligned}
$$

Training heart rate range = 132 to 162 bpm

Another common method used to monitor exercise intensity is based on an individual's rating of perceived exertion (RPE). RPE is derived from the Borg scale (see Table 30.1). A rating of 12 to 13 (using the 15-point scale) corresponds to approximately 60% of the heart rate range. Using the RPE scale is an easy and reliable way to monitor exercise intensity. The RPE scale is underused compared with heart rate when monitoring exercise intensity.

One of the simplest ways to monitor an individual's stress during exercise is the old talk test. During light and comfortable exercise, you should be able to carry on a normal conversation with your exercise partner. If not, you are probably exercising at too high an intensity.

Frequency. Frequency refers to the number of training sessions per week. It is recommended that individuals try to exercise 4 or 5 days per week. The frequency of exercise depends on the type of exercise performed and the fitness status and goals of the individual. For previously sedentary individuals or individuals with a medical or health limitation, the frequency of exercise may be daily, since their ability to exercise at a high intensity or long duration is limited, thereby decreasing the training stimulus.

Duration. Duration refers to the length of the training session. Duration and intensity are inversely related; that is, if the intensity of the exercise is high, the duration is generally low, and vice versa. From 30 to 40 minutes of continuous (aerobic) exercise is recommended per exercise session. Moreover, additional time must be dedicated to flexibility and muscular training. The duration of the exercise session can be affected by environmental factors (e.g., heat, humidity, altitude). It can also be affected by the present fitness level or energy supply of an individual.

Rate of progression. Rate of progression refers to how fast an individual progresses. Rate of progression is directly related to such factors as fatigue and dropout rate; that is, the faster the rate of progression, the greater the fatigue and probability of dropout. The intensity, duration, and frequency should all be gradually increased over time (weeks to months, not days). Rate of progression can be affected by chronic injury or illness. Rate of progression will need to be modified (reduced) if an injury or illness persists. As an individual adapts to training, the rate of progression can be increased.

Cool-down. The purpose of the cool-down period is to allow the body to return gradually to the resting state before exercise (homeostasis). A gradual cool-down period of rhythmic exercise also facilitates return of blood to the heart, thus reducing the risk of venous pooling. The cool-down period basically consists of the same exercises as the warm-up period. The cool-down period should last between 10 and 15 minutes. The same types of activities and stretches can be performed during the cool-down period.

Rest. The amount of rest between workouts is as important as the amount of time spent in workouts. Rest is needed between workouts to replace the energy stores in muscles (glycogen) and to let the overall body systems recover from training. If you push too hard and too long, your body will eventually break down. If exercising at high intensities or long durations, individuals need to be instructed to take at least 1 day off between training sessions. In addition, 1 or 2 minutes of rest is needed between resistance-training exercise sets. Certain training systems recommend that you take as little time as possible between sets to get the most out of your training; however, this technique is not recommended for young or sedentary individuals.

Programs for Muscular Strength and Endurance

The history of strength training probably dates back to the beginning of the Olympic games. It has been said that the great Olympic champion Milo of Crotono, who lived in Greece in the sixth century BC, used to carry around a newborn bull on his shoulders to improve his strength. As the bull grew heavier with age, Milo improved his strength. Since then, strength training has developed into a high-tech, billion dollar business. Strength training has become a popular way to improve athletic ability, look and feel better, relieve stress, and improve health.

Resistance Exercise and Weight Training

Strength can be defined as the ability to exert muscular force against resistance. Strength training is defined as the use of different progressive resistance exercise methods designed to increase muscular strength. Weight training typically uses common forms of equipment, such as free weights or machines, to provide the resistance needed to increase strength. As adaptations occur, more weight is added to provide additional resistance.

Weight training can also be performed by providing resistance in forms other than a weight load. Resistance can also be provided by opposing muscle groups, the individual's body weight, elastic bands or tubing, free weights, or machines. The intended outcome of resistance training is increased muscular strength and endurance. Instead of adding more weight to change the resistance as adaptation occurs, the intensity or duration of exercise is increased. Because resistance training is more comprehensive in scope and because strength or weight training usually assumes that free weights or weight machines are needed, the term *resistance* or *strength training* should be used in preference to weight training when applied to training for health and fitness.

Resistance-Training Programs

There are a variety of strength and weight-training systems. Unfortunately, many of these new and revolutionary programs have not been scientifically proved effective and thus should be viewed with caution. Virtually all strength and weight-training systems are based on a variation of the fundamental principles of strength and weight training (i.e., load, repetition, intensity, rest, and frequency).

Training for General Muscular Strength and Conditioning

A strength and weight-training program for general conditioning should consist of 2 to 3 days of strength training, in addition to cardiovascular conditioning (e.g., running, swimming, cycling) for at least 30 to 40 minutes, 3 days per week. For most people seeking a toned, well-defined body, simple calisthenics or exercises performed with rubber exercise tubing are enough. Unless the goal is to gain a great deal of muscle hypertrophy, the workouts described in the following paragraphs should be effective for toning muscles.

Calisthenic Exercises

Calisthenic exercises are one of the oldest forms of exercise. Such exercises use the weight of the body for the resistance. The resistance can be changed by changing body positions or by performing more repetitions. Calisthenic exercises are convenient because they do not require assistance or equipment. They are generally performed after a brief cardiovascular and stretching warm-up. They can also be performed before or after a cardiovascular workout, on alternating days from aerobic exercise, or in conjunction with other forms of resistance exercises. Examples of calisthenic exercises are provided in Focus Box 30.2.

Rubber-Tubing Exercises

Another safe, inexpensive, and effective way to develop strength is with the use of rubber tubing (see Focus Box 30.3). The rubber tubing provides resistance during the exercise movements. Tubing comes in different lengths and tensions so that young athletes of different ages and abilities can exercise safely and effectively.

Free Weights and Weight Machines

Strength training with weights and weight machines is the most common form of strength training. When an exercise is first performed the correct starting weight must be

FOCUS BOX 30.2

General guidelines for performing calisthenic exercises and examples of calisthenic exercise

Guidelines

1. Always warm up before performing calisthenic exercises.

2. Remember to breathe evenly during the exercises.

3. Perform each exercise slowly, using controlled movements.

4. Support the lower back at all times.

5. Try to perform each exercise through a full range of motion.

6. As with many of the routines described in this chapter, work the larger muscle groups first.

Upper Body Exercises

1. Straight-leg push-up

2. Bent-knee push-up

3. Elevated upper body push-up

4. Lower body push-up

5. Pull-ups

Arm Exercises

1. Upright dips

2. Bench dips

Abdominal Exercises

1. Hanging knee raise

2. Curl-up

3. Supported leg raise

4. Twists

Back Exercises

1. Knee press

2. Back lift

Lower Body Exercises

1. Quadriceps lift

2. Gluteal and hamstring lift

3. Leg abduction

4. Leg adduction

5. Calf raise

6. Lunge

FOCUS BOX 30.3

General guidelines for using exercise bands and tubing

1. Before using any tubing, check for tears, cuts, or abnormal wear and tear points.

2. Perform each exercise as illustrated. Perform the extension on a slow count of one, two and return on three, four.

3. On the return, the rubber tubing should not go completely slack. Always maintain slight tension.

4. The appropriate tension of tubing should allow you to perform a minimum of 10 repetitions.

5. Increase repetitions to 20 before you consider an increase in resistance.

6. For certain large muscle group exercises you may increase the resistance by doubling up the tubing.

7. Always make sure the tubing is centered under the shoe.

8. Most resistance training with rubber tubing is designed for high repetition and moderate resistance. This minimizes the chances of muscle overload, strain, or "snapping back."

9. Be aware that rubber exercise tubing is not a toy.

10. Keep your face turned slightly away from the direction of the exercise movement.

11. Always control the tubing during the return phase of the exercise movement.

12. If unable to complete an exercise for at least 10 repetitions, with correct technique, use a lighter resistance.

13. Always follow the recommendations of the manufacturer.

FOCUS BOX 30.4

General guidelines for training with weights

1. Always use collars on barbells and dumbbells.
2. Never perform one-repetition maximum lifts.
3. Always breathe out during the explosive part of the lift.
4. Always use proper form and technique.
5. Keep all lifting motions slow and controlled. Avoid fast or jerking motions.
6. Keep weights as close to your body as possible.
7. Lift with your knees and keep your back straight when picking up a weight from the ground.
8. Rest between exercises.
9. Lift with individual goals in mind.

established. Although there are a variety of ways to establish the correct starting weight for an exercise, the easiest and safest way is to have an individual perform the exercise for 10 to 12 repetitions. If that weight can be lifted without a great deal of exertion or fatigue, the weight is light enough for a starting weight. This method of establishing the starting weight is referred to as the 10 repetition maximum (10 RM). The starting weight should be changed if chronic fatigue is noticed 1 to 2 days later. Basic guidelines for training with weights are listed in Focus Box 30.4.

Programs for Cardiorespiratory Endurance

Aerobic exercise is defined as any activity that uses large muscle groups, rhythmically, for a continuous period. The most common forms of aerobic exercise are walking, jogging, swimming, and cycling. The selection of exercise mode should be based on the subject's past exercise experience, budget, current fitness level, and desires. One of the easiest programs for health and fitness is walking. Many different forms of exercise are beneficial for health, and it is not possible to cover all of them in detail in this book. Walking is discussed at some length because it is a convenient, safe, and effective form of exercise for health and fitness.

Walking for Fitness

Walking has become one of the most popular forms of aerobic exercise. It has been estimated that more that 77 million Americans walk on a serious basis. Walking is being hailed as perhaps the safest and most effective form of aerobic exercise for anyone, young or old. Medical and fitness experts routinely encourage people to get out and walk as a way to improve their cardiovascular endurance, recover from an injury, prevent heart disease, and lose weight.

Besides the increased publicity of the benefits of exercise, the reasons for the increased popularity of walking have to do with its ease, the ability to walk almost anywhere without the need for special equipment, and the low risk of injury.

FIGURE 30.2

Calculations of oxygen consumption and energy expenditure for different walking speeds, grades, and body weights. (Data are based on the equations of the American College of Sports Medicine.)

Walking speed						
m/min	50	60	70	80	90	100
km/hr	3.0	3.6	4.2	4.8	5.4	6.0
mi/hr	1.9	2.2	2.6	3.0	3.4	3.7
Oxygen consumption (ml/kg/min)						
0% grade	8.5	9.5	10.5	11.5	12.5	13.5
2% grade	10.3	12.1	13.0	14.4	15.7	17.1
4% grade	12.1	13.8	15.5	17.3	19.0	20.7
6% grade	13.9	16.0	18.1	20.1	22.2	24.3
Caloric expenditure (Kcal/min)						
0% grade						
50 kg	2.06	2.30	2.55	2.79	3.03	3.27
70 kg	2.88	3.22	3.56	3.90	4.24	4.58
90 kg	3.71	4.15	4.58	5.02	5.45	5.89
2% grade						
50 kg	2.50	2.93	3.15	3.49	3.81	4.15
70 kg	3.50	4.11	4.41	4.89	5.33	5.80
90 kg	4.50	5.28	5.67	6.29	6.85	7.46
4% grade						
50 kg	2.93	3.35	3.76	4.19	4.61	5.02
70 kg	4.11	4.68	5.26	5.87	6.45	7.03
90 kg	5.28	6.02	6.77	7.55	8.29	9.03
6% grade						
50 kg	3.37	3.88	4.39	4.87	5.38	5.89
70 kg	4.72	5.43	6.14	6.82	7.53	8.25
90 kg	6.07	6.98	7.90	8.77	9.69	10.61

FOCUS BOX 30.5

Beginning, intermediate, and advanced walking training programs

Individuals should complete the following at an intensity that will elicit a suitable training stimulus (that is, 60% to 80% HRR or RPE ≈ 13 to 15).

Week	Warm-up walk (min)	Training pace (min)	Cool-down walk (min)	Total exercise time (min)
Beginning Program				
1	5	7	5	17
2	5	9	5	19
3	5	11	5	21
4	5	13	5	23
5	5	15	5	25
6	5	18	5	28
7	5	20	5	30
8	5	23	5	33
9	5	26	5	36
10	5	28	5	38
12	5	30	5	40
Intermediate Program				
1	5-7	8	5-7	18-20
2	5-7	10	5-7	20-22
3	5-7	12	5-7	22-24
4	5-7	14	5-7	24-26
5	5-7	16	5-7	26-28
6	5-7	19	5-7	29-31
7	5-7	21	5-7	31-33
8	5-7	24	5-7	34-36
9	5-7	27	5-7	37-39
10	5-7	29	5-7	39-41
12	5-7	31	5-7	41-43
Advanced Program				
1	15-10	12	5-10	22-32
2	5-10	14	5-10	24-34
3	5-10	16	5-10	26-36
4	5-10	18	5-10	28-38
5	5-10	20	5-10	30-42

FOCUS BOX 30.5—Cont'd

Beginning, intermediate, and advanced walking training programs

| Week | Advanced Program | | | |
	Warm-up walk (min)	Training pace (min)	Cool-down walk (min)	Total exercise time (min)
6	5-10	23	5-10	33-43
7	5-10	25	5-10	35-45
8	5-10	29	5-10	38-49
9	5-10	32	5-10	41-52
10	5-10	33	5-10	43-53
12	5-10	35	5-7	45-55

From Roberts SO: *Fitness walking*, 1995, Masters Press.

Figure 30.2 lists the average caloric cost of walking for different body weights. Although the caloric cost of walking is relatively low compared with jogging at slow speeds, with brisk walking the movement becomes progressively less economical and the caloric cost approaches that of jogging. Because walking is less intense than jogging or running, longer sessions can be maintained with less likelihood of injury. Normal daily walking is an extremely easy task to perform. However, following some specific recommendation will help the fitness walker get the most benefit.

Sample Walking Programs

Listed in Focus Box 30.5 are three different walking programs. If an individual is currently sedentary, falls into the low to below-average fitness category after completing a fitness test, or has known medical or health limitations, he or she should start with the beginning walking program. If someone is currently somewhat active, falls into an average to above-average fitness category, and does not have or has only mild medical or health limitations, he or she can start with the intermediate program. If an individual is currently active, falls into a high fitness category, and does not have any medical or health limitations, he or she can start with the advanced program.

As individuals improve in fitness, they need to exercise for longer periods and possibly at a faster pace to continue to improve their fitness levels. In addition to the duration of the walking sessions, it is important to consider the frequency, intensity, and rate of progression of exercise. Generally, if an individual has been sedentary for several years, it is advisable to start with the beginning program, frequency, intensity, and

progression rate (i.e., 3 to 4 days per week at 55% to 65% of the maximal rate, progressing in exercise time at a rate of 3% to 5% per week).

Before starting a walking program, or any exercise program for that matter, individuals should remember three important points; (1) the need to be patient (improvement in the fitness level will not happen overnight), (2) improvements in fitness come in small increments (the most rapid improvements happen in the first months), and (3) the need to make small and infrequent increases in the program (i.e., increases in time, duration, frequency, and intensity). If individuals follow these simple guidelines, they will enjoy their walking program and the benefits that come along with it.

Programs for Developing Flexibility

Flexibility is defined as the range of motion (ROM) in a joint or combination of joints (Figure 30.3). Flexibility training is an important part of a balanced fitness program but is often overlooked even by experienced athletes. Flexibility training is often viewed as being unnecessary and time consuming. Although scientific evidence demonstrating the benefits of flexibility training is limited, most medical experts agree that such training is important for optimal health and peak athletic performance.

Flexibility training is used in athletics to improve performance and reduce the possibility of injury and in sports medicine fields (physical therapy) as a component of injury treatment and rehabilitation. It is well known that a decrease in flexibility is inevitable with age and physical inactivity. One

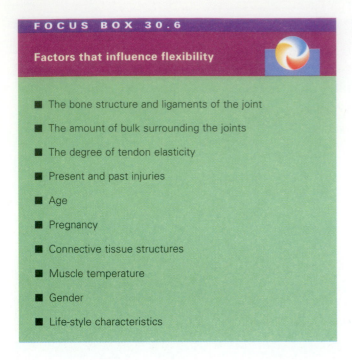

FOCUS BOX 30.6

Factors that influence flexibility

- The bone structure and ligaments of the joint
- The amount of bulk surrounding the joints
- The degree of tendon elasticity
- Present and past injuries
- Age
- Pregnancy
- Connective tissue structures
- Muscle temperature
- Gender
- Life-style characteristics

of the most common ailments for adults is chronic low-back pain, which is due primarily to a decrease in flexibility, along with inadequate strength. Some sports require movement patterns that demand a great deal of flexibility, for example, the butterfly stroke in swimming. The importance of superior flexibility in sports, such as basketball or football, is debatable. Regardless, adequate flexibility should help to reduce muscle tension, improve posture and coordination, reduce body stiffness, possibly reduce injury, and enhance athletic performance.

Factors Influencing Flexibility

A variety of factors influence flexibility (Focus Box 30.6). The bone structure and ligaments of the joint as well as the bulk surrounding the joints, affect flexibility. The elbow and knee joints limit ROM because of their structure, whereas the ankle and hip joints limit ROM because of connective tissue.

The type and location of connective tissue can limit the degree of flexibility. Although muscles are generally quite elastic, connective tissue is rather nonelastic. If connective tissue has recently been torn or injured, elasticity is further reduced. As we get older, the degree of flexibility is reduced. During pregnancy the hormone relaxin causes the elastic properties of ligaments and connective tissues to increase. Muscle temperature increases flexibility. Women generally have greater flexibility than men.

Benefits and Risks of Stretching

The potential benefits of stretching include increased performance, increased joint stability, increased joint range of motion, enhanced warm-up results, injury prevention and

increased recovery time. An average improvement in joint mobility after flexibility training is approximately 5% to 20%, and data have shown that adding flexibility to a training program can reduce injuries by as much as 75% for such sports as soccer, American football, and tennis.

Some risks are associated with stretching. Attention has recently been focused on the timing of stretching. Current theory suggests that stretching be performed after a brief warm-up period. The logic behind such practice is based on the fact that preliminary movement raises the temperature of connective tissue and collagen becomes softer and thus more elastic when heated. The potential for injury may be increased if stretching is performed before an active warm-up. The risk of injury from stretching is greatest when it is performed by poorly conditioned individuals or those with a preexisting injury, and when stretches are performed with poor technique.

Methods of Stretching

There are three forms of flexibility training—static, ballistic, and proprioceptive neuromuscular facilitation (PNF). **Static stretching** is the most common form of stretching and probably the oldest, dating back some 2000 years. With static stretching a muscle or group of muscles are slowly stretched and held for 8 to 12 seconds. During the period when the stretch is held, the muscle spindle is at rest and the stretch reflex is gradually diminished.

Static stretching is perhaps the safest and most effective form of stretching. Static stretching exercise should be performed after a mild warm-up period to increase the temperature of the muscles and connective tissue. The static stretch should be held for about 8 to 12 seconds. During the performance of a static stretch, the position should always be held just below the threshold for pain. Static stretching causes gradual inhibition of the muscle spindle activation, which allows greater long-term maintenance of ROM.

FIGURE 30.3

Static stretching.

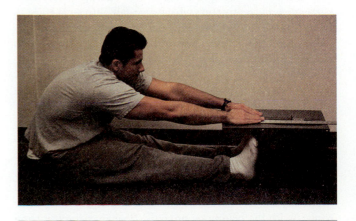

FOCUS BOX 30.7

General flexibility exercises

Exercise: Low-back stretch
In this stretch the individual lies on the back and pulls both knees into the torso until a sufficient stretch is achieved in the low back.

Exercise: Supine hamstring stretch
The individual lies on the back on the floor and pulls one leg up to a stretched position. The leg should remain as straight as possible. The opposite leg is bent with the heel on the floor. Alternate legs.

Exercise: Modified hurdler's stretch
Here the individual sits on the floor with one leg extended and the other leg bent and turned outward (heel against the thigh of the straight leg). The individual bends forward at the waist (leaning toward the straight leg) until a stretch is achieved and then holds this position for the required count. Alternate legs.

Exercise: Standing quadriceps stretch
The individual is standing (and may be supported by another person or an object) and grasps a leg by the ankle with the opposite arm. The leg is pulled to a stretched position, taking care not to allow the knee to drift away from the side of the adjoining leg. Alternate legs.

Exercise: Triceps stretch
The individual takes the opposite elbow and pulls the arm behind the head and down until a stretch is felt in the back of the arm. Hold for the desired time and repeat for the other arm as well.

Exercise: Shoulder and chest stretch
The individual places one arm parallel to the floor and back behind the torso. The individual may hold onto a wall, partner, or whatever is available. To further improve the effectiveness of this stretch, the individual may turn away from the side being stretched until the stretch is felt in the shoulder and lateral chest region. Alternate sides.

Exercise: Rotator cuff stretch
For this stretch to be effective the individual should grasp the elbow of the opposite arm (keeping it bent at a 90-degree angle) and pull it across the chest until the stretch is felt. Alternate arms.

Exercise: Achilles tendon and calf stretch
The individual should face the wall and place both palms on the wall. Then one foot should have the toes elevated against the wall, with the heel on the floor, until a sufficient stretch is accomplished. Alternate legs.

Proprioceptive neuromuscular facilitation (PNF) stretching uses a contract-stretch format in which a muscle is contracted for 4 to 6 seconds, followed by an immediate 8- to 12 second static stretch. The one drawback to PNF is that it requires a partner. The steps involved in PNF are as follows: (1) the muscle group is in the elongated position, (2) the muscle group is isometrically contracted and held for 6 to 10 seconds, and (3) the contracted muscles are then relaxed, immediately followed by a concentric contraction of the opposing group.

The PNF technique is based on reciprocal inhibition. When a muscle is contracted, the antagonist, or opposing, muscle is relaxing. This is a natural prerequisite for movement in a joint. In PNF stretching the agonist muscle is first contracted, followed by static stretching of the antagonist muscle. It is believed that by first contracting the agonist muscle, reflex contraction will be suppressed during the static stretching of antagonist muscle and allow a greater stretching capacity. The experimental evidence demonstrating the effectiveness of PNF over other methods of stretching is lacking.

Ballistic stretching is the least effective and most dangerous form of stretching because it uses high-force, quick movements to stretch the muscle or muscle group. Ballistic stretching is best described as a bouncing motion that may or may not be held for a brief period. The bouncing motion

causes activation of the muscle spindles, which are protective organs in the muscle. When muscle spindles are activated, muscles reflexively contract. If the main point of stretching is to cause the muscle to stretch, thereby stretching the connective tissue, ballistic stretching is inappropriate and may even cause tighter muscles and injury to the connective tissue. Examples of flexibility exercises are presented in Focus Box 30.7.

static stretching
when a muscle or group of muscles are slowly stretched and held for a short period (usually 8 to 12 seconds).

proprioceptive neuromuscular facilitation (PNF)
a type of stretching routine in which a muscle is contracted for 4 to 6 seconds, followed by an immediate 8- to 12-second static stretch.

ballistic stretching
the least effective and most dangerous form of stretching because it uses high-force, quick movements to stretch the muscle or muscle groups. Ballistic stretching is best described as a bouncing motion that induces a stretch that may or may not be held for a brief period.

Body Composition

*W*hat is the most effective exercise for losing or maintaining weight and increasing muscle mass? Unfortunately, there is no one or even best exercise to affect body composition. Obviously aerobic exercise is good because it expends additional calories and raises basal metabolic rate. Some form of resistance training is also good because it builds lean body mass, which helps expend calories at a higher rate and replaces the fat lost with muscle mass. A sensible exercise program of stretching, aerobic exercise, flexibility, and resistance training is the best overall exercise plan for modifying body composition. Exercise helps establish a negative caloric balance, essential to weight loss and weight maintenance.

SUMMARY

- Despite the mounting evidence of the benefits of regular exercise, only 22% of adults engage in leisure-time activities at or above the level recommended for health benefits in the United States Public Health Service's health and disease prevention goals and objectives for the nation. Instead of defining physical fitness in terms of athletic abilities (e.g., speed, power, balance), **health-related fitness** defines an individual's fitness status based on cardiorespiratory fitness, muscular strength, muscular endurance, flexibility, and body composition.

- Every adult should accumulate 30 minutes or more of moderate-intensity physical activity over the course of most days of the week. An exercise program is based on five key principles: screening, warm-up, exercise, cool-down, and rest.

- The purpose of the health appraisal is to establish the current health status of an individual and provide fitness professionals with baseline information that will be used to design an exercise program. An individual's **medical history** is an important component of the health screening. Baseline data collected from fitness tests can be used to plan safe, effective exercise; motivate a client; and change or modify an exercise program.

- Exercise intensity is best determined by measuring oxygen consumption, but indirect methods are by heart rate, breathing rate, or a **rating of perceived exertion.** To determine a training heart rate range, an individual's maximal heart rate (HR_{max}) must first be determined or estimated from $220 -$ age. Low-intensity exercise would be equal or 50% to 60% of an individual's maximal heart rate, whereas 85% to 90% would relate to high-intensity exercise. A range of heart rates during training can also be estimated by taking a percentage of an individual's heart rate reserve (HRR) using the Karvonen method.

- Three forms of flexibility training exist: **static, ballistic,** and **proprioceptive neuromuscular facilitation (PNF).** The potential benefits of stretching include increased performance, increased joint stability, increased joint range of motion, enhanced warm-up, injury prevention, and decreased recovery time.

REVIEW QUESTIONS

1. Why is there a distinction between health-related fitness and sports fitness?

2. How much exercise does an individual need to perform for health benefits?

3. What are some potential problems with the low amount of exercise required for health benefits?

4. Why is walking becoming a popular mode of exercise?

APPLICATIONS

1. List some patient populations that should benefit from multiple short-duration bouts of physical activity during the course of a day.

2. Explain why exercise would help these individuals.

Case Study

Joan is a 35-year-old executive who wants to start an exercise program to reduce stress and maintain good health. She has no risk factors for heart disease and has been quite active all her life. She likes to bike and swim and has about 1 hour, four times a week to exercise.

Mode—Swimming and cycling. Joan should also be encouraged to spend some additional time performing flexibility and weight-training exercises.

Intensity—Joan's maximal heart rate (MHR) is $220 - 35 = 185$. Since Joan has not been exercising recently, she should start out at a relatively low level, approximately 60% to 70% of her MHR. Joan's training heart rate (THR) is 111 to 130 beats per minute. Joan should be instructed to take her pulse several times during her initial training sessions to make sure she is within her training heart rate zone.

Frequency—Joan should exercise at least four times to five times per week. She may want to alternate days of swimming and cycling.

Duration—Joan should start out cycling and swimming for 25 to 30 minutes. Total exercise duration should be gradually increased to 30 to 60 minutes.

Rate of Progression—If she feels excessively fatigued initially, she should cut back on the intensity, duration, or frequency of her exercise program. With training, she will notice that she will be able to cover more miles on her bike and yards in the pool in less time, at which point she will need to modify her training program.

REFERENCES

1. American College of Sports Medicine: *Guidelines for exercise testing and prescription,* ed 5, Philadelphia, 1995, Williams & Wilkins.

2. Anspaugh DJ, Hamrick MH, Rosato FD: *Concepts and applications wellness,* St. Louis, 1994, Mosby.

3. Borg GAV: Psychophysical bases of perceived exertion, *Med Sci Sports Exerc* 14:377-381, 1982.

4. Roberts SO: Special populations and health concerns. In Cotton RT, editor: *Aerobics instructor manual,* San Diego, 1993, American Council on Exercise.

5. Shephard RJ, Thomas S, Weller I: The Canadian home fitness test: 1991 update, *Sports Med* 11:358, 1991.

6. American College of Sports Medicine: Summary statement—workshop on physical activity and public health, *Sports Med Bull* 28(4):7, 1993.

7. US Department of Health and Human Services: *Healthy people 2000—National health promotion and disease prevention objectives,* DHHS Publication No (PHS) 91-50212, 1991, US Government Printing Office, Washington, DC, 20402.

8. Roberts SO: *Fitness walking,* Indianapolis, 1995, Masters Press.

RECOMMENDED READINGS

▪ American College of Sports Medicine: *Guidelines for exercise testing and prescription,* ed 5, Philadelphia, 1995, Williams & Wilkins.

▪ US Department of Health and Human Services: *Healthy people 2000—national health promotion and disease prevention objectives,* DHHS Publication No (PHS) 91-50212, US Government Printing Office, Washington, DC, 20402.

Appendix A
Conversion Charts

In 1977 the World Health Organization recommended the world-wide adoption of the Systeme International d'Unites (SI units). This recommendation occurred amidst the use of different units for similar measurements in the medical and applied science communities around the world.

The adoption of different scientific units has a history that dates back to the 19th century. In 1800 the meter was officially introduced in France as a measure of length. At that time, the definition of a meter was the ten-millionth part of the earth's quadrant.[1] The units of the meter simply differed from each other by a factor of ten. At the same time, the weight of 1 cubic decimeter of water was accepted as a unit of weight called the kilogram.

The other common unit of length, the inch, was based on the size of three grains of dry round barley. The inch unit was historically favored in England by Royal decree, and the larger units of length (foot, yard, furlong, rod) were derived from the inch, with an area of 40 x 4 rods being named an acre. The English units for weight were also based on agriculture. The penney stirling weighed 32 grains of wheat, which was termed a pence. Twenty pence was termed an ounze, and 12 ounzes was termed one pound. An 8 pound volume of wine was termed a gallon, which could be divided into 8 pints and 4 quarts.

The English units of measure were introduced to North America by the early colonists, and were legislated by Congress in 1838. In 1860 North America legalized use of the meter system. In 1875 the meter and kilogram were proposed as established international units of measure, and the International Bureau of Weights and Measures (BIPM) was founded. The BIPM reported recommendations of units changes at the General Conference of Weights and Measures (CGPM).

In 1954 the 10th CGPM decided to introduce a system of six units, from which all other units could be derived. This system was named the Systeme International d'Unites (abbreviated SI). A seventh unit, the mole was added in 1971, and these units are presented in Table A.1. Tables A.2 through A.5 provide additional detailed conversion charts for various units of measure routinely used in exercise science and research.

TABLE A.1

The units of the International System of Units

QUANTITY	BASIC UNIT	SYMBOL
Length	meter*	m
Mass	kilogram	kg
Time	second	s
Electric current	ampere	A
Thermodynamic temperature	kelvin	K
Luminous intensity	candela	cd
Amount of substance	mole	mol

*American spelling. European spelling is metre.

Recommended rules for the use of measurement symbols are:

1.) Symbols should be written without a period (full stop; ".").
2.) Symbols that are not named after persons should be written in small letter (e.g., m for meter and W for Watt).
3.) For differing units that have the same name, unique symbols must be used (e.g., time minute [min] vs angle minute [']).

The adoption of the SI units of measurement enables scientific and medical communities to standardize test methods and units for reporting results, and to decrease errors associated with the need for conversion. In countries such as Germany, Australia, Canada, and India, the SI unit has been recommended by national legislation. In the United States, limited consensus has evolved over the use of the SI units, even though Congress passed the Metric Conversion Act in 1975, which endorsed the SI units of measurement.[2]

In the United States, the formation of the American National Metric Council (ANMC) has occurred to coordinate the conversion to SI units or measurement. The ANMC established the Medical and Health Coordinating Group to aid the reporting of clinical laboratory data in SI units during the 1980s.

TABLE A.2

Units pertinent to Exercise Science, recommended by the International Union of Pure and Applied Chemistry and the International Federation of Clinical Chemistry

QUANTITY	SYMBOL	UNIT	UNIT SYMBOL	NOT RECOMMENDED UNITS
Length	l	meter	m	cm, u, A
Area	A	square meter	m^2	cm^2, u^2
Volume	V	cubic meter	m^3	cc, u^3
Mass	m	kilogram	kg	kg/gr
Number	N	one	1	all other factors
Amount of substance	n	mole	mol	M, eq, mM, nM, µM
Mass concentration		kilogram per liter	kg/l	mg/dl, g/ml, g%, ppm
Substance concentration	c	mole per liter	mol/l	M, mM, meq/l
Molality	m	mole per kilogram	mol/kg	m, mol/g
Number concentration	C	reciprocal liter	l^1	ml^1
Thermodynamic temperature	T	kelvin	K	°K
Celsius temperature		degree Celsius	°C	C, °, C°
Pressure	p	pascal	$Pa = N/m^2$	atm, bar, mm Hg, torr
Time	t	second	s	min, m, sec, yr
Density	d	kilogram per liter	kg/l	g/ml, mg/ml

TABLE A.3

SI derived units with special names pertinent to Exercise Sciences

QUANTITY	SI UNIT		
	NAME	SYMBOL	EXPRESSION BY OTHER UNITS
Frequency	hertz	Hz	s^{-1}
Force	newton	N	$kg/m/s^2$
Pressure, stress	pascal	Pa	N/m^2
Energy, work, heat	joule	J	N/m
Power, radiant flux	watt	W	J/s
Electricity, electric charge	coulomb	C	A/s
Electric potential, difference, electromotive force	volt	V	W/A
Capacitance	farad	F	C/V
Electric resistance	ohm		V/A
Conductance	siemens	S	A/V
Surface tension	newton per meter	N/m	—
Specific energy	Joule per kilogram	J/kg	—
Enzyme catalytic activity	katal	kat	mol/s

TABLE A.4

Conversion factors for the different units of work, power, force, pressure, mass, length, volume, temperature, frequency, and ph*

WORK	Kjoule	Kcal	ft lb	kgm		
1 kilojoule	1.0	0.2388	737	1786.9		
1 Kcal	4.1868	1.0	3086	426.8		
1 ft lb	0.000077	0.000324	1.0	0.1383		
1 kgm	0.009797	0.002345	7.23	1.0		

POWER	Horsepower	kgm/min^{-1}	ft lb/min^{-1}	Watt	Kcal/min^{-1}	Kj/min^{-1}
1 Horsepower	1.0	4,564.0	33,000.0	745.7	10.694	44.743
1 kgm/min^{-1}	0.000219	1.0	7.233	0.16345	0.00234	0.0098068
1 ft lb/min^{-1}	0.00003	0.1383	1.0	0.0226	0.000324	0.0013562
1 Watt	0.001314	6.118	44.236	1.0	0.014335	0.060
1 Kcal/min^{-1}	0.0936	426.78	3086.0	69.697	1.0	4.186
1 Kj/min^{-1}	0.02235	101.97	737.30	16.667	0.2389	1.0

FORCE	lb	kg	N
1 lb	1.0	0.4545	0.04635
1 kilogram (kg)	2.2	1.0	0.10197
1 Newton (N)	19.614	9.807	1.0

PRESSURE	mm Hg	kPa	Torr	mBar
1 mm Hg	1.0	0.1333	1.0	0.7502
1 kPa	7.501	1.0	7.501	5.6272
1 Torr	1.0	0.1333	1.0	0.7502
1 mBar	1.333	0.1777	1.333	1.0

*For the following conversion tables, the conversion factors represent how many units listed down the page equals the units listed across the page. For example, 1 Kjoule equals 0.2388 Kcal and 0.0056 kgm.

T A B L E A . 4 — Cont'd

Conversion factors for the different units of work, power, force, pressure, mass, length, volume, temperature, frequency, and ph*

MASS	ounce	gram	pound	kilogram
ounce	1.0	28.35	0.0625	0.028
gram	0.0353	1.0	0.0022	0.001
pound	16.129	454	1.0	0.454
kg	35.714	1000	2.2	1.0

LENGTH	inch	cm	m m	feet	yard	meter	mile	km
inch	1.0	2.54	25.4	0.0833	0.0278	0.0254	63,360	39,283
cm	0.3937	1.0	10	0.0324	14.1732	100	1,610	100,000
mm	0.03937	0.1	1.0	0.4724	0.01312	0.001	6.21×10^{-7}	1.0×10^{-6}
feet	12	30.48	304.8	1.0	0.3333	0.304	1.894×10^{-4}	0.000394
yard	0.02778	91.44	914.4	3	1.0	0.912	1760	1093.17
meter	0.0254	100	1000	3.2895	1.0936	1.0	6.214×10^{-4}	0.001
mile	15840	40233.68	1.6094×10^{6}	5280	1760	1610	1.0	1.61
km	2.546×10^{-5}	0.0001	0.00001	0.0003055	0.000916	0.001	0.62112	1.0

VOLUME	fluid ounce	teaspoon	tablespoon	cup	ml	pint	liter	quart	gallon
fluid ounce	1.0	6	2	0.125	29.575	0.0625	33.8123	0.03125	0.007812
teaspoon	0.1667	1.0	0.3333	0.0208	4.97	0.01042	0.005	0.0052	0.0013
tablespoon	0.5	3	1.0	0.0625	14.8	0.03125	0.0149	0.0156	0.0039
cup	8	48	16	1.0	236.6	0.5	0.2366	0.25	0.0625
ml	0.0338	0.2012	0.0676	0.00423	1.0	0.0021	0.001	0.00106	2.64×10^{-4}
pint	16	96	32	2	473.2	1.0	0.473	0.5	0.125
liter	33.6	201.6	67.2	4.2265	1000	2.1	1.0	0.961	0.246
quart	32	192	64	4	946.4	2	1.057	1.0	0.25
gallon	128	768	256	16	3785.6	8	4.065	4	1.0

TABLE A.4—Cont'd

Conversion factors for the different units of work, power, force, pressure, mass, length, volume, temperature, frequency, and ph*

TEMPERATURE	°F	°C	°K
Farenheit (°F)	1.0	(°F-32) x 0.5556	—
Celsius (°C)	(°C x 1.8) +32	1.0	—
Kelvin (°K)	273 °K = 32 °F	273 °K = 0 °C	1.0

FREQUENCY	Hz	1/min	
Hertz (Hz)	1.0	60	
1/min	0.01667	1.0	

PH	PH	[H+]	
pH	1.0	10^{-pH}	
[H+] (mol/l)	$-(\log_{10})$	1.0	

Adapted from Lippert H, Lehmann HP: *SI units in medicine: an introduction to the international system of units with conversion tables and normal ranges*, Baltimore, 1978, Urban & Schwarzenburg; and Young DS: *Annal Intern Med* 106: 114-120, 1987.

The application of the SI system has some difficulties for reporting clinical laboratory data, as is the case in exercise physiology related research. For example, hematologic measurements such as hemoglobin concentration have been reported as gm/dl (or gm%), but according to the SI system should be reported as mmol/L. Because there are several forms of hemoglobin (monomer–HbFe, or tetramer $Hb(Fe_4)$, reporting a concentration based on a molar amount is difficult, and the recommended unit by the Medical and Health Coordinating Group is g/L. The units and conversions to SI for clinical measurements pertinent to exercise physiology research are presented in Table A.5.

TABLE A.5

Conversion factors between non-SI and SI recommended units for measurements routinely performed in exercise and health-related research

MEASUREMENT	PRESENT UNIT	NORMAL RANGE	CONVERSION FACTOR	SI UNIT	SI NORMAL RANGE
HEMATOLOGY					
erythrocyte count (B)					
female	$10^6/mm^3$	3.5-5.0	1	$10^{12}/L$	3.5-5.0
male	$10^6/mm^3$	4.3-5.9	1	$10^{12}/L$	4.3-5.9
hematocrit (B)					
female	%	33-43	0.01	1	0.33-0.43
male	%	39-49	0.01	1	0.39-0.49
hemoglobin mass concentration (B)					
female	g/dL	12.0-15.0	10	gm/L	120-150
male	g/dL	13.6-17.2	10	gm/L	136-172
leukocyte count (B)	mm^3	3200-9800	0.001	$10^9/L$	3.2-9.8
mean corpuscular hemoglobin (MCH) mass	pg	27-33	1	pg	27-33
mean corpuscular volume (MCV)	μm^3	76-100	1	fL	76-100
platelet count (B)	$10^3/mm^3$	130-400	1	$10^9/L$	130-400
reticulocyte count (adults) (B)					
number	mm^3	10,000-75,000	0.001	$10^9/L$	10-75
fraction	0/00	1-24	0.001	1	0.001-0.024
per 1000 erythrocytes	%	0.1-2.4	0.001	1	0.001-0.024
Metabolites/Proteins/Lipoproteins					
acetoacetate (S)	mg/dL	0.3-3.0	97.75	$\mu mol/L$	30-300
albumin (S)	g/dL	4.0-6.0	10.0	g/L	40-60
bilirubin (S)					
total	mg/dL	0.1-1.0	17.10	$\mu mol/L$	2-18
conjugated	mg/dL	0-0.2	17.10	$\mu mol/L$	0-4

TABLE A.5—Cont'd

Conversion factors between non-SI and SI recommended units for measurements routinely performed in exercise and health-related research

MEASUREMENT	PRESENT UNIT	NORMAL RANGE	CONVERSION FACTOR	SI UNIT	SI NORMAL RANGE
cholesterol (P)					
<29 years	mg/dL	<200	0.02586	mmol/L	<5.2
30-39 years	mg/dL	<225	0.02586	mmol/L	<5.85
40-49 years	mg/dL	<245	0.02586	mmol/L	<6.35
>50 years	mg/dL	<265	0.02586	mmol/L	<6.85
citrate (B)	mg/dL	1.2-3.0	52.05	µmol/L	60-160
creatine (S)					
female	mg/dL	0.35-0.93	76.25	µmol/L	30-70
male	mg/dL	0.17-0.50	76.25	µmol/L	10-40
creatine (U)					
female	mg/24 h	0-80	7.625	µmol/d	0-600
male	mg/24 h	0-40	7.625	µmol/d	0-300
creatinine (S)	mg/dL	0.6-1.2	88.40	µmol/L	50-110
creatinine (U)	g/24 h	variable	8.840	mmol/day	variable
free fatty acids (P)	mg/dL	8-20	10.0	80-200	mg/L
ferritin (S)	ng/mL	18-300	1	µg/L	18-300
fibrinogen (P)	mg/dL	200-400	0.01	g/L	2.0-4.0
fructose (P)	mg/dL	<10	0.05551	mmol/L	<0.6
glucose (P)	mg/dL	70-110	0.05551	mmol/L	2.8-4.4
glycerol, free (S)	mg/dL	<1.5	0.1086	mmol/L	<0.16
beta-hydroxybutarate (S)	mg/dL	<1.0	96.05	µmol/L	<100
iron (S)					
female	µg/dL	60-160	0.1791	µmol/L	11-29
male	µg/dL	80-180	0.1791	µmol/L	14-32
iron binding capacity (S)	µg/dL	250-460	0.1791	µmol/L	45-82
lactate (P) rest	mEq/L	0.5-2.0	1.0	mmol/L	0.5-2.0
	mg/dL	5-20	0.1110	mmol/L	0.5-2.0
lipoproteins (as cholesterol) (P)					
low density (LDL) or					
high density (HDL)	mg/dL	50-190	0.02586	mmol/L	1.3-4.9
protein-Total (S)	g/dL	6-8	10	g/L	60-80
pyruvate (B)	mg/dL	0.30-0.90	113.6	µmol/L	35-100

TABLE A.5—Cont'd

Conversion factors between non-SI and SI recommended units for measurements routinely performed in exercise and health-related research

MEASUREMENT	PRESENT UNIT	NORMAL RANGE	CONVERSION FACTOR	SI UNIT	SI NORMAL RANGE
lipoproteins (as cholesterol) (P) —Cont'd					
uric acid (S)	mg/dL	2.0-7.0	59.48	µmol/L	120-420
Urea nitrogen (S)	mg/dL	8-18	0.3570	mmol/L	3.0-6.5
ELECTROLYTES					
calcium (S)					
female <50	mg/dL	8.8-10.0	0.2495	mmol/L	2.20-2.50
female >50	mg/dL	8.8-10.2	0.2495	mmol/L	2.20-2.56
male	mg/dL	8.8-10.3	0.2495	mmol/L	2.20-2.58
chloride (S)	mEq/L	95-105	1	mmol/L	95-105
magnesium (S)	mEq/L	1.6-2.4	0.5	mmol/L	0.8-1.2
osmolality (P)	mOsm/kg	280-300	1	mmol/kg	280-300
osmolality (U)	mOsm/kg	50-1200	1	mmol/kg	50-1200
phosphate (S)	mg/dL	2.5-5.0	0.3229	mmol/L	0.8-1.60
potassium (S)	mEq/L	3.5-5.0	0.2558	mmol/L	3.5-5.0
sodium (S)	mEq/L	135-147	1	mmol/L	135-147
BLOOD GASES/ACID BASE					
carbon dioxide					
content (B, P, S)					
(bicarbonate + CO2)	mEq/L	22-28	1	mmol/L	22-28
partial pressure	mm Hg	33-44	0.1333	kPa	4.4-5.9
carbon monoxide (B)					
proportion COHb	%	<15	0.01	1	<0.15
oxygen					
partial pressure	mm Hg	75-105	0.1333	kPa	10.0-14.0
ENZYMES					
aldolase (S)	U/L	0-6	16.67	nkat/L	0-100
creatine kinase (CK) (S)	U/L	0-130	0.01667	µkat/L	0-2.16
lactate dehydrogenase (LDH) (S)	U/L	50-150	0.01667	µkat/L	0.82-2.66
HORMONES					
adrenocorticotrophin (P)					
(ACTH)	pg/mL	20-100	0.2202	pmol/L	4-22
aldosterone (S)	ng/dL	8.1-15.5	27.74	pmol/L	220-430

TABLE A.5—Cont'd

Conversion factors between non-SI and SI recommended units for measurements routinely performed in exercise and health-related research

MEASUREMENT	PRESENT UNIT	NORMAL RANGE	CONVERSION FACTOR	SI UNIT	SI NORMAL RANGE
adrenocorticotrophin (P)—Cont'd					
androstenedione (S)					
female (>18 years)	μg/L	0.8-3.0	3.492	nmol/L	3.0-10.5
male (>18 years)	μg/L	0.2-3.0	3.492	nmol/L	0.5-10.5
calcitonin (S)	pg/mL	<100	1	ng/L	<100
epinephrine (P)					
after 15 min rest	pg/mL	31-95	5.458	pmol/L	170-520
estradiol (S)					
male >18 years	pg/mL	15-40	3.671	pmol/L	55-150
estriol (U) female-nonpregnant					
menstruation	μg/24 h	4-25	3.468	nmol/d	15-85
ovulation peak	μg/24 h	28-99	3.468	nmol/d	95-345
luteal peak	μg/24 h	22-105	3.468	nmol/d	75-365
menopausal	μg/24 h	1.4-19.6	3.468	nmol/d	5-70
estriol (U) male	μg/24 h	5-18	3.468	nmol/d	15-60
estrogens (S)					
female	pg/mL	20-300	3.671	pmol/L	
female peak	pg/mL	200-800	3.671	pmol/L	
male	pg/mL	<50	3.671	pmol/L	
follicle stimulating hormone (FSH) (U)					
female					
follicular phase	IU/24 h	2-15	1.0	IU/d	2-15
midcycle	IU/24 h	8-40	1.0	IU/d	8-40
luteal phase	IU/24 h	2-10	1.0	IU/d	2-10
menopause	IU/24 h	35-100	1.0	IU/d	35-100
male	IU/24 h	2-15	1.0	IU/d	2-15
glucagon (S)	pg/mL	50-100	1	ng/L	50-100
growth hormone (fasting) (P,S)					
female	ng/mL	0-10.0	1	μg/L	0-10.0
male	ng/mL	0-5.0	1	μg/L	0-5.0

TABLE A.5—Cont'd

Conversion factors between non-SI and SI recommended units for measurements routinely performed in exercise and health-related research

MEASUREMENT	PRESENT UNIT	NORMAL RANGE	CONVERSION FACTOR	SI UNIT	SI NORMAL RANGE
leutinizing hormone (S)					
female	mIU/mL	2-20	1	IU/L	2-20
female peak	mIU/L	30-140	1	IU/L	30-140
male	mIU/L	3-25	1	IU/L	3-25
norepinephrine (P)					
at rest	pg/mL	15-475	0.005911	nmol/L	1.27-2.81
norepinephrine (U)	µg/24 h	<100	5.911	nmol/d	<590
progesterone (P)					
follicular phase	ng/mL	<2	3.180	nmol/L	<6
luteal phase	ng/mL	2-20	3.180	nmol/L	6-64
prolactin (P)	ng/mL	<20	1	µg/L	<20
renin (P)	ng/mL/h	1.1-4.1	0.2778	ng/(L•s)	0.30-1.14
testosterone (P)					
female	ng/mL	0.6	3.467	nmol/L	2.0
male	ng/mL	4.6-8.0	3.467	nmol/L	14.0-28.0
TSH (S)	µU/mL	2-11	1	mU/L	2-11
thyroxine (T4) (S)	µg/gL	4-11	12.87	nmol/L	51-142
triiodothyronine (T3)	ng/dL	75-220	0.01536	nmol/L	1.2-3.4

Adapted from Young DS; *Annal Intern Med* 106:114-120, 1987.
B, Whole blood; *P*, plasma; *S*, serum.

REFERENCES

1. Lippert H, Lehmann HP: *SI units in medicine: An introduction to the international system of units with conversion tables and normal ranges,* Baltimore, 1978, Urban & Schwarzenberg.

2. Young DS: Implementation of SI units for clinical laboratory data. Style specifications and conversion tables, *Annal Intern Med* 106:114–120, 1987.

Appendix B
Gas Laws and Indirect Calorimetry

This appendix presents the gas laws and equations necessary for converting gas volumes to standard conditions, provides a summary of the equations of indirect calorimetry, and presents example data from which to calculate ventilation volumes, oxygen consumption, carbon dioxide production, the respiratory exchange ratio, and caloric expenditure.

In biologic systems, like the human body, other animals, and plants, knowledge of the volume of gas production or consumption is essential for a thorough understanding of physiology. Consequently, it is important to understand the factors that can affect gas volumes, other than metabolic production and consumption, and to account for them in calculations of volumes.

The conditions known to affect a given gas volume are temperature, pressure, and water vapor. Each of these conditions can change from day to day, and from one geographic location to another. To solve for these fluctuations, gas volumes are converted to standard temperature, pressure, and water vapor conditions. The different gas volume conditions are summarized below:

Standard Temperature and Pressure Dry (STPD)

Temperature = 273°K (0°C); Pressure = 760 mm Hg;
Water Vapor = 0 mm Hg

Atmospheric Temperature and Pressure Saturated (ATPS)

Temperature = measured °K; Pressure = measured mm Hg;
Water Vapor = measured mm Hg (at measured temperature)

Body Temperature and Pressure Saturated (BTPS)

Temperature = 310°K (=37°C); Pressure = measured mm Hg;
Water Vapor = 47 mm Hg (at body temperature of 37°C)

Generally, gas volumes are measured under ATPS conditions and the main conversion of interest is that from ATPS to STPD. However, in pulmonary function and lung volume measurements, it is of interest to know these volumes under BTPS conditions, and the conversion from ATPS to BTPS is necessary.

Gas Laws

To be able to complete these conversions, knowledge of the laws that govern changes in gas volumes for given changes in pressure and temperature is necessary.

Temperature

Gas volumes change in direct proportion to changes in temperature. An increase in temperature of a given gas volume will increase the volume of that gas. This relationship is known as Charle's Law.

$$T \propto V$$

Charle's Law exists because the kinetic motion of a given number of gas molecules is influenced by temperature. An increased temperature causes an increased motion, which expands the gas volume, and vice versa. If a given volume of gas is exposed in a finite volume, and the temperature of the gas increases, the pressure of the gas increases. It is for this reason that gas tanks should not be left in the sun!

Charle's Law can be applied to calculating the volume of a gas that has undergone a change in temperature. For example, the change in gas temperature from T_1 to T_2 will cause a proportionate change in gas volume from V_1 to V_2. These changes can be mathematically represented by the following equation.

B.1
$$T_1/T_2 = V_1/V_2$$

B.2
$$V_2 = T_2 V_1/T_1$$

B.3
$$V_2 = V_1(T_2/T_1)$$

To convert expired minute ventilation (V_E) from ATPS to STPD for temperature;

B.4
$$V_{ESTPD} = V_{EATPS} * [273/(273 + T_{room})]$$

The common unit for gas volumes is liters per minute ($L \cdot min^{-1}$).

Equation 4 reveals that unless the absolute measured temperature is less than 273°K (less than freezing), the correction factor will be less than one, thus lowering the measured gas volume. In a typical exercise physiology laboratory, the correction of gas volumes to standard temperature conditions will always produce a correction factor less than one, and lower the gas volume.

Pressure

The gas law governing the relationship between gas volume and pressure is called Boyle's Law. Gas volumes are inversely proportional to pressure. Thus an increase in pressure will decrease the volume of a gas and vice versa.

$$P \propto 1/V$$

This relationship exists because pressure determines the degree of compression of gas molecules. A given number of gas molecules will be packed closer together and occupy a smaller volume when exposed to increased pressure and vice versa.

Boyle's Law can be applied to calculating the volume of a gas that has undergone a change in pressure. For example, the change in gas pressure from P_1 to P_2 will cause an inversely proportional change in gas volume from V_1 to V_2. These changes can be mathematically represented by the following equation.

B.5 $$P_1/P_2 = V_2/V_1$$

B.6 $$V_2 = P_1V_1/P_2$$

B.7 $$V_2 = V_1(P_1/P_2)$$

Atmospheric air not only contains oxygen, carbon dioxide and nitrogen, but also water vapor. To account for the air pressure contributed by water vapor, the pressure of water vapor must be removed in the conversion of gas volume to STPD conditions. To calculate a water vapor pressure, the humidity of the air must be determined. For ATPS conditions, air is saturated with water vapor, and therefore is at 100% relative humidity. Table B.1 provides water vapor pressures for saturated air at temperatures ranging from 14°C to 40°C, and clearly shows that the maximal amount of water vapor in air is a function of temperature. For example, at 14°C fully saturated air can only hold 12.9 mm Hg of water vapor pressure. At 37°C saturated air can hold 47.1 mm Hg in water vapor pressure. The difference in water vapor pressure for air of different temperatures is the reason why we have a relative scale for humidity, and the reason why both the temperature of the gas and the relative humidity must be known for a calculation of water vapor pressure.

For air not saturated with water vapor, relative humidity can be calculated from wet and dry thermometers using Table B.2, or of course, be obtained from a hydrometer. Relative humidity can be used to determine water vapor pressure for air of a given temperature using Figure B.1. This figure provides curves for a variety of temperatures revealing the change in water vapor pressure with a change in relative humidity.

FIGURE B.1

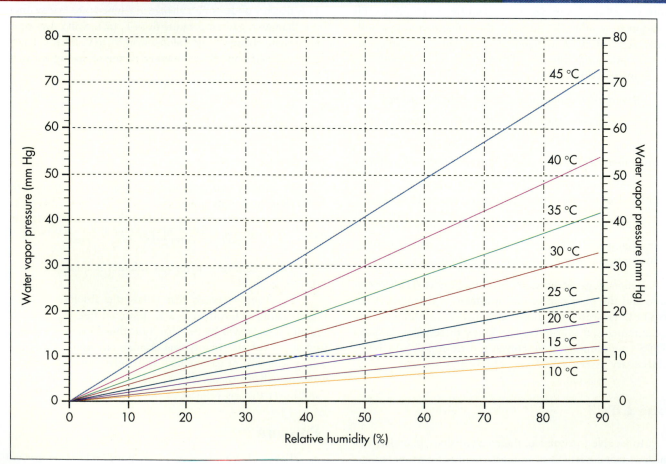

TABLE B.1

Water vapor pressure (P_{H_2O}) at selected gas temperatures

AMBIENT TEMPERATURE (°C)	P_{H_2O} (mm HG)
14	12.9
15	13.5
16	14.1
17	14.9
18	15.5
19	16.5
20	17.5
21	18.7
22	19.8
23	21.1
24	22.4
25	23.8
26	25.2
27	26.7
28	28.3
29	30.0
30	31.8
31	33.7
32	35.7
33	37.7
34	39.9
35	42.2
36	44.6
37	47.1
38	49.4
39	52.0
40	54.7

Calculations are based on the formula: $P_{H_2O} = (13.955 - 0.6584T) + 0.419T^2$.

Correcting from ATPS to STPD conditions

To convert expired minute ventilation (V_E) from ATPS to STPD for pressure;

B.8
$$V_{ESTPD} = V_{EATPS} * [P_B - P_{H_2O}) / 760]$$

Equation B.8 reveals that unless the barometric pressure adjusted for water vapor pressure exceeds 760 mm Hg (impossible unless exposed to hyperbaric conditions; below sea level or in a hyperbarometric chamber), the correction factor will be less than one, thus lowering the measured gas volume. In a typical exercise physiology laboratory, the correction of gas volumes to standard pressure conditions will always produce a correction factor less than one and lower the gas volume.

The combined correction factors for converting a gas volume from ATPS to STPD conditions is as follows;

B.9
$$V_{ESTPD} = V_{EATPS} * [273 / (273 + T_{room})] * [(P_B - P_{H_2O}) / 760]$$

It is recommended that both corrections be combined as in equation B.9, since this will prevent potential calculation errors in making two separate corrections for gas volume.

Correcting from ATPS to BTPS conditions

It is helpful to apply the principles of Charle's and Boyle's Laws before proceeding further with these corrections. For most situations, body temperature with be greater than environmental temperature, so this will cause the correction factor to be greater than one, and increase gas volume. Hence,

B.10
$$V_{EBTPS} = V_{EATPS} * [(273 + 37) / 273 + T_{room}]$$

For pressure, atmospheric pressure is the same, but because temperature is greater in the body there will be a larger water vapor pressure in the lungs of the body, slightly increasing volume, and therefore producing a correction factor greater than one. Hence,

B.11
$$V_{EBTPS} = V_{EATPS} * [(P_B - P_{H_2O} @T_{room}) / (P_B - P_{H_2O} @T_{body})]$$

Indirect Calorimetry

The equations presented in Chapter 7 are listed below to provide a concise summary of the calculations required in indirect calorimetry

Oxygen consumption and inspired ventilation

B.1
$$VO_2 = V_I O_2 - V_E O_2$$

B.2
$$VO_2 = V_I F_I O_2 - V_E FEO_2$$

B.3
$$V_I N_2 = V_E N_2$$

B.4 and
$$V_I F_I N_2 = V_E F_E N_2$$

B.5 thus,
$$V_I = V_E F_E N_2 / F_I N_2$$

B.6
$$V_I = V_E (F_E N_2 / F_I N_2)$$

TABLE B.2

Relative humidity values from temperatures from wet and dry bulb thermometers*

T_{dry} (°C)					$T_{dry} - T_{wet}$ (°C)										
	1	2	3	4	5	6	7	8	9	10	11	12	13	14	15
	RELATIVE HUMIDITY (RH)														
16	90	81	71	63	54	46	38	30	23	15	8				
17	90	81	72	64	55	47	40	32	25	18	11				
18	91	82	73	65	57	49	41	34	27	20	14	7			
19	91	82	74	65	58	50	43	36	29	22	16	10			
20	91	83	74	66	59	51	44	37	31	24	18	12	6		
21	91	83	75	67	60	53	46	39	32	26	20	14	9		
22	92	83	76	68	61	54	47	40	34	28	22	17	11	6	
23	92	84	76	69	62	55	48	42	36	30	24	19	13	8	
24	92	84	77	69	62	56	49	43	37	31	26	20	15	10	5
25	92	84	77	70	63	57	50	44	39	33	28	22	17	12	8
26	92	85	78	71	64	58	51	46	40	34	29	24	19	14	10
27	92	85	78	71	65	58	52	47	41	36	31	26	21	16	12
28	93	85	78	72	65	59	53	48	42	37	32	27	22	18	13
29	93	86	79	72	66	60	54	49	43	38	33	28	24	19	15
30	93	86	79	73	67	61	55	50	44	39	35	30	25	21	17
31	93	86	80	73	67	61	56	51	45	40	36	31	27	22	18
32	93	86	80	74	68	62	57	51	46	41	37	32	28	24	20
33	93	87	80	74	68	63	57	52	47	42	38	33	29	25	21
34	93	87	81	75	69	63	58	53	48	43	39	35	30	26	23
35	94	87	81	75	69	64	59	54	49	44	40	36	32	28	24
36	94	87	81	75	70	64	59	54	50	45	41	37	33	29	25
37	94	87	82	76	70	65	60	55	51	46	42	38	34	30	26
38	94	88	82	76	71	66	61	56	51	47	43	39	35	31	27
39	94	88	82	77	71	66	61	57	52	48	43	39	36	32	28
40	94	88	82	77	72	67	62	57	53	48	44	40	36	33	29

*From U.S. Weather Bulletin No. 1071.

Example: T_{dry} = 22°C; T_{wet} = 17°C; $T_{dry} - T_{wet}$ = 5°C; RH = 61%

B.7 $V_I = V_E * \dfrac{[1-(F_ECO_2 + F_EO_2)]}{0.7903}$

B.8 $VO_2 = (V_E * \dfrac{[1-(F_ECO_2 + F_EO_2)]}{0.7903} * F_IO_2) - (V_E * F_EO_2)$

When indirect calorimetry is performed with inspired volume measured rather than expired volume, equation B.4 must be solved for VE rather than VI.

B.4 $V_I F_I N_2 = V_E F_E N_2$

B.9 $V_E = V_I F_I N_2 / F_E N_2$

B.10 $V_E = V_I (F_I N_2 / F_E N_2)$

B.11 $V_E = V_I * \dfrac{0.7903}{[1-(F_ECO_2 + F_EO_2)]}$

B.12 $VO_2 = (V_I * F_IO_2) - V_I * [(\dfrac{0.7903}{[1-(F_ECO_2 + F_EO_2)]})] * F_EO_2$

Carbon Dioxide Production

B.13 $VCO_2 = V_E F_E CO_2 - V_I F_I CO_2$

Respiratory Exchange Ration

B.14 $RER = VCO_2 / VO_2$

Caloric Expenditure

B.15 Kcals = VO_2 (L/min^{-1}) × RER caloric equivalent
(Kcals/L^{-1}) × time (min)

Calculation Examples

The following data were obtained in a laboratory, under the specific environmental conditions listed with each data set:
Two sets of data are listed.

Data set #1: 5 min of seated rest, with data computed in 30 second intervals.

barometric pressure = 730 mm Hg
room temperature = 19°C
relative humidity = 55%
inspired volume measured via a flow meter from "fresh" air at 19°C

Rest	V_EATPS	F_EO_2	F_ECO_2
30	14.94	0.1681	0.0368
60	13.23	0.1676	0.0366
90	13.46	0.1673	0.0370
120	14.14	0.1668	0.0371
150	15.62	0.1661	0.0388
180	12.64	0.1653	0.0386
210	14.28	0.1650	0.0380
240	14.44	0.1657	0.0377
270	14.82	0.1653	0.0390
300	14.17	0.1660	0.0377

Data set #2: 3 min of seated rest, followed immediately by cycle ergometry exercise at 150 Watts for 5 min. Data are computed in 30 second intervals.

barometric pressure = 630 mm Hg
(i.e.: 5,000 feet above sea level)
room temperature = 19°C
relative humidity = 55%
expired volume measured via a pneumotach from saturated expired air at 19°C

Rest	V_EATPS	F_EO_2	F_ECO_2
30	21.1380	0.1626	0.0359
60	16.4630	0.1642	0.0362
90	14.6809	0.1647	0.0370
120	17.7484	0.1659	0.0360
150	16.9581	0.1651	0.0367
180	18.0029	0.1654	0.0330
Exercise			
30	32.7106	0.1648	0.063
60	40.9753	0.1644	0.0418
90	63.6664	0.1565	0.0466
120	85.2860	0.1533	0.0479
150	91.3941	0.1559	0.0477
180	90.7511	0.1586	0.0491
210	87.4560	0.1586	0.0484
240	95.8278	0.1602	0.0469
270	87.3220	0.1607	0.0470
300	94.0463	0.1602	0.0471
Recovery			
30	75.4272	0.1603	0.0470
60	51.5574	0.1595	0.0470
90	38.8723	0.1621	0.0455
120	25.2898	0.1649	0.0430
150	27.7277	0.1665	0.0421
180	24.1521	0.1677	0.0413
210	21.5660	0.1688	0.0401
240	20.7345	0.,1692	0.0398
270	20.0255	0.1691	0.0396
300	18.5787	0.1694	0.0360

Appendix C
Nutrient Recommendations for Canadians

TABLE C.1

Recommended Nutrient Intake

Age	Sex	Weight (kg)	Pro-tein (g)	Vit. A (RE*)	Vit. D (µg)	Vit. E (mg)	Vit. C (mg)	Folate (µg)	Vit. B₁₂ (µg)	Cal-cium (mg)	Phos-phorus (mg)	Mag-nesium (mg)	Iron (mg)	Iodine (µg)	Zinc (mg)
MONTHS															
0-4	Both	6.0	12†	400	10	3	20	25	0.3	250‡	150	20	0.3§	30	2§
5-12	Both	9.0	12	400	10	3	20	40	0.4	400	200	32	7	40	3
YEARS															
1	Both	11	13	400	10	3	20	40	0.5	500	300	40	6	55	4
2-3	Both	14	16	400	5	4	20	50	0.6	550	350	50	6	65	4
4-6	Both	18	19	500	5	5	25	70	0.8	600	400	65	8	85	5
7-9	M	25	26	700	2.5	7	25	90	1.0	700	500	100	8	110	7
	F	25	26	700	2.5	6	25	90	1.0	700	500	100	8	95	7
10-12	M	34	34	800	2.5	8	25	120	1.0	900	700	130	8	125	9
	F	36	36	800	2.5	7	25	130	1.0	1100	800	135	8	110	9
13-15	M	50	49	900	2.5	9	30	175	1.0	1100	900	185	10	160	12
	F	48	46	800	2.5	7	30	170	1.0	1000	850	180	13	160	9
16-18	M	62	58	1000	2.5	10	40ǁ	220	1.0	900	1000	230	10	160	12
	F	53	47	800	2.5	7	30ǁ	190	1.0	700	850	200	12	160	9
19-24	M	71	61	1000	2.5	10	40ǁ	220	1.0	800	1000	240	9	160	12
	F	58	50	800	2.5	7	30ǁ	180	1.0	700	850	200	13	160	9
25-49	M	74	64	1000	2.5	9	40ǁ	230	1.0	800	1000	250	9	160	12
	F	59	51	800	2.5	6	30ǁ	185	1.0	700	850	200	13	160	9
50-74	M	73	63	1000	5	7	40ǁ	230	1.0	800	1000	250	9	160	12
	F	63	54	800	5	6	30ǁ	195	1.0	800	850	210	8	160	9
75+	M	69	59	1000	5	6	40ǁ	215	1.0	800	1000	230	9	160	12
	F	64	55	800	5	5	30ǁ	200	1.0	800	850	210	8	160	9

*Retinol equivalents.

†Protein is assumed to be from breast milk and must be adjusted for infant formula.

‡Infant formula with high phosphorus should contain 375 mg calcium.

§Breast milk is assumed to be the source of the mineral.

ǁSmokers should increase vitamin C by 50%.

From Scientific Review Committee: *Nutrition Recommendations,* Ottawa, Canada, 1990, Health and Welfare. Reproduced with permission of the Minister of Supply and Services Canada, 1996.

TABLE C.1—Cont'd

Recommended Nutrient Intake

Age	Sex	Weight (kg)	Pro-tein (g)	Vit. A (RE*)	Vit. D (µg)	Vit. E (mg)	Vit. C (mg)	Folate (µg)	Vit. B₁₂ (µg)	Cal-cium (mg)	Phos-phorus (mg)	Mag-nesium (mg)	Iron (mg)	Iodine (µg)	Zinc (mg)
PREGNANCY (ADDITIONAL)															
1st Trimester			5	0	2.5	2	0	200	0.2	500	200	15	0	25	6
2nd Trimester			20	0	2.5	2	10	200	0.2	500	200	45	5	25	6
3rd Trimester			24	0	2.5	2	10	200	0.2	500	200	45	10	25	6
Lactation (additional)			22	400	2.5	3	25	100	0.2	500	200	65	0	50	6

TABLE C.2

Energy Expressed as Daily Rates

Age	Sex	Energy (cal)	Thiamin (mg)	Riboflavin (mg)	Niacin (NE[†])	n-3 PUFA[*] (g)	n-6 PUFA (g)
MONTHS							
0-4	Both	600	0.3	0.3	4	0.5	3
5-12	Both	900	0.4	0.5	7	0.5	3
YEARS							
1	Both	1100	0.5	0.6	8	0.6	4
2-3	Both	1300	0.6	0.7	9	0.7	4
4-6	Both	1800	0.7	0.9	13	1.0	6
7-9	M	2200	0.9	1.1	16	1.2	7
	F	1900	0.8	1.0	14	1.0	6
10-12	M	2500	1.0	1.3	18	1.4	8
	F	2200	0.9	1.1	16	1.2	7
13-15	M	2800	1.1	1.4	20	1.5	9
	F	2200	0.9	1.1	16	1.2	7
16-18	M	3200	1.3	1.6	23	1.8	11
	F	2100	0.8	1.1	15	1.2	7
19-24	M	3000	1.2	1.5	22	1.6	10
	F	2100	0.8	1.1	15	1.2	7
25-49	M	2700	1.1	1.4	19	1.5	9
	F	1900	0.8	1.0	14	1.1	7
50-74	M	2300	0.9	1.2	16	1.3	8
	F	1800`	0.8[‡]	1.0[‡]	14[‡]	1.1[‡]	7[‡]
75+	M	2000	0.8	1.0	14	1.1	7
	F[§]	1700	0.8[‡]	1.0[‡]	14[‡]	1.1[‡]	7[‡]
PREGNANCY (ADDITIONAL)							
1st Trimester		100	0.1	0.1	1	0.05	0.3
2nd Trimester		300	0.1	0.3	2	0.16	0.9
3rd Trimester		300	0.1	0.3	2	0.16	0.9
Lactation (additional)		450	0.2	0.4	3	0.25	1.5

[*]PUFA, polyunsaturated fatty acids.
[†]Niacin equivalents.
[‡]Level below which intake should not fall.
[§]Assumes moderate physical activity.
From Scientific Review Committee: *Nutrition Recommendation*, Ottawa, Canada, 1990, Health and Welfare. Reproduced with permission of the Minister of Supply and Services Canada, 1996.

Glossary

1 repetition maximum (1 RM): the maximum strength from one contraction. Typically, the 1 Rm is obtained during dynamic contractions. When the contraction is isometric, this strength measure is termed the maximal voluntary contraction (MVC)

17-ß estradiol (17-ß): the most biologic active estrogen steroid hormone that influences lipid metabolism, bone growth, and the development of female secondary sex characteristics. Estrogens are produced by the ovary of the female, and to a lesser extent by the adrenal cortex and testes of the male

3-methylhistidine (3-meth'il-his'ti-deen): methylated amino acid that is used as a urine marker for muscle protein catabolism

A

acclimation (a'kli-ma'shun): the process of chronic adaptation to an artificially imposed environmental stress

acclimatization (a'kly-ma-ty-za'shun): the process of chronic adaptation to a given environmental stress

accumulated oxygen deficit: the amount of energy able to be generated by contracting skeletal muscle that did not involve mitochondrial respiration

Acetyl-CoA: molecule produced from carbohydrate and FFA catabolism that enters into the TCA cycle

acidosis (as'i-do'sis): the decrease in pH (increase in free hydrogen ion concentration)

actin (ac'tin): a contractile protein of skeletal muscle

activation energy: the amount of energy required to convert 1 mole of substrate to the transition state

active site: the location on/within an enzyme responsible for the reaction mechanism

activity ratio: in vitro ratio of glycogen synthetase activity with zero G6P divided by maximally saturating G6P concentrations

acute (a-kut): immediate

acute mountain sickness: the illness that accompanies acute altitude exposure, typically expressed by symptoms of headache and lethargy

adaptation (ad-ap-ta'shun): a modification in structure or function that benefits life in a new or altered environment

adaptation (ad-ap-ta'shun): change in function or structure in response to changing conditions

adenylate charge: the ratio between the phosphate bound to adenylate molecules that can be used in chemical transfer to the total adenylate phosphate molecule concentrations

adolescence (ad'o-les'ens): the duration where there is the most rapid growth and development of children

aerobic metabolism: reactions that are involved in the use of oxygen. However, this term loosely refers to mitochondrial respiration and in particular the combined reactions of pyruvate oxidation, the TCA cycle, and electron transport chain

afterload (af'ter-load): the blood pressure exposed to the aortic valve immediately before ventricular contraction

aging (a'jing): the process of growing old, involving the inability to reverse the gradual deterioration of cells important to the life process.

alanine cycle: the release of alanine from muscle into the circulation for uptake by the liver and conversion to glucose

all-cause mortality: the rate of death from all causes

allosteric enzymes: enzymes that have increased activity at a given substrate concentration when bound to specific molecules

alpha-gamma coactivation: the interaction between alpha and gamma motor nerves and type I and II afferent nerves of skeletal muscle and muscle spindles that results in smooth and controlled dynamic muscle contractions

alveolar ventilation: that part of ventilation that reaches the respiratory zone of the lung

amino acid oxidation: the catabolism of amino acids involving the removal of the amine group and subsequent oxidation of the remaining carbon chain in the TCA cycle

amino acids: amine (NH_2) containing molecules that are the primary components of proteins

ammonia (a-mo'ni-ah): a bi-product of the AMP deaminase reaction, forming IMP

amphetamines (am'fet-a'meen): drugs that overcome the discomfort and some of the neuromuscular recruitment limitations experienced during intense exercise

anabolic-androgenic steroids: hormones that stimulate growth and the development of secondary sex characteristics

anabolism (a-nab'o-lizm): the reactions of the body that involve the synthesis of molecules

anaerobic capacity: the capacity of skeletal muscle to regenerate ATP from non-mitochondrial respiration pathways

anaerobic capacity: the maximal amount of ATP able to be regenerated from creatine phosphate hydrolysis and glycolysis during intense exercise

anaerobic metabolism: reactions of metabolism that do not require the presence of oxygen. However, this term is also used to loosely refer to the reactions of creatine kinase, adenylate kinase, and glycolysis

anaerobic threshold: the term used to denote the intensity of exercise when there is an abrupt increase in creatine phosphate hydrolysis and glycolysis, resulting in increased lactate production and the decrease in muscle creatine phosphate

anatomic dead space: the conducting zone of the lung; typically 150 ml in the average-sized individual

android obesity: the storage of fat on the upper part of the body around the abdominal area

anemia (a-ne′mi-ah): abnormally low erythrocyte content, hemoglobin concentration, or hematocrit of the blood

angina pectoris: is severe pain about the heart, usually radiating to the left shoulder and down the left arm. Angina pectoris is caused by ischemia resulting from a temporary blockage or permanent blockage in one or more coronary arteries

anthropometery: the study of body and body part dimensions

anti-oxidants (an′ti-ok′si-dant): substance that provides electrons to reduce free radicals, thus preserving other, more important molecules

antibodies (an′ti-bod′ys): immune protein that binds to an antigen to invoke an immune response

antidiueretic (an′ti-di′u-re′sis): a reduction in urine volume

antigen (an′ti-jen): substance that induces an immune response

aortic bodies: the mechano-receptors and chemical receptors located in the wall of the aorta artery, which respond to stretch of artery wall, as well as PCO_2 and PO_2

apoprotein (apo-pro′teen): the regulatory protein constituents of lipoproteins

appendicular skeleton: the skeletal structures comprising the bones of the legs, pelvis, and arms

applied research: uses physiology to further understand exercise

arrhythmia (a-rith′mi-ah): abnormal cardiac rhythm; many different cardiac arrhythmias exist

artificial electrical stimulation: the application of needle or surface electrodes that provide small electrical stimulations to skeletal muscle, resulting in muscle contraction

asthma (az′mah): the condition of hypersensitivity of the smooth muscle lining the bronchioles of the lung, causing constriction of these airways and increased difficulty in ventilating the lung

atherosclerosis (ath′er-o-skle-ro′sis): the condition of irregularly distributed lipid deposits in the intima of large and medium sized arteries

athletic amenorrhea: the absence of a menstrual cycle induced by endocrinologic responses from exercise training that inhibit the release of follicle stimulating hormone from the anterior pituitary gland

athletic amenorrhea: the loss of the menstrual cycle as a result of excessive exercise training

augmented (awg′men′ted): a description of the leads that measure the electrical activity at one electrode

autologous transfusion: the reinfusion of red blood cells that were removed from the same individual

autoregulation (aw′to-reg-u-la′shun): the ability of a tissue bed to retain near normal blood flow despite changes in systemic blood pressure

axial skeleton: the skeletal structure comprising the bones of the head, thoracic cage, and vertebral column

axon of Hillock: the region of a cell body near the axon that is responsible for the development of an action potential

---

B

ß-oxidation: the reactions of the oxidation of FFA molecules to acetyl-CoA

ballistic stretching: the least effective and most dangerous form of stretching because it uses high-force, quick movements to stretch the muscle or muscle groups. Ballistic stretching is best described by a bouncing motion that induces a stretch that may or may not be held for a brief period of time

binding site: the location on or within an enzyme responsible for the noncovalent binding of substrate(s)

bioelectrical impedance (BIA): the method of determining body fat, fat free body mass, and total body water by measuring the resistance to current passed through the body

bioenergetics (bi′o-en-er-jet′iks): the study of energy transfer in chemical reactions within living tissue

biologic age: the functional age of an individual, based on physiologic conditioning

biologic catalyst: molecules that enhance the rate of chemical reactions

bipolar (bi-pole′ar): a description of the leads that compare the electrical difference between two electrodes

blood (blud): the fluid medium that contains cells that function to transport oxygen and carbon dioxide, cells involved in immunity, certain proteins involved in blood clotting and the transport of nutrients, and electrolytes necessary for optimal cell function

blood doping: the term used for the removal of blood from the body, and its eventual reinfusion at a later date for the purpose of increasing hematocrit and blood oxygen carrying capacity

body composition: the science of determining the absolute and relative contributions of specific components of the body

body density: the density of the body when submerged in water, expressed in gm/ml

body mass index: body weight expressed relative to stature (BMI = weight $[kg]/height^2[m]$)

Bohr effect: the shift in the O_2-hemoglobin dissociation curve down and to the right by increases in temperature, PCO_2, and acidosis

bone remodeling: the dynamic exchange between mineral deposition and resorption in bone

bradycardia (brad-i-kar′di-ah): a heart rate below 60 bpm

bronchitis (brong-ki′tis): a form of obstructive pulmonary disease involving an inflammation of the mucous membranes or bronchial tubes

buffering capacity: the capacity to remove free hydrogen ions from solution

C

caffeine (kaf'een): a naturally occurring substance that acts as a central nervous system (CNS) stimulant and a competitive antagonist for adenosine receptors in the CNS and periphery

calmodulin (cal'mod-u'lin): an intracellular protein that binds 4 calcium ions, and when bound to calcium can activate specific enzymes within the cell.

calorimeter (kal'o-rim'eter): an instrument that measures heat release from the body

calorimetry (kal'o-ri-met'ri): the measurement of body metabolism from heat release from the body

calveoli (kal-ve'ol'i): small circular invaginations located on sarcolemma of smooth muscle that transmit the depolarization to sarcoplasmic reticulum

cancellous bone: spongy, or trabecular bone, devoid of a Haversion system

carbonic anhydrase: the enzyme located on the surface of red blood cells that catalyzes the conversion of CO_2 and water (H_2O) to carbonic acid (H_2CO_3)

cardiac catheterization: the procedure where a catheter is passed into the heart (ventricle or coronary artery) and dye is infused to visualize coronary blood vessels, and the presence of any coronary occlusions

cardiac cycle: the events in a functional heart that occur between successive heart beats

cardiac output: the blood volume pumped by the heart each minute

cardiac rehabilitation: restoring and maintaining the person with cardiovascular disease to optimal physiologic, social, vocational, and emotional status

cardiac rhythm: the electrical pattern of the electrocardiograph. The rhythm can be normal or abnormal. When normal, it is usually described as normal sinus rhythm

cardiovascular system: the heart and blood vessels of the body

carnitine (kar'ni-teen): a molecule required for the transport of medium to long chain fatty acids in the mitochondria

carnitine shuttle: the enzyme-catalyzed transfer of activated long chain free fatty acid molecules from the cytosol into the mitochondria

carotid bodies: the chemical receptors located in the walls of the carotid arteries

catabolism (ca-tab'o-lizm): a part of metabolism that involves the breakdown of relatively complex molecules with the release of energy

cause-specific mortality: the rate of death from specific causes

cell-mediated immune response: that is triggered by the activation of phagocytes and lymphocytes and specifically directed towards infected cells

central fatigue: fatigue caused by alterations in the central nervous system processing and execution of motor patterns

central limitations: cardio-respiratory or central nervous system functions/conditions that limit the ability of skeletal muscle to consume oxygen during exercise

cerebrovascular accident (CVA): a general term used to describe cerebrovascular symptoms caused by an ischemic or hemorrhagic lesion

chemoreceptors (kem'o-re-sep'tor): cells that can generate action potentials in response to changes in the chemical composition of its surroundings (usually blood)

cholesterol (kol-ester'ol): a steroid lipid that is produced by almost all cells, and whose production is regulated by a receptor mediated mechanism in both hepatic and extrahepatic tissues

chronic (kron'ik): long term

chronic obstructive pulmonary disease (COPD): a term used to classify and group chronic respiratory disorders that obstruct airflow

chronologic age: the age of a person expressed relative to time (usually years)

chronotropic (kron'o-trop'ik): pertaining to the rate of myocardial contraction (heart rate)

clinical (klin'i-kl): pertaining to a medical issue

clinical exercise physiology: study of how exercise alters the structure and function of the human body

coenzymes (co-en'zyms): cofactors that are organic molecules

cofactors (co-fak-tors): additional chemical compounds that are required to bind to enzymes to give catalytic activity

collaterals (co-lat'er'al): coronary blood vessels that grow as a result of chronic exposure of a region to ischemia

compact bone: dense bone characterized by the cellular arrangement of mineral and cells into Haversion systems

complement proteins: proteins that exist in the blood and other body fluids that become activated during an immune response and assist in the destruction of the pathogen

complete proteins: proteins that contain all of the essential amino acids

compliance (kom-pli'ans): the measure of the ease at which a structure can increase it's volume capacitance. The reciprocal of elasticity

concentric (kon-sen'trik): in reference to skeletal muscle contraction; a contraction involving the shortening of muscle

conducting zone: the regions of the lung, comprising the trachea, bronchi, and bronchioles, that allow for the bulk flow of air into the lung yet are not involved in gas exchange

contractility (kon-trak'til i-ti): the ability of muscle to contract and generate tension, at the expense of metabolic energy, when adequate stimulus is received

contraction cycling: the repeated cycling of actin and myosin binding, movement, and release during contraction

contraindication (kon-tra-in'di-ka'shun): a condition that prevents the use or application of something

Cori cycle: the release of lactate from muscle into the circulation for uptake by the liver and conversion to glucose

coronary angiogram: the resulting image of the coronary artery network following dye infusion during cardiac catheterization

coronary artery bypass grafting (CABG): a major surgical procedure whereby grafts of veins are harvested from the leg or arm and "grafted" from the aorta to a point past the blockage of one or more of the coronary arteries

coronary artery disease (CAD): a common disease resulting from a process known as atherosclerosis

creatine phosphate shuttle: the transfer of phosphate from mitochondrial ATP to cytosolic creatine and ADP

criterion variable: the variable that is being predicted. The criterion variable is also known as the dependent variable

criterion-referenced fitness standards: fitness standards that are based on an established fitness and health relationship

cross-training: the practice of exercise training with more than one exercise mode

cyclic AMP (cAMP): the second messenger produced by the activation of adenylate cyclase in response to the binding of certain hormones to their cell receptor

D

dehydration (de-hi-dra'shun): a decreased water content of the body below normal

deinnervation (de-in'er-va'shun): the complete removal of neural connections to skeletal muscle

detraining (de-tray'ning): the absence of training, usually occurring after the attainment of training adaptations

diabetes mellitis: the condition characterized by the decreased ability to regulate blood glucose concentrations via insulin

diagnostic (di-ag-nos'tik): having a value in diagnosing/detecting a medical condition

dichloracetate (di-klor'o-ass'e-tate): an artificial chlorinated derivative of acetyl-CoA that stimulates the activity of pyruvate dehydrogenase, reduces lactate accumulation in the blood, and decreases peripheral vascular resistance

diffusion capacity: the capacity for a gas the diffuse down a concentration gradient in the acqueous environment of the body

diuresis (di'u-re'sis): an increase in urine volume

down-regulation: a decreased biologic response to a given compound; usually involves a decrease in receptor numbers, or an impaired cellular response to the binding of a hormone to it's receptor

dual x-ray absorptiometry (DEXA): a method used for measuring the mineral density of bone

dynamometer (di-na-mom'e-ter): an instrument for the measurement of muscle force application

E

eccentric (e-sen'trik): in reference to skeletal muscle contraction; a contraction involving the lengthening of muscle

echocardiography (ek'o-kar-di-og'ra-fi): the process of recording the movement and dimensions of the heart and its structures by rebounding high frequency (nonaudible) sound waves

economy (e-kon'o-mi): the concept pertaining to the oxygen consumption required to perform a given task

efficiency (e-fish'en-si): when applied to exercise; the ratio (expressed as percentage) between the mechanical energy produced during exercise and the energy cost of the exercise

Einthoven's triangle: the law that equates the limb leads of the 12-lead ECG, where the average electrical potential of lead II equals the sum of leads I and III

ejection fraction: the volume of blood pumped by the heart per beat, expressed relative to the end diastolic volume of the ventricle

elasticity (e-las'tis-i-ti): the ability of muscle to resume its resting length after being stretched or contracted

electrical axis: the average direction of depolarization, expressed as a degree based on the hexaxial arrangement of the leads

electrocardiogram (e'lek'tro-kar-di'o-gram): the recording from an electrocardiograph

electrocardiograph (ECG) (e'lek'tro-kar-di'o-graf): the equipment used to detect and record the electrical activity of the heart

electron transport chain: the series of electron receivers located along the inner mitochondrial membrane that sequentially receive and transfer electrons to the final electron receiver—molecular oxygen

emphysema (em-fi-se'mah): another form of chronic pulmonary disease caused by over-inflation and damage of the alveoli

endergonic (en-der-gon'ik): referring to a reaction that takes place with absorption of free energy from its surroundings

endogenous opioids: hormones released from the anterior pituitary gland that exert a biologic response similar to morphine

endothermic (end-o-ther'mik): denotes a chemical reaction that absorbs heat

energetics (en-er-jet'iks): the study of energy transfer in physical and chemical changes

enthalpy (en'thal'py): a thermodynamic function concerning heat content

entropy (en'tro-pi): the fraction of energy from a reaction that is unable to be used to perform work because of its use in increasing randomness or disorder

epidemiology (ep-i-de-mi-ol'o-ji): the study of the presence and spread of disease in a community

epiphyseal plate: the cartilagenous region of the end of long bones responsible for bone growth relative to a change in length

epiphysis (e-pif'i-sis): the end regions of long bones

EPOC: the abbreviation for excess post exercise oxygen consumption

equilibrium (e'kwi-lib'ri-um): a state of dynamic balance in one or more reactions that proceed in opposing directions

equilibrium constant (Keq): the product of product concentrations divided by the product of substrate concentrations for a reaction when at equilibrium

ergogenic aid: a physical, mechanical, nutritional, psychologic, or pharmacologic substance or treatment that either directly improves physiologic variables associated with exercise performance or removes subjective restraints which may limit physiologic capacity

ergolytic (er-go-lit'ik): the term used for substances that impair exercise performance

ergometer (er-gom'e-ter): a device used to measure work

ergometry (er-gom'e-tree): the science of the measurement of work and power

erythrocyte (e-rith'ro-syt): red blood cell

erythrocythemia (e-rith'ro-si-the'mi-ah): artificially increased red blood cell concentrations in the blood

erythropoietin (e'rith-ro-poy'e-tin): a hormone released from the kidney that is responsible for stimulating red blood cell production (erythropoiesis)

essential fat: fat and lipid component of the body that comprises cell membranes, bone marrow, intramuscular fat, etc.

excitability (ex-si'ta-bil'i-ti): the ability to respond to a stimulus (e.g., neurotransmitter or hormone) by the generation and conduction of a reversal in membrane potential (action potential)

exercise induced hypoxemia: the hypoxemia that occurs in highly endurance-trained individuals during intense exercise, even at sea level barometric pressures

exercise physiology: the study of how exercise alters the structure and function of the human body

exergonic (eks-er-gon'ik): referring to a reaction that takes place with a release of free energy to its surroundings

exothermic (eks-o-ther'mik): denotes a chemical reaction that releases heat

extensibility (ex-ten'si-bil-i-ti): the ability of muscle to be stretched

external respiration: gas exchange that occurs in the lung between the respiratory zone and blood

F

fat free body mass: the component of the body that is not storage and essential fat

fatigue (fa'teeg): when concerned with exercise fatigue can be generally defined as the inability to continue to exercise at a given intensity

fatty acids: the lipid components of triacylglycerols, which are catabolized in tissues

ferritin (fer-i'tin): an iron protein complex, mainly found in the liver, small intestine, and spleen, but also present in blood

fiber type: a categorization of muscle fibers based on their enzymatic and metabolic characteristics

fibers (fi'bers): muscle cells

fitness (fit'ness): a state of well being that provides optimal performance

follicular phase: the phase of the menstrual cycle beginning with the onset of menstruation and ending at the start of ovulation; usually 9 to 23 days in duration

fractional velocity: similar to activity ration, but the numerator is the glycogen synthetase activity measured with a physiologic G6P concentration

free energy: the energy from a reaction that can be used to perform work

free radicals: small molecules within the body that have an extremely high affinity for electrons

fructose (fruc-tos): the form of sugar predominantly found in fruit and honey

G

ganglia (gang-gli-ah): an aggregation of nerve cell bodies located in the peripheral nervous system

gastric emptying: the emptying of stomach contents into the small intestine

gland: a organ that secretes a substance(s)

gluconeogenesis (glu'ko-ne-o-jen'e-sis): formation of glucose from noncarbohydrates, such as amino acids or alcohol

glucose (glu-kos): the form of sugar by which carbohydrate is metabolised in animals

glucose polymers: glucose residues connected together to form a chain structure

glucose-fatty acid cycle: the proposed inhibition of glucose uptake by skeletal muscle by high circulating concentrations of fatty acid molecules

GLUT proteins: the predominant glucose transport protein on the sarcolemma of skeletal muscle

glycemic index: a rating of the increase in blood glucose after the ingestion of a standard amount of carbohydrate. The rating is based on a comparison with the blood glucose response following the ingestion of an equivalent amount of carbohydrate in the form of white bread

glycerol (gli-ser-ol): an alcohol, which is the structural backbone of triacylglycerols

glycerol (glis'er-ol): a bi-product of glycolysis that is used in triacylglycerol synthesis. During the mobilization of fatty acids in lipolysis, glycerol is released and is often used as an indirect reflection of the mobilization of fatty acids in blood and adipose tissue

glycogen (gli'ko-jen): a sugar polysaccharide that is the form of carbohydrate storage in animal tissues

glycogen supercompensation: a regimen of increased carbohydrate ingestion and modified exercise training that results in maximal storage of glycogen in skeletal muscle

glycogen synthetase: the enzyme catalyzing the addition of glucose residues from UDP-glucose to glycogen

glycogenolysis (gli-ko-jen-ol-is-is): the removal of glucose units from glycogen, producing glucose 1-phosphate

glycolysis (gli-kol'i-sis): reactions involving the catabolism of glucose to pyruvate

glycolytic metabolism: reactions of the glycolytic pathway

growth hormone: a hormone that functions to primarily regulate blood glucose, and secondarily function in concert with somatomedins to stimulate bone and muscle growth

gynoid obesity: the storage of fat in the lower half of the body around the hip and thigh area, whereas men tend to store fat on the upper part of the body around the abdominal area (android obesity)

H

Haldane effect: the increasing affinity between hemoglobin and CO_2 during conditions of low PO_2

Haldane transformation: the use of equal inspired and expired nitrogen volumes to solve for either inspired or expired ventilatory volumes

haversian canal: the central vascular component of the Haversian system

haversian system: the organized circular cellular and vascular structure of compact bone

health-related fitness: fitness that provides benefits to health and well being

heat exhaustion: decreased exercise tolerance because of a combination of dehydration, a reduced plasma volume and cardiovascular compromise, and hyperthermia

heat stroke: the progression from heat exhaustion; when body core temperature increases to values that impair central nervous system and damages peripheral tissues

helium dilution: the method used to measure the functional residual capacity (FRC) of the lung that is based on the dilution of a known amount of helium

hematocrit (hem'a-to-krit): the ratio of the volume of blood cells and formed elements of blood to total blood volume. Usually expressed as a percentage

hematopoiesis (hem'a-to-poy-e'sis): increased blood cell production

hemoconcentration (he'mo-kon'sen-tra'shun): increased hematocrit as a result of the loss of plasma volume

hemodynamics (he'mo-di-nam'iks): the study of the dynamics of the blood circulation

hemoglobin (he-mo-globe'in): the globular protein on red blood cells that contains four iron containing heme groups that can bind oxygen and carbon dioxide

hemolysis (he-mol'i-sis): destruction of red blood cells causing the release of hemoglobin into solution

homologous transfusion: the reinfusion of red blood cells that were removed from a different individual

hormone (hor'mone): a substance secreted from a tissue or cell that exerts a biologic response on itself or other cells located locally or distant

humoral immune response: that which is triggered by the presence of free pathogens in the blood or interstitial spaces of the body

hydrodensitometry (hi'dro-den'si-tom'e-tri): the method of determining body density by under water weighing

hydrogen bond: a weak bond formed by the electrostatic attraction between a weak negatively charges atom and a weak positively charged atom in the same of another molecule

hydrostatic force: force exerted by a column of water

hydroxyapatite (hi-droks'i-ap-a'tite): the mineral structure of the bone matrix

hyperbaria (hi-per-bar'i-ah): increased barometric pressure

hypercapnia: increased arterial partial pressure of carbon dioxide ($PaCO_2$) above normal (40 mm Hg)

hyperemia (hi-per-e'mi-ah): increased blood flow above normal. Usually expressed relative to a particular tissue

hyperglycemia (hi-per-gli-se'mi-ah): abnormally high blood glucose concentrations (>5 mmol/L)

hyperhydration (hi'per-hy'dra-shun): the increase in body water content above normal values

hyperplasia (hi'per-pla'zi-ah): the increase in muscle fiber number in skeletal muscle

hyperplastic obesity: a classification of obesity in which an individual has a greater number of fat cells, which are also larger than normal. This type of obesity begins at an early age and results in severe obesity. Hypertrophic obesity is caused by a normal number of fat cells that have increased in size

hypertension (hi'per-ten'shun): abnormally high blood pressure

hyperthermia (hi'per-ther-mi'ah): a body core temperature above 37°C

hypertrophic obesity: a classification of obesity in which a normal number of fat cells have increased in size

hypertrophy (hi-per'tro-fi): the increase in size of skeletal muscle resulting from the increased size of individual muscle fibers

hypobaria (hi-po-bar'i-ah): decreased barometric pressure

hypobaric hypoxia: decreased oxygen availability due to decreased barometric pressure

hypoglycemia (hi-po-gli-se'mi-ah): abnormally low blood glucose concentrations (<3.5 mmol/L)

hyponatremia (hi'po-na-tre'mi-ah): a decrease in the serum concentration of sodium below 135 mEq/L

hypotension (hi'po-ten'shun): abnormally low blood pressure

hypothermia (hi'po-ther-mi'ah): a decreased body temperature below 37°C

hypoxemia (hi-pok-se'mi-ah): the decrease in the oxygen saturation of hemoglobin below normal

hypoxic ventilatory response (HVR): the increase inventilation for given changes in oxyhemoglobin saturation. The HVR is expressed as the slope of this linear relationship, and by convention is reported as a positive value

I

immunoglobulins (im'un-o-glob'u-lins): an antibody, and is abbreviated Ig. They are grouped into 5 different classes-IgD, IgM, IgG, IgA, IgE

incremental exercise: exercise performed at intensities that progressively increase over time

inosine monophosphate (IMP): the product of the AMP deaminase reaction

inotropic (in-o-trop'ik): pertaining to the contractility of the myocardium

insulin responsiveness: refers to the ability of the pancreas to release insulin in response to hyperglycemia

insulin sensitivity: refers to the ability of the body (usually related to skeletal muscle) to be stimulated by insulin to increase glucose uptake

intercalated discs: low resistance-high conduction velocity tissue dispersed through the myocardium, causing a rapid depolarization of the myocardium when stimulated

interferon (inter-fer'on): a glyco-protein released by infected cells, which functions to increase the resistance to infection of "healthy" cells

internal respiration: gas exchange that occurs by tissues for the purpose of energy metabolism

international unit: the recognized unit of enzyme activity

intestinal absorption: the absorption of water organic and inorganic nutrients from the small intestine

intrinsic rhythmicity (in'trin-sik rith-miss i'ti): the ability of a tissue to develop its own depolarization, usually at some consistent rate

ionization state: the charge characteristics of a molecule; usually used for amino acid molecules within proteins

isokinetic (i-so-ki-net'ik): in reference to skeletal muscle contraction; a contraction involving a constant velocity

isometric (i-so-met'rik): in reference to skeletal muscle contraction; a contraction involving no change in the length of muscle

isozymes (i'so-zymes): different structures of a specific enzyme that often have different kinetic characteristics

J

J-point: the end of the QRS complex and the beginning of the baseline portion of the s-t segment

K

ketone bodies: the molecules produced by the liver from acetyl-CoA derived from ß-oxidation when TCA cycle activity is compromised from a lack of carbohydrate

ketone bodies: the product of the liver during conditions of low carbohydrate and high lipid catabolism

kinesthesis (kin'es-the'sis): the sense of awareness of moving body parts

kymograph (ki'mo-graf): the rotating drum component of an instrument (e.g., spirometer) that is used to record wave-like modulations (e.g., ventilation)

L

lactate (lac'tate): product of the reduction of pyruvate

lactate paradox: the decreased maximal lactate production by contracting skeletal muscle after chronic altitude exposure

lactate threshold: the term used to denote the intensity of exercise when there is an abrupt increase in lactate accumulation in blood or muscle

lead (leed): the electrical arrangement of specific electrodes when placed in the body during electrocardiography

lean body mass: the component of the body that is not storage fat

left ventricular hypertrophy: the increased mass of the myocardium of the left ventricle

leukocytosis (lu'ko-si-to-sis): increased leukocyte concentration in the blood

life expectancy: the average, statistically predicted, length of life for an individual

lipolysis (li-pol'i-sis): catabolism of triacylglycerol releasing FFA and glycerol

lipoprotein (lip'o-pro'teen): blood compounds containing lipid and protein

longevity (lon-jev'i-ti): the duration of a life beyond the norm

luteal phase: the phase of the menstrual cycle beginning with the end of ovulation and ending at the start of menstruation; usually 13 days in duration

lymph (limf): the fluid of the lymphatic system

lymph nodes: an aggregation of lymph tissue that forms and stores lymphocytes

lymphatic system: the combined fluid, cells, tissues, and organs that form the vascular system external to the systemic circulation. The lymphatic system is responsible for fluid distribution in the body, as well as the body's immune capabilities

lymphocytes (lim'fo-site): class of leukocytes formed in the lymphoid tissue that are subgrouped as B and T cells

M

macronutrients (ma-kro-nu'tri-ents): essential food component required in large quantities

magnetic resonance (MR): the ability of objects to precess when forced out of alignment in a magnetic field

magnetic resonance imaging (MRI): the detection of different frequencies of precessing objects in a magnetic field, and the processing of this information to provide a visual two-dimensional picture of the anatomical distribution of these frequencies

magnetic resonance spectroscopy (MRS): the detection of differing frequency sound waves from precessing objects in a magnetic field, and the processing of these signals allowing the graphical illustration and quantification of the different signals, and their respective intensities

malonyl CoA: the first product of free fatty acid synthesis

Mason-Likar lead system: the location of the limb electrodes on the torso, rather than wrists and ankles during the 12-lead ECG

mass action effect: lactate production caused by an increased rate of glycolytic metabolism

mass action ratio: the product of product concentrations divided by the product of substrate concentrations for a reaction under physiologic conditions

maximal oxygen consumption (VO$_2$max): the maximal rate of oxygen consumption by the body

medical history: the medical records of an individual

menstrual cycle: the monthly variation in gonadal hormones of the female that result in the release of an ovary and the eventual expulsion of the ovary and developing placenta during menstruation

metabolism (me-tab'o-lizm): the sum of all reactions of the body

microgravity (mi-kro-grav'i-ti): conditions of decreased gravitational force

micronutrients (my-kro-nu'tri-ents): essential food component required only in small quantities

mineral (min'er-al): inorganic micronutrients, essential for normal bodily functions

mitochondrial respiration: reactions of the mitochondria that ultimately lead to the consumption of oxygen

mortality (mor-tal'i-ti): death rate

motor unit: an alpha motor nerve and the muscle fibers that it innervates

multiple regression: the use of multiple variables (independent) in the prediction of a criterion variable. Multiple regression results in the formulation of an equation that contains variables that best combine to predict the criterion variable

muscle biopsy: the procedure of removing a sample of skeletal muscle from an individual

muscle fatigue: fatigue resulting from altered function of skeletal muscle

muscle power: the mechanical power during dynamic by muscle contractions

muscle pump: the action of contracting muscles that forces venous blood flow against gravity towards the heart

muscle spindle: the sensory receptor within skeletal muscle that is sensitive to static and dynamic changes in muscle length

muscular endurance: the ability of muscle to contract repeatedly over time

muscular strength: the maximal force generated by contracting skeletal muscle for a given contractile velocity

myocardial infarction: the injury to myocardium because of lack of oxygen caused by ischemia

myocardial ischemia: decreased blood flow to the myocardium

myofibrils (mi'o-fi'bril): the longitudinal anatomic unit within skeletal and cardiac muscle fibers that contains the contractile proteins

myoglobin (my'o-globe'in): the globular protein of muscle that contains one iron containing heme group that can bind oxygen

myosin (mi'o-sin): the largest of the contractile proteins of skeletal muscle

N

NADPH: one of the main products of the Pentose Phosphate Pathway. NADPH provides reducing power and free energy during anabolic reactions

natural killer cells (NK cells): a leukocyte that assists in the destruction of foreign substances in the body

neural adaptation: the decrease in discharge frequency of action potentials that leave a sensory receptor

neuro-endocrinology (nu'ro-end'o-kri-nol'o-ji): study of the anatomy and function of the endocrine system, and components of the nervous system that regulate endocrine function

neuromuscular junction: the connection between a branch of an alpha motor nerve and a skeletal muscle fiber

neurotransmitter (nu'ro-trans-mit'er): a chemical released at a synapse in response to the depolarization of the presynaptic membrane

nitrogen balance: equal nitrogen intake versus excretion from the body

nitrogen washout: a method used to measure residual FRC that is based on the dilution of the nitrogen fraction of air in the lung with pure oxygen

normobaric hypoxia: decreased oxygen availability at normal barometric pressure resulting from a lowered oxygen fraction of inspired air

nutrients (nu'tri-ent): a food component that can be utilized by the body

nutrition (nu-trish'un): the science involving the study of food and liquid requirements of the body for optimal function

O

obesity (o-bee-si'ti): having "excess fat" relative to body weight. Body fat percentages greater than 20% for men or 30% for women are considered an indication of obesity

orthostatic tolerance: the ability to withstand gravitational force in opposing blood flow back to the heart

osmolality (oz'mo-lal'i-ti): the number of particles per kg of solvent

osmoreceptor (oz'mo-re-sep'tor): cells that can generate an action potential in response to changes in the osmolality of the blood

osseous tissue: bone

ossification (ox'i-fik-a'shun): the replacement of cartilagenous bone with bone mineral

osteoarthritis (os-te-o-ar-thri'tis): also referred to as degenerative joint disease, is a degenerative process caused by the wearing away of cartilage, leaving two surfaces of bone in contact with each other

osteocyte (os'te-o-site): bone cell

osteoporosis (os'te-o-po-ro'sis): the clinical condition of decreased bone mineral content

overfat (o'ver-fat): a condition of excess body fat, as determined from body composition analysis

overload (o'ver-lode): exposure of the body to unaccustomed stress

overtraining (o'ver-tray'ning): training that causes excess overload that the body is unable to adapt to, resulting in decreased exercise performance

overweight (o'ver-wate): a condition of excess weight based on either a height-weight relationship, or computed from body composition analysis

ovulatory phase: the phase of the menstrual cycle involved with ovulation; usually 3 days in duration

oxidation (ok-si-da'shun): the process of removing electrons from a molecule during a chemical reaction

oxidative phosphorylation: the production of ATP from the coupled transfer of electrons to the generation of a H^+ gradient between the two mitochondrial membranes

oximetry (ok'sim'e-tri): indirect measurement of the oxygen saturation of hemoglobin in blood

oxygen deficit: the difference between oxygen consumption and the oxygen demand of exercise during non-steady state exercise conditions

oxygen drift: the increase in oxygen consumption during presumably "steady state" exercise when it is performed for extended periods of time

P

pathogen (path'o-jen): foreign substance in the body

peak height velocity: the period of rapid growth during the adolescent period, usually occurring 2 years earlier for girls than boys

pediatric exercise science: a specialized sub-field of exercise physiology dealing with the unique aspects of the effects of exercise on children and adolescents

pediatrician (pe-di-a-trish'an): a medical doctor who specializes in the care of children

Pentose Phosphate Pathway: a side branch of glycolysis resulting in the conversion of glucose-6-phosphate to NADPH and ribose-5-phosphate

peripheral limitations: conditions within skeletal muscle that decrease the cellular ability to take up and utilize oxygen during exercise

peripheral vascular disease (PVD): a condition caused by atherosclerotic lesions in one or more peripheral (usually in the legs) arterial and/or venous blood vessels

phagocytes (fag'o-site): a type of leukocyte that engulfs foreign or damaged substances in the body

phosphagen system: the regernation of ATP via creatine phosphate hydrolysis, and ADP

phosphate loading: the practice of ingesting phosphate for the purpose of improving exercise performance

phosphatidate (fos-fa-ti'date): the product formed after two FFA additions to glycerol-3-phosphate

phosphorylation potential: the ratio between ATP to ADP

pneumotachometer (nu'mo-ta-kom'e-ter): an instrument for measuring the instantaneous flow during ventilation

polycythemia (pol'i-si-the'mi-ah): above normal increase in the erythrocyte content of the blood

polycythemia (pol'i-si-the'mi-ah): increased red blood cell concentrations in the blood

pores of Kohn: small holes between neighboring alveoli that allow for the even distribution of surfactant over the respiratory membranes

power (pow'er): the application of force relative to time

pre-capillary sphincter: region of smooth muscle that surrounds blood vessels before the capillary bed

prediction (pre-dic'shun): the estimation of one variable from the measurement of others

predictive value: a measure of how accurately an exercise test correctly identifies an individual with coronary artery disease (positive test) or without it (negative test)

preload (pre'load): the load to which a muscle is subjected to before shortening. Preload is usually explained as the stretch induced on the myocardium by the filling of the ventricles of the heart

primary risk factors: those proven by research to directly cause atherosclerosis, and include cigarette smoking, hyperlipidemias, inactivity, hypertension and diabetes

primary structure: the sequence of amino acids that forms the covalent back bone structure of proteins

progesterone (pro-jes'ter-own): a steroid hormone synthesized by the developing follicle of the ovary, and released during the luteal phase of the menstrual cycle

proprioception (pro'pri-o-sep'shun): the sense of awareness of body part positions in space

proprioceptive neuromuscular facilitation (PNF): a type of stretching routine where a muscle is contracted for 4 to 6 seconds, followed by an immediate 8 to 12 second static stretch

puberty (pu'ber-ti): the period of growth and development where the secondary sex characteristics that differentiate genders develop

pulmonary circulation: the circulation between the right ventricle and left atrium

pulmonary circulation: the vasculature that connects the heart to the lungs

pulmonary transit time: the time required for a red blood cell to pass through the pulmonary capillary; essentially the time available for gas exchange between the alveoli and blood circulating through the lung

pure research: uses exercise to further understand physiology

purine nucleotide cycle: conversion of AMP to IMP, which is reconverted back to AMP during recovery

Q

Q_{10} value: the relative increase in enzyme activity with a 10°C increase in temperature

R

rating of perceived exertion: a rating based on an individuals perception of exercise intensity

rebound hypoglycemia: the decrease in blood glucose when exercising at least 30 min after the ingestion of carbohydrate

receptor (re-sep'tor): a protein located within a membrane that is able to bind another molecule

redox potential: the ratio of NAD^+ to NADH

reduction (re-duk'shun): the process of adding electrons to a molecule during a chemical reaction

reduction potential: a measure of the propensity for a molecule to receive electrons

rehydration (re-hi-dra'shun): the process of returning fluids to the body

rehydration (re-hi-dra'shun): the return of water to the body during recovery from dehydration

residual volume: the volume remaining in the lungs after a forced maximal exhalation

resistance exercise: muscle contractions performed against a resistance, typically in the form of external loads like that used in weight lifting

respiration (res'pi-ra'shun): gas exchange at the tissue level; usually refers to the consumption of oxygen for use in oxidative phosphorylation

respiratory exchange ratio: the ratio of carbon dioxide production to oxygen consumption, as measured from expired gas analysis indirect calorimetry

respiratory quotient: the ratio of carbon dioxide production to oxygen consumption during metabolism

respiratory zone: the regions of the lung, comprising the respiratory bronchioles and alveoli, that are involved in gas exchange

reversability (re-ver'si-bil'i-ti): the loss of training adaptations when exercise training ceases

rheumatoid arthritis: caused by an inflammation of the membrane surrounding joints

ribonucleic acid: the nucleic aid bases that complement those of DNA

ribose-5-phosphate: one of the main products of the Pentose Phosphate Pathway. Ribose-5-phosphate is a precursor of both RNA and DNA synthesis

ribosome (ri'bo-som): the cytosolic organelle involved in protein synthesis

S

S0.5: the substrate concentration at half Vmax for a given reaction condition

sarcolemma (sar'ko-lem'ah): the cell membrane of a muscle fiber

sarcomere (sar'ko-mere): the smallest contractile unit of skeletal muscle, consisting of the contractile proteins between the two Z-lines

sarcoplasmic reticulum (sar'ko-plas-mik re-tik'u-lum): extensive intracellular membrane compartment that stores calcium

second messenger: a compound within a cell that increases in concentration during the amplification response to the binding of a hormone to it's cell receptor

secondary risk factors: those not yet proven to directly cause atherosclerosis, but contribute to the disease, and include obesity, gender, family history, and age

sensory receptor: a specialized region of an afferent nerve that is receptive to a specific stimuli that can result in the change in receptor membrane potential and the eventual generation of an action potential

set point theory: the theory that explains an individual's body fat content to be based on a genetically predetermined regulation of food intake to several physiologic stimulii such as blood glucose, fatty acids, and adipocyte number and size

sodium bicarbonate: the molecule in blood that provides the greatest buffer power of acid

somatosensory cortex: the three dimensional region of the cerebral cortex responsible for receiving afferent nerves from peripheral receptors

specific activity: enzyme activity expressed relative to total protein

specificity (spes'i-fis'i-ti): having a fixed relation to a single cause or definite result

spirometry (spi-rom'e-tri): the measurement of human lung volumes and functional capacities with a spirometer

ST-segment depression: the lowering of the ST segment, usually because of myocardial ischemia. However, pharmacologic and ventilation conditions can also lower the ST segment

static stretching: when a muscle, or group of muscles are slowly stretched and held for a short period of time (usually 8 to 12 seconds)

storage fat: fat and lipid stored in adipose tissue

striated (stri-ate'ed): pertaining to the highly organized dark and light stained pattern of skeletal muscle fibers, as seen through microscopy

stroke: a condition caused by an embolus or thrombus that occludes one or more arteries leading to the brain

stroke volume: the volume of blood ejected from the ventricle each beat

summation (sum-a'shun): the increase in muscle force during contraction caused by the frequent stimulation of the same or multiple motor units

surfactant (sur-fak'tant): a lipoprotein secreted by tissue of the lung that reduces surface tension of the alveolar membranes

synapse (sin'aps): the junction between two nerves

synthesis (sin-the'sis): the formation of larger molecules

systemic circulation: the vasculature of the body other than the pulmonary circulation

T

t-tubules (t tu'bul): transverse tubule system connecting the sarcolemma to the sarcoplasmic reticulum in skeletal and cardiac muscle

tachycardia (tak-i-kar'di-ah): a heart rate above 100 bpm

taper (tape'er): a period of reduced training before athletic competition

tetanus (tet'a-nus): sustained maximal contraction of a muscle

thallium-201 stress test: the procedure of injecting an isotope into the circulation immediately after exhausting exercise to determine whether there are any blockages to coronary arteries

thermodynamics (ther'mo-di-nam'iks): the branch of physicochemical science concerned with energy transfer between heat and mechanical work

thermogenesis (ther'mo-jen'e-sis): energy expenditure

tidal volume: the volume of air inhaled and exhaled each breath; typically 500 ml at rest in the average-sized individual

torque (tork): force applied to a lever system that causes rotational movement

training (tray'ning): an organized program of exercise designed to stimulate chronic adaptations

transamination (trans-amin'a-shun): the removal of an amino group from one amino acid and its placement on a carbon chain that forms another amino acid

transcription (trans-krip'shun): the duplication of specific DNA regions in the form of RNA

transferrin (trans-fer'in): an iron transporting ß-globulin of the blood

transient ischemic attacks (TIAs): temporary disruption of blood flow to the brain

transition state: the temporary activated structure of a substrate that exists before product formation

translation (trans-la'shun): the formation of amino acids from the enzymatic association between ribosomes, RNA, and tRNA

transluminal coronary angioplasty (PTCA): an invasive procedure where by a specialized catheter is advanced through an artery (usually femoral), into a coronary artery to the atherosclerotic plaque. Once placed correctly, a small balloon is inflated until the plaque is compressed against the walls of the artery

triacylglycerol (tri-as'il-glis'er-ol): a lipid consisting of a glycerol backbone and three free fatty acid molecules, which is the principle form of fat storage in the body

triad (tri'ad): junction between a t-tubule and the sarcoplasmic reticulum

tricarboxylic acid cycle: mitochondrial reactions involving the addition of acetyl-CoA to oxaloacetate, and the eventual release of carbon dioxide, electrons, and protons during the reformation of oxaloacetate

tropomyosin (tro'po-my'osin): a contractile protein of striated muscle

troponin (tro'po'nin): the regulatory calcium binding contractile protein of striated muscle

U

up-regulation: an increased biologic response to a given compound

V

vasoconstriction (vas'o-kon-strik'shun): narrowing of the lumen diameter of blood vessels

vasodilation (vas'o-di-la'shun): widening of the lumen diameter of blood vessels

vasomotor center: the neural region within the medulla responsible for regulating central and peripheral cardiovascular function

ventilation (ven'til-a'shun): the bulk flow of air into and out of the lung

ventilation-perfusion ratio: the ratio between ventilation and blood flow for the lung, or for specific regions of the lung

ventilatory threshold: the increase in ventilation corresponding to the development of metabolic acidosis; usually detected during an incremental exercise test

vitamins (vi'ta-min): organic micronutrient of food, essential for normal body functions

Vmax: the maximal rate of catalysis of an enzyme

VO$_2$peak: the largest VO$_2$ during an incremental exercise test

voluntary dehydration: the progressive development of dehydration despite the availability of fluid to drink ad libitum

W

waist-to-hip ratio: waist circumference divided by hip circumference

warm-up: a general term used for practices performed before exercise for the purpose of preparing the body for the exercise

water intoxication: excess drinking of fluid (typically plain water) that lowers the concentration of serum sodium, increasing the risk for developing hyponatremia

water intoxication: water ingestion that causes decreased blood concentrations of electrolytes, especially sodium

weight cycling: the increasing and decreasing body weight experienced by individuals who attempt to lose weight by diet alone

wet bulb globe index (WBGI): an abbreviation for the Wet Bulb Globe Index, used to rate the relative risk of heat injury associated with given environmental conditions

work (wer'k): the product of an applied force exerted over a known distance against gravity

Index

N

O

P

Q

R

Credits

CHAPTER 27

p. 687, Table 27.1, Used with permission of Williams & Wilkins, a Waverly Company; p. 691, Figure 27.3, Copyright 1976, Massachusetts Medical Society; p. 692, Figure 27.4, Used with permission of W.B. Saunders Company; p. 695, Figure 27.5, Used with permission of the American Heart Association.

CHAPTER 28

p. 722, Figure 28.5 and p. 735, Figure 28.10, Used with permission of Mosby-Year Book, Inc.; p. 734, Figure 28.9 and p. 736, Figures 28.11 and 28.12, Used with permission of Williams & Wilkins, a Waverly Company.

CHAPTER 29

p. 756, Figure 29.4, Used with permission of Mosby-Year Book, Inc.; pp. 758-759, Focus Box 29.5 and Focus Box 29.6, Used with permission of Williams & Wilkins, a Waverly Company.

CHAPTER 30

p. 768, Figure 30.1, Reprinted by special permission from the Canadian Society for Exercise Physiology, Inc., Copyright 1994, CSEP; pp. 774-775, Focus Box 30.5, Reproduced with permission of the publisher, Masters Press, Division of Howard W. Sams, a Bell Atlantic Company, Indianapolis, IN, Fitness Walking by Scott O. Roberts © 1995.

ELEMENTS IMPORTANT TO CELLULAR BIOCHEMISTRY

Element	Symbol	Atomic Number	Atomic Weight (gm)
Hydrogen	H	1	1.00794
Carbon	C	6	12.011
Nitrogen	N	7	14.00674
Oxygen	O	8	15.9994
Sodium	Na	11	22.989768
Magnesium	Mg	12	24.305
Phosphorus	P	15	30.973762
Sulfur	S	16	32.066
Chlorine	Cl	17	35.4527
Potassium	K	19	39.0983
Calcium	Ca	20	40.078
Iron	Fe	26	55.847
Copper	Cu	29	63.546
Zinc	Zn	30	65.39

MOLECULES IMPORTANT TO SKELETAL MUSCLE BIOCHEMISTRY

Molecule	Molecular Weight (gm/M)	Function(s)
ATP	507.2	Chemical energy exchange
Creatine phosphate	209.1	Rapid regeneration of ATP
Glucose	180.1	Glycolytic substrate
Glycogen*	—	Glucose polymer stored in muscle and the liver
Palmitate	255.0	Main free fatty acid of metabolism
Lactate	89.0	By-product of glycolysis; helps maintain cytosolic redox
Pyruvate	87.0	Final product of glycolysis
Acetyl-CoA	582.1	Branch molecule in CHO and lipid catabolism
NAD+	663.4	Proton and electron transfer
Alanine	89.1	Amino acid involved in transamination reactions
Histidine	155.0	Main amino acid that contributes to the muscle buffer capacity
Bicarbonate	61.0	Main buffer in blood

*Assayed as glucose units per tissue weight.

IMPORTANT CONSTANTS AND FORMULA

Constant	Symbol	Formula
Avogadro constant	N_A	6.02214×10^{23} / mol
Faraday constant	F	95485.31 C / mol
Molar gas constant	R	1.98589 cal / mol • °K
Acceleration of gravity	ga	9.80665 m / s²
Gibbs free energy		
-Standard	ΔG	$-RT \ln ([prod] / [sub])$
-Absolute	$\Delta G^{\circ\prime}$	$\Delta G + RT \ln ([prod] / [sub])$